Intraoperative and Interventional Echocardiography

Atlas of Transesophageal Imaging

Intraoperative and Interventional Echocardiography

Atlas of Transesophageal Imaging

SECOND EDITION

Donald C. Oxorn, MD
Professor of Anesthesiology
Adjunct Professor of Medicine
School of Medicine
University of Washington
Seattle, Washington

Catherine M. Otto, MD
Professor of Medicine
J. Ward Kennedy-Hamilton Endowed Chair in Cardiology
Associate Director, Echocardiography
Department of Medicine
School of Medicine
University of Washington
Seattle, Washington

ELSEVIER

ELSEVIER

1600 John F. Kennedy Blvd.
Ste 1800
Philadelphia, PA 19103-2899

INTRAOPERATIVE AND INTERVENTIONAL ECHOCARDIOGRAPHY: ATLAS OF TRANSESOPHAGEAL IMAGING, SECOND EDITION

ISBN: 978-0-323-35825-5

Library of Congress Cataloging-in-Publication Data

Names: Oxorn, Donald C., author. | Otto, Catherine M., author.
Title: Intraoperative and interventional echocardiography: atlas of transesophageal imaging / Donald C. Oxorn, Catherine M. Otto.
Other titles: Atlas of intraoperative transesophageal echocardiography | Atlas of transesophageal imaging
Description: Second edition. | Philadelphia, PA: Elsevier, [2018] | Preceded by Atlas of intraoperative transesophageal echocardiography / Donald C. Oxorn, Catherine M. Otto. 2007. | Includes bibliographical references and index.
Identifiers: LCCN 2016046687 | ISBN 9780323358255 (hardcover: alk. paper)
Subjects: | MESH: Echocardiography, Transesophageal–methods | Heart Diseases–diagnostic imaging | Heart–diagnostic imaging | Intraoperative Care–methods | Atlases | Case Reports
Classification: LCC RC683.5.U5 | NLM WG 17 | DDC 616.1/207543–dc23 LC record available at https://lccn.loc.gov/2016046687

International Standard Book Number: 978-0-323-35825-5

Content Strategist: Maureen Iannuzzi
Content Development Specialist: Lisa Barnes
Publishing Services Manager: Catherine Jackson
Senior Project Manager: Rachel E. McMullen
Design Direction: Julia Dummitt

Printed in China

Last digit is the print number: 9 8 7 6 5 4 3 2 1

FOREWORD

During the past 25 years, advances in technology have made intraoperative TEE indispensable in monitoring cardiac function, and in helping to guide all forms of cardiac surgery—coronary artery bypass, valve repair and replacement, congenital disease, pericardial disease, cardiomyopathy, mechanical circulatory support, and transplantation. There is no better way to learn more about this technique than by illustration with cases.

Dr. Donald Oxorn was a member of the Department of Anesthesia at Sunnybrook Health Sciences Centre in Toronto from 1990 to 1998. I am a cardiologist, and have been the Medical Director of the Echocardiography Laboratory at Sunnybrook since 1984. We acquired our first monoplane TEE probe in 1989. In the early days of TEE, cardiologists performed the TEE examinations in our cardiac Operating Rooms (ORs). There was great interest from our anesthesia group to learn the technique. Dr. Oxorn trained in transthoracic echocardiography and TEE in our lab in 1991 and has made performing this procedure a large part of his professional career. His curiosity and enthusiasm for the technology were remarkable and he quickly excelled in obtaining optimal TEE images. Within a few short years, our anesthesia colleagues including Dr. Oxorn took over the practice of intraoperative TEE at our institution. Dr. Oxorn enjoyed reviewing the images of challenging cases with us and the collaborative relationship with our anesthesia colleagues has continued.

The second edition of the *Atlas of Intraoperative Transesophageal Echocardiography* (now *Intraoperative and Interventional Echocardiography: Atlas of Transesophageal Imaging,* second edition) is timely. Since the first edition was published in 2007, TEE technology has advanced, and there have been many changes in cardiac procedures. 3D TEE images showing the "surgeon's view" of the mitral valve have had a major impact on the preop and in intraop assessment of mitral valve prolapse and the repair of this disorder. 3D TEE color assessment of mitral regurgitation is still evolving, but provides a significant advance over 2D color in many cases. A number of new cardiac procedures have become the standard of care and others are evolving. Transcatheter valve therapies (TAVR and MitraClip) are well established. Percutaneous mitral valve replacement procedures are evolving. Tricuspid valve procedures are on the horizon. Transcatheter device closures now include the left atrial appendage as well as septal and paravalvular defects. Many advances in CT and MRI imaging are complementary to echocardiography. Dr. Oxorn has done an excellent job incorporating these images into his new atlas. Many of our complex patients are managed by a "Heart Team" and the team members rely more than ever on advanced imaging to make decisions about patient selection and management. A cardiac surgeon, interventional cardiologist, and anesthesiologist now work together in the same interventional suite or OR with a procedure guided in large part by TEE, a situation unheard of 10 years ago.

Dr. Donald Oxorn and Dr. Catherine Otto are in a unique situation as they work together in the same institution and both have authored state-of-the-art echocardiography textbooks. Dr. Otto's, *The Practice of Clinical Echocardiography* is, I believe, the definitive reference textbook in echocardiography, and her shorter book, *The Textbook of Clinical Echocardiography*, is a favorite among residents and fellows doing their training in transthoracic and transesophageal echocardiography. *Intraoperative and Interventional Echocardiography: Atlas of Transesophageal Imaging,* second edition, with its excellent echo images as well as images of additional imaging modalities will make a fascinating learning experience for anesthesiologists, intensive care specialists, cardiologists, trainees, and individuals preparing for echo examinations. The surgical images and videos should especially appeal to individuals who do not see what actually goes on in the OR.

It has been a pleasure for me to have known Dr. Oxorn since 1990, and to be one of his teachers of this incredible technology that has evolved so much over the past 25 years.

Campbell D. Joyner, MD, FRCPC, FACC, FASE
Medical Director, Echocardiography Laboratory
Sunnybrook Health Sciences Centre
Professor of Medicine, University of Toronto
Toronto, Ontario, Canada

PREFACE

The complexity of cardiac surgical procedures has increased dramatically in recent decades. In addition to surgery for coronary artery disease, the typical cardiac center now provides all types of valve surgery, including complex mitral valve repairs, newer types of aortic valve replacement, and aortic root procedures. Now there are increasing numbers of adults who have survived congenital heart disease presenting for reoperation, patients requiring mechanical circulatory support for end-stage heart failure, and those requiring cardiac transplantation. All these procedures require transesophageal echocardiography (TEE) for procedural guidance, typically performed with simultaneous interpretation by a qualified anesthesiologist or cardiologist. The practitioner performing TEE procedural guidance is often called upon to confirm or refute the preprocedure diagnosis or to evaluate a previously unsuspected abnormality. In addition, TEE is used to evaluate the success of the procedure and to detect any acute complications. TEE procedural guidance is not confined to the operating room (OR), with many procedures now performed in the cardiac interventional suite with a Heart Team that includes cardiac anesthesiologists, interventional cardiologists, cardiac surgeons, noninvasive cardiologists, and other imaging experts.

This atlas will be of interest to all the Heart Team health care providers involved in the preoperative, intraoperative, and postoperative care of patients undergoing cardiac surgical procedures and interventions. The primary audience for this book is cardiac anesthesiologists, but this book also will be useful to cardiac surgeons seeking to understand echocardiography, cardiologists and cardiology fellows interested in expanding their knowledge of cardiac surgery, radiologists with a particular interest in cardiovascular disease, and to the rest of the Heart Team including cardiac sonographers, cardiac perfusionists, nurse practitioners, and physician assistants, especially those who are not familiar with what actually transpires in the OR. Primary care physicians with an interest in cardiology will also find this atlas helpful.

In the OR and interventional suite, the TEE practitioner does not just acquire echocardiographic images, but is actively involved in clinical decision making. Thus, the TEE practitioner needs to be knowledgeable about the clinical presentation of cardiac conditions, indications for intervention, and expected outcomes. Supplemental information from other imaging and diagnostic modalities, reviewed before surgery, assists the practitioner in the interpretation of intraoperative TEE.

The impetus to write this book came out of our personal experiences of TEE practice in the setting of cardiac anesthesia and surgery and acute care medicine. What we found lacking was a method of conveying to students and colleagues the correlation between findings on TEE, results of other diagnostic modalities, and what was actually seen in the OR. This book provides a unique integration of the clinical presentation, intraoperative and intraprocedural transesophageal echocardiographic images, other diagnostic modalities, surgical procedure, and cardiac pathology.

This book is formatted as an atlas using a case-based format, each with a different clinical focus. Cases are grouped into chapters defined by the clinical diagnosis including coronary artery disease, mitral valve disease, aortic valve disease, endocarditis, prosthetic valves, right-sided valve disease, adult congenital heart disease, hypertrophic cardiomyopathy, pericardial disease, diseases of the great vessels, and masses. In this second edition, all these chapters have undergone extensive revision with new echocardiographic and surgical images, more 3D and advanced imaging, updated text, and new suggested reading material. Entirely new chapters have been added on transcatheter interventions and mechanical circulatory support, reflecting the increased scope of practice for the practitioner providing TEE procedural guidance. In addition, most still images now are accompanied by video images that can be viewed online or on any smart device by simply clicking on the image, ensuring a seamless viewing experience for readers.

In each chapter, approximately 15 cases—some common, some esoteric—are presented. Each case includes the clinical presentation; multiple TEE images (both still and video); and images from other diagnostic modalities such as the ECG, standard radiographs, cardiac catheterization, radionuclide perfusion studies, cardiac magnetic resonance imaging, and computed tomography where applicable, images from the surgical procedure itself, along with gross and microscopic pathology, are included. Each case is accompanied by explanatory text discussing the acquisition, interpretation, and clinical significance of the TEE findings, along with suggestions for further reading.

This atlas is not a substitute for training in performance and interpretation of TEE for procedural guidance; instead, it is designed to serve as an adjunct in furthering or testing the individual's knowledge. The case-based format allows integration of multiple types of data but does not provide comprehensive coverage of all topics in echocardiography. We expect that readers already have studied standard textbooks of clinical echocardiography and have some clinical

(Continued)

experience with echocardiography. Clinical TEE practitioners should adhere to guidelines for education as detailed in accreditation standards for each medical specialty, levels of supervised training as established by professional medical societies, certification as provided by board examinations for each medical specialty with added qualification in echocardiography, and the credentialing standards set by each medical institution. This atlas will accelerate education and training for those early in their career and will enhance clinical experience and skills for the active TEE practitioner.

Donald C. Oxorn, MD
Professor of Anesthesiology
Adjunct Professor of Medicine
School of Medicine
University of Washington
Seattle, Washington

Catherine M. Otto, MD
Professor of Medicine
J. Ward Kennedy-Hamilton Endowed Chair in Cardiology
Associate Director, Echocardiography
Department of Medicine
School of Medicine
University of Washington
Seattle, Washington

ACKNOWLEDGMENTS

For their contributions and assistance, we would like to acknowledge our colleagues in:

Cardiothoracic Anesthesiology (Faculty)

T. Andrew Bowdle
Jorg Dziersk
Renata Ferreira
Michael Hall
Srdjan Jelacic
Denise Joffe
Stefan Lombaard
G. Burkhard Mackensen
Kris Natrajan
Carly Peterson
Richard Sheu
Kei Togashi
Peter Von Homeyer

Cardiothoracic Anesthesiology (Fellows)

Winston Choi
Paul Jacobs
Stephanie Jones
Sean McLean
Heather Reed
Tatyana Shkolnikova

Cardiac Surgery

Gabriel Aldea
Joshua Hermsen
Nahush Mokadam
Jay Pal
Jason Smith
Edward Verrier

Interventional Cardiology

Larry Dean
Creighton Don
Thomas Jones
James McCabe
Mark Reisman
Douglas Stewart

Cardiac Pathology

Dennis Reichenbach

We would also like to thank Valerie Oxorn and Starr Kaplan for their artwork, and Dolores Meloni and Lisa Barnes from Elsevier for their constant help and encouragement.

The patience and encouragement of our families, including (DCO) my wife Susan Murdoch and my children, Jonathan Oxorn, Sean Murdoch-Oxorn, and Alexandra Murdoch-Oxorn and (CMO) my husband, daughter and granddaughter was ever present and much appreciated.

I (DCO) would like to thank two individuals from the University of Toronto: my friend and mentor Gerald Edelist, and Cam Joyner, my first and foremost teacher in echocardiography.

ABBREVIATIONS

2D	two dimensional
3D	three dimensional
A1, A2, A3	anterior mitral leaflet sections
A-COM	anterior commissure
AICD	automatic implantable cardioverter defibrillators
AML	anterior mitral leaflet
Ao	aorta
AP	anteroposterior
AR	aortic regurgitation
ARDS	adult respiratory distress syndrome
AS	aortic stenosis
ASA	atrial septal aneurysm
ASD	atrial septal defect
ATL	anterior tricuspid leaflet
AV	aortic valve
AVR	aortic valve replacement
CABG	coronary artery bypass graft
CPB	cardiopulmonary bypass
CS	coronary sinus
CT	computed tomography
CVA	cerebrovascular accident
CW	continuous wave (Doppler)
Cx	circumflex coronary artery
DA	descending aorta
ECG	electrocardiogram
ECMO	extracorporeal membrane oxygenation
FAC	fractional area of change
FO	fossa ovalis
IABP	intraaortic balloon pump
IAS	interatrial septum
ICD	implantable cardioverter defibrillator
IVC	inferior vena cava
IVS	interventricular septum
LA	left atrium
LAA	left atrial appendage
LAD	left anterior descending coronary artery
LCC	left coronary cusp
LCX	left circumflex artery
LIMA	left internal mammary artery
LLPV	left lower pulmonary vein
LMCA	left main coronary artery
LPA	left pulmonary artery
LUPV	left upper pulmonary vein
LV	left ventricle
LVOT	left ventricular outflow tract
MAIVF	mitral aortic intervalvular fibrosa
MI	myocardial infarction
MPR	multiplanar reconstruction
MR	mitral regurgitation
MRI	magnetic resonance imaging
MS	mitral stenosis
MV	mitral valve
MVA	mitral valve area
MVR	mitral valve replacement
NCC	noncoronary cusp
OR	operating room
P1, P2, P3	posterior mitral leaflet sections
PA	pulmonary artery
P-COM	posterior commissure
PDA	patent ductus arteriosus
PE	pericardial effusion
PFO	patent foramen ovale
PG	pressure gradient
PISA	proximal isovelocity surface area
PLSVC	persistent left superior vena cava
PM	papillary muscle
PML	posterior mitral leaflet
PMN	polymorphonuclear leukocytes
PR	pulmonic regurgitation
PTL	posterior tricuspid leaflet
PVR	pulmonic valve replacement
PW	pulsed wave (Doppler)
RA	right atrium
RAA	right atrial appendage
RBC	red blood cells
RCA	right coronary artery
RCC	right coronary cusp
RLPV	right lower pulmonary vein
ROA	regurgitant orifice area
RPA	right pulmonary artery
RUPV	right upper pulmonary vein
RV	right ventricle
RVH	right ventricular hypertrophy
RVOT	right ventricular outflow tract
SAM	systolic anterior motion
SP	septum primum
SS	septum secundum
STJ	sinotubular junction
STL	septal tricuspid leaflet
STS PROM	Society of Thoracic Surgeons 30-day Predicted Risk of Mortality
SV	stroke volume
SVC	superior vena cava
TAPSE	tricuspid annular plane systolic excursion

TAVR (TAVI)	transcatheter aortic valve replacement
TEE	transesophageal echocardiography
THV	transcatheter heart valve
TMR	transmyocardial revascularization
TR	tricuspid regurgitation
TTE	transthoracic echocardiography
TV	tricuspid valve
TVR	tricuspid valve replacement
V-A ECMO	veno-arterial extracorporeal membrane oxygenation
VC	vena contracta
VIV	valve in valve
VSD	ventricular septal defect
VTI	velocity time integral
V-V ECMO	veno-venous extracorporeal membrane oxygenation

CONTENTS

1 Coronary Artery Disease

Visualization of the Coronary Arteries and Regional Wall Motion

CASE 1-1
Normal Coronary Arteries

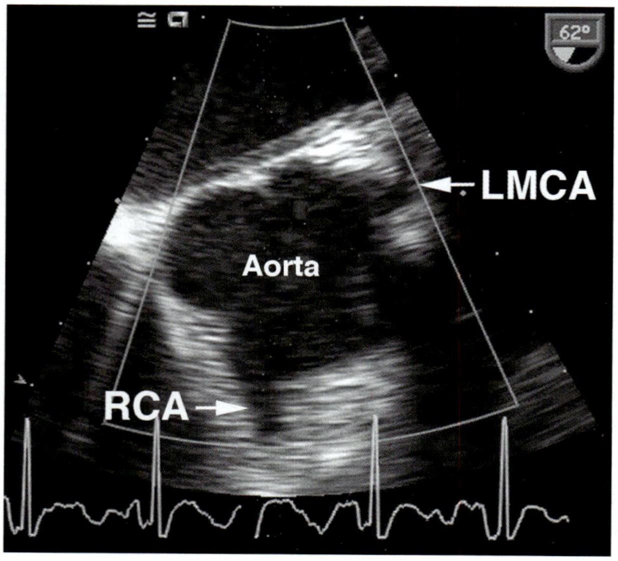

Fig 1.1 In a magnified short-axis view of the aorta slightly cephalad to the valve plane, the right coronary artery (RCA) and left coronary artery (LCA) ostia are seen arising from the right and left coronary sinuses of Valsalva, respectively. The left main coronary artery is easily visualized in nearly all patients. The right coronary is visualized less often.

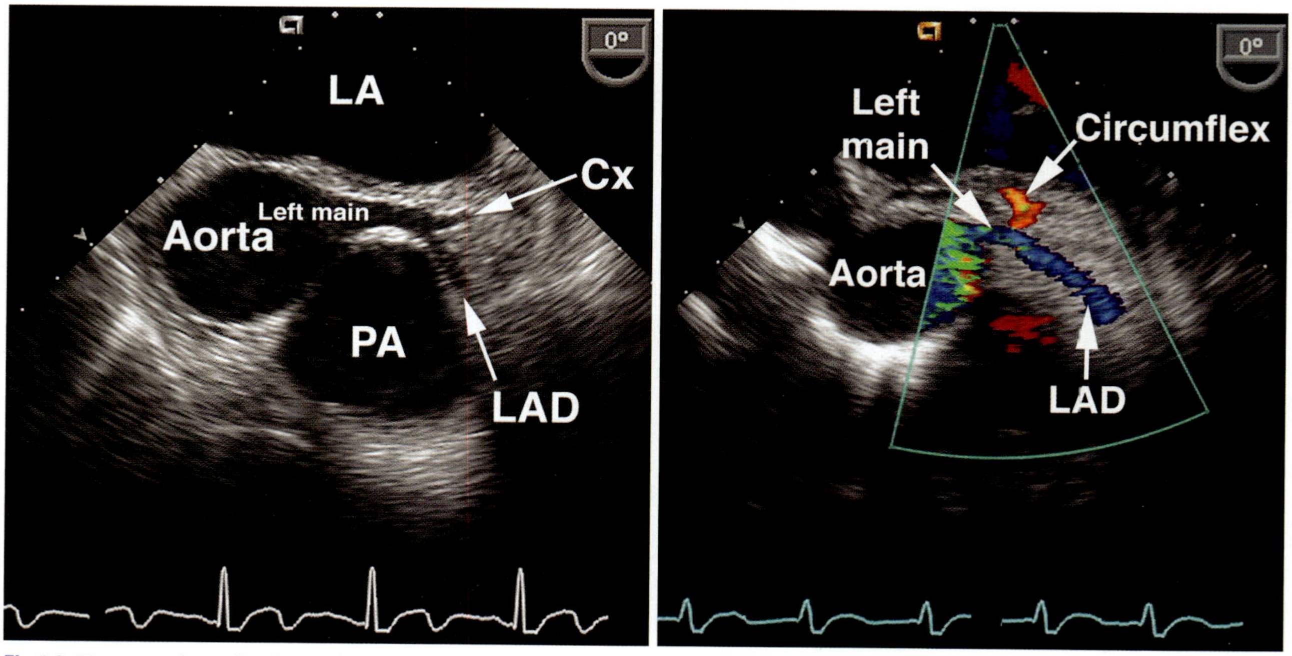

Fig 1.2 Transesophageal echocardiography (TEE) images in a different patient demonstrate the course of the left main coronary artery as it passes behind the main pulmonary artery and bifurcates into the posterior direct circumflex (Cx) and more anteriorly the direct left anterior descending (LAD) coronary artery. This view was obtained starting in a short-axis view of the aorta to visualize the left main coronary ostium and then rotating the image plane until the bifurcation was seen. On the right, color Doppler demonstrates the predominantly diastolic flow in the left main, circumflex, and left anterior descending (LAD) coronary arteries.

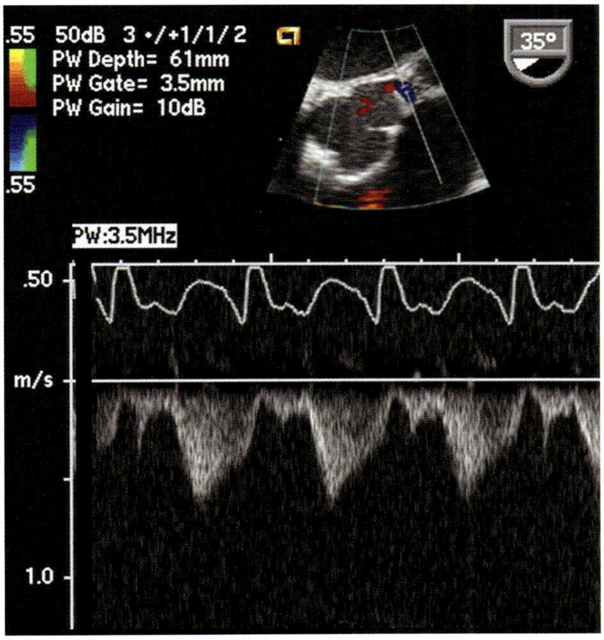

Fig 1.3 A pulsed Doppler sample volume is positioned in the left anterior descending coronary artery. The spectral tracing shows low-velocity diastolic flow, with small systolic component, typical for normal coronary blood flow.

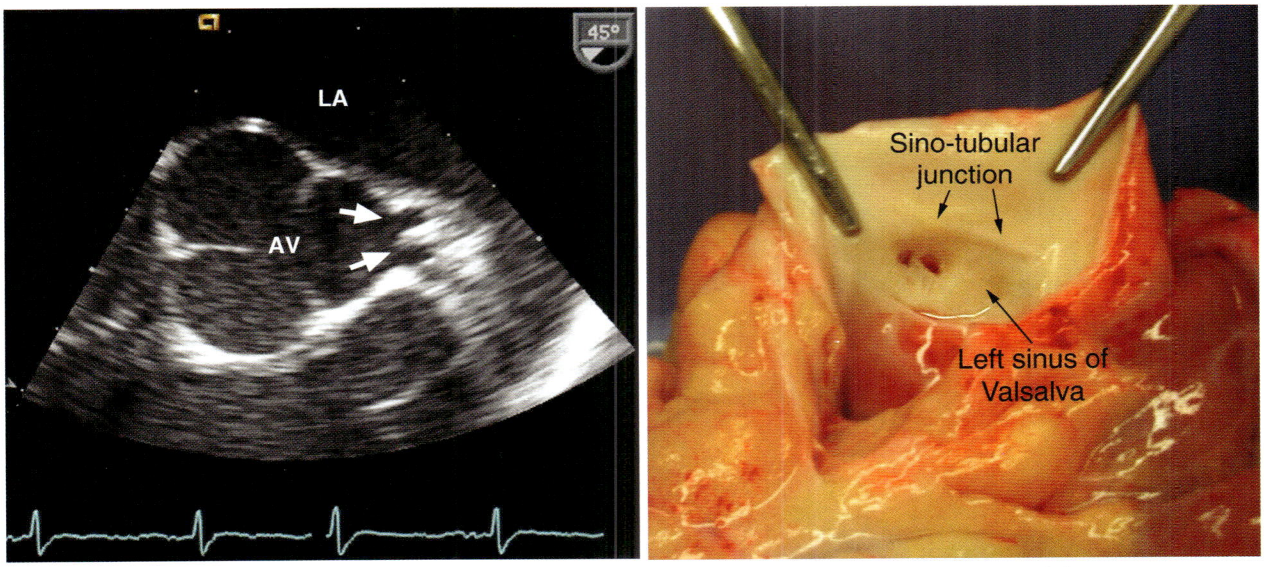

Fig 1.4 In this patient with an idiopathic dilated cardiomyopathy undergoing heart transplantation, the left main coronary artery is absent, and both the circumflex and left anterior descending arteries arise from the left coronary sinus of Valsalva as seen on TEE *(left)* and in the explanted heart *(right)*.

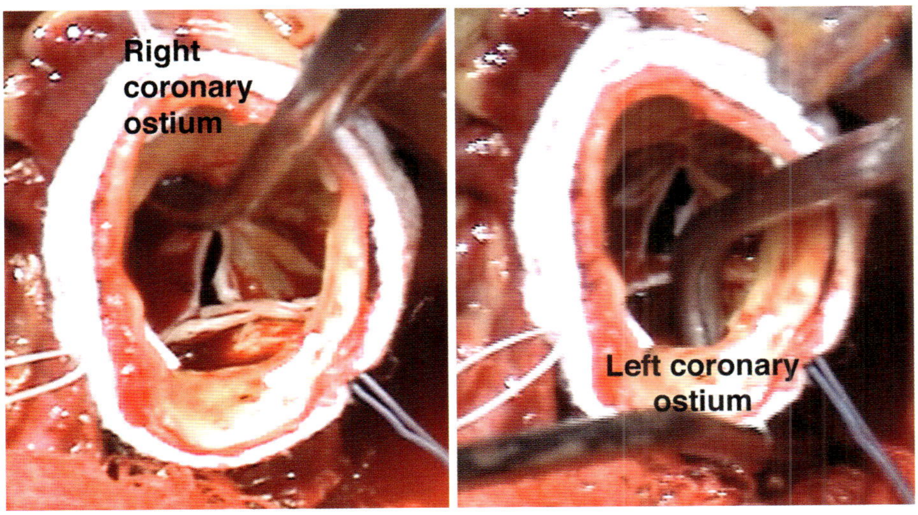

Fig 1.5 In this intraoperative photograph of the aortic valve from the aortic root side, the forceps tip is at the ostium of the right coronary artery *(left)*. The right coronary ostium is anterior and slightly more cephalad than the left main coronary artery *(right)*. The photograph is taken from the head of the operating table, and is therefore rotated 180 degrees from what is seen in TEE imaging.

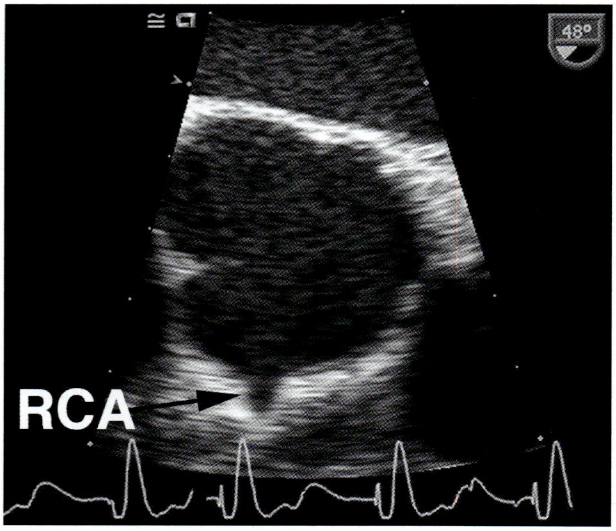

Fig 1.6 In a magnified short-axis TEE image, the ostium of the right coronary artery (RCA) is seen.

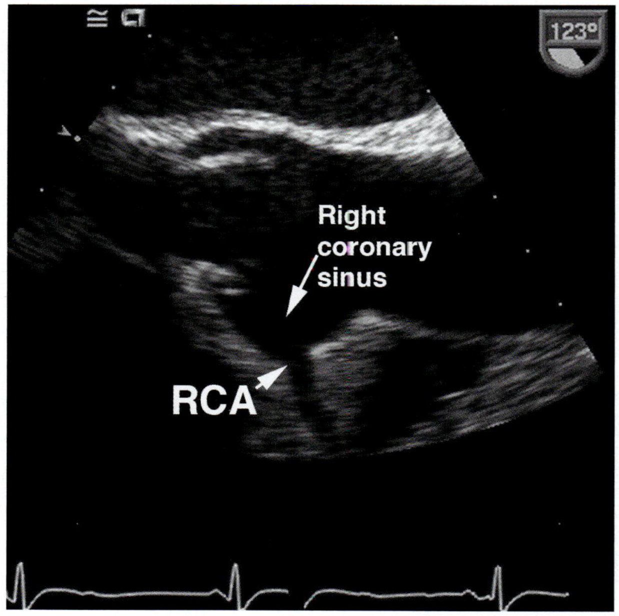

Fig 1.7 The RCA is often more easily visualized in a long-axis view of the aortic root, as shown in this example.

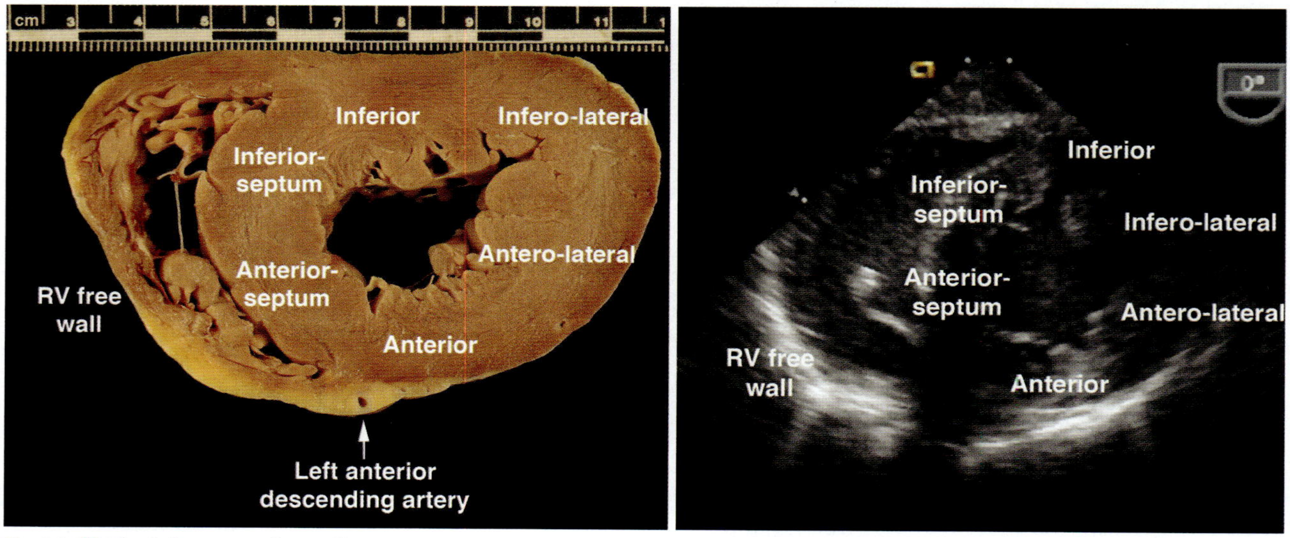

Fig 1.8 The left ventricular wall segments are shown for an anatomic specimen in the same orientation as a transgastric short-axis view of the ventricle. The ventricle is divided into six segments at the base and midventricular level, as shown. The posterior wall is also called the inferior–lateral wall, using the standard nomenclature for regional wall motion analysis.

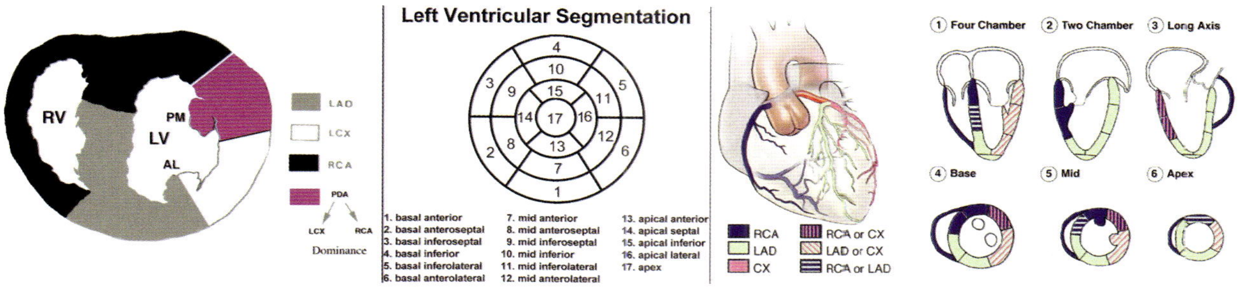

Fig 1.9 This schematic diagram of a short-axis view of the left (LV) and right ventricle (RV) in the same orientation as the transgastric short-axis views *(left-side frame)* illustrates the correlation between coronary anatomy and regional myocardial function. In the middle frame, the 17-segment model of the LV is seen, and in the right-side frame, the coronary perfusion of these segments is shown. There is some variability in the region supplied by the left circumflex artery (LCX), even at the base and midventricular levels. The apical region of the ventricle may be supplied by either the left anterior descending (LAD) or the right coronary artery (RCA) so that identification of the culprit vessel becomes problematic when only an apical abnormality is present. (Reproduced with permission from Oxorn D, Edelist G, Smith MS. An introduction to transoesophageal echocardiography: II clinical applications. Can J Anaesth 1996; 43:278-294 [left-side frame], and from Lang R, Badano L, Victor Mor-Avi V et al. Recommendations for cardiac chamber quantification by echocardiography in adults: An update from the American Society of Echocardiography and the European Association of Cardiovascular Imaging. J Am Soc Echocardiogr 2015; 28:1–39 [middle and right-side frames]).

Comments

As shown in these examples, the proximal coronary arteries can often be visualized on TEE. The left main coronary artery arises from the left coronary sinus of Valsalva, is easily visualized in over 85% of patients and has a normal diameter of 4.2 ± 0.7 mm, with a slightly smaller average diameter in women (3.5 mm) compared with men (4.3 mm). The left main coronary artery bifurcates into the left anterior descending coronary, with a normal proximal diameter of 3.5 ± 1.0 mm, which supplies the anterior wall and anterior septum, and the circumflex coronary artery, with a normal diameter of 3.0 ± 0.6 mm, which supplies the lateral left ventricular wall. The right coronary artery arises from the right coronary sinus, with an average diameter of 3.6 ± 0.8 mm. The right coronary artery gives rise to the posterior descending coronary artery, supplying the inferior and posterior walls, in about 80% of patients (e.g., a right-dominant coronary circulation). The right coronary artery is not always visualized on TEE, being seen in about 50% of cases in one series.

The apical segments of the ventricle are often supplied by the left anterior descending artery, although the posterior descending coronary artery may extend to the inferior apex in some cases. The posterior (or inferior–lateral) left ventricular wall is variably supplied by either the circumflex or the posterior descending coronary artery. Coronary blood flow can be recorded using pulsed Doppler in many patients, with the typical pattern showing prominent diastolic flow, with a velocity about 0.6 cm/s, with little flow in systole. Although an increased velocity (>1 m/s) suggests stenosis and Doppler evaluation of coronary flow reserve is possible, these data are rarely used clinically.

TEE evaluation of the coronary arteries is most useful for detection of coronary artery aneurysms, coronary fistula, and anomalous origins from a different sinus of Valsalva or from the pulmonary artery. Although some studies have shown that TEE evaluation is sensitive and specific for detection of significant left main or proximal coronary stenosis, TEE has not gained clinical acceptance as an approach to evaluation of atherosclerotic coronary disease. In addition to variable image quality, the inability to visualize distal vessel anatomy is a major limitation. Echocardiographic evaluation of coronary disease currently relies on evaluation of regional myocardial function at rest and with stress.

Suggested Reading

1. Lenter C, editor: Geigy Scientific Tables, Vol. 5: Heart and Circulation, Basel, Switzerland, 1990, CIBA-GEIGY Limited, pp 173–181.
2. Oxorn D, Edelist G, Smith MS: An introduction to transoesophageal echocardiography: II Clinical applications, Can J Anaesth 43:278–294, 1996.
3. Lang R, Badano L, Victor Mor-Avi V, et al: Recommendations for cardiac chamber quantification by echocardiography in adults: An update from the American Society of Echocardiography and the European Association of Cardiovascular Imaging, J Am Soc Echocardiogr 28:1–39, 2015.

CASE 1-2
Right Coronary Artery Dissection

This 71-year-old man had severe symptomatic calcific aortic stenosis. When undergoing diagnostic coronary angiography, he suffered a spiral dissection of the right coronary artery that was initially treated with multiple stents. Despite efforts to reperfuse the right coronary distribution, he suffered a ventricular fibrillation arrest. TEE at the outside hospital showed a proximal ascending aortic dissection. He was airlifted to our medical center and brought directly to the operating room.

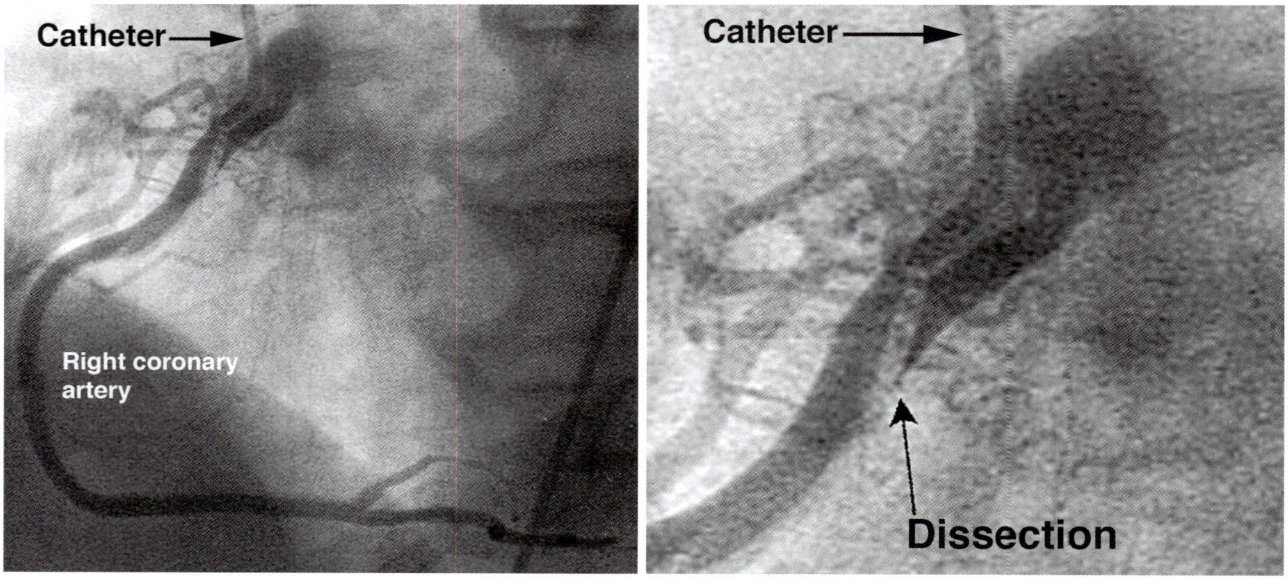

Fig 1.10 The right coronary angiogram demonstrates extravasation of contrast near the vessel origin in the proximal aorta. The close-up view *(right)* shows the spiraling echolucency in the right coronary consistent with a dissection.

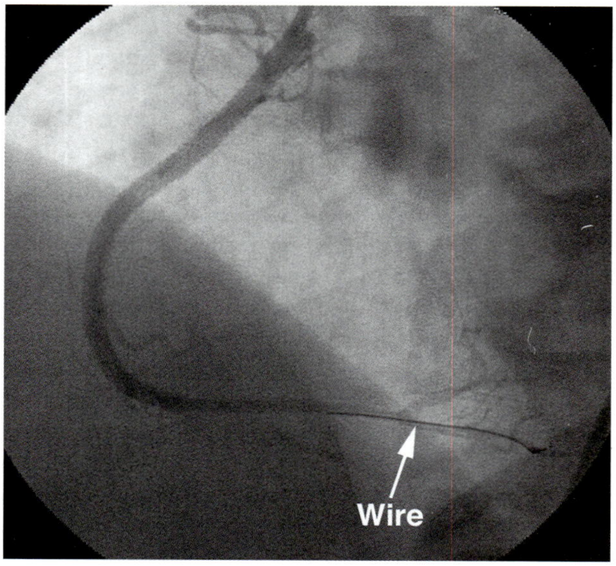

Fig 1.11 After completion of the angioplasty, the right coronary artery appears widely patent, with the distal end of the guidewire seen in the posterior descending coronary branch.

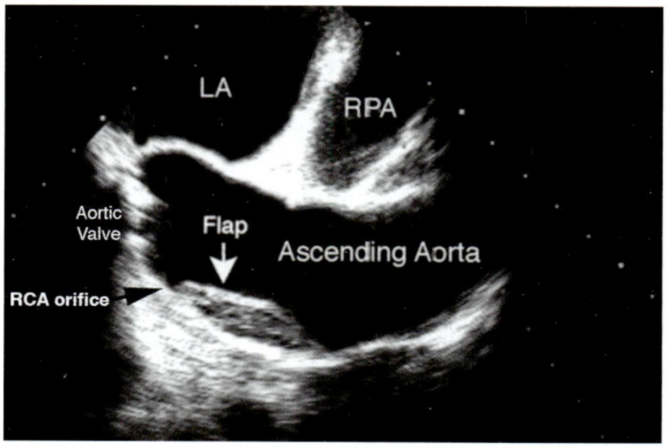

Fig 1.12 On intraoperative TEE, the long-axis view of the ascending aorta demonstrates a luminal flap, originating near the right coronary ostium. The echo density in the false lumen suggests thrombus formation. Note that the aortic valve is heavily calcified.

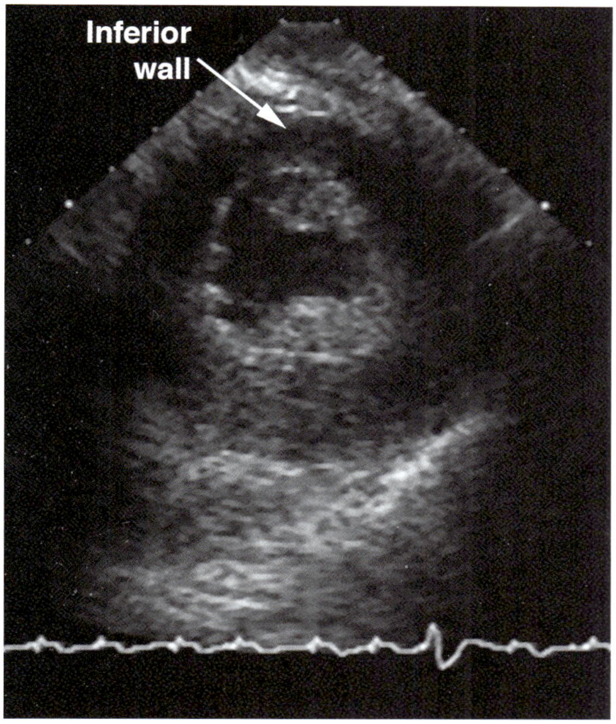

Fig 1.13 The transgastric short-axis view of the left ventricle shows severe hypokinesis of the inferior wall, consistent with ischemia in the distribution of the right coronary artery.

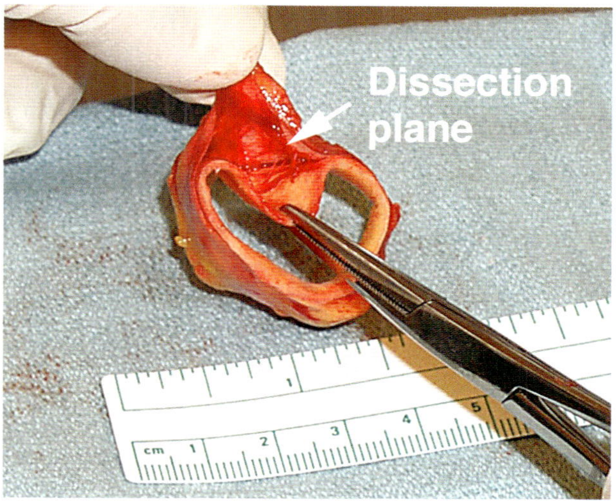

Fig 1.14 The patient underwent replacement of the aortic valve and ascending aorta with a composite valve and conduit. The left main coronary artery was reimplanted into the graft and a bypass graft was placed to the distal right coronary artery, with the proximal right coronary artery oversewn. A small segment of the resected aorta shows the dissection plane between the endothelium and media of the vessel. The patient had an uneventful hospital course and was discharged home on the sixth postoperative day.

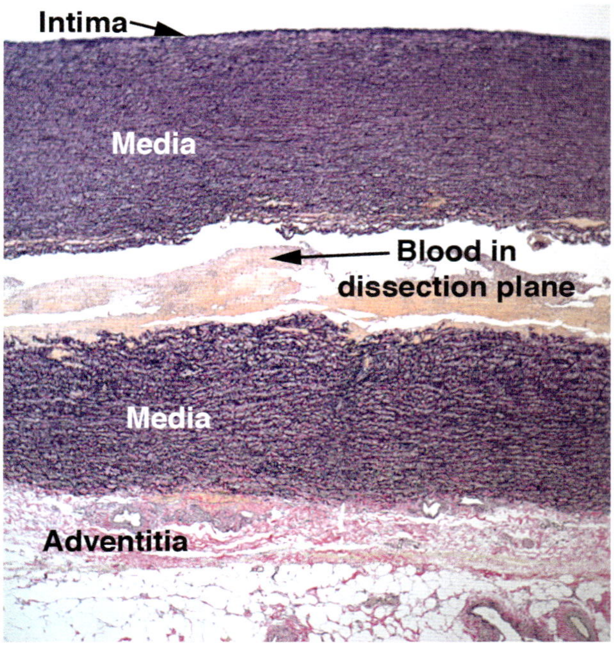

Fig 1.15 Microscopic examination of the aortic specimen shows the dissection plane through the media, filled with blood.

Comments

Coronary artery dissection can occur spontaneously or as a complication of cardiac catheterization. Coronary dissection is a rare cause of acute myocardial infarction in younger patients. Although there are no specific clinical predictors of spontaneous coronary dissection, it is more common in women than in men and the risk is increased during pregnancy.

Coronary dissection owing to diagnostic cardiac catheterization is rare but can result in acute severe myocardial ischemia, as in this case. The overall incidence of myocardial infarction with diagnostic coronary angiography is 0.06%, with infarction more often due to vessel thrombosis or embolization rather than to coronary dissection. When coronary dissection complicates a diagnostic or therapeutic percutaneous coronary procedure, the dissection flap may propagate retrograde into the aorta, as in this case.

Suggested Reading

1. Saw J: Spontaneous coronary artery dissection, Can J Cardiol 29(9):1027–1033, 2013.
2. Crea F, Battipaglia I, Andreotti F: Sex differences in mechanisms, presentation and management of ischaemic heart disease, Atherosclerosis 241(1):157–168, 2015.
3. Alfonso F, Bastante T, Cuesta J, et al: Spontaneous coronary artery dissection: Novel insights on diagnosis and management, Cardiovasc Diagn Ther 5(2):133–140, 2015.
4. Lou X, Mitter SS, Blair JE, et al: Intraoperative coronary artery dissection in fibromuscular dysplasia, Ann Thorac Surg 99(4): 1442–1444, 2015.

CASE 1-3
Right Coronary Artery Air

After cardiac surgery (especially when cardiac chambers have been opened), and in preparation for separation from cardiopulmonary bypass, the cardiac chambers are imaged to determine the presence of intracardiac air. If substantial air is present, there is concern that air entering the coronary ostia might interrupt coronary blood flow, resulting in myocardial ischemia. The surgeon will therefore make attempts to "de-air" the heart by applying suction to the ascending aorta in order to evacuate air as it passes through the aortic valve, and before it enters the coronary ostia. In extreme cases, actual needle aspiration of the left ventricular cavity may be undertaken.

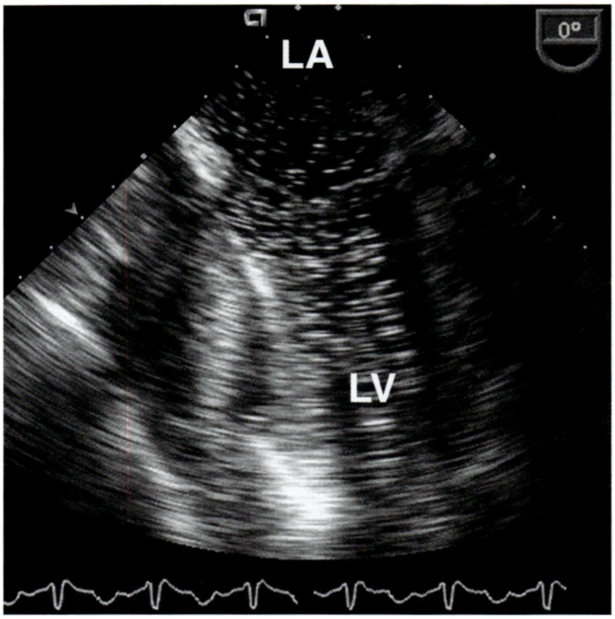

Fig 1.16 In the TEE four-chamber view at 0 degrees rotation, there are multiple bright mobile echodensities (termed echocardiographic contrast) in all four chambers of the heart, suggesting that microbubbles are present in the left- and right-sided circulations. A pocket of air *(bright density at the LV apex)* is frequently enmeshed in the left ventricular apex.

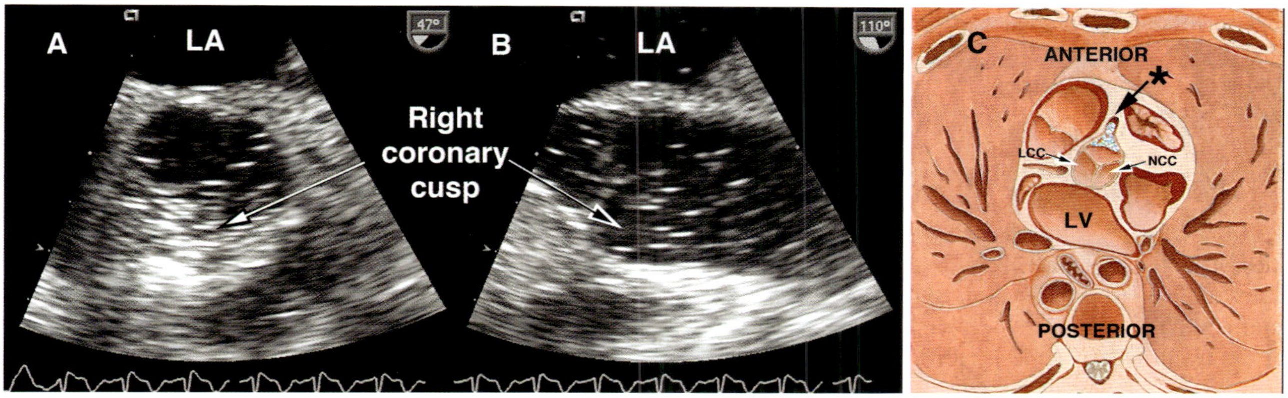

Fig 1.17 In both short- *(left)* and long-axis *(center)* views of the aortic valve, microbubbles are seen in the aortic root. Microbubbles tend to accumulate in the sinus of Valsalva adjacent to the right coronary cusp (RCC), with preferential flow into the right coronary artery; this occurs because when the patient is lying supine, the right coronary artery is the most superior *(right)*.

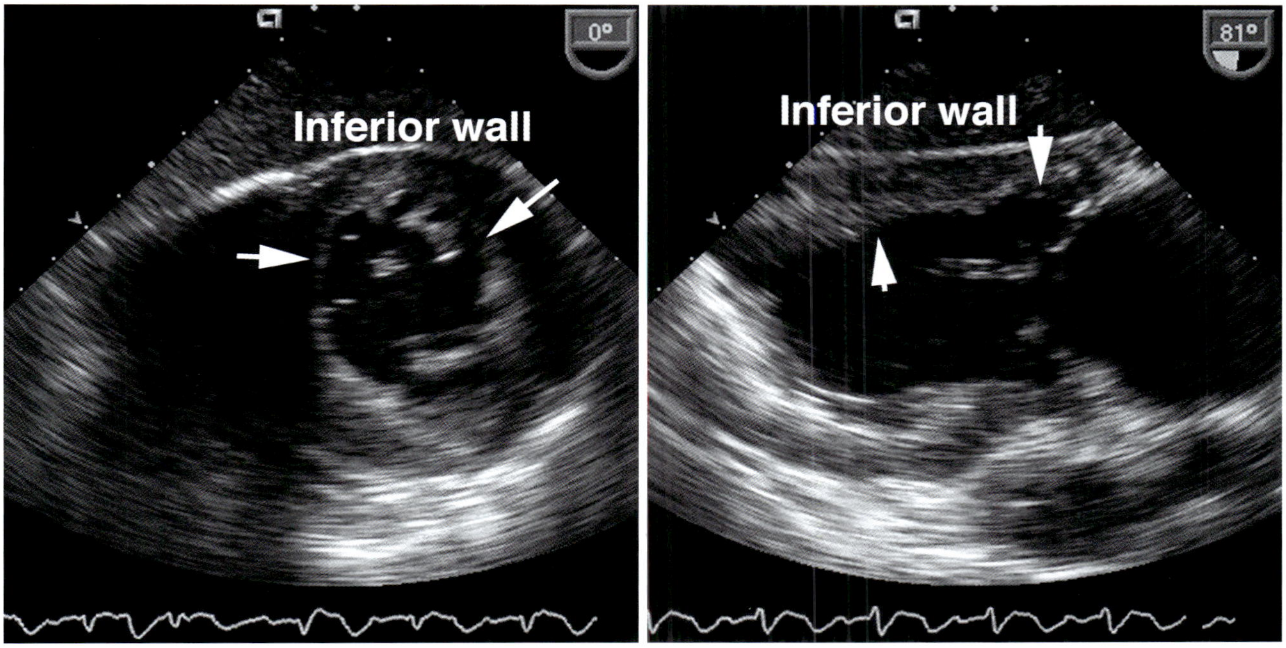

Fig 1.18 Transgastric views of the left ventricle in a short-axis *(left)* and two-chamber *(right)* view show that the inferior wall segments between the arrows are akinetic, but not thinned.

Comments

On echocardiography, air in the cardiac chambers appears as mobile echodensities, e.g., echo contrast. The echocardiographer may be asked to evaluate residual air as the patient is weaned from cardiopulmonary bypass. Air detected by TEE is associated with transient ST-segment elevation on the electrocardiogram (ECG) and wall motion abnormalities on two-dimensional (2D) imaging. The association between intracardiac air and neurologic events after cardiac surgery is less clear, with some studies suggesting that left-sided microbubbles are not predictive of neurologic recovery, but other studies showing better postoperative cognitive function in patients with fewer microbubbles after surgery.

Suggested Reading

1. Jha AK, Malik V, Hote M: Minimally invasive cardiac surgery and transesophageal echocardiography, Ann Card Anaesth 17(2):125–132, 2014.
2. Akiyama K, Arisawa S, Ide M, et al: Intraoperative cardiac assessment with transesophageal echocardiography for decision-making in cardiac anesthesia, Gen Thorac Cardiovasc Surg 61(6):320–329, 2013.

Myocardial Infarction

CASE 1-4
Anterior Myocardial Infarction

This 56-year-old man with no previous cardiac history presented with a 3-hour history of intermittent chest pain and anterior ST-segment elevation on ECG. He was taken directly to the cardiac catheterization laboratory where he was found to have an occluded proximal right coronary artery, with filling of the distal vessel by left-to-right collaterals, and an acute occlusion of the left anterior descending coronary artery. The left anterior descending occlusion could not be crossed. An intraaortic balloon pump was placed and he was referred for emergency coronary bypass grafting surgery. Preoperative echocardiography demonstrated a left ventricular ejection fraction of 29% with severe hypokinesis of the inferior wall and akinesis of the mid and apical segments of the anterior wall.

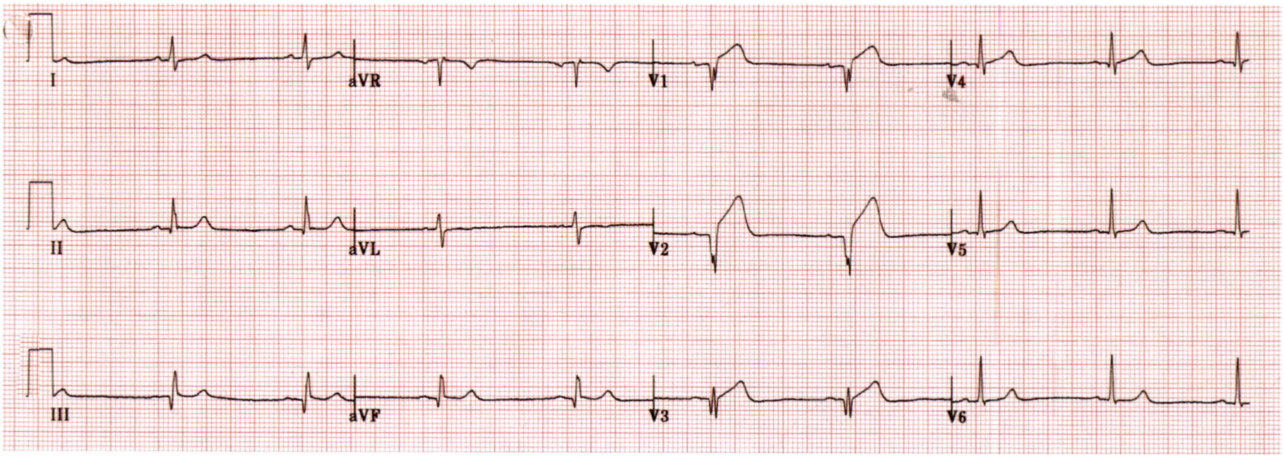

Fig 1.19 The ECG demonstrates Q-waves and ST elevation in leads VI–V3 consistent with an acute anteroseptal myocardial infarction. There also are small Q-waves in III and AVR without associated ST changes.

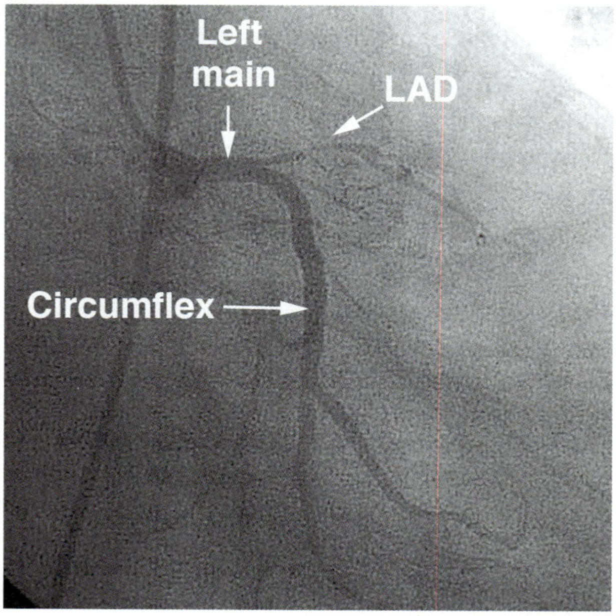

Fig 1.20 At coronary angiography there was an old occlusion of the right coronary artery. The left main and left circumflex showed only mild diffuse disease, but there was a complete proximal occlusion of the left anterior descending coronary (LAD) with contrast filling only a small diagonal branch to the basal anterior wall.

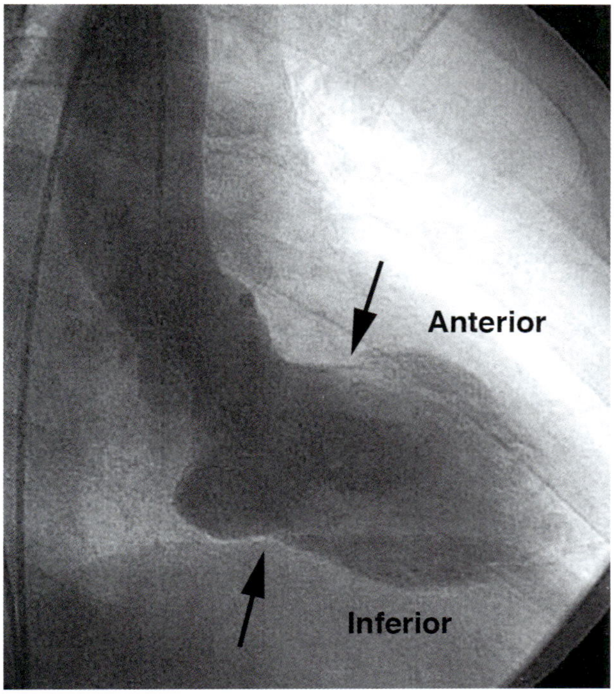

Fig 1.21 The left ventriculogram in a right anterior oblique view demonstrates normal endocardial motion at the ventricular base *(arrows)* with akinesis of the anterior wall, consistent with the acute event, and akinesis of the inferior wall, consistent in turn with the old myocardial infarction.

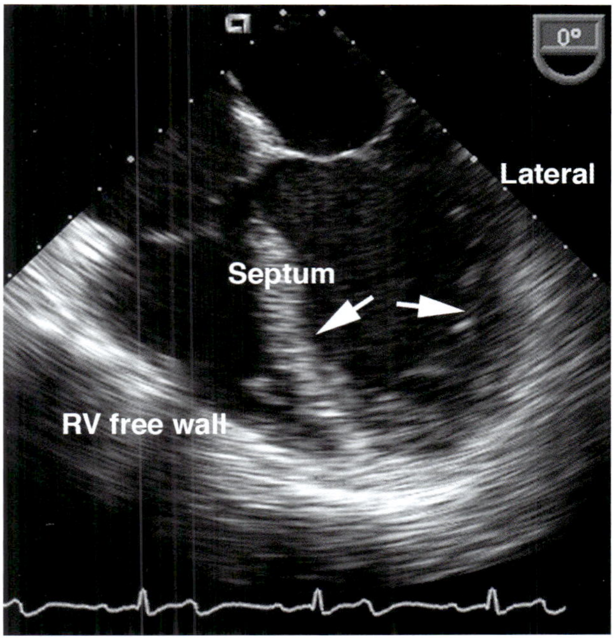

Fig 1.22 In the TEE four-chamber view at 0 degrees, the apical segments of the lateral wall and septum under the arrows are akinetic.

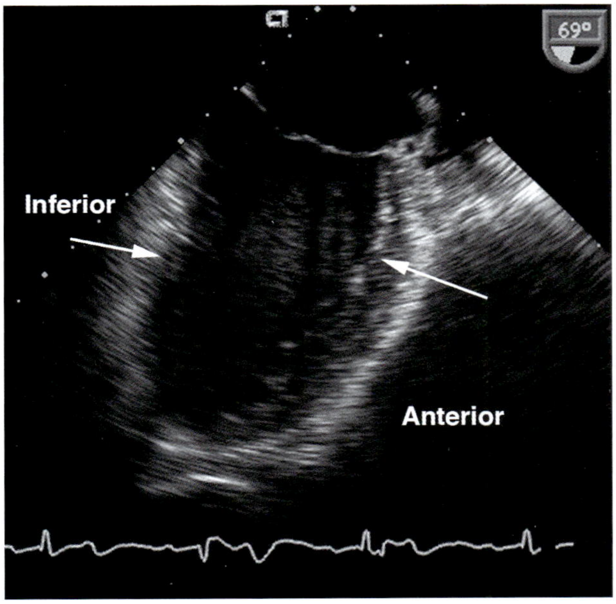

Fig 1.23 The image plane is rotated to 69 degrees to obtain a two-chamber view. The arrows indicate "hinge points" in the inferior and anterior walls; the myocardium below these points is akinetic.

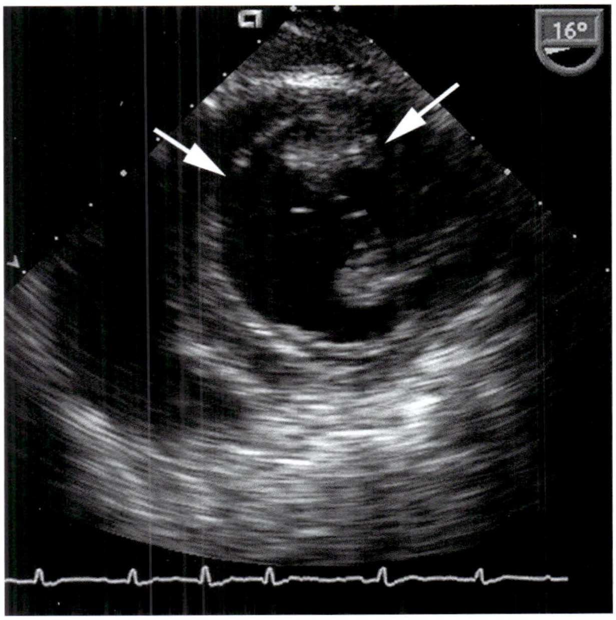

Fig 1.24 In the transgastric short-axis view, the area of basal hypokinesis of the inferior wall *(between the arrows)* is seen.

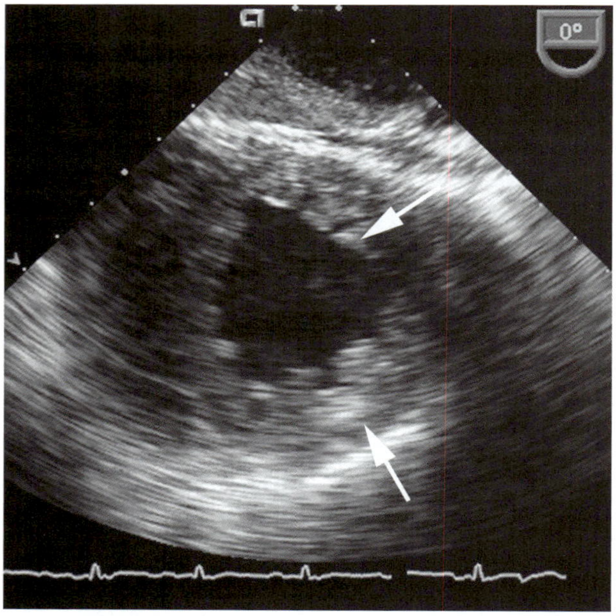

Fig 1.25 In a short-axis view more apical than in Fig 1.24, the lateral wall is the only functioning segment *(between the arrows).*

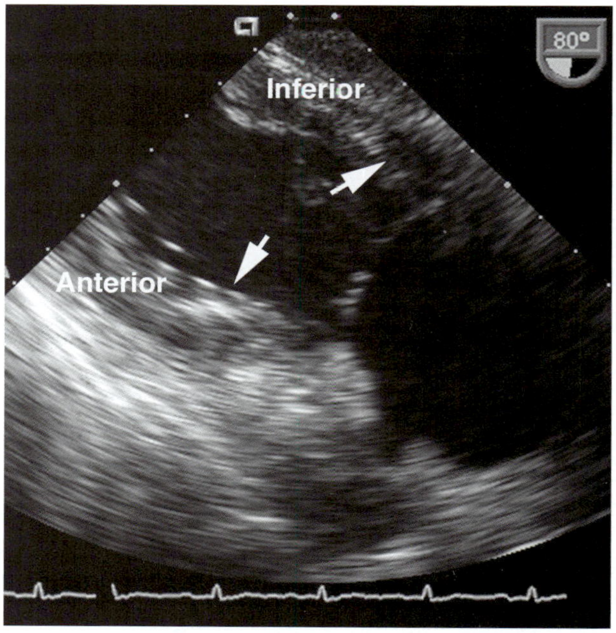

Fig 1.26 From the transgastric short-axis view, the image plane is rotated to 80 degrees to obtain a two-chamber view of the ventricle. As in the midesophageal TEE two-chamber view, this image plane shows the anterior and inferior walls, and "hinge points" *(arrows).*

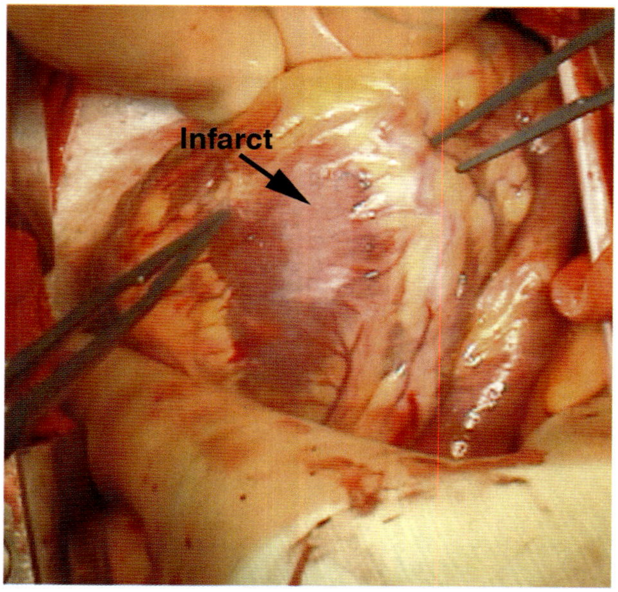

Fig 1.27 At surgical inspection, the infarct of the anterior wall is seen as an area of pallor, or "bullseye." The patient underwent three-vessel coronary-bypass grafting. His postoperative course was complicated by atrial fibrillation and a prolonged need for inotropic support. However, by the tenth postoperative day, he had an ejection fraction of 45% on oral medications and was discharged home.

Comments

Assessment of coronary disease by echocardiography is most often based on the pattern of wall motion abnormalities, rather than by direct visualization of the coronary vessels. In order to fully evaluate all segments of the ventricular myocardium, multiple image planes are used, with the standard views being the four-chamber, two-chamber, and long-axis views from a high transesophageal position and the midventricular, short-axis view from a transgastric position, with each wall divided into thirds—basal, midventricular, and apical. The lateral wall and inferior septum are seen in the four-chamber view, the inferior and anterior walls in the two-chamber view, and the anterior septum and posterior (or inferior–lateral) wall in the long-axis view. The short-axis view provides an orthogonal view of these same segments. A transgastric two-chamber view can also be obtained by rotating 90 degrees from the short-axis view. In some patients, transgastric apical views can also be obtained. However, on both TEE and transgastric views, the true ventricular apex may be foreshortened so that apical wall motion abnormalities may be missed.

A full-volume 3D acquisition from a high TEE position allows accurate measurement of LV volumes and ejection fraction. In addition, multiple short-axis views, or simultaneous apical four-, two-, and long-axis views can be reconstructed from the 3D data set. This 3D approach likely will become more useful in the intraoperative patient care settings as image acquisition and display become increasingly automated.

In patients undergoing cardiopulmonary bypass, regional wall motion is evaluated before and after the bypass run. In patients undergoing off-pump coronary bypass surgery, the majority of wall segments can be evaluated during the procedure, although cardiac displacement may limit visualization of some segments.

Suggested Reading

1. De Mey N, Couture P, Laflamme M, et al: Intraoperative changes in regional wall motion: Can postoperative coronary artery bypass graft failure be predicted? J Cardiothorac Vasc Anesth 26(3):371–375, 2012.
2. Swaminathan M, Morris RW, De Meyts DD, et al: Deterioration of regional wall motion immediately after coronary artery bypass graft surgery is associated with long-term major adverse cardiac events, Anesthesiology 107:739–745, 2007.
3. American Society of Anesthesiologists and Society of Cardiovascular Anesthesiologists, Task Force on Transesophageal Echocardiography: Practice guidelines for perioperative transesophageal echocardiography: An updated report by the American Society of Anesthesiologists and the Society of Cardiovascular Anesthesiologists Task Force on Transesophageal Echocardiography, Anesthesiology 112:1084–1096, 2010.

CASE 1-5
Inferior Wall Myocardial Infarction with Dyskinesis (True Aneurysm)

This 68-year-old man presented to his family doctor with waxing and waning exertional chest pain over the previous month. Physical examination was unremarkable. 12-Lead ECG showed evidence of an inferior wall myocardial infarction. Coronary angiography showed three-vessel disease and he was referred for bypass surgery.

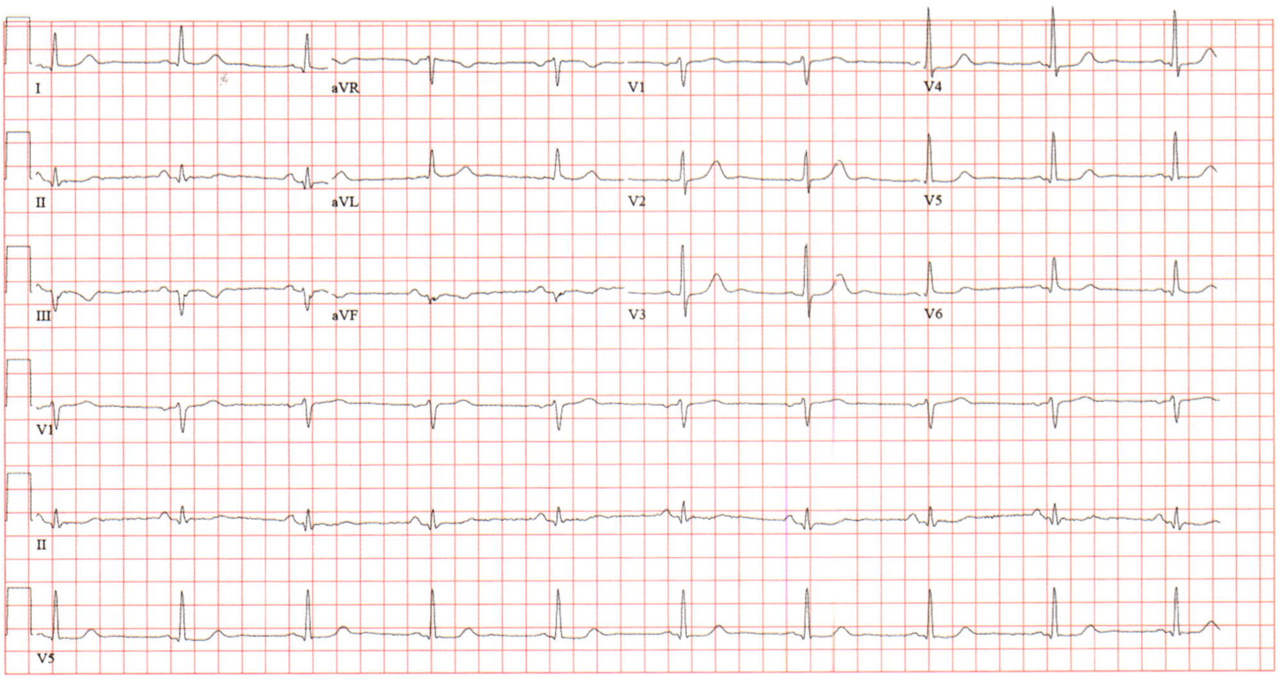

Fig 1.28 In this 12-lead ECG taken at the time of coronary angiography shows evidence of a remote inferior myocardial infarction.

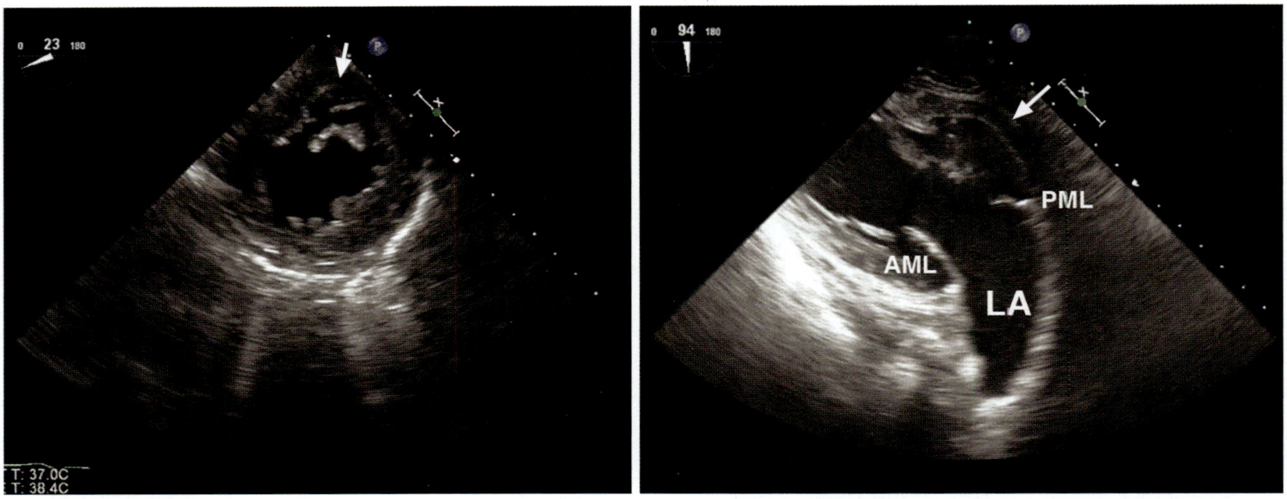

Fig 1.29 On the left is a transgastric short-axis view at the basal end of the papillary muscles. The white arrow indicates the basal inferior wall, which in real time is seen to move in a dyskinetic fashion. On the right is a transgastric long-axis view, which again shows the abnormal basal inferior septum.

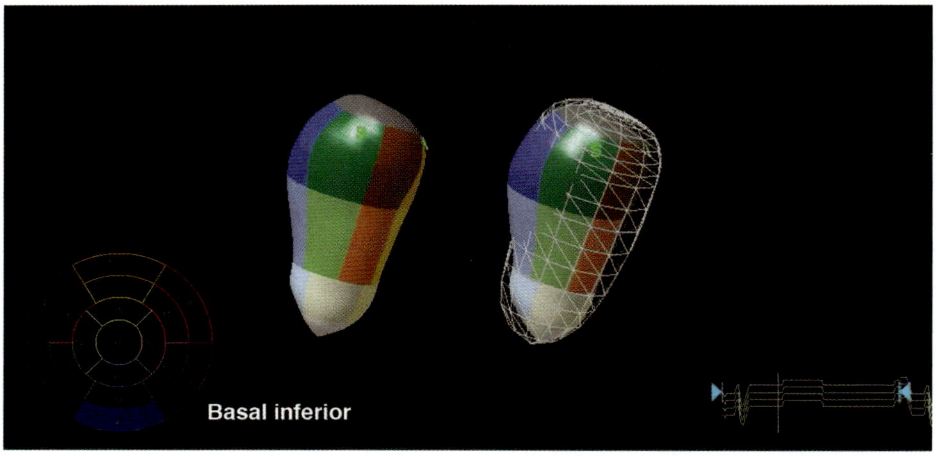

Fig 1.30 Volumetrics are acquired by manual definition of the septal, lateral, anterior, inferior, and apical endocardial borders of the end systolic and the end diastolic frames, followed by an automated border-tracking algorithm (Philips, Bothell, Washington, USA). It can be seen that the basal inferior segment is dyskinetic. The shell in the right-side image defines end diastolic volume.

CASE 1-6
Lateral Wall Myocardial Infarction

This 56-year-old man presented to hospital with multiple episodes of chest pain, which became constant approximately 2 hours before his admission.

ECG evidence of an MI prompted cardiac catheterization, which showed a proximal circumflex occlusion and severe stenosis of the posterior descending artery that originated from the RCA. Attempts at PCI were unsuccessful. A surgical consult was obtained.

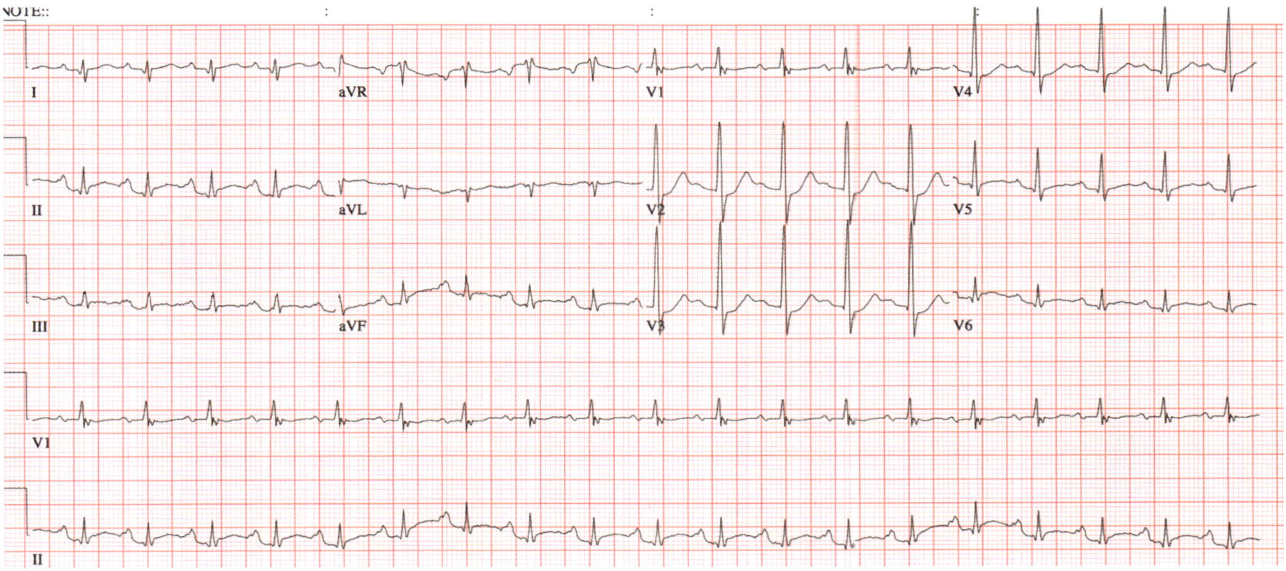

Fig 1.31 ECG revealed putative evidence of both a lateral and posterior wall myocardial infarction.

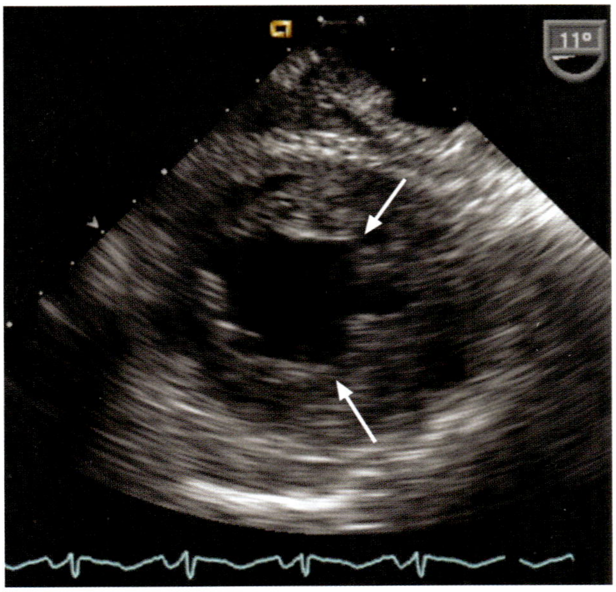

Fig 1.32 In real time, a transgastric short-axis view reveals akinesis in the antero-lateral and infero-lateral walls, between the two arrows or hinge points, as seen in the figure.

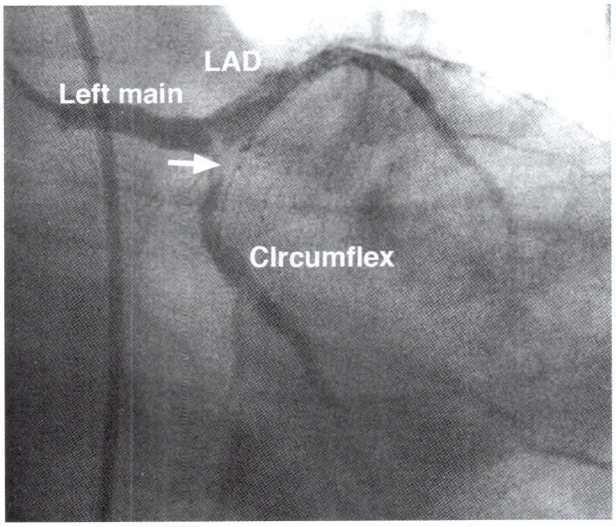

Fig 1.33 Cardiac catheterization showed evidence of thrombus at the origin of the circumflex artery *(arrow)*.

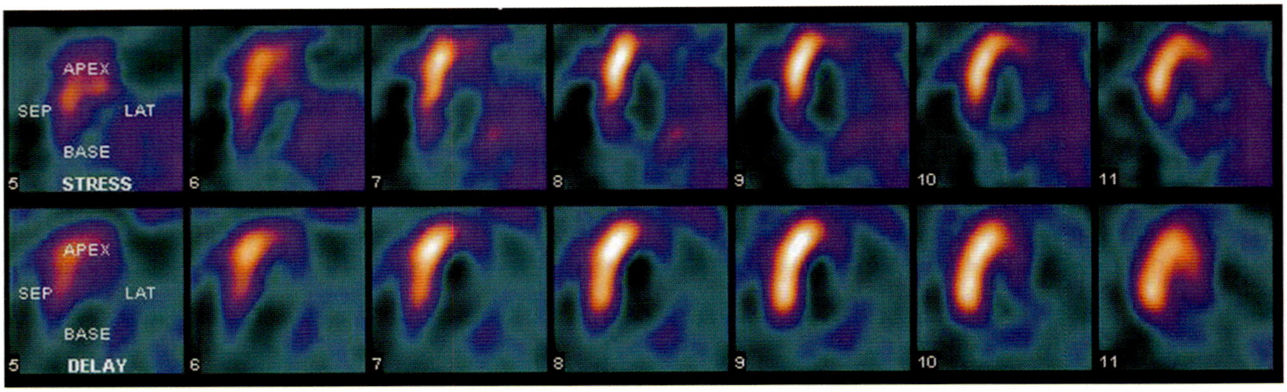

Fig 1.34 A nuclear viability study showed absent perfusion of the lateral wall with stress and little evidence of viability.

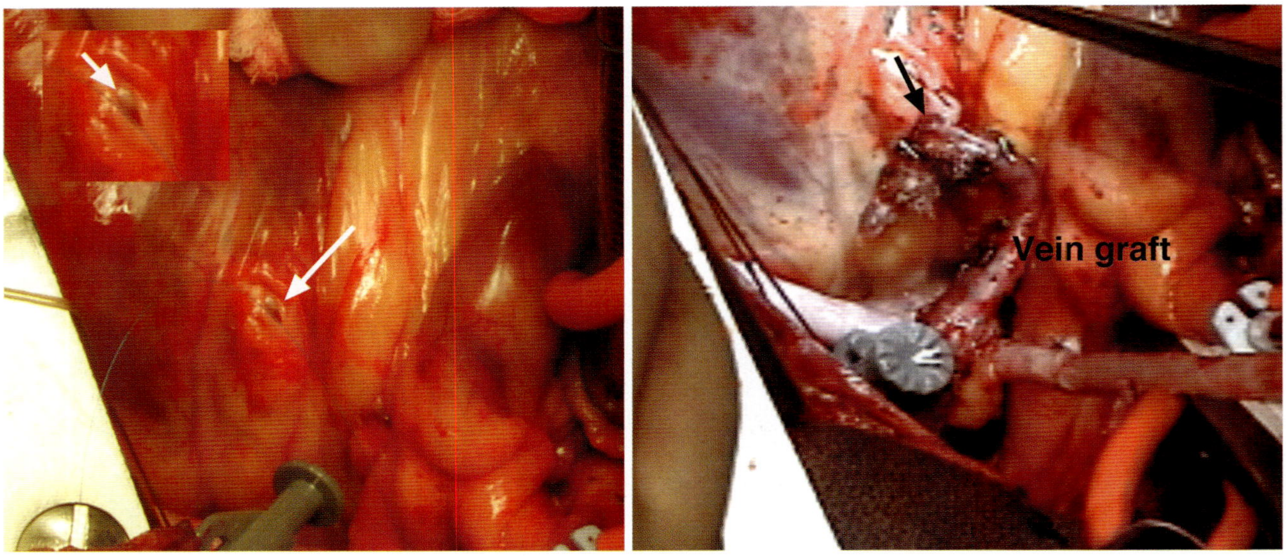

Fig 1.35 At surgery, the surgeon performs an arteriotomy of the circumflex artery *(left)* and the inset *(arrow)* shows some calcium. On the right, a vein graft has been placed from the ascending aorta to the circumflex ostium *(arrow)*.

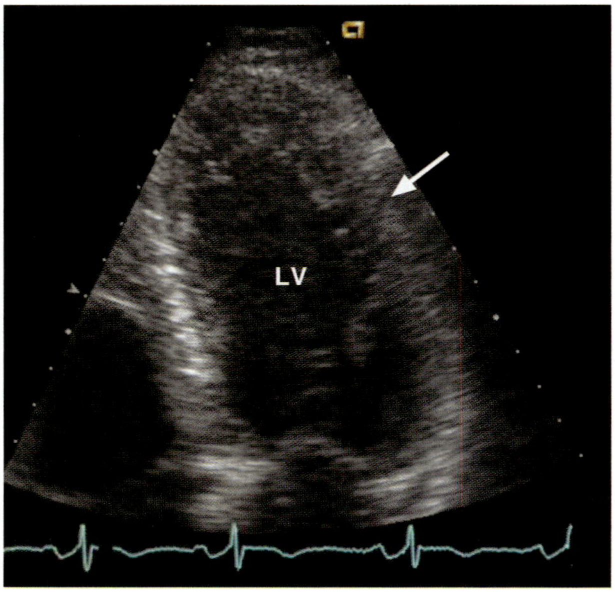

Fig 1.36 Outpatient TTE was performed. The lateral wall *(arrow)* was still akinetic, which can be appreciated in the video.

CASE 1-7
Myocardial Infarction Followed by Heart Transplantation

This 58-year-old woman suffered an acute aortic dissection complicated by a perioperative anterior myocardial infarction 18 months ago. Because of an episode of ventricular tachycardia, she was treated with amiodarone and an automatic implanted defibrillator was placed. Because of her arrhythmias and low left ventricular ejection fraction (about 35%), she was undergoing evaluation for heart transplantation. She was now admitted with recurrent ventricular tachycardia, resistant to medical therapy. A donor became available, and she was taken to the operating room for heart transplantation.

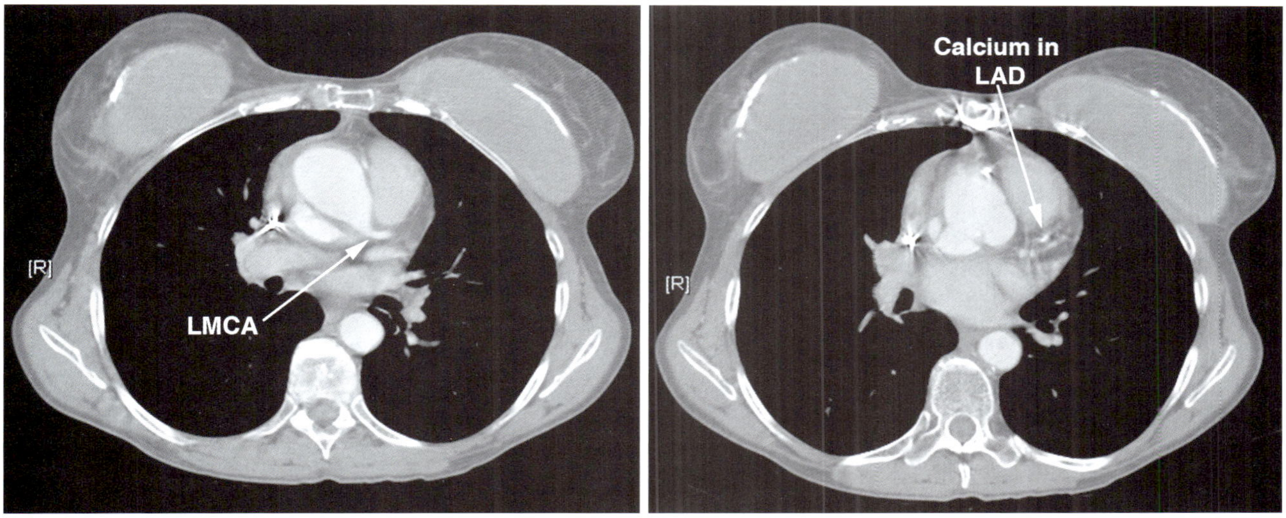

Fig 1.37 Chest CT shows the origin of the left main coronary artery (LMCA) from the enlarged aortic root *(left)*. There is calcification of the left anterior descending (LAD) coronary artery *(right)*.

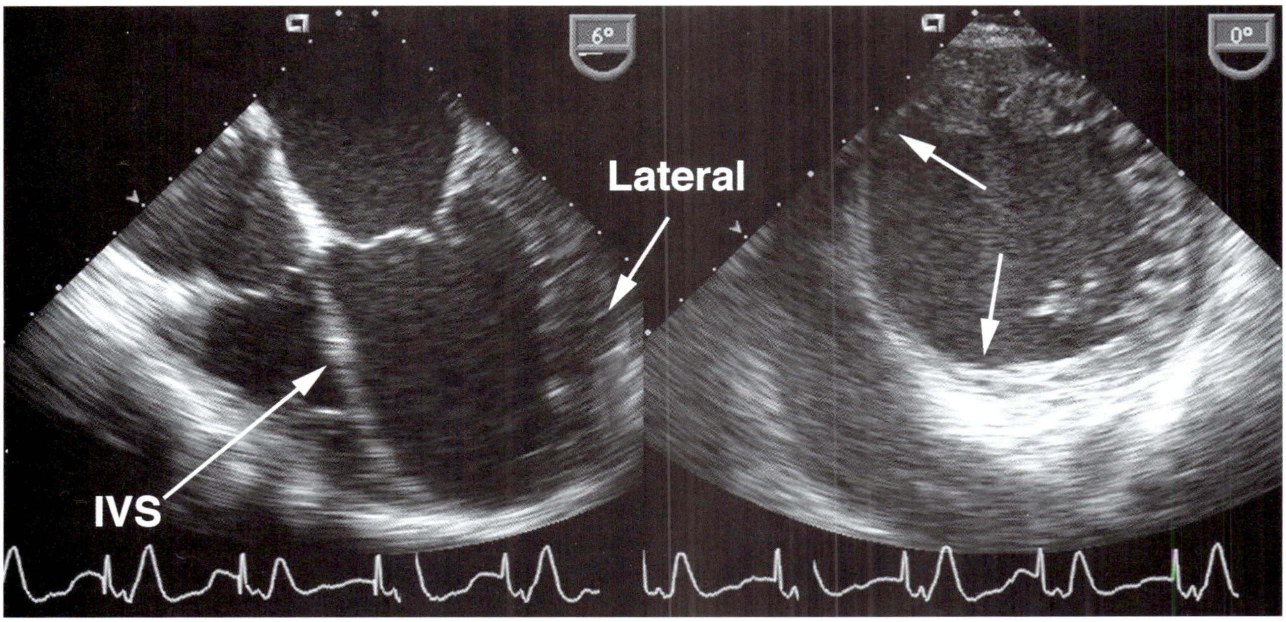

Fig 1.38 In the TEE four-chamber view *(left)* the interventricular septum (IVS) is thin and akinetic, with relatively normal wall thickness and function of the lateral wall. The transgastric short-axis view *(right)* shows the thinned and akinetic anterior and inferior walls *(arrows)*.

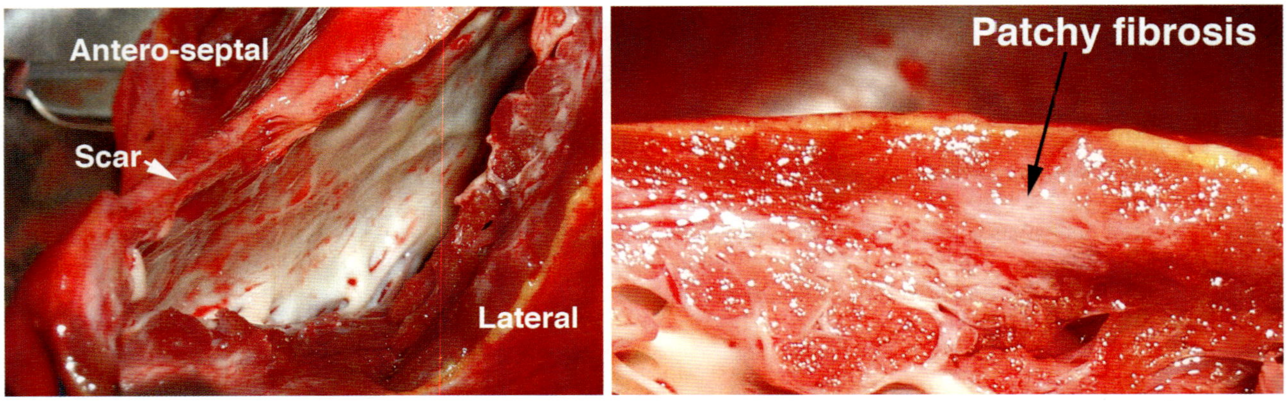

Fig 1.39 The endocardium of the explanted heart shows the scar area along the septum *(left).* A transverse section of the anterior wall of the myocardium shows areas of patchy fibrosis *(right).*

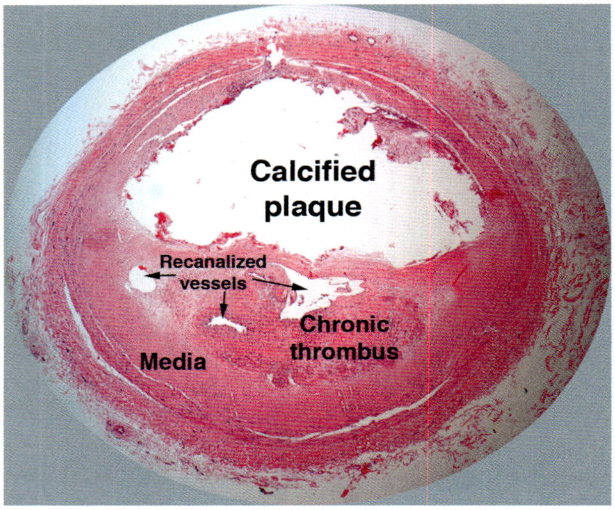

Fig 1.40 Microscopic section of the left anterior descending artery shows a calcified plaque, chronic thrombus, and a small amount of recanalization.

Comments (Cases 5 to 7)

In patients with coronary artery disease, myocardial wall thickness and systolic thickening are normal at rest if there has been no prior myocardial infarction, even when there is a significant degree of coronary stenosis. However, with ischemia there is a prompt decrease in endocardial motion and wall thickening in the myocardial segments supplied by the affected vessel. Wall motion returns to normal with relief of ischemia. This sequence of events is the basis of echocardiographic stress testing, with exercise or dobutamine. However, acute ischemia may also be seen in the operating room.

With myocardial infarction, the irreversible changes in the myocardium correspond to a persistent wall motion abnormality. Wall motion is graded as hypokinetic, akinetic, or dyskinetic with consideration of both the degree of wall thickening and endocardial motion in this grading system. As in Cases 5 and 6, the location of wall motion abnormalities corresponds to the region of myocardium supplied by the affected coronary artery. Wall motion abnormalities in a "noncoronary" distribution often are due to conditions other than coronary artery disease. After myocardial infarction, wall thickness initially is normal but, over time, scarring occurs, with decreased wall thickness and increased echogenicity. The degree of wall thinning corresponds to the transmural extent of the infarction.

In Case 7, the echocardiographic findings were consistent with a large transmural anterior myocardial infarction with the thin akinetic segments on echocardiography corresponding to the scar area on pathology. The lateral wall showed relatively normal function, even though patchy nontransmural infarction was found on pathology.

Suggested Reading

1. Siegel R, Rader F: Exercise echocardiography for diagnosis of coronary disease. In Otto CM, editor: The practice of clinical echocardiography, ed 5, Philadelphia, 2016, Elsevier.
2. Freeman RV: The comprehensive diagnostic transesophageal echocardiogram: Integrating 2D and 3D imaging, Doppler quantitation and advanced approaches. In Otto CM, editor: The practice of clinical echocardiography, ed 5, Philadelphia, 2016, Elsevier.

Complications of Myocardial Infarction

CASE 1-8
Postmyocardial Infarction Ventricular Septal Defect (Anterior)

This 75-year-old woman presented to an outside hospital 3 weeks prior to admission to our institution with an acute anterior myocardial infarction. Because she presented late after symptom onset, she did not receive reperfusion therapy and her postmyocardial infarction echocardiogram showed severely reduced left ventricular systolic function with an apical aneurysm. She was treated with warfarin for an apical thrombus. Ten days later, she presented with a large pericardial effusion and tamponade physiology. After removal of 600 ml of hemorrhagic pericardial fluid, hemodynamics improved, but a new murmur was noted and echocardiography showed an apical ventricular septal defect (VSD). She was then transferred to our medical center for possible surgical intervention.

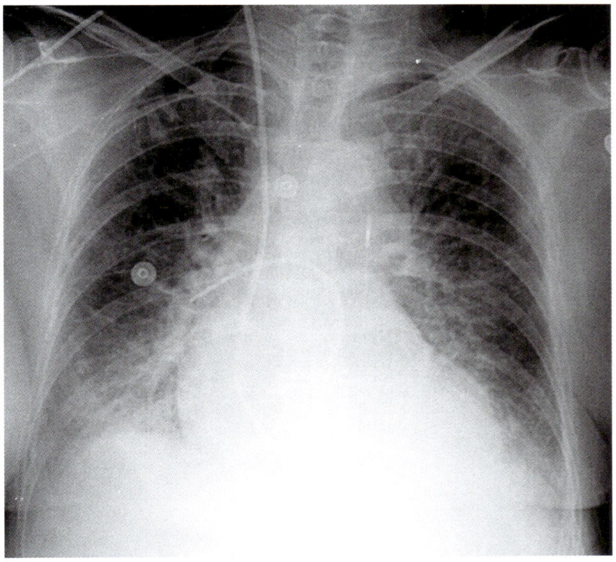

Fig 1.41 Chest radiography shows enlargement of the cardiac silhouette and pulmonary edema.

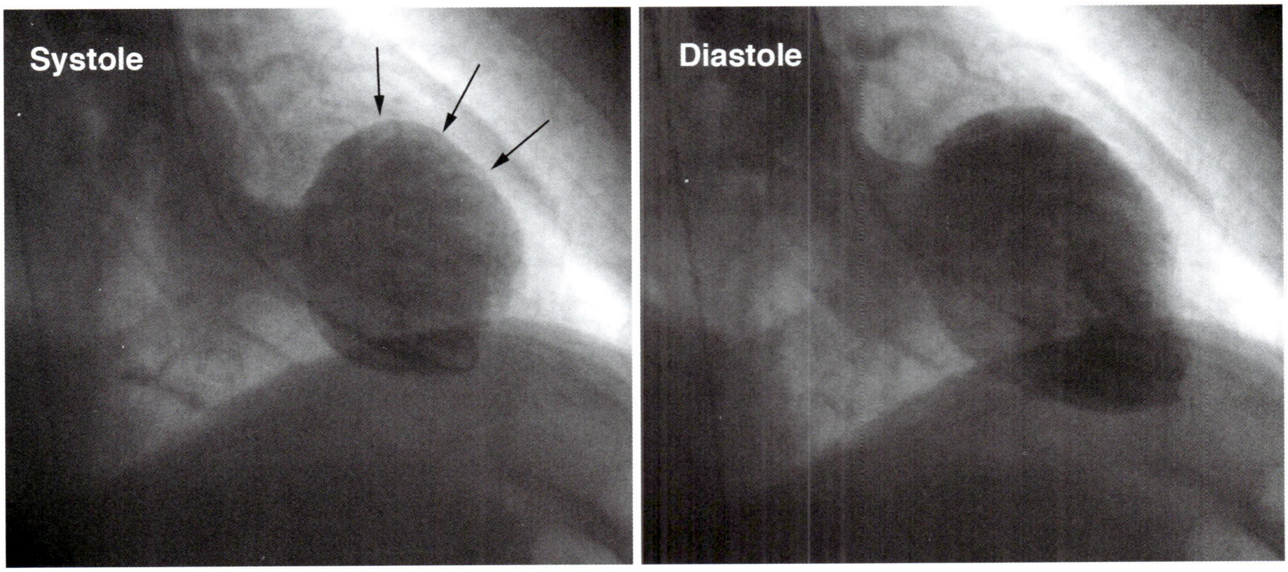

Fig 1.42 Left ventricular angiography in a right anterior oblique projection shows the dilation of the anterior wall of the left ventricle in diastole *(right)* and the akinetic segment in systole *(arrows, left)*.

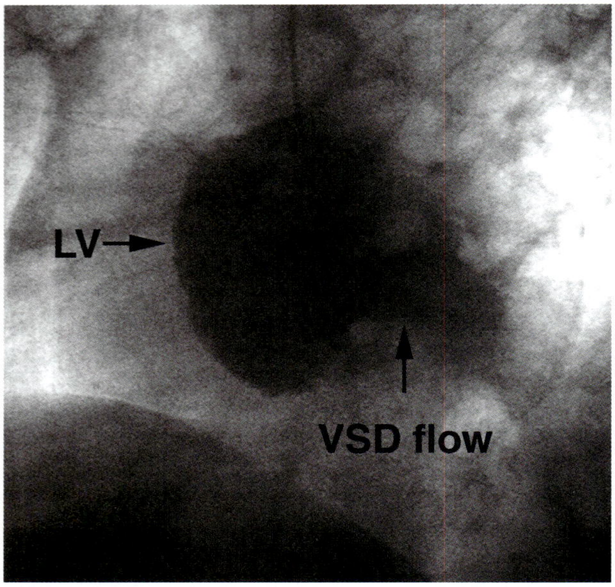

Fig 1.43 Left ventricular angiography was also performed in the less traditional right posterior oblique projection to show contrast entering the right ventricle via the septal defect.

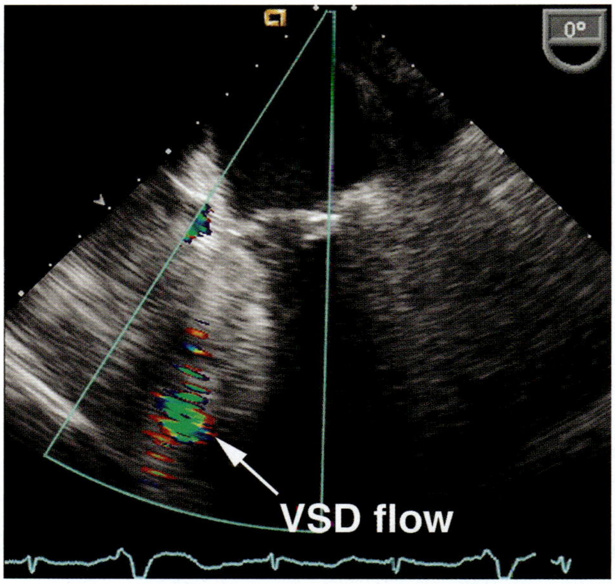

Fig 1.44 In the transesophageal four-chamber view, color Doppler demonstrates turbulent systolic flow in the right ventricular apex.

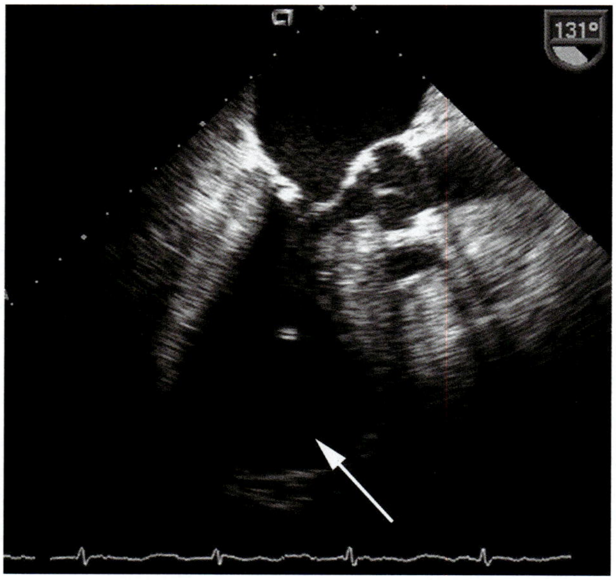

Fig 1.45 In the transesophageal long-axis view, the diastolic contour abnormality and dyskinesis of the midventricular and apical segments of the anterior septum are seen. The arrow indicates the akinetic LV apex.

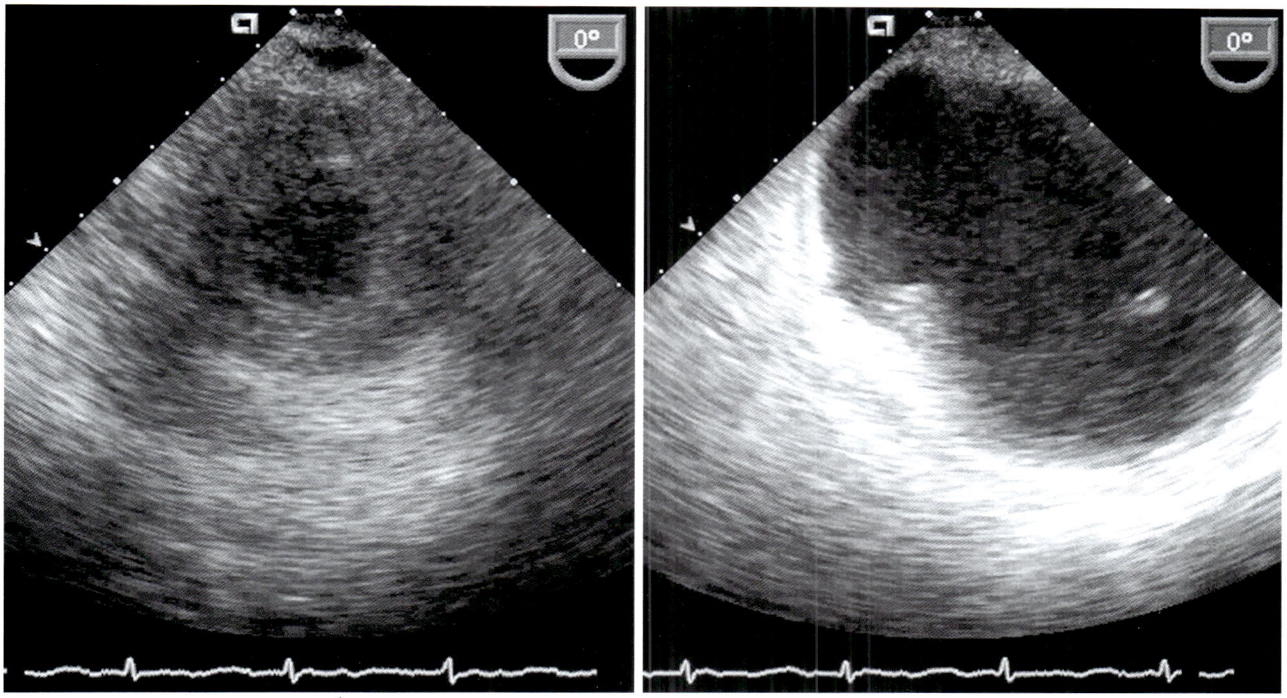

Fig 1.46 In this transgastric short-axis view of the left ventricle, function at the midpapillary level is hyperdynamic *(left)*, whereas the apex *(right)* is aneurysmal and akinetic.

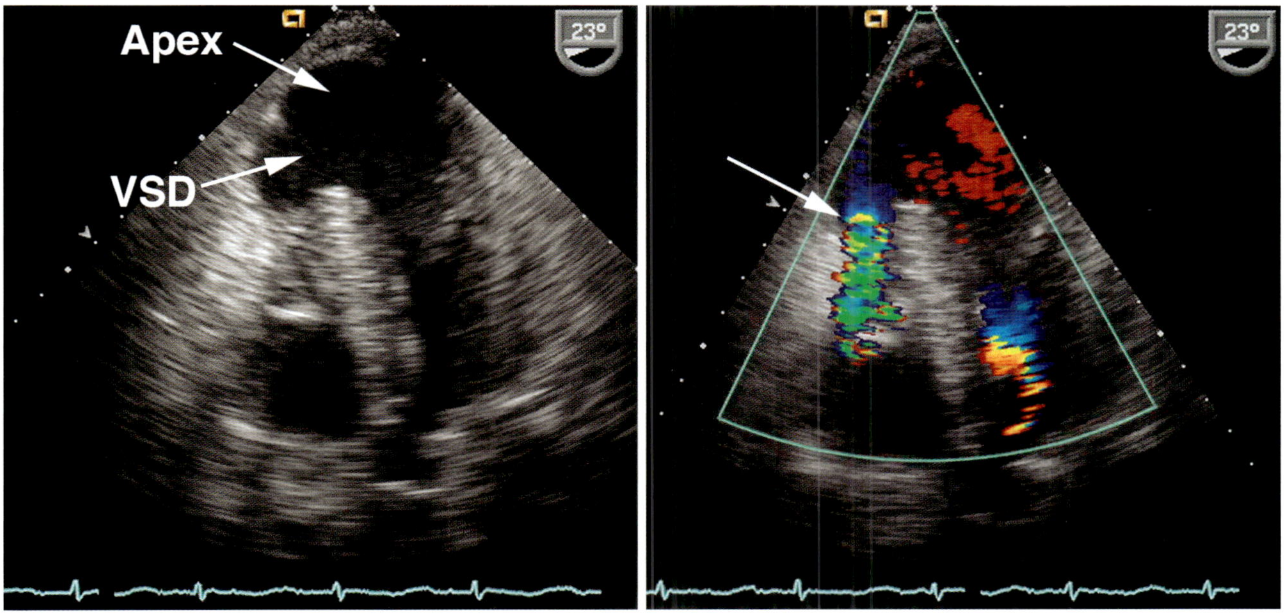

Fig 1.47 In a transgastric apical view with anteflexion of the probe tip, the aneurysm of the apical septum is seen with an area of discontinuity in the septum. Color Doppler *(arrow, right)* confirms flow across the septum consistent with a postmyocardial-infarction ventricular septal defect.

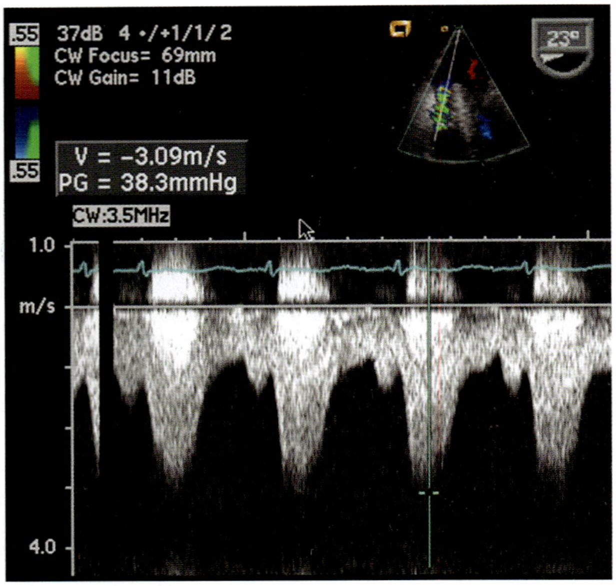

Fig 1.48 Continuous wave Doppler of the flow through the ventricular septal defects shows high-velocity flow in systole, consistent with the systolic pressure difference between the right and left ventricles. The velocity of 3.1 m/s (pressure difference of only 38 mm Hg) is lower than expected with a chronic small ventricular septal defect; thus, it may be underestimated due to a nonparallel intercept angle. However, the patient's systolic blood pressure at the time of this recording was only 100 mm Hg and pulmonary artery pressure was about 50 mm Hg, indicating that velocity is only slightly underestimated. The persistent low-velocity flow in diastole is due to the slightly higher left than right ventricular diastolic pressure.

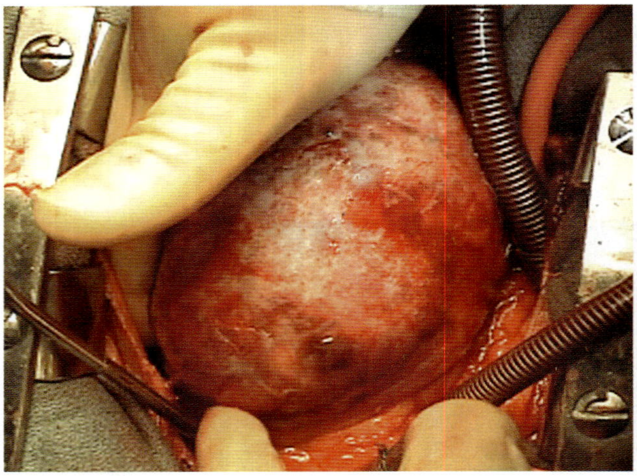

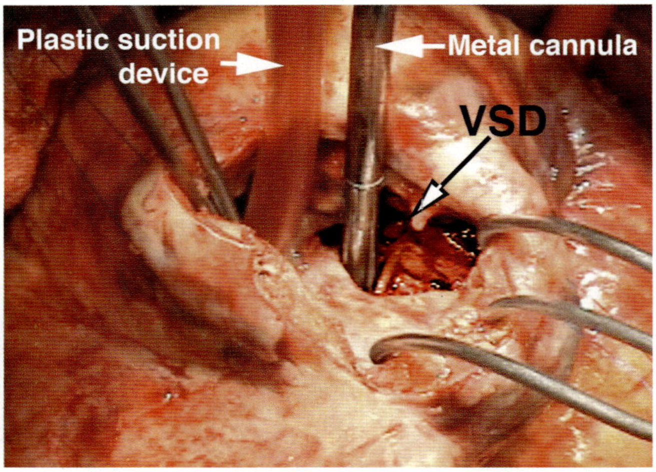

Fig 1.49 On direct inspection at surgery, the anterior left ventricular wall is aneurysmal *(left)*. The left ventricle has been opened through the apical scar with the metal suction cannula in the VSD *(right)*.

CASE 1-9
Postmyocardial Infarction Ventricular Septal Defect (Posterior)

This 58-year-old man with hypertension as his only risk factor for coronary artery disease presented to another hospital with cardiogenic shock. He notes that about 7 days before admission, he developed abdominal and left-sided chest pain, which he attributed to gastrointestinal disease. Over the next several days the pain progressed and radiated to the back. On presentation to the emergency room, he was found to have had elevated troponins and inferior Q-waves on his ECG, consistent with an inferior wall myocardial infarction. An TTE earlier in the morning suggested a VSD. He was transferred to our hospital for management. A right heart catheterization was performed, with the following results:

1. Low cardiac index (Qs) by Fick equation with severely elevated systemic vascular resistance
2. Severely elevated right-sided filling pressures. Mildly elevated left sided filling pressures. Hemodynamics c/w RV infarction
3. Mildly elevated pulmonary artery pressures with normal pulmonary vascular resistance
4. Qp:Qs of 2.6:1. Shunt at the level of the RV

An intraaortic balloon pump was placed and he was taken to the OR. The inferior septal defect was repaired by an inferior left ventriculotomy and endocardial patch placement with infarct exclusion.

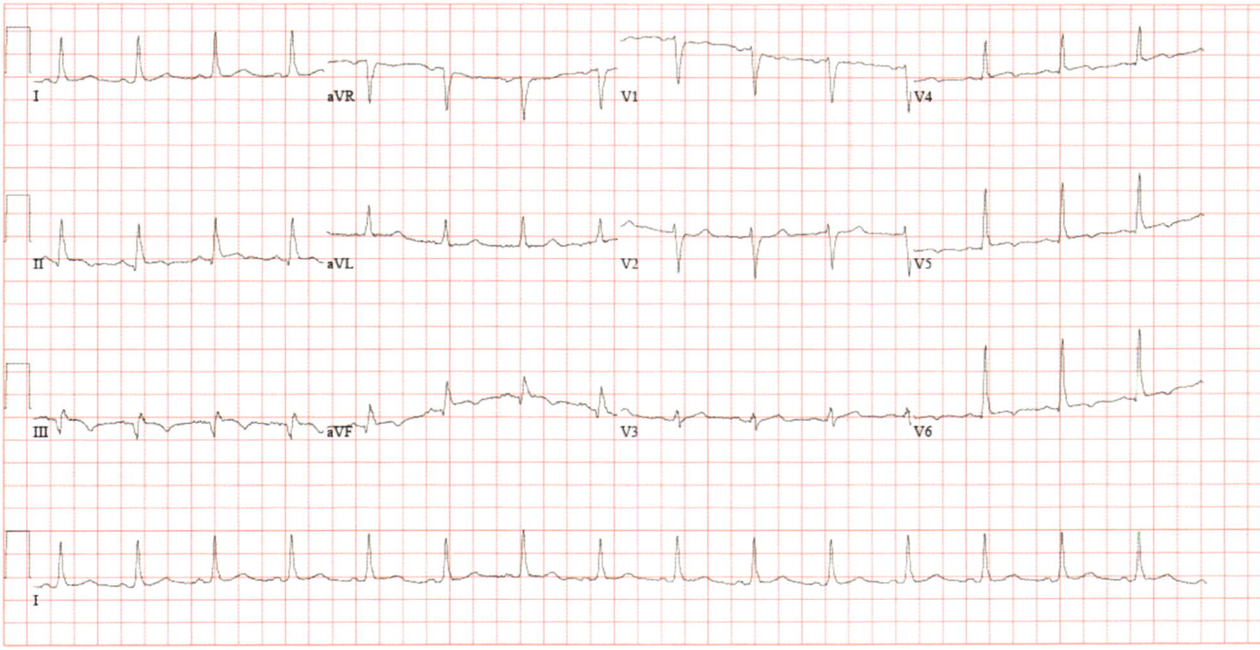

Fig 1.50 ECG on admission to our hospital showed evidence of an inferior wall myocardial infarction.

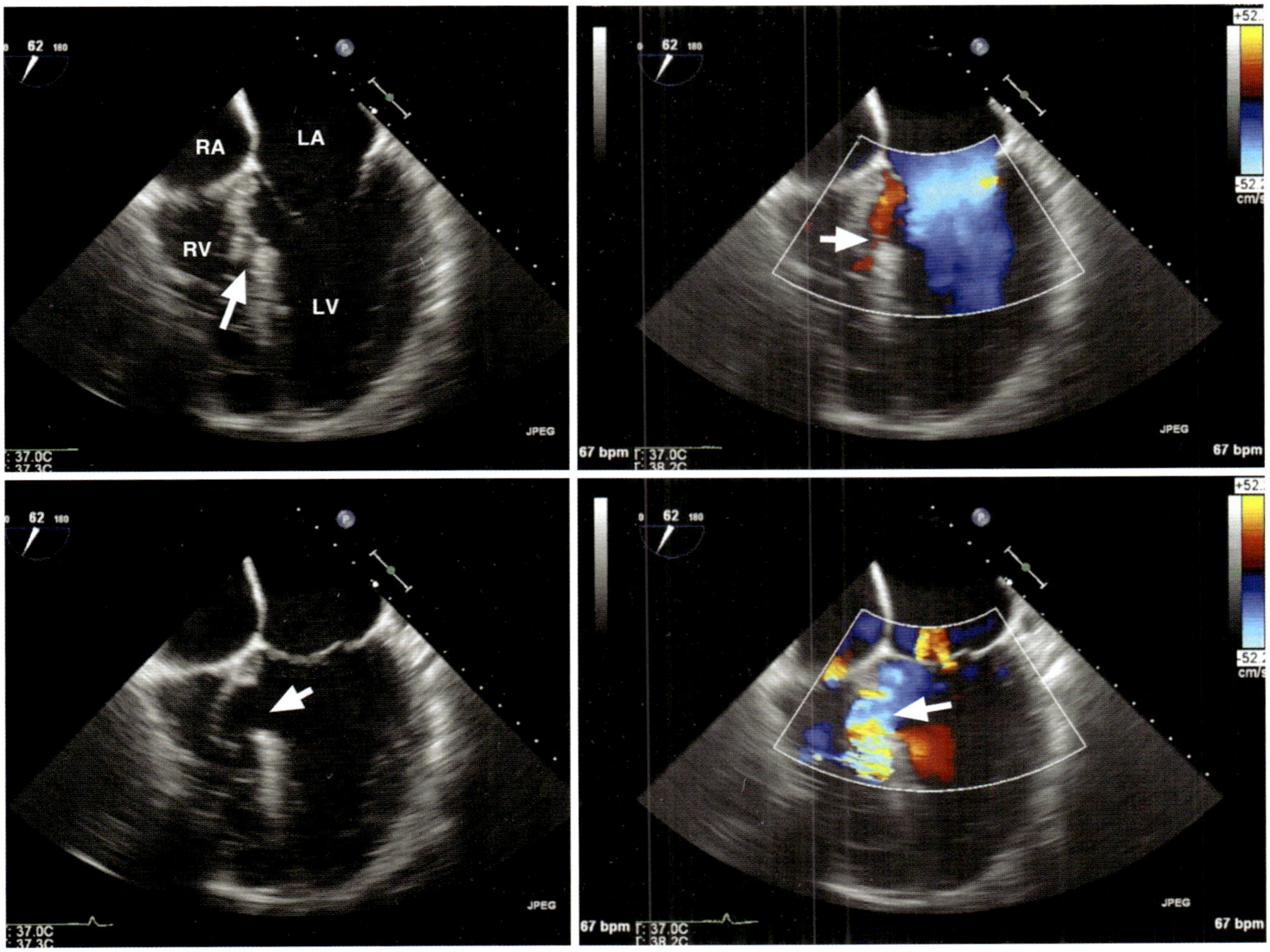

Fig 1.51 This image is a midesophageal four chamber with retroflexion of the probe tip. The upper two images are in diastole, and there appears to be a small amount of flow through a small basal defect in the interventricular septum *(white arrows)*. In the lower two images during systole, the basal defect is more pronounced and the flow between the ventricles is evident *(arrows)*.

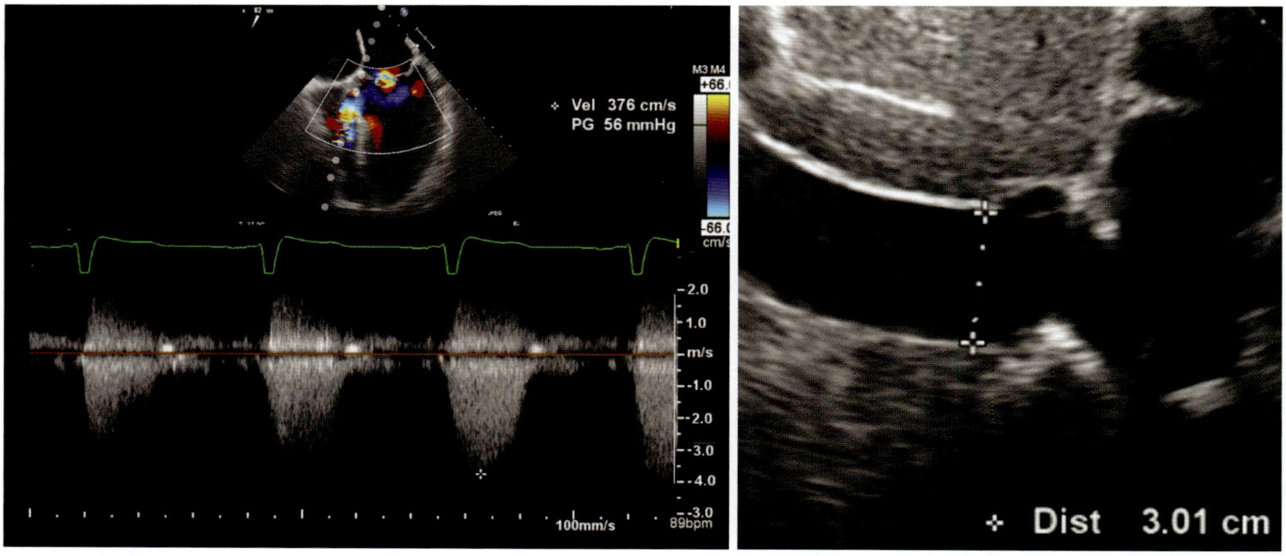

Fig 1.52 On the left, CW Doppler confirms this as left-to-right shunt. On the right, the IVC diameter is increased to 3.01 cm, indicative of increased right atrial pressure.

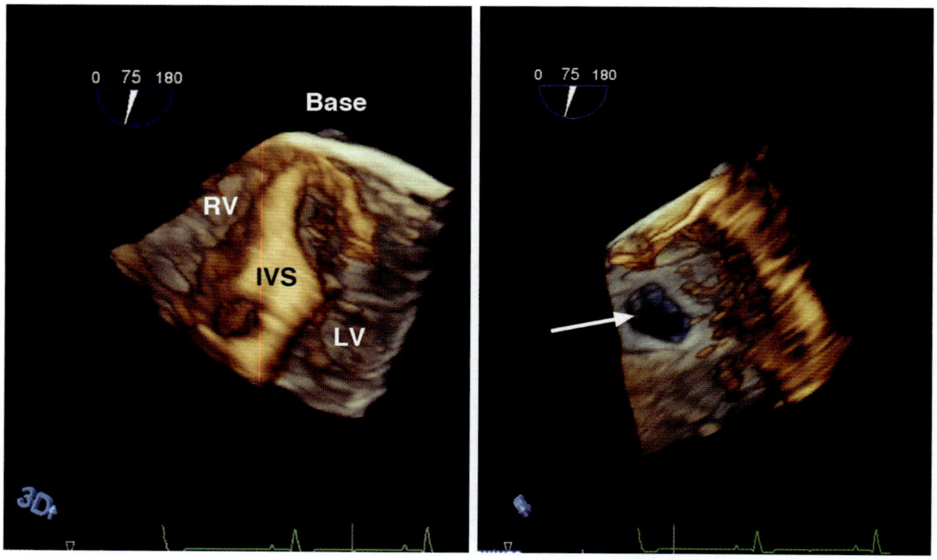

Fig 1.53 3D TEE imaging. On the left, the two ventricles and the interventricular septum are seen. On the right, with the image rotated in a clockwise fashion, the left ventricular aspect of the septum is seen, as is the VSD *(arrow)*.

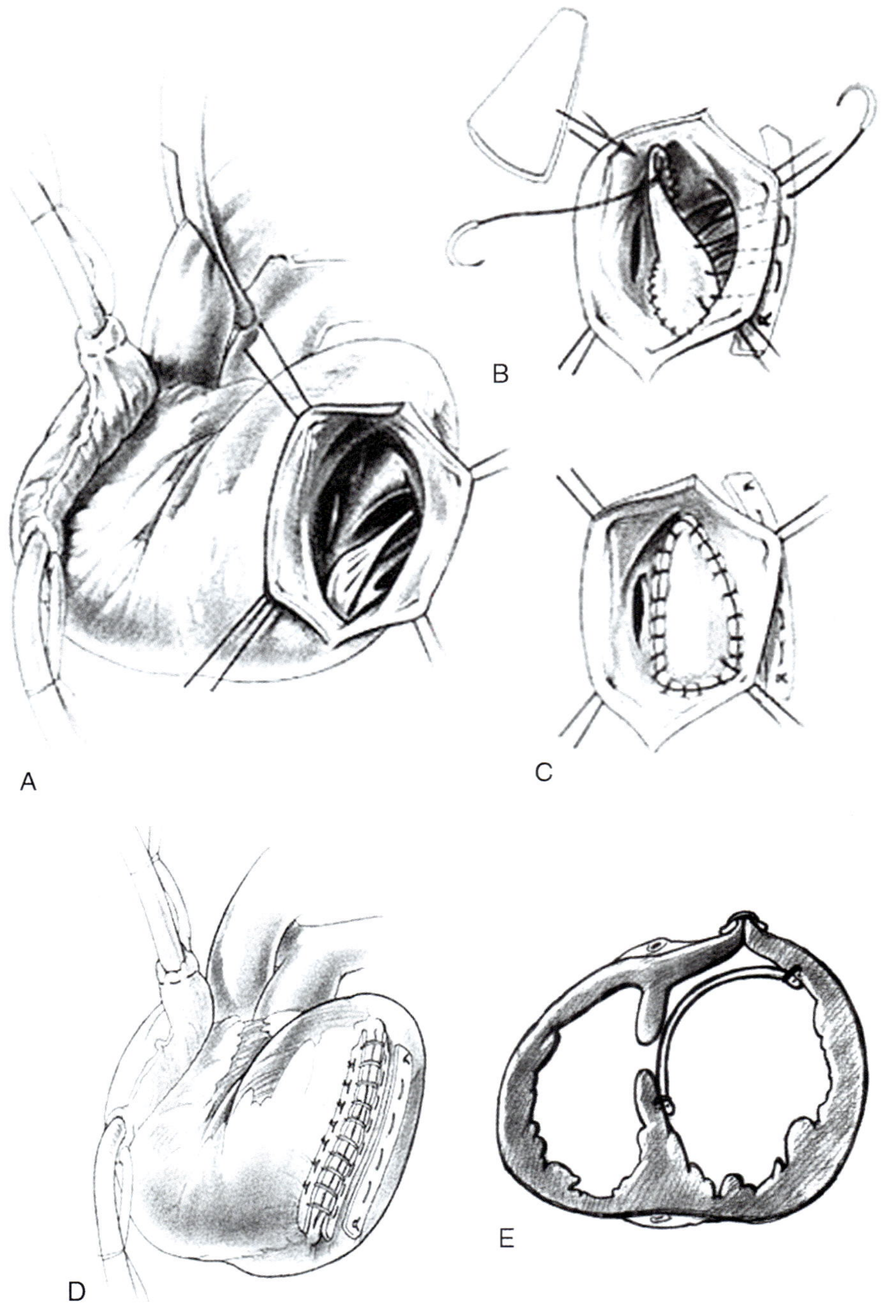

Fig 1.54 Repair of posterior VSD. After the left ventricle is opened inferiorly (**A**), a pericardial patch is sutured to the mitral annulus, septum, and posterior wall, and the left ventricular incision closed (**B** through **D**). In (**E**), the endocardial patch is seen to exclude the septal infarct. (Reproduced with permission from David TE, Dale L, Sun Z. Postinfarction ventricular septal rupture: Repair by endocardial patch with infarct exclusion. J Thorac Cardiovasc Surg 1995;110:1315–1322.)

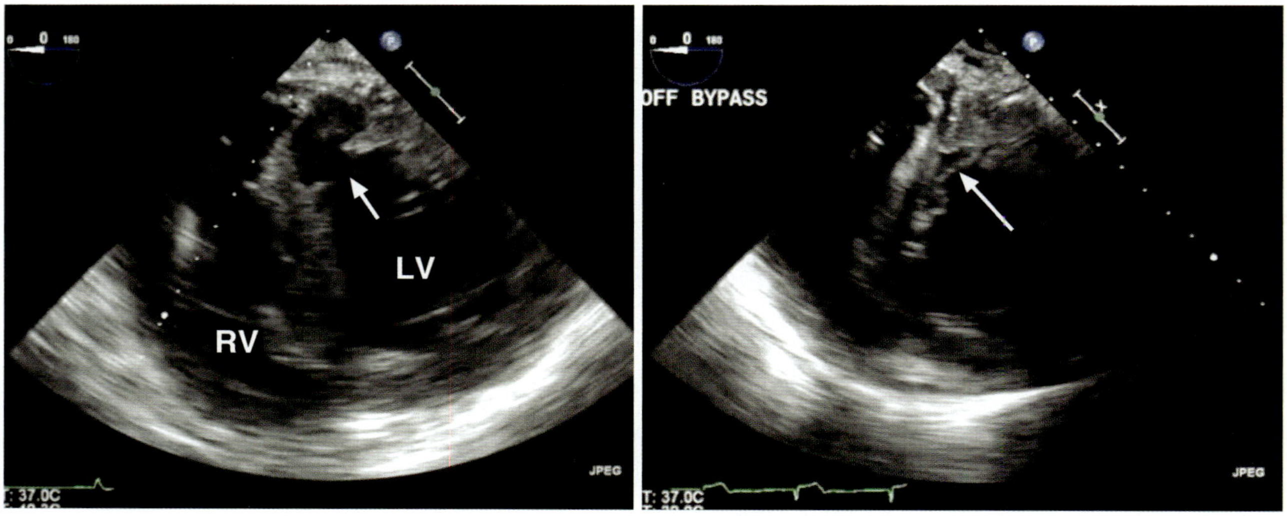

Fig 1.55 On the left is a transgastric prebypass image, with the arrow indicating the VSD. On the right, the arrow indicates a portion of the exclusion patch, which in real time is redundant, minimizing tension on the patch.

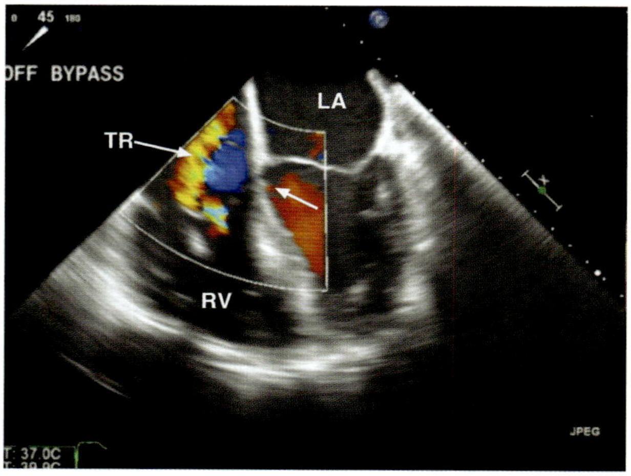

Fig 1.56 A midesophageal four-chamber view, postbypass, shows absence of flow between the ventricles *(arrow)*.

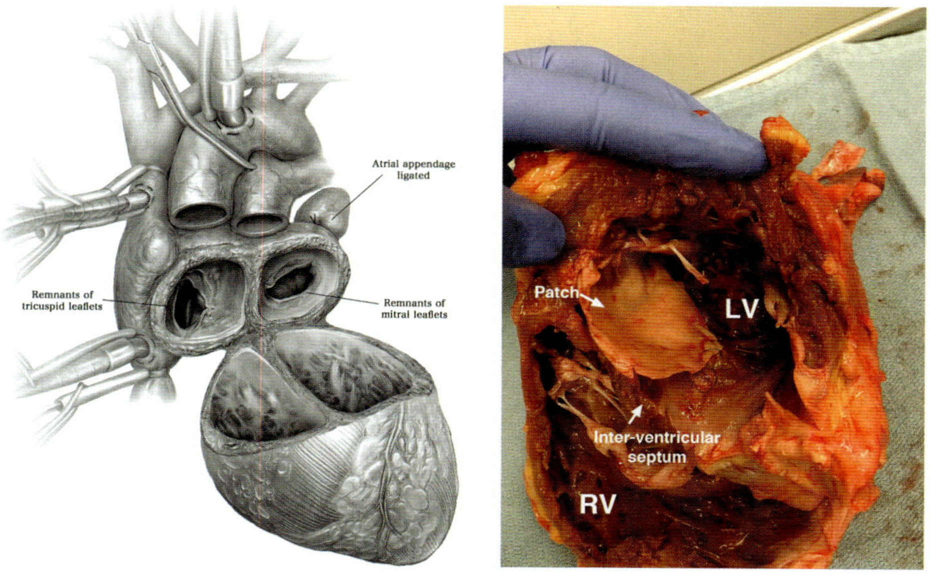

Fig 1.57 The patient developed biventricular failure, and 3 weeks later was scheduled for a total artificial heart. The image on the left shows the procedure by which the surgeon excised both ventricles; on the right is the patient's explanted specimen with the VSD patch clearly visible. (Reproduced with permission from Morris RJ. The SynCardia total artificial heart: implantation technique. Oper Tech Thorac Cardiovasc Surg 2012; 17:154–164.)

Comments (Cases 8 and 9)

Rupture of the myocardium is a rare but life-threatening complication of acute myocardial infarction (MI). Rupture of the left ventricular free wall leads to acute tamponade or a contained rupture with pseudoaneurysm formation (<1% of acute MI patients), rupture of the papillary muscle results in acute mitral regurgitation, and rupture of the septum leads to a VSD (2% of all MIs). Rupture occurs equally in the anterior and inferior septum and may be basal or apical. Risk factors for ventricular rupture include first myocardial infarction, transmural infarction (ST elevation or Q-wave formation), and a greater rise in cardiac enzymes. These factors suggest that the key parameters leading to rupture are the absence of collateral vessels and a larger infarction. Reperfusion therapy decreases the likelihood of rupture, although the clinical presentation may be earlier in those who do suffer this complication.

The clinical presentation in this patient is consistent with a postmyocardial infarction VSD, as clearly demonstrated on echocardiography. The history of pericardial tamponade is of concern, suggesting that she may also have had a contained free wall rupture. Outcome with a postmyocardial infarction VSD is poor, with a 30-day mortality as high as 74%. Treatment includes medical stabilization followed by surgical repair, although the timing of surgery remains controversial. Currently, many patients are treated with a transcatheter closure of the VSD, either as definitive therapy or as stabilization before elective surgery after myocardial healing has occurred.

Suggested Reading

1. Foster E, Gerber I: Echocardiography in the coronary care unit: Management of acute myocardial infarction, detection of complications and prognostic implications. In Otto CM, editor: The practice of clinical echocardiography, ed 5, Philadelphia, 2016, Elsevier.
2. Egbe AC, Poterucha JT, Rihal CS, et al: Transcatheter closure of postmyocardial infarction, iatrogenic, and postoperative ventricular septal defects: The Mayo Clinic experience, Catheter Cardiovasc Interv 2015.
3. Cossor W, Cui VW, Roberson DA: Three-dimensional echocardiographic en face views of ventricular septal defects: Feasibility, accuracy, imaging protocols and reference image collection, J Am Soc Echocardiogr 28(9):1020–1029, 2015.
4. Liu Y, Frikha Z, Maureira P, et al: 3D transesophageal echocardiography is a decision-making tool for the management of cardiogenic shock following a large postinfarction ventricular defect, J Cardiothorac Surg 10:8, 2015.

CASE 1-10
Left Ventricular Reconstructive Surgery (Dor Procedure)

This 65-year-old woman was referred for ventricular endoaneurysmorrhaphy, mitral valve repair, and an atrial Maze procedure. Four months ago she suffered an anterior wall myocardial infarction. Despite thrombolytic therapy and emergency stent placement, she developed an akinetic anterior wall and apex. Over the ensuing 3 months of hospitalization, she had multiple complications, including intermittent congestive heart failure requiring several intubations, renal insufficiency, mitral regurgitation, pulmonary hypertension, anemia, a gastrointestinal bleed, pulmonary hypertension, and paroxysmal atrial fibrillation. Serial echocardiograms demonstrated an akinetic anterior wall and apex with moderate to severe mitral regurgitation and pulmonary hypertension. A nuclear scan demonstrated no viability in the anterior wall. After an extensive discussion with the cardiology service, heart failure team, arrhythmia service, and cardiac surgery service, the decision to proceed with surgical intervention was undertaken.

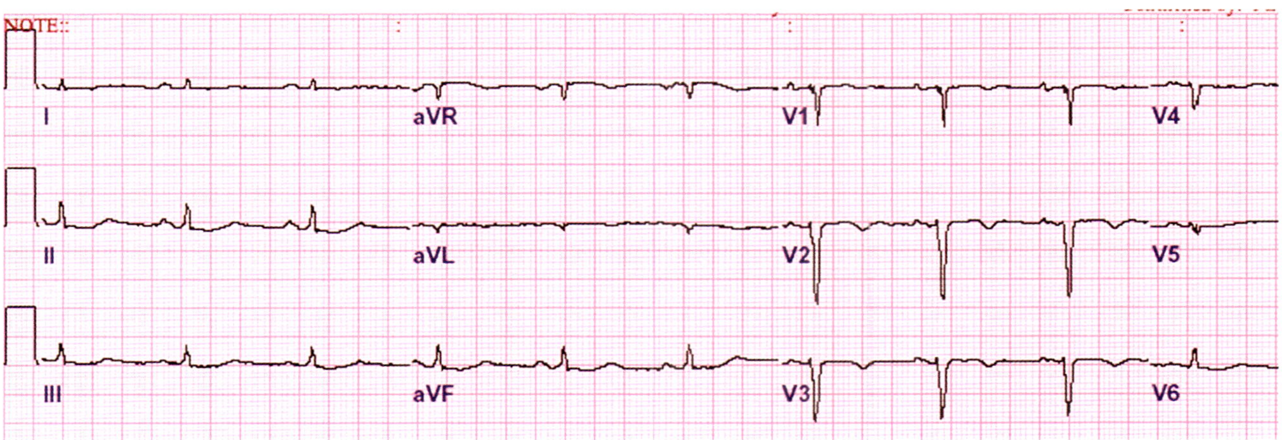

Fig 1.58 The ECG shows Q-waves in leads V1–V5, with T-wave inversion but no acute ST changes, consistent with an old anterior myocardial infarction.

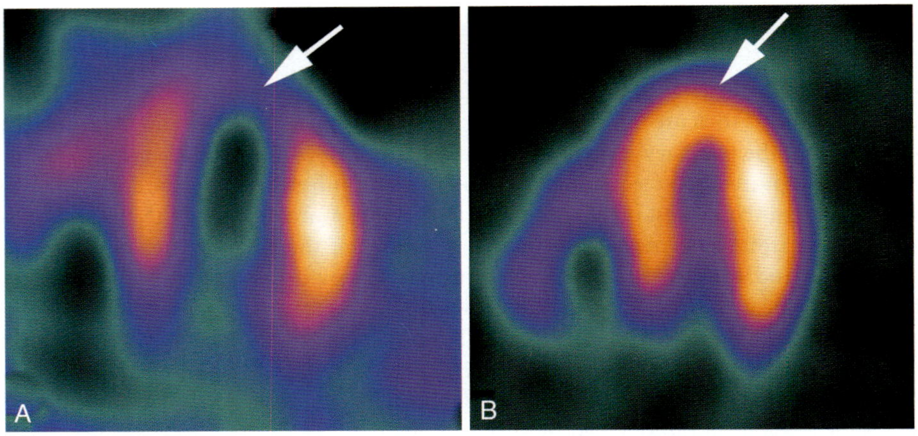

Fig 1.59 On the patient's resting radionuclide perfusion scan **(A)** in a four-chamber orientation, there is no uptake in the apical one third of the ventricle *(arrow)*, consistent with a large area of infarction. Late redistribution images showed no change in the pattern of perfusion, indicating that the apical region of the ventricle is not viable. A normal perfusion image from a different patient is shown **(B)** for comparison.

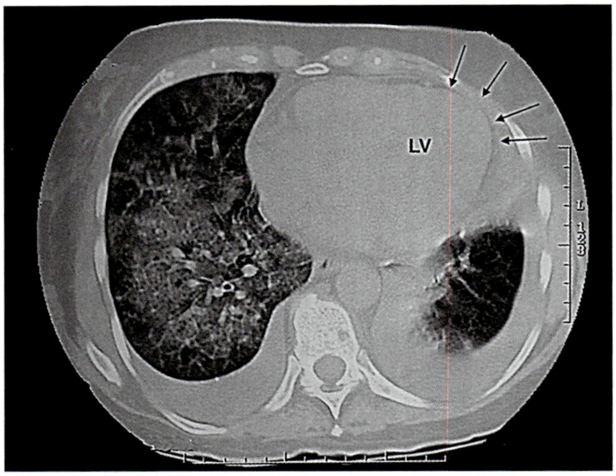

Fig 1.60 This chest computed tomographic (CT) scan at the LV level shows the apical aneurysm *(arrows)*.

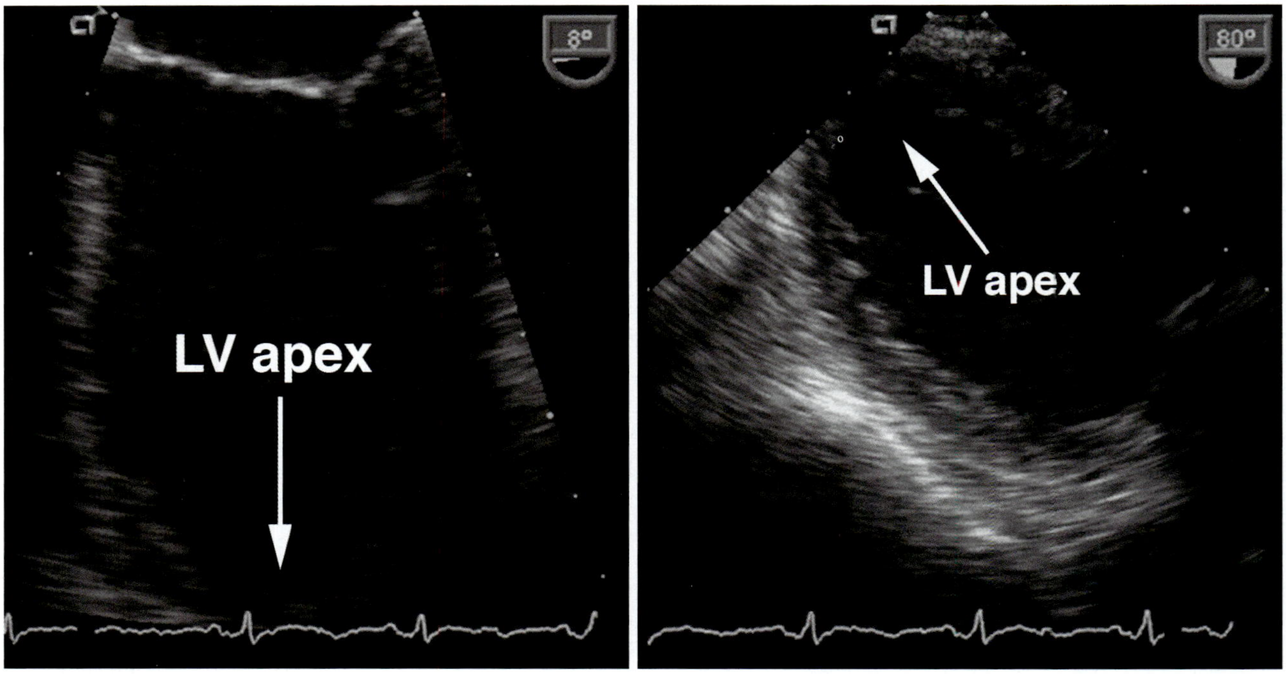

Fig 1.61 The left ventricular apex (LV apex) is seen in close up in a midesophageal four-chamber view *(left)* and a transgastric two-chamber view *(right)*. In real time, the apex is seen to be dyskinetic.

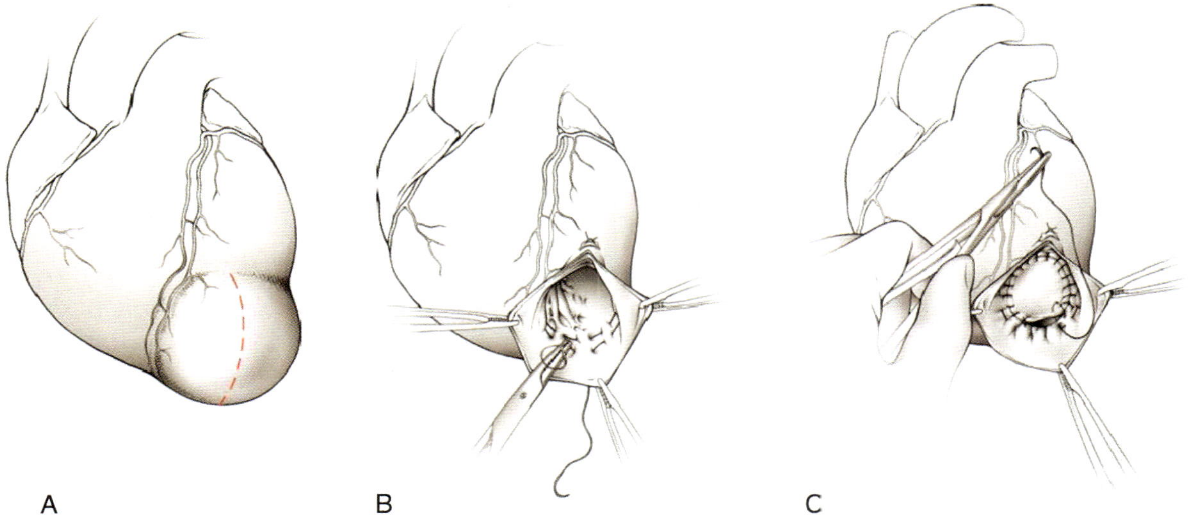

Fig 1.62 The Dor procedure is designed to exclude the akinetic scarred segment of the ventricle to restore normal left ventricular geometry and improve overall ventricular performance. The left ventricular cavity is opened in the middle of the aneurysm **(A).** One or more sutures of 2-O Prolene monofilament are placed circumferentially approximately 1 cm above the border between the scarred and normal myocardium to restore the apex of the contracting ventricle **(B).** Then a circular fabric (usually Dacron) patch, about 2 cm in diameter, is fixed inside the ventricle along this suture line to close the ventricular cavity **(C).** The scarred myocardium is closed over the patch. (Reproduced with permission from Franco KL, Verrier ED. Advanced Therapy in Cardiac Surgery 2e. Hamilton: BC Decker Inc., 2003.)

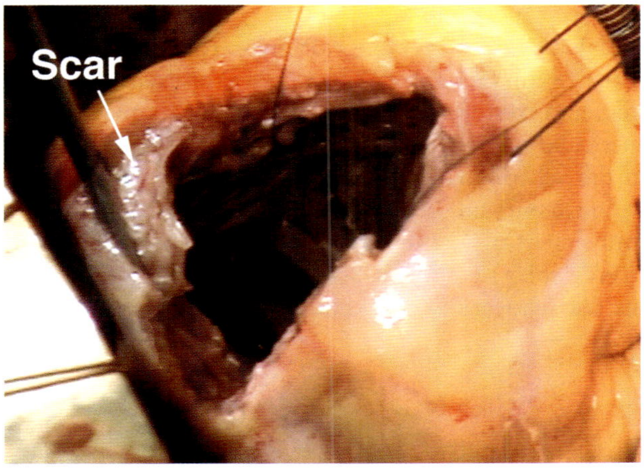

Fig 1.63 At surgery the apical scar was opened, corresponding to step A in Fig 1.62 Normal trabeculations are seen in the ventricular chamber.

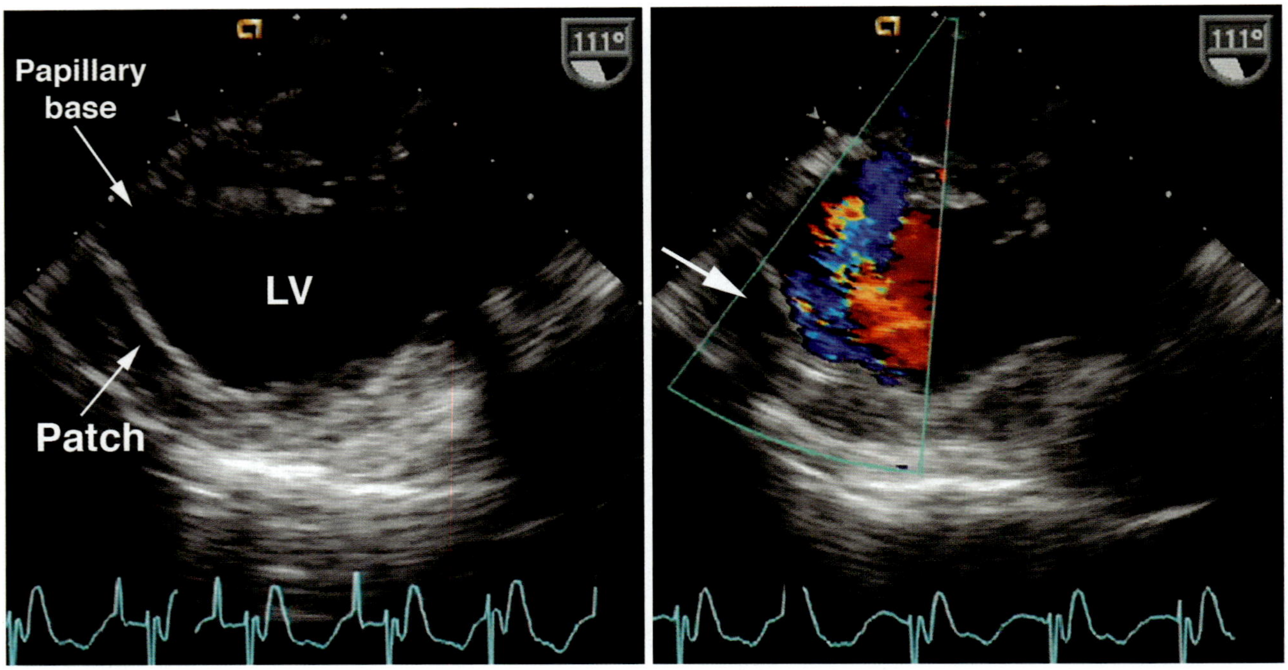

Fig 1.64 The transgastric transesophageal image in a long-axis orientation, after completion of the procedure, shows the Dacron patch in the apical region. Color Doppler *(right)* demonstrates the patch to be intact, with no flow entering the excluded apex *(arrow)*.

Comments

This patient developed a large apical aneurysm after anterior myocardial infarction. The concept behind the Dor procedure is that ventricular performance can be improved by removal or exclusion of the scarred akinetic segment. The proposed mechanism of improvement is restoration of normal ventricular geometry, which leads to a decrease in wall stress because of the smaller ventricular diameter. With the Dor procedure, instead of excising the aneurysm, the aneurysmal area is excluded from the ventricular chamber with a patch closure of the residual opening between the normal part of the ventricle and the aneurysm, as detailed in the figures. Overall, operative mortality for this procedure is 8% with an average improvement in ejection fraction from 33% preoperatively to 50% 1 week after surgery, with sustained improvement in ventricular function at 1-year follow-up. The benefit of this procedure depends on the size of the myocardial scar. Thus the echocardiographic examination focuses on defining the extent and location of wall thinning, akinesis, and dyskinesis.

Suggested Reading

1. Dor V, Saab M, Coste P, et al: Endoventricular patch plasties with septal exclusion for repair of ischemic left ventricle: Technique, results and indications from a series of 781 cases, Jpn J Thorac Cardiovasc Surg 46(5):389–398, 1998.
2. Singh SP, Narula J, Malhotra P: Video Commentary 1: Tee for endoventricular patch plasty/dor procedure, Ann Card Anaesth 18(3):392, 2015.
3. Cho Y, Ueda T, Inoue Y, et al: Long-term results and mid-term features of left ventricular reconstruction procedures on left ventricular volume, geometry, function and mitral regurgitation, Eur J Cardiothorac Surg 42(3):462–469, 2012.

CASE 1-11
Postmyocardial Infarction Pseudoaneurysm

This 63-year-old male presented to an outside hospital with an ST-segment-elevation myocardial infarction (STEMI), and had his RCA stented. He was discharged home with residual inferior wall motion abnormalities consistent with myocardial infarction. Eleven days later he was readmitted with shortness of breath; a TTE showed a larger circumferential pericardial effusion. Subsequently 900 ml were removed at pericardiocentesis, and a presumptive diagnosis of postmyocardial infarction, or Dressler's syndrome. On routine follow-up 4 years later, an inferior wall pseudoaneurysm was seen, and the patient was referred for surgical consultation.

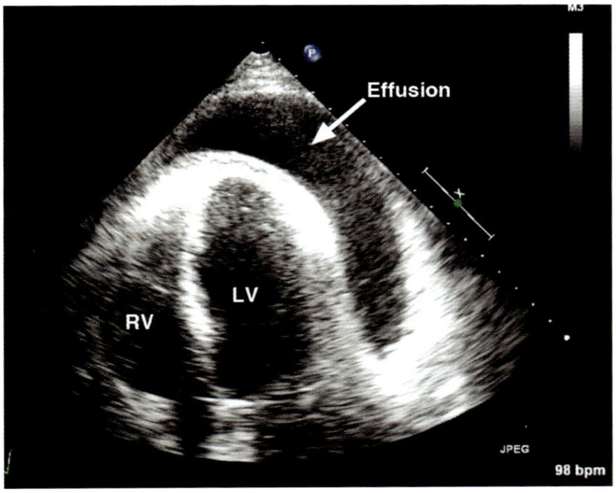

Fig 1.65 An apical four-chamber TTE showed a large pericardial effusion that was successfully drained.

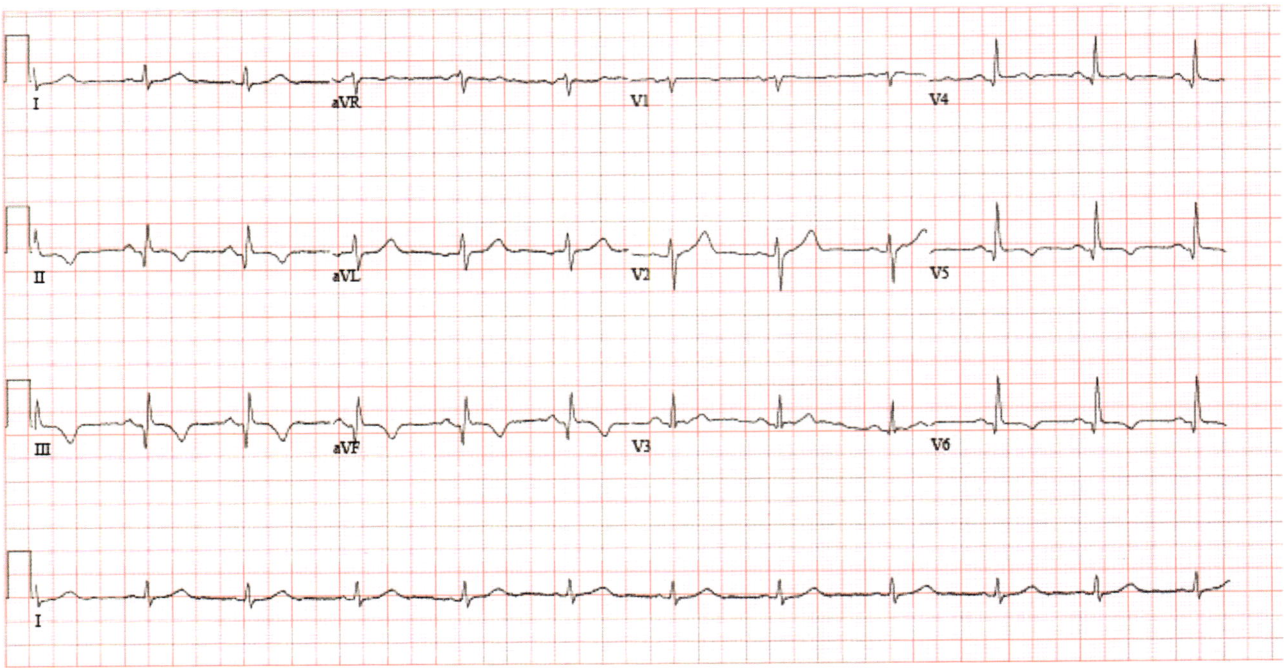

Fig 1.66 This ECG taken after pericardiocentesis shows evidence of an inferior myocardial infarction. The ECG was unchanged just before surgery.

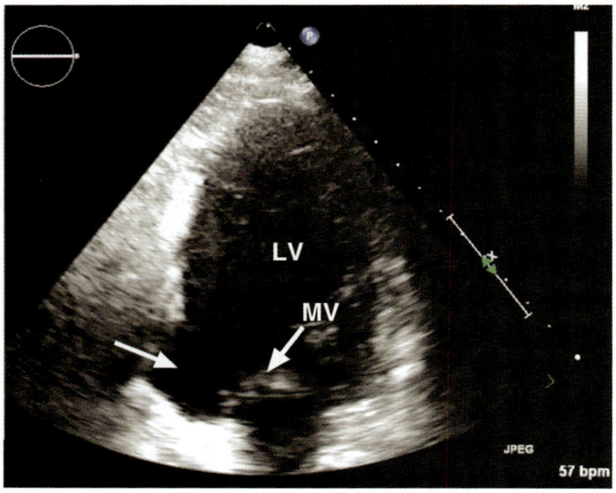

Fig 1.67 An apical two-chamber TTE before surgery shows the basal inferior pseudoaneurysm *(arrow)*.

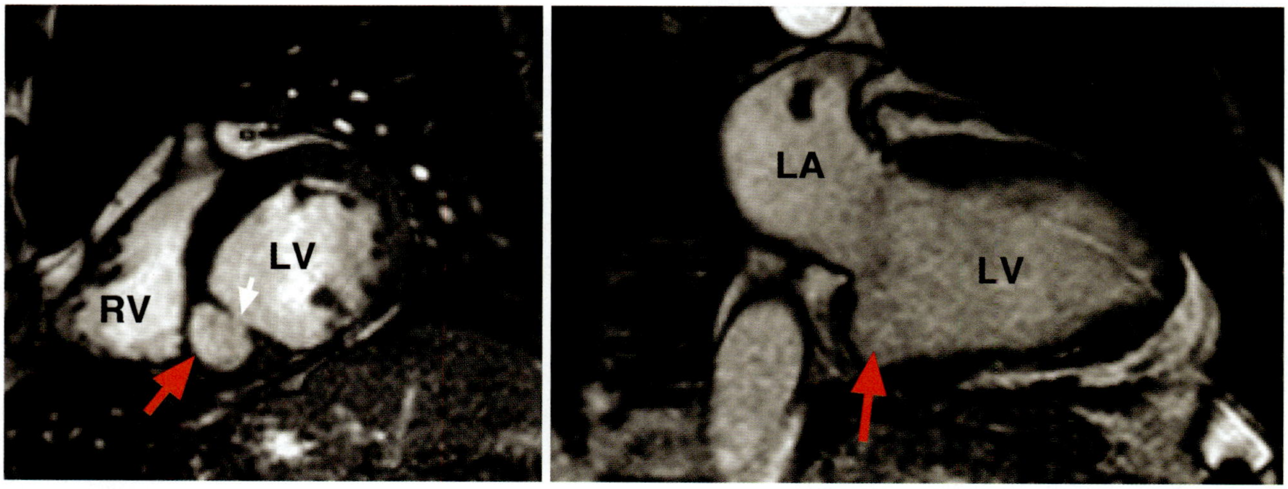

Fig 1.68 In the left-side panel, a short-axis MRI shows the inferior wall defect *(white arrow)* leading to the pseudoaneurysm *(red arrow)*. On the right, a two-chamber view also shows the pseudoaneurysm *(red arrow)*.

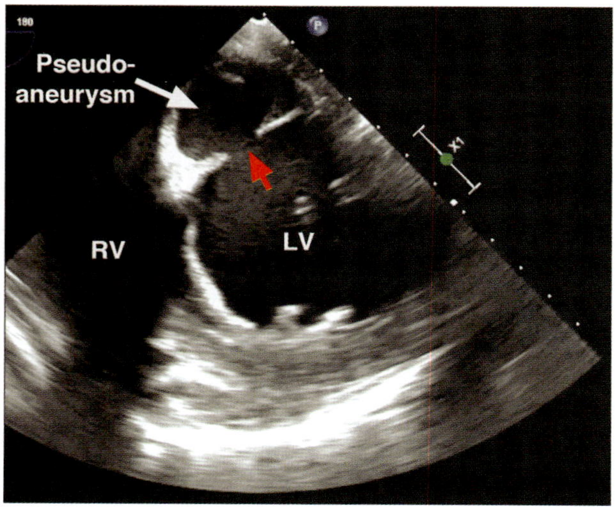

Fig 1.69 In the OR, basal transgastric short-axis TEE shows the inferior wall defect *(red arrow)* and the pseudoaneurysm.

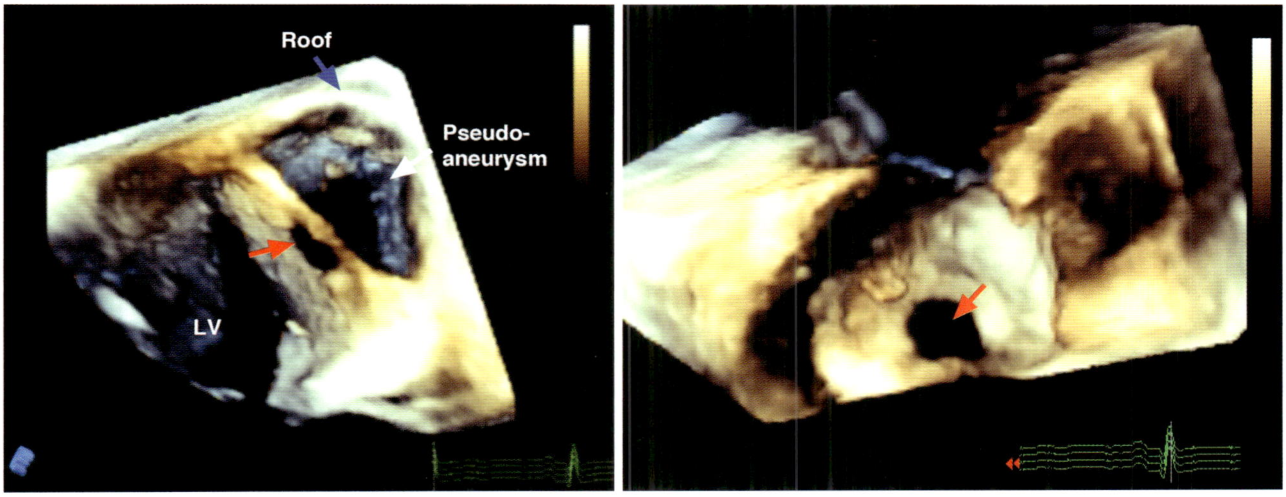

Fig 1.70 In the left-side panel, 3D TEE shows the defect *(red arrow)* and pseudoaneurysm. On the right, with the roof of the pseudoaneurysm "cropped away," the 3D nature of the inferior wall defect is appreciated.

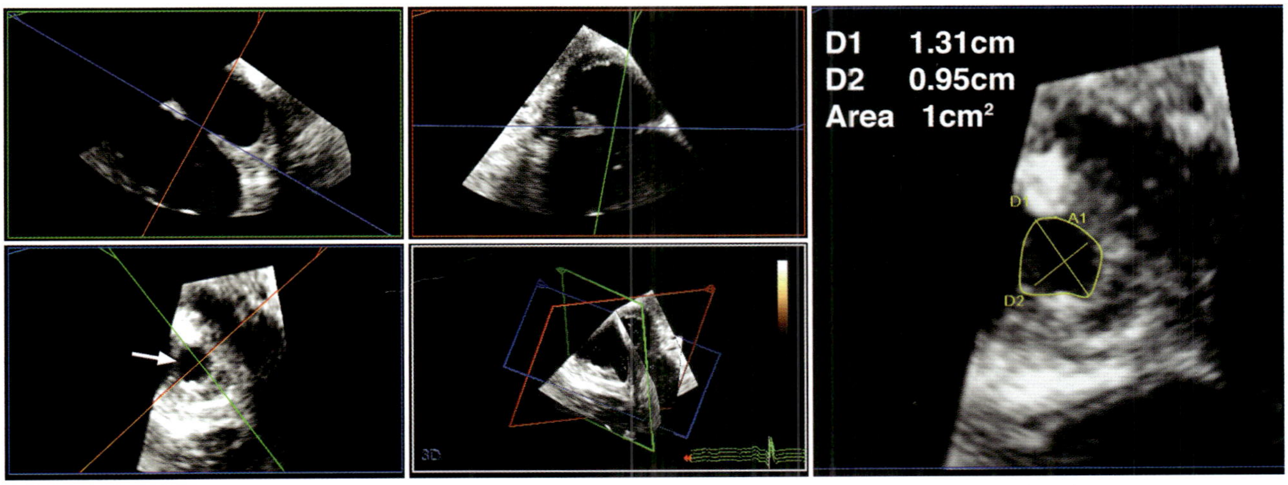

Fig 1.71 Multiplanar reconstruction of the defect in the inferior wall allows measurement of its dimensions.

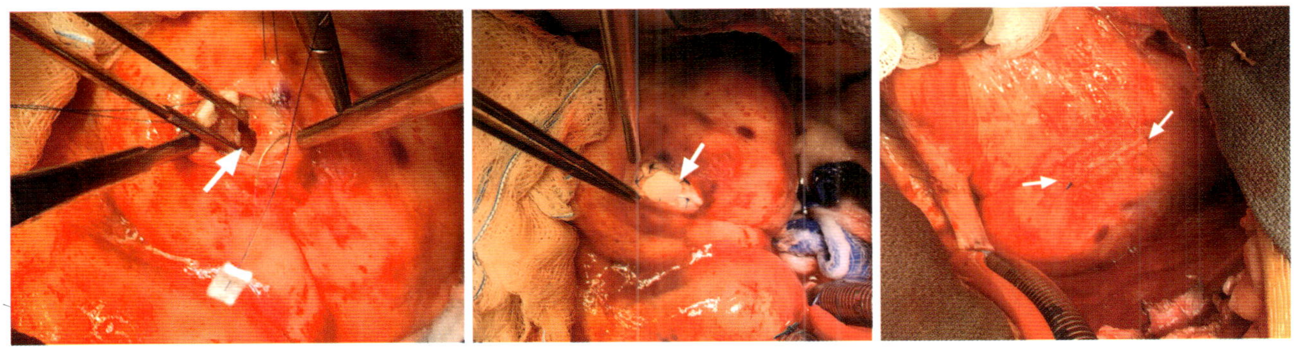

Fig 1.72 In the OR, the surgeon has unroofed the epicardium covering the pseudoaneurysm revealing the defect in the inferior wall *(left, arrow)*. The defect is patched with Dacron *(center, arrow)*, and the epicardium closed with a second patch *(right, between arrows)*.

Commentary

An LV pseudoaneurysm is due to rupture of the free LV wall with the rupture contained by pericardial adhesions. In this patient, the initial effusion likely was due to LV rupture that was sealed by pericardial adhesions after removal of the pericardial fluid. Over the ensuing years, the area of pericardium sealing the myocardial rupture gradually enlarged, resulting in the saccular pseudoaneurysm seen at surgery. Surgical repair is recommended, even late after the initial incident, because recurrent rupture can occur with a high mortality rate. In addition to postmyocardial infarction cases, LV pseudoaneurysm may be seen after mitral valve surgery. In patients with a postmyocardial infarction ventricular septal defect, there may be an associated pseudoaneurysm if the septal rupture occurred adjacent to the junction of the septum with the LV free wall.

Pathologically, a true LV aneurysm has walls that consist of thinned and scarred myocardium versus a pseudoaneurysm that has walls with no myocardial tissue. On echocardiography there are several features that distinguish a pseudoaneurysm from a true aneurysm. The neck of a pseudoaneurysm is narrow, compared with the size of the aneurysm, with an abrupt transition from normal myocardial thickness to absent myocardium. A true aneurysm typically has a tapering thickness of the LV wall with a wide opening compared with the maximum aneurysm diameter.

Suggested Reading

1. Vargas-Barron J, Molina-Carrion M, Romero-Cardenas A, et al: Risk factors, echocardiographic patterns, and outcomes in patients with acute ventricular septal rupture during myocardial infarction, Am J Cardiol 95(10):1153–1158, 2005.
2. McMullan MH, Maples MD, Kilgore TL Jr, et al: Surgical experience with left ventricular free wall rupture, Ann Thorac Surg 71(6):1894–1898, 2001.

2 Mitral Valve Disease

Normal Mitral Valve

CASE 2-1
Normal Mitral Valve Anatomy

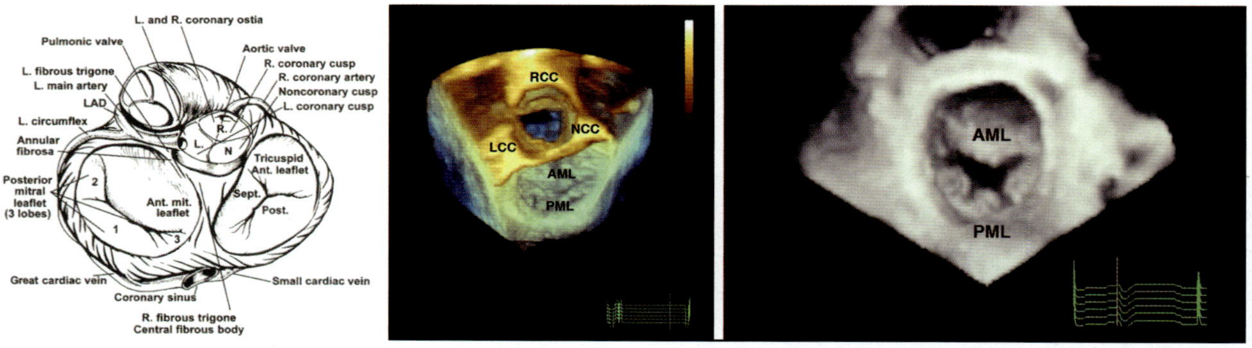

Fig 2.1 Anatomic view of the cardiac valves from the perspective of the base of the heart with the atria cut away and the great vessels transected. All four valves have a close anatomic relationship. In particular, the aortic valve is adjacent to the mitral valve along the midsegment of the anterior mitral leaflet. In the center frame a 3D image shows the mitral aortic relationship. In the right frame, the valve is seen from the ventricular aspect, and the three scallops of the posterior leaflet are appreciated. (Reproduced with permission from Otto CM. Valvular Heart Disease 2e. Philadelphia: WB Saunders, 2004. ©2004, Elsevier Inc.)

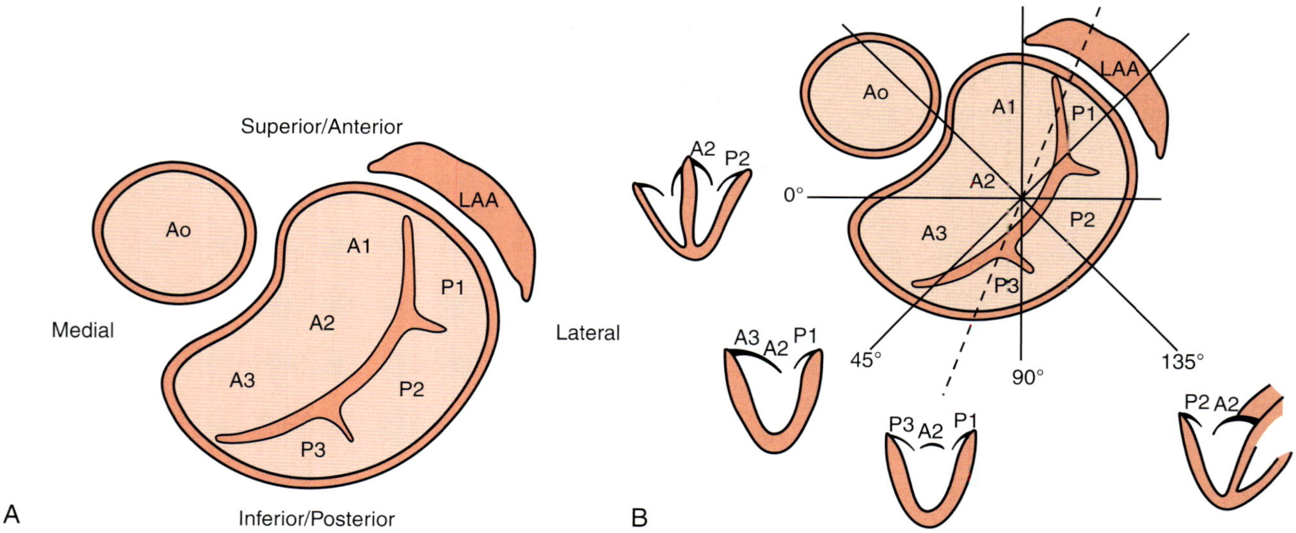

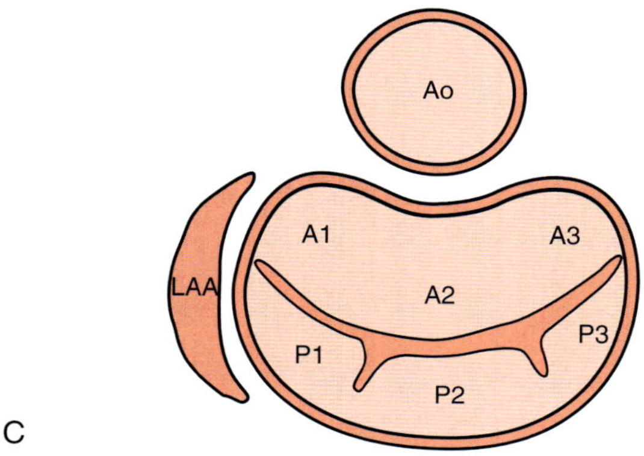

Fig 2.2 Reference view displaying the mitral valve and its anatomic relationship to the aortic root **(A)** and the left atrial appendage (LAA) as seen from the left ventricular apex or TEE short-axis view. **(B)** Reference view demonstrating the relationship of the TEE imaging planes to the mitral valve with the probe positioned in the standard midesophageal position. **(C)** Surgical view of the mitral valve as seen from left atrium with the heart rotated. A1, A2, A3 = anterior leaflet sections; P1, P2, P3 = posterior leaflet sections. (Reproduced with permission from Foster GP et al. Accurate localization of mitral regurgitant defects using multiplane transesophageal echocardiography. Ann Thoracic Surg 1998; 65:1025-1031. ©1998 Elsevier Inc.)

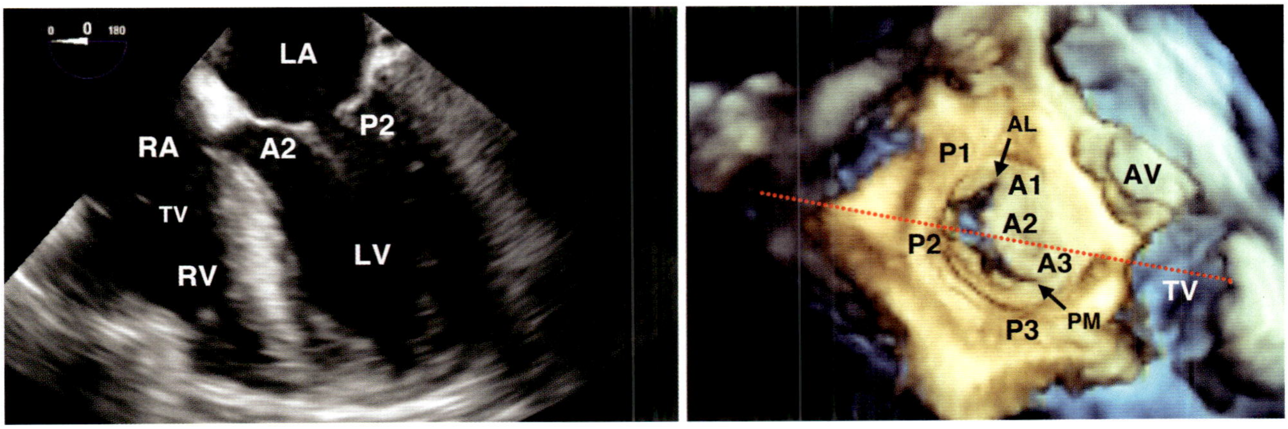

Fig 2.3 TEE in a four-chamber view at 0 degrees demonstrating the central section of the anterior leaflet (A2) and the central scallop of the posterior leaflet (P2). In the right frame, 3D TEE of the mitral valve is shown, illustrating how the view is developed.

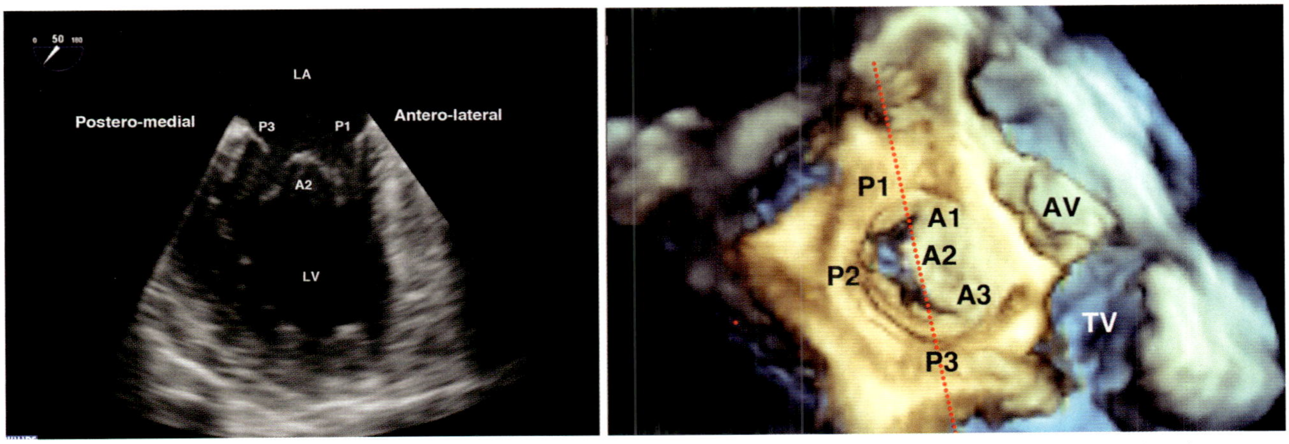

Fig 2.4 TEE mitral commissural view, obtained here at 50 degrees by slight backward rotation from the two-chamber view, demonstrates the central segment of the anterior leaflet (A2) and the medial (P3) and lateral (P1) segments of the posterior leaflet.

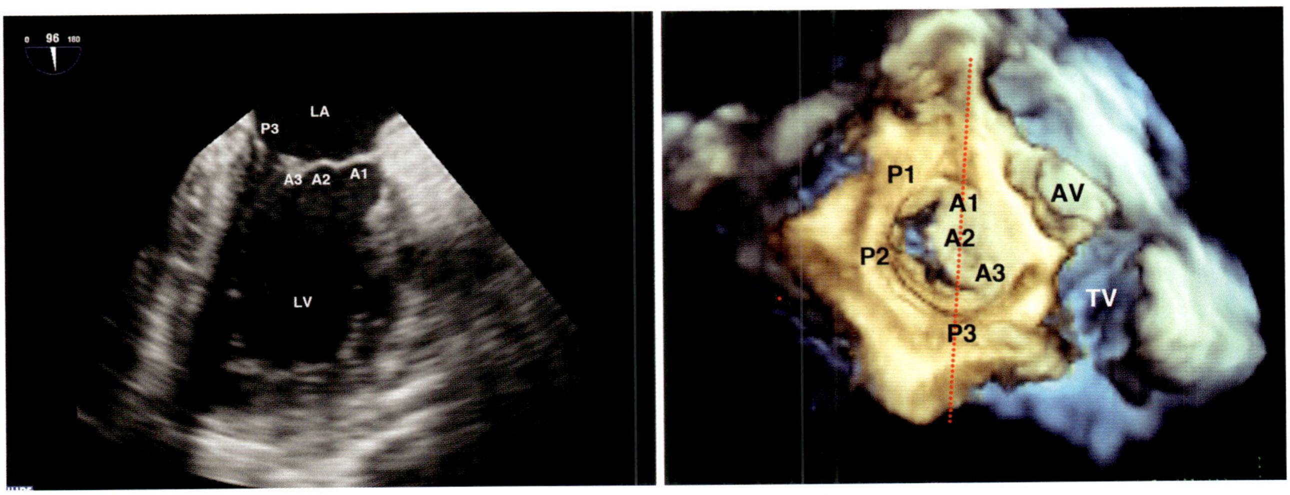

Fig 2.5 TEE two-chamber view, obtained at 96 degrees, shows A1, A2, A3, and P3.

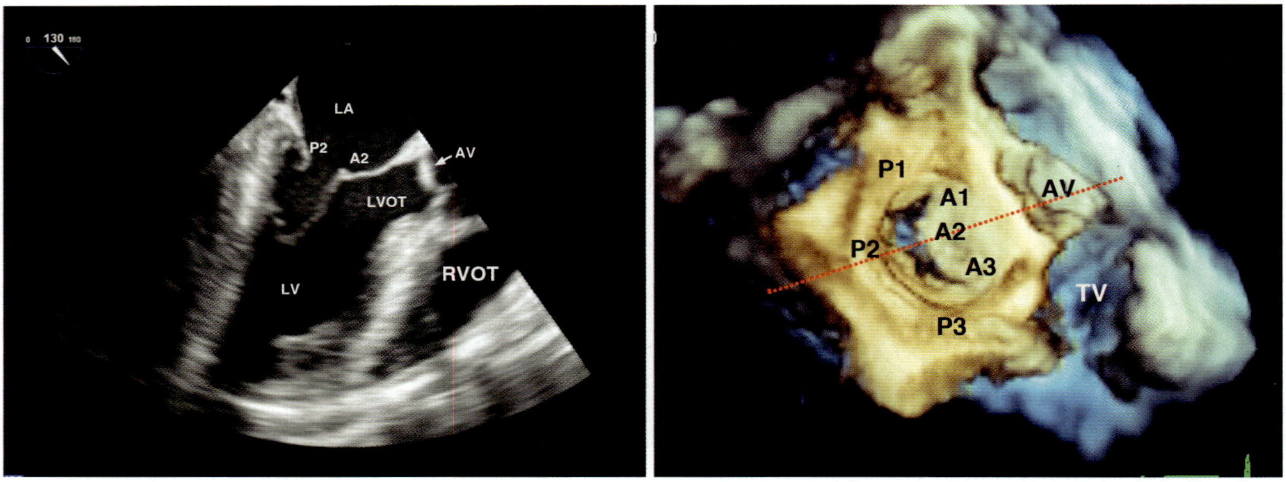

Fig 2.6 Further rotation to 130 degrees results in a long-axis view, again showing the central section of the anterior leaflet (A2) and the central scallop of the posterior leaflet (P2).

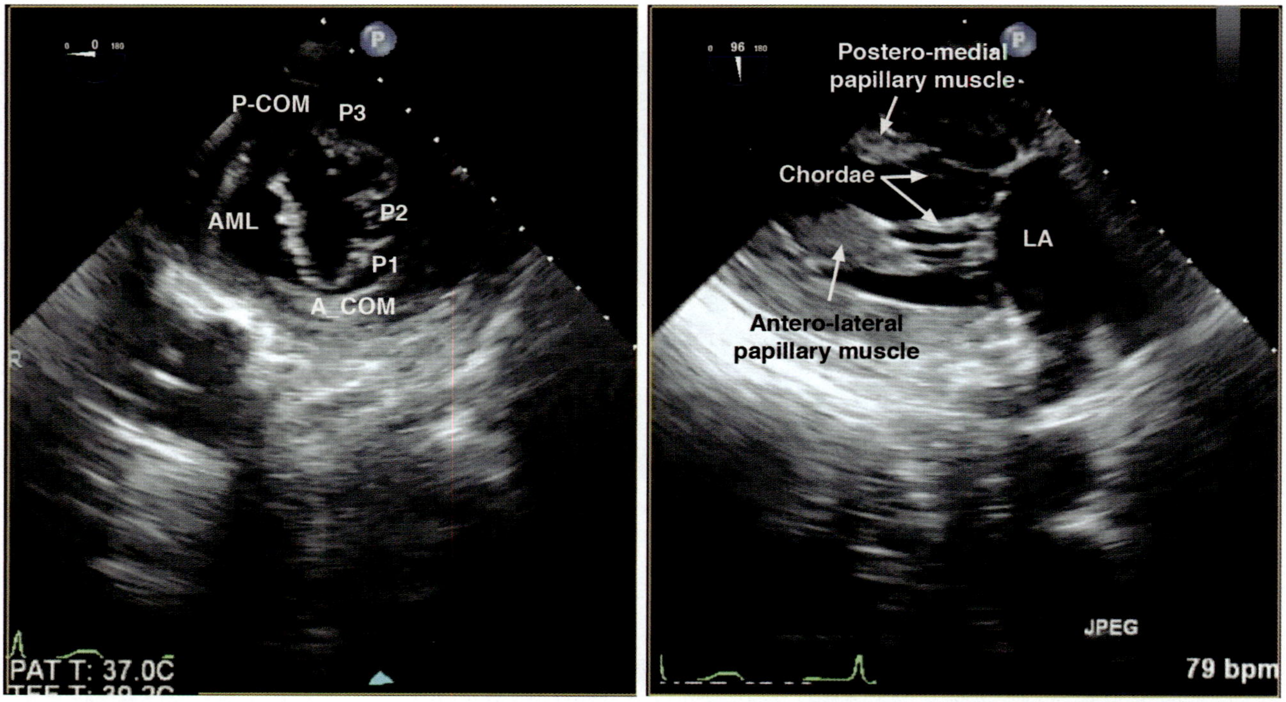

Fig 2.7 The transgastric short-axis view at the level of the mitral valve demonstrates the anterior mitral leaflet (AML) and the three scallops of the posterior leaflet (PML), along with the posterior (P-COM) and anterior commissures (A-COM). Rotation to about 90 degrees (96 degrees in this case) from the transgastric short axis provides a two-chamber view with visualization of the mitral leaflets, chords, and papillary muscles.

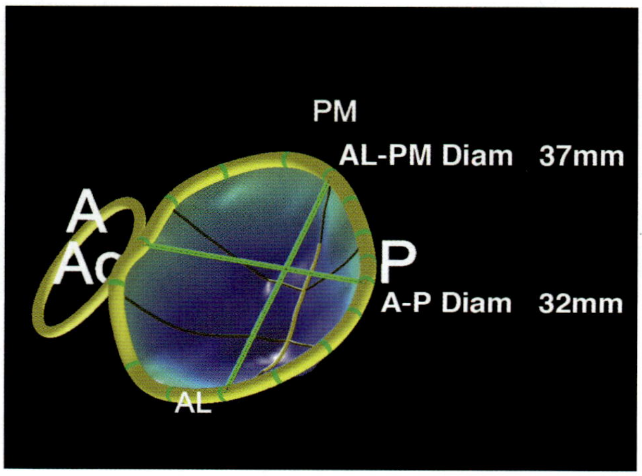

Fig 2.8 A model of the mitral valve with corresponding annular measurements is shown. A = anterior, P = posterior, AL = antero-lateral, PM = postero-medial.

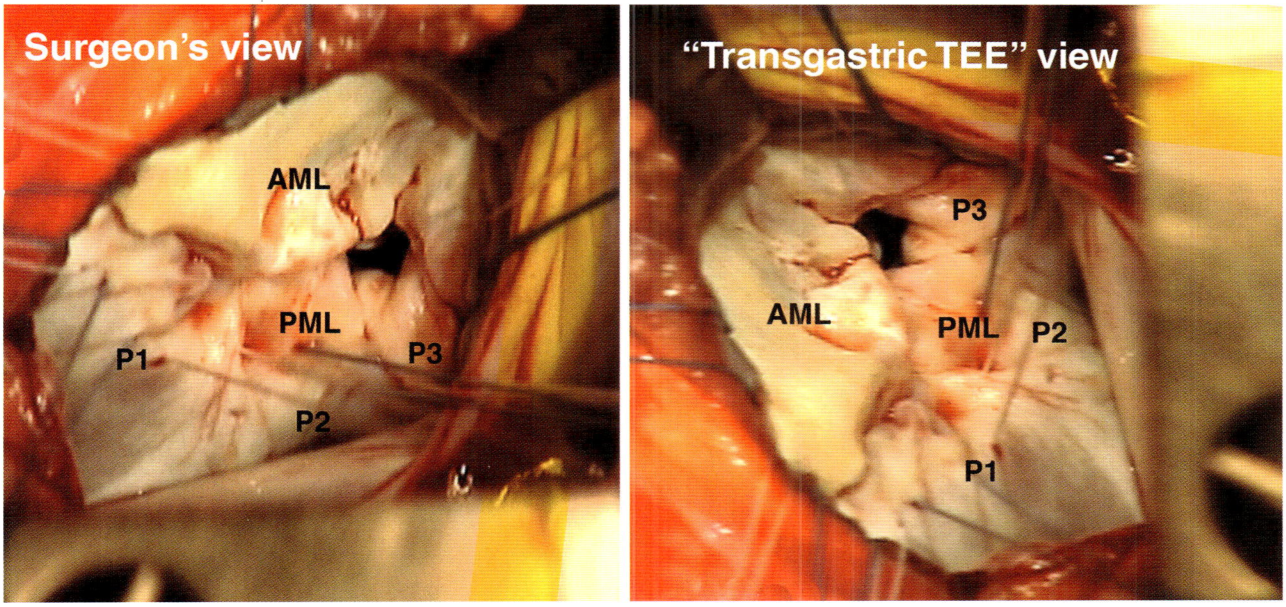

Fig 2.9 The normal mitral valve in vivo, as seen after incisions in the right atrium, and the interatrial septum. On the left is the surgeon's view from the right side of the operating table. On the right is the valve as it would appear on a basal transgastric short-axis TEE, as in Fig 2.7.

Comments

The mitral valve apparatus is a complex structure in three dimensions that includes the saddle-shaped mitral annulus, leaflets, chords, and papillary muscles. The anterior leaflet is longer than the posterior leaflet but extends only about one third of the distance around the annulus circumference. The anterior leaflet does not have anatomically discrete segments, but location can be described as the lateral (A1), central (A2), and medial (A3) aspects of the leaflet. The posterior leaflet is shorter but extends a greater distance around the mitral annulus. The posterior leaflet typically has three discrete scallops: lateral (P1), central (P2), and medial (P3). Standard 2D and 3D TEE images are summarized in Table 2-1.

TABLE 2-1
The Systematic Mitral Valve Examination

Name of View	Description of View	See Case 2-1, Normal Mitral Valve Anatomy
ME four-chamber view (0 degrees)	• AML is on left side, adjacent to aortic valve. • PML is on right side. • Area of PML and AML that are visible are mostly P2 and A2.	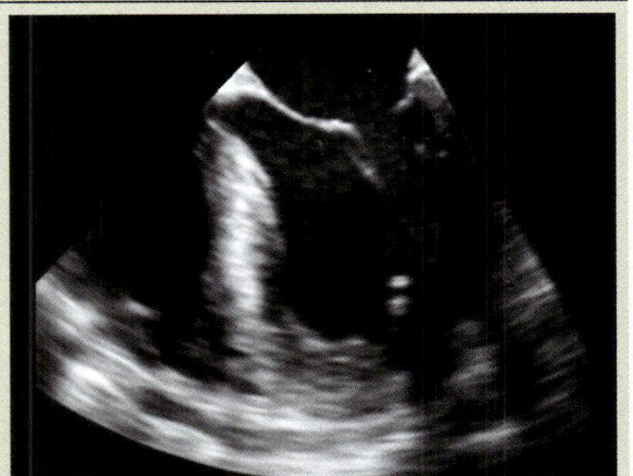
ME commissural view (60 degrees)	• Two apparent coaptation points. • From left to right, visible mitral segments are P3, A2, and P1.	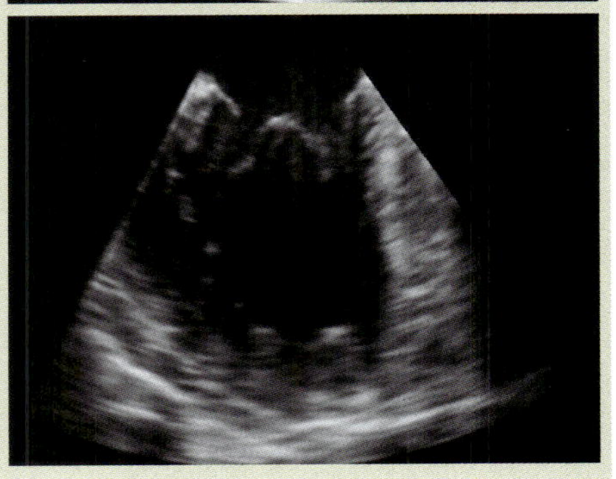

Continued

TABLE 2-1
The Systematic Mitral Valve Examination—cont'd

Name of View	Description of View	See Case 2-1, Normal Mitral Valve Anatomy
ME two-chamber view (90 degrees)	• Small P3 on left side and large AML on right side. • Segment that coapts with P3 is A3. • Rest of visible AML is variable.	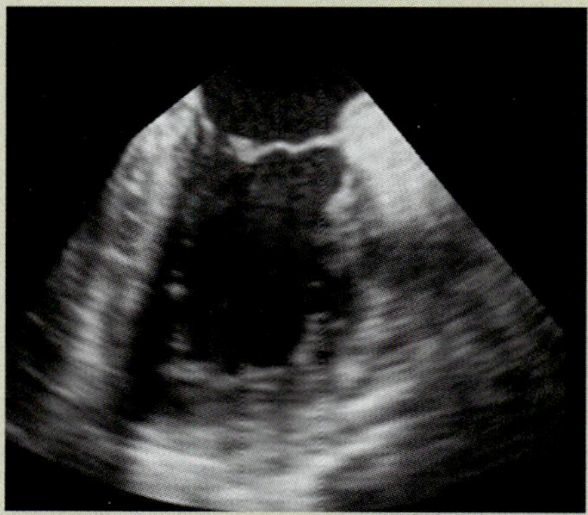
ME long-axis view (130–150 degrees)	• PML on left side and AML on right side. • If plane of scan is centered, P2 and A2 visible. • May scan from side to side.	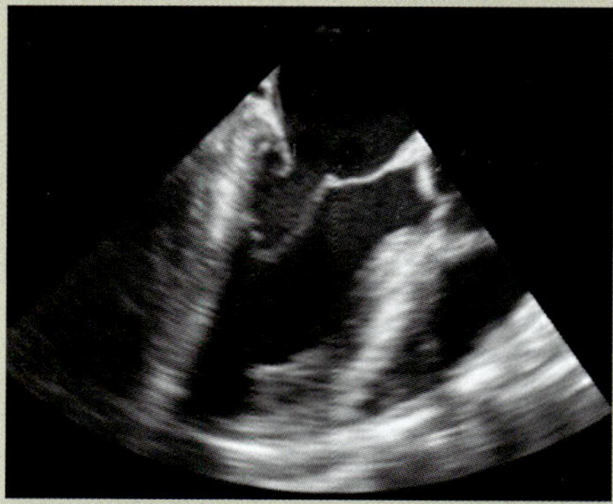
TG short-axis view (0 degree)	• AML on left side and PML on right side. • Posterior commissure at top, anterior commissure at bottom.	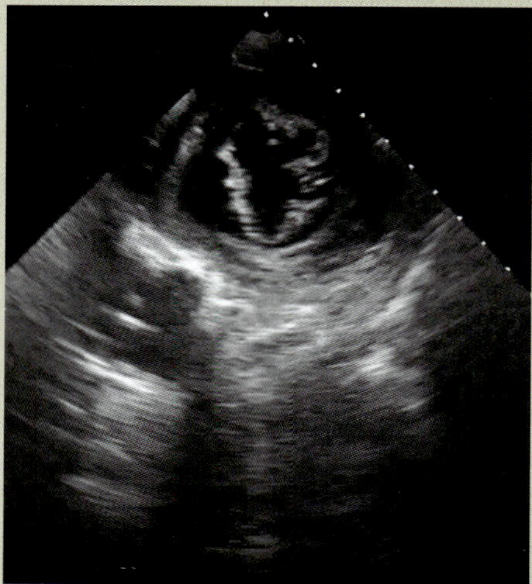
TG two-chamber view (90 degrees)	• Inferior wall at top. • Anterior wall at bottom. • Slight movement from side to side will reveal both papillary muscles.	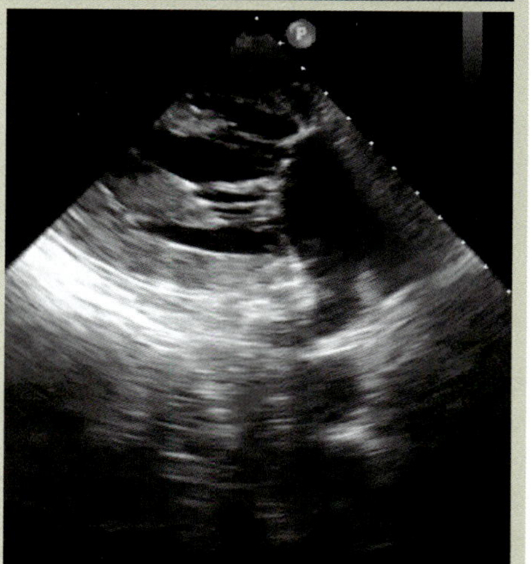

TABLE 2-1
The Systematic Mitral Valve Examination—cont'd

Name of View	Description of View	See Case 2-1, Normal Mitral Valve Anatomy
3D LA view	• This view looks "down" at valve from LA and is closest to surgeon's actual view of valve. • By convention, AML is at top, and PML is at bottom.	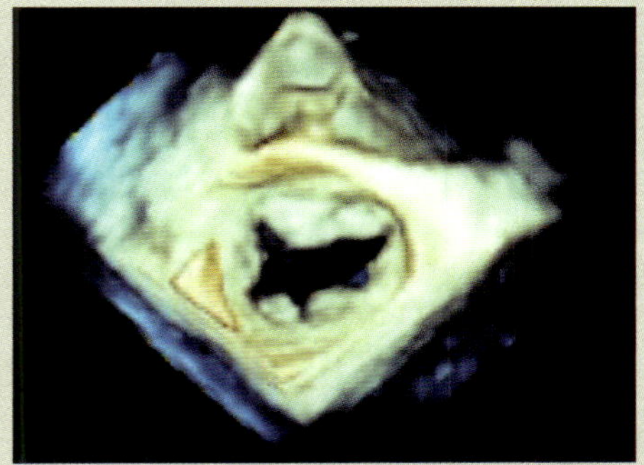
3D LV view	• This view looks "up" at valve from LV apex. • The AML is at top, and PML is at bottom.	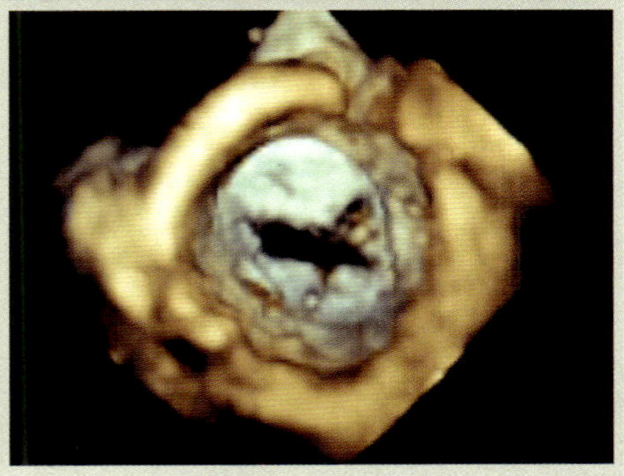

Mitral regurgitant severity is best evaluated using multiple Doppler measures on a preoperative complete transthoracic echocardiogram (TTE). Decisions about timing of surgery are based not only on severity of regurgitation, but on clinical status and serial changes in left ventricular dimensions and systolic function. When regurgitant severity is reevaluated in the operating room (OR), regurgitant severity may be less than expected because of a lower afterload in the anesthetized versus awake patient. Useful measures of regurgitant severity in the OR include:

- Vena contracta width—narrowest diameter of the regurgitant jet at the valve orifice or just distal to it; for the mitral valve, best measured in the antero-posterior diameter (midesophageal long axis.)
- Proximal isovelocity surface area (PISA)—region of flow convergence on the ventricular side of the valve. The instantaneous regurgitant flow rate is the area of a hemisphere ($2\pi r^2$) times the aliasing velocity.
- Continuous wave (CW) Doppler—intensity and time course of the regurgitant velocity signal
- Regurgitant orifice area (ROA)—calculated from PISA and CW Doppler velocity as the instantaneous flow rate (cm^3/s) divided by the maximum regurgitant jet velocity (cm/s) to yield the cross sectional area of regurgitant flow
- With primary MR, a ROA of 0.4 cm^2 or greater is consistent with severe MR. For secondary MR, a ROA of 0.2 cm^2 or greater is severe.
- Regurgitant volume can be calculated as the ROA times the velocity time integral of the MR jet: RV (mL or cm^3) = ROA (cm^2) × VTIMR (cm).
- The direction, size, and shape of the regurgitant jet are less useful for quantitation of severity but often help identify the mechanism of regurgitation because the direction of the jet typically is opposite the prolapsing leaflet; for instance, posterior leaflet prolapse results in an anteriorly directed jet. With severe leaflet restriction, the regurgitant jet is typically directed towards the restricted leaflet; for instance, posterior leaflet restriction results in a posteriorly directed jet.

Suggested Reading

1. Otto CM: Valvular regurgitation. In textbook of clinical echocardiography, ed 5, Philadelphia, 2013, Elsevier Saunders, pp 305–341.
2. Hung J: Mitral regurgitation: Valve anatomy, regurgitant severity and timing of intervention. In Otto CM, editor: The practice of clinical echocardiography, ed 5, Philadelphia, 2016, Elsevier, Chapter 18.
3. Zoghbi WA, Enriquez-Sarano M, Foster E, et al: Recommendations for evaluation of the severity of native valvular regurgitation with two-dimensional and Doppler echocardiography, J Am Soc Echocardiogr 16:777–802, 2003.
4. Nishimura RA, Otto CM, Bonow RO, et al. 2014 AHA/ACC Guideline for the Management of Patients With Valvular Heart Disease: A Report of the American College of Cardiology/American Heart Association Task Force on Practice Guidelines. J Am Coll Cardiol. 63:e57-e185, 2014.

Myxomatous Mitral Valve Disease

CASE 2-2
Posterior Leaflet Prolapse with Flail Central (P2) Scallop

A 46-year-old man with a 20-year history of a murmur was transferred from another hospital with increasing shortness of breath and hemoptysis of 1 month's duration. A loud holosystolic murmur at the apex was noted on physical examination. Because the patient also had a long history of intravenous drug use, blood cultures were obtained and the patient was started on empiric intravenous antibiotics for possible endocarditis.

Transthoracic echocardiography showed severe mitral regurgitation with a posterior leaflet flail segment and an anteriorly directed regurgitant jet. Left ventricular size was at the upper limits of normal (end-systolic dimension 39 mm) with an ejection fraction of 60%. The left atrium was moderately enlarged and pulmonary pressures were severely elevated with an estimated systolic pressure of 70 mm Hg. Transesophageal echocardiography was performed to evaluate for possible vegetations. This study demonstrated a flail central scallop of the posterior leaflet with severe mitral regurgitation. He was referred for mitral valve surgery.

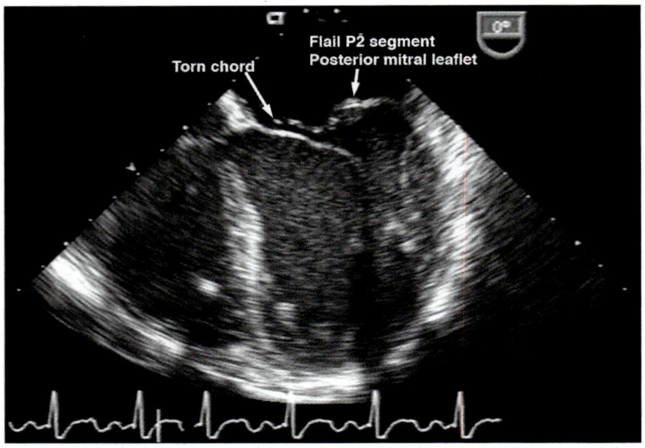

Fig 2.10 Intraoperative 2D images of the mitral valve from a high esophageal position at 0 degrees rotation show the relatively thin anterior leaflet with normal motion and a thickened, redundant posterior leaflet. The flail segment of the posterior leaflet is seen on the atrial side of the annulus with the tip of the leaflet pointing away from the left ventricular apex. In contrast, with severe prolapse but intact chordae, there is bowing of the leaflet into the atrium, with the leaflet tip still pointing toward the ventricular apex.

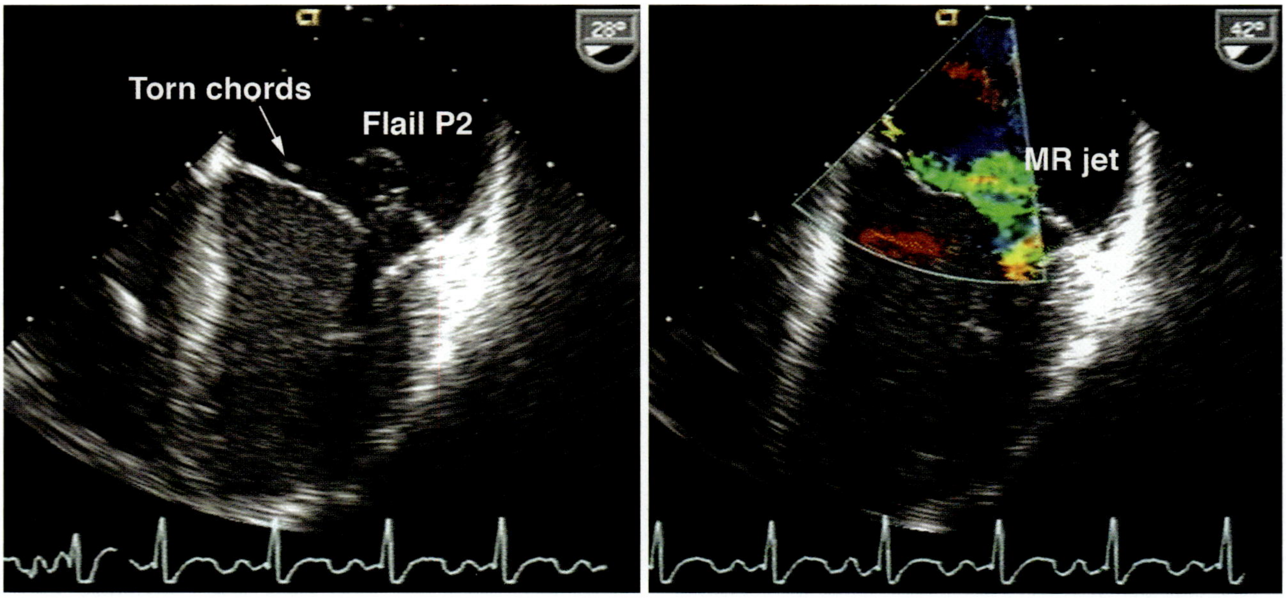

Fig 2.11 Rotation of the 2D-image plane to 28 degrees *(left)* more clearly demonstrates the flail middle scallop of the posterior leaflet (P2) with a torn chord on the left atrial side of the valve in systole. Color flow Doppler at 42 degrees rotation *(right)* demonstrates a wide eccentric mitral regurgitant (MR) jet with flow acceleration on the ventricular side of the valve. The jet is directed away from the affected leaflet; for example, an anteriorly directed jet with posterior leaflet disease.

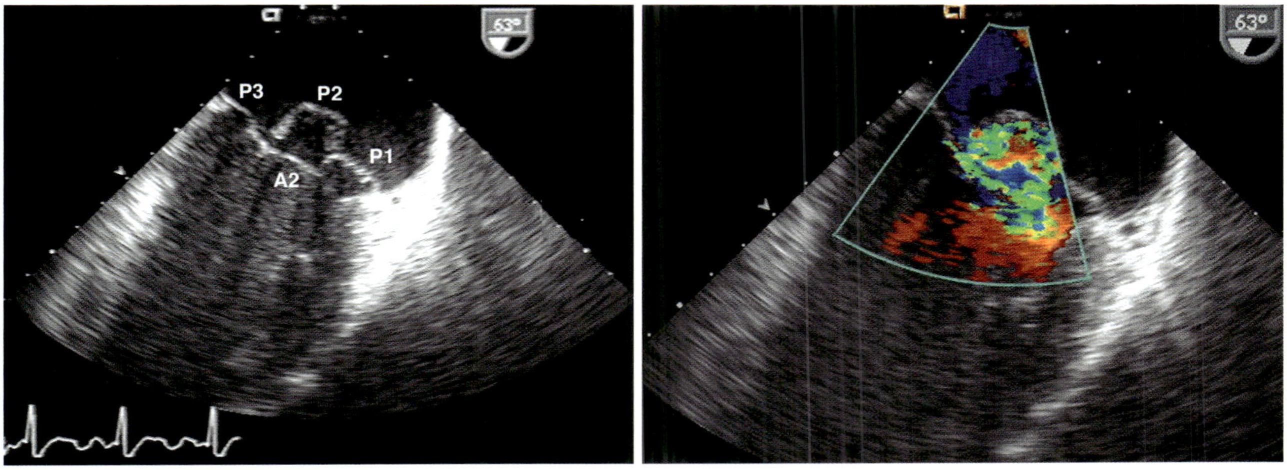

Fig 2.12 Further rotation of the image plane to the mitral commissural view (63 degrees) shows the severe prolapse and partial flail of the central scallop of the posterior leaflet (P2). Color Doppler *(right)* in the mitral commissural plane shows significant mitral regurgitation.

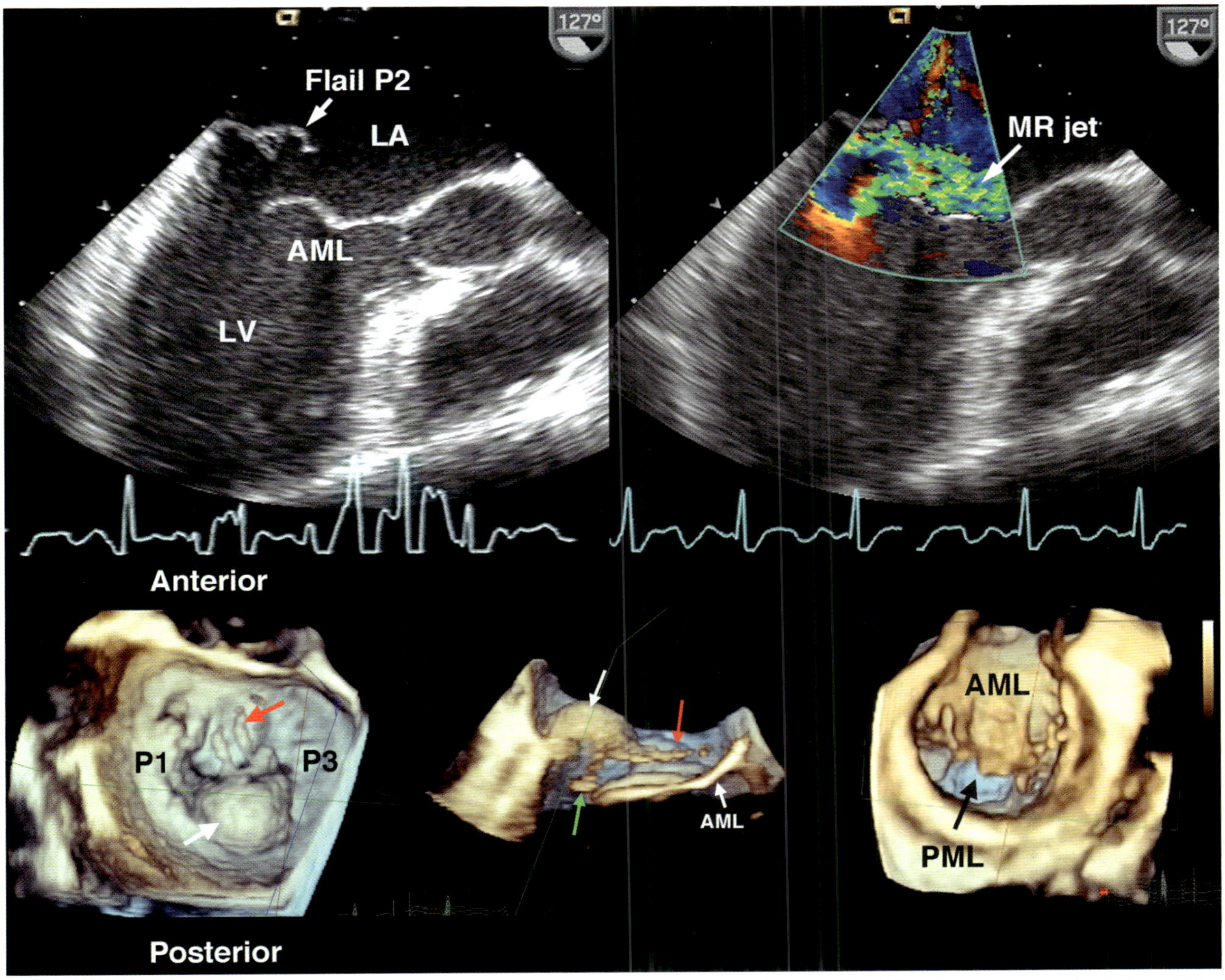

Fig 2.13 In the upper two frames, rotation of the 2D-image plane to 127 degrees *(left)* also demonstrates the flail middle scallop of the posterior leaflet (P2). Color flow Doppler at 127 degrees rotation *(right)* also demonstrates a wide eccentric mitral regurgitant (MR) jet with flow acceleration on the ventricular side of the valve and a vena contracta width of 9 mm. The jet is directed away from the affected leaflet—for example, an anteriorly directed jet with posterior leaflet disease. In the lower three frames 3D TEE of the mitral valve is illustrated from the left atrial perspective *(left)*, from the medial side of the mitral valve with the most medial aspect cropped away *(center)*, and from the left ventricular perspective *(right)*. The white arrows indicate the flail P2 segment, the red arrows indicate torn chordae, and the green arrows indicate thickened subvalvular chordae.

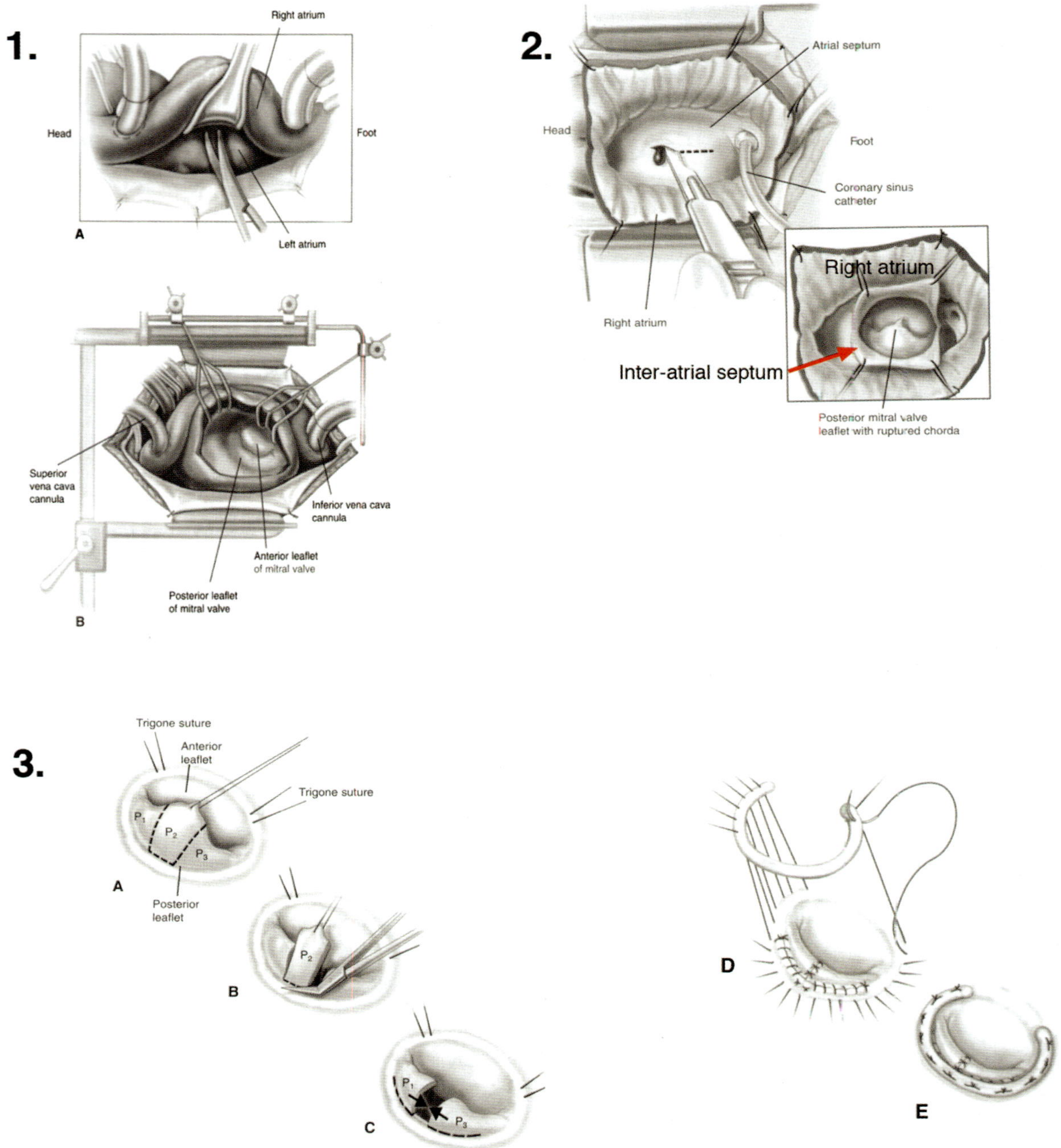

Fig 2.14 Approach to mitral valve repair. (1) The mitral valve may be approached through the dome of the left atrium, having developed Sondergaards's plane by blunt and sharp dissection. (2) The mitral valve may also be approached through the right atrium and interatrial septum. (3) The diseased P2 is excised, the remainder of the posterior leaflet reapproximated, and an annuloplasty ring secured **(A–E).** (Cohn L. Mitral valve repair: Operative techniques in thoracic and cardiovascular surgery 1998; 3(2):109–125. Reprinted with permission.)

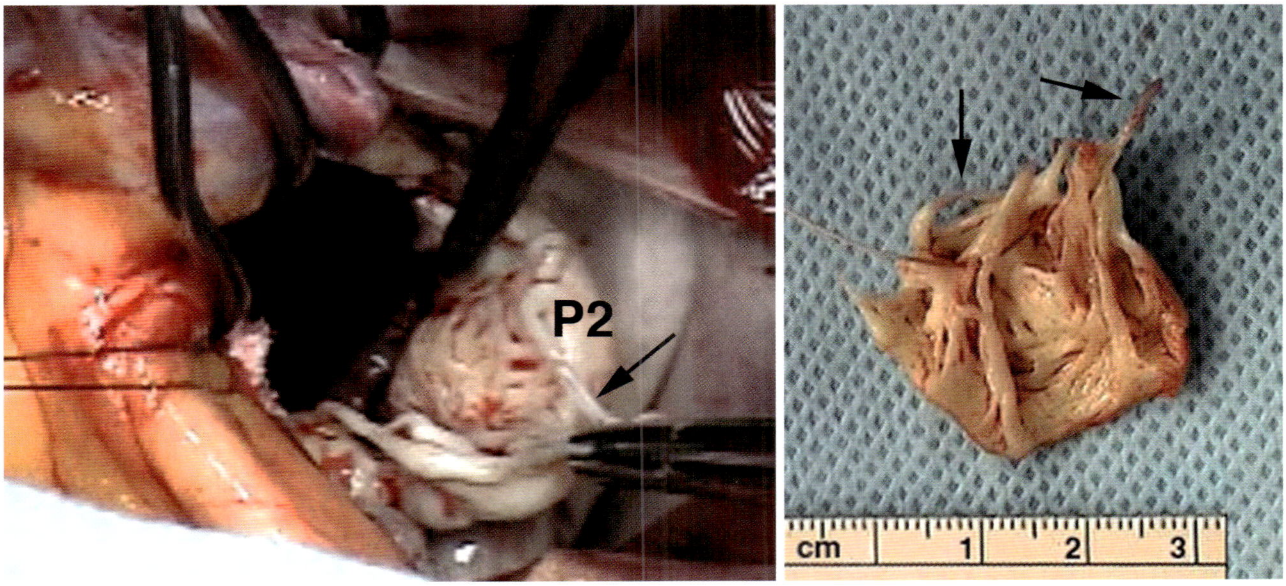

Fig 2.15 Intraoperative visualization of the valve confirmed the flail middle scallop of the posterior leaflet with the surgical view shown on the left and the resected leaflet segment shown on the right. The anterior mitral leaflet was normal but there were three sets of ruptured chords to the central scallop of the posterior leaflet (P2) *(arrows)*. There was no evidence for vegetation or abscess. The video shows that after resection of the flail leaflet segment and reapproximation of the leaflet edges, an annuloplasty ring was placed with the sutures positioned in the annulus and then the ring positioned.

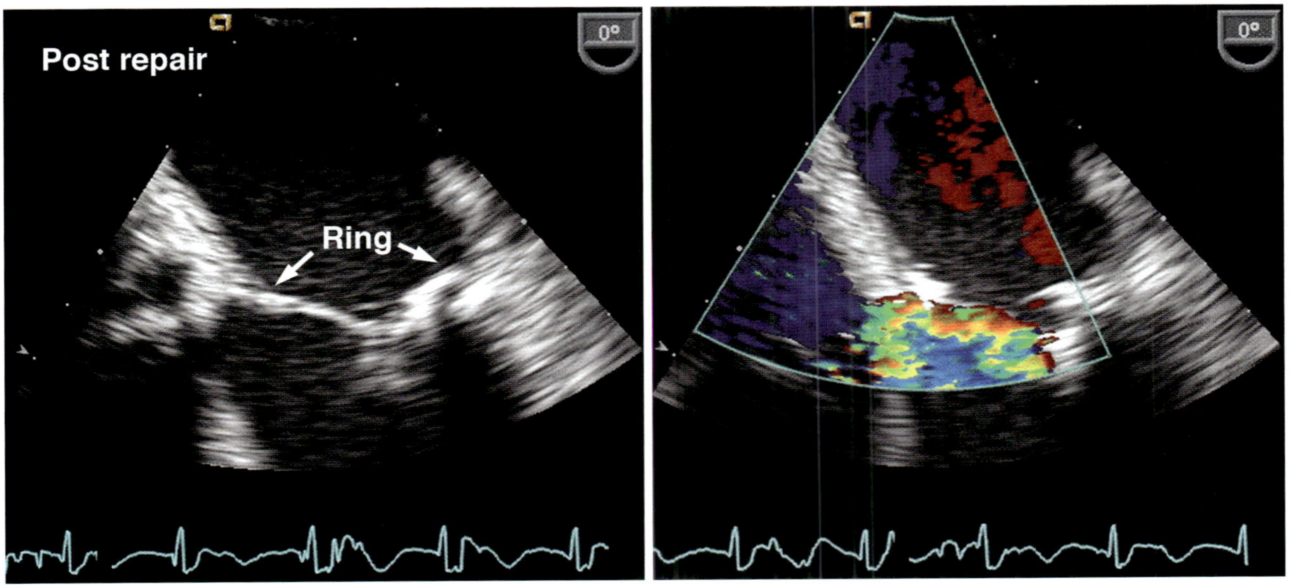

Fig 2.16 Postrepair images at 0 degrees show increased echogenicity of the posterior leaflet and the annuloplasty ring, with normal leaflet closure in systole on 2D imaging *(left)* and the absence of mitral regurgitation on color flow imaging *(right)*.

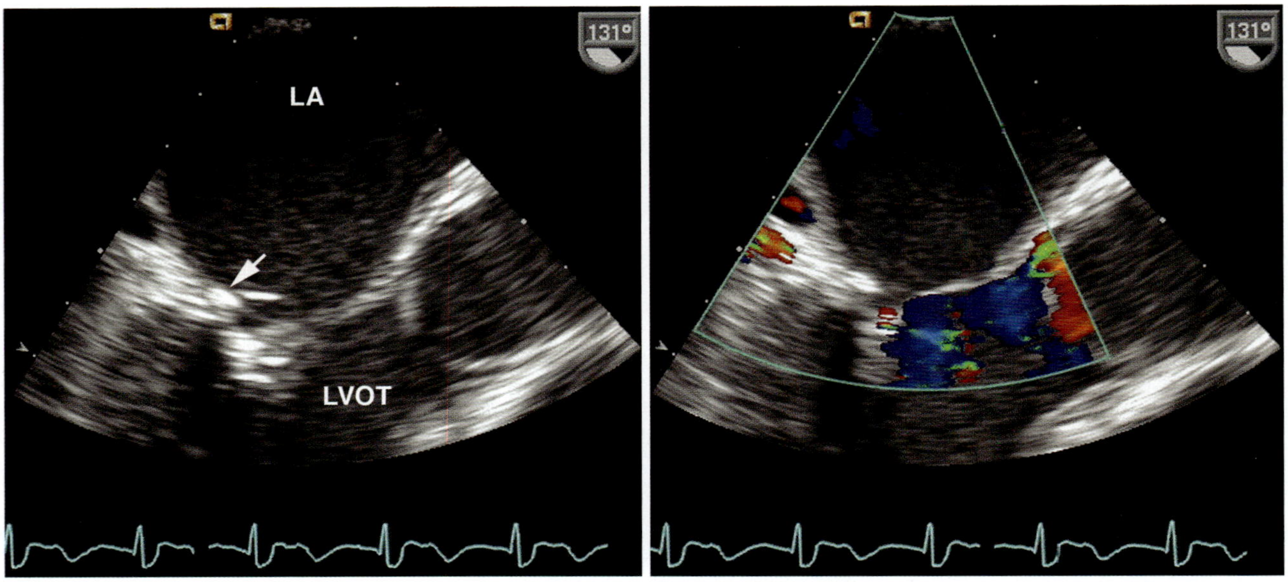

Fig 2.17 Postrepair images in a long-axis view (131 degrees) show the annuloplasty ring *(arrow)* and the site of the posterior leaflet resection and repair *(left)*. It is important to evaluate for regurgitation in multiple views; no regurgitation is seen with color flow imaging in this view *(right)*.

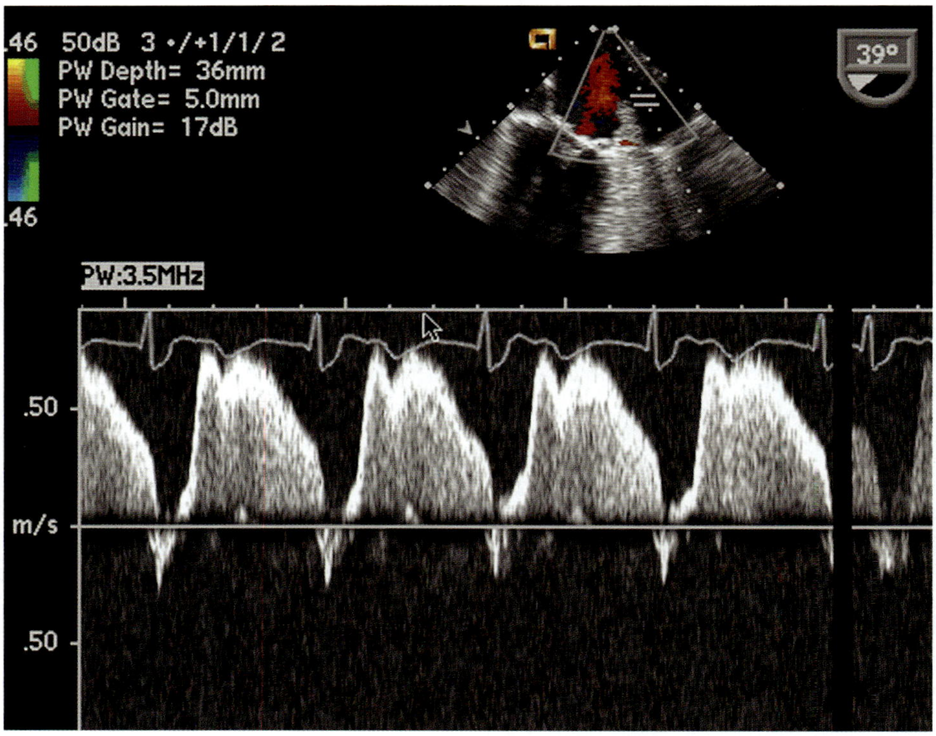

Fig 2.18 Pulsed Doppler evaluation of flow in the left upper pulmonary vein shows normal diastolic and systolic atrial inflow *(top)*. In contrast, the prerepair pulmonary venous flow *(bottom)* shows holosystolic reversal of flow *(arrow)* consistent with severe mitral regurgitation.

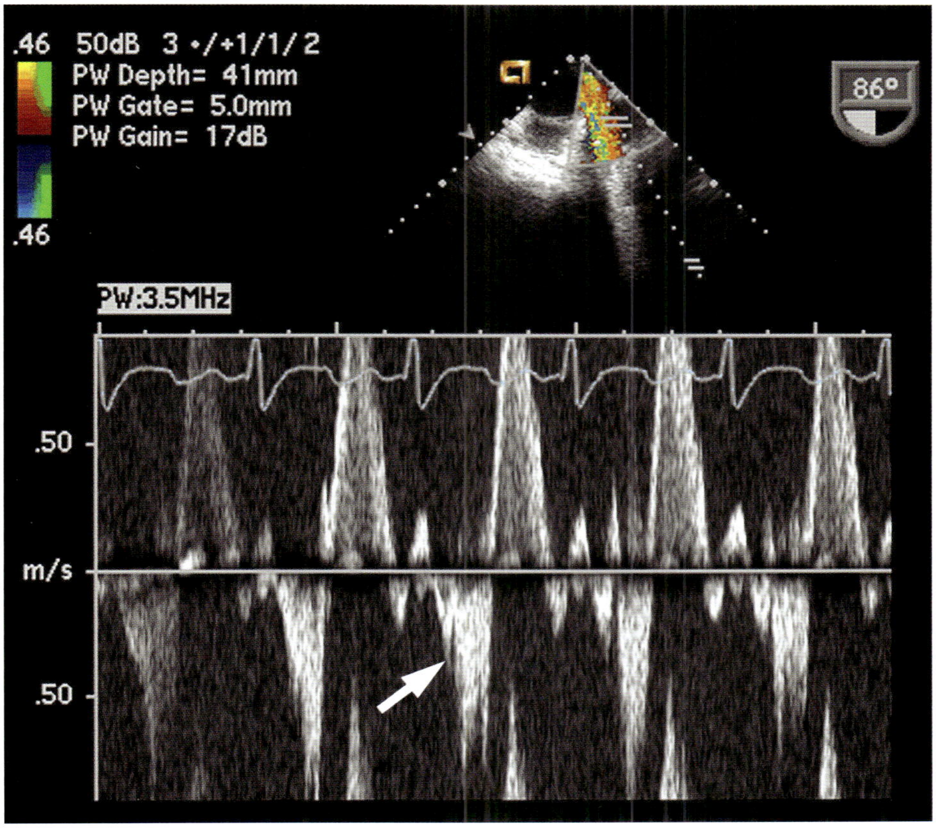

Fig 2.18, cont'd

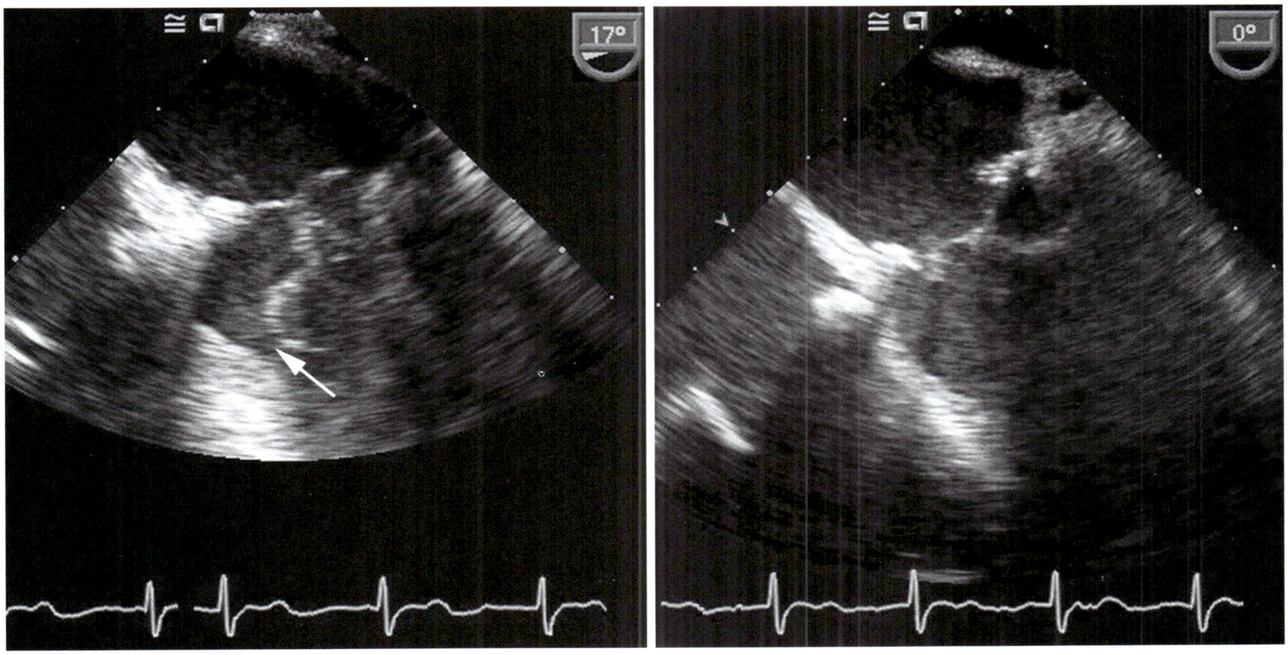

Fig 2.19 In another patient with similar pathology and an identical procedure, postoperative TEE in the four-chamber view showed systolic anterior motion (SAM) of the anterior mitral leaflet *(arrow) (left)*. After adjustment of loading conditions, the SAM resolved *(right)*.

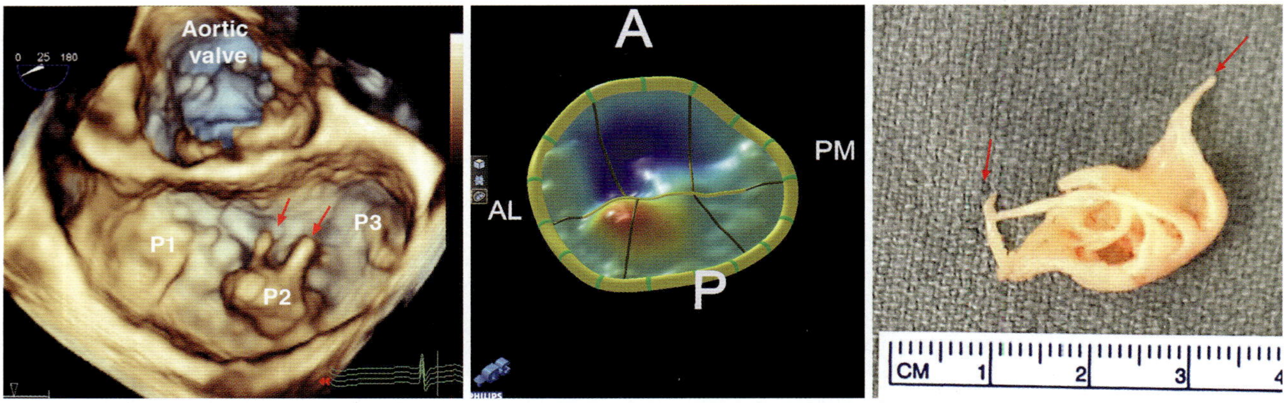

Fig 2.20 In a case with a similar clinical presentation, 3D TEE en face view in systole shows torn chordae *(red arrows)* and a flail P2 segment. There appears to be prolapse of P1 *(left)*. In the middle, software reconstruction shows the prolapsing P2 and P1 segments. On the right the excised segment with torn chordae *(red arrows)* is seen. A = anterior, P = posterior, AL = antero-lateral, PM = postero-medial.

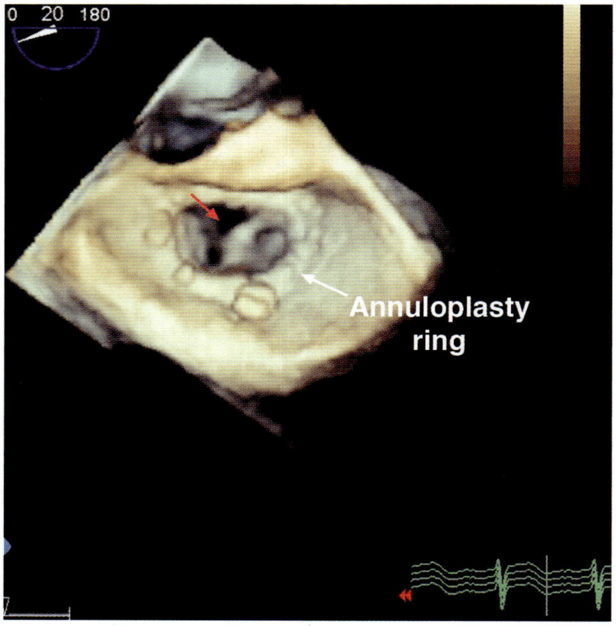

Fig 2.21 The flail segment was resected, and an annuloplasty ring placed. The anterior leaflet has a dropout defect *(red arrow)* but functions as a monocusp, and completely covers the mitral orifice during systole; in real time it can be appreciated that the posterior leaflet is much reduced in size.

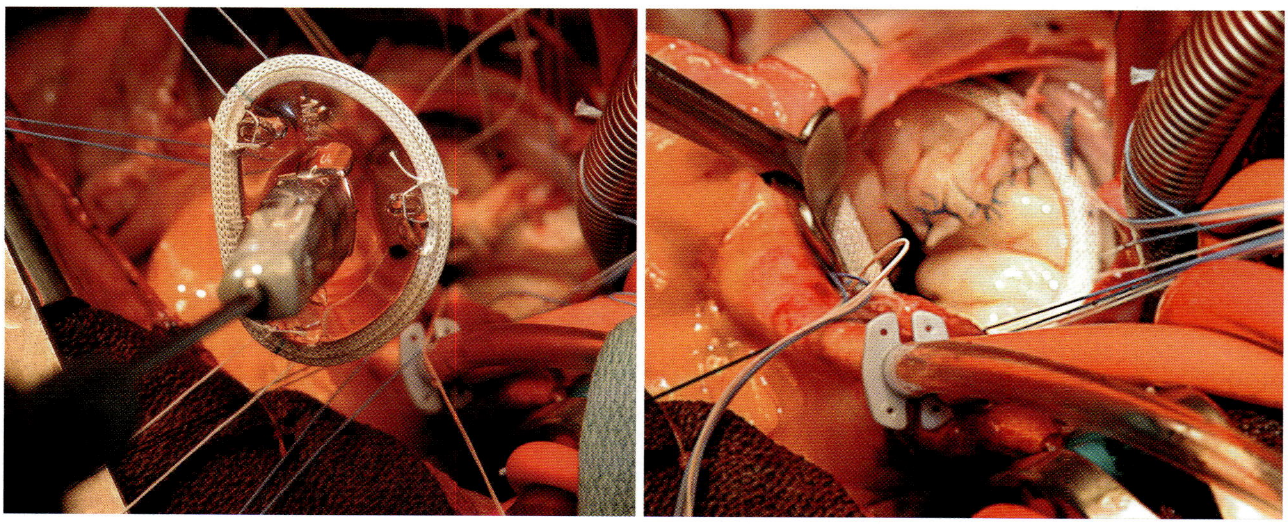

Fig 2.22 In a similar case, a complete annuloplasty ring is chosen, as opposed to the C-shaped ring used in the first case.

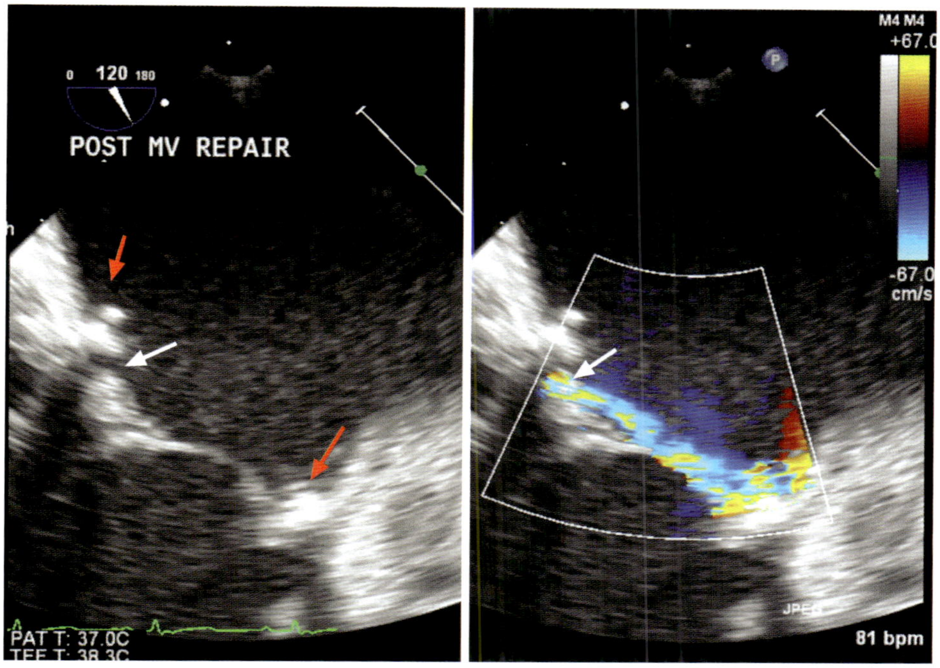

Fig 2.23 In another patient with an excision of the P3 scallop, postoperative imaging revealed a very eccentric jet *(white arrow)* through the repaired posterior leaflet *(white arrow)*, suggesting that the posterior leaflet closure was not intact. This was confirmed on reexploration, and re-repaired. (The annuloplasty ring is indicated by the *red arrows.)*

CASE 2-3
Posterior Leaflet Prolapse of Medial (P3) Scallop

The patient is a 79-year-old woman who states that she was in reasonable health until 3 months before admission, when she was admitted to an outside hospital with severe shortness of breath and was found to have heart failure. An echocardiogram showed severe mitral regurgitation and a massively enlarged left atrium, an enlarged left ventricle and ejection fraction of 55%. Based on the presence of severe mitral regurgitation with heart failure symptoms and an ejection fraction over 30%, she had an ACC/AHA Class I indication for intervention; thus she was referred for mitral valve surgery.

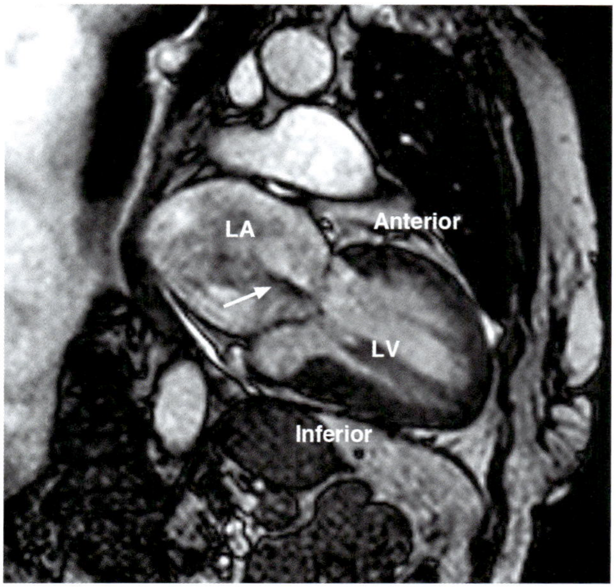

Fig 2.24 Preoperative MRI. In this two-chamber view, a jet of MR *(arrow)* as well as an enlarged left atrium is seen.

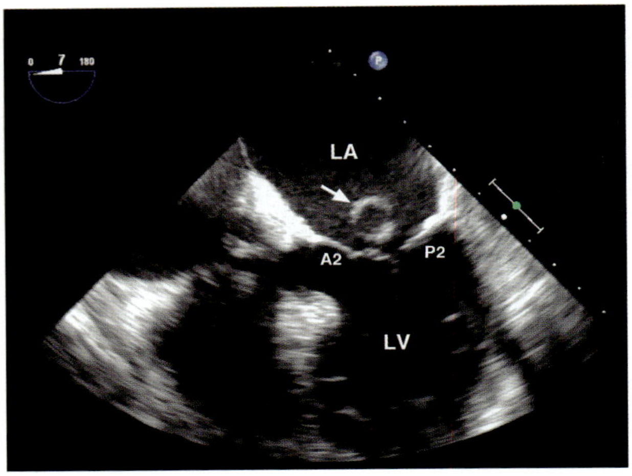

Fig 2.25 In this midesophageal, four-chamber view, A2 and P2 are seen coapting during systole; however, an apparent echolucent circular mass is seen in the left atrium, which does not appear to connect to the mitral valve in this tomographic view. The left atrium is enlarged.

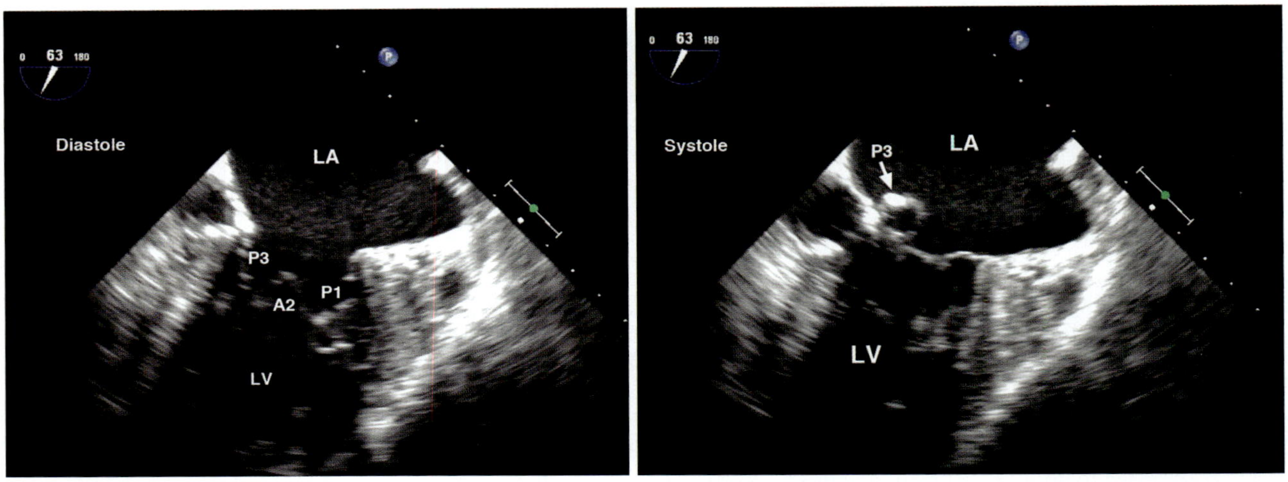

Fig 2.26 In this midesophageal commissural view, the mitral leaflets move normally during diastole; however, during systole, P3 prolapse occurs; therefore, this view confirms that the apparent "mass" seen in the left atrium in the four-chamber view is in fact the P3 scallop.

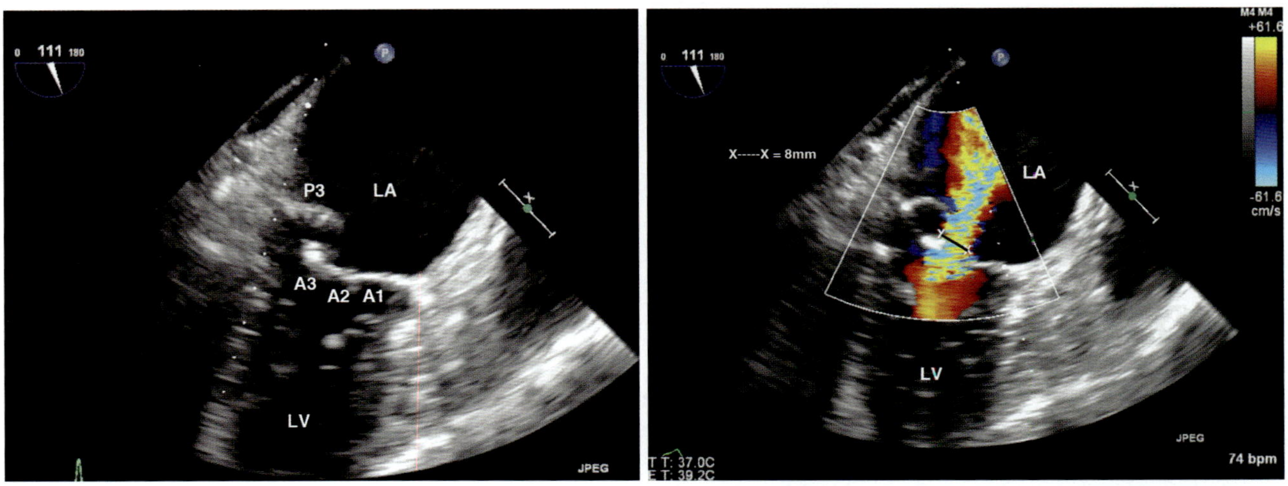

Fig 2.27 The multiplane angle is rotated to obtain a two-chamber view, in which P3 is again seen to be prolapsing; in the right frame, a broad jet of MR with a vena contract width of 8 mm is seen.

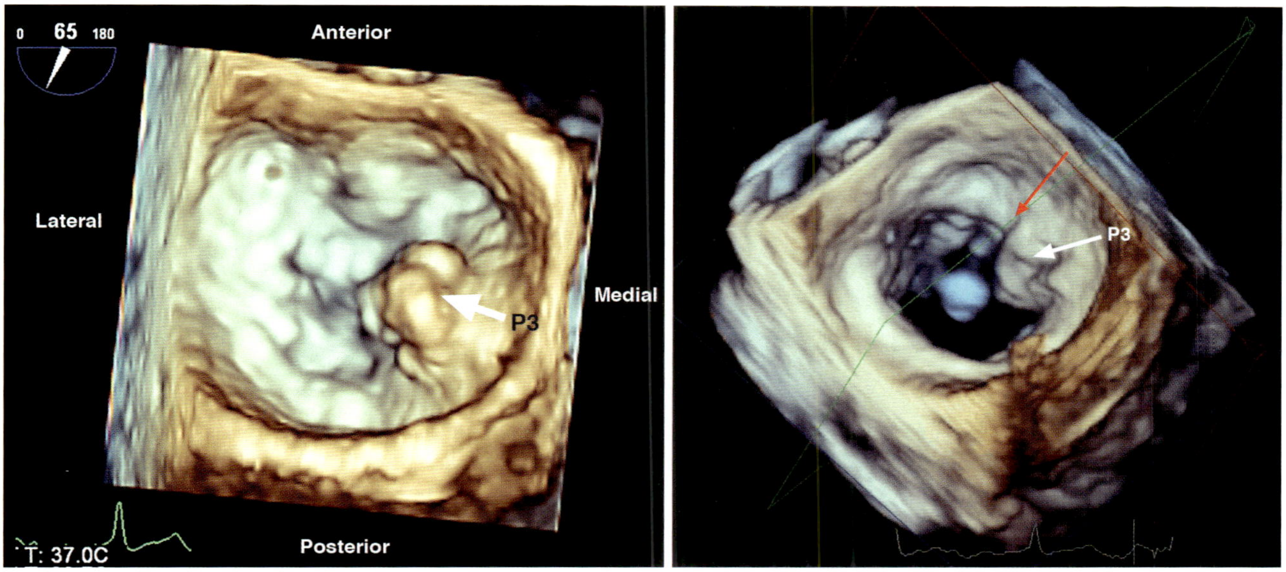

Fig 2.28 3D TEE of the mitral valve from the LA perspective. In systole, a thickened and prolapsing P3 scallop is seen *(left)*; on the right, during diastole, with the image slightly rotated, the P3 segment moves very little, and is seen to be encroaching on the medial commissure *(red arrow)*. Because of this, the valve was deemed irreparable, and was replaced with a bileaflet mechanical prosthesis.

CASE 2-4
Anterior Leaflet Prolapse of Medial (A3) Scallop

Two years before admission, when still living in Mexico, this 27-year-old male presented with left-sided chest pain, progressive shortness of breath on exertion, and tingling in his fingers. An echocardiogram was done, which showed that he had mitral valve prolapse with at least moderate mitral regurgitation. Although surgery was contemplated, the patient declined. He was doing relatively well and moved to this region approximately 4 months ago. However, recently he began to have some more chest discomfort, as well as tingling in his fingers. He saw his primary care doctor who referred him for echocardiography which showed severe MR with normal LV systolic function but with significant LV dilation. The decision was made to proceed with mitral valve surgery.

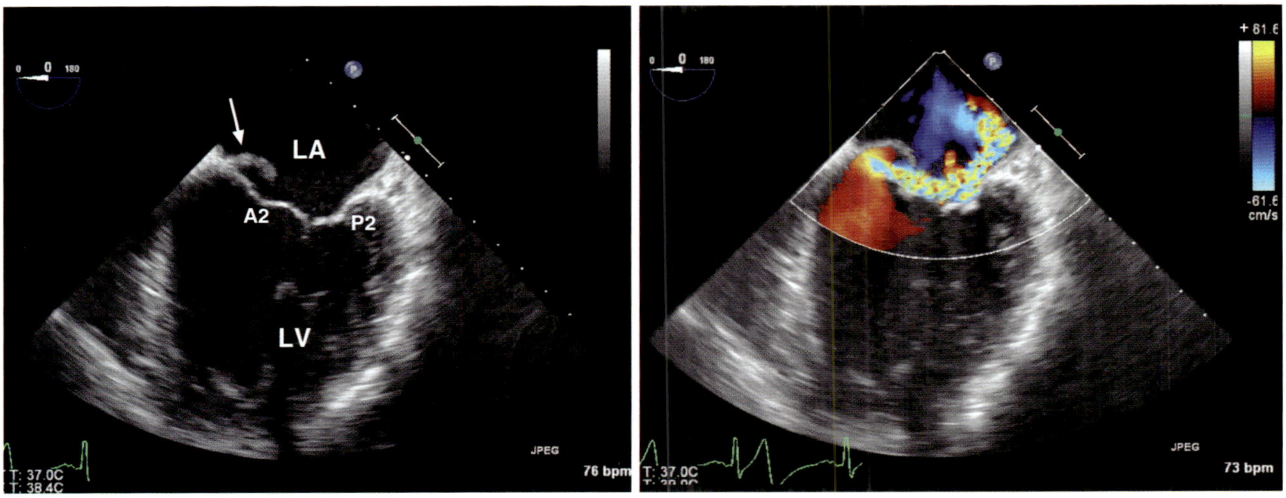

Fig 2.29 2D imaging in a posteriorly angulated four-chamber view at 0-degrees rotation during systole demonstrates normally functioning A2 and P2 segments; however, there is presumably a flail segment of one of the mitral leaflets *(arrow)*. Color flow imaging showed a posteriorly directed mitral regurgitant jet, which is most consistent with anterior leaflet disease.

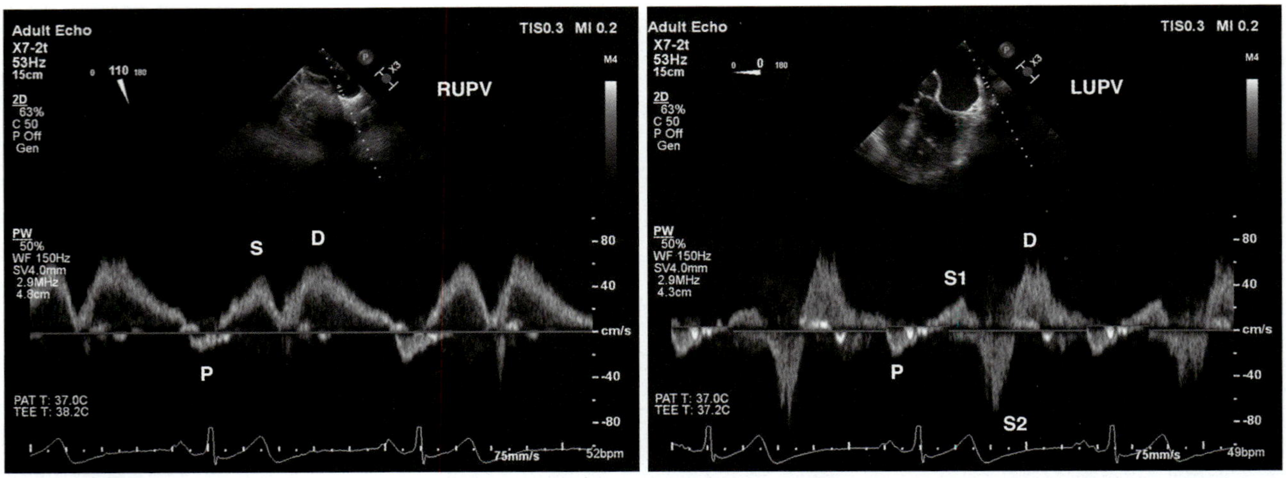

Fig 2.30 Pulsed wave Doppler in the right upper pulmonary vein (RUPV) is normal. In the left upper pulmonary vein (LUPV), two components of the systolic (S) wave are evident—the S1 wave is a result of atrial relaxation, and the reversed S2 wave is a result of severe MR.

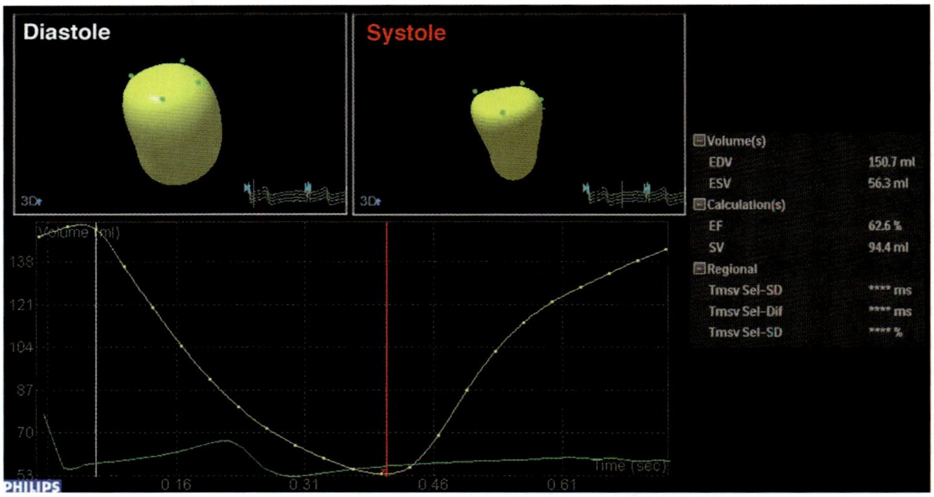

Fig 2.31 3D volume analysis shows a preserved ejection fraction of 63% but with increased end-diastolic and end-systolic volumes.

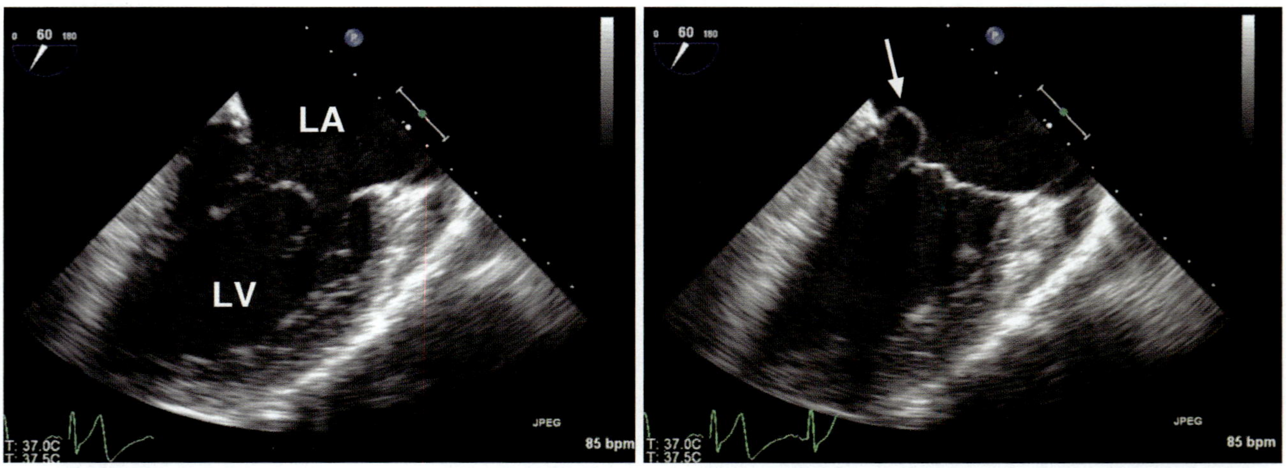

Fig 2.32 In a commissural view at 60 degrees, the valve opens normally in diastole *(left)*. During systole, there is prolapse *(arrow)* of what would appear to be the P3 scallop. This is contradicted, however, by the posterior direction of the MR jet as seen in Fig 2.29, suggesting that the medial segment of the anterior leaflet may be visualized because of a slight anterior angulation of the image plane.

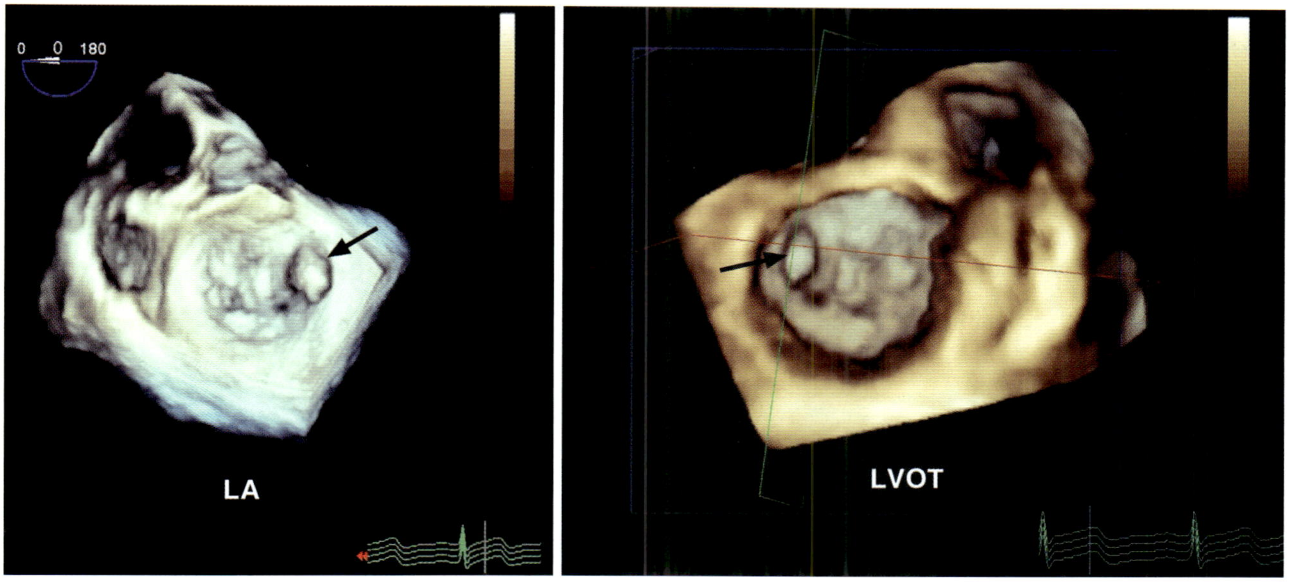

Fig 2.33 3D TEE from the LA perspective *(left)* and the LVOT perspective *(right)* shows prolapse of the A3 segment *(arrows)*, which is better appreciated in real time. The posterior leaflet is normal with no prolapse of P3, but the A3 prolapsing segment overlies the P3 segment.

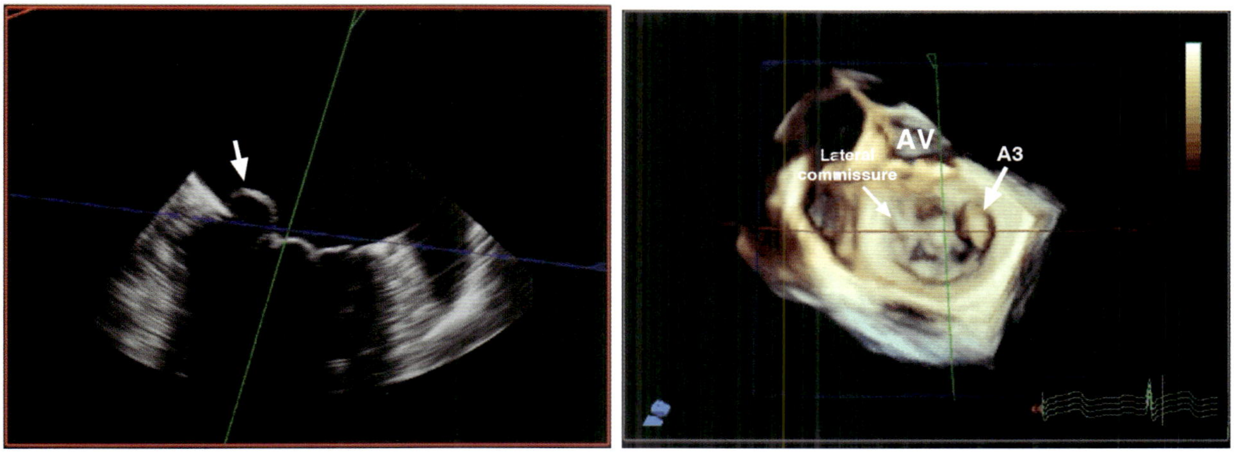

Fig 2.34 3D quantification shows how this paradox can arise. In the right frame, the red line approximates the commissural plane; however, P3 and the medial commissure are obscured by the abnormal motion of the A3 segment *(left frame, arrow)*.

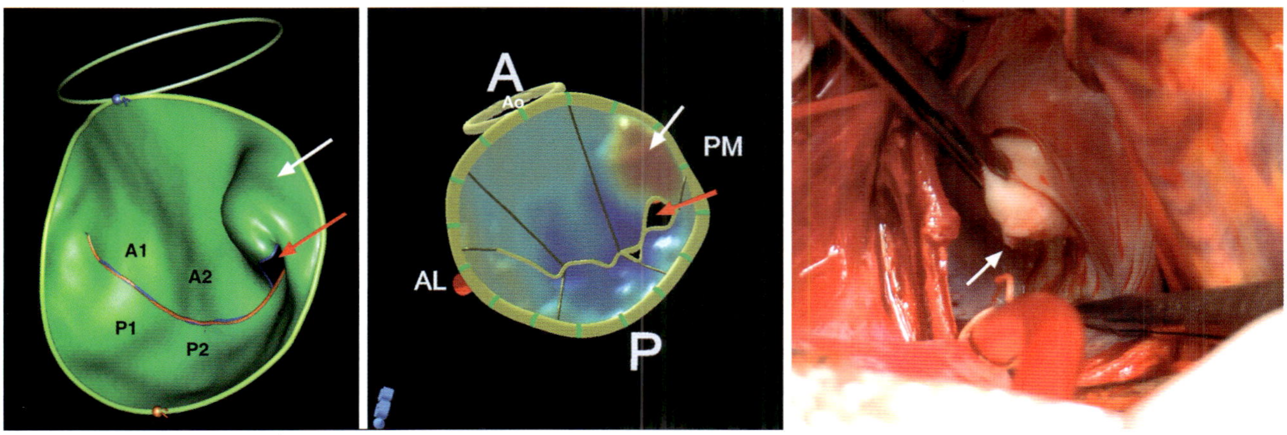

Fig 2.35 In the left and center frames, mitral valve quantification shows prolapse in the A3 region *(white arrow)* and the regurgitant orifice *(red arrow)*. On the right, the surgeon grasps the A3 segment; the arrow indicates a torn chord. A = anterior, P = posterior, AL = antero-lateral, PM = postero-medial.

CASE 2-5
Bileaflet Mitral Valve Prolapse

This 58-year-old male with a known history of mitral valve prolapse presented with increasing shortness of breath, and frequent runs of ventricular tachycardia. TTE showed severe mitral valve prolapse. He was referred for mitral valve surgery for symptomatic severe MR. Despite involvement of both leaflets, valve anatomy was favorable for valve repair, and a quadrangular resection of P2 and ring annuloplasty were performed under TEE guidance.

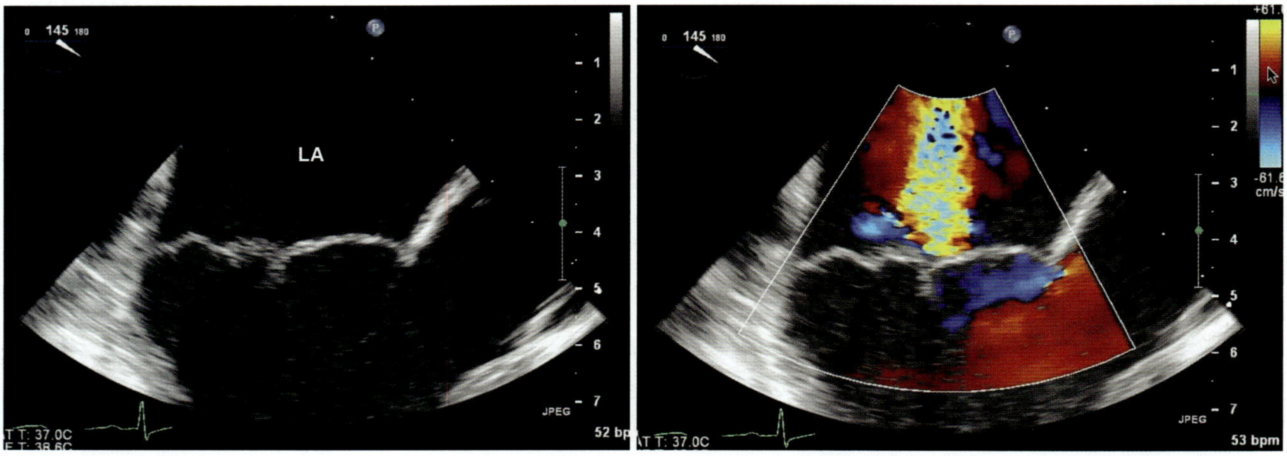

Fig 2.36 In a midesophageal long-axis view, both mitral leaflets are seen to prolapse into the LA. With color Doppler *(right)*, a large central jet of MR is seen.

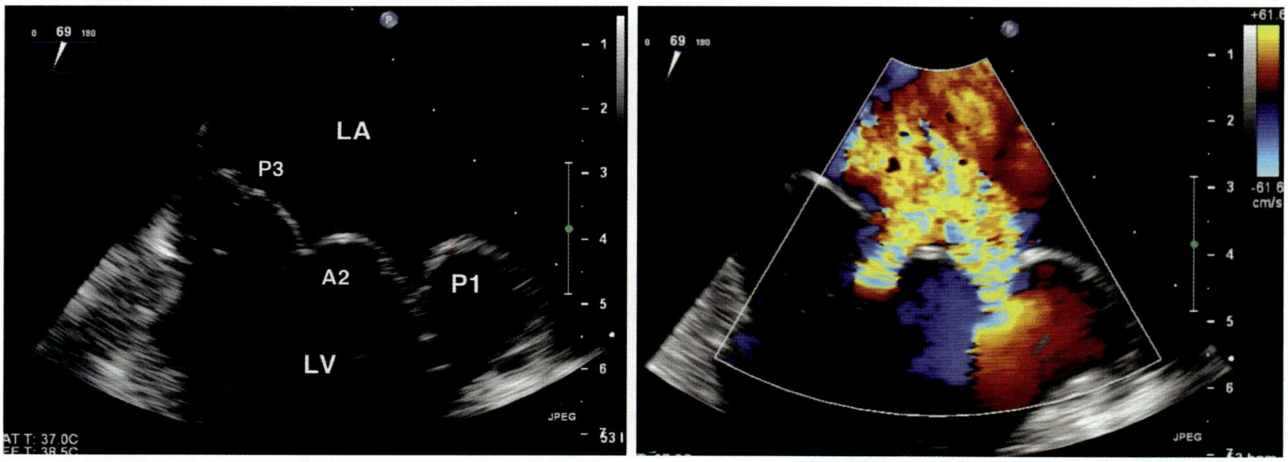

Fig 2.37 In a midesophageal commissural view, there is prolapse of all visualized segments. Color Doppler *(right)* shows two components of the jet of MR.

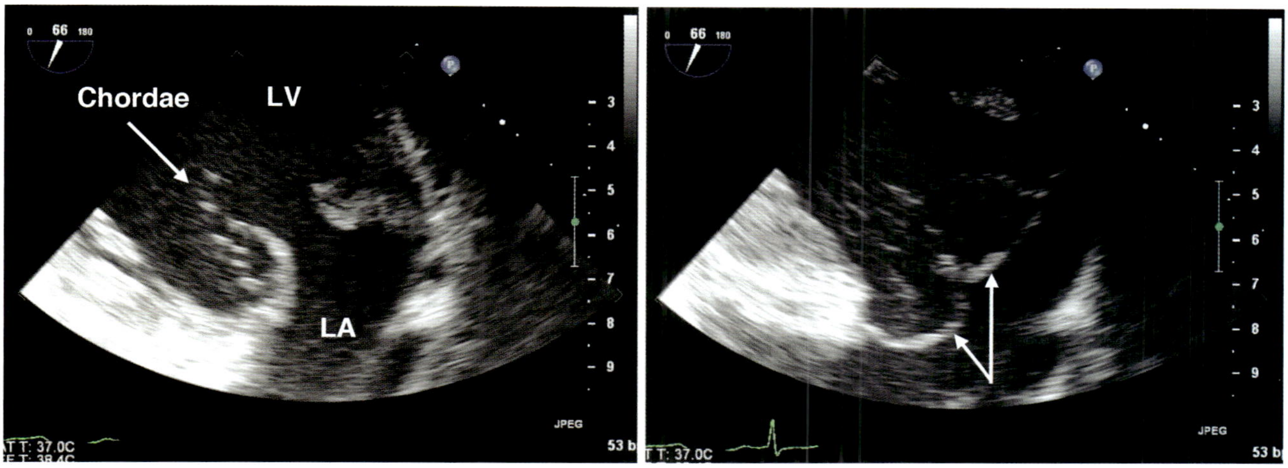

Fig 2.38 Transgastric imaging is especially helpful when examining the submitral apparatus. This two-chamber view shows thickened leaflets and multiple chordae during diastole *(left)* and leaflet prolapse during systole *(arrows, right)*.

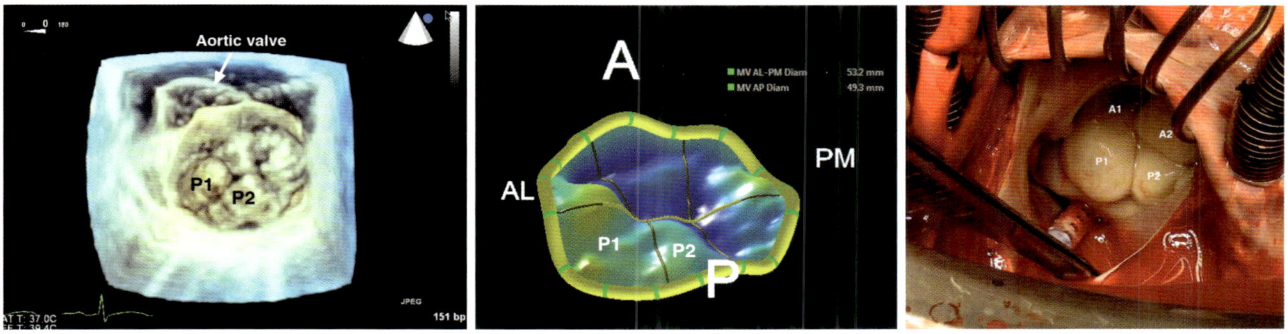

Fig 2.39 3D TEE en face imaging of the mitral valve from the left atrial perspective shows fullness and prolapse of all segments, but especially of P1 and P2 *(left)*. This is also seen in the mitral valve reconstruction *(middle)*. Exposure of the valve confirms these findings. A = anterior, P = posterior, AL = antero-lateral, PM = postero-medial.

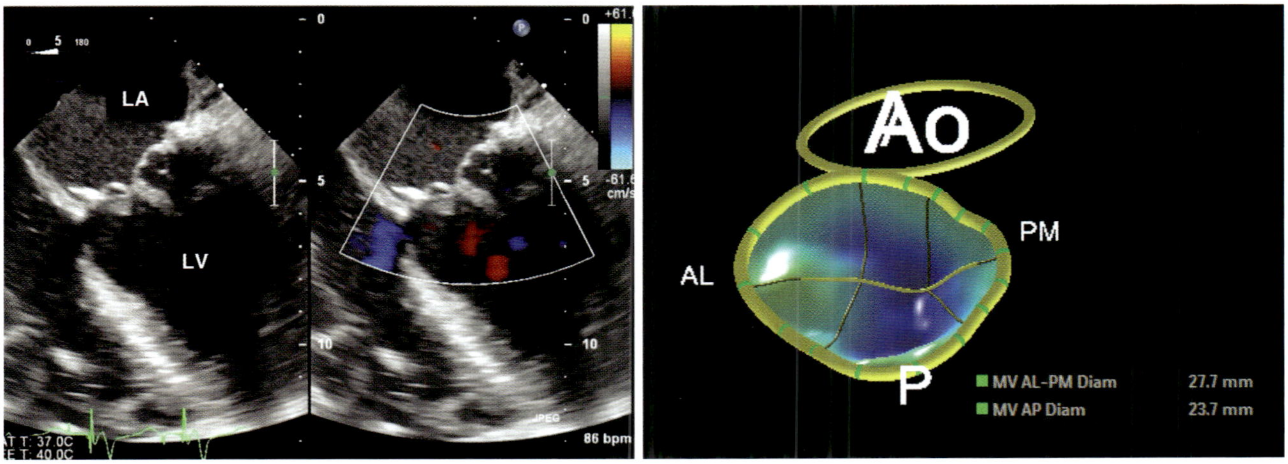

Fig 2.40 Resection of the P2 portion of the posterior leaflet was performed as well as ring annuloplasty. Postoperative imaging in the midesophageal four-chamber view showed no residual regurgitation. Mitral valve reconstruction reveals that the bulk of the prolapse has been eliminated. A = anterior, P = posterior, AL = antero-lateral, PM = postero-medial.

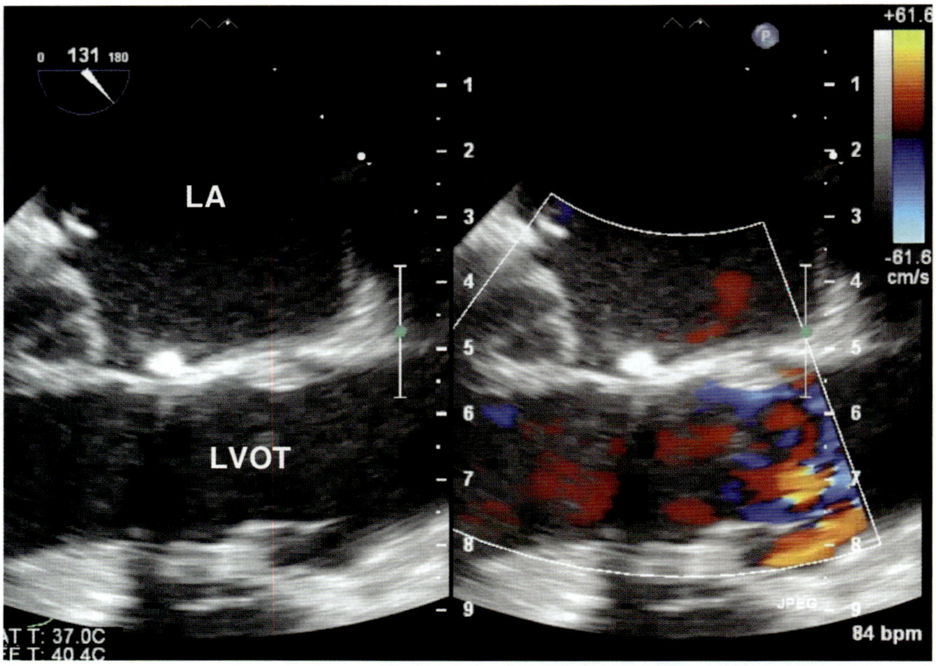

Fig 2.41 Postoperative imaging in the midesophageal long-axis view demonstrates no regurgitation, as well as the absence of systolic anterior motion (SAM) of the anterior mitral leaflet.

CASE 2-6
Mitral Valve Prolapse and Aortic Valve Fibroelastoma

This 87-year-old female with severe mitral regurgitation and persistent heart failure symptoms despite medical therapy was referred for mitral valve surgery. An extensive resection of the posterior leaflet was performed, with ring annuloplasty. The aortic mass was resected and pathologic diagnosis was papillary fibroelastoma.

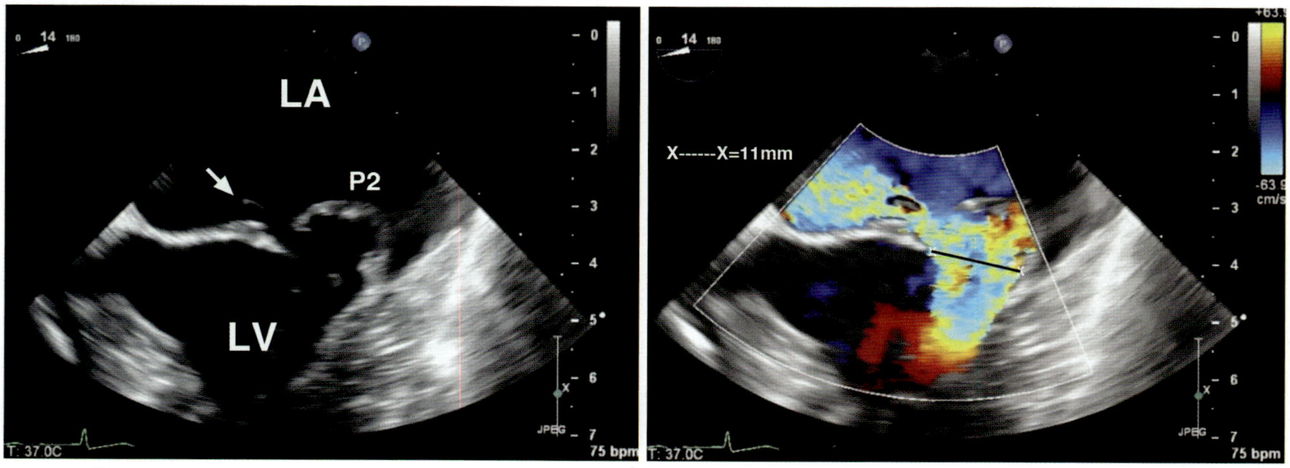

Fig 2.42 In this midesophageal four-chamber view, there is prolapse of the P2 scallop. The arrow indicates a torn chord. In the right frame, a large, anteriorly directed jet of mitral regurgitation, with a vena contracta width of 11 mm, is seen.

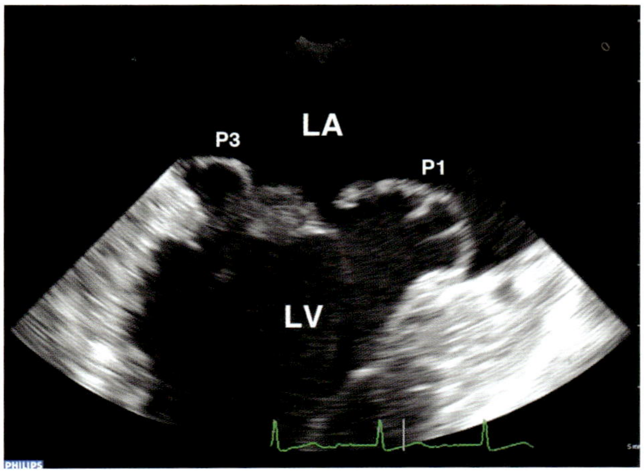

Fig 2.43 In this midesophageal commissural view, there appears to be prolapse in the P1 and P3 scallops, especially prominent in the P1 scallop.

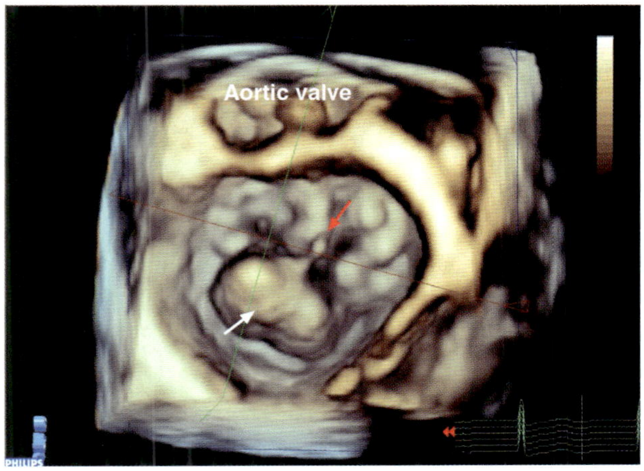

Fig 2.44 This 3D TEE is an en face view of the mitral valve from the left atrial perspective. There is redundancy of both leaflets, and gross prolapse of a large portion of the posterior leaflet *(white arrow)*. The red arrow indicates a torn chord.

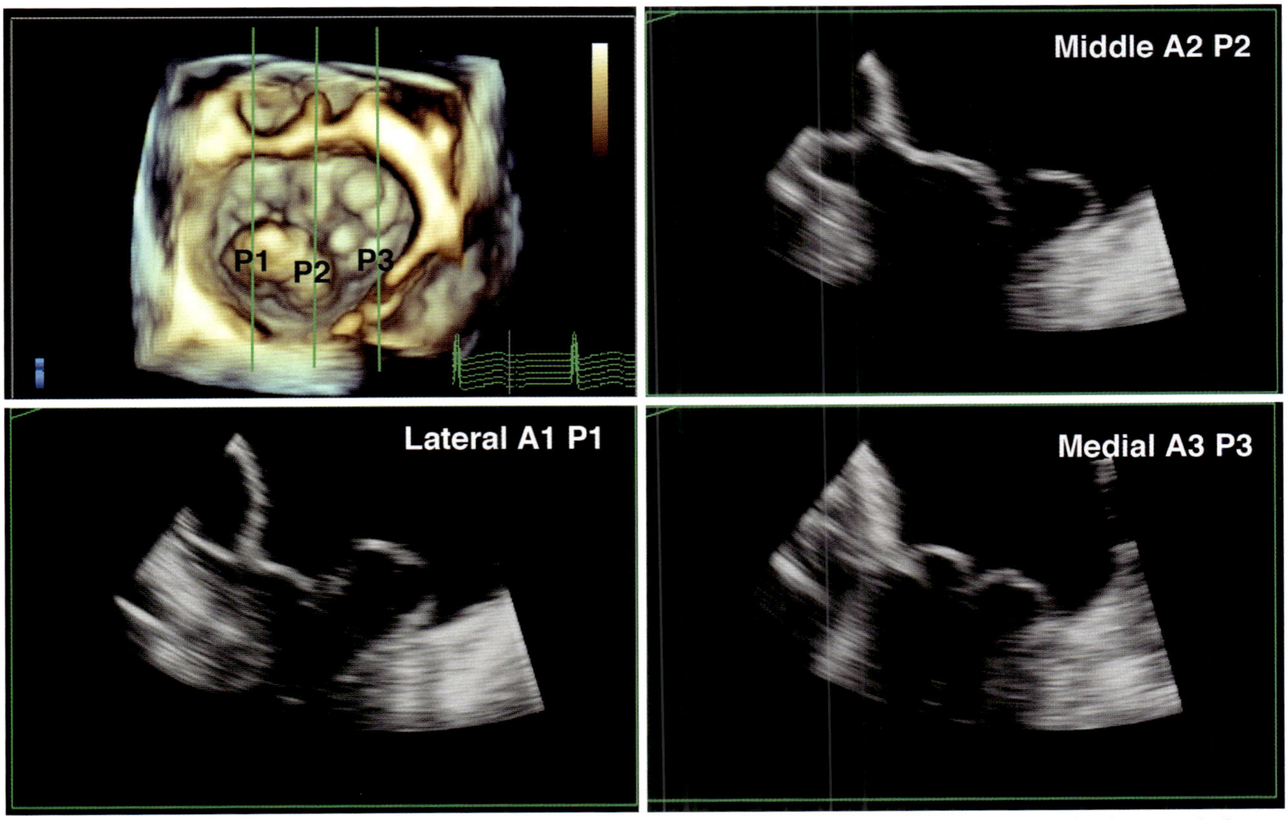

Fig 2.45 3D quantification can sometimes help in determining which portions of the mitral valve are involved in a pathologic process. The green lines indicate cuts through the lateral, middle, and medial portions of the valve. The disease is most prominent in the P1 and P2 segments, and less so in the A2 and P2 segments. The A3 and P3 segments are largely uninvolved.

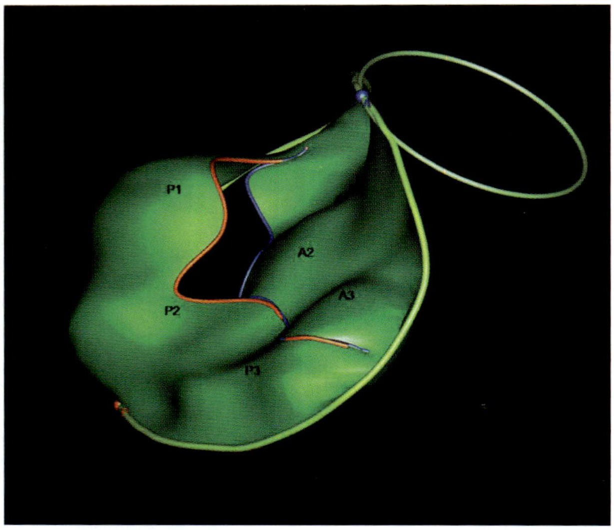

Fig 2.46 Anatomic mitral quantification supports the findings of the 3D TEE, with prominent prolapse of the P1 and P2 segments. There appears to be a large regurgitant orifice, although this finding may be unreliable because of ultrasound drop-out in some cases.

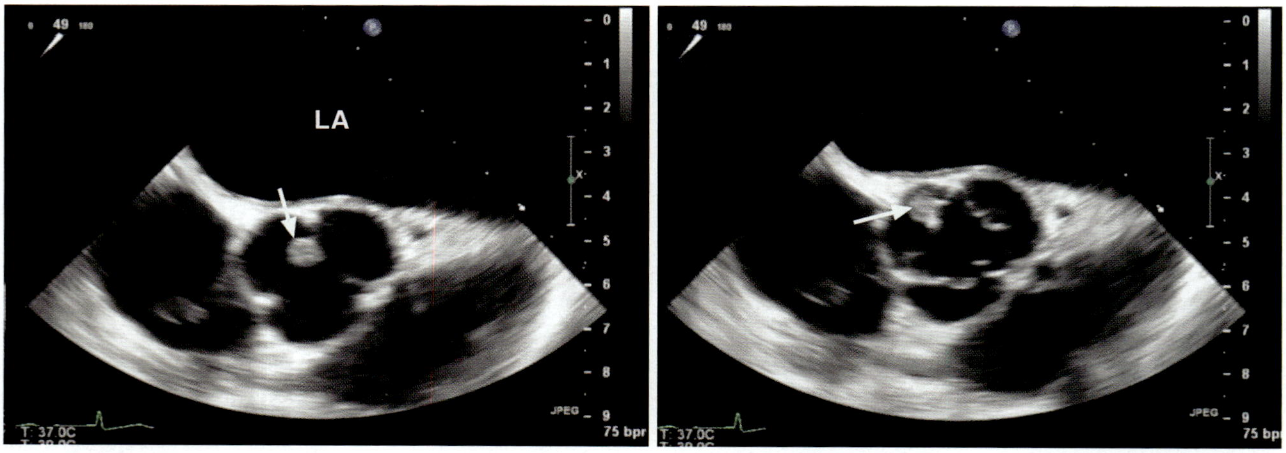

Fig 2.47 In addition to the mitral valve pathology, a small mass was seen on the aortic valve. In this midesophageal short-axis view of the aortic valve, a small mass is seen in diastole *(left)*, whereas in systole *(right)*, the lesion appears attached to the noncoronary cusp. The video clip compares 2D *(left)* and 3D imaging.

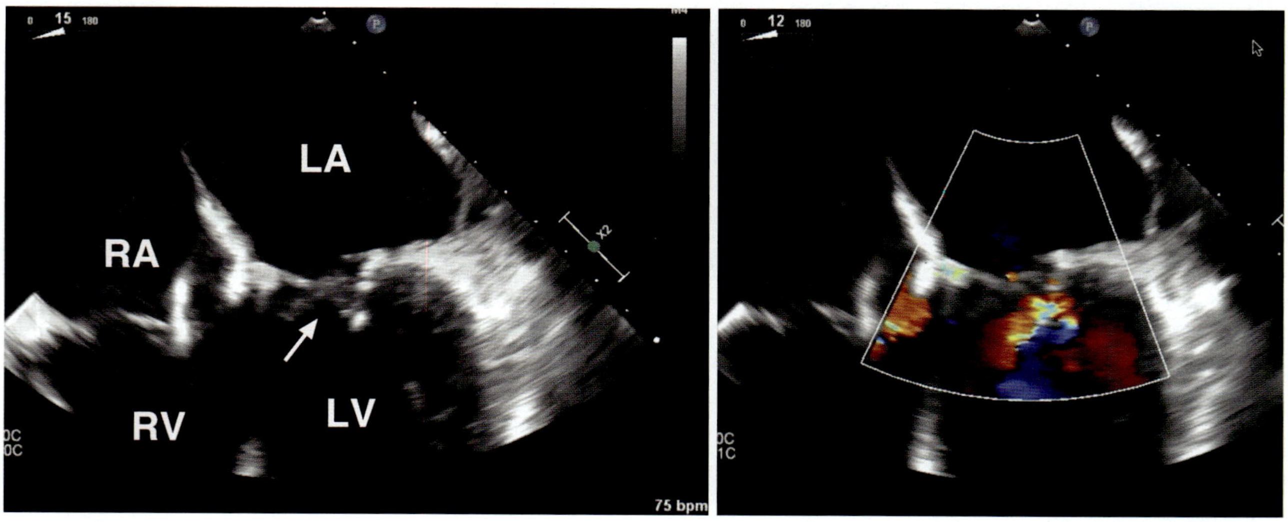

Fig 2.48 After an extensive quadrangular resection of the posterior leaflet and ring annuloplasty, there is no residual MR seen with color Doppler *(right)*. The aortic lesion was removed, and postoperatively, no aortic regurgitation was seen.

Comments

The first step in evaluation of a patient with mitral regurgitation is to establish the cause of valve dysfunction. Causes of mitral regurgitation are divided into primary anatomic abnormalities of the valve apparatus and secondary regurgitation resulting from left ventricular dilation and dysfunction with an anatomically normal valve. Common causes of primary mitral regurgitation include myxomatous mitral valve disease (e.g., mitral valve prolapse), rheumatic valve disease, and endocarditis. In the patients presented here, the etiology of valve dysfunction was myxomatous mitral valve disease. Differentiation of a valvular vegetation from a flail leaflet can be difficult, even with TEE imaging, as both have a similar echocardiographic appearance.

In patients with myxomatous mitral valve disease, attention is next focused on defining the exact anatomy of the valve leaflets and chords. The likelihood of a successful valve repair is highest with posterior leaflet involvement, particularly when the problem is isolated to the central (or P2) scallop. With severe prolapse, the leaflet bows into the left atrium in systole but the tip of the leaflet still points toward the LV apex because the chords are intact. In contrast, with chordal rupture and a flail leaflet segment, the leaflet tip points away from the LV apex, often with small mobile chords attached. With the typical anatomy of regurgitation caused by dysfunction of the central scallop of the posterior leaflet, quadrangular or triangular resection of the flail segment followed by placement of an annuloplasty ring usually results in a functional valve apparatus. The two broad categories of annuloplasty rings that have been used in the current era of mitral valve repair have been the C-shaped ring, and the complete ring. The former was used when it was assumed that there was no chance of dilation in the intertrigonal area, but some surgeons prefer a complete ring as distention in the intertrigonal area can occur.

In patients with mitral valve repair, systolic anterior motion (SAM) of the anterior leaflet can result in significant dynamic left ventricular outflow tract obstruction. In many cases, SAM is transient as cardiopulmonary bypass is weaned and resolves with restoration of normal loading conditions. When significant outflow obstruction persists after normalization of loading conditions, a second pump run for correction of this abnormality should be considered. Systolic anterior motion can often be prevented by use of the "sliding-leaflet" technique where the posterior leaflet is separated from the mitral annulus at the time of posterior leaflet quadrangular resection and then reattached after reducing annular size with a flexible ring.

Intraoperative TEE by an experienced echocardiographer for evaluation of the adequacy of mitral valve repair and for detection of any complications such as circumflex artery or aortic valve injury, is indicated in all patients undergoing valve repair surgery. A second bypass pump run with revision of the repair or valve replacement is needed in about 5% to 10% of cases because of residual significant mitral regurgitation.

Baseline images provide a standard of reference for postrepair evaluation of valve function. However, it is important to ensure that the loading conditions, as measured by systemic blood pressure, heart rate, and forward cardiac output, are similar on the prevalve and postvalve repair studies. A lower blood pressure or cardiac output on the postrepair study may result in underestimation of regurgitant severity. The echocardiographic instrument settings also should be similar, including image depth, frame rate, 2D and color gain, wall filters, and color map. The valve should be carefully evaluated in multiple image planes after the repair, and the direction and shape of any residual mitral regurgitation may be different than shown on the prerepair images.

The surgeon may also assess the adequacy of repair by direct visual inspection of the amount of backflow across the valve when the ventricle is filled.

Suggested Reading

1. Delling FN, Vasan RS: Epidemiology and pathophysiology of mitral valve prolapse: new insights into disease progression, genetics, and molecular basis, Circulation 129(21):2158–2170, 2014.
2. Faletra F, Demertzis S, et al: Three dimensional transesophageal echocardiography in degenerative mitral regurgitation, J Am Soc Echocardiogr 28:437–448, 2015.
3. Clavel MA, Mantovani F, Malouf J, et al: Dynamic phenotypes of degenerative myxomatous mitral valve disease: quantitative 3-dimensional echocardiographic study, Circ Cardiovasc Imaging 8:e002989–e002998, 2015.
4. Sidebotham DA, Drake DH, Zimmerman KG: Surgical mitral valve repair: Patient selection, operative planning and intra-operative monitoring. In Otto CM, editor: The practice of clinical echocardiography, ed 5, Philadelphia, 2016, Elsevier, Chapter 19.
5. Lancellotti, P, Moura. L, Pierard, LA, et al. European Association of Echocardiography recommendations for the assessment of valvular regurgitation. Part 2: mitral and tricuspid regurgitation (native valve disease). Eur J Echocardiogr 11:307–32, 2010.

Rheumatic Mitral Valve Disease

CASE 2-7
Rheumatic Mitral Stenosis

This 56-year-old man presented with severe symptomatic mitral stenosis and atrial fibrillation and was initially considered for percutaneous balloon valvotomy. The preoperative TEE showed typical rheumatic mitral valve disease with superimposed calcification and an immobile posterior leaflet with overall mitral valve morphology that was suboptimal for a percutaneous procedure. In addition, there was a large laminated left atrial thrombus. Thus he was referred for surgical intervention.

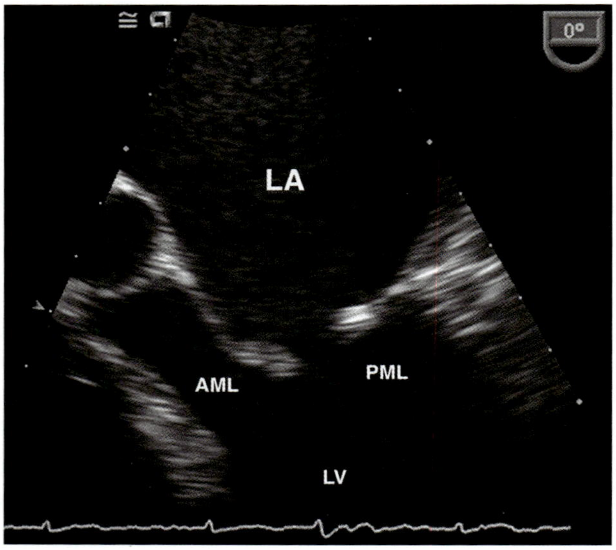

Fig 2.49 In a high TEE view, a middiastolic frame shows the mitral leaflets with thickening and tethering of the leaflet tips, resulting in the "doming" of the valve in diastole that is typical of rheumatic valve disease. This appearance is caused by commissural fusion, along with chordal thickening and shortening.

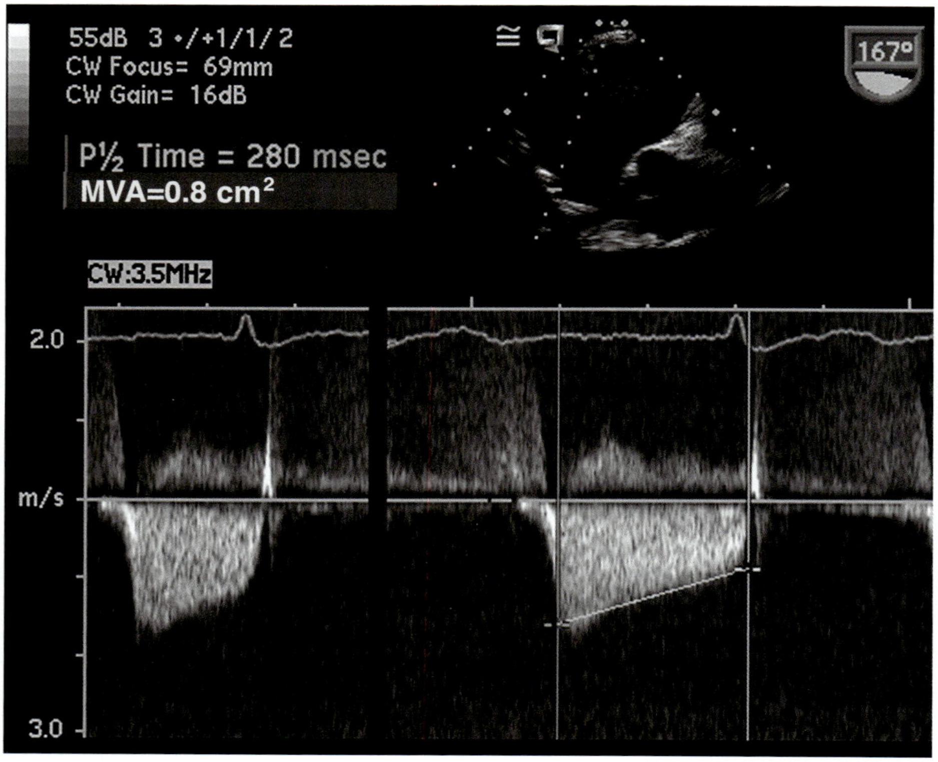

Fig 2.50 With the image plane rotated to provide a long-axis view of the mitral valve with the direction of the CW Doppler beam parallel to the jet through the narrowed mitral valve, the diastolic flow signal is recorded. The patient is in atrial fibrillation with variation in R-R interval and no a-velocity. The line shows the diastolic slope of the velocity curve with calculation of the pressure half-time. The pressure half-time is the time interval from the peak transmitral gradient to the point where the gradient is half the peak gradient. Mitral valve area is the empiric constant 220 divided by the pressure half-time.

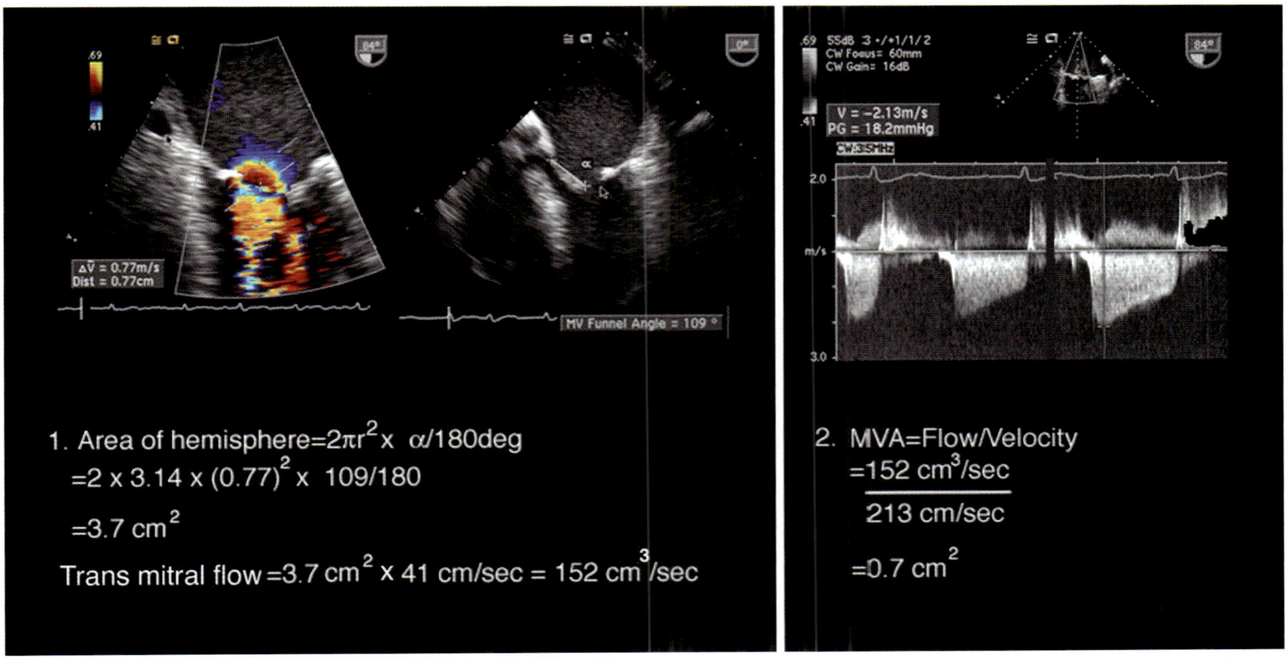

Fig 2.51 Mitral valve area (MVA) can also be calculated using the continuity principle. The maximal transmitral volume flow rate is calculated from a color flow image of the proximal acceleration of flow as shown (Equation 1), analogous to the PISA calculation of regurgitation flow rate. The maximum flow rate is then divided by maximum velocity to estimate MVA (Equation 2). This method assumes that maximal velocity and maximal flow rate occur at the same point in time.

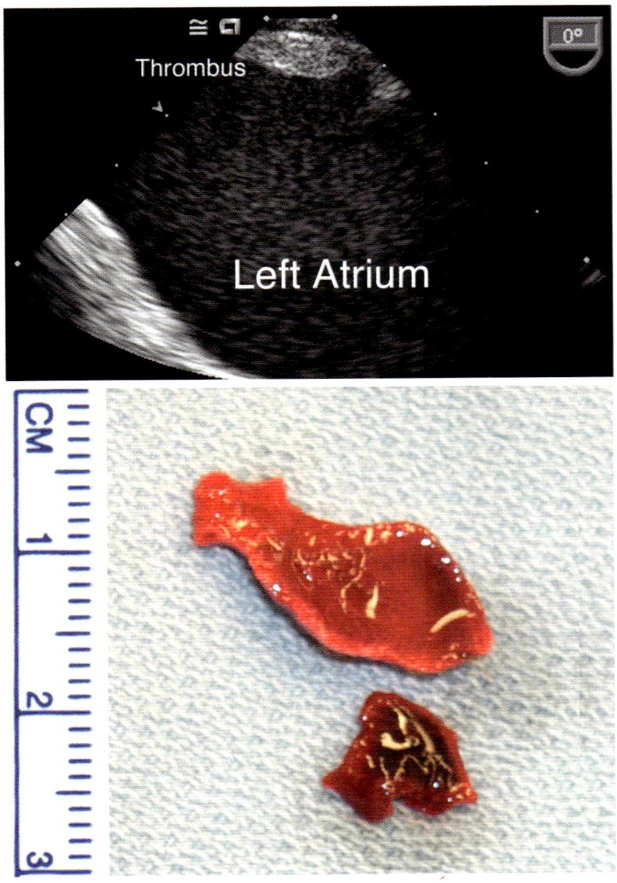

Fig 2.52 *(Top)* A mass in the dome of the left atrium. *(Bottom)* Fragments of the mass that pathologically was identified as platelets and fibrin, consistent with recent thrombus.

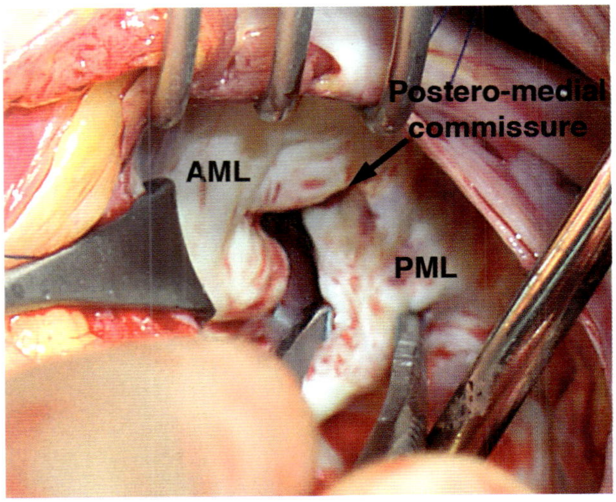

Fig 2.53 Intraoperative visualization of the valve shows leaflet thickening that is characteristic of rheumatic disease. There was dense fusion of the anterior and posterior leaflets at the commissures, with retraction and calcification of the central scallop of the posterior leaflet. A repair was performed with a commissurotomy and placement of an annuloplasty ring. Although initial postoperative TEE images showed only mild regurgitation, when loading conditions returned to the preoperative baseline, moderate to severe regurgitation was seen. The patient then underwent a second pump run with mitral valve replacement.

CASE 2-8
Rheumatic Mitral Stenosis and Regurgitation

This 39-year-old female with a history of rheumatic heart disease and mitral valve involvement presented with progressive fatigue and shortness of breath. She had a history of atrial fibrillation complicated by a cerebral embolic event 4 years before this visit. She was referred for mitral valve replacement for mixed mitral stenosis and regurgitation with worsening clinical symptoms. She also underwent pulmonary vein isolation and ablation (maze procedure for atrial fibrillation).

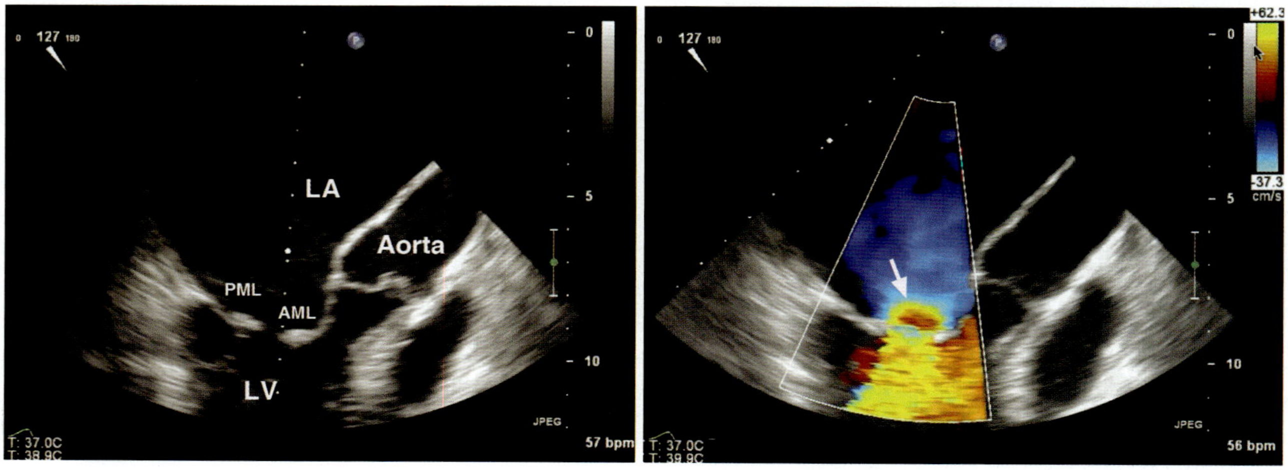

Fig 2.54 In this midesophageal long-axis view during diastole, the left frame demonstrates an enlarged left atrium, thickened aortic valve leaflets, and restricted mitral leaflets, with the anterior leaflet doming, sometimes described as having the appearance of a "hockey stick," secondary to commissural fusion. On the right, with the Nyquist limit reduced to 37 cm/s, color Doppler reveals flow acceleration as the stenotic orifice is approached. The PISA, or proximal isovelocity surface area, will be used to calculate mitral valve area.

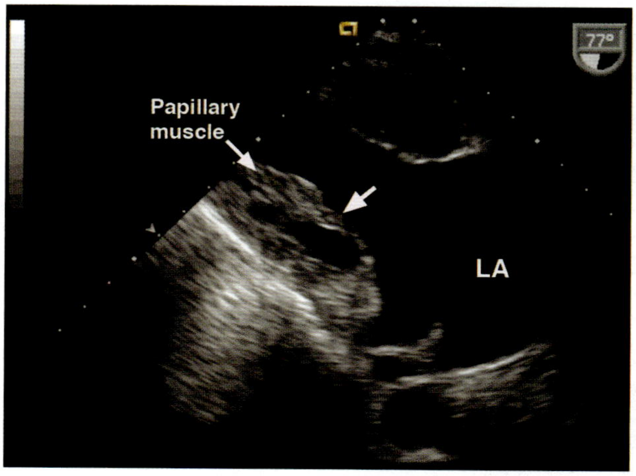

Fig 2.55 In another patient with a similar clinical presentation, transgastric long-axis imaging shows thickened and shortened chordae *(arrow)*, as is commonly found in rheumatic mitral disease.

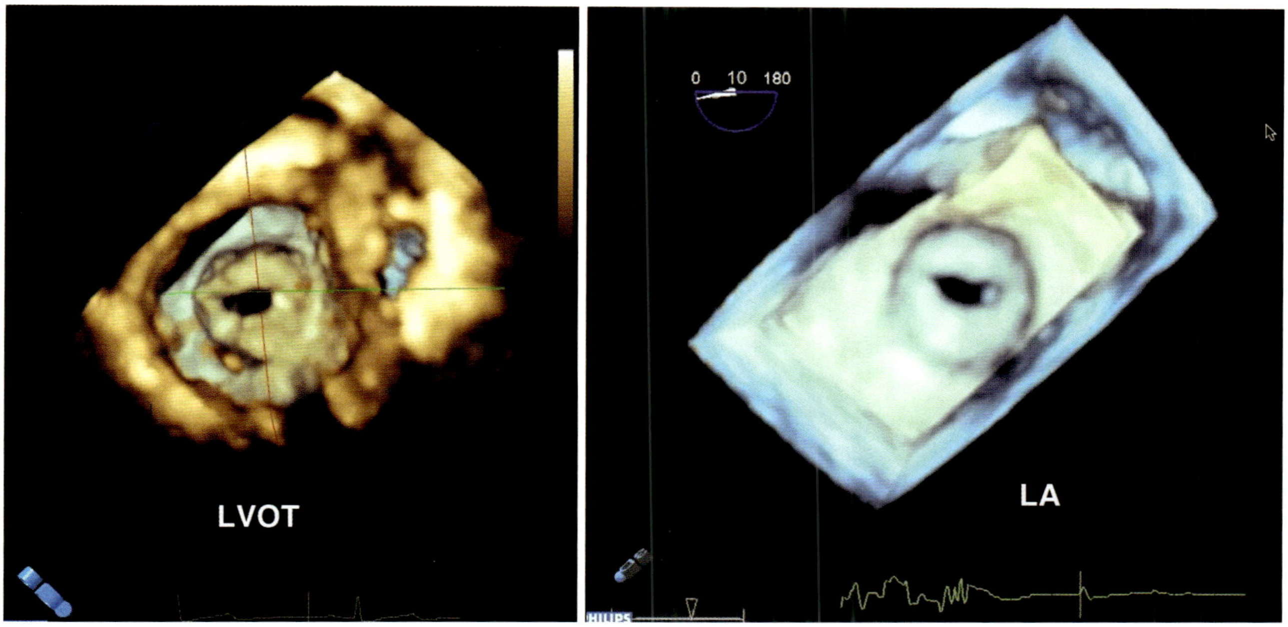

Fig 2.56 3D TEE from the LVOT perspective *(left)* and LA perspective *(right)* shows grossly thickened leaflets during diastole, giving a "fish mouth" appearance. Measurement of anatomic mitral valve orifice area from a 3D full-volume acquisition is very accurate and is a standard element in the evaluation of a patient with rheumatic mitral valve disease.

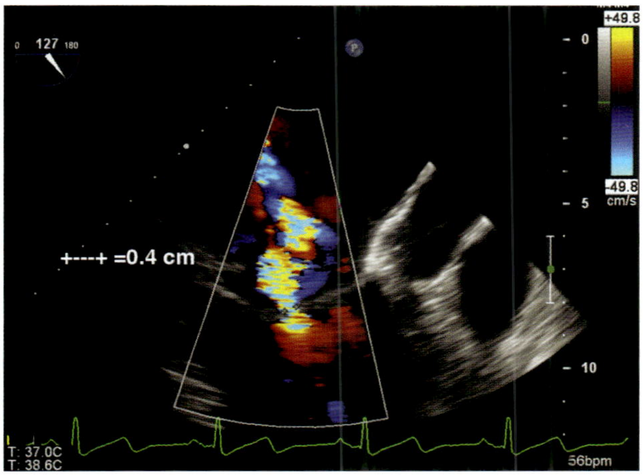

Fig 2.57 In the midesophageal long-axis view, color Doppler shows a vena contracta of 0.4 cm, consistent with moderate mitral regurgitation.

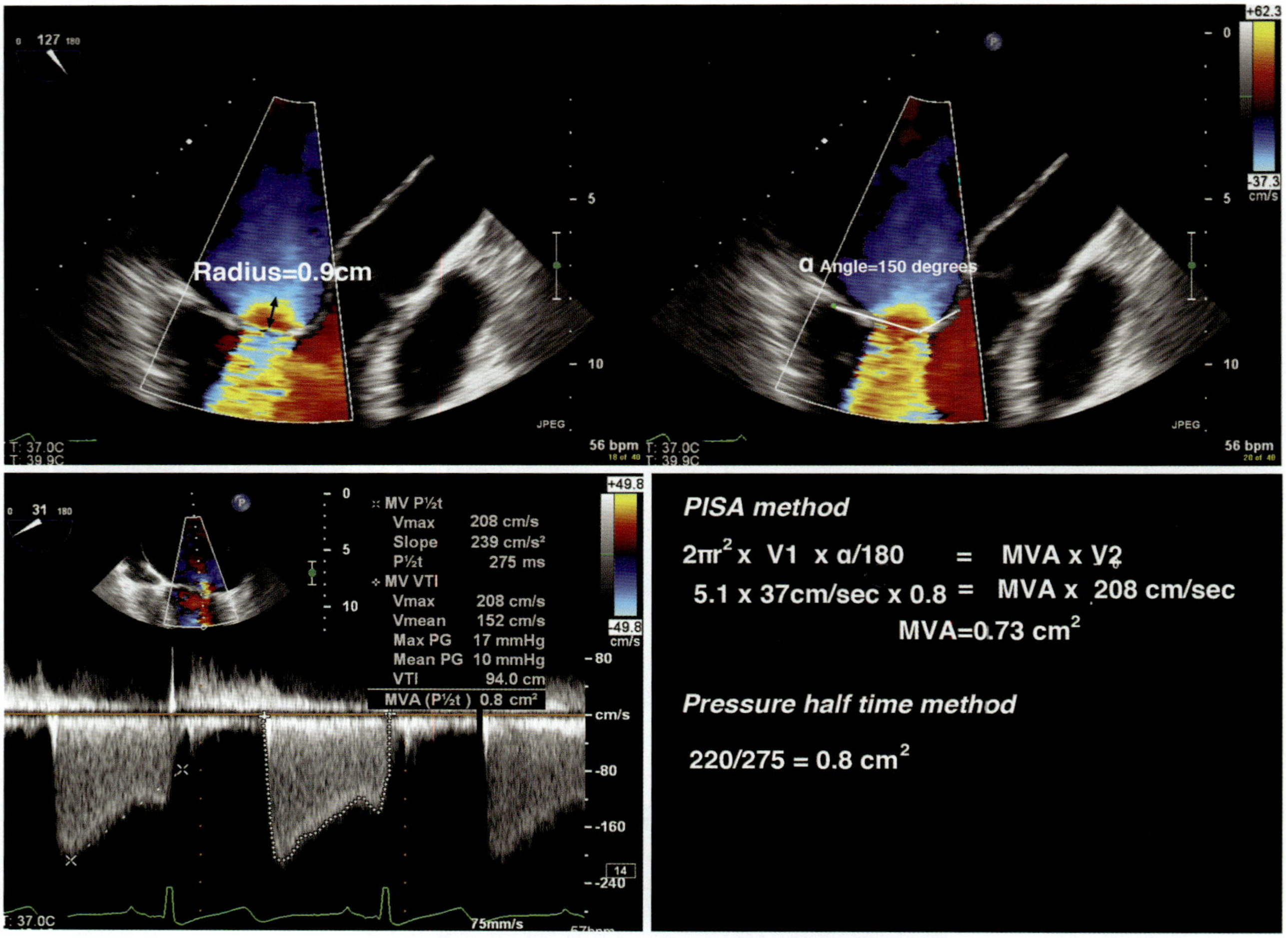

Fig 2.58 MVA calculation using PISA. Using a radius of 0.9 cm, a valve opening angle of 150 degrees, a peak velocity of mitral inflow of 210 cm/s, MVA is equal to 0.73 cm². By the pressure half-time method, MVA = 0.8 cm².

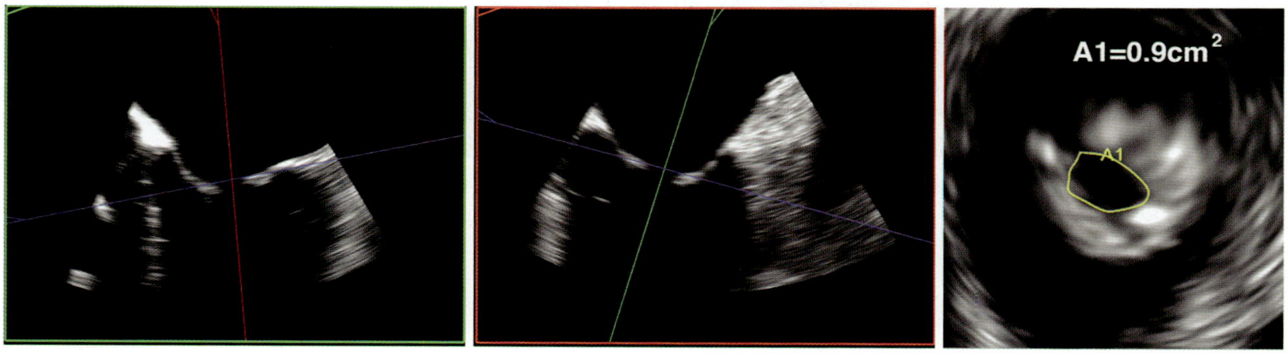

Fig 2.59 Using multiplanar reconstruction, planimetry of the mitral orifice yields a MVA of 0.9 cm².

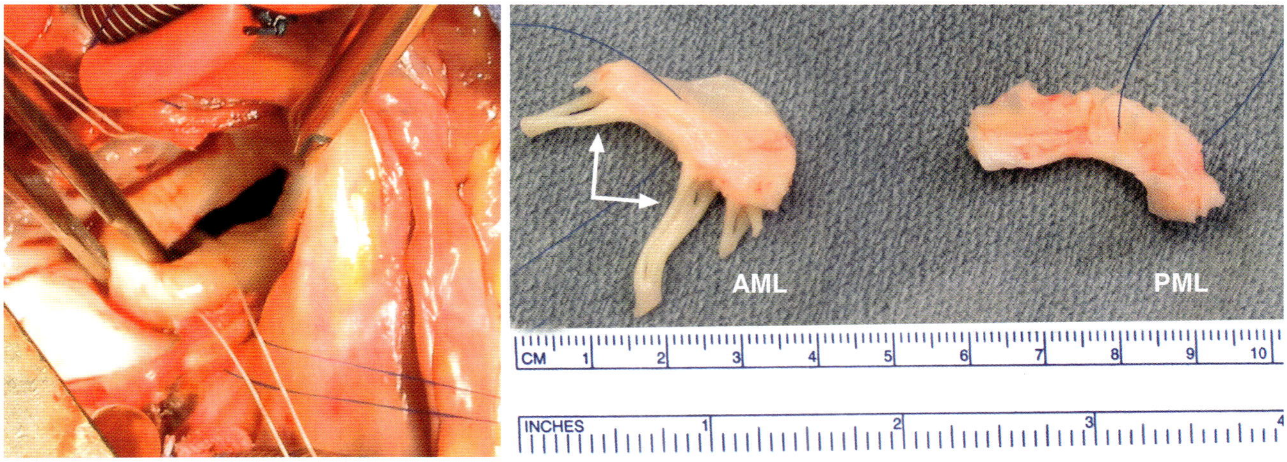

Fig 2.60 At surgery, the thickness of both leaflets of the mitral valve is seen. After explantation, the thickened chordae *(arrows)* of the AML are seen.

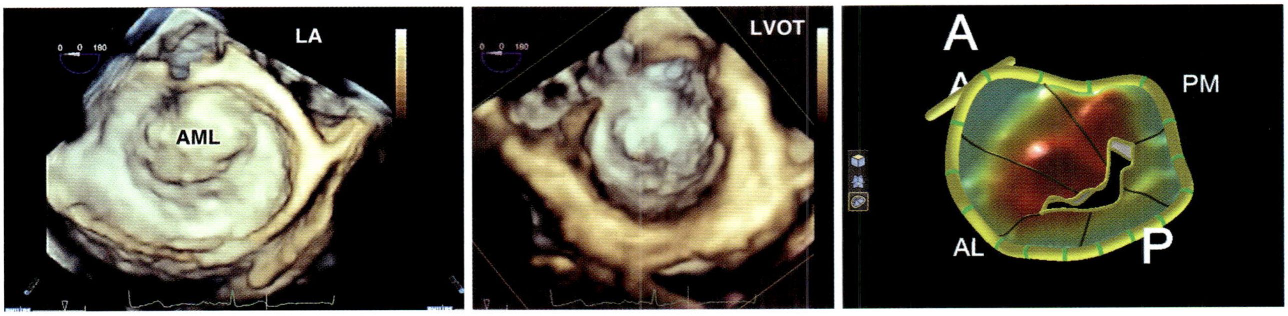

Fig 2.61 3D TEE from the LA perspective *(left)* and LVOT perspective *(middle)* show leaflet thickening and AML prolapse. This is also illustrated by the red areas seen with mitral valve quantification *(right)*.

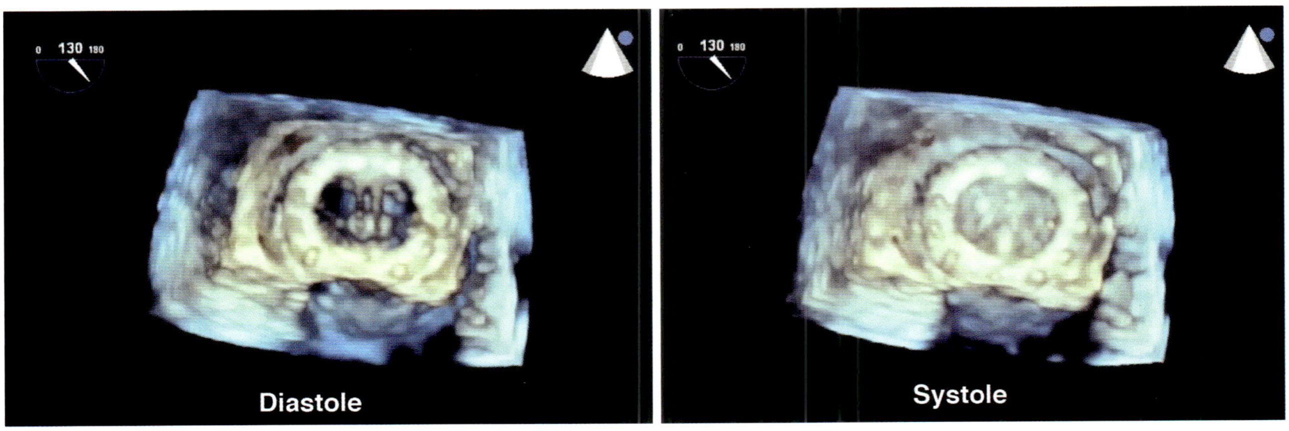

Fig 2.62 A bileaflet mechanical prosthesis was placed. Normal leaflet motion is seen in diastole *(left)* and systole *(right)*.

Comments (for Cases 2-7 and 2-8)

The hallmark of rheumatic valve disease is commissural fusion of the mitral leaflets with the typical echocardiographic appearance of diastolic doming of the leaflets. The standard approach to measurement of mitral valve area on transthoracic imaging is 2D planimetry of the orifice. However, this view can rarely be obtained on transesophageal imaging, as it is difficult to obtain a short-axis view at the leaflet tips. With 3D imaging, a full volume acquisition allows accurate measurement of the anatomic orifice area, and thus is recommended on both TTE and TEE imaging. The 3D volume allows the measurement plane to be located at the leaflet tips (where the narrowest area occurs) and to be aligned to avoid an oblique image plane.

The mitral pressures half-time method, based on the Doppler velocity curve, is useful in the OR because the mitral jet is directed away from the transducer and it is relatively easy to obtain a parallel intercept angle between the ultrasound beam and mitral stenosis jet.

The continuity equation valve area can be estimated from maximal flow rate and velocity as shown. Alternatively, stroke volume can be calculated by measurement of flow from the pulmonary artery. Then valve area in cm^2 is calculated by dividing stroke volume (cm^3) by the velocity time integral of the mitral stenosis CW Doppler signal (cm). These alternate methods for evaluation of mitral stenosis severity should show reasonable agreement. Agreement between anatomic and Doppler measures of mitral stenosis severity increases the confidence in the accuracy of these data. Most patients with rheumatic mitral valve disease also have coexisting mitral regurgitation. The severity of mitral regurgitation is assessed by standard approaches although pulmonary vein systolic flow may be abnormal when atrial fibrillation is present, even in the absence of significant mitral regurgitation. TEE evaluation of a patient with rheumatic mitral stenosis also should include a thorough examination for thrombus in the left atrial appendage or body of the left atrium.

Suggested Reading

1. Otto CM: Valvular stenosis. In Textbook of clinical echocardiography, ed 5, Philadelphia, 2012, Elsevier Saunders.
2. Marijon E, Mirabel M, Celermajer DS, et al: Rheumatic heart disease, Lancet 379(9819):953–964, 2012.
3. de Agustin JA, Mejia H, Viliani D, et al: Proximal flow convergence method by three-dimensional color Doppler echocardiography for mitral valve area assessment in rheumatic mitral stenosis, J Am Soc Echocardiogr 27(8):838–845, 2014.
4. Min SY, Song JM, Kim YJ, et al: Discrepancy between mitral valve areas measured by two-dimensional planimetry and three-dimensional transoesophageal echocardiography in patients with mitral stenosis, Heart 99(4):253–258, 2013.

Mitral Regurgitation Due to Coronary Artery Disease

CASE 2-9
Ischemic Mitral Regurgitation

This 83-year-old man with severe aortic stenosis and a left ventricular ejection of 7% was also found to have severe mitral regurgitation. Coronary angiography showed a 60% stenosis of the left anterior descending coronary artery and an 80% stenosis of a large first obtuse marginal branch of the circumflex coronary artery. Mitral leaflet anatomy was normal but there was thinning and akinesis of the posterior–lateral left ventricular wall, suggesting that the etiology of mitral regurgitation was ischemic. After aggressive medical management and placement of an intraaortic balloon pump, he was referred for aortic valve replacement, coronary bypass grafting, and mitral valve repair.

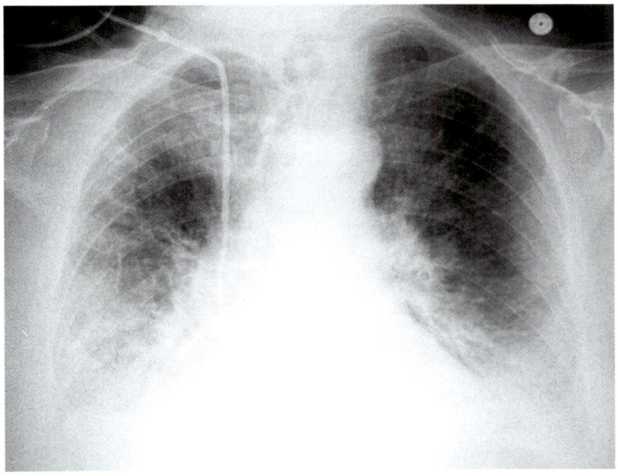

Fig 2.63 The portable PA chest radiograph shows cardiomegaly with increased pulmonary vascularity and pulmonary edema.

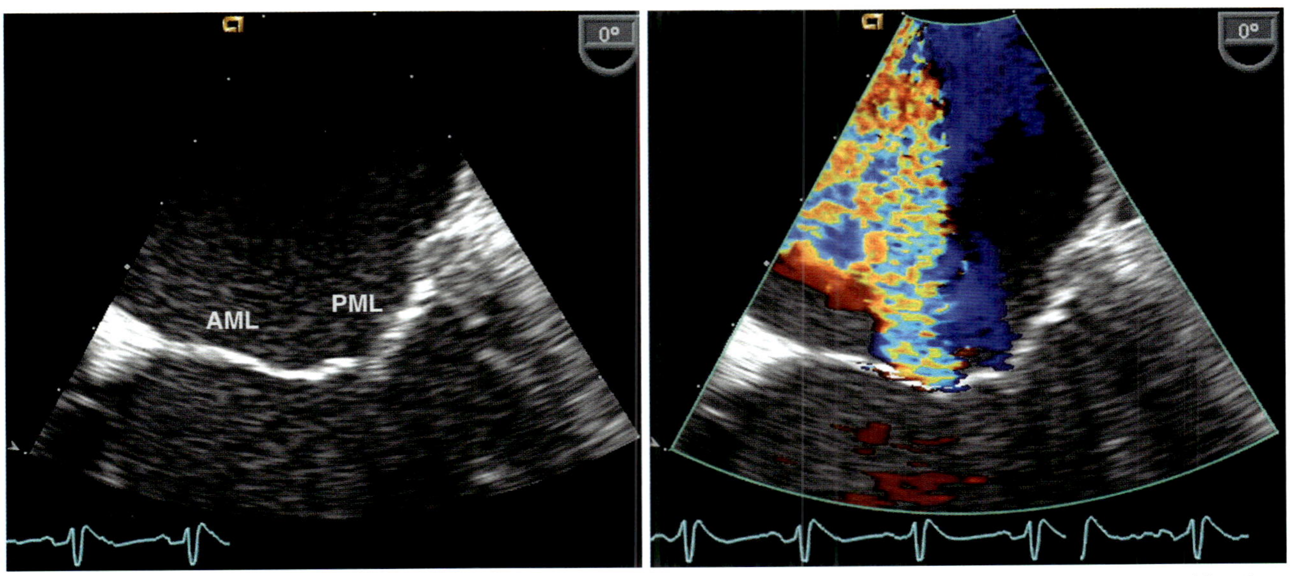

Fig 2.64 In a four-chamber TEE view, the mitral leaflets and chords appear anatomically normal but the annulus is dilated and during systole the anterior leaflet appears to "slide" behind the posterior leaflet caused by tethering (or inadequate closure) of the posterior leaflet. Color Doppler demonstrates a central jet of regurgitation.

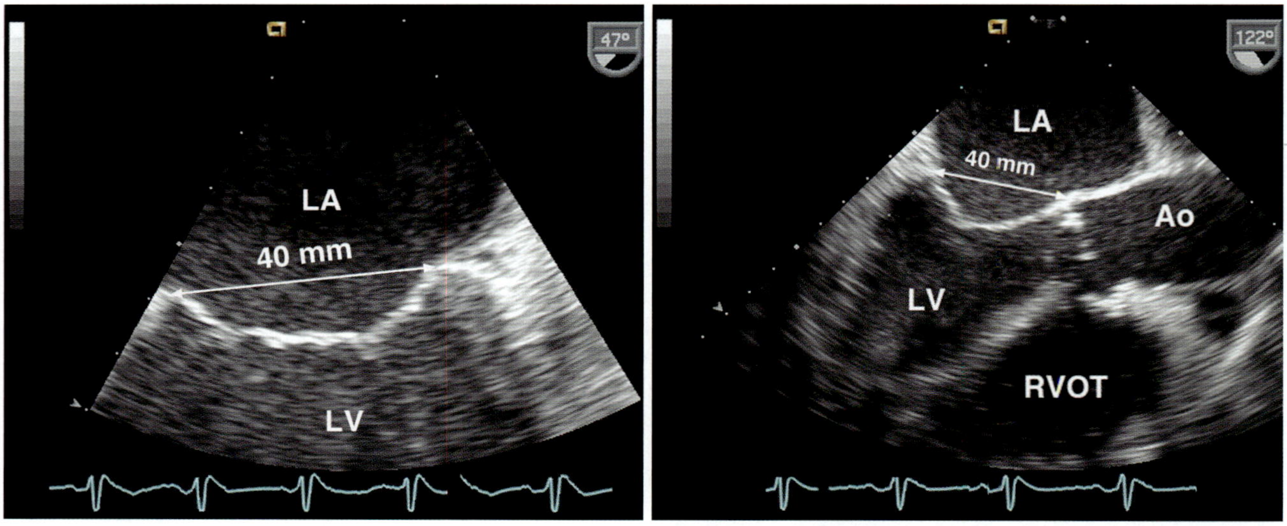

Fig 2.65 Because an annular ring is often used in the surgical approach to ischemic mitral regurgitation, it is helpful to obtain an annulus dimension for surgical planning. Typically, this measurement is made in midsystole in two views: *(1)* The commissural view, between the junctions of the left atrium and mitral annulus *(left)*; and *(2)* The midesophageal long-axis view between the junction of the posterior annulus and left atrium, and the junction of the left atrium and aortic root *(right)*. AML = anterior mitral leaflet, PML = posterior mitral leaflet, LA = left atrium.

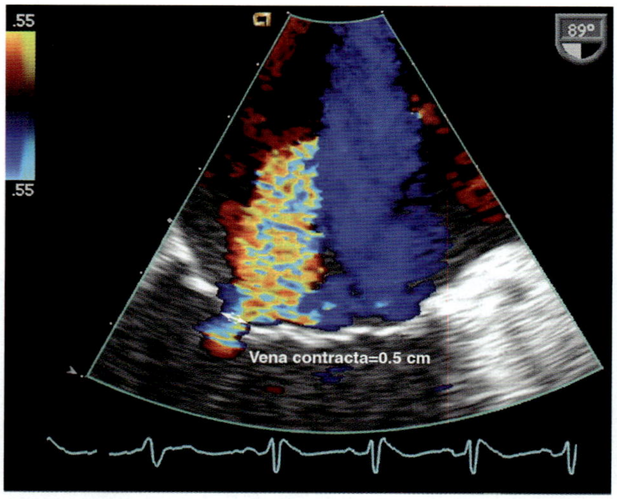

Fig 2.66 Quantitation of mitral regurgitant severity begins with measurement of vena contracta width. The vena contracta is measured at the narrowest jet width with a clearly defined "waist" between the proximal flow acceleration and distal jet expansion. The width of 0.5 cm is consistent with moderate mitral regurgitation and indicates that further quantitation is needed.

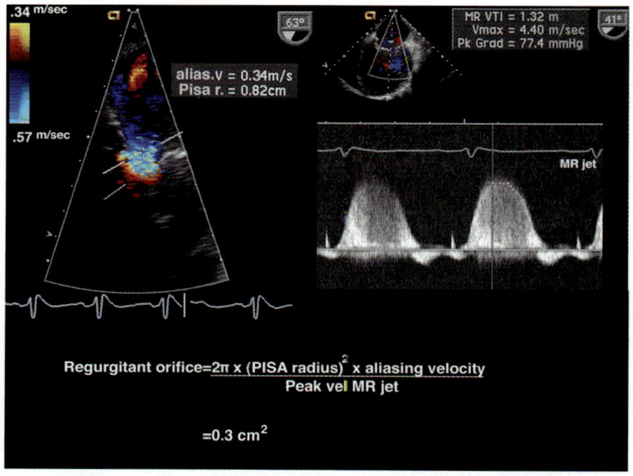

Fig 2.67 Using the PISA approach for quantitation of regurgitant severity, a PISA radius of 0.8 cm is measured at an aliasing velocity of 0.34 m/s. Multiplying the surface area of a hemisphere with a radius of 0.8 cm times the aliasing velocity yields a maximum regurgitant flow rate of 137mL/s. Maximum regurgitant orifice area (ROA) is then determined by dividing by the CW Doppler MR jet velocity. An ROA of 0.3 cm^2 is consistent with moderate mitral regurgitation. Regurgitant volume can then be calculated either from the difference between stroke volume across the mitral versus aortic valve or by multiplying the velocity time integral (VTI) by the ROA, as shown in Fig 2.68.

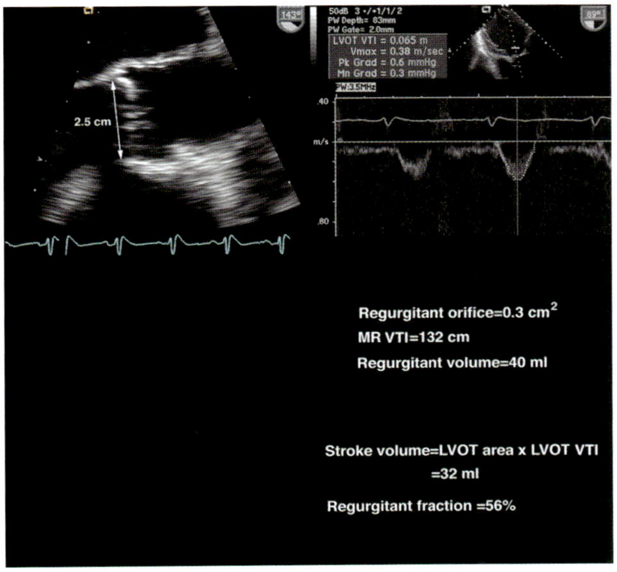

Fig 2.68 The regurgitant fraction is the ratio of regurgitant stroke volume to total stroke volume (RSV + antegrade flow in the LVOT). Both the regurgitant volume of 40 mL and the regurgitant fraction of 56% are consistent with moderate mitral regurgitation. It is likely that regurgitation is more severe when the patient is not under general anesthesia.

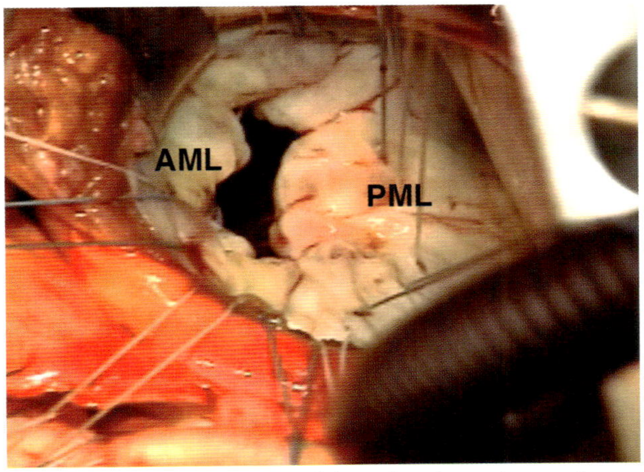

Fig 2.69 Surgical inspection of the valve shows incomplete valve closure with relatively normal valve leaflets. Sutures have been placed in the mitral annulus for securing the annuloplasty ring. AML = anterior mitral leaflet, PML = posterior mitral leaflet.

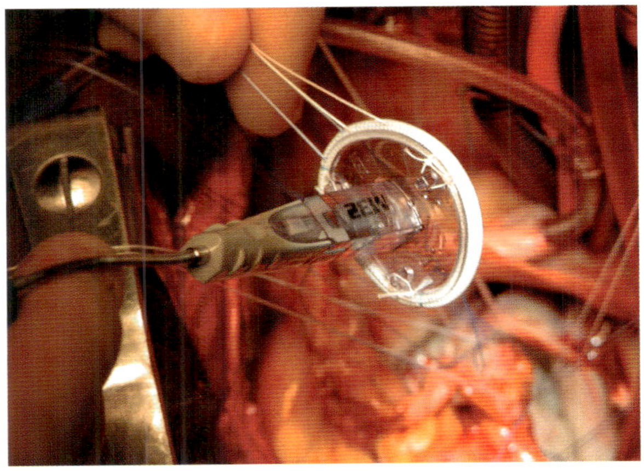

Fig 2.70 The annuloplasty ring being prepared for placement.

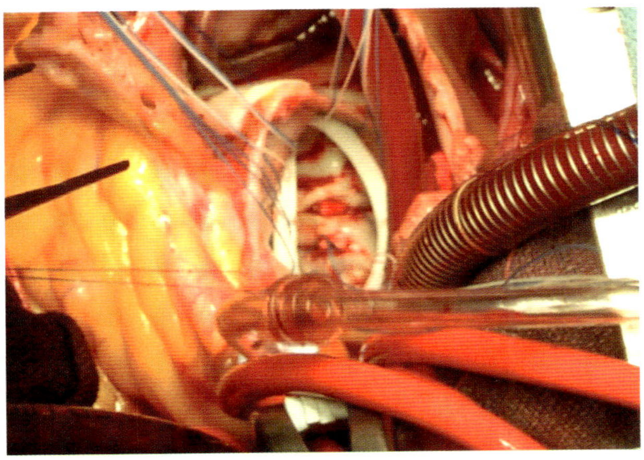

Fig 2.71 The annuloplasty ring in position.

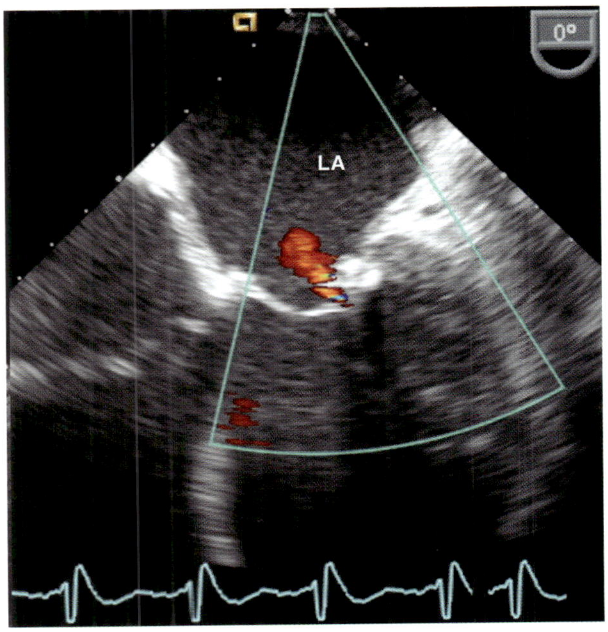

Fig 2.72 Immediate postoperative images show the annuloplasty ring in position and the normal coaptation of the mitral leaflets in systole. There was trace mitral regurgitation on color Doppler examination.

Comments

Ischemic mitral regurgitation may be caused by several different mechanisms. Wall motion abnormalities localized to the regions underlying the papillary muscles result in mitral regurgitation at rest when the myocardium is infarcted, or only with stress, when there is intermittent ischemia. In patients with left ventricular dilation and systolic dysfunction resulting from coronary artery disease, regurgitation has a mechanism similar to that seen in patients with dilated cardiomyopathy. The most catastrophic form of ischemic mitral regurgitation is papillary muscle rupture.

With ischemic mitral regurgitation caused by a regional wall motion abnormality, "tethering" of the posterior leaflet is typical, as seen in this case. The posterior leaflet appears relatively immobile and fails to move completely toward the mitral annulus in systole, so that the normal motion of the anterior leaflet results in the appearance that it is "sliding" behind the coaptation point with the posterior leaflet. Revascularization alone has variable effects on the severity of ischemic mitral regurgitation, so that many surgeons will place an annuloplasty ring to reduce the size of the posterior aspect of the annulus, resulting in more complete leaflet coaptation in systole.

Recent studies indicate that valve repair and valve replacement for moderate ischemic MR at the time of coronary artery bypass grafting are associated with similar clinical outcomes.

Suggested Reading

1. Grayburn PA, Carabello B, Hung J, et al: Defining "severe" secondary mitral regurgitation: Emphasizing an integrated approach, J Am Coll Cardiol 64(25):2792–2801, 2014.
2. Acker MA, Parides MK, Perrault LP, et al: Mitral-valve repair versus replacement for severe ischemic mitral regurgitation, N Engl J Med 370:23–32, 2014.
3. Smith PK, Puskas JD, Ascheim DD, et al: Surgical treatment of moderate ischemic mitral regurgitation, N Engl J Med 371(23): 2178–2188, 2014.
4. Kron IL, Hung J, Overbey JR, et al: CTSN Investigators. Predicting recurrent mitral regurgitation after mitral valve repair for severe ischemic mitral regurgitation, J Thorac Cardiovasc Surg 149(3):752–761, e1, 2015.

CASE 2-10
Papillary Muscle Rupture

This 64-year-old man presented with chest pain and an abnormal ECG. His past medical history was remarkable for hypertension, hypercholesterolemia, and smoking. Coronary angiography showed diffuse disease in the left anterior descending artery, a chronically occluded right coronary artery, and a 95% stenosis in the first obtuse marginal branch, which was considered to be the "culprit" lesion. The left ventricular angiogram showed an ejection fraction of 45% with akinesis of the inferior and lateral walls.

He underwent percutaneous angioplasty of the obtuse marginal vessel with only a small residual stenosis. However, because of progressive hypotension and pulmonary congestion, an intraaortic balloon pump was inserted and an echocardiogram was requested.

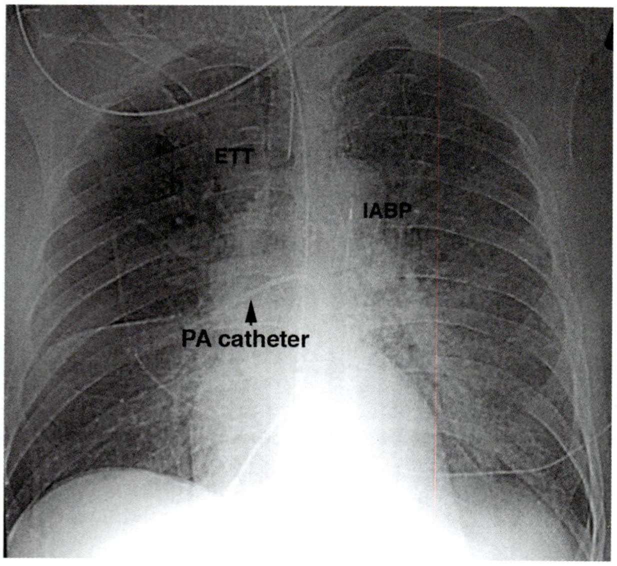

Fig 2.73 The portable bedside chest radiograph shows a normal size heart with mild pulmonary congestion. The endotracheal tube (ETT), intraaortic balloon pump (IABP), and pulmonary artery (PA) catheter are seen.

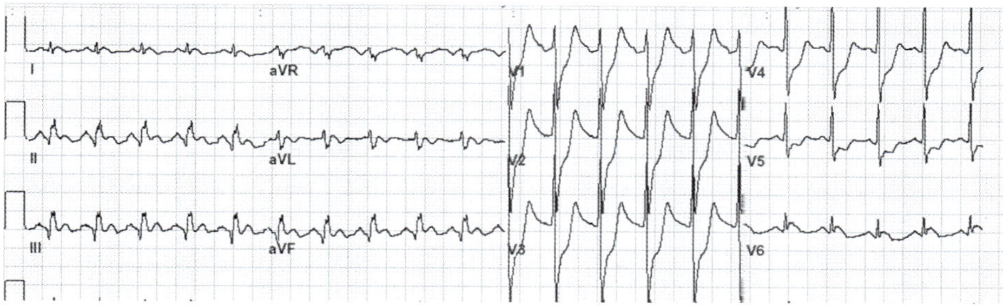

Fig 2.74 The ECG shows inferior Q waves and marked ST depression in the anterior and lateral leads.

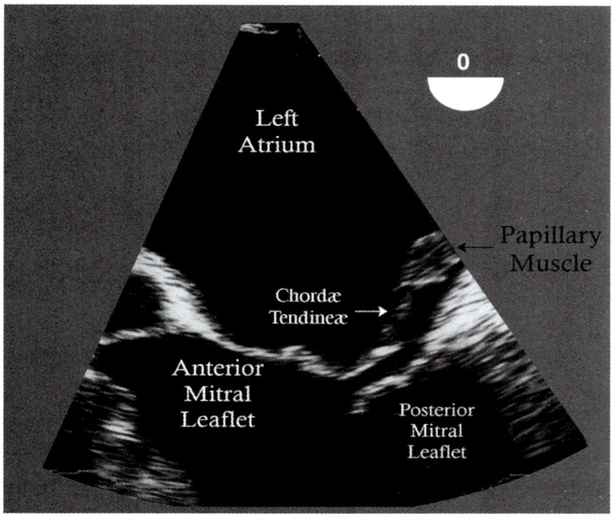

Fig 2.75 The four-chamber view shows a ruptured papillary muscle attached to the anterior leaflet, with the head of the papillary muscle prolapsing into the left atrium in systole, with corresponding severe mitral regurgitation.

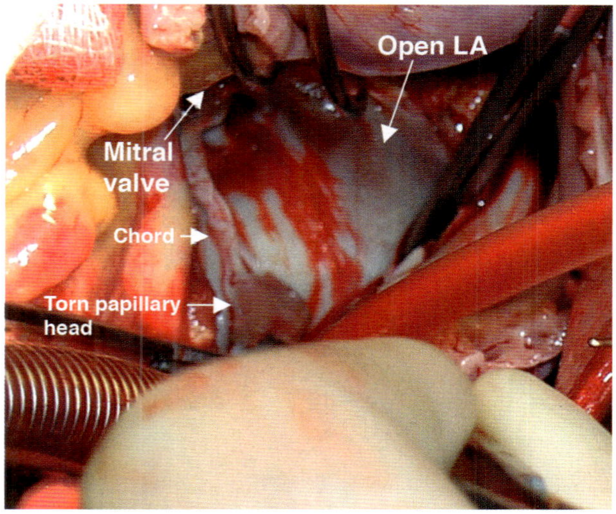

Fig 2.76 Operative findings showed papillary muscle rupture with disruption of chordal attachments to the anterior mitral leaflet resulting in a partial flail leaflet. The anatomy was not amenable to repair so that mitral valve replacement was performed.

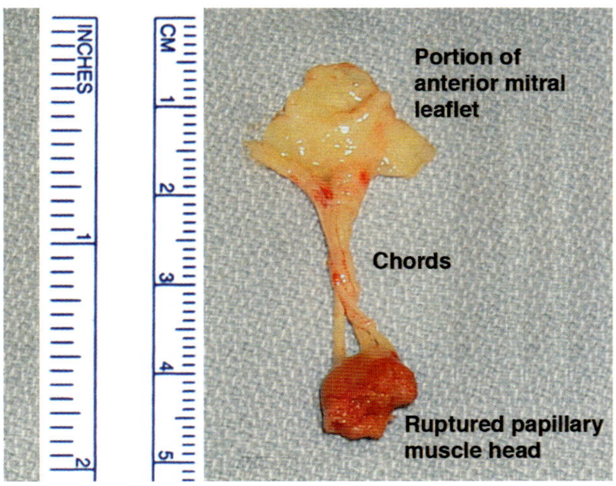

Fig 2.77 The excised leaflet and papillary muscle head.

CASE 2-11
Another Case of Papillary Muscle Rupture

This 67-year-old male, with a history of hypertension treated with lisinopril, was seen 2 days before admission at an outside hospital with cough and green sputum. He was sent home with a diagnosis of acute bronchitis. The next day, he developed chest burning which gradually intensified over the next 24 hours, and was accompanied by worsening shortness of breath at rest. On admission to hospital, an acute coronary syndrome was suspected. He underwent left heart catheterization that showed diffuse LAD disease, 100% RCA, and 100% OM occlusions, and TTE revealed severe MR with suspicion for a papillary muscle rupture. A chest x-ray showed pulmonary edema. His respiratory symptoms worsened, and arrangements were made to transfer to our hospital, after endotracheal intubation and intraaortic balloon pump placement. At surgery, the anterior papillary muscle was partially ruptured giving rise to a flail posterior leaflet.

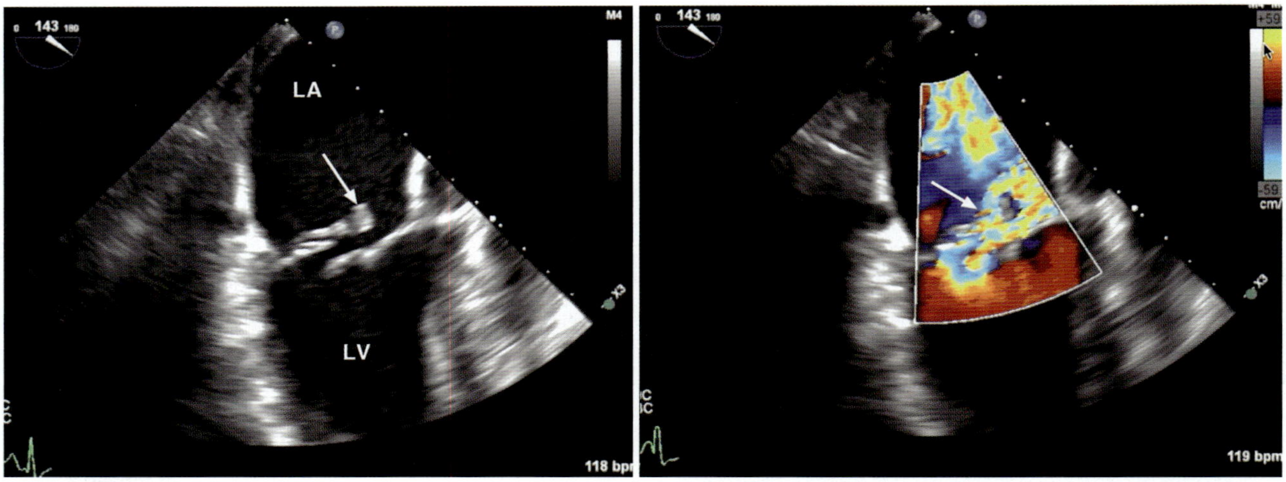

Fig 2.78 A midesophageal long-axis view shows what appears to be a flail posterior mitral leaflet. The thickness at the leaflet is suspicious for a ruptured papillary muscle. Color Doppler shows an anteriorly directed jet of MR *(arrow)*, which further suggests that the posterior leaflet is the culprit.

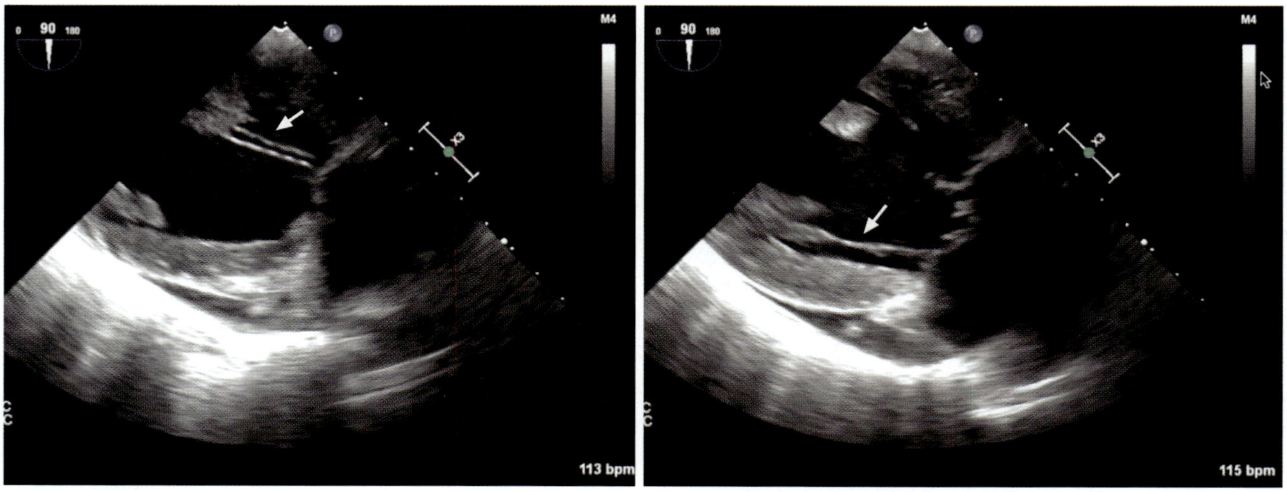

Fig 2.79 These transgastric long-axis views of the LV are both obtained at 90 degrees, the only difference between them being slight rotation of the probe. These images underscore the difficulty that sometimes arises in deciding which papillary muscle is necrotic, as the tears are often subtotal. In the left frame chordae are seen from the postero-medial muscle and the anterior muscle seems incomplete; the opposite holds for the right frame.

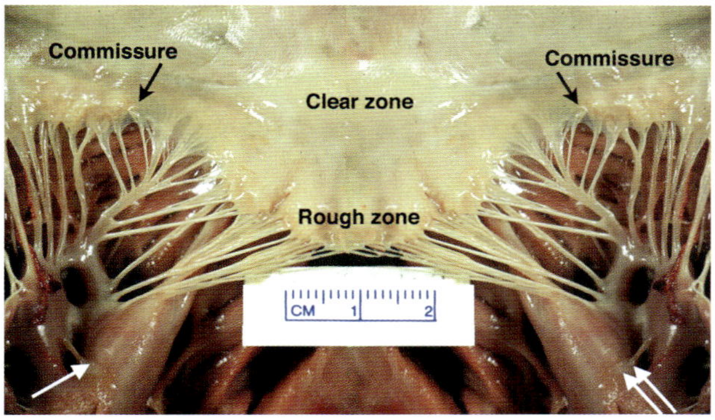

Fig 2.80 In this pathologic specimen, the posterior leaflet has been sectioned at its midpoint. The commissures, and the clear and rough zones of the anterior mitral leaflet are seen. It is noted that the anterolateral *(single arrow)* and the posteromedial *(double arrow)* papillary muscle both give chords to both leaflets, which explains why rupture of a papillary muscle may lead to prolapse of either of the mitral leaflets. (Image courtesy of Dr. Dennis Reichenbach.)

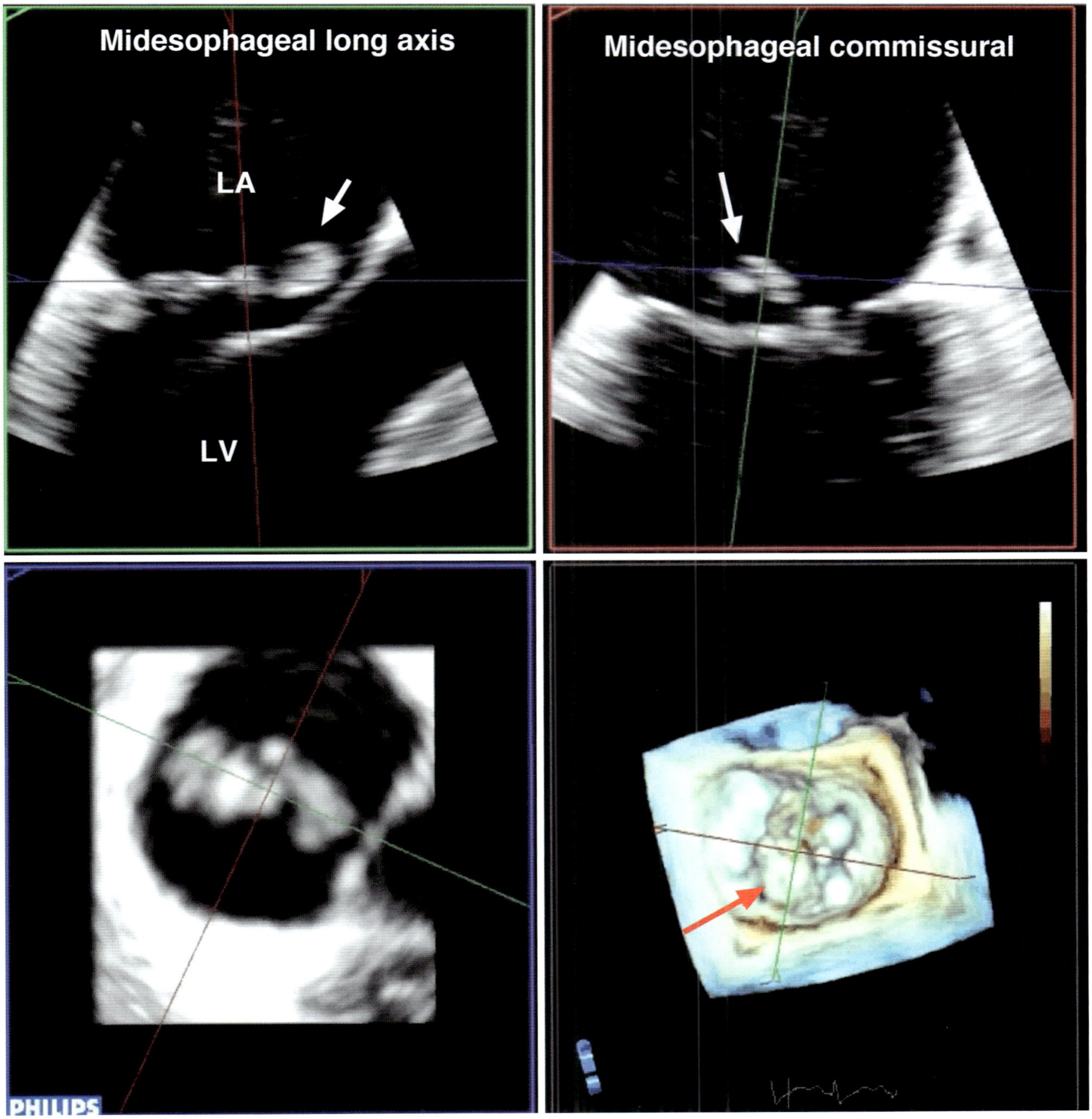

Fig 2.81 Multiplanar reconstruction of the mitral valve. In the bottom right frame, a 3D TEE image of the mitral valve is seen from the LA perspective, with the red arrow indicative of the prolapsing segment. The green plane sections the valve in antero-posterior direction, and the red plane sections the valve in the commissural plane. The white arrows indicate the putative portion of the ruptured papillary muscle.

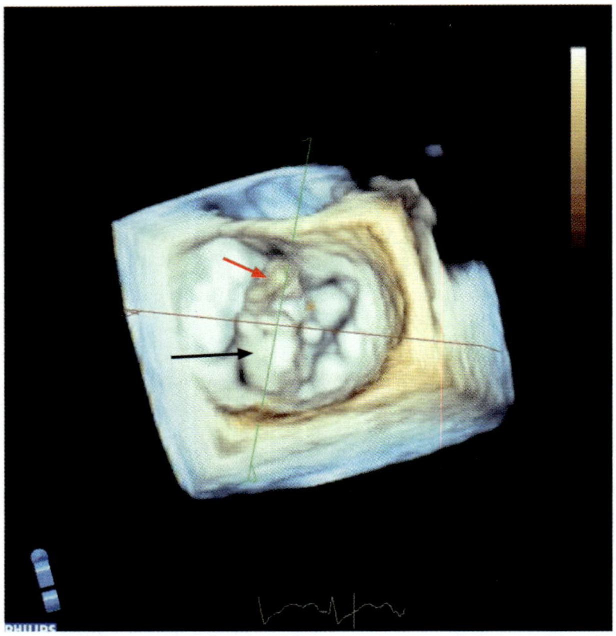

Fig 2.82 3D TEE image of the mitral valve seen from the LA perspective. The black arrow indicates what is likely the portion of the posterior leaflet that is subtended by the torn papillary muscle, and the red arrow indicates what is likely the head of the torn papillary muscle.

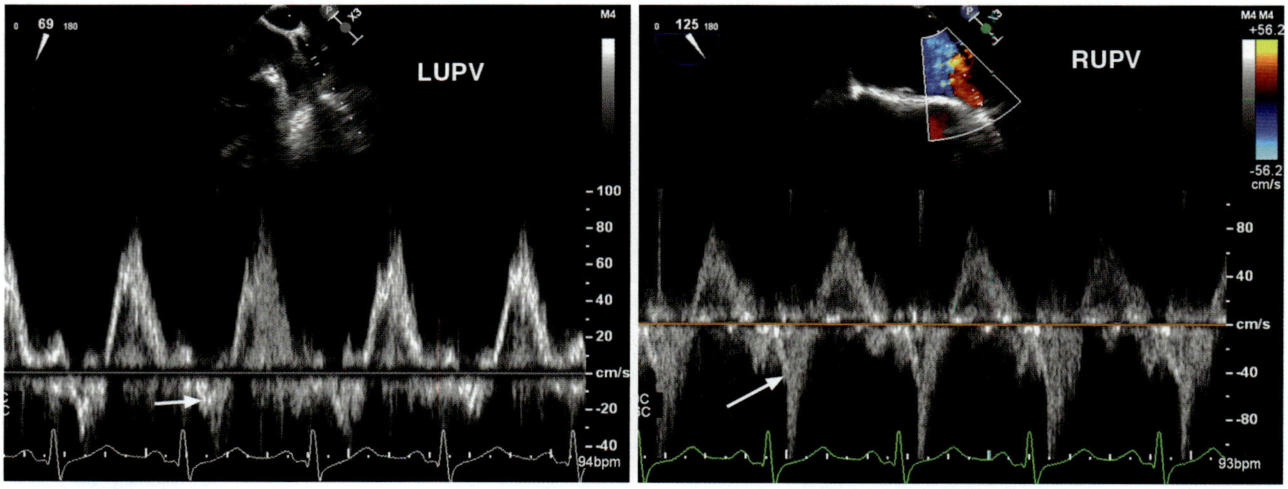

Fig 2.83 There is systolic reversal *(arrows)* in both left upper (LUPV) and right upper (RUPV) pulmonary veins.

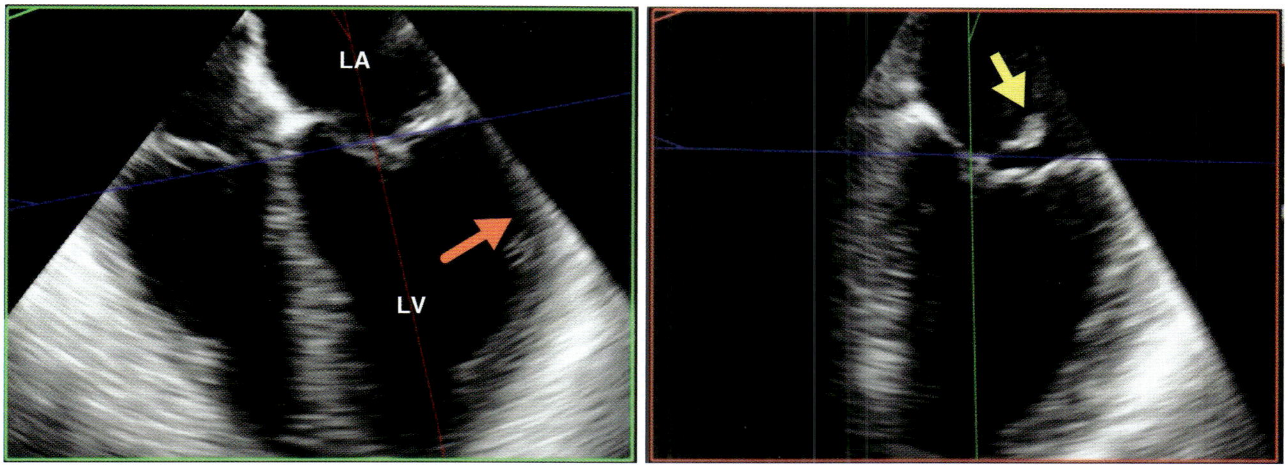

Fig 2.84 On the left, a midesophageal four-chamber view is seen with the red arrow indicating the lateral wall. In real time, the lateral wall appears hypokinetic. On the right, the yellow arrow indicates the flail segment. See comments (for Cases 2-10 and 2-11).

Comments (for Cases 2-10 and 2-11)

Papillary muscle rupture is a rare (<0.1%) but often fatal (95% mortality within 2 weeks) complication of acute myocardial infarction. The onset of papillary muscle rupture is usually several days after the infarction and typically occurs with small, localized transmural myocardial damage, rather than with a large infarction. The patient presents with heart failure symptoms ranging from acute pulmonary edema to frank cardiogenic shock, depending on how much of the papillary muscle has ruptured, and consequent mitral regurgitant severity.

Although echocardiography is the optimal approach to diagnosis, care is needed in the examination as overall left ventricular systolic function may appear relatively normal and the rupture of papillary muscle is often not visualized on transthoracic examination. A complete TEE examination is usually diagnostic with demonstration of the flail leaflet, with the detached papillary muscle head prolapsing into the left atrium in systole.

Suggested Reading

1. Foster E, Gerber I: Echocardiography in the coronary care unit: Management of acute myocardial infarction, detection of complications and prognostic implications. In Otto CM, editor: The practice of clinical echocardiography, ed 5, Philadelphia, 2016, Elsevier, Chapter 12.
2. Kutty RS, Jones N, Moorjani N: Mechanical complications of acute myocardial infarction, Cardiol Clin 31(4):519–531, vii–viii, 2013.
3. Flueckiger PB, Cheng AC, Patton JM, et al: Partial papillary muscle rupture: A cause of acute mitral regurgitation, Am J Med Sci 345:478–481, 2013.
4. Jayawardena S, Renteria, Burzyantseva O, et al: Anterolateral papillary muscle rupture caused by myocardial infarction: A case report, Cases J 1:172–175, 2008.
5. Fradley MG, Picard MH: Rupture of the posteromedial papillary muscle leading to partial flail of the anterior mitral leaflet, Circulation 123:1044–1045, 2011.

Mitral Regurgitation Secondary to Dilated Cardiomyopathy

CASE 2-12
Mitral Regurgitation Associated with Dilated Cardiomyopathy

This 35-year-old woman with heart failure caused by dilated cardiomyopathy was referred for surgical intervention for severe mitral regurgitation. Her TTE showed mild left ventricular dilation, with an end-diastolic dimension of 59 mm, but with moderate global hypokinesis, with an end-systolic dimension of 52 mm and an ejection fraction of 44%. The left atrium was severely dilated at 58 mm and pulmonary systolic pressure was mildly elevated at 35 mm Hg. Severe mitral regurgitation was present, with a vena contracta width of 10 mm and a regurgitant fraction of 78%.

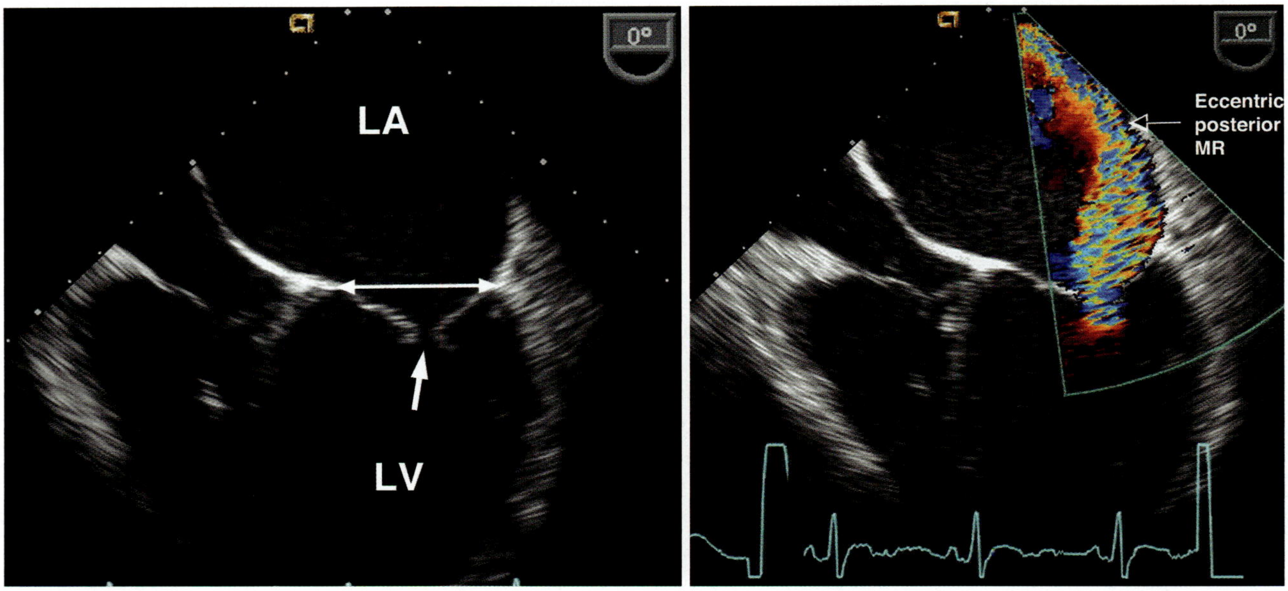

Fig 2.85 In a four-chamber view, the severely dilated left atrium and left ventricle are seen. The mitral annulus is dilated at 4.2 cm. During systole, the mitral leaflets fail to coapt *(left, arrow)*. Color Doppler shows a large eccentric posteriorly directed mitral regurgitant (MR) jet in the left atrium *(right)*.

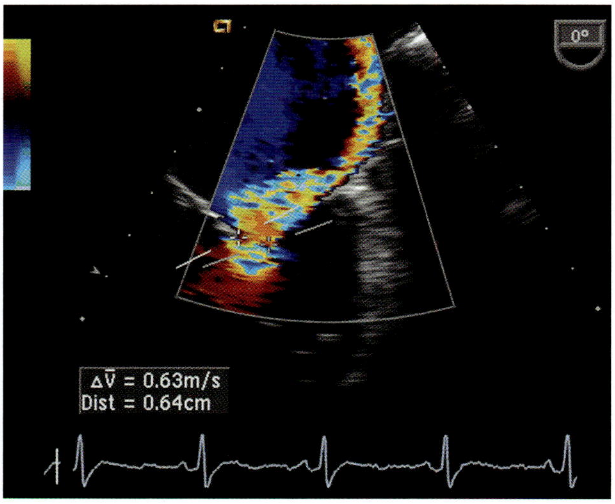

Fig 2.86 The vena contracta is optimized by decreasing the interrogation depth and enlarging the area of interest to minimize error in measurement. The vena contracta is seen as the narrow waist between the PISA and the expansion of the jet in the atrium. This vena contracta width of 0.6 cm is consistent with moderate regurgitation.

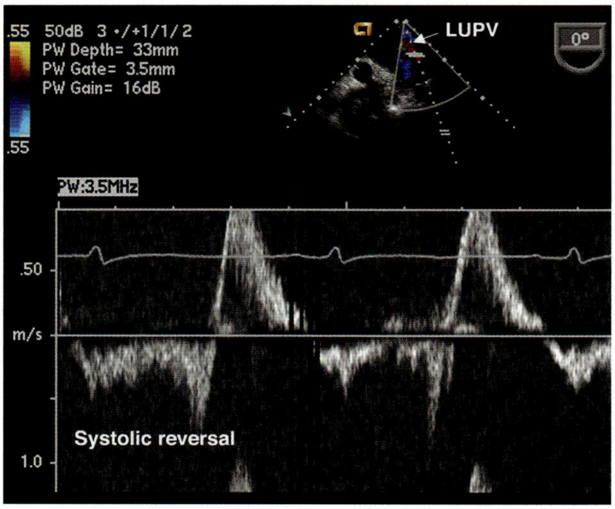

Fig 2.87 Pulsed Doppler evaluation of pulmonary vein flow provides an additional approach to evaluation of regurgitant severity. This image shows holosystolic flow reversal in the left upper pulmonary vein (LUPV) as expected, given the direction of the regurgitant jet.

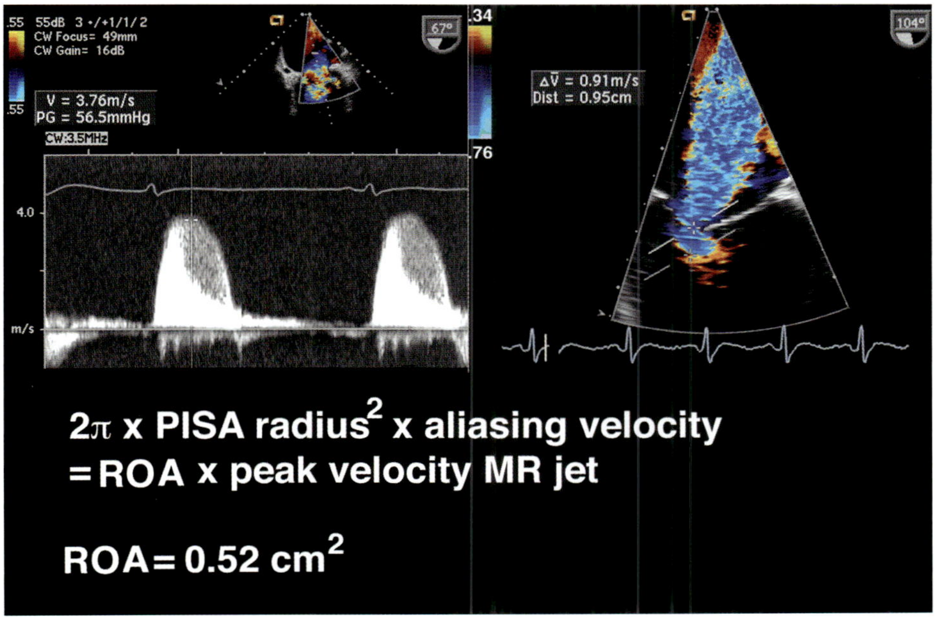

Fig 2.88 The PISA is visualized by decreasing depth, enlarging the image and adjusting the Nyquist limit to optimize the image. The maximum regurgitant flow rate (cm^3/s) is calculated by multiplying the PISA ($2\pi(0.95\ cm)^2$) by the aliasing velocity (34 cm/s). Maximal regurgitant orifice area (ROA) is then estimated by dividing by the peak regurgitant jet velocity (376 cm/s). The ROA of 0.5 cm^2 is consistent with severe regurgitation.

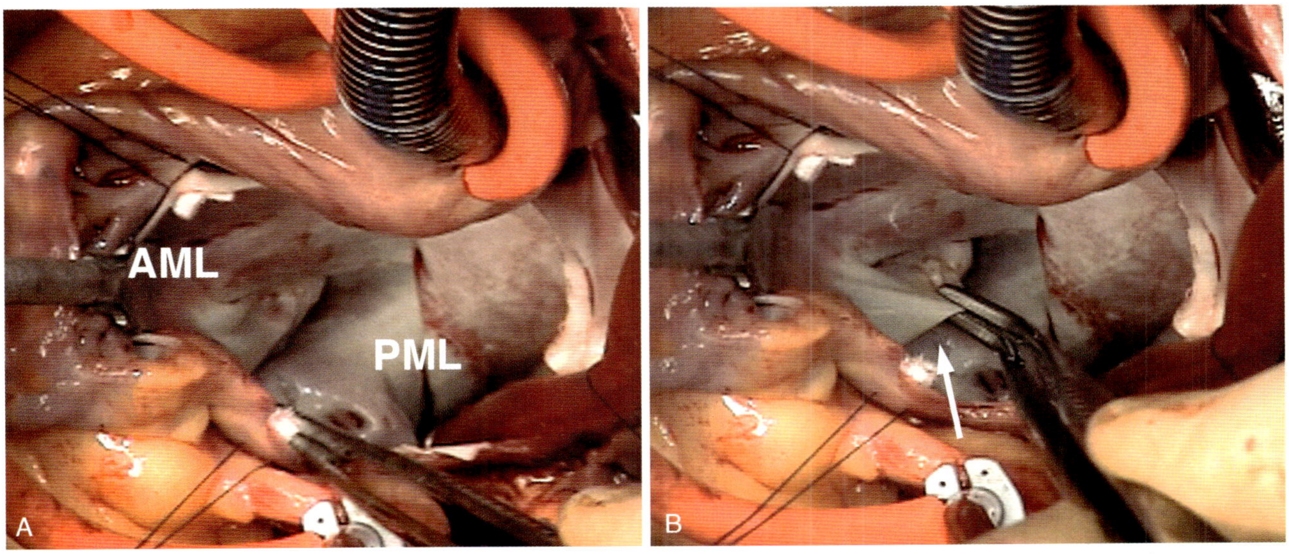

Fig 2.89 At surgery, the mitral annulus was enlarged with normal mitral leaflets and chordae (**A**). The thinness of the anterior leaflet *(arrow)* is demonstrated during retraction (**B**).

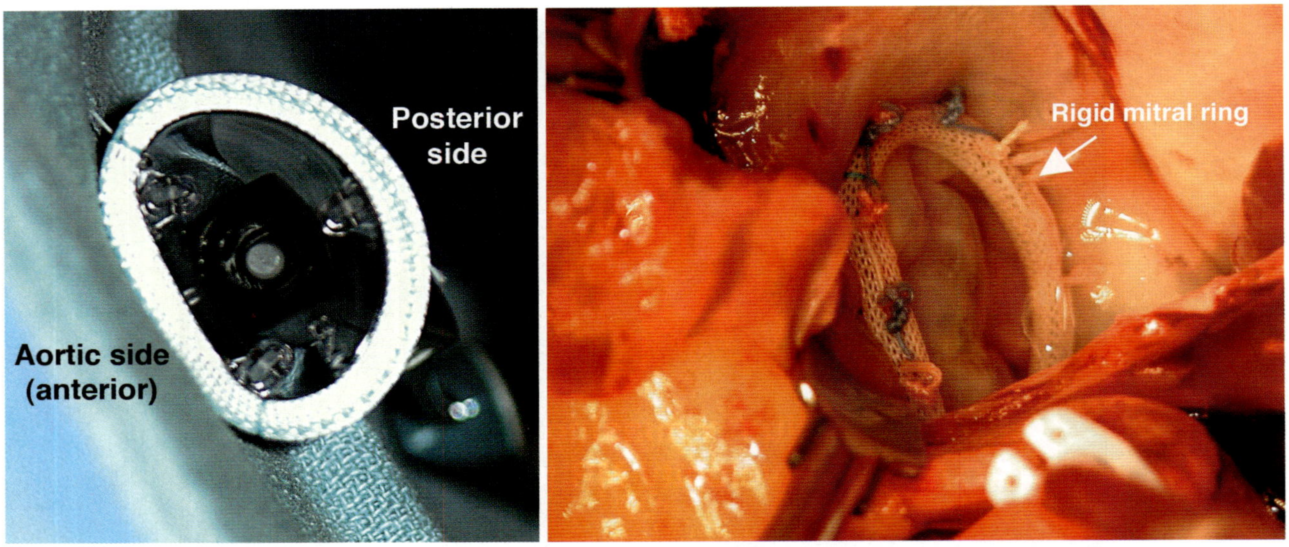

Fig 2.90 An annuloplasty was performed, with this image showing the positioning of the mitral annuloplasty ring *(right)*. On the left, the ring is shown before implantation.

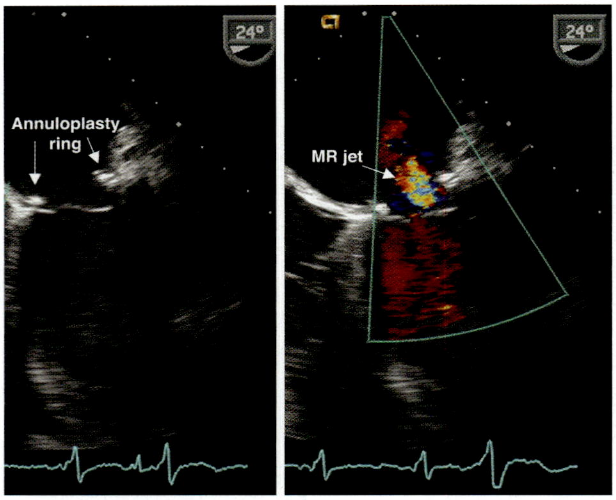

Fig 2.91 Postannuloplasty images show the ring on the left atrial side of the valve at the junction of the leaflets with the annulus *(left)*, with color Doppler showing only mild residual regurgitation.

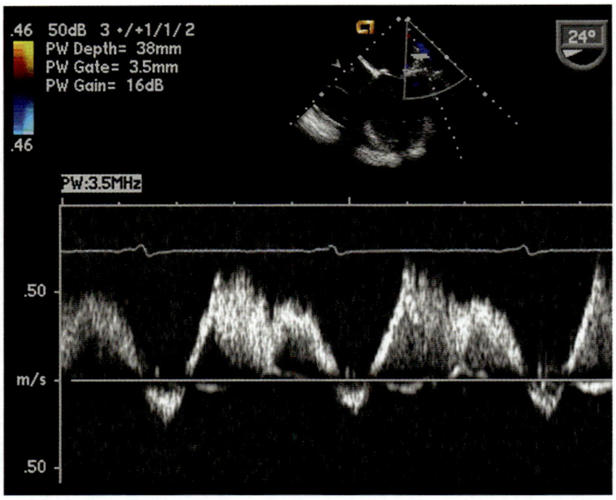

Fig 2.92 Post annuloplasty, the left upper pulmonary vein flow pattern now shows normal antegrade flow in systole (compare with Fig 2.87).

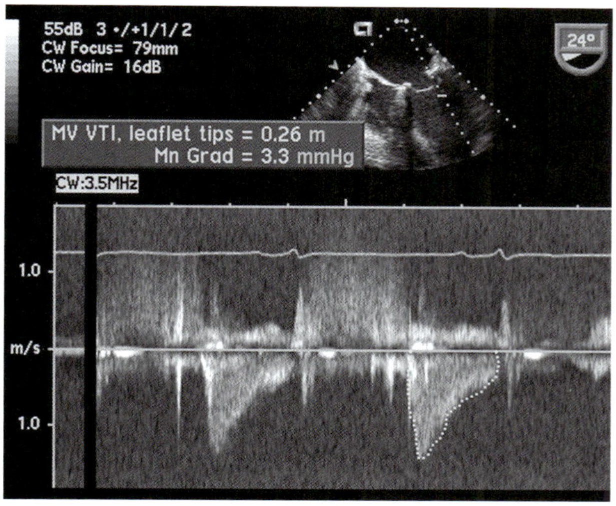

Fig 2.93 The antegrade velocity across the mitral valve is rechecked after the procedure to ensure that there is no significant functional stenosis by measurement of the mean gradient (now 3 mm Hg) and visual examination of the deceleration slope (note the steep slope on the first beat).

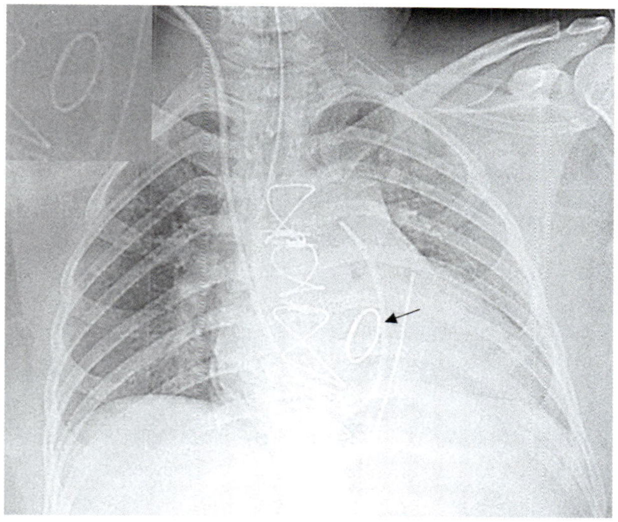

Fig 2.94 The postoperative chest radiography shows the sternotomy wires, the pulmonary artery catheter, the endotracheal tube, a chest tube, and the semicircular annuloplasty ring *(arrow)*, also seen in the inset.

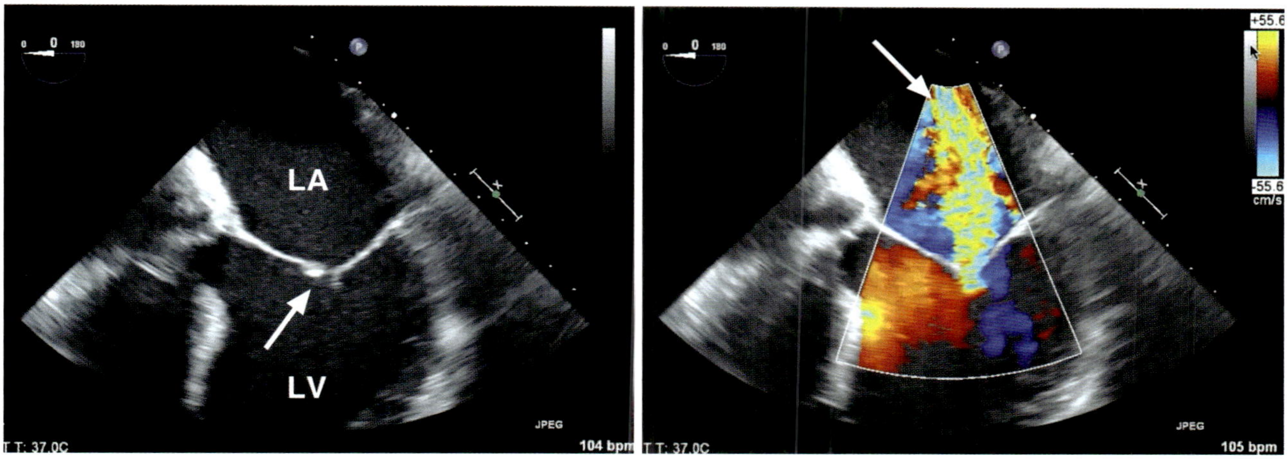

Fig 2.95 In a patient with a similar case history, four-chamber midesophageal imaging shows left atrial and left ventricular enlargement, incomplete mitral systolic coaptation, and a central jet of mitral regurgitation.

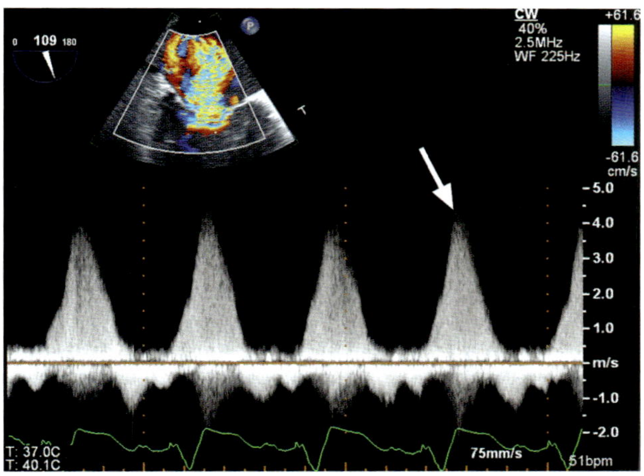

Fig 2.96 Continuous wave Doppler of the MR jet is dense, peaks early in systole, and is triangular shaped, all indicative of severe MR.

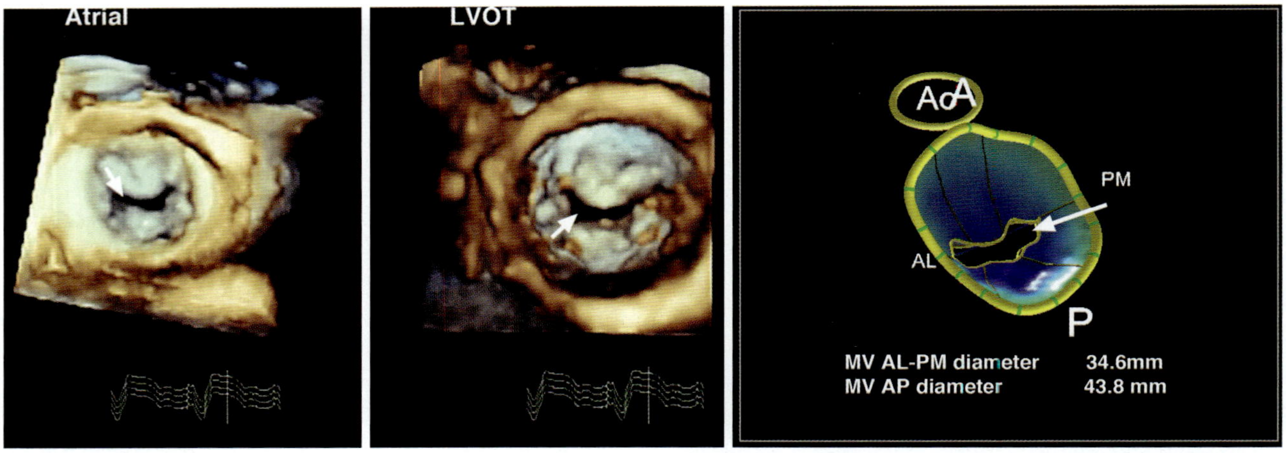

Fig 2.97 3D TEE in the left and central panels show incomplete mitral systolic coaptation *(white arrow)*. Mitral valve quantification in the right frame again shows the regurgitant defect and a dilated mitral annulus. A = anterior, P = posterior, AL = antero-lateral, PM = postero-medial.

Comments

Mitral regurgitation often accompanies dilated cardiomyopathy and contributes to heart failure symptoms. The mechanisms of secondary mitral regurgitation remain controversial with proposed alterations in the 3D anatomy of the mitral apparatus, including an altered angle between the papillary muscles and mitral annulus, altered left ventricular curvature and strain patterns, and mitral annular dilation; the MR jet may either be central or directed towards the restricted leaflet, depending on the predominant mechanism. Mitral regurgitation resulting from dilated cardiomyopathy often responds to medical therapy for the underlying left ventricular systolic dysfunction. However, some patients with refractory regurgitation are referred for surgical intervention. Because the surgical approach usually includes placement of a mitral annuloplasty ring, measurement of mitral annular dimensions is helpful; most often measurements are made in the midesophageal bicommissural and long-axis planes. It is important to identify the point where the anterior mitral leaflet joins the annulus (or aortic root) for each leaflet for an accurate measurement.

Suggested Reading

1. Hung J: Ischemic (functional) mitral regurgitation, Cardiol Clin 31:231–236, 2013.
2. Hung J, Capoulade R: Therapy for secondary mitral regurgitation: Time to 'cut the chord'?, Heart 101(13):996–997, 2015.
3. Song JM, Kim JJ, Ha TY, et al: Basal chordae sites on the mitral valve determine the severity of secondary mitral regurgitation, Heart 101:1024–1031, 2015.
4. Grayburn PA, Carabello B, Hung J, et al: Defining "severe" secondary mitral regurgitation: emphasizing an integrated approach, J Am Coll Cardiol 64:2792–2801, 2014.

3 Aortic Valve Disease

Aortic Valve Anatomy

CASE 3-1a
Normal Trileaflet Aortic Valve

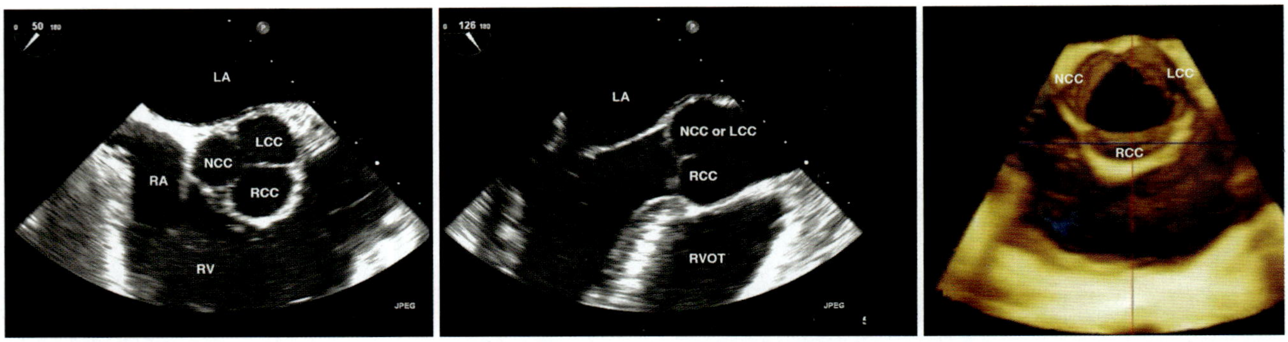

Fig 3.1 Intraoperative TEE in a short-axis view *(left)* shows the closed aortic valve and the orientation of the three cusps: noncoronary cusp (NCC), left coronary cusp (LCC), and right coronary cusp (RCC). The long-axis view *(middle)* shows the RCC and NCC; these are the cusps most often seen in the long-axis orientation, although occasionally the LCC is seen instead of the NCC. A 3D TEE image of an aortic valve *(right)* is demonstrated, and in real time, artifactual dropout is seen in the NCC. LA = left atrium, RA = right atrium, RV = right ventricle, RVOT = right ventricular outflow tract.

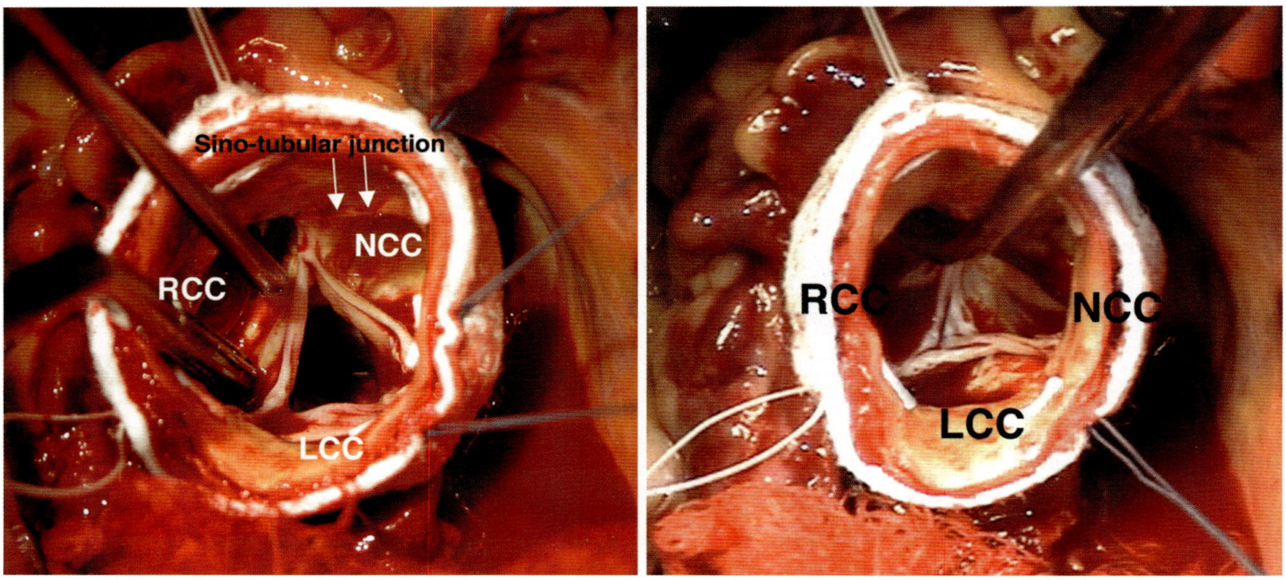

Fig 3.2 At surgery, in an image taken from the head of the operating table, a normal aortic valve is seen. The leaflets are thin and noncalcified. The commissural attachments to the sinotubular junction are visible.

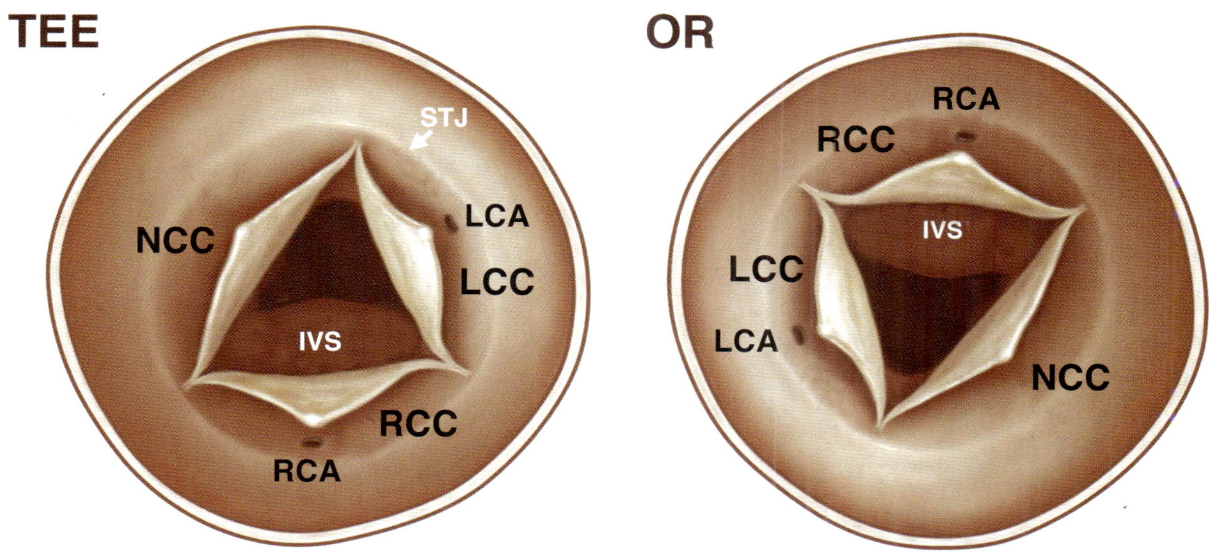

Fig 3.3 This illustration shows the relationship between the normal aortic valve and associated structures as seen on TEE, and as seen in the OR from the patient's head.

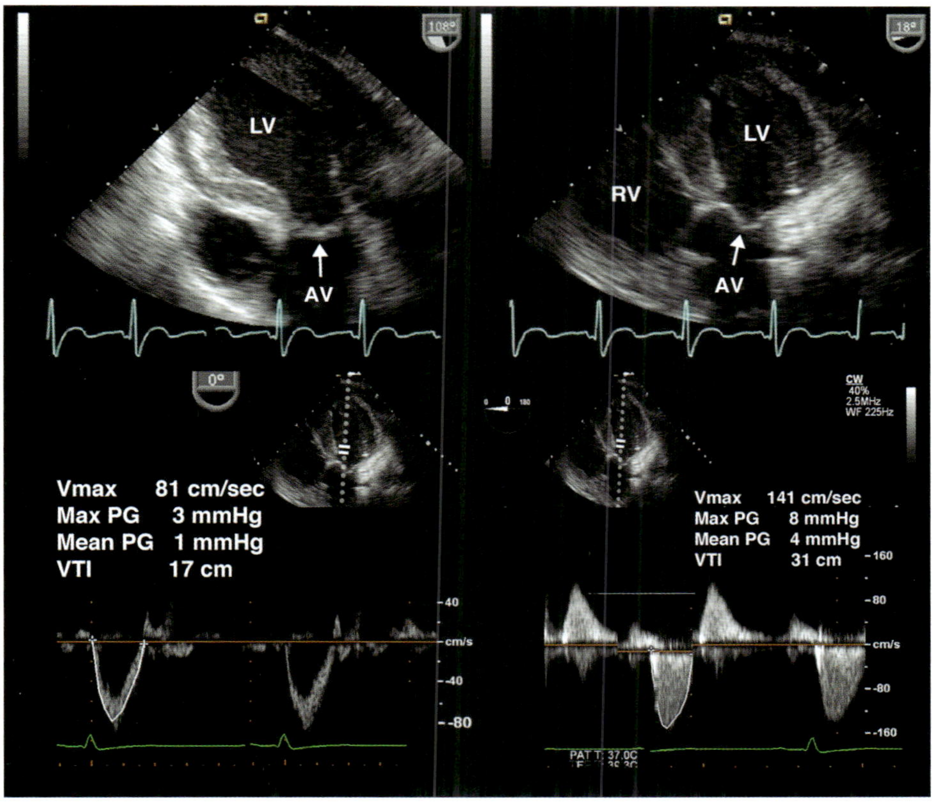

Fig 3.4 The deep transgastric *(right top panel)* and transgastric long-axis *(left top panel)* views of the aortic valve. These may be used for assessment of LVOT and transvalvular gradients. The bottom left panel shows a pulse wave Doppler tracing from the LVOT, and the bottom right panel shows a continuous wave Doppler through the aortic valve. There is little pressure gradient in this patient with a normal aortic valve. The two diastolic waves seen in the bottom right panel are the velocities of transmitral LV filling picked up by continuous wave Doppler.

CASE 3-1b
Bicuspid Aortic Valve

This 47-year-old male presented to the OR for mitral valve repair. Incidentally, a bicuspid aortic valve was detected; however, the systolic opening was normal with a normal antegrade flow velocity, and only mild aortic regurgitation was present.

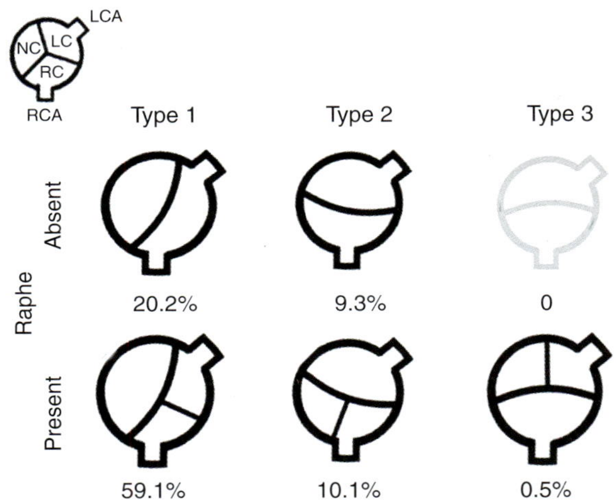

Fig 3.5 Bicuspid aortic valve leaflet morphology. Schematic of BAV phenotypes, with this figure modified to correspond to a TEE midesophageal short-axis view. Small inset at top left depicts a normal aortic valve in the same orientation with right coronary cusp (RC), left coronary cusp (LC), noncoronary cusp (NC), right coronary artery (RCA), and left coronary artery (LCA). Valve phenotypes and their frequencies are shown: type 1, "fusion" between right and left coronary cusp; type 2, "fusion" between right and noncoronary cusp; type 3, "fusion" between left and noncoronary cusp. Top row, without a raphe; bottom row, with raphe. Type 3 with without a raphe was not seen in the study group. Numbers indicate the observed frequency in the authors' cohort. (Adapted with permission from Schaefer BM, Lewin MB, et al. The bicuspid aortic valve: An integrated phenotypic classification of leaflet morphology and aortic root shape. Heart 2008; 94:1634–1638.)

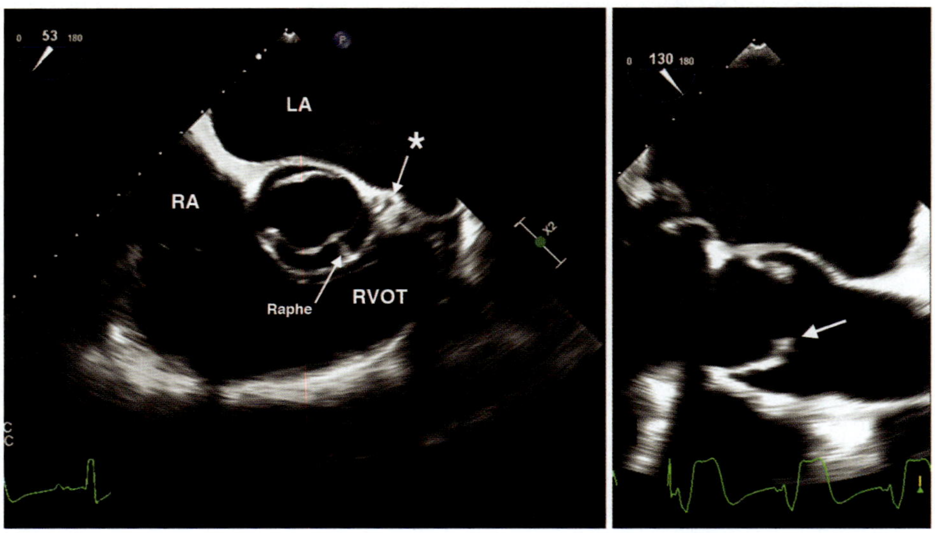

Fig 3.6 The left panel is a midesophageal short-axis view demonstrating a raphe at the fusion of the right and left coronary cusps. The asterisk indicates the left main coronary artery. The right panel is a midesophageal long-axis view demonstrating doming of the fused cusp *(arrow)*.

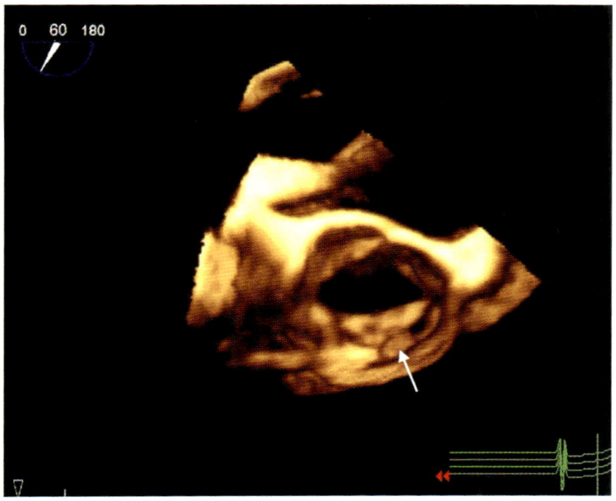

Fig 3.7 A 3D image of the bicuspid aortic valve from the ascending aortic perspective. The arrow indicates the raphe. In real time, Dropout is noted in the region of the anterior cusp.

CASE 3-1c
Unicuspid Aortic Valve

This 22-year-old male with a known unicuspid valve had mild and slightly progressive dyspnea on exertion, but was otherwise well. Serial echocardiographic imaging showed only mild regurgitation and moderate stenosis; however, because of progressive aortic root dilation (7 cm), he was referred for aortic valve and aortic root replacement.

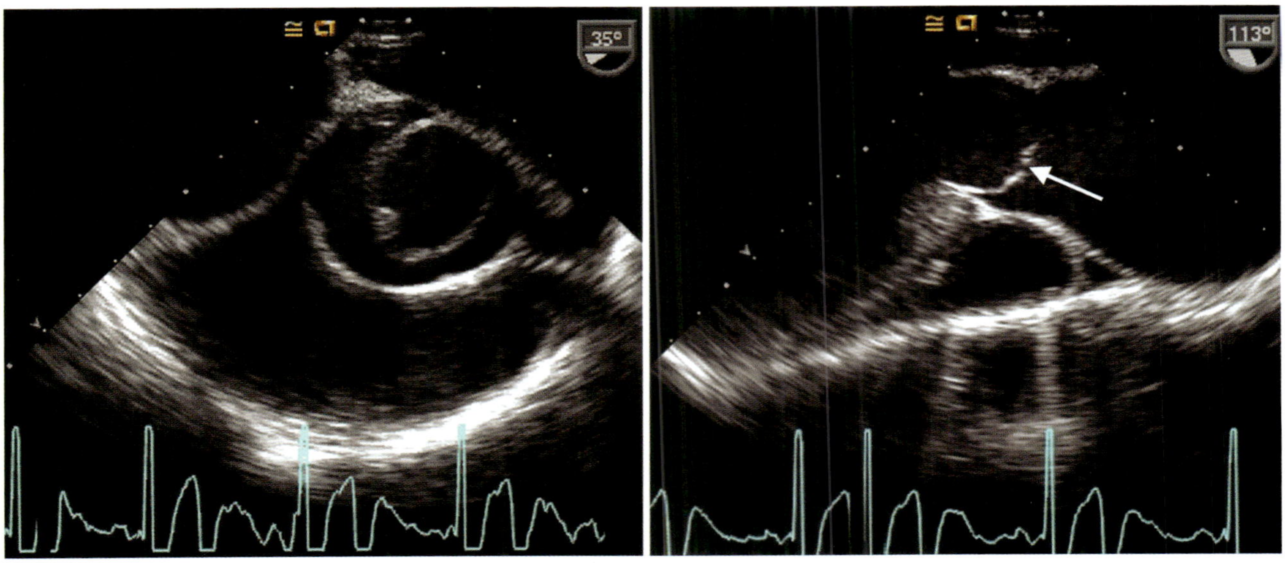

Fig 3.8 The left panel is a midesophageal short-axis image of a unicuspid aortic valve with only a single postero-lateral attachment. The right panel midesophageal long-axis image of the unicuspid aortic valve reveals doming *(arrow)* in the anterior portion of the leaflet.

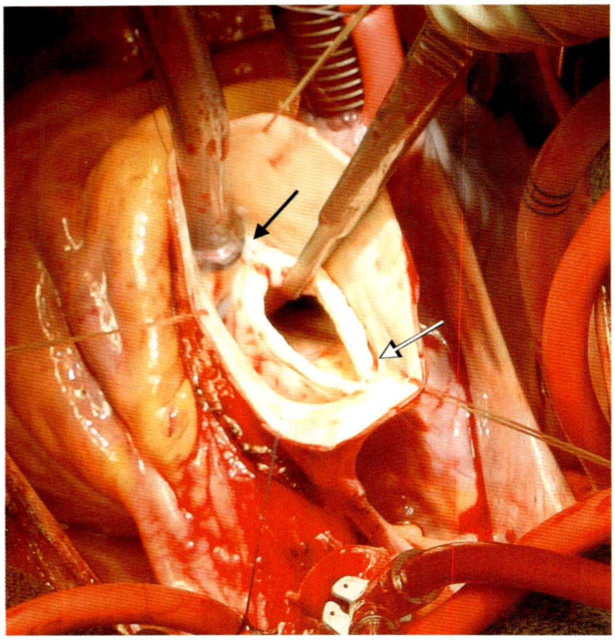

Fig 3.9 Intraoperative exposure of the unicuspid aortic valve demonstrates a thick leaflet. There is posterior attachment *(white arrow)* but no anterior attachment *(black arrow)*, which distinguishes it from a bicuspid valve.

CASE 3-1d
Quadricuspid Aortic Valve

This 39-year-old female had a repair of tetralogy of Fallot as an infant and was also known to have a quadricuspid aortic valve. She developed increasing dyspnea on exertion and fatigue. Noninvasive imaging showed severe pulmonic and aortic regurgitation with increasing right and left ventricular volumes so she was referred for aortic and pulmonic valve replacements.

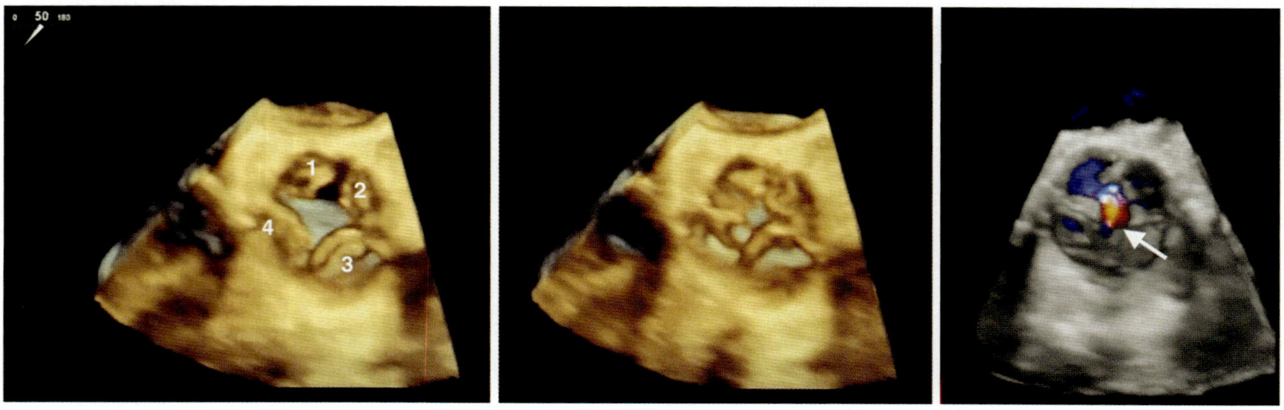

Fig 3.10 3D TEE images from the aortic perspective show four aortic leaflets in systole *(left)* and diastole *(center)*. The addition of color Doppler *(right)* during diastole shows central regurgitation *(arrow)*.

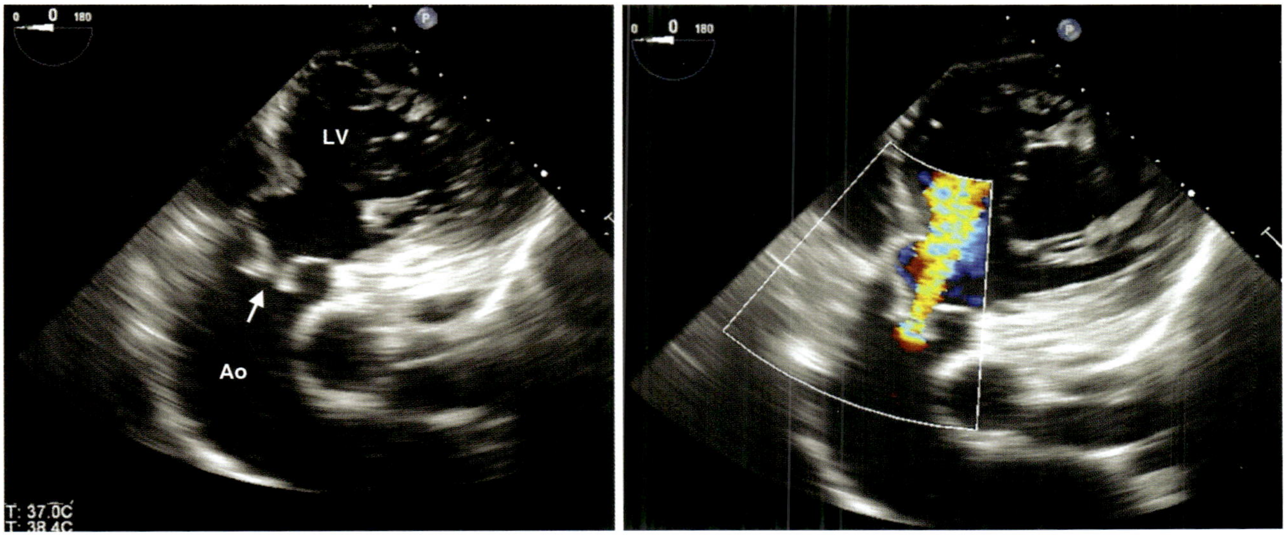

Fig 3.11 In the left panel, a deep transgastric image shows thickened and poorly coapting leaflets *(arrow)*. In the right panel, a deep transgastric image with the addition of color Doppler shows aortic regurgitation.

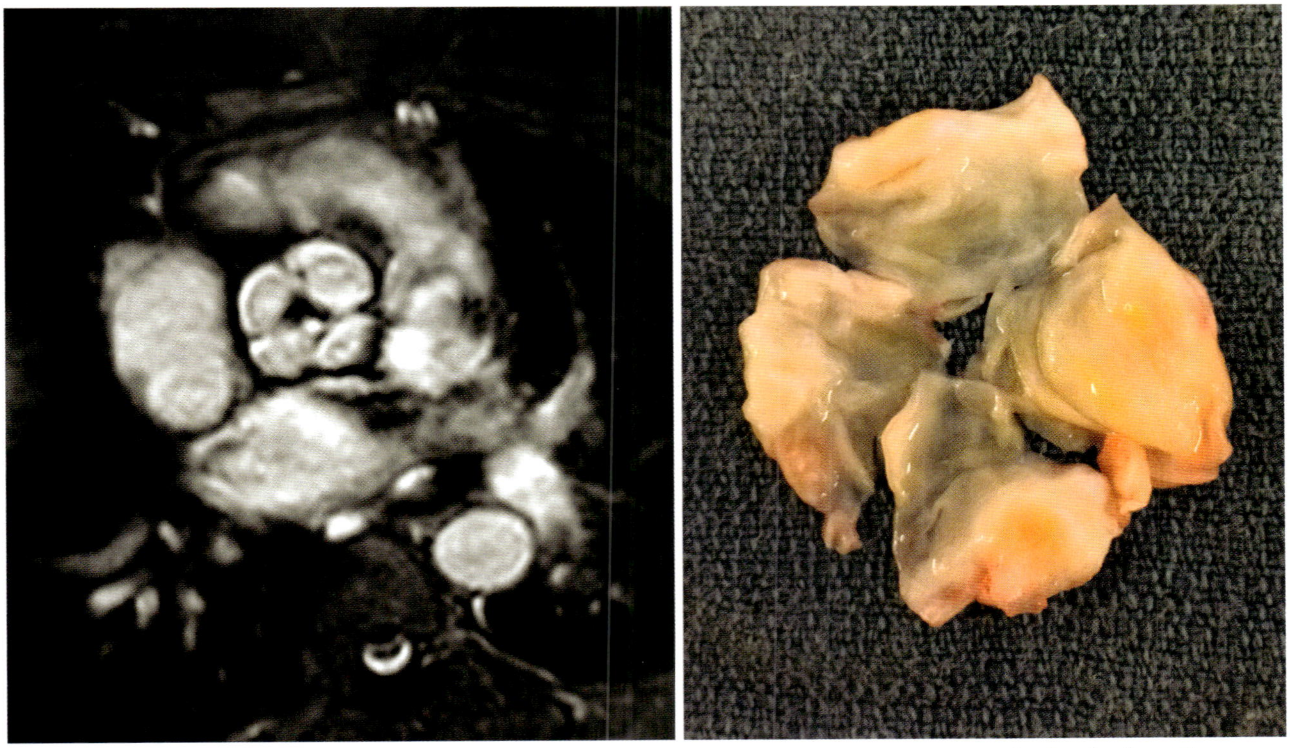

Fig 3.12 Magnetic resonance imaging (MRI) of the aortic valve in a short-axis plane demonstrates the four leaflets. The explanted aortic valve leaflets are arranged to show the anatomic positions.

TABLE 3-1
Optimal TEE Views for Assessing the Aortic Valve

Midesophageal short-axis aortic valve view	Relative to the heart, the aortic valve plane is oblique. A 30- to 60-degree transducer angle is necessary to show symmetrical imaging of all valve cusps (Fig 3.1). During systole, cusp opening is normally unrestricted with the orifice shape identifying the number of cusps and planimetry of the edges determining the anatomic valve area. During diastole, the three cusps of the normal valve close and color Doppler may be added to show AR. Withdrawing the probe slightly in the esophagus reveals the left and right coronary ostia, whereas advancing the probe yields a short-axis view of the LV outflow tract.
Midesophageal long-axis aortic valve view	Rotating the transducer angle to 120 to 140 degrees from the short-axis view with slight probe advancement shows a long-axis view of the LV outflow tract, aortic valve, and ascending aorta (see Fig 3.1). The normal aortic valve leaflets appear as thin, parallel lines within the sinuses of Valsalva, the RCC is always anterior adjacent to the RV outflow tract, and the posterior cusp is either the LCC or, more often, the NCC. Aortic annular dimensions are measured during systole, whereas color Doppler demonstrates the presence and site of disturbed flow related to obstruction or AR.
Transgastric view of aortic valve	In the transgastric long-axis view at 90 to 120 degrees, the aortic valve is displayed on the right side of the screen. From a deep transgastric view at 0 degrees the image plane is angled anteriorly from the foreshortened four-chamber view to display the aortic valve (Fig 3.4). Although assessment of aortic valve anatomy may be imprecise in transgastric views, they may be useful for spectral Doppler alignment to measure optimal transvalvular velocity.
3D echocardiographic aortic valve imaging	3D TEE can assess valvular morphology in more detail compared with 2D TTE. In some cases, 3D planimetry of the anatomic aortic valve orifice may be helpful.

AR, aortic regurgitation; LCC, left coronary cusp; LV, left ventricular; NCC, noncoronary cusp; RCC, right coronary cusp; RV, right ventricular; TEE, transesophageal echocardiography; TTE, transthoracic echocardiography; 2D, two-dimensional. (From Oxorn D. Intraoperative Echocardiography, Practical Echocardiography Series, Elsevier, 2012.)

Aortic Stenosis

CASE 3-2
Severe Calcific Aortic Stenosis

A 71-year-old man presented to a local ED with shortness of breath and dyspnea on exertion. His symptoms had progressed over the past 6 months and now were consistent with NYHA class III. TTE revealed severe aortic stenosis (AS) with an aortic velocity of 4.1 m/s, valve area of 0.9 cm^2 by continuity equation, a significantly dilated LV, and an ejection fraction of 35%. He was sent for surgical consultation for potential aortic valve replacement.

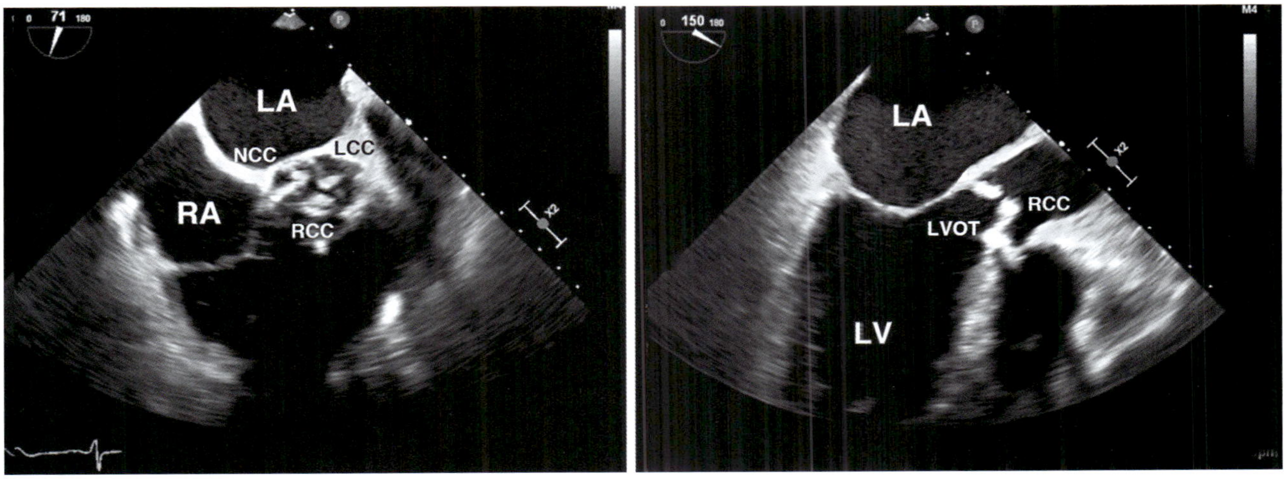

Fig 3.13 Intraoperative TEE in a midesophageal short-axis view, obtained with rotation of the image plane to 71 degrees and slight flexion of the probe, shows a heavily calcified trileaflet aortic valve with reduced systolic opening. Although this short-axis image is correctly aligned, planimetry of the valve area is not possible because of shadowing and reverberations from the valve calcium and the irregular shape of the orifice. In addition, the stenotic valve often has a complex 3D shape with a nonplanar orifice that may not be visualized in a single 2D-image plane. With rotation of the image plane to 150 degrees and leftward turning of the probe, a long-axis view of the aortic valve, aortic root, and left ventricular outflow tract is obtained. This long-axis view shows severe leaflet calcification with reduced systolic motion.

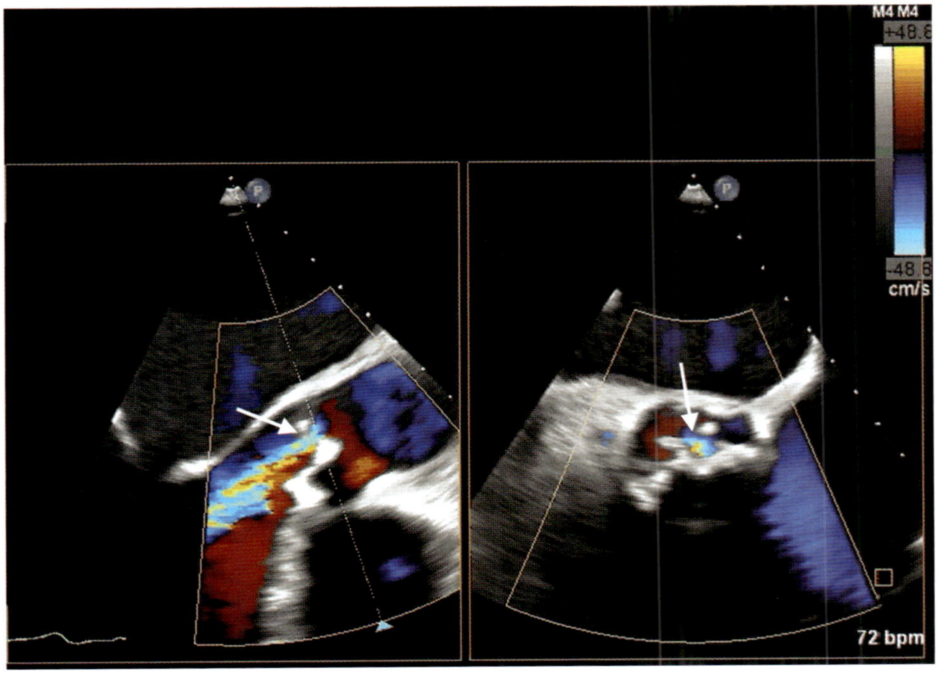

Fig 3.14 Color Doppler flow imaging in the long and short axis views shows a small amount of aortic regurgitation *(arrows)*.

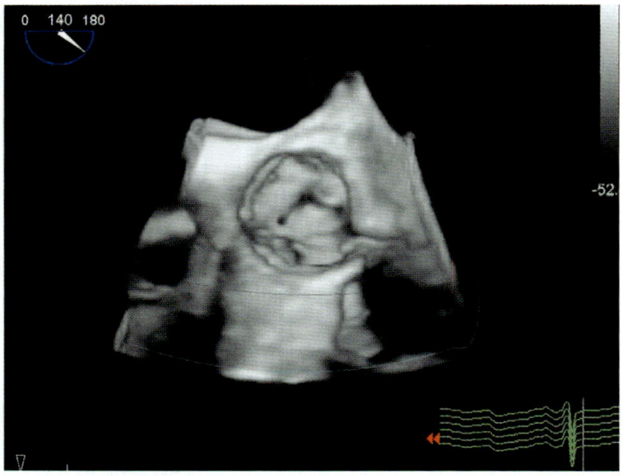

Fig 3.15 In this 3D image of the aortic valve, from the ascending aortic perspective, the leaflets are noted to be extremely thick, with minimal opening in systole and an irregular-shaped orifice but no commissural fusion.

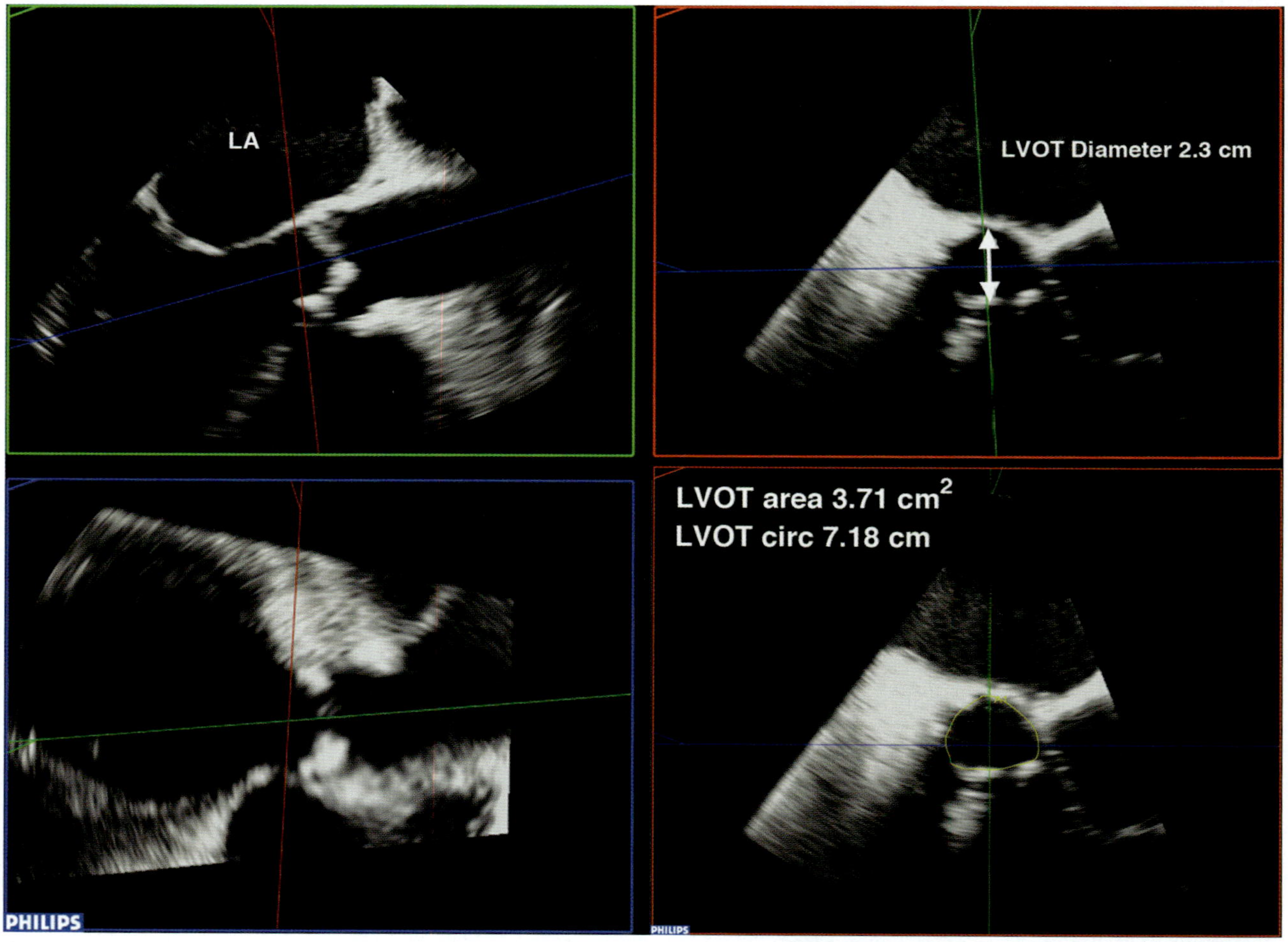

Fig 3.16 Multiplanar reconstruction of the aortic valve allows measurement of the LVOT diameter at 2.3 cm, area at 3.71 cm^2, and circumference at 7.18 cm.

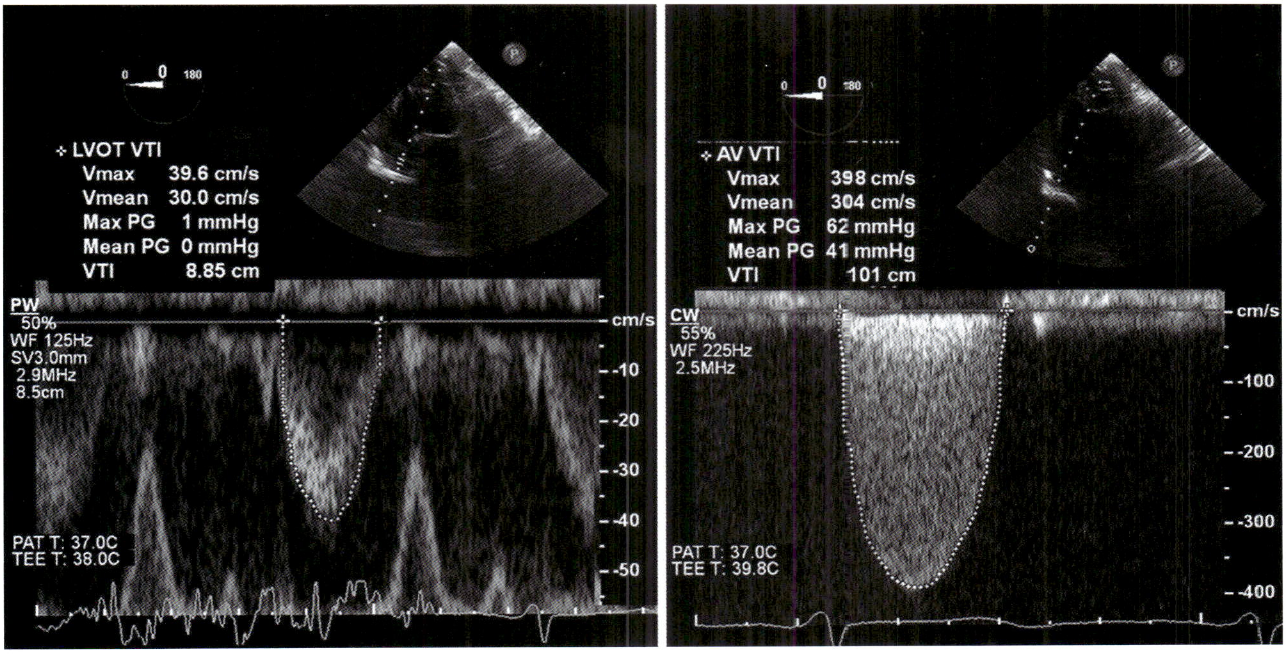

Fig 3.17 Continuous wave Doppler obtained in the deep transgastric position of the LVOT *(left panel)* and the aortic valve *(right panel)*. The maximum velocity is 3.9 m/sec. The mean gradient (40 mm Hg) is calculated by tracing the velocity curve with averaging of the instantaneous pressure gradients over the systolic ejection period. Although this velocity and mean gradient might be underestimated because of a nonparallel intercept angle, both are consistent with severe aortic stenosis.

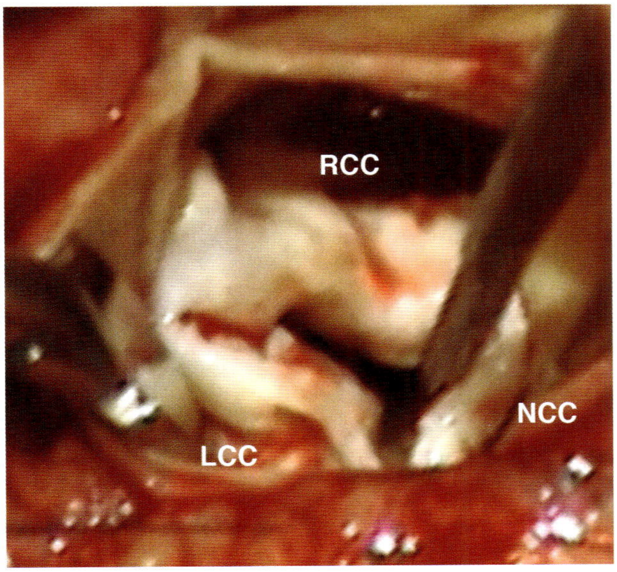

Fig 3.18 At surgery, the valve was heavily calcified and stenotic. The leaflets were nonpliable as demonstrated by the surgeon, who is grasping the noncoronary cusp. The valve was replaced with a 23-mm tissue valve.

Comments

In current clinical practice, aortic stenosis is best evaluated by transthoracic echocardiography. The standard evaluation of stenosis severity is based on:

1. 2D or 3D imaging of valve anatomy, the extent of calcification, and leaflet motion.
2. Continuous wave Doppler measurement of the antegrade velocity across the valve (the aortic "jet") with calculation of maximum and mean pressure gradients.
3. Calculation of valve area using the continuity equation.

On 2D imaging the number of valve leaflets is identified, although severe calcification of a bicuspid valve may be indistinguishable from a severely calcified trileaflet valve. TEE 3D imaging may provide better visualization of the number of valve leaflets and degree of valve opening when TTE imaging is suboptimal. Accurate planimetry of valve area is possible on 3D TEE imaging in many cases.

The aortic jet velocity is recorded from the acoustic window that shows the highest velocity signal. This is especially important, as accurate velocity data (and calculated pressure gradients) depend on a parallel intercept angle between the ultrasound beam and the high-velocity jet. Because the 3D direction of the jet is unpredictable, in practice the jet velocity is recorded from multiple windows with careful patient positioning to ensure that a parallel intercept angle is obtained. The most useful windows are apical and suprasternal, but in some cases the highest velocity is recorded from a subcostal or high right parasternal position. The most common error in assessment of aortic stenosis severity is failure to obtain a parallel intercept angle, which results in underestimation of stenosis severity. TEE transgastric views may allow measurement of aortic velocity but the possibility of underestimation resulting from a nonparallel intercept angle always should be considered.

Transaortic pressure gradients (ΔP in mmHg) are calculated with the simplified Bernoulli equation using the aortic jet velocity (V_{AS}) as:

$$\Delta P = 4(V_{AS})^2$$

The simplified Bernoulli equation assumes that the proximal velocity can be ignored, a reasonable assumption when velocity is <1 m/s because squaring a number <1 makes it even smaller. The maximum instantaneous gradient is calculated from the maximum velocity; the mean gradient is calculated by averaging the instantaneous gradients over the ejection period, or can be approximated by the formula:

$$\Delta P_{mean} = 2.4(V_{AS})^2$$

The physiologic cross-sectional area of flow across the stenotic valve is calculated using the continuity equation, based on the principle that the stroke volume (SV) proximal to and in the orifice must be equal. Volume flow rate at any site equals the 2D cross-sectional area × the velocity time integral of flow (mean velocity × ejection period) through that site.

Stroke volume in the left ventricular outflow tract (LVOT) and in the narrowed aortic stenotic (AS) orifice are equal:

$$SV_{LVOT} = SV_{AS}$$

Thus,

$$CSA_{LVOT} \times VTI_{LVOT} = AVA \times VTI_{AS}$$

Solving for aortic valve area (AVA):

$$AVA = (CSA_{LVOT} \times VTI_{LVOT})/VTI_{AS}$$

In clinical practice, this equation is often simplified by using maximum velocities, instead of velocity time integrals:

$$AVA = (CSA_{LVOT} \times V_{LVOT})/V_{AS}$$

Clinical decision making is primarily based on the patient's symptoms, and there are no absolute values for stenosis severity that define symptom onset. Aortic stenosis severity is classified as Stage A in patients at risk of AS but with no obstruction to outflow, as in a normally functioning bicuspid aortic valve. Progressive AS (Stage B) is present with an abnormal aortic valve and velocity between 2 and 4 m/s. Severe AS is present when the velocity is >4 m/s and is classified as Stage C in asymptomatic patients and Stage D in symptomatic patients. Valve area typically is <1.0 cm^2, but this is not required to diagnose severe AS. Severe AS also may be present with a low flow rate, resulting in a lower velocity and gradient despite severe valve obstruction (see suggested reading).

When Doppler data are diagnostic for aortic stenosis, invasive evaluation of stenosis severity is not indicated, although coronary angiography may be needed to evaluate for possible coronary disease. Intraoperative TEE provided visual confirmation of the diagnosis and was useful in monitoring ventricular function.

Suggested Reading

1. Otto CM: Valve stenosis. In textbook of clinical echocardiography, ed 5, Philadelphia, 2012, Elsevier, pp 271–304.
2. Otto CM, Prendergast B: Aortic-valve stenosis—from patients at risk to severe valve obstruction, N Engl J Med 371(8):744–756, 2014.
3. von Homeyer P, Oxorn, D: Aortic Stenosis: Echocardiographic Diagnosis, Anesth Analg 115: 517–521, 2012.

CASE 3-3
Aortic Stenosis with Epiaortic Scanning

This 41-year-old woman with multiple sclerosis had a history of a bicuspid aortic valve. She presented with increasing dyspnea on exertion, presyncope, and chest pain. Transthoracic echocardiography showed a bicuspid aortic valve with secondary calcification. The antegrade velocity was 4.9 m/s and continuity equation valve area was 0.8 cm^2. Left ventricular systolic function was normal, with an ejection fraction of 75% measured by the apical biplane method.

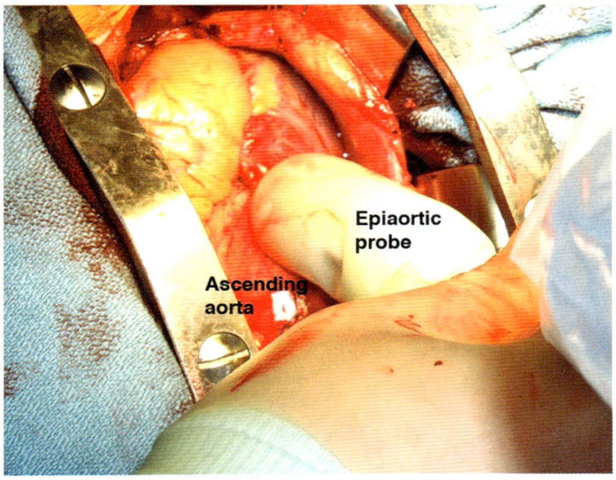

Fig 3.19 An epiaortic probe was used to examine the aortic valve at the time of surgery, which illustrates the use of alternate transducer positions in the operating room for evaluation of aortic stenosis severity. The probe (in a sterile sleeve) is positioned by the surgeon or echocardiographer directly on the ascending aorta, as shown here. The probe position is then adjusted, with rotation and angulation as needed, to obtain standard image planes of the aortic valve. In some cases, improved images are obtained by using a stand-off (such as a fluid-filled glove) or repositioning the transducer so that the area of interest is in the focal zone of the ultrasound beam instead of in the near field of the image.

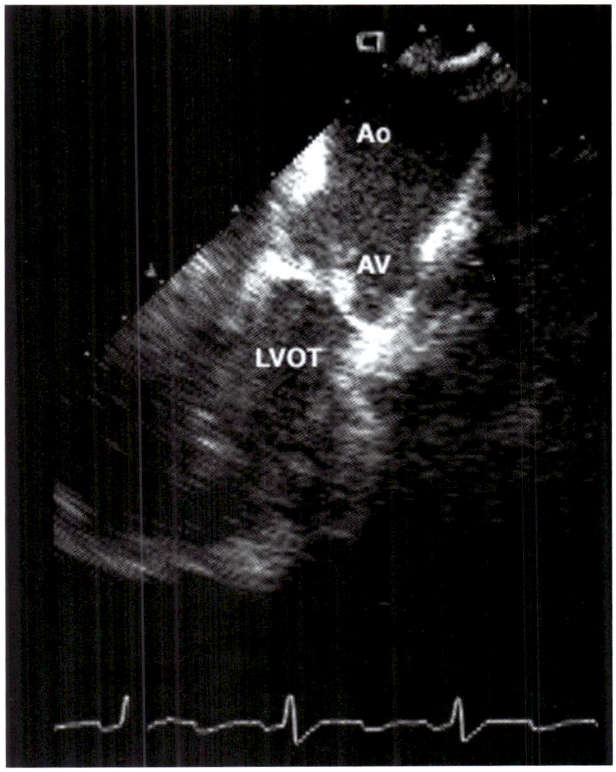

Fig 3.20 The epiaortic long-axis images of the aortic valve show the ascending aorta with the sinotubular junction. The aortic valve leaflets are severely calcified with reduced mobility.

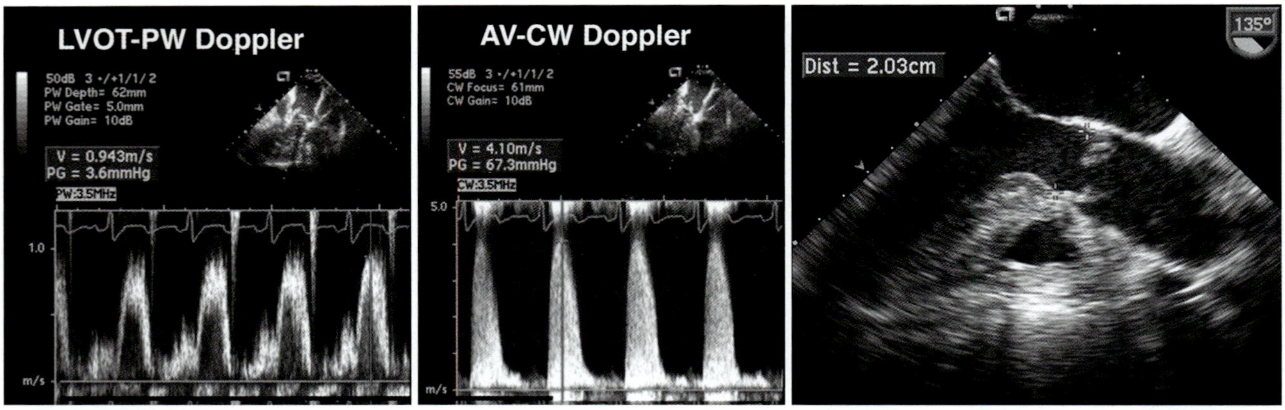

Fig 3.21 This composite image shows calculation of the continuity equation valve area using epiaortic scanning to obtain Doppler flows and a transesophageal long-axis view of the left ventricular outflow tract (LVOT) for measurement of outflow tract diameter (2.0 cm). The pulsed wave (PW) Doppler sample volume was positioned just on the ventricular side of the aortic valve to obtain a smooth velocity curve with a narrow band of velocities and a well-defined peak at 0.9 m/s. Continuous wave (CW) Doppler of the aortic valve (AV) showed an aortic jet velocity of 4.1 m/s. The aortic valve area (AVA) calculated with the continuity equation is 0.7 cm^2. The Doppler aortic jet velocity is lower than the 4.9-m/s jet obtained on transthoracic examination, most likely the outcome of a lower cardiac output during anesthesia, although a nonparallel intercept angle between the ultrasound beam and aortic jet is also a possibility. However, the LVOT velocity is similarly lower, so that the continuity equation valve area of 0.7 is similar to the value obtained preoperatively.

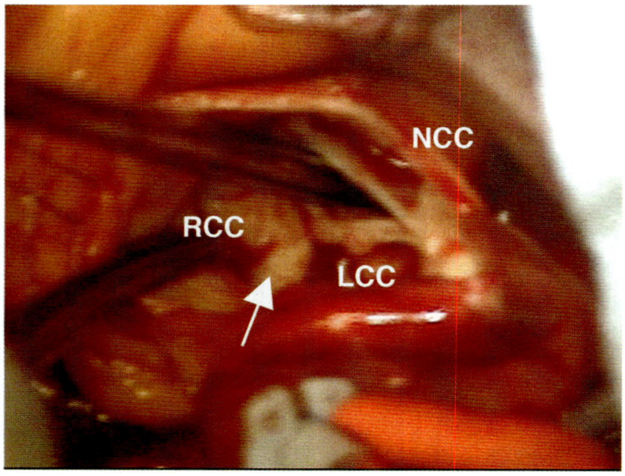

Fig 3.22 Direct inspection of the valve through the aortotomy shows a bicuspid aortic valve with severe calcification of the leaflets. The arrow indicates the raphe in the congenitally fused right and left coronary cusps (RCC, LCC). She underwent valve replacement with a 21-mm bioprosthetic valve. Her postoperative course was uneventful and she was discharged 6 days after surgery.

Comments

Evaluation of the severity of aortic stenosis on TEE with 2D imaging is problematic. In many cases, 3D imaging allows accurate planimetry of orifice area in systole but shadowing and reverberations from valve calcification may limit this approach. Planimetry from 2D images is not recommended because valve area may be overestimated if areas of calcification in the body of the leaflet are mistaken for the leaflet edge or if the image plane is not at the level of the narrowest valve orifice.

Doppler evaluation of stenosis severity is suboptimal because of the limited acoustic windows available from the transesophageal approach. Unlike transthoracic imaging, transducer positioning is constrained to the narrow window provided by the esophagus and stomach. It is rarely possible to align the Doppler beam parallel to ventricular outflow from either a transesophageal or transgastric probe position. Occasionally, the aortic jet can be accurately recorded from a transgastric apical view, although alignment in the elevational plan cannot be evaluated. Deviations from a parallel intercept angle result in substantial errors: for example, with an actual jet velocity of 5 m/s, the measured velocity is only 4.3 m/s at an intercept angle of 30 degrees and 2.5 m/s at a 60-degree intercept angle. This corresponds to an actual maximum pressure gradient of 100 mm Hg being underestimated at 75 or even 25 mm Hg.

Thus we recommend that all patients with suspected aortic stenosis undergo a careful and complete TTE examination as part of the preoperative evaluation. If an unsuspected abnormal aortic valve is noted during the intraoperative echocardiogram and no prior evaluation is available, the possibility that intraoperative Doppler may underestimate stenosis severity should be taken into consideration.

Suggested Reading

1. Baumgartner H, Hung J, Bermejo J, et al: American Society of Echocardiography; European Association of Echocardiography. Echocardiographic assessment of valve stenosis: EAE/ASE recommendations for clinical practice, J Am Soc Echocardiogr 22(1):1–23, 2009.
2. Machida T, Izumo M, Suzuki K, et al: Value of anatomical aortic valve area using real-time three-dimensional transesophageal echocardiography in patients with aortic stenosis: a comparison between tricuspid and bicuspid aortic valves, Eur Heart J Cardiovasc Imaging 16(10):1120–1128, 2015.

CASE 3-4
Moderate Aortic Stenosis in a Patient Undergoing Coronary Bypass Surgery

A 70-year-old man with coronary artery disease is noted to have a systolic murmur on preoperative examination. Transthoracic echocardiography shows an aortic jet velocity of 3.4 m/s, a mean transaortic gradient of 26 mm Hg and a continuity equation valve area of 1.3 cm^2.

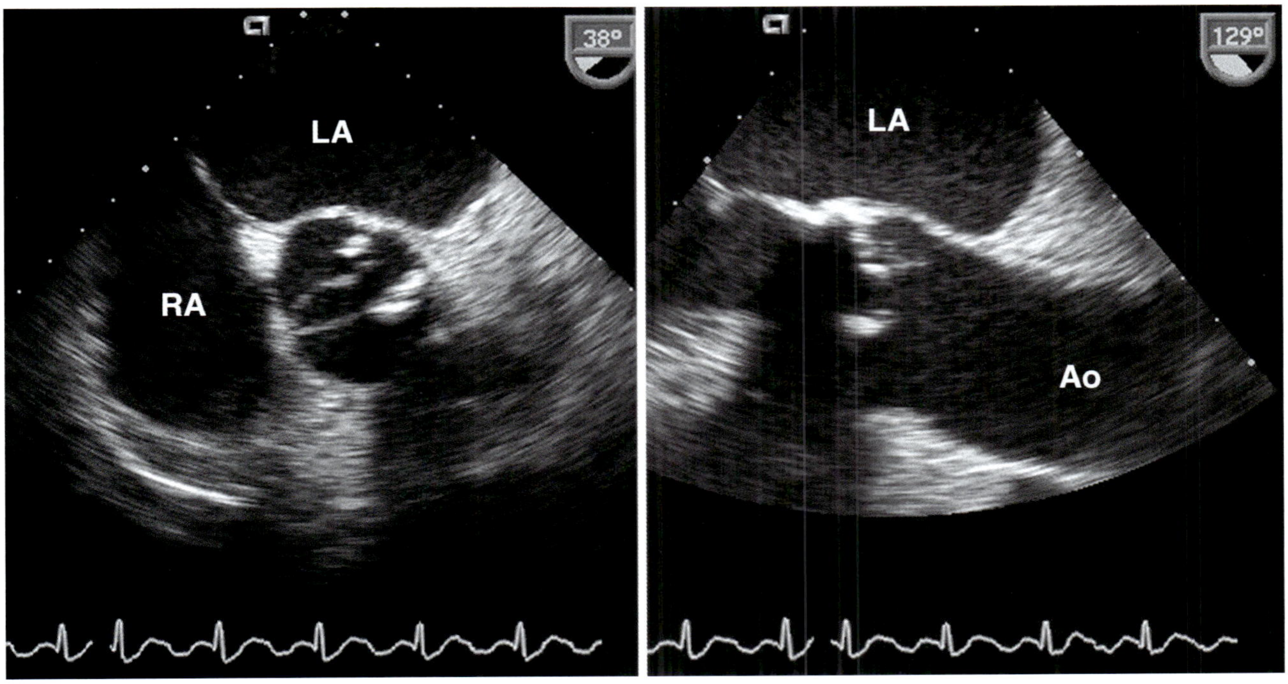

Fig 3.23 Intraoperative imaging in a long-axis *(right)* and short-axis *(left)* view of the aortic valve shows a bicuspid valve with moderate leaflet calcification and moderately reduced systolic motion.

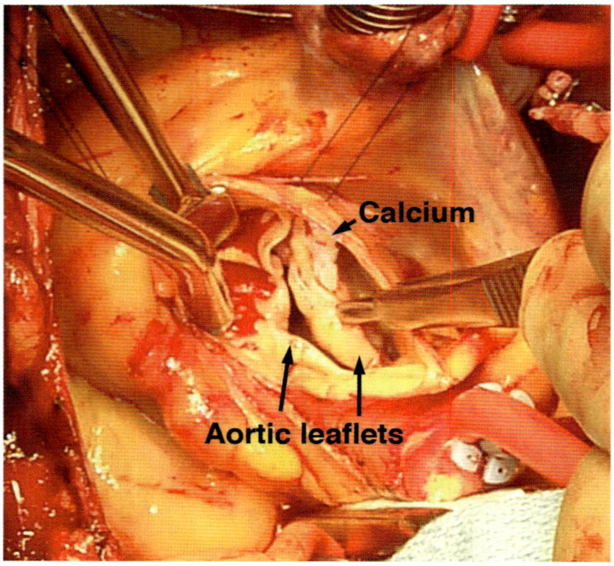

Fig 3.24 Direct visualization of the valve by the surgeon confirms the moderately calcified bicuspid aortic valve with increased leaflet stiffness. The leaflets were resected in preparation for valve replacement.

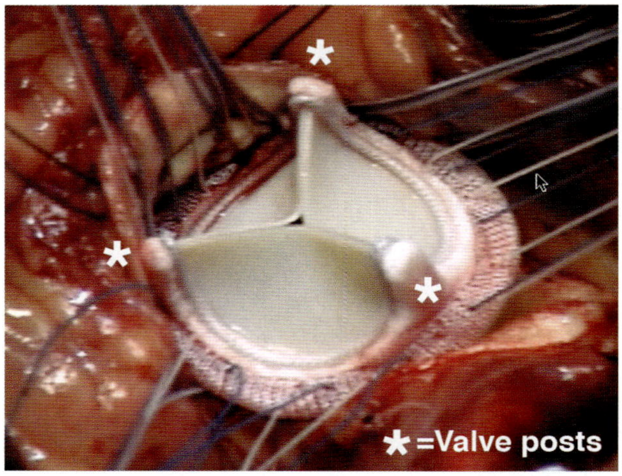

Fig 3.25 This intraoperative photograph shows implantation of the stented tissue valve.

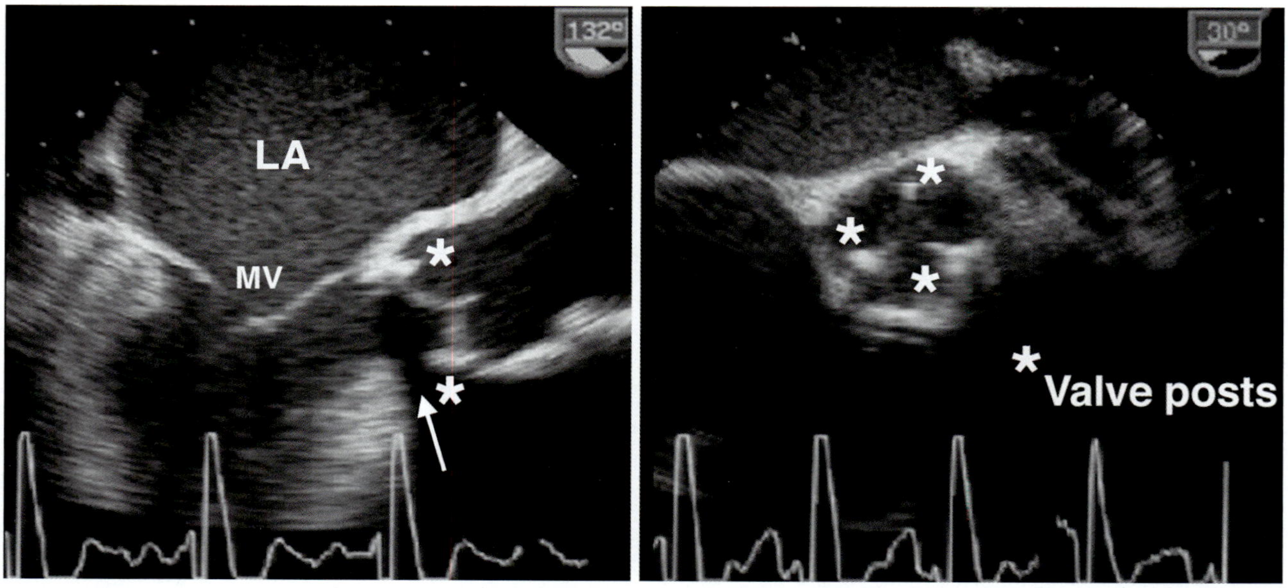

Fig 3.26 After weaning from cardiopulmonary bypass, long-axis *(left)* and short-axis *(right)* images of the aortic valve in diastole show the prosthetic valve posts and the thin leaflets. Note the shadowing by the prosthetic valve *(arrow)*.

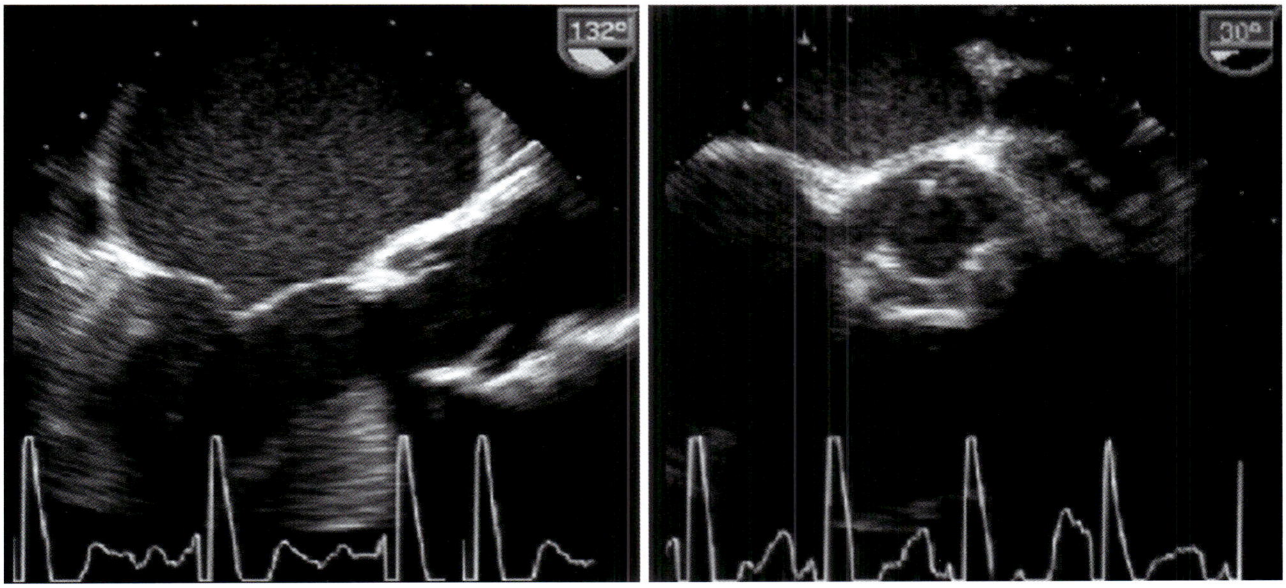

Fig 3.27 Systolic images of the stented tissue prosthesis show the open leaflets in a long-axis *(left)* and short-axis *(right)* view. In real time the normal motion of the thin prosthetic leaflets is seen.

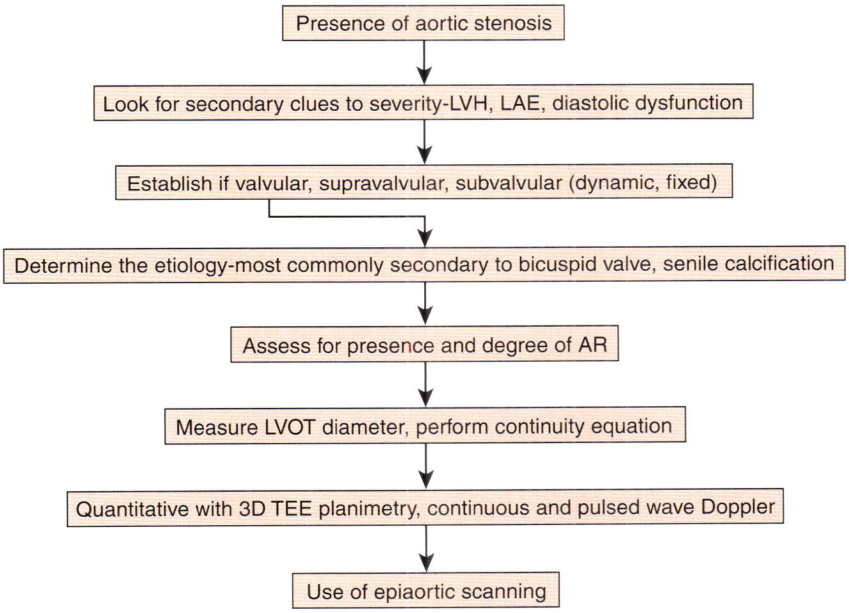

Fig 3.28 Algorithm for intraoperative assessment of AS discovered during other cardiac surgery. LAE = left atrial enlargement.

Comments

In patients with asymptomatic aortic valve stenosis who are undergoing surgery for coronary artery, aortic root, or mitral valve disease, the option of concurrent aortic valve replacement should be considered. The rationale for aortic valve replacement in these patients is that progression of aortic stenosis leading to symptoms is predictable and inevitable and the risk of repeat surgery is high. Balanced against these potential benefits are the additional surgical time and risk for the current procedure and the durability, suboptimal hemodynamics, and potential complications of a prosthetic valve.

Recent prospective Doppler echocardiography studies have improved our understanding of the natural history of asymptomatic aortic stenosis. In patients with mild stenosis (jet velocity <3.0 m/s), progression to severe symptomatic aortic stenosis occurs in only 10% to 15% by 2 to 3 years, compared with 80% in those with severe stenosis (jet velocity >4.0 m/s). Thus there now is general agreement that valve surgery for asymptomatic disease may not be needed when stenosis is mild but is appropriate when stenosis is severe. Decision making is more difficult in patients with moderate stenosis, as in this case, with a progression to severe symptomatic disease in about 30% at 3 years.

In patients with moderate stenosis, other factors that are taken into account include patient age, preferences and comorbidities, the expected hemodynamics and durability of available prosthetic valves, and the degree of valve calcification. Significant valve calcification is associated with rapid disease progression. In this case example, the decision to proceed with valve replacement was based on the finding of significant calcification of a bicuspid valve with moderate obstruction to outflow. As our choices for valve replacement improve, with durable valves that have favorable hemodynamics and do not require anticoagulation, the balance may shift toward valve replacement at the time of other cardiac surgery in more patients with aortic valve disease.

Suggested Reading

1. Nishimura RA, Otto CM, Bonow RO, et al: ACC/AHA Task Force Members. 2014 AHA/ACC Guideline for the Management of Patients with Valvular Heart Disease: A report of the American College of Cardiology/American Heart Association Task Force on Practice Guidelines, Circulation 129(23):e521–643, 2014.
2. Vahanian A, Alfieri O, Andreotti F, et al: Joint Task Force on the Management of Valvular Heart Disease of the European Society of Cardiology (ESC); European Association for Cardio-Thoracic Surgery (EACTS). Guidelines on the management of valvular heart disease (version 2012), Eur J Cardiothorac Surg 42(4): S1–S44, 2012.

CASE 3-5
Rheumatic Aortic Stenosis

This 56-year-old man presented 3 months ago with shortness of breath and atrial fibrillation. Physical examination showed a grade IV/VI systolic murmur at the base and he was referred for echocardiography. The transthoracic examination showed severe aortic stenosis with a jet velocity of 4.3 m/s, a mean gradient of 40 mm Hg, and a valve area of 0.9 cm^2. There was moderate aortic regurgitation. In addition, the mitral valve had changes consistent with rheumatic disease, with mild mitral stenosis.

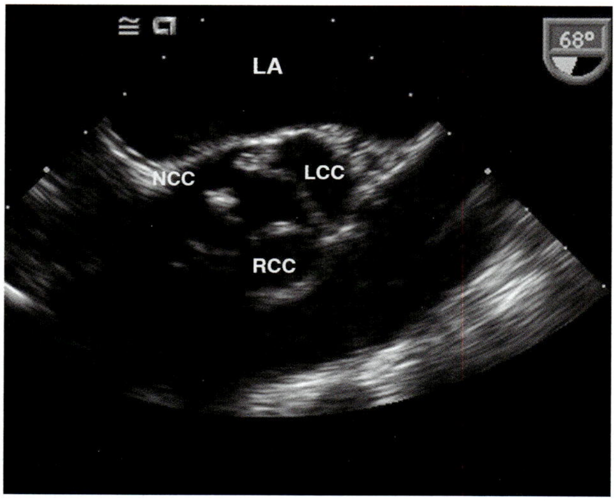

Fig 3.29 This short-axis image of the aortic valve in systole shows a trileaflet valve with a triangular orifice resulting from commissural fusion, as is typical with rheumatic valve disease. The video shows the reduced systolic opening of the leaflets on 2D imaging *(left)* and with color Doppler *(right, video)* showing only mild aortic regurgitation.

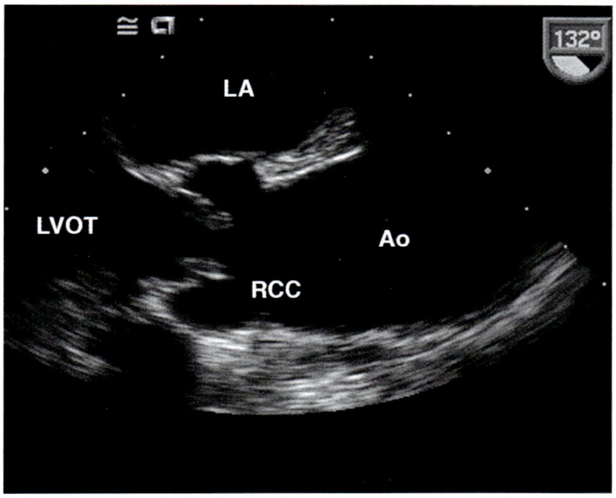

Fig 3.30 The long-axis view of the aortic valve and ascending aorta shows doming of the leaflets in systole, again typical for rheumatic disease. The anterior cusp of the aortic valve in this view is the RCC. The posterior cusp is usually the NCC, although the LCC may be seen, depending on the exact position of the valve relative to the transducer in the esophagus (see the short-axis view for reference).

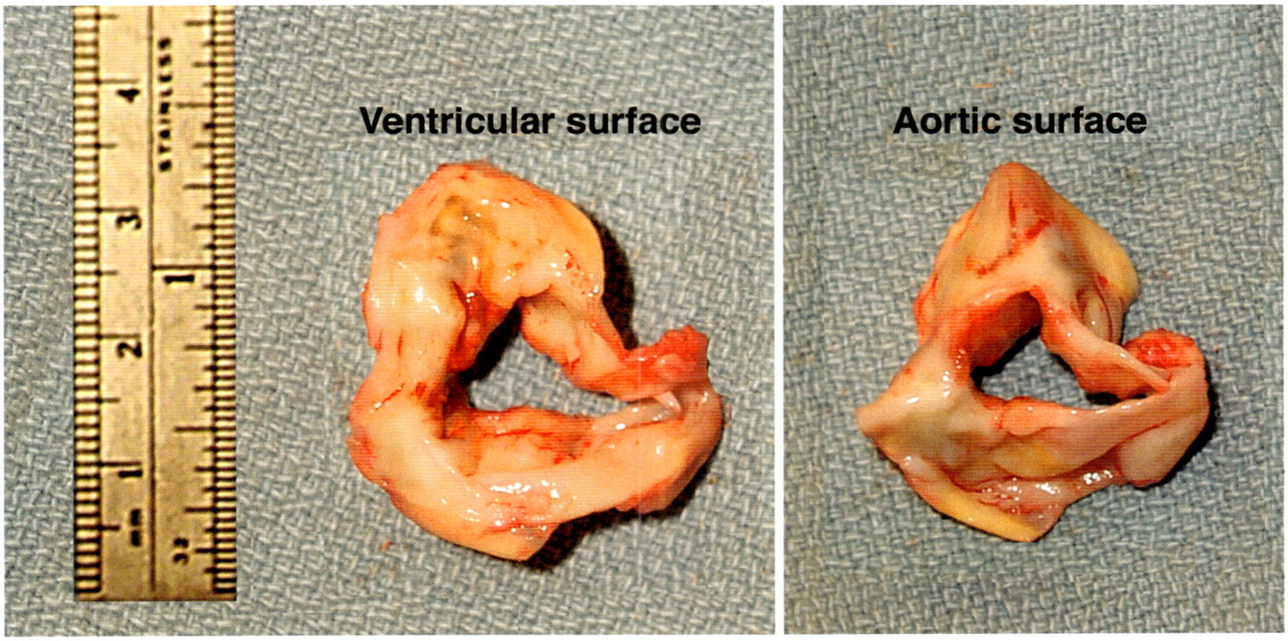

Fig 3.31 The explanted valve shows dramatic commissural fusion with a triangular orifice at the leaflet tips, seen both from the ventricular and aortic aspects. The leaflets are diffusely thickened, including the leaflet edges, with a smooth surface and only mild superimposed calcification, in contrast to the irregular calcific masses seen in the central part of the leaflets with calcific valve disease.

Comments

Although calcific valve disease is the most common cause of aortic stenosis in Europe and North America, rheumatic valve disease is highly prevalent in Asia, Africa, and the Pacific Islands, and sporadic cases are seen in every country. Rheumatic valve disease is the long-term sequela of acute rheumatic fever. The pathognomonic features of rheumatic valve disease are primary involvement of the mitral valve, with characteristic commissural fusion and chordal fusion and shortening. The aortic valve is affected in about 40% of cases, with involvement of the tricuspid valve in only 6% of those patients with rheumatic mitral valve disease. Rheumatic aortic valve disease can be recognized by the characteristic mitral valve changes and evidence for commissural fusion and diffuse leaflet thickening, particularly along the leaflet edges of the aortic valve. In systole, a central triangular orifice is seen, in contrast to the complex stellate orifice of calcific aortic stenosis.

Suggested Reading

1. Iung B, Vahanian A: Epidemiology of acquired valvular heart disease, Can J Cardiol 30(9):962–970, 2014.
2. Rosenhek R, Baumgartner H: Aortic stenosis. In Otto CM, Bonow RO, editors: Valvular Heart Disease, ed 4, Philadelphia, 2014, Elsevier, pp 139–162.

Aortic Regurgitation

CASE 3-6
Acute on Chronic Aortic Regurgitation

This 67-year-old male with a known history of aortic valve disease presented with a month-long history of increasing orthopnea and dyspnea on exertion. After treatment at an outside hospital, he was transferred for definitive management. Transthoracic echocardiography revealed severe aortic regurgitation, as well as deterioration in left ventricular systolic function.

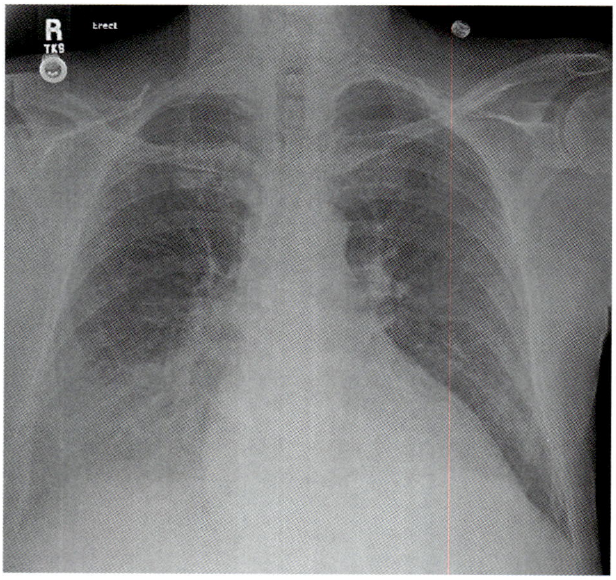

Fig 3.32 A chest x-ray reveals cardiomegaly and pulmonary edema.

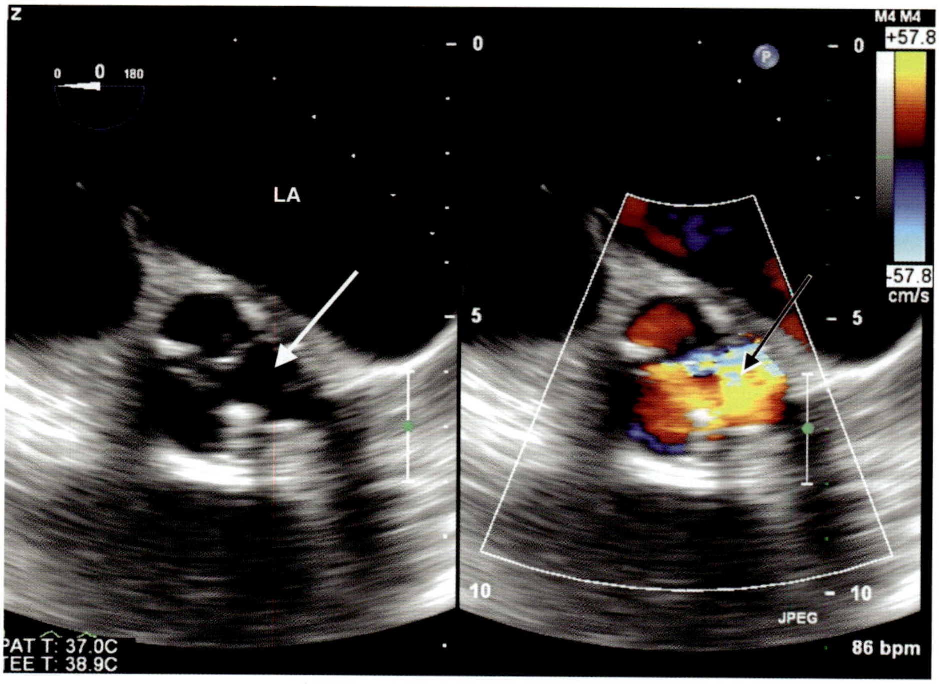

Fig 3.33 A midesophageal short-axis of the aortic valve reveals leaflet thickness and destruction. Color Doppler shows severe aortic regurgitation. The arrows indicate where the LCC would be.

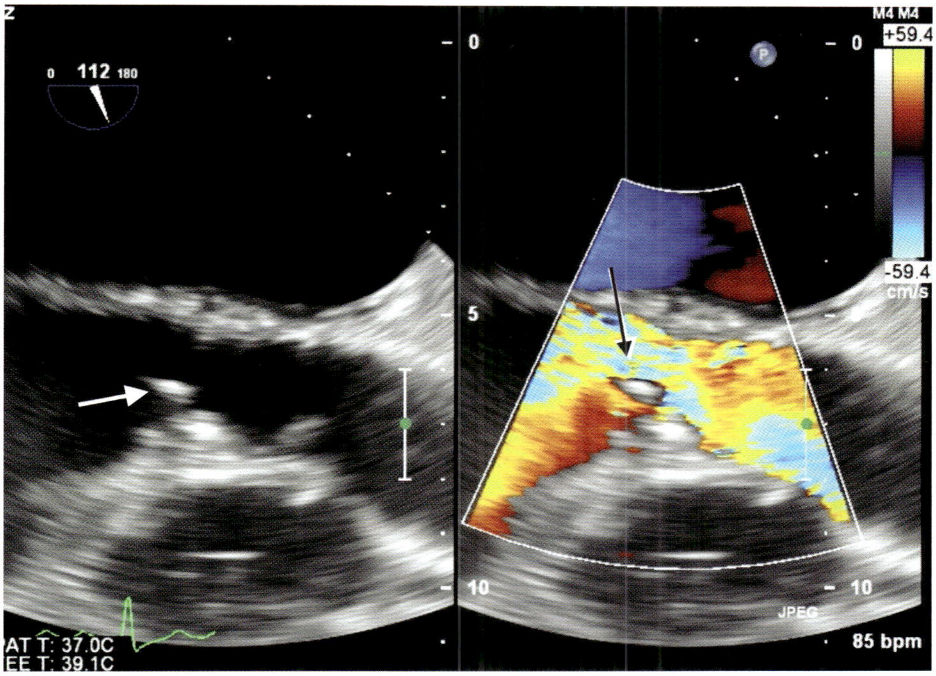

Fig 3.34 A midesophageal long-axis of the aortic valve reveals a thickened and prolapsing RCC *(arrow, left panel)*. Color Doppler shows the regurgitant jet filling the whole LVOT *(arrow, right panel)*.

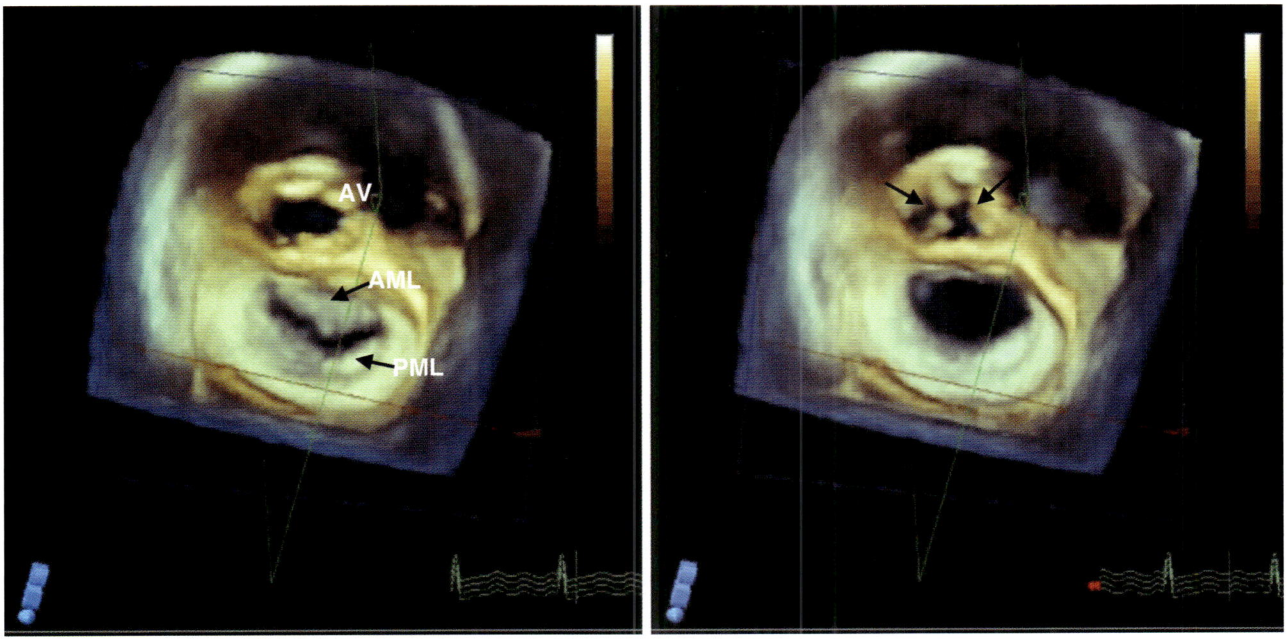

Fig 3.35 3D TEE in systole and diastole *(left and right panels, respectively)*. There is lack of coaptation of the mitral leaflets during systole, which resulted in significant "functional" MR. During diastole leaflet destruction of the aortic valve is seen, with defects in the vicinity of the LCC and NCC *(arrows)*.

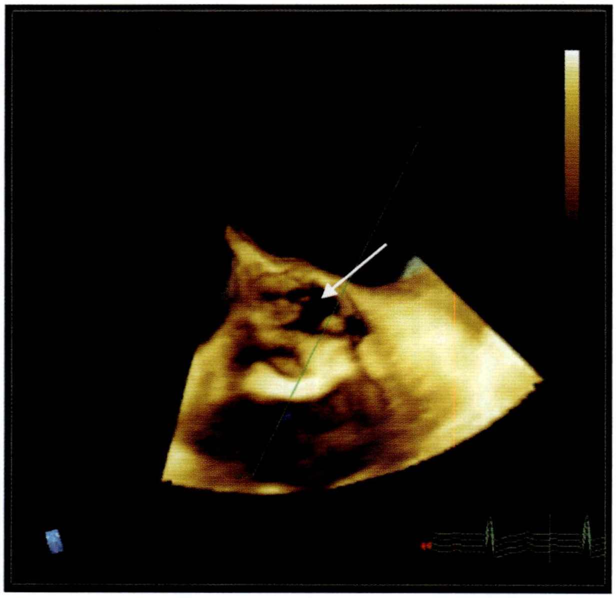

Fig 3.36 A short-axis 3D image of the aortic valve is seen. Leaflet destruction is evident, and the arrow indicates where the LCC would ordinarily be seen.

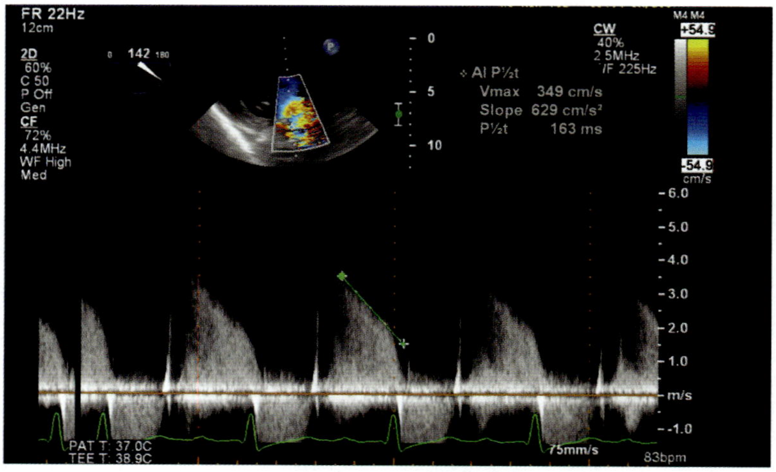

Fig 3.37 CW Doppler shows an extremely short pressure half time consistent with severe AR.

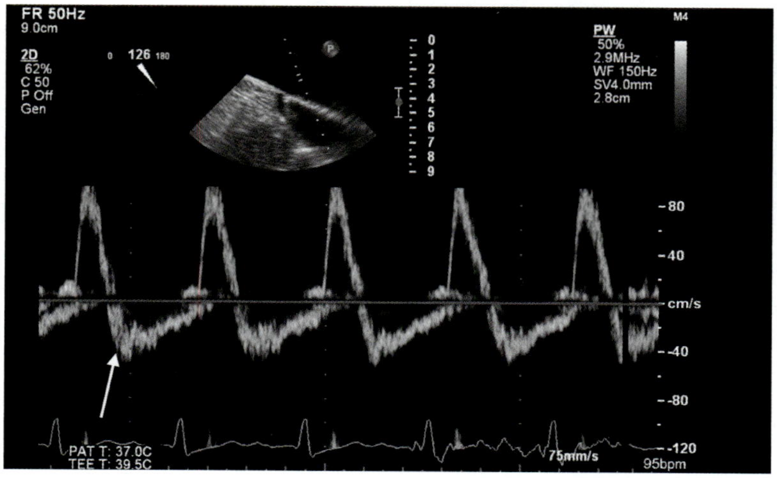

Fig 3.38 PW of the descending aorta shows holodiastolic reversal, also consistent with severe AR.

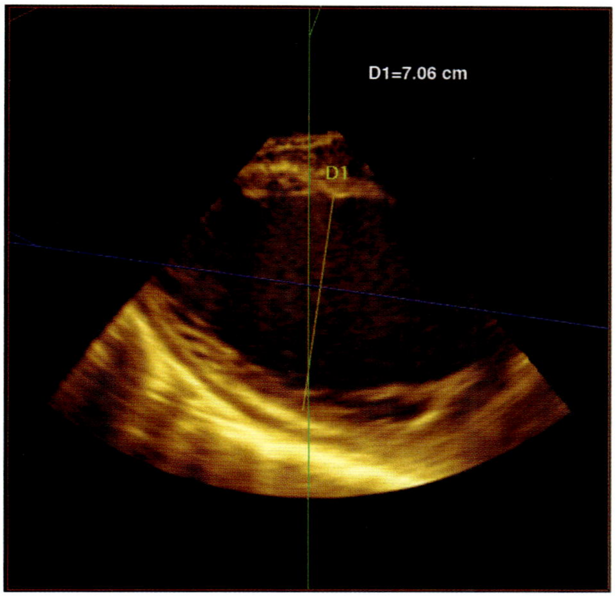

Fig 3.39 The LV in diastole is dilated (7.06 cm), as seen in a transgastric long-axis view.

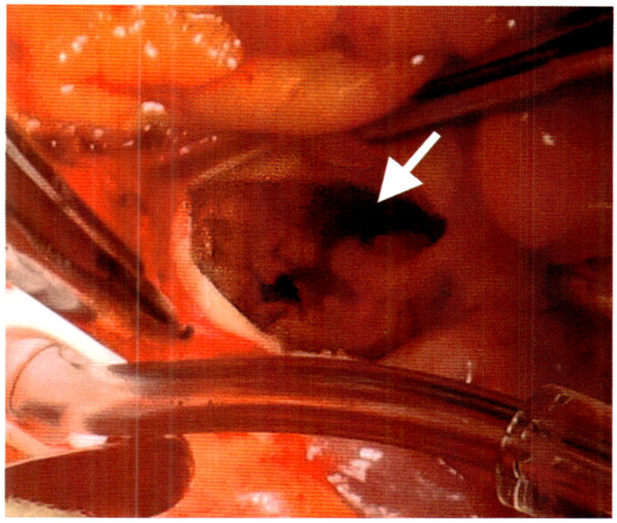

Fig 3.40 The surgeon exposes the valve. There is obvious leaflet thickening. The arrow indicates where the LCC would have been. LCC = left coronary cusp.

Comments

Chronic aortic regurgitation may be caused by disease of the valve leaflets or the aortic root. Examples of aortic root disease include Marfan syndrome and cystic medial necrosis. The most common primary diseases of the valve leaflets producing regurgitation are a congenitally bicuspid aortic valve and rheumatic disease. Congenital valve fenestrations, as seen in this case, are unusual but there are several reports of similar cases. It has been proposed that when congenital fenestrations are in the overlapping part of the valve closure plane, valve function is normal. With an increase in aortic size, possibly related to aging, these overlap regions become load-bearing, resulting in stretching of the fenestration and aortic regurgitation.

Myxomatous valve disease usually primarily involves the mitral valve, with involvement of the aortic valve leaflets seen in only 2% of patients with mitral valve prolapse. Isolated myxomatous changes of the aortic valve are unusual.

The timing of surgery in chronic aortic regurgitation is based on the response of the left ventricle to chronic volume overload and clinical symptoms. Surgery is recommended for patients with severe aortic regurgitation at symptom onset, with the initial symptom typically dyspnea on exertion, as in this case. Patients who remain asymptomatic are at risk of developing irreversible left ventricular systolic function so that annual echocardiography is recommended for monitoring. The parameters that are most useful for predicting a decline in left ventricular contractility are left ventricular size and systolic performance. The most useful echocardiographic parameters are left ventricular end-systolic and end-diastolic dimension and ejection fraction. Although some clinicians prefer left ventricular volume calculations, dimension measurements are more widely used because of their simplicity and reproducibility.

The ACC/AHA Guidelines for Valvular Heart Disease recommend aortic valve surgery for chronic aortic regurgitation when symptoms are present or, in asymptomatic patients, when ejection fraction is <50%, end-systolic dimension is >50 mm, or end-diastolic dimension is >65 mm. The indication for surgery in the case presented here was symptom onset, although the change in ejection fraction and left ventricular dimensions was also worrisome.

Suggested Reading

1. Nishimura RA, Otto CM, Bonow RO, et al: ACC/AHA Task Force Members. 2014 AHA/ACC Guideline for the Management of Patients with Valvular Heart Disease: A report of the American College of Cardiology/American Heart Association Task Force on Practice Guidelines, Circulation 129(23):e521–643, 2014.
2. Vahanian A, Alfieri O, Andreotti F, et al: Joint Task Force on the Management of Valvular Heart Disease of the European Society of Cardiology (ESC); European Association for Cardio-Thoracic Surgery (EACTS). Guidelines on the management of valvular heart disease (version 2012), Eur Heart J 33(19):2451–2496, 2012.
3. Zoghbi WA, Enriquez-Sarano M, Foster E, et al: Recommendations for evaluation of the severity of native valvular regurgitation with two-dimensional and Doppler echocardiography, J Am Soc Echocardiogr 16(7):777–802, 2003.
4. Schäfers HJ, Langer F, Glombitza P, et al: Aortic valve reconstruction in myxomatous degeneration of aortic valves: are fenestrations a risk factor for repair failure? J Thorac Cardiovasc Surg 139(3):660–664, 2010.
5. von Homeyer P, Oxorn D: Aortic Regurgitation: Echocardiographic Diagnosis, Anesth Analg 122: 37–42, 2016.

CASE 3-7
Rheumatic Aortic Regurgitation

This 44-year-old man had a long history of rheumatic valvular heart disease. Four years ago he had an episode of endocarditis caused by *Streptococcus viridans* and was treated with 6 weeks of intravenous antibiotics. Four months ago he had another episode of endocarditis with blood cultures positive for *Haemophilus segnis* and was again treated with 6 weeks of intravenous antibiotics. However, he had the onset of congestive heart failure symptoms, as a result of increasing aortic regurgitation. Echocardiography showed a left ventricular end-systolic dimension of 59 mm, an end-diastolic dimension of 72 mm, and an ejection fraction of 44%. Coronary angiography was normal.

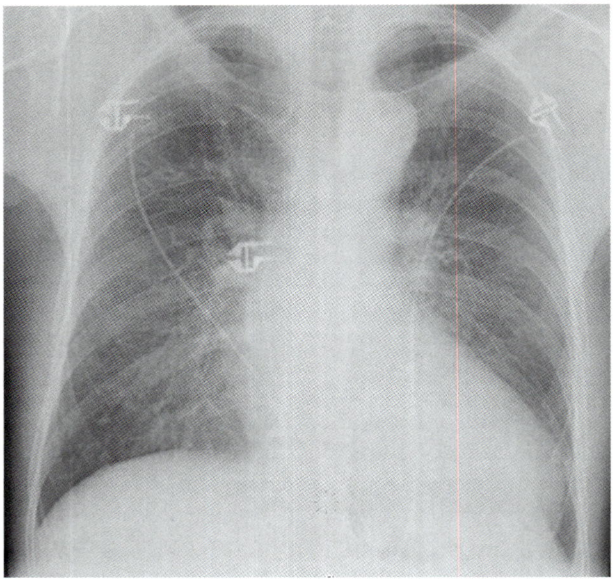

Fig 3.41 Chest radiography shows severe left ventricular enlargement with clear lung fields.

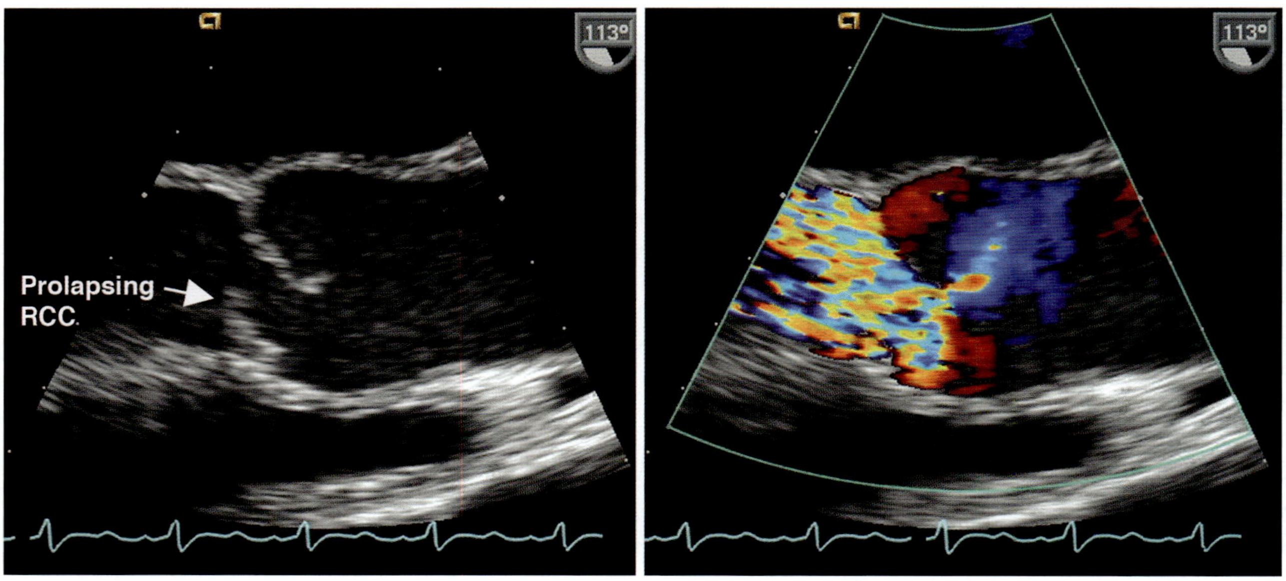

Fig 3.42 Long-axis images *(left)* of the aortic valve were obtained by rotating the image plane to 113 degrees. The aortic leaflets are thickened with slight systolic doming and with partial prolapse of the more anterior leaflet (RCC) into the outflow tract in diastole. Color flow images *(right)* show severe aortic regurgitation with a wide (vena contracta width = 8 mm) eccentric jet through the area of noncoaptation of the leaflets.

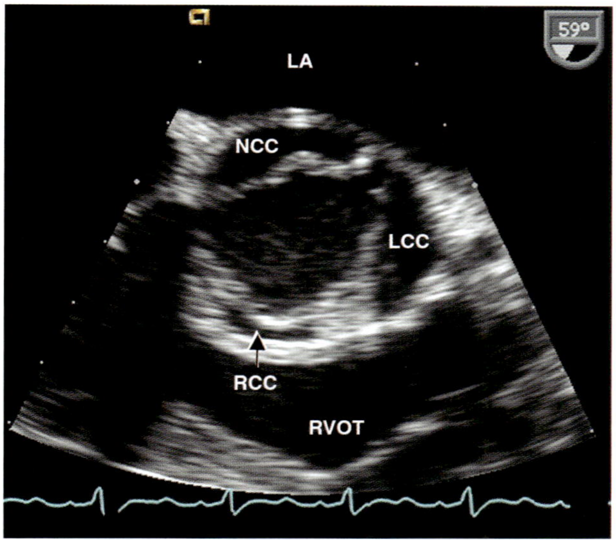

Fig 3.43 Short-axis images of the aortic valve obtained at 59-degree rotation of the image plane show a trileaflet valve with thickening and fusion at the commissures typical for rheumatic disease.

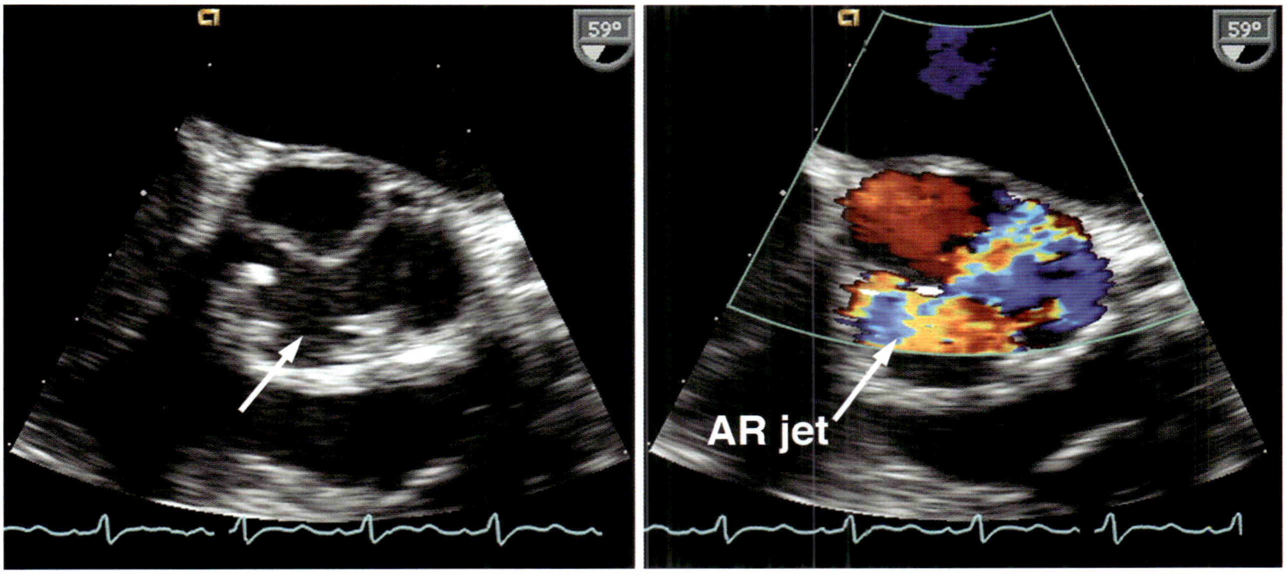

Fig 3.44 Short-axis images of the aortic valve in diastole demonstrate partial destruction of the right coronary cusp resulting from endocarditis *(arrow, left)* with color Doppler *(right)* demonstrating the aortic regurgitant (AR) jet in cross section.

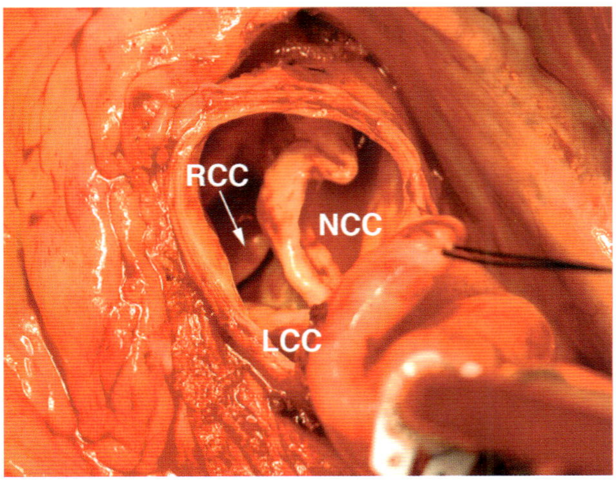

Fig 3.45 At surgery, the valve was trileaflet with commissural fusion typical of rheumatic valve disease and with evidence of destruction of the RCC resulting from previous endocarditis, but no evidence of active infection.

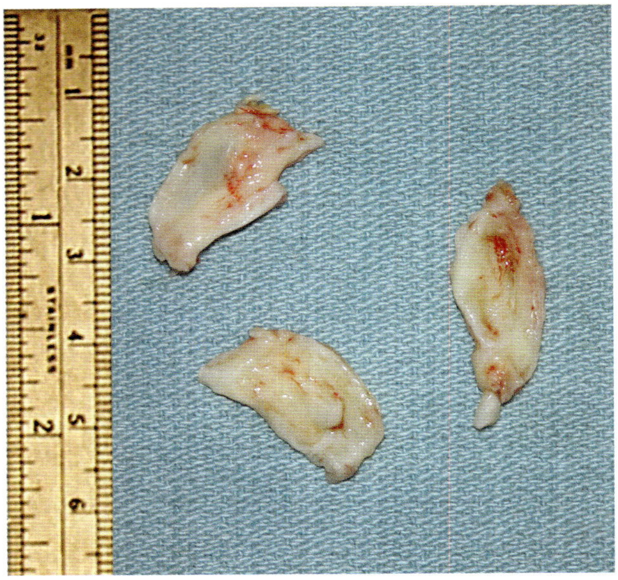

Fig 3.46 The explanted valve shows thickened and deformed valve leaflets, especially along the leaflet edges. Microscopic examination of the valve leaflets demonstrated diffuse leaflet thickening with focal neovascularization consistent with a postinflammatory process, which is typical for rheumatic valve disease.

Comments

This patient, with valve destruction resulting from endocarditis superimposed on chronic rheumatic valve disease, illustrates the issues in establishing the etiology of aortic regurgitation by echocardiography. Evaluation of aortic root anatomy is essential, as surgical intervention for aortic regurgitation caused by root disease differs from the management of primary valve disease. The long-axis image of the ascending aorta demonstrates the sites needed for aortic measurements in patients undergoing aortic valve and/or root surgery:

1. Diameter measurements just proximal to the valve (e.g., the left ventricular outflow tract) are used for continuity equation valve area calculations and correspond to the sewing ring size of stented tissue and mechanical valves.
2. Aortic root enlargement is often most severe at the sinuses of Valsalva.
3. The normal contour of the sinotubular junction is absent in patients with Marfan syndrome, and this measurement site becomes especially important upon implantation of a stentless valve.
4. It is important to visualize and measure ascending aortic diameter in patients with aortic valve disease as the aorta is often abnormal as well.

The physiology in this patient is consistent with a combination of chronic and acute regurgitation. Chronic regurgitation caused by rheumatic disease led to significant left ventricular dilation, with preserved systolic function. However, the additional volume of aortic regurgitation resulting from valve destruction with endocarditis led to clinical decompensation with symptoms of heart failure and a decline in ejection performance.

Suggested Reading

1. Iung B, Vahanian A: Epidemiology of acquired valvular heart disease, Can J Cardiol 30(9):962–970, 2014.
2. Stout KK, Verrier ED: Acute valvular regurgitation, Circulation 119(25):3232–3241, 2009.

CASE 3-8
Traumatic Acute Aortic Regurgitation

This previously healthy 73-year-old woman was transferred directly from the ED to the OR with a diagnosis of acute severe aortic regurgitation. She had been kicked by a horse on her left upper chest and fell backward, hitting a metal pole, with loss of consciousness. She was intubated in the field and then underwent emergency transthoracic and transesophageal echocardiography that showed severe aortic regurgitation and a pericardial effusion.

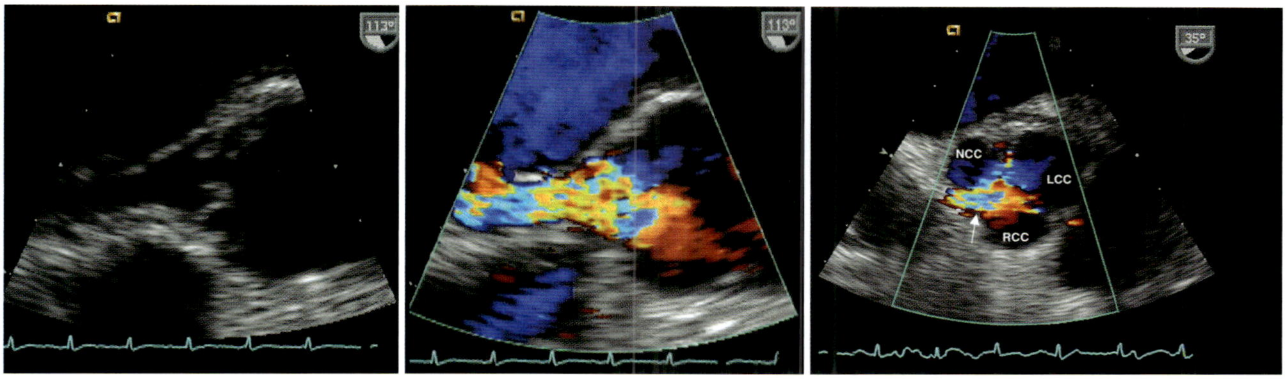

Fig 3.47 TEE in a long-axis view of the aortic valve shows apparent thickening and prolapse of the aortic valve leaflets. On real-time imaging, the flail trileaflet valve is seen. On color Doppler, the regurgitant jet *(arrow)* nearly fills the outflow tract in both long- and short-axis views with a vena contracta diameter $>$15 mm.

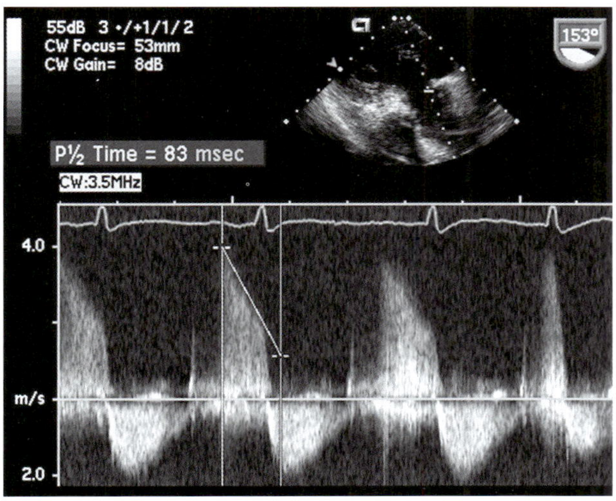

Fig 3.48 Continuous wave Doppler was recorded from a transgastric long-axis view. Although the intercept angle between the ultrasound beam and aortic regurgitant jet may result in underestimation of velocity, the intensity of the velocity curve relative to antegrade flow indicates severe regurgitation. In addition, the steep deceleration slope indicates rapid equilibration of aortic and ventricular diastolic pressures consistent with acute regurgitation.

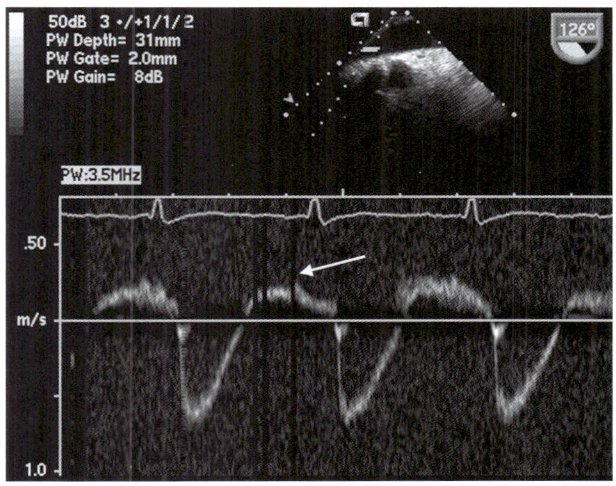

Fig 3.49 Pulsed Doppler recording of flow in the descending thoracic aorta shows holodiastolic flow reversal *(arrow)* confirming the presence of severe aortic regurgitation. This signal is best recorded starting from a short-axis view of the descending thoracic aorta, rotating the image plane to a long-axis view and then placing the pulsed Doppler sample volume as distal as possible in the aorta, to obtain a relatively parallel intercept angle. If the Doppler beam is perpendicular to the direction of flow, there will be no Doppler signal, because the cosine of 90 degrees (in the Doppler equation) is zero.

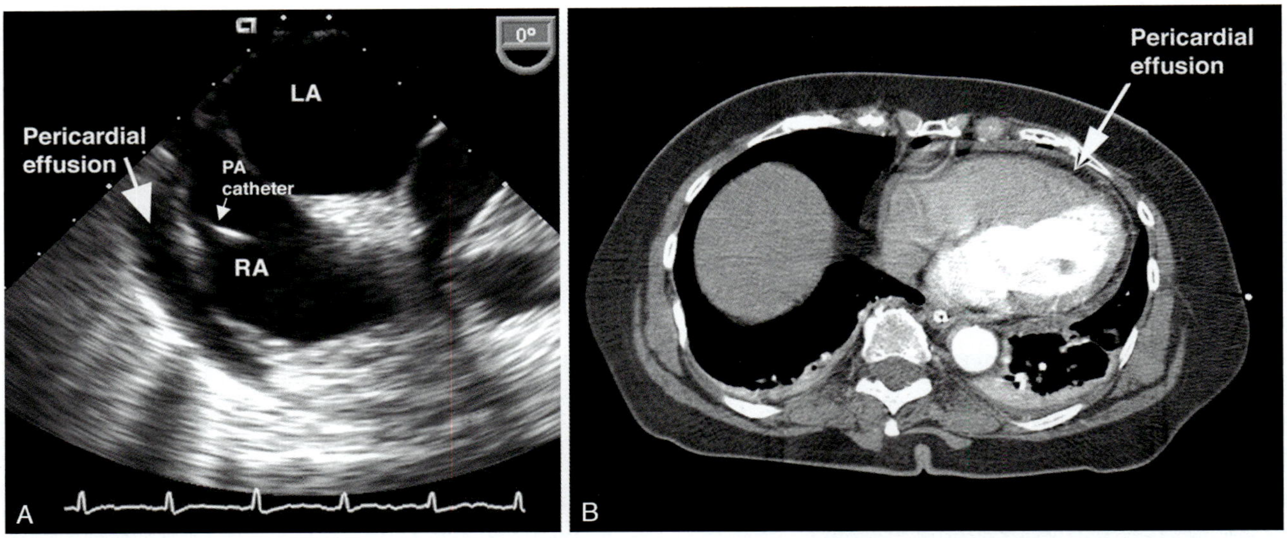

Fig 3.50 A small pericardial effusion is present adjacent to the right atrium in this high transesophageal view, and on CT scanning. The pulmonary artery catheter is seen in the right atrium. On opening of the pericardium at surgery, there was evidence of high pericardial pressures with a moderate amount of pericardial fluid.

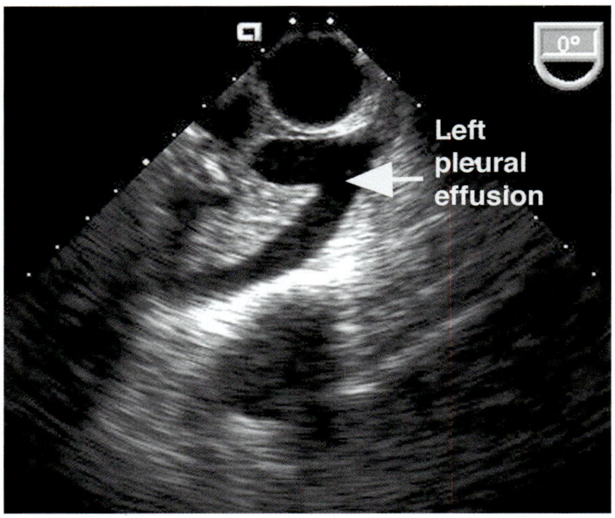

Fig 3.51 A left pleural effusion is noted when the image plane is oriented toward the descending thoracic aorta.

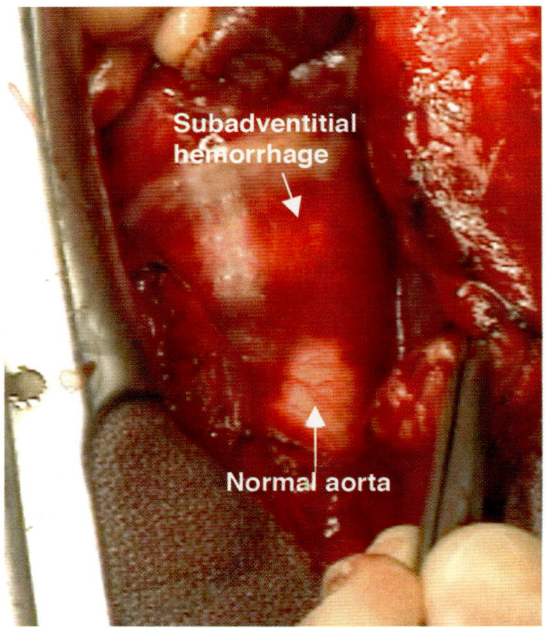

Fig 3.52 After sternotomy, aortic subadventitial hemorrhage was noted.

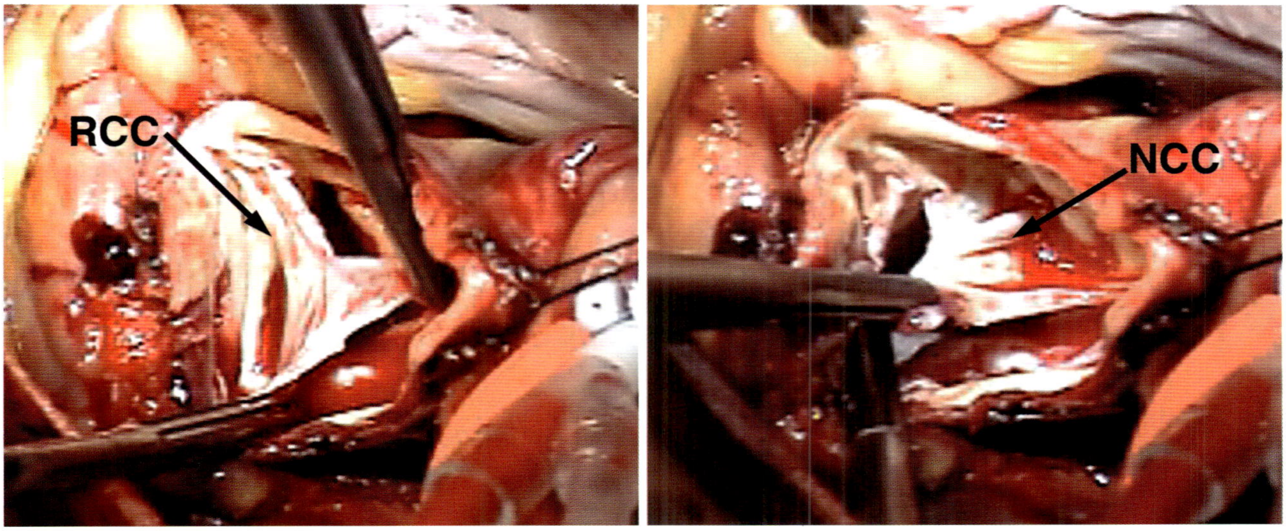

Fig 3.53 On direct inspection of the aortic valve at surgery, there was disruption of the commissure between the right and noncoronary cusps, resulting in flail motion of both leaflets.

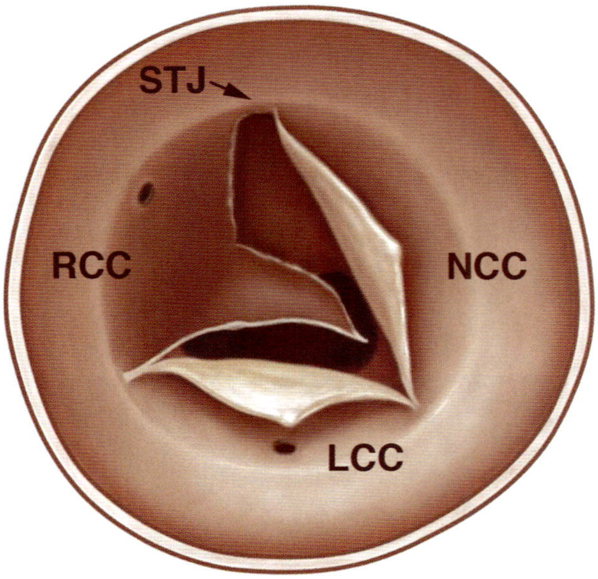

Fig 3.54 This drawing shows how disruption of the attachment of the RCC to the sinotubular junction (STJ) and tearing of the body of the leaflet would result in valvular incompetence. The torn NCC is not illustrated here.

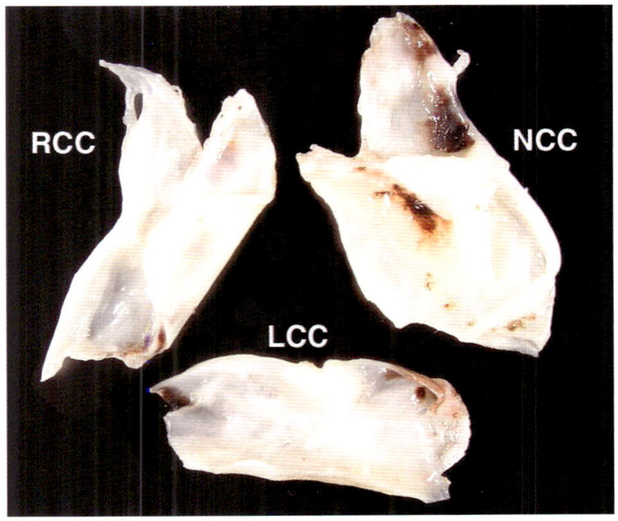

Fig 3.55 The explanted valve shows the tearing and disruption of the right and noncoronary cusps. The aortic valve was replaced with a tissue prosthesis and the patient had a successful recovery.

Comments

Blunt trauma to the chest can cause a range of cardiac disorders, including myocardial contusion and disruption of the thoracic aorta related to deceleration and traction. Valve injury is less common, with most cases involving the anteriorly located tricuspid valve. However, some valve damage is postulated to be related to sudden changes in ventricular or aortic pressure and may affect the left-sided valves. For example, in early diastole the closed aortic valve may be damaged by a sudden increase in aortic pressure, resulting in increased mechanical force on the valve leaflets. The acute onset in this case is consistent with either direct compression of the heart by the horse kick or a sudden rise in aortic pressure resulting in a flail aortic leaflet.

There are several approaches to quantitation of aortic regurgitation severity by echocardiography. A simple and useful approach is to measure the narrowest diameter of the regurgitant jet, or the vena contracta. Ideally, both the proximal flow convergence region and distal expansion of the jet are seen, with the vena contracta being the narrow segment just beyond the valve orifice. A vena contracta width >6 mm indicates severe regurgitation, 3 to 6 mm indicates moderate and <3 mm is consistent with mild aortic regurgitation. Another simple measure is evidence for holodiastolic flow reversal in the descending thoracic aorta. A small amount of early diastolic flow reversal is normal, but retrograde flow in the aorta throughout diastole is consistent with severe regurgitation. The signal strength of the continuous wave Doppler aortic regurgitation jet, relative to antegrade flow, provides a qualitative evaluation of regurgitant severity. In addition, the diastolic slope of the aortic regurgitation jet can be measured with a pressure half-time <200 (i.e., a steeper slope) consistent with severe regurgitation. This patient met all these criteria for severe aortic regurgitation with a wide vena contracta width, a dense continuous wave signal with a steep deceleration slope and dramatic holodiastolic flow reversal in the aorta. When the severity of regurgitation is less clear, regurgitant volume, fraction, and orifice area can be calculated based on measurement of volume flow at two intracardiac sites.

Suggested Reading

1. Linefsky JP, Otto CM: Emergency valve disorders. In Fink MP, Vincent JL, Abraham E, et al, editors: Textbook of Critical Care, ed 7, Philadelphia, 2015, Elsevier, Chapter 88.
2. Pretre R, Chilcott M: Blunt trauma to the heart and great vessels, N Engl J Med 336:626–632, 1997.
3. Zoghbi WA, Enriquez-Sarano M, Foster E, et al: Recommendations for evaluation of the severity of native valvular regurgitation with two-dimensional and Doppler echocardiography, J Am Soc Echocardiogr 16(7):777–802, 2003.
4. Anselmino M, Andria A, Lusardi P: Acute traumatic disruption of a bicuspid aortic valve, Eur J Echocardiogr 7(2):109–111, 2006.

CASE 3-9
Perforated Aortic Valve with Regurgitation

This 49-year-old man presented with new-onset heart failure and a diastolic murmur on examination. Six months ago he suffered an inferior myocardial infarction that was treated with a percutaneous coronary intervention. Transthoracic echocardiography showed severe left ventricular dilation with a large area of inferior akinesis and an ejection fraction of 29%. There was moderate central mitral regurgitation caused by abnormal left ventricular geometry resulting in tethering of the posterior leaflet. The estimated pulmonary systolic pressure was 75 mm Hg. In addition, severe aortic regurgitation was present on Doppler examination, although the etiology of valve dysfunction was uncertain.

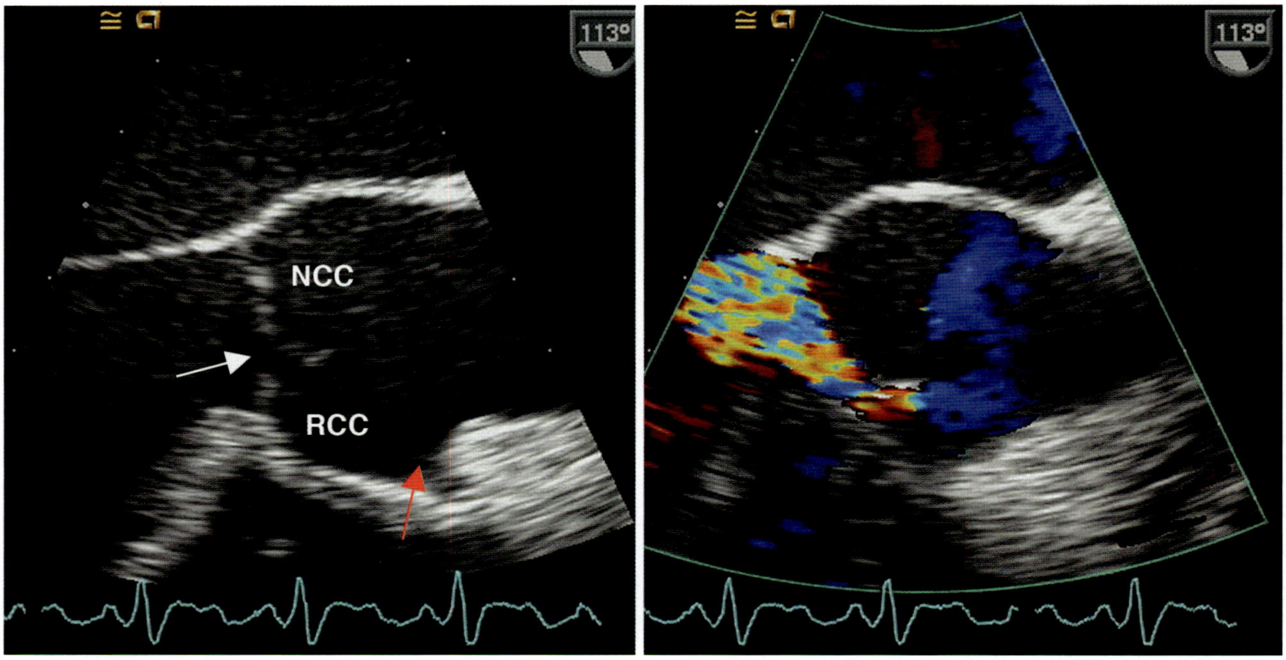

Fig 3.56 The 2D midesophageal long-axis view *(left)* shows the normal aortic root size and anatomy with the NCC (less likely the LCC) and RCC of the aortic valve. Discontinuity is noted in the RCC *(white arrow)* with an eccentric jet of aortic regurgitation through this region on color flow imaging *(right)*. The red arrow indicates the orifice of the right coronary artery.

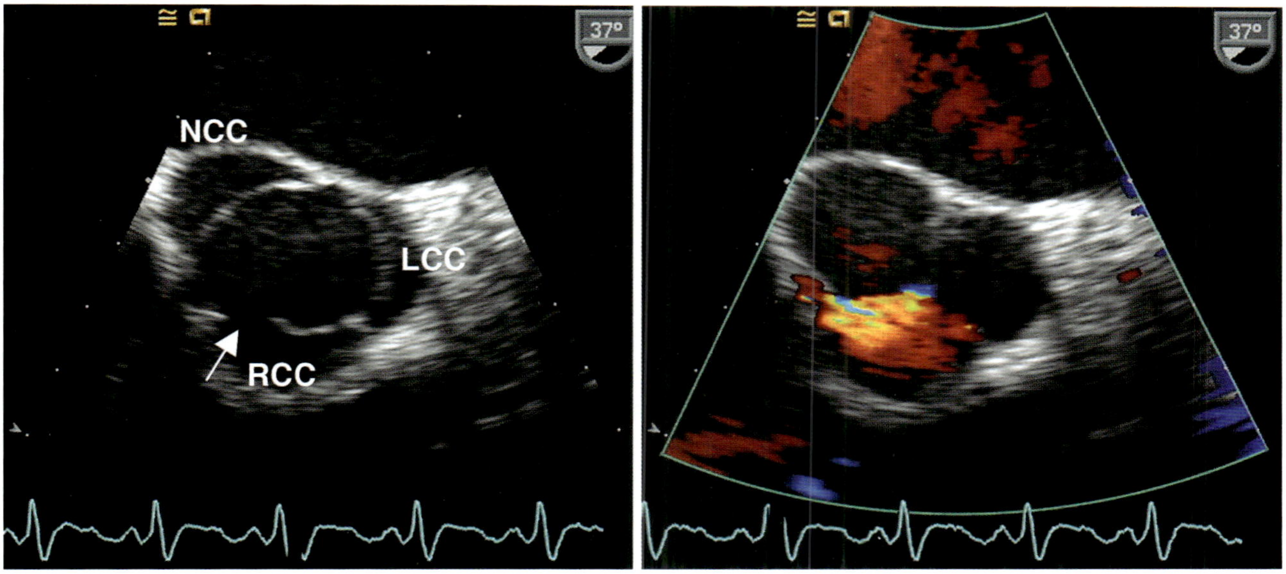

Fig 3.57 The corresponding short-axis view of the aortic valve shows a trileaflet valve with normal systolic motion. Color flow imaging *(right)* shows a wide jet of aortic regurgitation in the region of the RCC. These findings are consistent with a perforation of the RCC *(arrow, left)*.

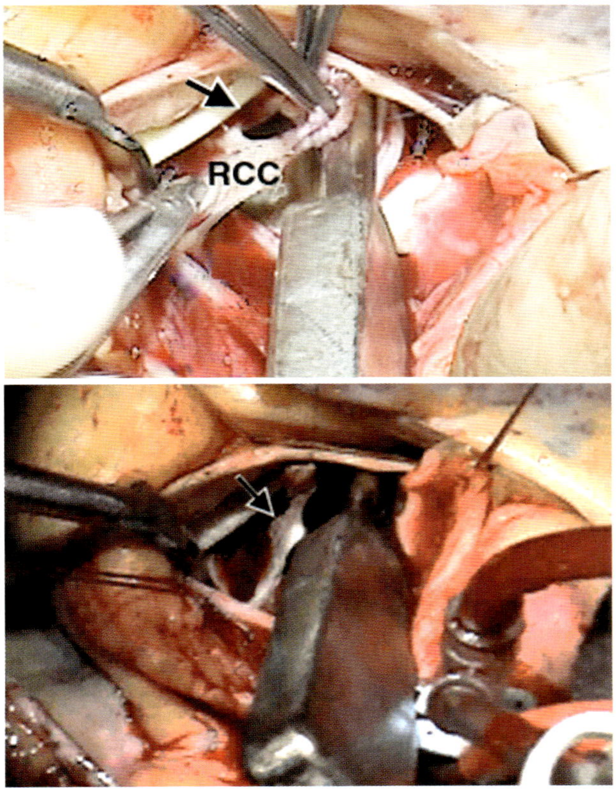

Fig 3.58 *(Top)* Inspection of the valve at surgery showed a perforation in the RCC, as shown by the arrow. *(Bottom)* The valve was repaired with a pericardial patch on the RCC, as shown by the arrow.

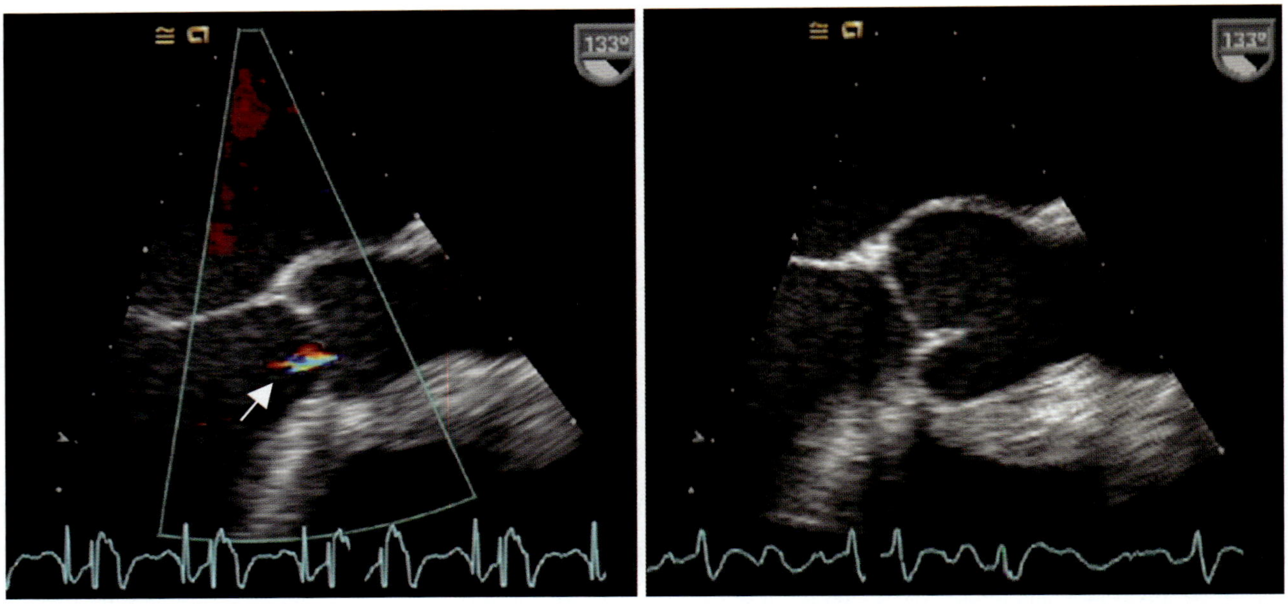

Fig 3.59 After weaning from cardiopulmonary bypass, long-axis images of the repaired valve show normal motion and only trace central aortic regurgitation *(arrow)*.

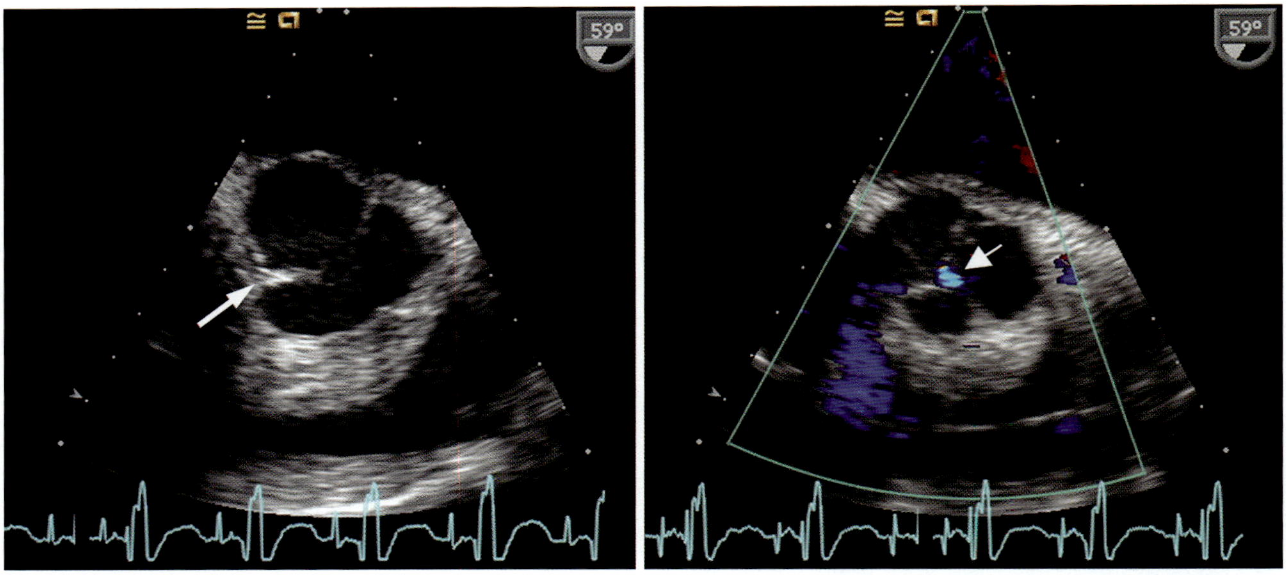

Fig 3.60 Short-axis views of the aortic valve after RCC repair *(left, arrow)* show only a small jet of central aortic regurgitation *(right, arrow)*.

Comments

Traumatic injury of the aortic valve resulting from a percutaneous coronary intervention is rare but is the most likely cause of aortic regurgitation in this patient given the perforation in the right coronary cusp and the normal tissue characteristics of the other valve leaflets. This patient tolerated the aortic regurgitation for several months before presenting with congestive heart failure symptoms, which suggests that an initial small tear in the leaflet may have gradually increased in size, resulting in subacute aortic regurgitation with time for ventricular compensation. The severe ventricular enlargement, which had improved by 6 months after surgery, is consistent with chronic volume overload of the left ventricle.

Suggested Reading

1. Hill AC, Bansal RC, Razzouk AJ, et al: Echocardiographic recognition of iatrogenic aortic valve leaflet perforation, Ann Thorac Surg 64(3):684–689, 1997.
2. Tuluca A, Omer S, Cornwell L, et al Aortic valve leaflet entrapment by a percutaneous closure device, Ann Thorac Surg 98(1):e23–25, 2014.

The Bicuspid Aortic Valve

CASE 3-10
Combined Stenosis and Regurgitation

A 52-year-old woman with a bicuspid aortic valve was referred for valve replacement. Fourteen years ago she underwent resection of a benign cardiac tumor that was located in the LVOT just proximal to the aortic valve. At that time, direct inspection of the aortic valve showed a bicuspid valve with thin leaflets and echocardiography showed normal valve function. Over the past 3 months she noted increasing dyspnea on exertion, with physical examination showing a 3/6 aortic stenosis murmur, a 2/6 aortic regurgitant murmur, and diminished carotid upstrokes.

TTE results were as follows: There was moderate coexisting aortic regurgitation with mild left ventricular dilation, moderate concentric hypertrophy and an ejection fraction of 61%. Dilation of the ascending aorta was present with a maximum diameter on chest CT of 5.0 cm.

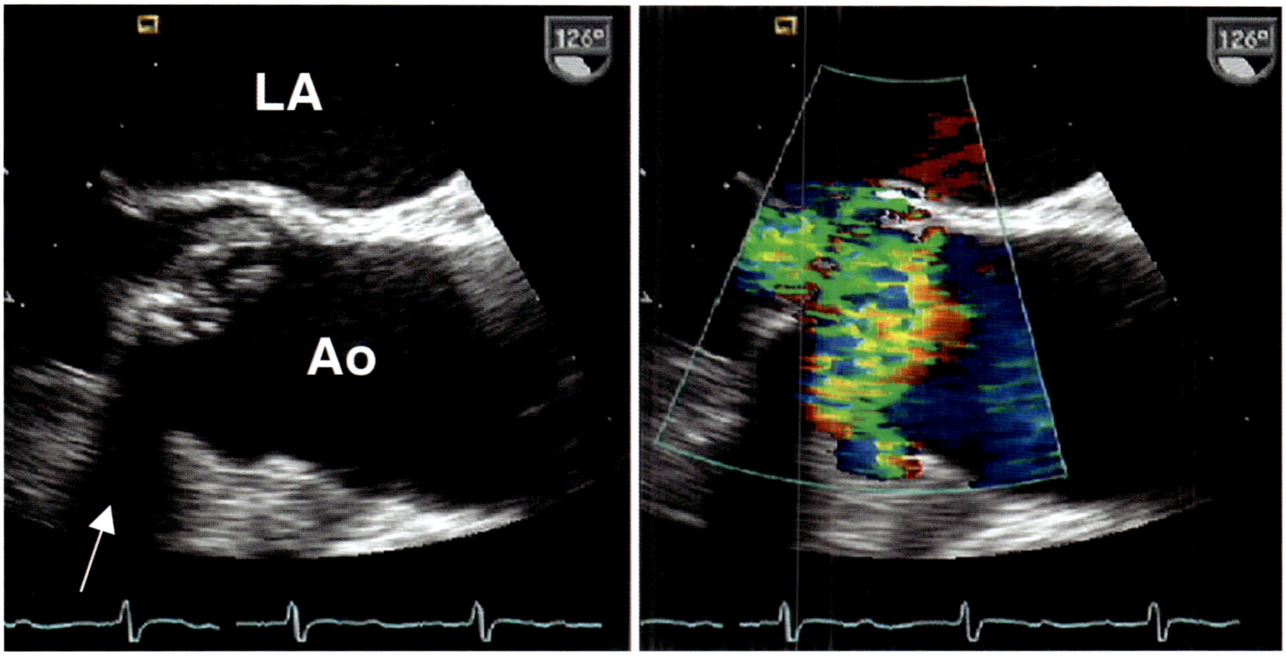

Fig 3.61 Intraoperative TEE in a midesophageal long-axis view of the aortic valve in diastole with 2D images *(left)* and color flow Doppler *(right)*. Note the thickening and calcification of the aortic valve with prominent shadowing *(arrow)*. A broad jet of aortic regurgitation is seen, filling about 60% of the diameter of the outflow tract, with a vena contracta width >12 mm. On this frame, which best demonstrates the maximum width of the vena contracta of the aortic regurgitant jet, a flow disturbance (in green mosaic) is seen on the aortic side of the valve caused by flow acceleration into the regurgitant orifice. The flow dynamics of the aortic regurgitation are better appreciated on the video images.

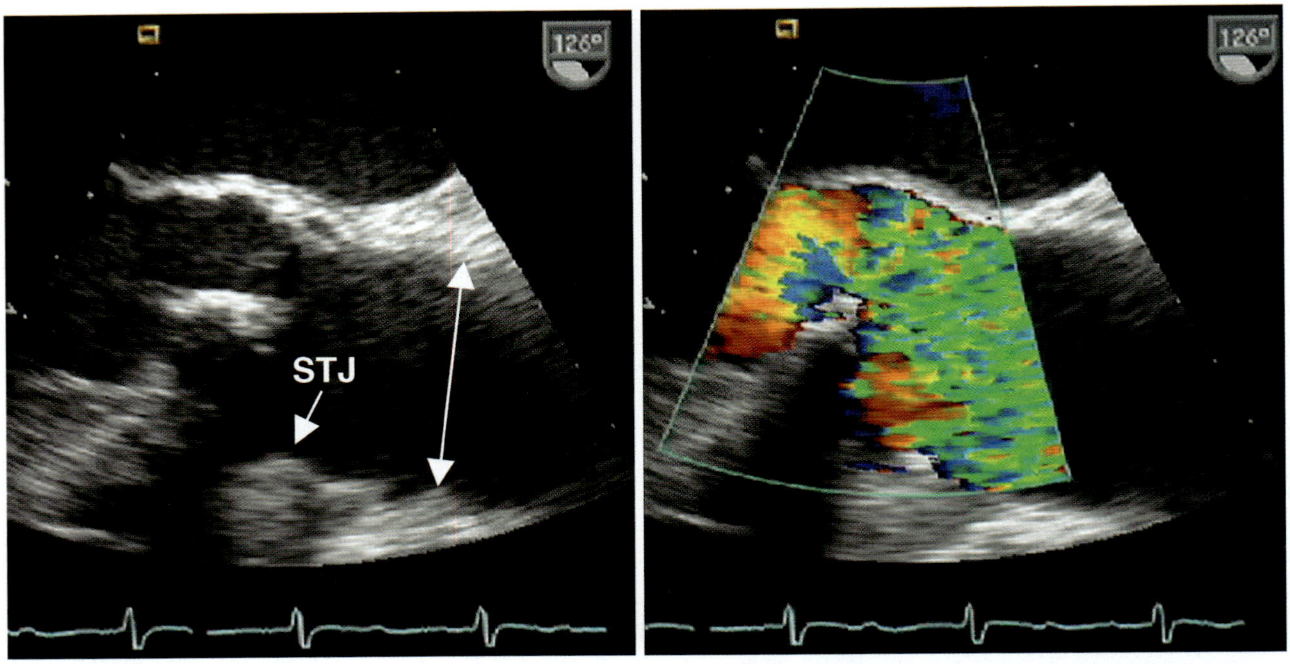

Fig 3.62 Long-axis view of the aortic valve in systole, with 2D images showing a restricted valve opening *(left)* with an eccentric antegrade jet of flow on color Doppler *(right)*. The bicuspid valve shows systolic "doming" with the smallest valve orifice at the leaflet tips. Also note the dilated ascending aorta *(arrows)* but with a normal contour of the sinotubular junction (STJ).

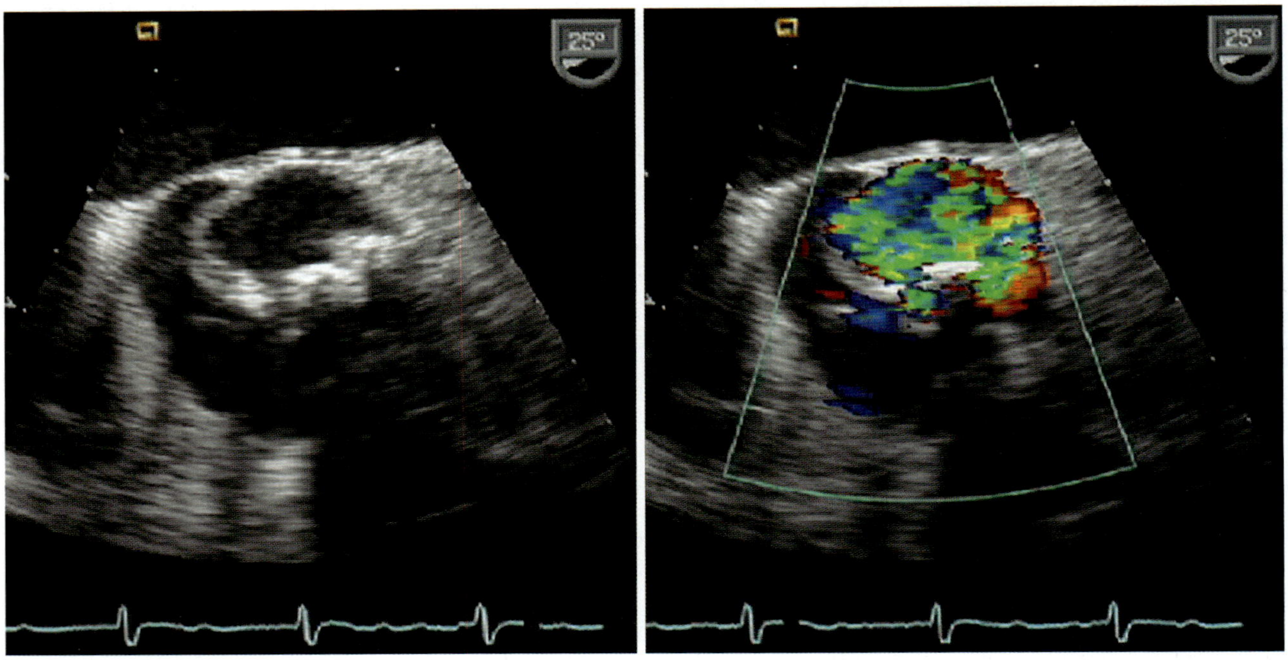

Fig 3.63 Short-axis views of the aortic valve in midsystole showing eccentric valve opening with only one commissure evident on 2D imaging *(left)*. Color Doppler confirms that antegrade flow is confined to this eccentric orifice *(right)*. With the doming of this bicuspid congenitally abnormal aortic valve, planimetry of valve area in short-axis views is problematic as the tomographic plane may be through the base of the doming leaflets, rather than at the leaflet tips. Thus the apparent large opening seen on this image does not represent the smallest valve area and should not be measured. The continuity equation valve area is a more accurate descriptor of functional valve area in this situation.

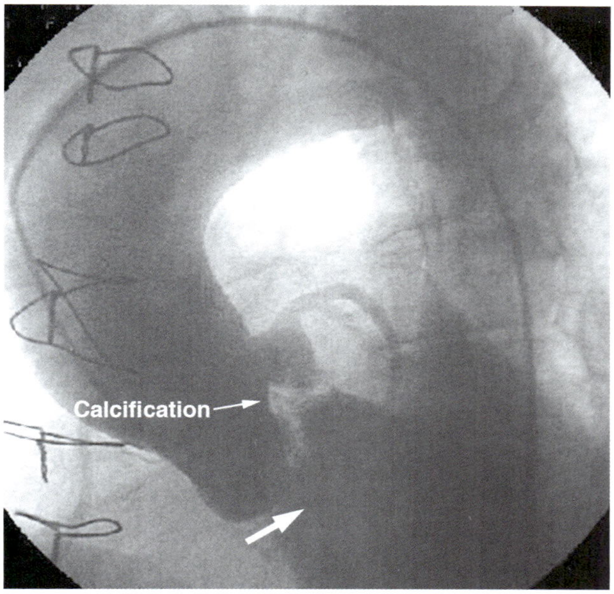

Fig 3.64 Aortogram with contrast injected into the ascending aorta shows severe valve calcification and dilation of the ascending aorta. Moderate aortic regurgitation is evident with contrast refluxing into the left ventricle, with an equal density of contrast in the left ventricle *(arrow)* and aorta after several beats.

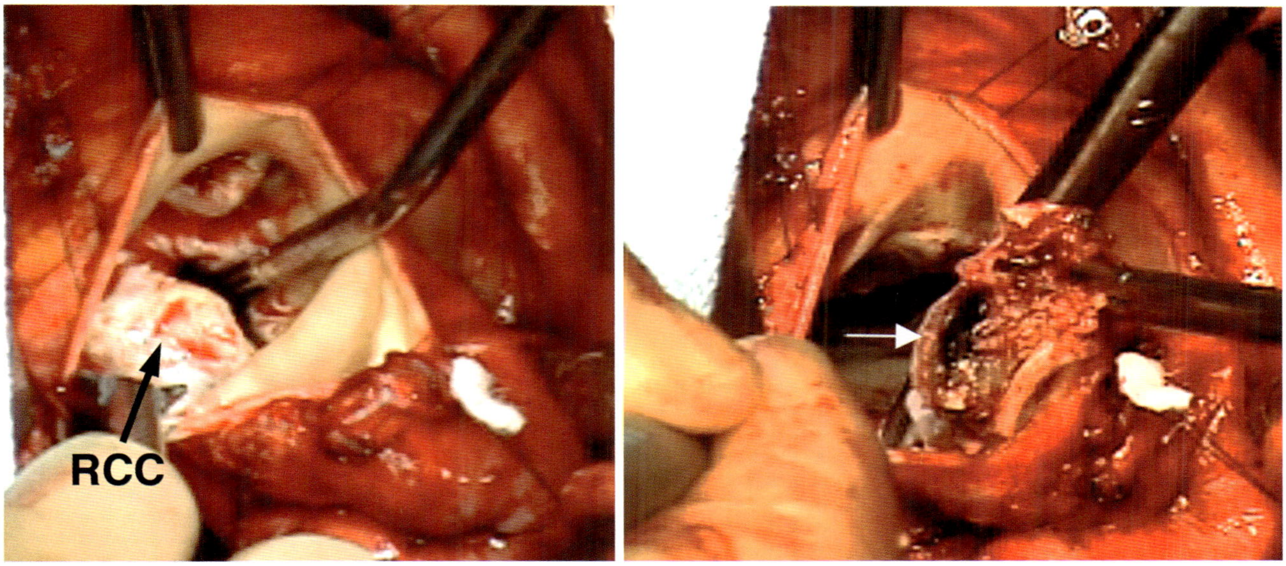

Fig 3.65 Inspection of the valve at surgery showed a bicuspid valve with severe fusion of two cusps resulting in a functional unicuspid valve *(left)*. The valve was heavily calcified with evidence of chronic inflammation beneath the right coronary cusp *(right, arrow)*, possibly caused by a jet lesion related to her previous outflow tract tumor. The aortic valve was resected and replaced with a 27-mm Carpentier-Edwards pericardial valve and the dilated ascending valve was replaced with a woven polyester aortic graft.

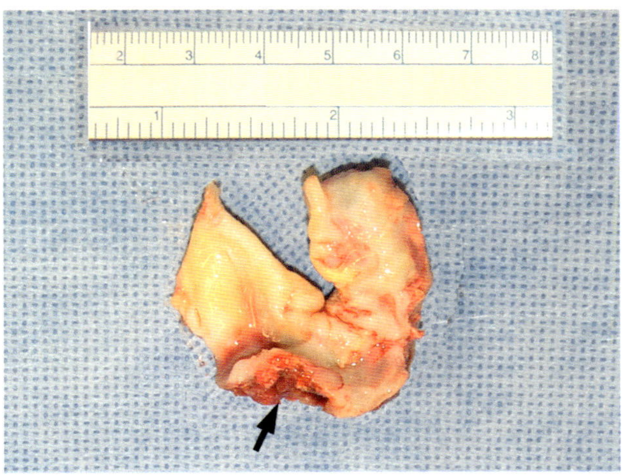

Fig 3.66 The excised valve appears unicuspid with severe calcification. The valve has been oriented to match the short-axis view in Fig 3.63. Note how the shape and size of the valve opening and the appearance of calcification on the pathology specimen correspond to the echocardiographic image. The arrow indicates the chronic inflammation beneath the right coronary cusp.

Comments

Some patients with a congenital bicuspid aortic valve develop severe aortic regurgitation with left ventricular dilation, requiring valve surgery in young adulthood. However, most patients have normal valve function until the fifth or sixth decade of life when progressive valve calcification results in outflow obstruction, often with some degree of coexisting aortic regurgitation. When severe stenosis results in symptoms, aortic valve replacement is needed. In this case the extent of valve deformity may have been affected by abnormal subvalvular hemodynamics related to the woman's outflow tract tumor.

Aortic stenosis presents with symptoms at a younger age in patients with a bicuspid valve rather than a trileaflet valve, presumably related to earlier calcification secondary to the abnormal shear and tensile stresses of the bicuspid valve leaflets. However, once mild stenosis is present, the rate of hemodynamic progression is similar, regardless of underlying valve anatomy. Over the past 6 years, this woman's progression was typical, with an increase in jet velocity of 0.3 m/s per year and a decrease in valve area of $0.1 cm^2$ per year.

Suggested Reading

1. Otto CM, Prendergast B: Aortic-valve stenosis—from patients at risk to severe valve obstruction, N Engl J Med 371(8):744–756, 2014.
2. Tzemos N, Therrien J, Yip J, et al: Outcomes in adults with bicuspid aortic valves, JAMA 300(11):1317–1325, 2008.
3. Michelena HI, Desjardins VA, Avierinos JF, et al: Natural history of asymptomatic patients with normally functioning or minimally dysfunctional bicuspid aortic valve in the community, Circulation 117(21):2776–2784, 2008.

CASE 3-11
Bicuspid Valve with an Aortic Aneurysm

An asymptomatic 47-year-old man was referred for repair of an ascending aortic aneurysm. Chest CT showed dilation of the ascending aorta, extending into the proximal arch, with a maximum dimension of 58 mm. On TTE, a bicuspid aortic valve with mild-to-moderate aortic regurgitation was seen with normal left ventricular size and systolic function. Cardiac catheterization showed normal coronary arteries, mild–moderate aortic regurgitation, and a dilated ascending aorta.

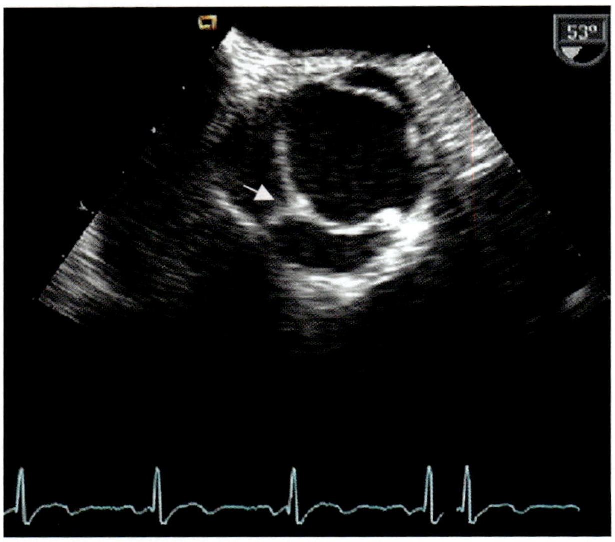

Fig 3.67 The intraoperative TEE short-axis view of the aortic valve shows two leaflets open in systole with a raphe in the larger, anterior cusp *(arrow)*.

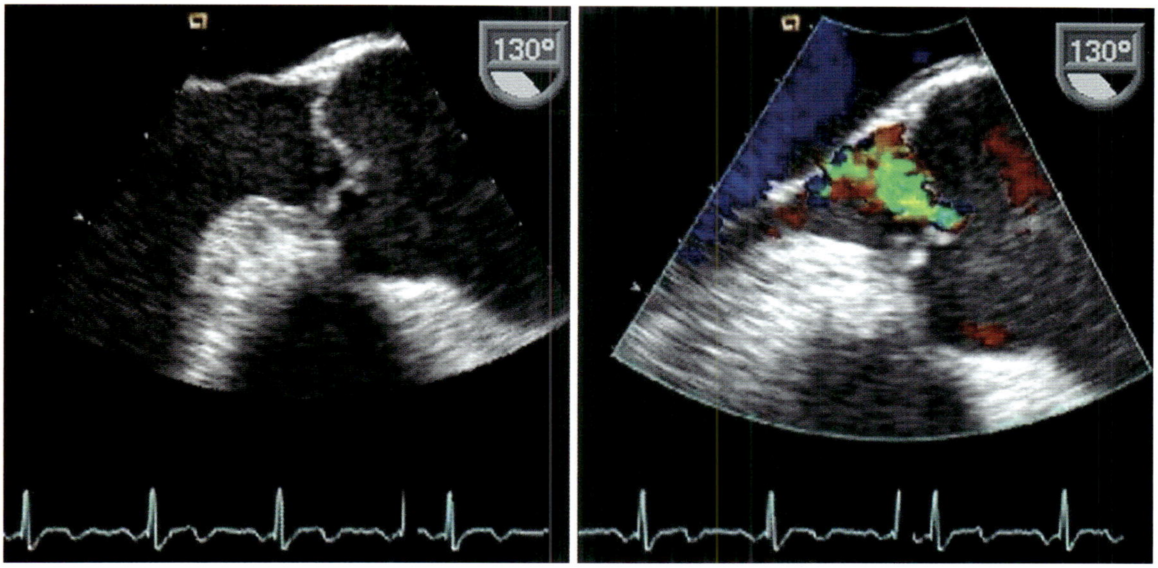

Fig 3.68 A midesophageal long-axis view of the aortic valve in diastole with 2D imaging showing the slight thickening of the closed leaflets *(left)* and color Doppler *(right)* showing mild aortic regurgitation with a vena contracta width of 3 mm. The aortic regurgitation originates centrally, which is consistent with stretched leaflets resulting in inadequate central coaptation caused by aortic root dilation.

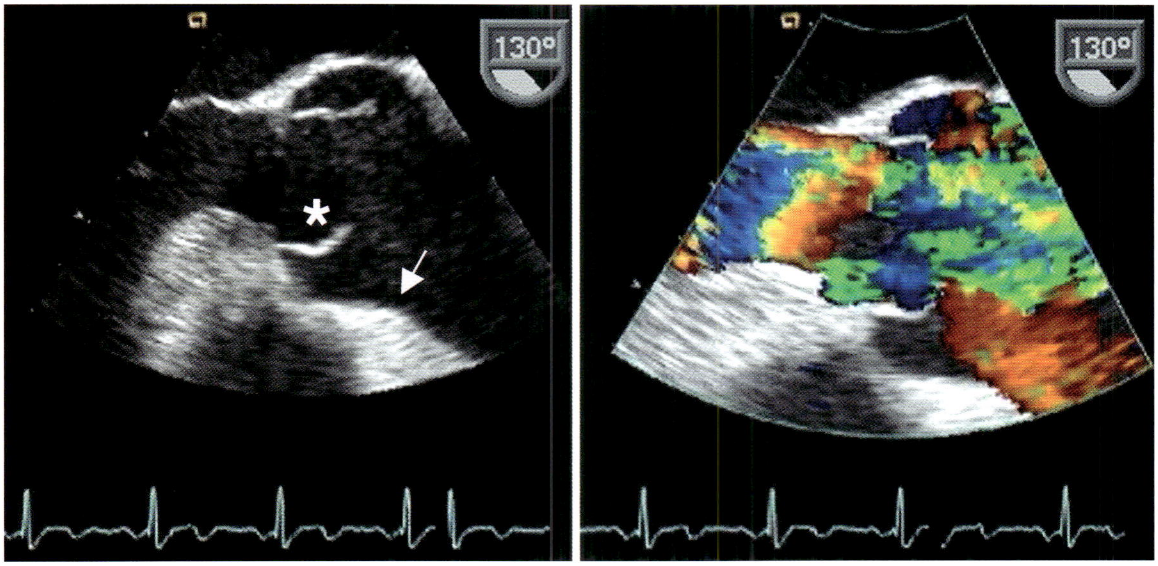

Fig 3.69 Long-axis view in systole with 2D imaging showing the open aortic leaflets *(left)* and color Doppler showing no outflow obstruction *(right)*. The more anterior right coronary cusp is "domed" *(asterisk)*. Note that the sinotubular junction *(arrow)* and contour of the sinuses of Valsalva appear normal despite the ascending aortic aneurysm.

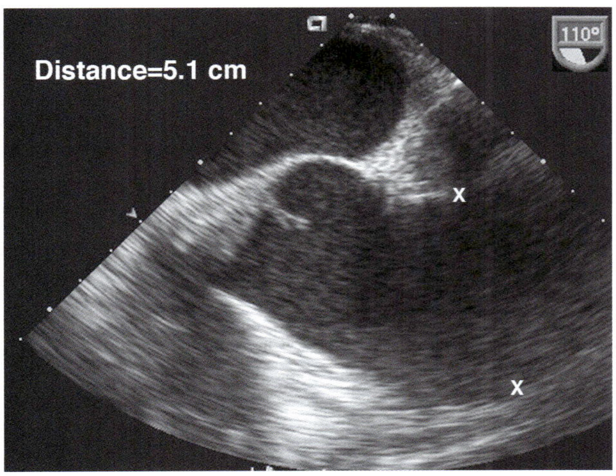

Fig 3.70 Long-axis view of the ascending aorta reveals the aneurysmal dilation.

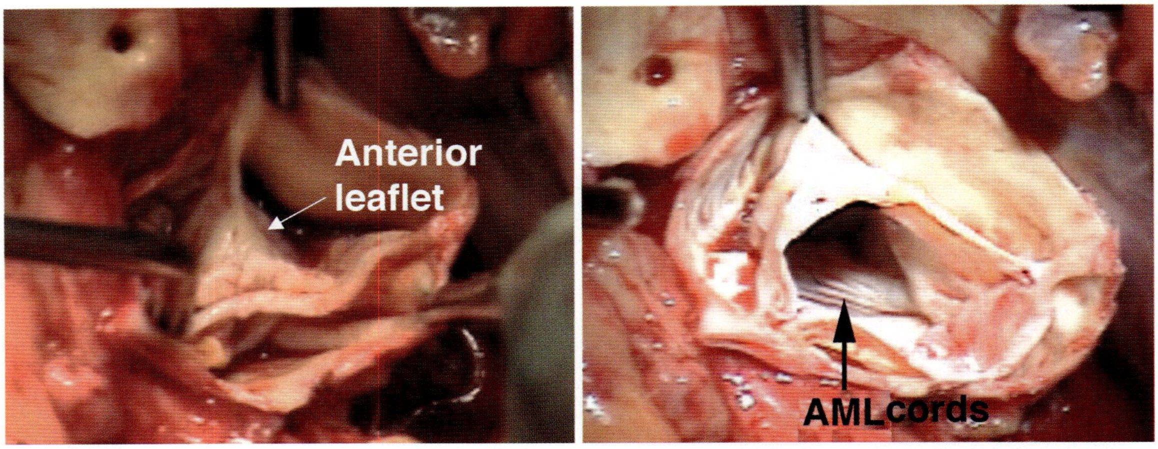

Fig 3.71 Surgical view of the bicuspid aortic valve *(left)*. The larger anterior leaflet is excessively redundant and thinned *(right)*. Chords of the anterior mitral leaflet (AML) are seen through the aortic valve orifice.

Comments

Although this patient presented primarily with an ascending aortic aneurysm, some degree of aortic dilation is common in patients with a bicuspid aortic valve. Even when the dilation is not as severe as in this case, the presence of a bicuspid aortic valve is associated with an increased risk of aortic dissection, even after valve replacement. Thus evaluation of the ascending aorta and consideration of the surgical approach is essential in patients with a bicuspid aortic valve.

In this patient, the clinical presentation was similar to Marfan syndrome but can be differentiated based on the lack of associated clinical findings (e.g., ocular, musculoskeletal) and the preservation of the sinotubular junction seen on echocardiography.

Suggested Reading

1. Verma S, Siu SC: Aortic dilatation in patients with bicuspid aortic valve, N Engl J Med 370(20):1920–1929, 2014.
2. Detaint D, Michelena HI, Nkomo VT, et al: Aortic dilatation patterns and rates in adults with bicuspid aortic valves: A comparative study with Marfan syndrome and degenerative aortopathy, Heart 100(2):126–134, 2014.

CASE 3-12
Chronic Aortic Regurgitation

The patient was a 60-year-old male who had presented 1 year previously with shortness of breath on exertion, which he ascribed to lack of conditioning. He began a fitness regimen but found that after a year he was only getting more symptomatic and was now developing exertional chest tightness. His primary care physician then sent him for echocardiogram, which revealed a bicuspid aortic valve, and severe aortic regurgitation. Cardiac catheterization showed normal coronary arteries. He was referred for surgery.

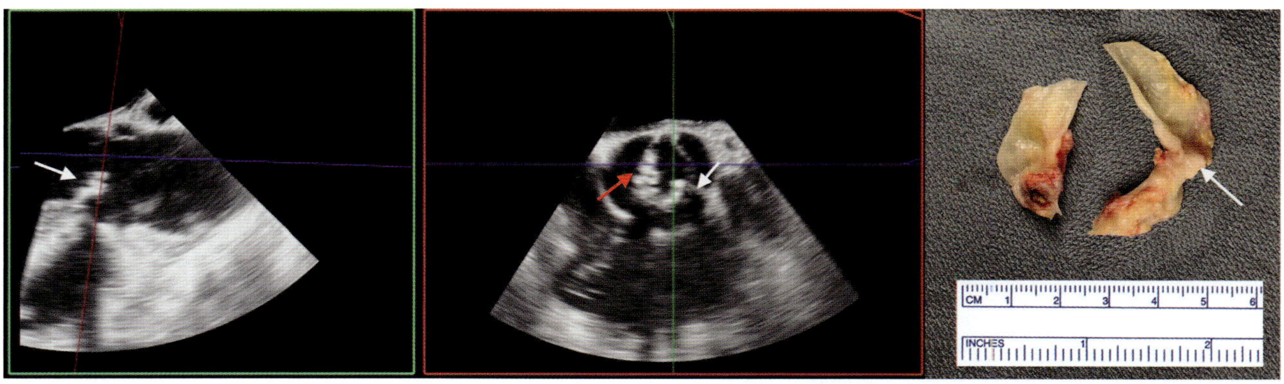

Fig 3.72 In the left panel, a midesophageal long-axis view shows a heavily calcified anterior cusp. The middle panel, a midesophageal short-axis view, shows that the valve is bicuspid, with fusion of the right and left coronary cusps and a raphe *(white arrow)*; the red arrow shows a heavily calcified noncoronary cusp. The right panel shows the explanted leaflets in the same orientation as the midesophageal short-axis view, with the white arrow again indicating the raphe.

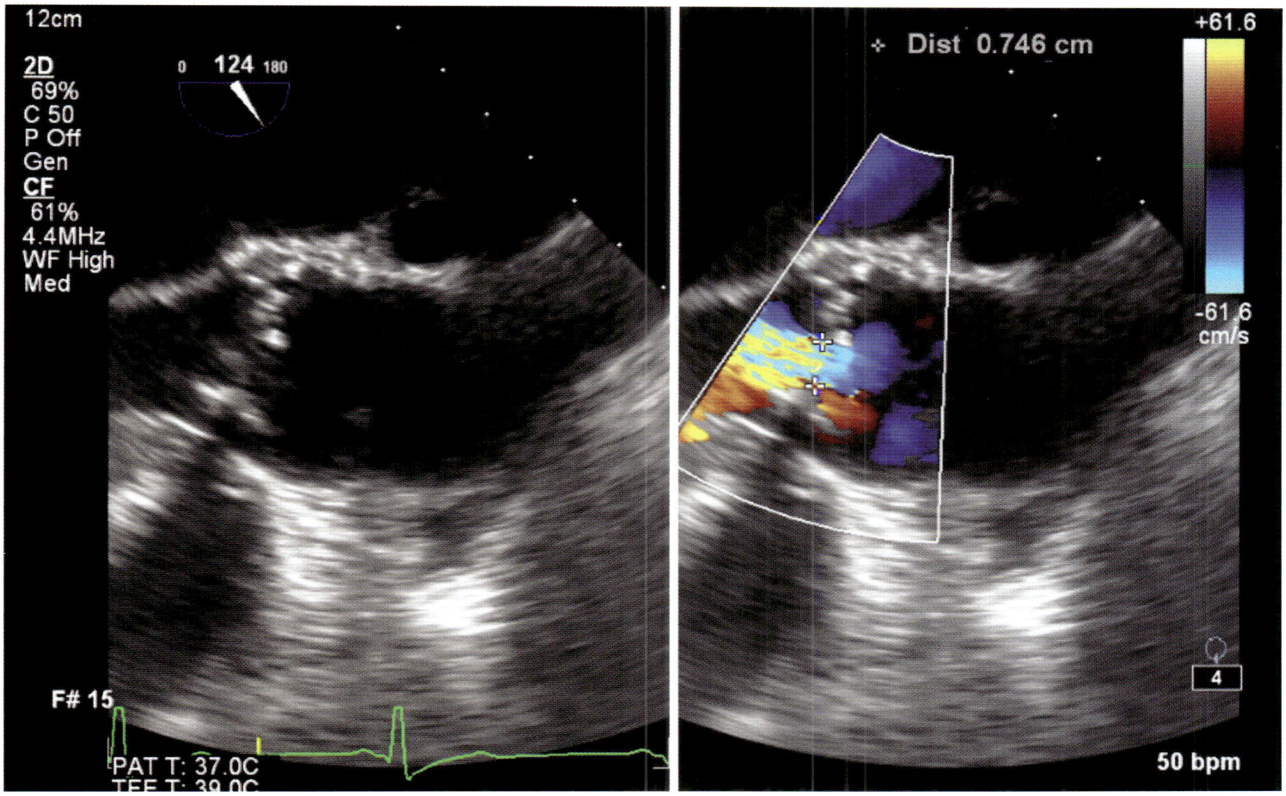

Fig 3.73 A midesophageal long-axis view with color Doppler shows a vena contracta width of 0.75 cm.

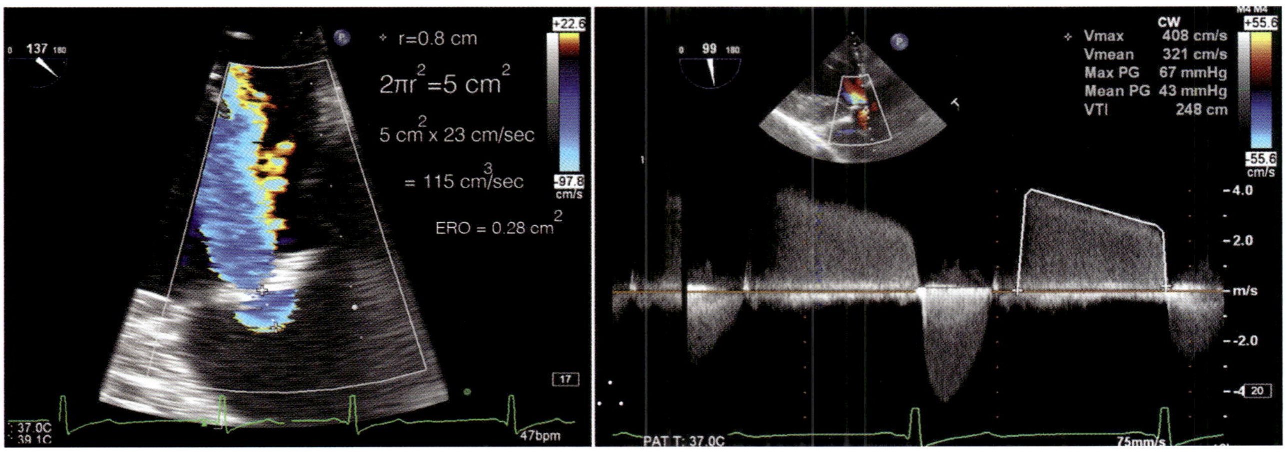

Fig 3.74 Images were obtained from the transgastric long-axis view. In the left panel, the Nyquist baseline has been shifted, yielding a PISA radius of 0.8 cm; thus the PISA is 5 cm^2. Multiplying by the aliasing velocity of 23 cm/s gives a flow of 115 cm^3/s. The right panel shows that the peak velocity of the AR jet is 408 cm/s; applying the continuity equation yields an ERO of 0.28 cm^2. PISA = proximal isovelocity surface area, ERO = effective regurgitant orifice.

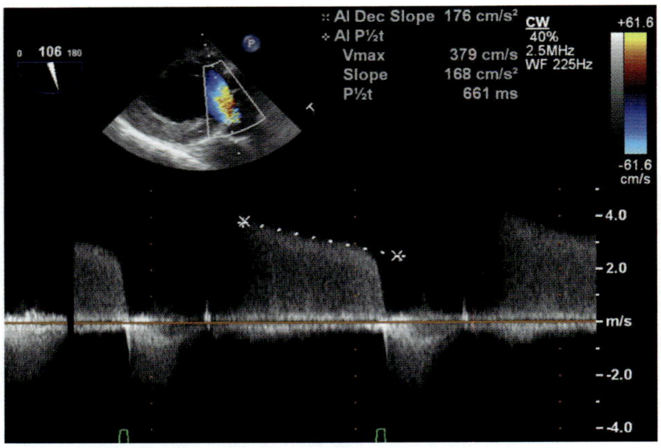

Fig 3.75 From the same view as Fig 3.74, the pressure half-time of the AR jet is 661 m/s.

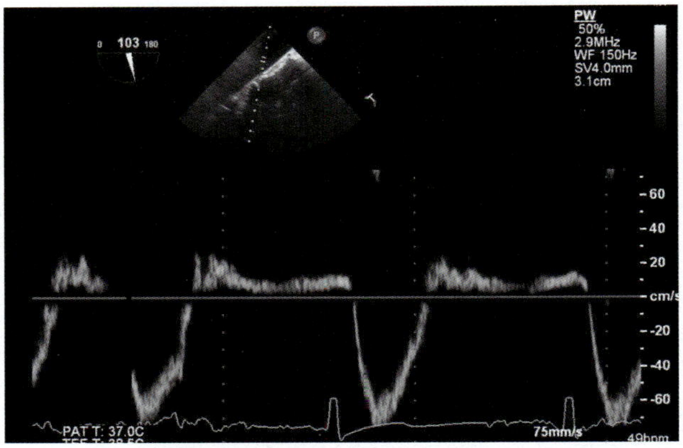

Fig 3.76 From a midesophageal long-axis view, pulse wave Doppler shows pandiastolic flow reversal.

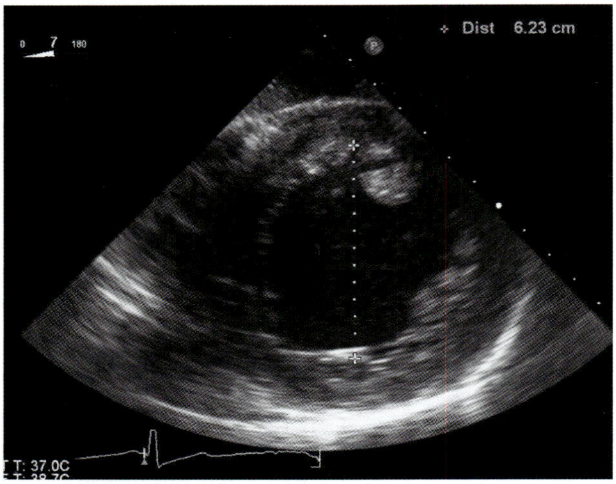

Fig 3.77 From a transgastric short-axis view, the end diastolic diameter of the LV was 6.2 cm.

Comments

This case illustrates several approaches to quantitation of aortic regurgitant severity. Typically, clinical evaluation is based on the vena contracta measurement and density of the CW Doppler signal. The presence of holodiastolic flow reversal in the proximal abdominal aorta indicates that regurgitation is severe whereas holodiasaotlic flow reversal in the descending thoracic aorta, as seen here, may be seen with either moderate or severe aortic regurgitation. Flow reversal in the descending aorta may be seen in the absence of aortic regurgitation (a "false positive" finding) if the aorta communicates with a different low pressure chamber, such as a congenital patent ductus arteriosus or a surgical aorto-pulmonary window. The proximal isovelocity surface area (PISA) approach to quantitation of regurgitation is rarely used for 2 reasons: (1) visualization of a PISA is rarely possible and (2) precise quantitation typically is not needed for clinical decision making. However, when a PISA is visualized, as in this case, effective regurgitant orifice (ERO) area can be calculated and then used to determine regurgitant volume by multiplying by the aortic regurgitant jet velocity time integral (69 ml in this example).

Suggested Reading

1. Otto CM. Valvular Regurgitation. In Otto CM, Textbook of clinical echocardiography, ed 5, Philadelphia, 2013, Elsevier.
2. Evangelista A, Gallian L: Aortic valve regurgitation: Quantitation of disease severity and timing of surgical intervention. In Otto CM, editor: The practice of clinical echocardiography, ed 5, Philadelphia, 2016, Elsevier.

4 Endocarditis

Native Valve Endocarditis

CASE 4-1
Aortic Valve Endocarditis

This 39-year-old female with a history of intravenous drug use, uncontrolled diabetes, and chronic pancreatitis had recently undergone a 21-day course of antibiotics for a soft tissue infection of her hand. In the 2 days before admission she had become severely fatigued and more short of breath on exertion. Auscultation of a murmur prompted a transthoracic echocardiogram that showed vegetations on the aortic valve, severe eccentric aortic regurgitation (AR), and biventricular dysfunction. She was referred for aortic valve surgery for acute heart failure resulting from severe aortic regurgitation secondary to presumptive endocarditis. Postop pathologic examination of the native aortic leaflets showed evolving endocarditis with gram-positive organisms, consistent with treated endocarditis.

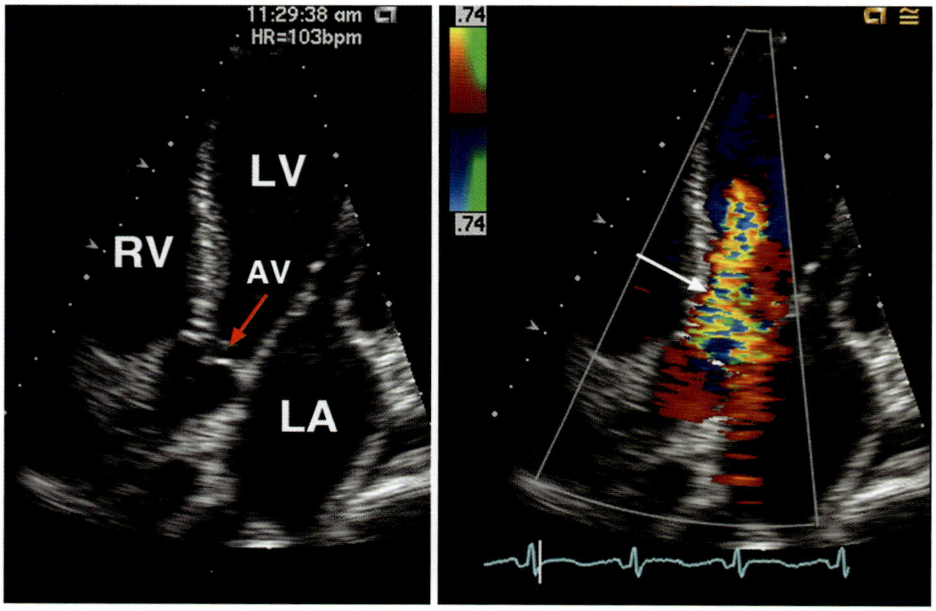

Fig 4.1 Preoperative TTE apical five-chamber view showed a broad jet of AR *(white arrow)*.

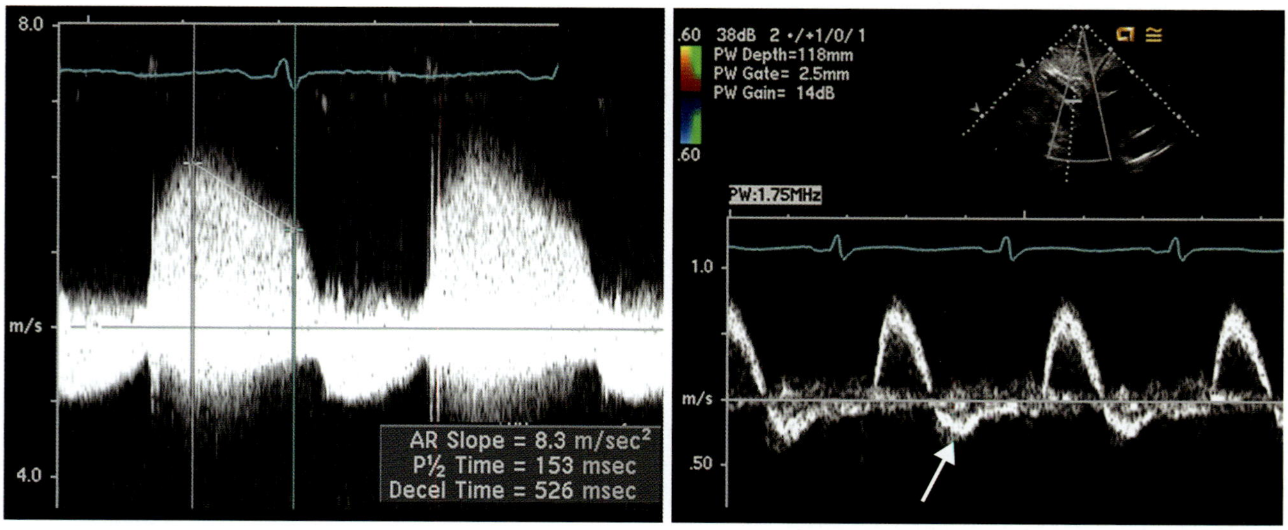

Fig 4.2 Preoperative TTE showed a pressure half-time of the AR jet to be 153 ms *(left)*, and diastolic flow reversal in the abdominal aorta. Both parameters are consistent with severe AR.

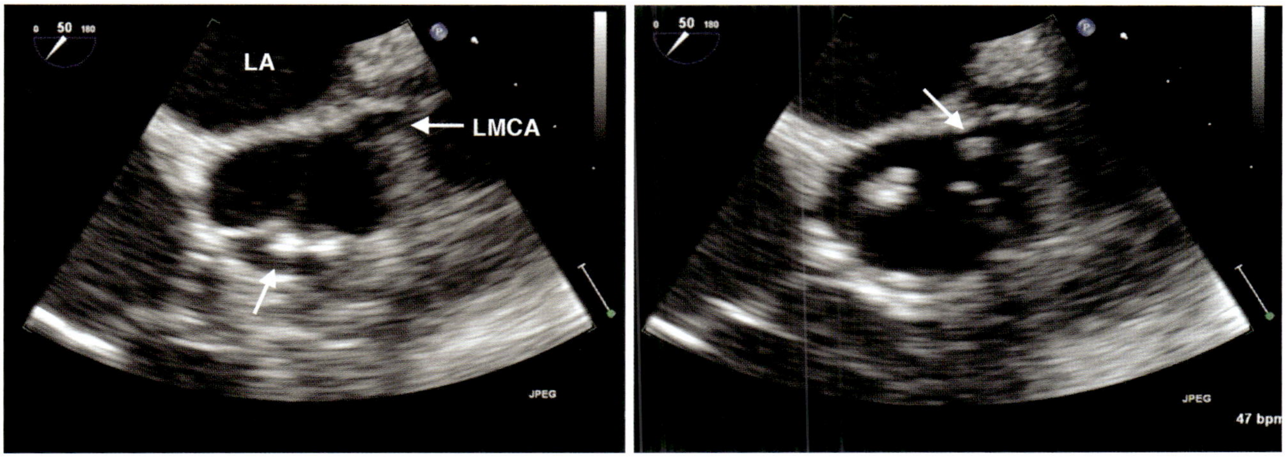

Fig 4.3 In this midesophageal short-axis image in diastole *(left panel)*, there are multiple echo-dense masses attached to the valve leaflets but with independent mobility, consistent with aortic valve vegetations *(arrow)*. There is no evidence for paravalvular abscess. The systolic image *(right panel)* shows one of the vegetations engaging the left main coronary artery (LMCA) orifice *(arrow)*, illustrating how embolization from an aortic valve vegetation can result in myocardial infarction as well as mycotic aneurysm of the coronary artery.

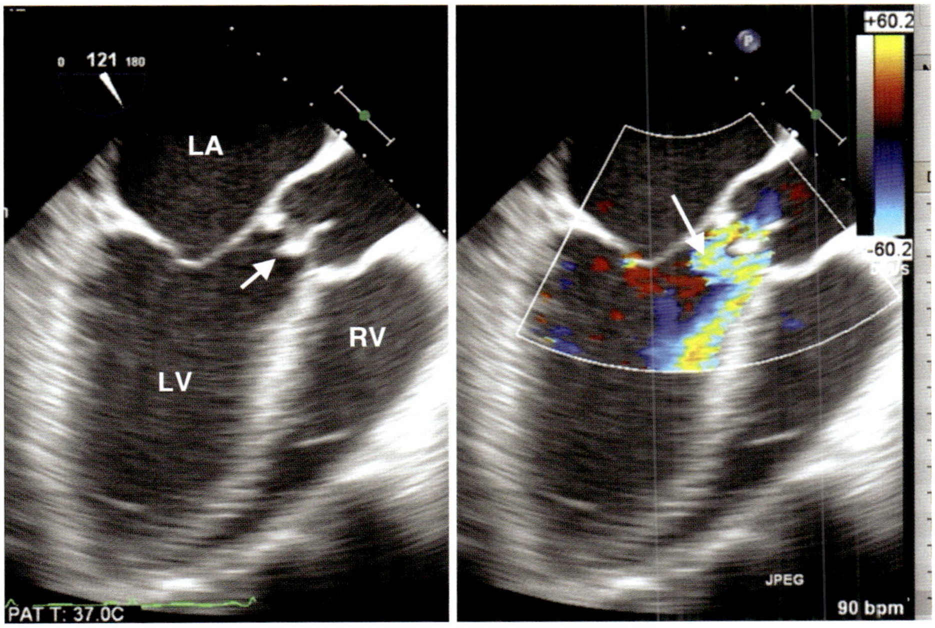

Fig 4.4 In this midesophageal long-axis image in diastole, multiple echodensities with independent motion consistent with aortic valve vegetations are again seen *(left panel, arrow)*. Color Doppler flow imaging *(right)* shows eccentric aortic regurgitation. Vena contracta is difficult to measure on this image as the jet courses obliquely across the outflow tract so that the minor axis diameter of the flow stream cannot be identified.

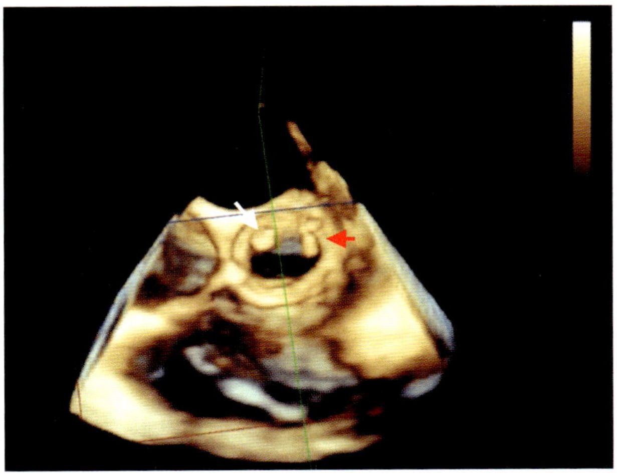

Fig 4.5 In this 3D view of the aortic valve from the perspective of the ascending aorta, vegetations are seen at the left *(red arrow)* and noncoronary *(white arrow)* cusps.

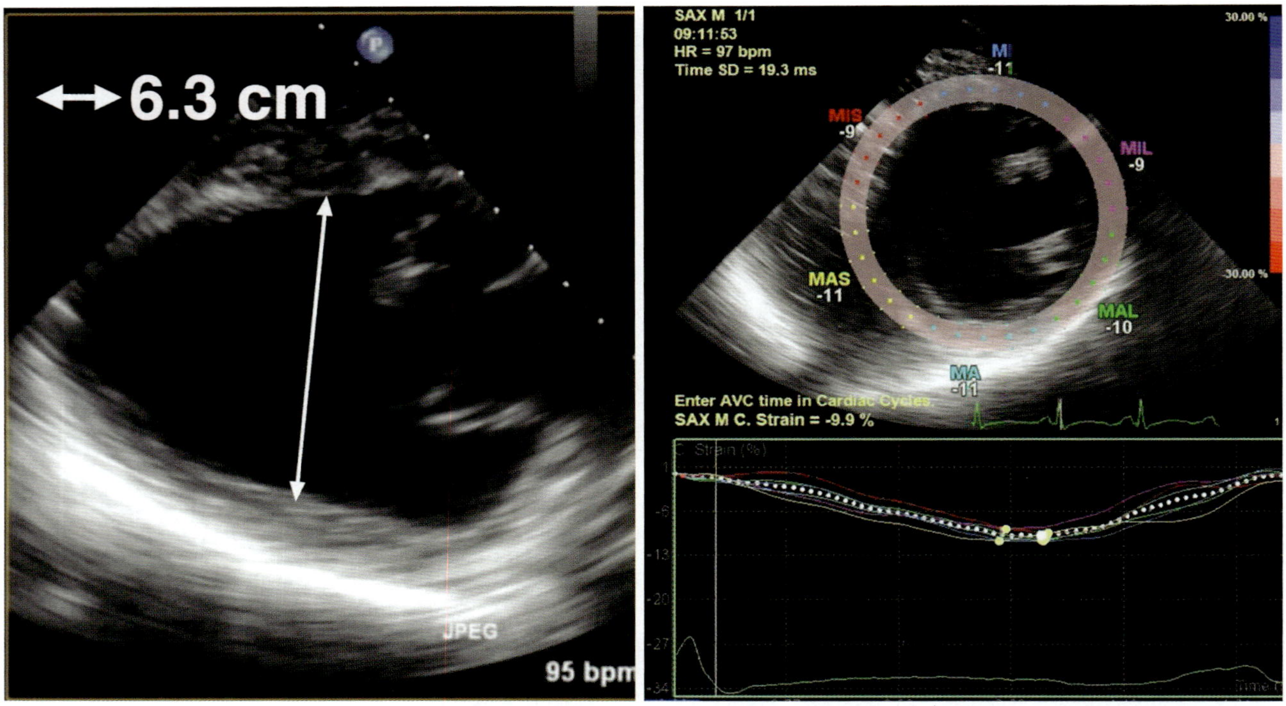

Fig 4.6 The transgastric two-chamber image *(left)* demonstrates significant LV dilation with an end-diastolic diameter of 6.3 cm. Speckle tracking in a midpapillary short-axis view shows a reduced circumferential strain of –9.9% consistent with moderately reduced overall systolic function. The biplane ejection fraction (EF) was 34%. These findings are unusual for acute severe aortic regurgitation, suggesting that chronic aortic regurgitation was present or that there is concurrent primary myocardial dysfunction.

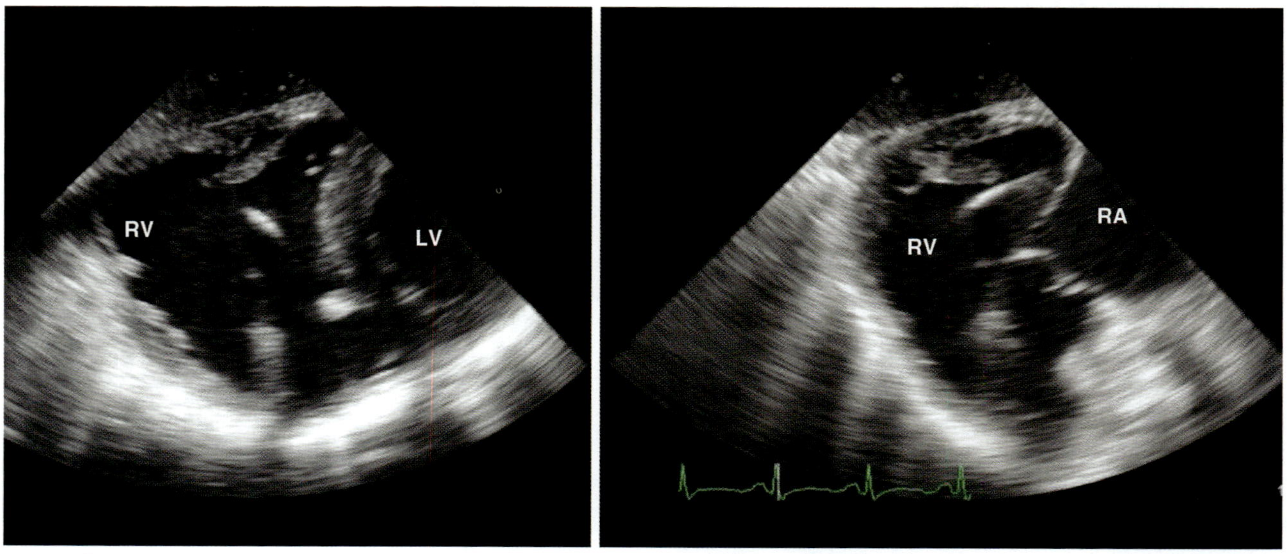

Fig 4.7 These transgastric short-axis *(left)* and long-axis *(right)* views show RV dilation. In real time there is mildly reduced RV function.

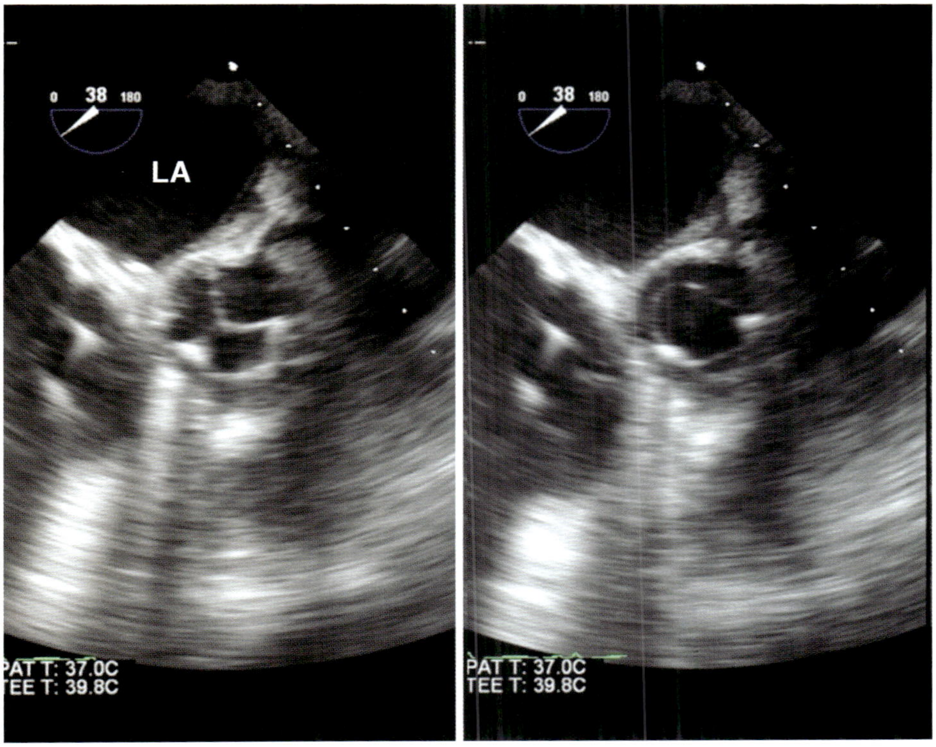

Fig 4.8 This midesophageal short-axis image in diastole *(left)* and systole *(right)* of the bioprosthetic aortic valve replacement shows thin leaflets with normal systolic opening. There was no aortic regurgitation on color Doppler imaging.

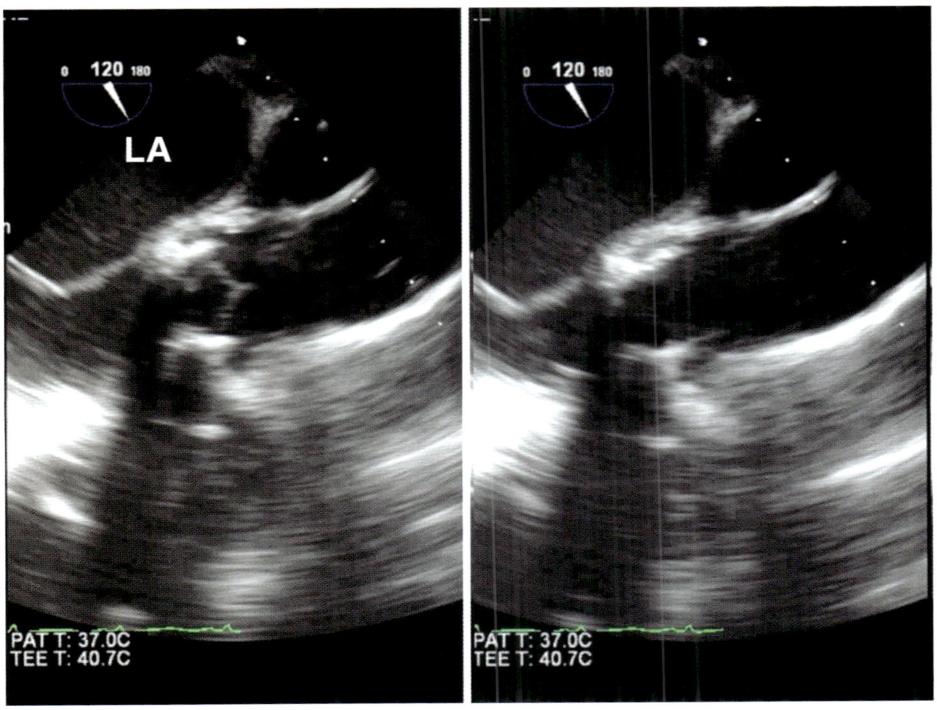

Fig 4.9 This midesophageal long-axis image in diastole *(left)* and systole *(right)* of the bioprosthetic valve replacement shows normal thin leaflets with diastolic closure and no regurgitation on color Doppler imaging. There was normal systolic opening.

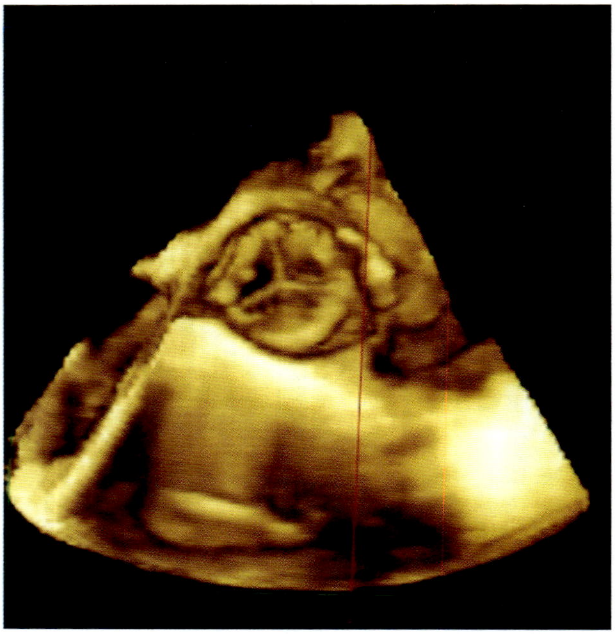

Fig 4.10 A 3D image of the bioprosthetic valve as seen from the perspective of the ascending aorta. In real time, there is some artifactual dropout of the leaflets.

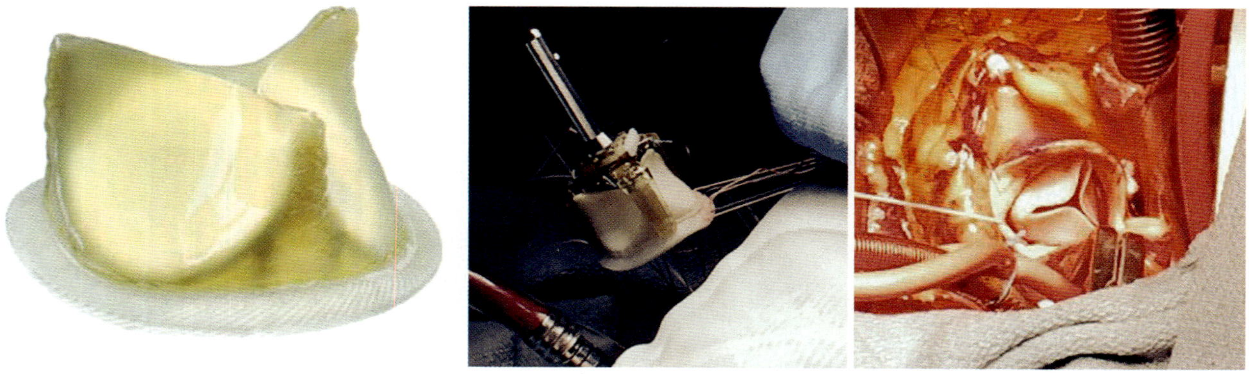

Fig 4.11 The Trifecta bioprosthesis (St. Jude Medical, St. Paul, Minnesota). In the left panel, the valve as it appears before implantation. The center panel shows the valve just before lowering into position. In the right panel, the valve has been sutured down to the annulus.

Comments

The clinical diagnosis of endocarditis is based on a combination of clinical, bacteriologic, and echocardiographic findings, known as the Duke criteria. In brief, definite endocarditis is present when there is evidence of persistent bacteremia plus echocardiographic findings consistent with endocardial infection. When only one rather than both of these criteria is present, other minor clinical criteria are used to support the diagnosis of endocarditis. A vegetation is recognized with echocardiography as an irregular mass attached to a valve leaflet but with motion independent of the normal valve motion. Vegetations are typically located on the upstream side of valves, such as the ventricular side of the aortic valve and the atrial side of the mitral valve. This case is atypical with vegetations seen on the aortic side of the valve, which is more typical for nonbacterial endocarditis.

Valvular regurgitation is present in over 90% of cases, due either to the vegetation interfering with normal valve closure or, more often, to tissue destruction with loss of leaflet tissue or perforation. Stenosis caused by a large vegetation is rare. Transesophageal echocardiography has a very high (nearly 100%) sensitivity and specificity for detection of valvular vegetations. Other echocardiographic findings that may be mistaken for a valvular vegetation include beam width artifact, normal valve tissue (i.e., myxomatous valve disease, Lambl's excrescence), prosthetic valve thrombus, papillary fibroelastoma, and nonbacterial thrombotic endocarditis.

Suggested Reading

1. Wang A, Samad Z: Endocarditis: the role of echocardiography in diagnosis and decision-making. In Otto CM, editor: The practice of clinical echocardiography, ed 5, Philadelphia, 2016, Elsevier.
2. Thuny F, Grisoli D, Cautela J, et al: Infective endocarditis: prevention, diagnosis, and management, Can J Cardiol 30(9): 1046–1057, 2014.
3. Thanavaro KL, Nixon JV: Endocarditis 2014: An update, Heart Lung 43(4):334–337, 2014.
4. Kaku K, Takeuchi M, Tsang W, et al: Age-related normal range of left ventricular strain and torsion using three-dimensional speckle-tracking echocardiography, J Am Soc Echocardiogr 27:55–64, 2014.

CASE 4-2
Aortic and Mitral Valve Vegetations

This 35-year-old man presented with a 6-week history of malaise and a 2-week history of fevers, chills, and right upper quadrant abdominal pain. After an abdominal ultrasound, he was started on antibiotics for ascending cholangitis. However, he continued to deteriorate clinically with sepsis and multiple blood cultures positive for *Haemophilus influenzae.* After further respiratory and hemodynamic compromise, he underwent echocardiography, which was consistent with aortic and mitral valve endocarditis, severe aortic regurgitation, and moderate mitral regurgitation. He developed cardiogenic shock and his mental status declined. Head CT showed focal right frontal lobe hypodensities consistent with embolic stroke. Because of his hemodynamic instability, he was taken to the OR for emergency aortic valve replacement.

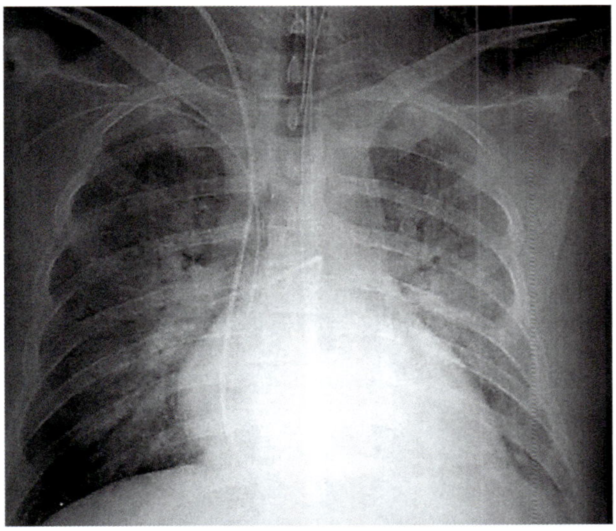

Fig 4.12 Posterior-anterior chest radiography shows cardiac enlargement and pulmonary edema.

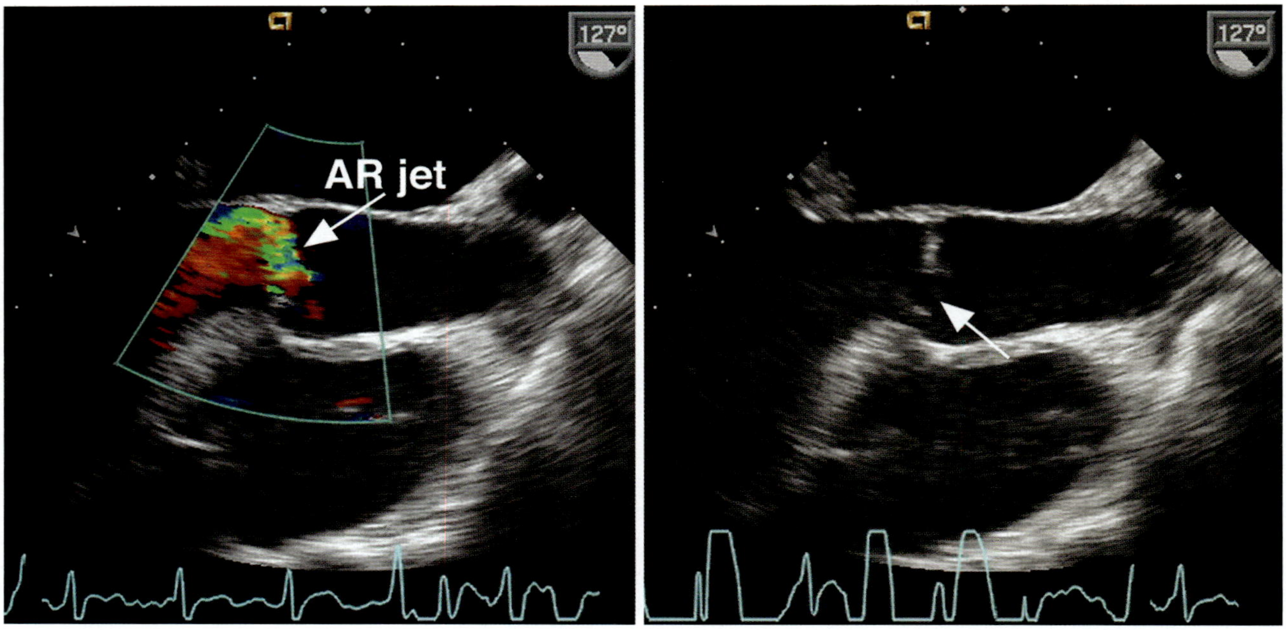

Fig 4.13 Long-axis TEE view of the aortic valve and ascending aorta demonstrates normal aortic root size and anatomy. However, there is a discontinuity in the anterior leaflet of the aortic valve *(arrow)* with color Doppler showing a wide jet of aortic regurgitation through this region.

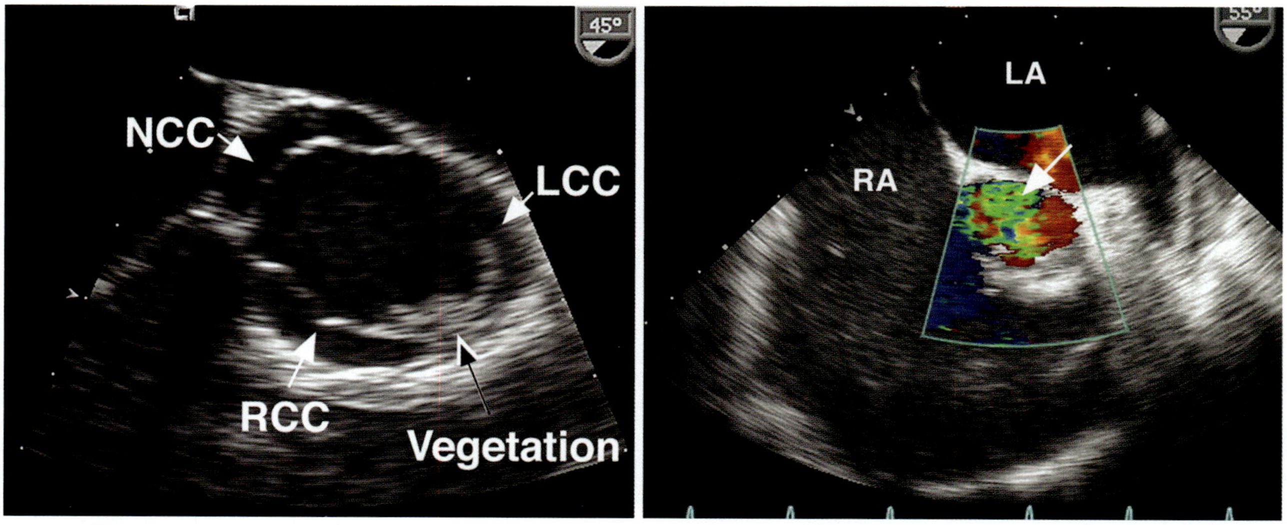

Fig 4.14 In the left panel, the midesophageal short-axis TEE view of the aortic valve demonstrates a valvular vegetation at the junction between the right (RCC) and left coronary cusps (LCC). The posteriorly located noncoronary cusp (NCC) appears normal in this view. Color Doppler in a short-axis view of the left ventricular outflow tract shows aortic regurgitation *(mosaic green pattern, arrow)* filling about two-thirds of the cross-sectional area of flow *(right panel)*.

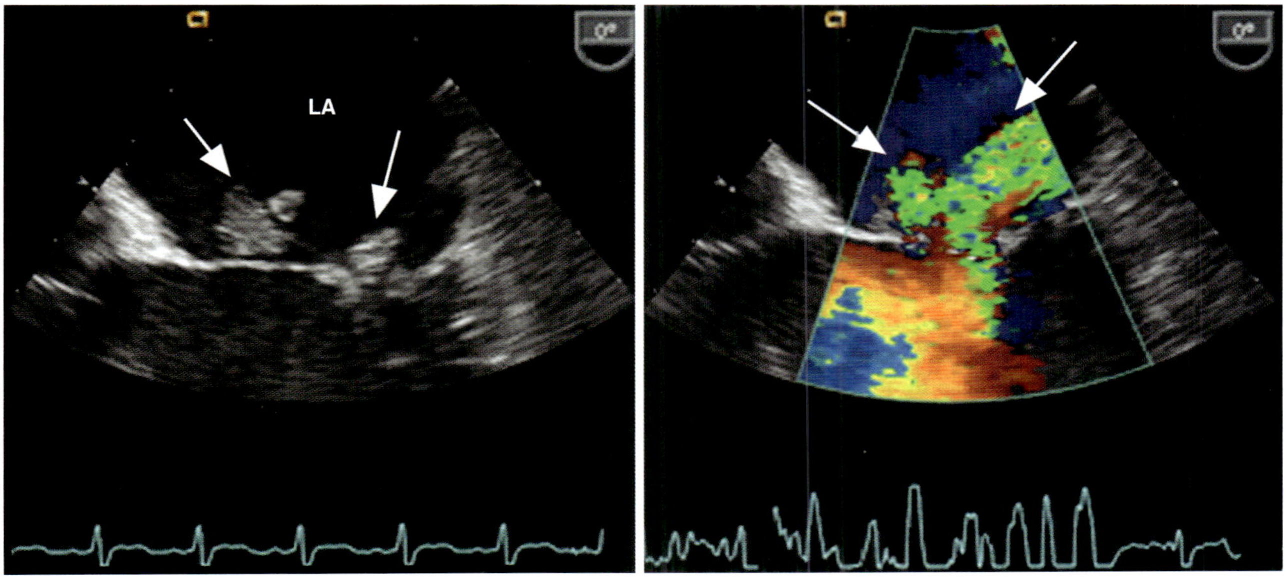

Fig 4.15 Images of the mitral valve at 0 degrees demonstrate large mobile masses on both leaflets. In real time, these masses move independently from the valve leaflets and are consistent with vegetations. Color Doppler shows a wide jet of mitral regurgitation with both anteriorly and posteriorly directed jets *(arrows)*.

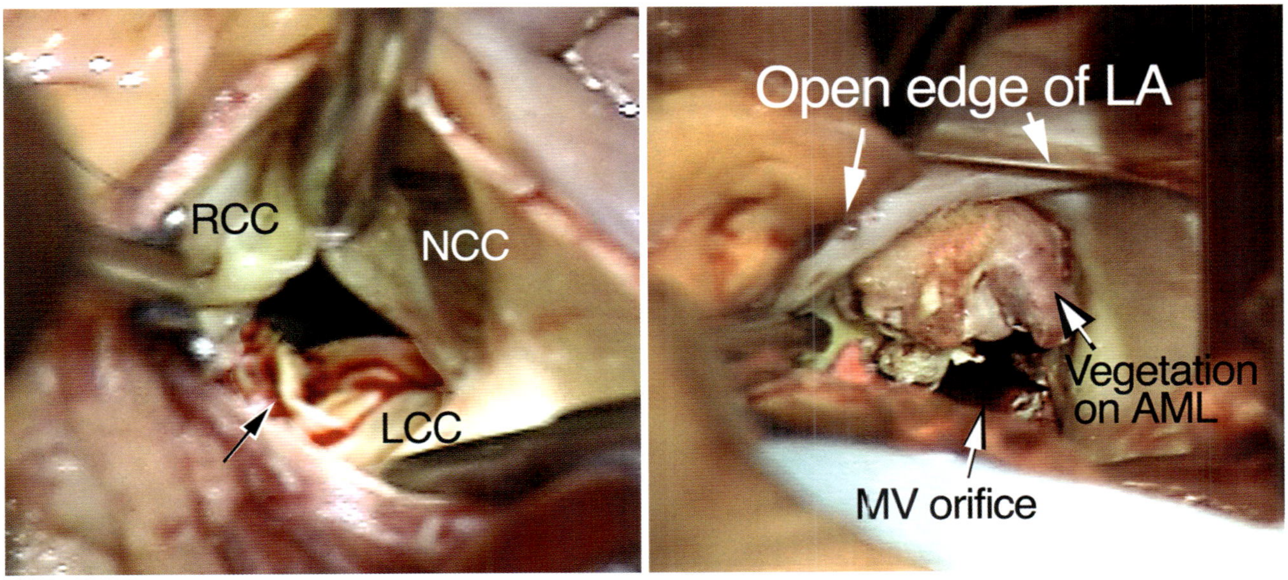

Fig 4.16 At surgical inspection, the 1-cm diameter vegetation at the junction of the left and right coronary cusps of the aortic valve is seen *(arrow, left panel)*. With the LA opened, the large vegetation on the anterior mitral leaflet can be appreciated *(right panel)*. Both anterior and posterior leaflets were extensively destroyed by the infectious process. The man underwent mechanical aortic and mitral valve replacements. Although his postoperative course was complicated, 2 years after surgery he is doing well clinically on medical therapy for a left ventricular ejection fraction of 36% with moderate paravalvular aortic regurgitation.

Comments

Vegetations are described on echocardiography in terms of location, size, mobility, and echodensity. The exact location on the valve may help determine whether valve repair, rather than replacement, is possible. Vegetation size and mobility are markers of increased risk of complications of endocarditis. The density of a vegetation may provide clues about the chronicity of disease, with denser, calcified vegetations suggesting chronic or healed endocarditis.

In patients with underlying valve disease, bacteremia may result in direct infection at more than one site. Even when one valve is primarily infected, vegetations may occur on other valves resulting from direct extension of the infection. An example is an aortic annular abscess eroding into the base of the anterior mitral leaflet. Infection of one valve may also damage an adjacent valve, leading to subsequent infection. For example, aortic regurgitation impinging on the anterior mitral leaflet results in endothelial disruption with a higher likelihood of bacterial adherence at that site. Thus one of the primary goals of intraoperative TEE in patients undergoing valve surgery for endocarditis is to exclude infection on the other "uninvolved" valves.

Suggested Reading

1. Bruun NE, Habib G, Thuny F, et al: Cardiac imaging in infectious endocarditis, Eur Heart J 35(10):624–632, 2014.
2. Bedeir K, Reardon M, Ramlawi B: Infective endocarditis: Perioperative management and surgical principles, J Thorac Cardiovasc Surg 147(4):1133–1141, 2014.

CASE 4-3
Mitral Valve Endocarditis with Perforated Anterior Leaflet

The patient is a 29-year-old male who presented to his primary care provider complaining of several months of chills, fatigue, and a 25-lb unintentional weight loss. Evaluation revealed a prominent new systolic murmur. He was sent for an echocardiogram that revealed a 1.7 × 1.4 cm mitral valve vegetation with significant mitral regurgitation.

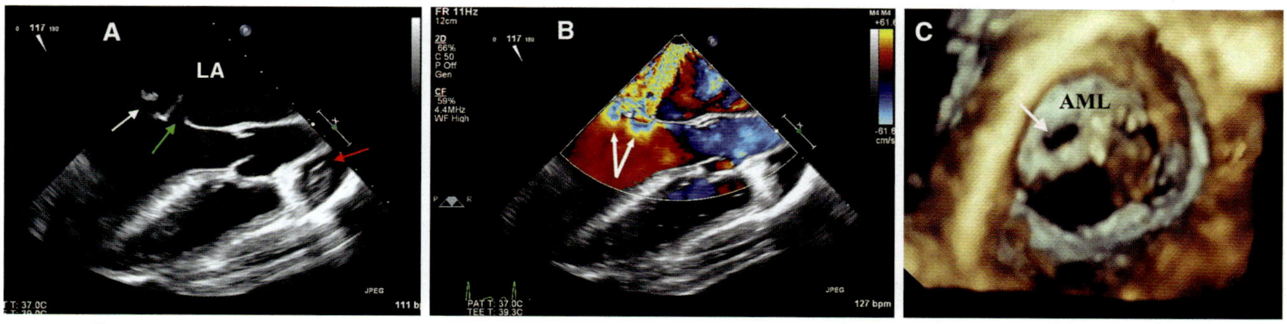

Fig 4.17 In the left panel, a midesophageal long-axis view demonstrates a perforation of the anterior mitral leaflet *(green arrow)*. The white arrow indicates the mitral orifice. The red arrow indicates fluid in the transverse pericardial sinus with a "mass" that is the normal left atrial appendage. The surgeon confirmed that there was no abnormal mass in the pericardial space. In the middle panel, two jets of mitral regurgitation are seen with proximal isovelocity surface areas (PISAs) on the LV side of the valve, as indicated by the white arrows. The location of the PISAs helps identify the exact site of leaflet perforation. In the right panel, a 3D image of the mitral valve from the left atrial perspective illustrates a perforation in the anterior mitral leaflet *(arrow)*.

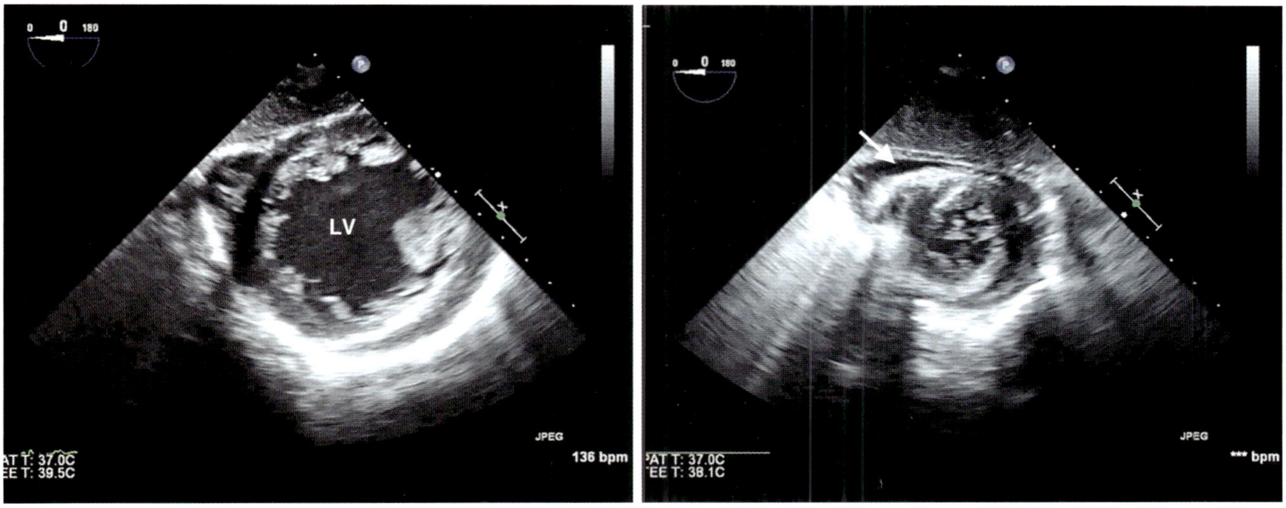

Fig 4.18 The left panel is a transgastric midesophageal short-axis view of the LV. By retroflexing and advancing the probe, the apex of the heart is visible, as well as a small pericardial effusion *(arrow)*.

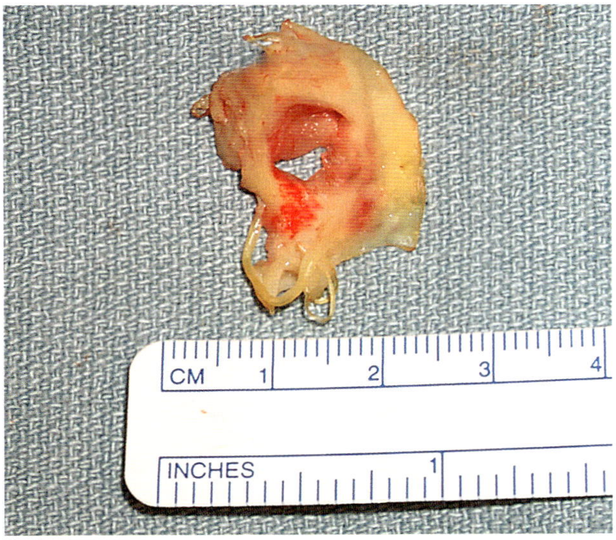

Fig 4.19 In a surgical specimen from a different patient with mitral valve endocarditis, there is a clear perforation in the anterior mitral leaflet.

Comments

The clinical sequelae of endocarditis are caused by two primary processes: tissue destruction and embolization. Tissue destruction leads to valve regurgitation and paravalvular abscess formation, whereas embolization leads to cerebrovascular events. Cerebral embolization occurs in 10% to 30% of patients with endocarditis, and coronary artery embolism occurs in about 10% of patients. Risk factors for embolization are infection with *Staph aureus*, fungal endocarditis, and mitral valve involvement. Several studies also have suggested that larger (>1 cm in diameter) and more mobile vegetations are at higher risk of embolization. However, earlier surgical intervention based on the appearance of the vegetation remains controversial.

Suggested Reading

1. Chu VH, Park LP, Athan E, et al: Association between surgical indications, operative risk, and clinical outcome in infective endocarditis: A prospective study from the International Collaboration on Endocarditis, Circulation 131(2):131–140, 2015.
2. Berdejo J, Shibayama K, Harada K, et al: Evaluation of vegetation size and its relationship with embolism in infective endocarditis: A real-time 3-dimensional transesophageal echocardiography study, Circ Cardiovasc Imaging 7(1):149–154, 2014.

CASE 4-4
Mitral Valve Endocarditis with Perforated Posterior Leaflet

The patient is a 67-year-old male with dialysis-dependant end-stage renal disease secondary to diabetes, known coronary artery disease, and a past history of admission to hospital for congestive heart failure. One month before admission he developed a dialysis catheter line infection. The line was removed, and was culture positive for *Staph aureus.* He was treated with appropriate antibiotics, and after an echocardiogram excluded valvular vegetations, he was discharged 2 weeks after admission.

On the day before surgery he presented to the ER with fever, confusion, a systolic BP of 60, and a white cell count of 21. Blood cultures grew gram-positive cocci clusters in several bottles. Urgent TTE showed severe MR, and a mass on the mitral valve. The patient was transferred to our medical center with worsening congestive heart failure in the setting of *Staph aureus,* coagulase-negative, mitral valve endocarditis.

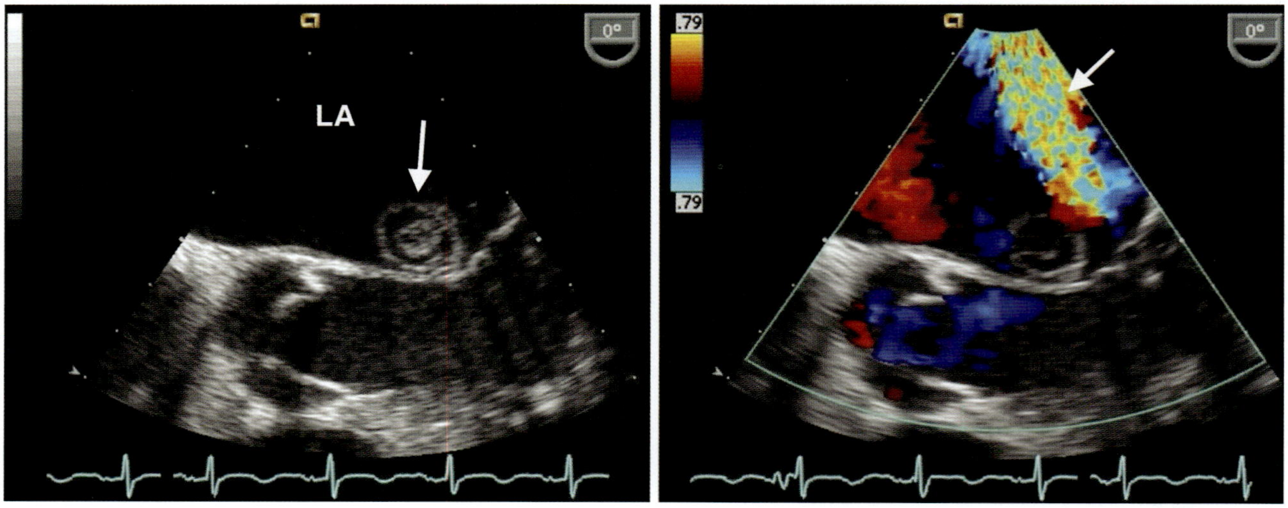

Fig 4.20 In this midesophageal view, a complex mass *(arrow, left panel)* is seen attached to some component of the mitral valvular apparatus. In the right panel, the arrow indicates a large regurgitant jet, presumably mitral regurgitation, although the origin of the jet is not visible in this view.

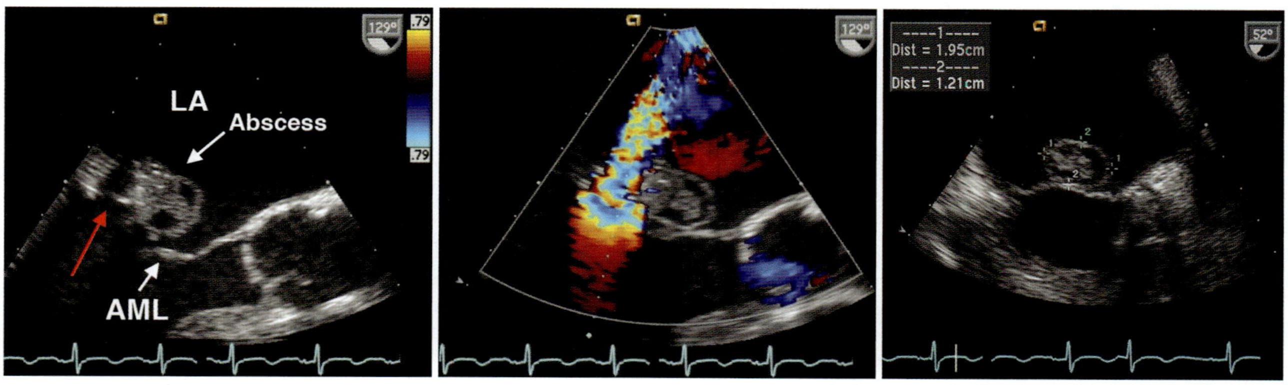

Fig 4.21 At the same probe depth, the angle of interrogation is rotated to a long-axis view. Here the mass attaches to the atrial side of the posterior mitral leaflet (PML), whereas in this view, the anterior mitral leaflet (AML) appears free of disease. The mass has the appearance of an abscess, possibly extending from the annulus into the posterior leaflet. In addition, there is a perforation of the PML *(red arrow)*, and in the middle frame, the jet of mitral regurgitation is seen traversing the defect. In the right frame, the dimensions of the mass are measured.

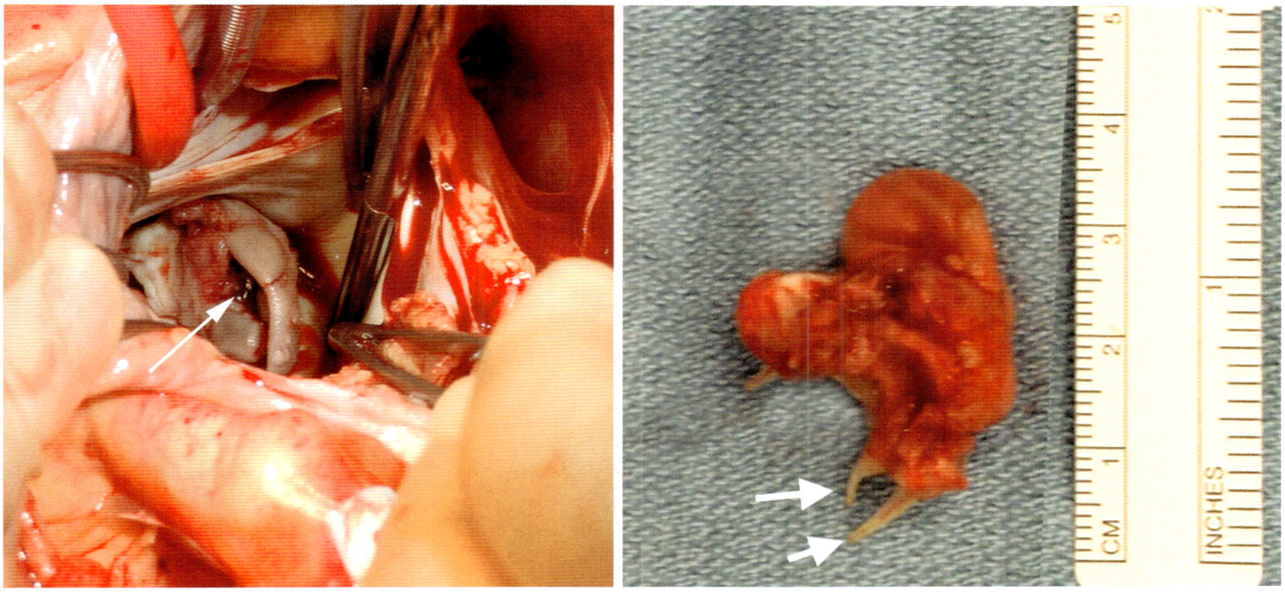

Fig 4.22 In the left frame, the LA has been opened, and the perforation through the vegetation on the posterior mitral leaflet is visible *(arrow)*. The excised mass is seen in the right frame. The arrows indicate chordae tendinea.

Comments

The treatment of endocarditis is based on antibiotic therapy and surgical intervention. Despite these therapies, overall mortality from endocarditis remains high at approximately 30% of all patients. Although decision making in each patient integrates multiple factors, there are three generally accepted indications for surgical intervention in patients with endocarditis: heart failure caused by valve regurgitation, persistent infection (abscess or persistent positive blood cultures), and recurrent embolic events. There is increasing clinical evidence to support early surgical intervention in many patients to prevent further tissue destruction and embolic events. This case illustrates that determining the involved leaflet, as well as the origin and direction of the regurgitant jet, requires interrogation of the valve with multiple transducer angles, depths, and degrees of flexion and extension.

Suggested Reading

1. Kang DH, Kim YJ, Kim SH, et al: Early surgery versus conventional treatment for infective endocarditis, N Engl J Med 366(26):2466–2473, 2012.

CASE 4-5
Pulmonic Valve Vegetation

This 39-year-old man with a history of IV drug use was transferred to our medical center with *Staph aureus* endocarditis involving the tricuspid and pulmonic valves resulting in severe regurgitation of both valves and clinical evidence of heart failure. The patient underwent tricuspid valve replacement with a pericardial bioprosthesis and pulmonic valve replacement with a pulmonic root homograft prosthesis. At surgery, both the tricuspid and pulmonic valves had large vegetations with severe valve destruction.

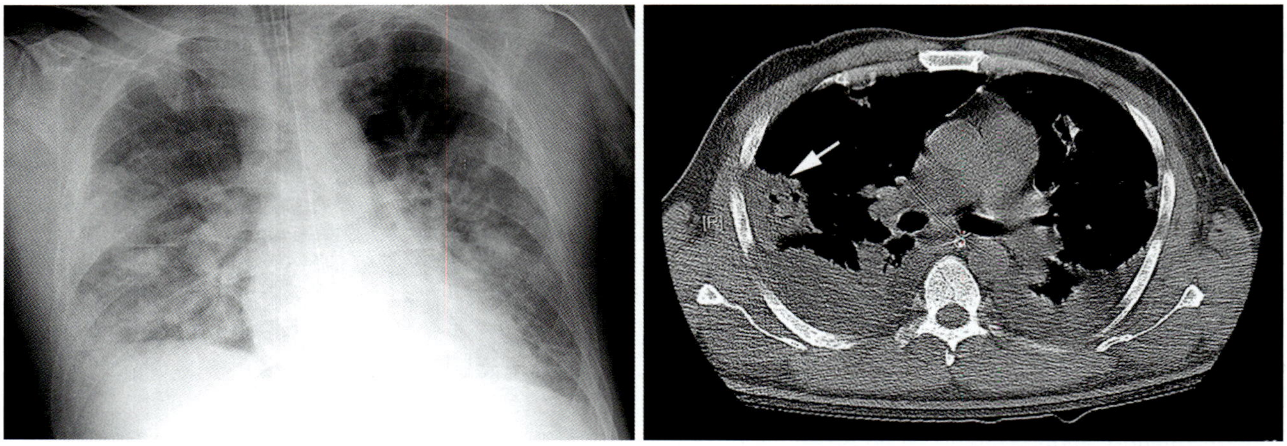

Fig 4.23 Chest x-ray *(left)* shows bilateral patchy lung consolidation. CT scan *(right)* reveals bilateral scattered densities with gas collections *(arrow)*, most compatible with septic emboli.

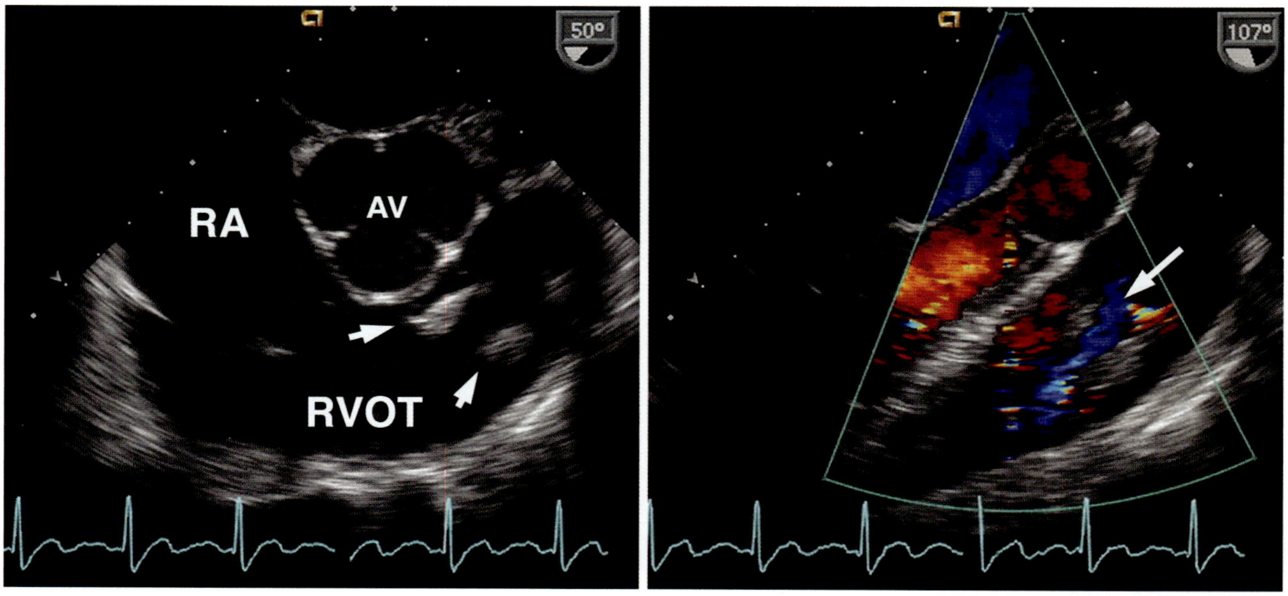

Fig 4.24 In a short-axis view of the aortic valve *(left)*, pulmonic valve vegetations are seen *(arrows)* in the RV outflow tract. In a view at 107-degrees rotation *(right)*, the pulmonic valve vegetations are visible, with color Doppler evidence of pulmonic regurgitation *(arrow)*.

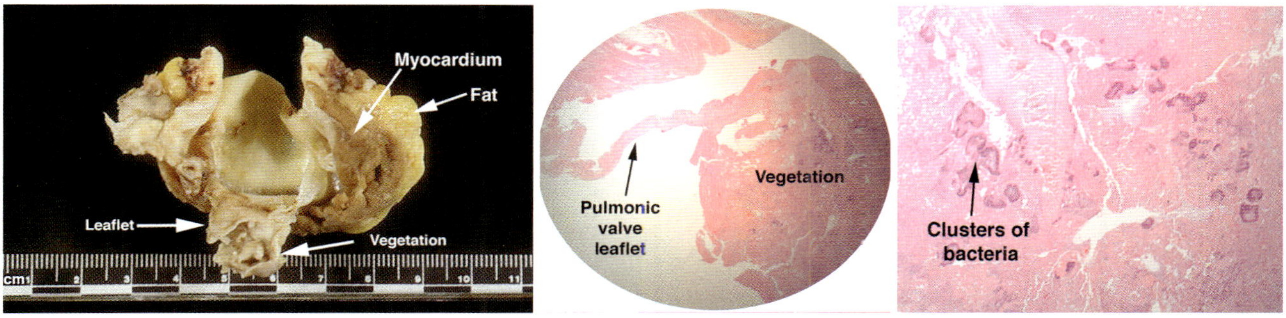

Fig 4.25 The excised pulmonic valve is accompanied by myocardium and epicardial fat. There is a vegetation attached to one of the pulmonic leaflets, which has ruptured *(left panel)*. Pathologic examination shows attachment of the vegetation to the pulmonic leaflet *(center panel)*. Clusters of bacteria are seen in the leaflet tissue *(right panel)*.

Comments

Endocarditis caused by intravenous drug use affects the tricuspid valve in 75% of cases, with pulmonic valve involvement being much less common. Over 50% of cases of right-sided endocarditis are the result of *Staph aureus*. With uncomplicated right-sided endocarditis, a shorter course of intravenous antibiotics is needed, compared with left-sided endocarditis. However, about 25% of patients also have involvement of left-sided heart valves so that TEE to evaluate for left-sided valve involvement is prudent. Complications of tricuspid valve endocarditis include septic pulmonary emboli and valve destruction leading to tricuspid regurgitation. The initial clinical prognosis is good with an in-hospital mortality of only 3% to 9%. However, long-term outcomes are poor, related to other medical and social issues, with a 10-year survival of only 10%. Tricuspid regurgitation may be well tolerated in the short term, but most patients eventually develop right heart failure and low output symptoms with uncorrected severe tricuspid regurgitation.

Suggested Reading

1. Ortiz-Bautista C, López J, García-Granja PE, et al: Current profile of infective endocarditis in intravenous drug users: The prognostic relevance of the valves involved, Int J Cardiol 187:472–474, 2015.

CASE 4-6
Tricuspid Valve Endocarditis

The patient, a 29-year old female with a history of intravenous drug use, developed severe, sudden onset of rigors lasting 30 min to 1 hr followed by severe headaches and generalized weakness. In the emergency department, a systolic murmur was heard, and TTE revealed a mass on the tricuspid valve.

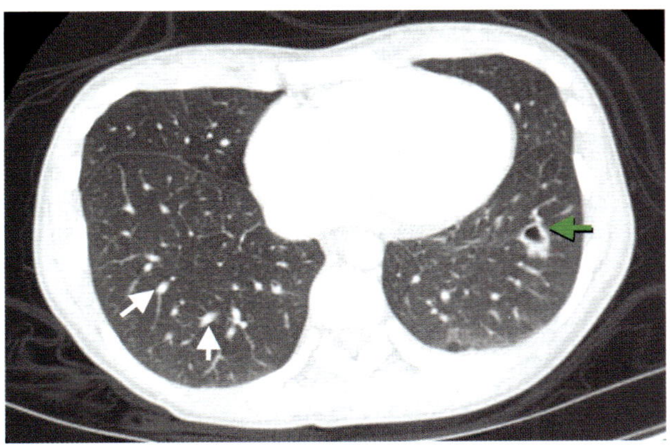

Fig 4.26 A chest CT showed multiple lesions in the lower lobes, suggesting septic emboli *(white arrows)*. In the left lower lobe cavitation one of the lesions is visible *(green arrow)*.

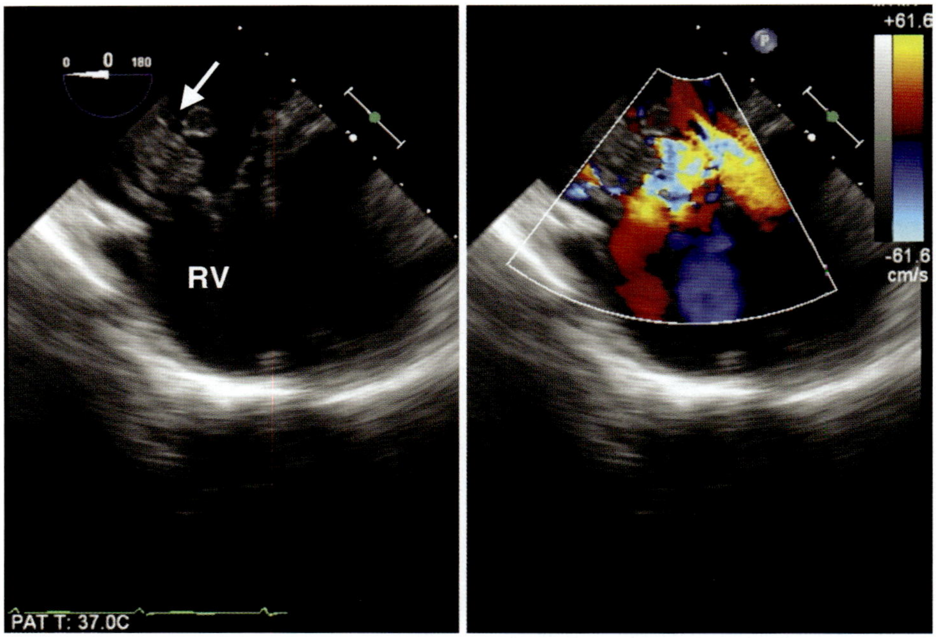

Fig 4.27 From a four-chamber position, the probe is rotated to the patient's right. A large mass *(arrow)* is seen attached to the atrial side of the tricuspid valve, but with independent motion, prolapsing into the RA in systole, consistent with vegetations. On the video images, the vegetation appears attached to the anterior leaflet of the tricuspid valve. Color Doppler *(right)* shows severe tricuspid regurgitation.

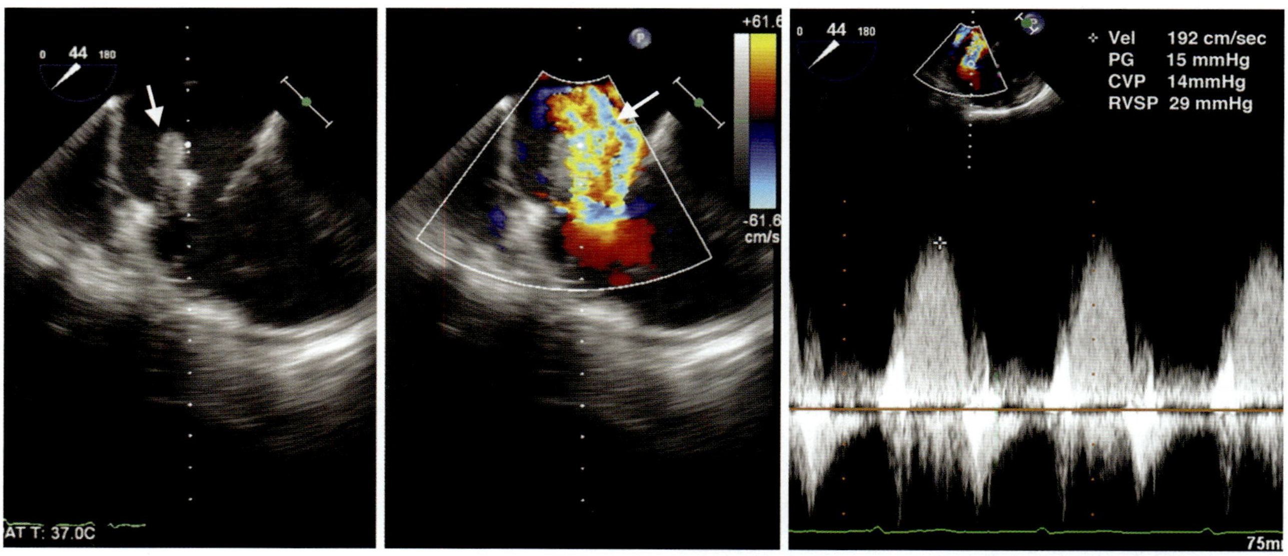

Fig 4.28 Rotating the image plane to 44 degrees to obtain an RV inflow view indicates that the vegetation is most likely attached to the anterior leaflet of the tricuspid valve. In the center panel, a wide jet of tricuspid regurgitation is seen *(arrow)* with a vena contracta width of 18 mm, diagnostic for severe regurgitation. In the right panel, CW Doppler shows a dense jet (relative to antegrade flow) that confirms severe regurgitation. The triangular shape suggests elevated RA pressures with an RA "v-wave" peak in early systole, both indicative of severe tricuspid regurgitation. The low peak velocity (Vel) in the regurgitant jet reflects normal pulmonary and RV systolic pressures. The RV systolic pressure (RVSP) of 29 mm Hg is estimated by adding the peak gradient (PG) between the RV and RA (using the simplified Bernoulli equation) to the directly measured central venous pressure (CVP) in this patient.

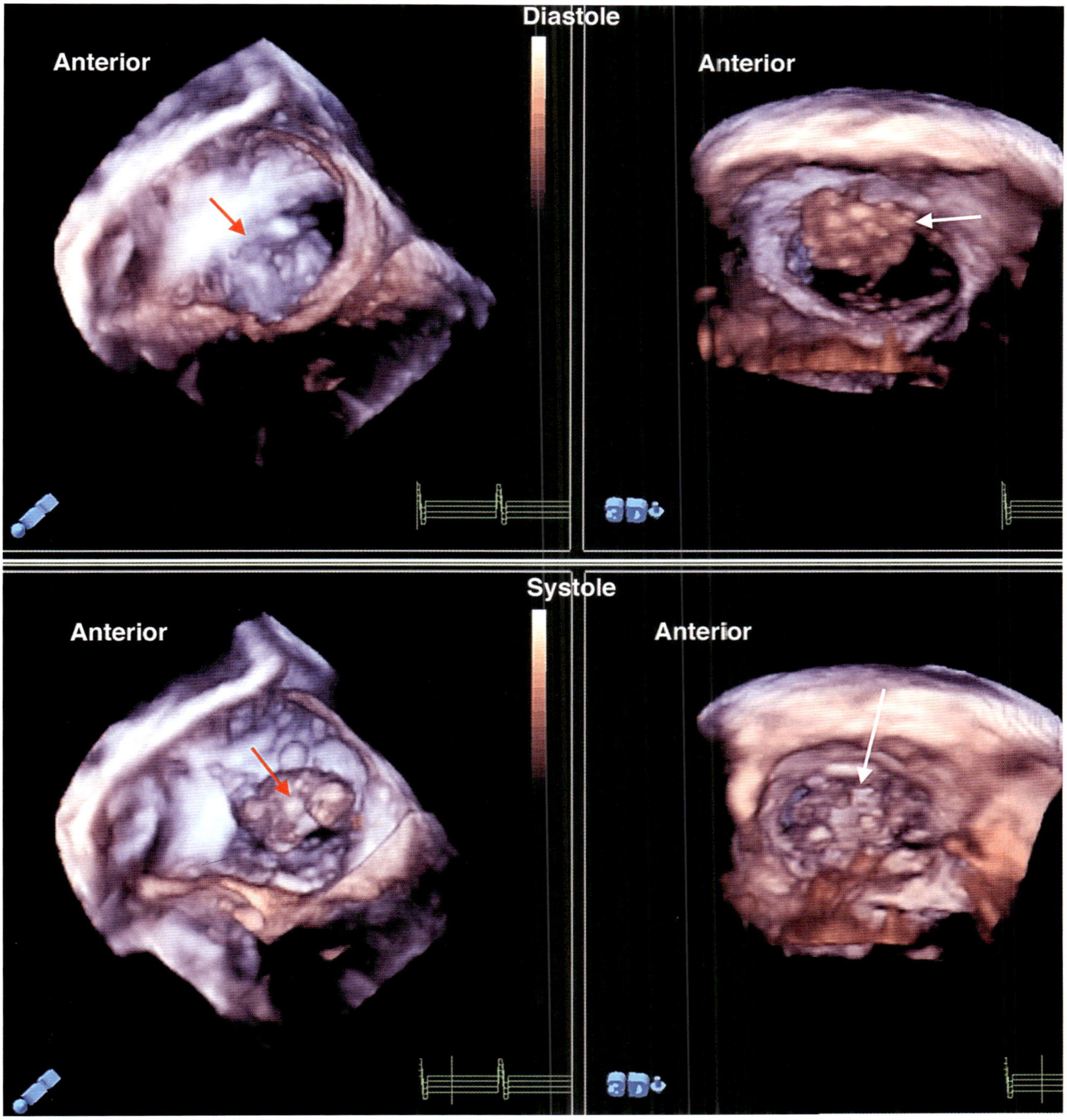

Fig 4.29 3D TEE of the tricuspid valve. A diastolic image of the valve is seen from the right atrial *(upper left)* and right ventricular *(upper right)* perspectives. The mass is indicated by the arrows. Similarly, the valve is seen in systole from the RA *(lower left)* and RV *(lower right)* perspectives with the mass, which is attached to the anterior leaflet, prolapsing into the RA.

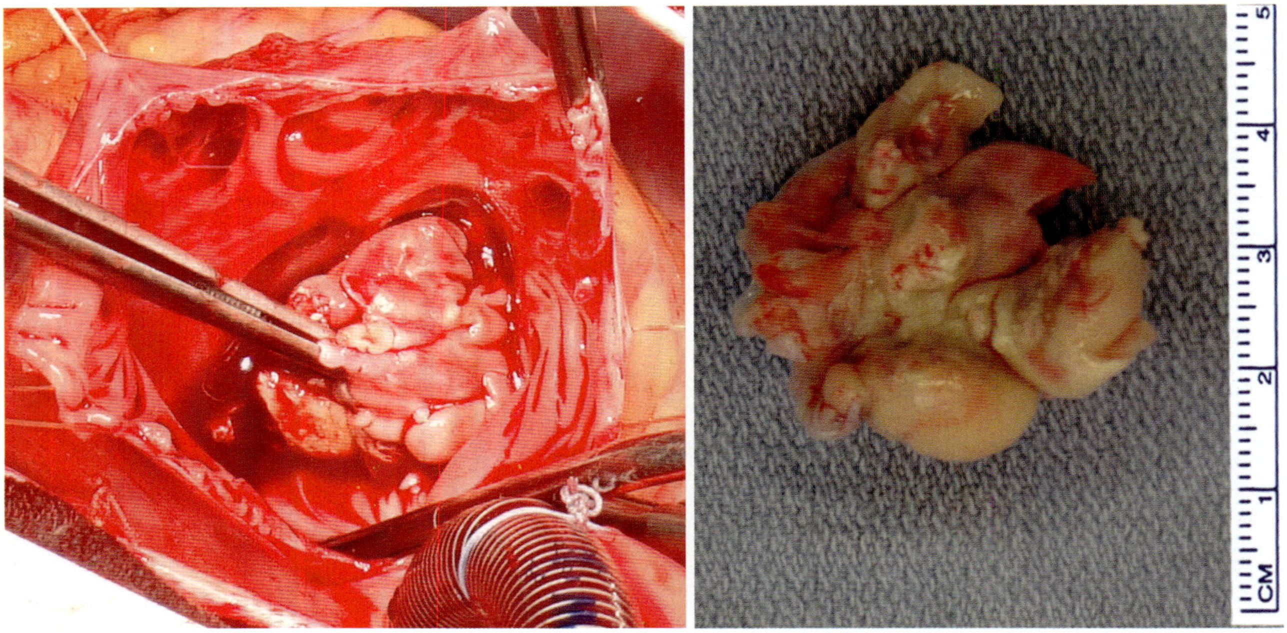

Fig 4.30 In the left panel, the RA has been opened, and the mass is visible firmly attached to the anterior leaflet of the tricuspid valve. The right panel shows the explanted mass.

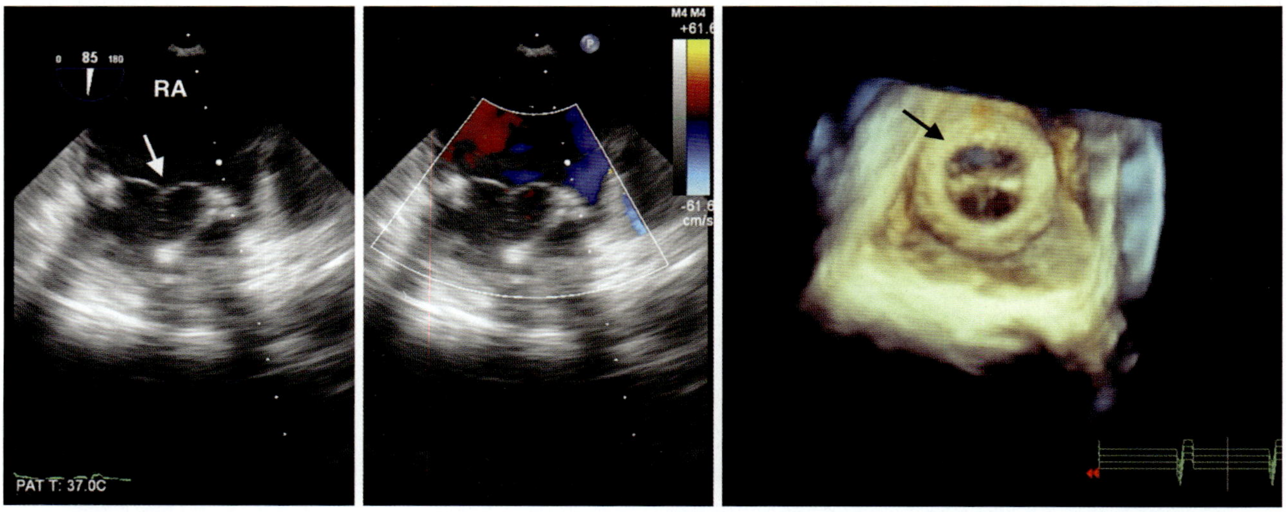

Fig 4.31 The patient underwent bioprosthetic tricuspid valve replacement. The closed leaflets of the stented bioprosthetic valve seen in systole on 2D imaging *(left)* and color Doppler imaging *(middle)* show no evidence of valve regurgitation. A 3D TEE image of the prosthetic valve from the right atrial perspective *(right)* shows the sewing ring *(arrow)*, and the thin leaflets are seen opening normally in diastole. Gram stain of the resected valve showed 2 + polymorphonuclear cells 4 + gram-positive Cocci. Subsequent culture was positive for *Staph aureus*.

Comments

Treatment of right-sided endocarditis in injection drug users (IDU) should include a commitment to a drug rehabilitation program to reduce the likelihood of future infection of the prosthetic valve. Some centers advocate simple removal of the valve and infected tissue, without valve replacement, in IDU patients with recurrent infective endocarditis but long-term severe valve regurgitation is not well tolerated. In some patients valve repair may be possible but tissue destruction of the tricuspid valve typically is so extensive as to require a prosthetic valve. Long-term survival after surgery for endocarditis in IDU patients is lower than in patients with no history of IDU. Long-term outcomes with bioprosthetic valves in IDU patients suggest this valve type is a reasonable choice.

Suggested Reading

1. Rabkin DG, Mokadam NA, Miller DW, et al: Long-term outcome for the surgical treatment of infective endocarditis with a focus on intravenous drug users, Ann Thorac Surg 93:51–57, 2012.

Complications of Native Valve Endocarditis

CASE 4-7
Aortic Annular Abscess

This 30-year-old man with no prior cardiac history transferred to our hospital with streptococcal aortic valve endocarditis and a possible paravalvular abscess.

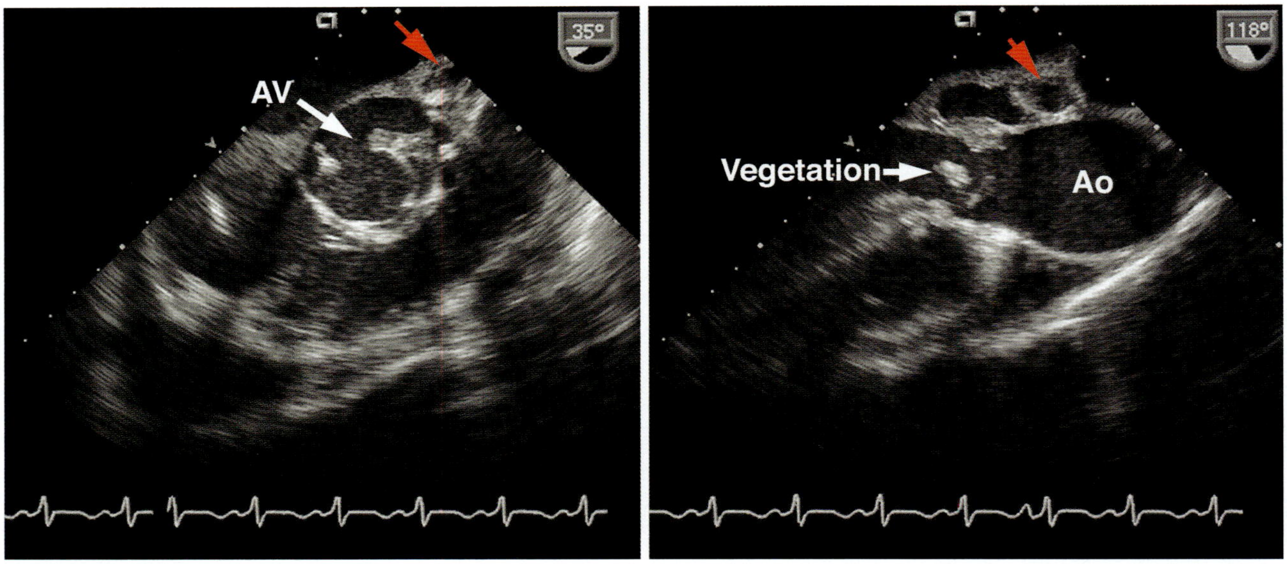

Fig 4.32 Midesophageal short-axis *(left)* and long-axis *(right)* views of the aortic valve demonstrate thickened valve leaflets and a complex echo-free space *(red arrows)* consistent with an abscess.

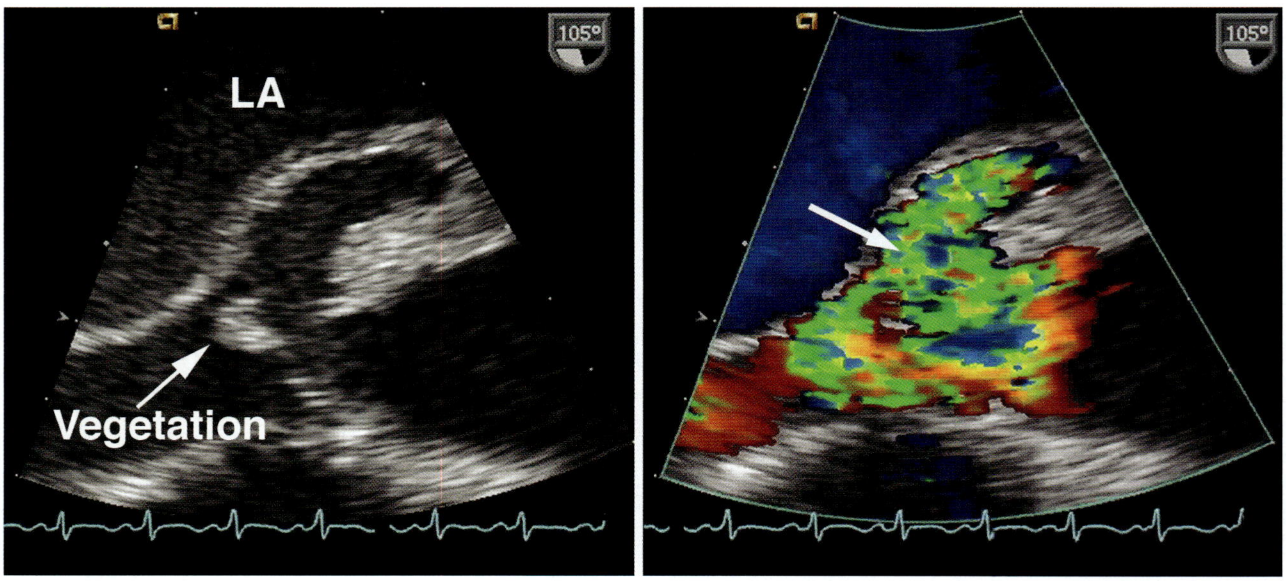

Fig 4.33 A close-up view with slight rotation of the image plane demonstrates the connection between the echo-free space posterior to the aorta with the aortic root, just distal to the aortic valve. Color Doppler *(right)* shows flows in and out of this cavity *(arrow)*.

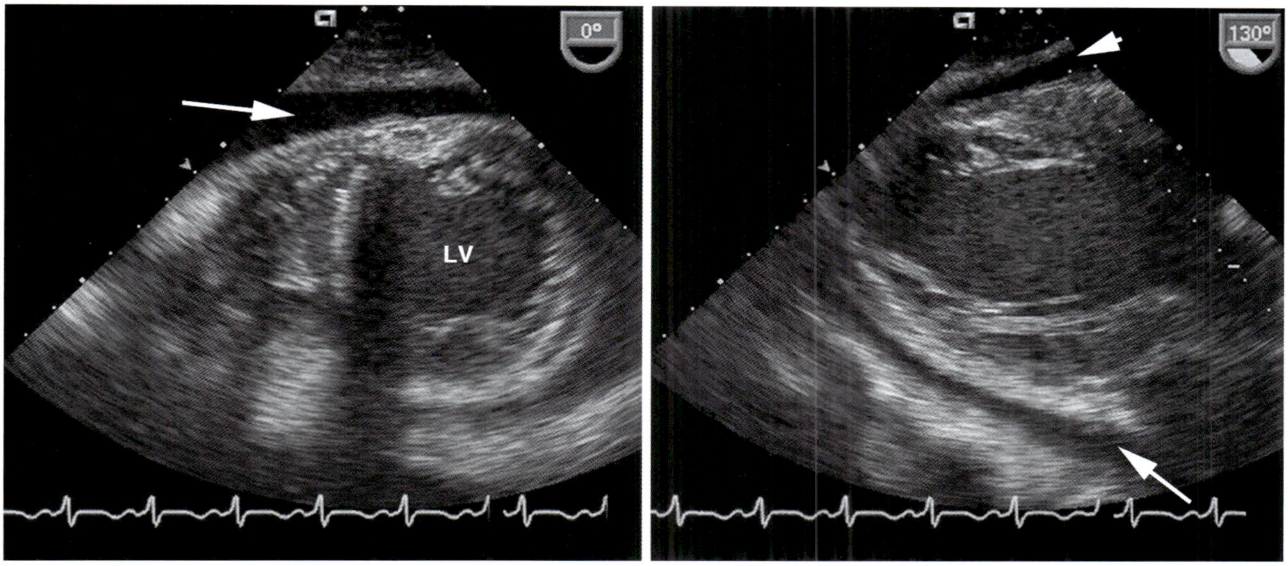

Fig 4.34 The transgastric short-axis *(left)* and two-chamber *(right)* views show a small to moderate pericardial effusion *(arrows)*. In real time, biventricular systolic function is reduced.

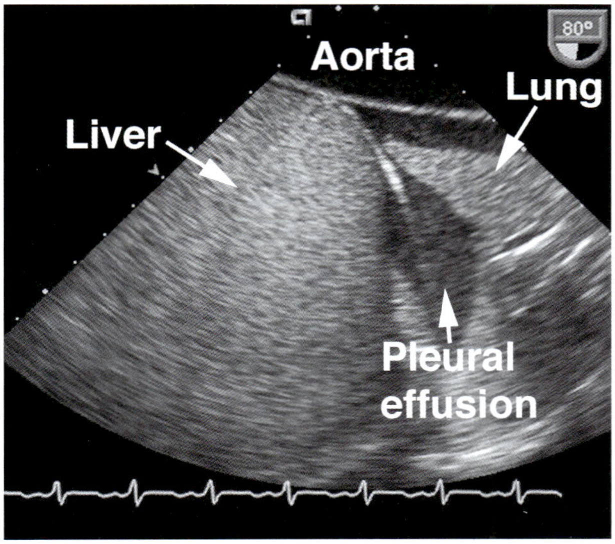

Fig 4.35 This image recorded with the transducer at the gastroesophageal junction with the transducer turned posteriorly toward the descending aorta shows compressed lung, with a surrounding pleural effusion, and the liver.

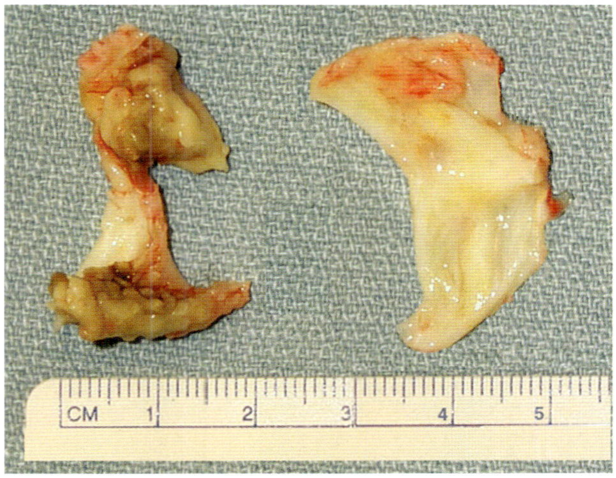

Fig 4.36 At surgery, there were large valve vegetations with a paravalvular abscess. A strip of pericardium was used to reconstruct the annulus and a 24-mm cryopreserved aortic allograft was implanted. The coronary buttons were anastomosed to the side of the graft. The resected bicuspid aortic valve shows diffuse thickening of the leaflet on the right. The leaflet on the left shows severe valve destruction caused by endocarditis.

Comments

Paravalvular abscess formation complicates 20% to 25% of aortic valve and about 15% of mitral valve endocarditis cases. With echocardiography, an intracardiac abscess may appear either echodense or echolucent, depending on whether the abscess cavity communicates with the bloodstream. For example, when aortic valve infection spreads to the sinuses of Valsalva, the sinus dilates and may be irregular in contour. Abscess may also appear as increased thickening in the paravalvular region, which can be difficult to distinguish from normal tissue. The sensitivity of transesophageal echocardiography for detection of abscess is about 90%, compared with <50% for transthoracic imaging. Clinically, patients with paravalvular abscess have evidence of persistent infection, including fever and persistently positive blood cultures. An aortic paravalvular abscess at the base of the septum may result in prolongation of the PR interval on ECG, or higher degrees of heart block caused by infection or edema of the conduction system. Mitral paravalvular abscess may rupture into the pericardium, resulting in purulent pericarditis.

Suggested Reading

1. Hoen B, Duval X: Infective endocarditis, N Engl J Med 369:785, 2013.
2. Murdoch DR, Corey GR, Hoen B, et al: Clinical presentation, etiology, and outcome of infective endocarditis in the 21st century: The International Collaboration on Endocarditis-Prospective Cohort Study, Arch Intern Med (169):463–473, 2009.

Prosthetic Valve Endocarditis

CASE 4-8
Bioprosthetic Tricuspid Valve Endocarditis

This 47-year-old woman, with a history of tricuspid valve replacement for severe regurgitation caused by Ebstein's anomaly and placement of a permanent pacer for complete heart block 10 years ago, presented with fever and chills. Blood cultures were positive for *Staph aureus.* She had progressive clinical deterioration in her status, with respiratory failure, renal failure, and pancreatitis. Echocardiography showed vegetations on the tricuspid valve and pacer leads. She was transferred to our medical center for surgical intervention.

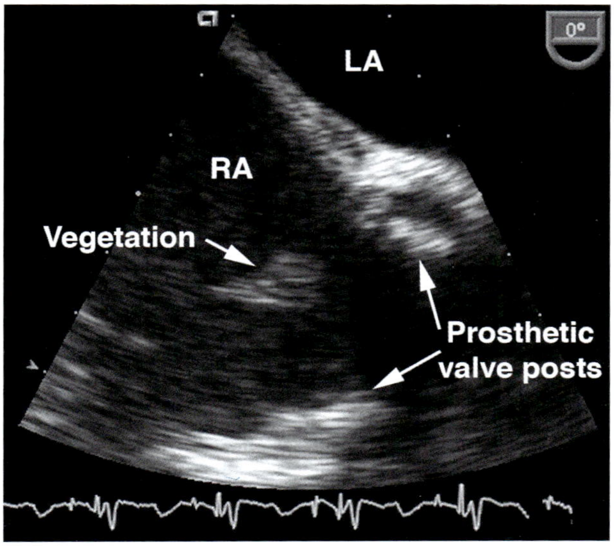

Fig 4.37 In a close-up image from a high TEE four-chamber view, a mobile mass consistent with a vegetation is seen on the atrial side of a tissue tricuspid valve prosthesis.

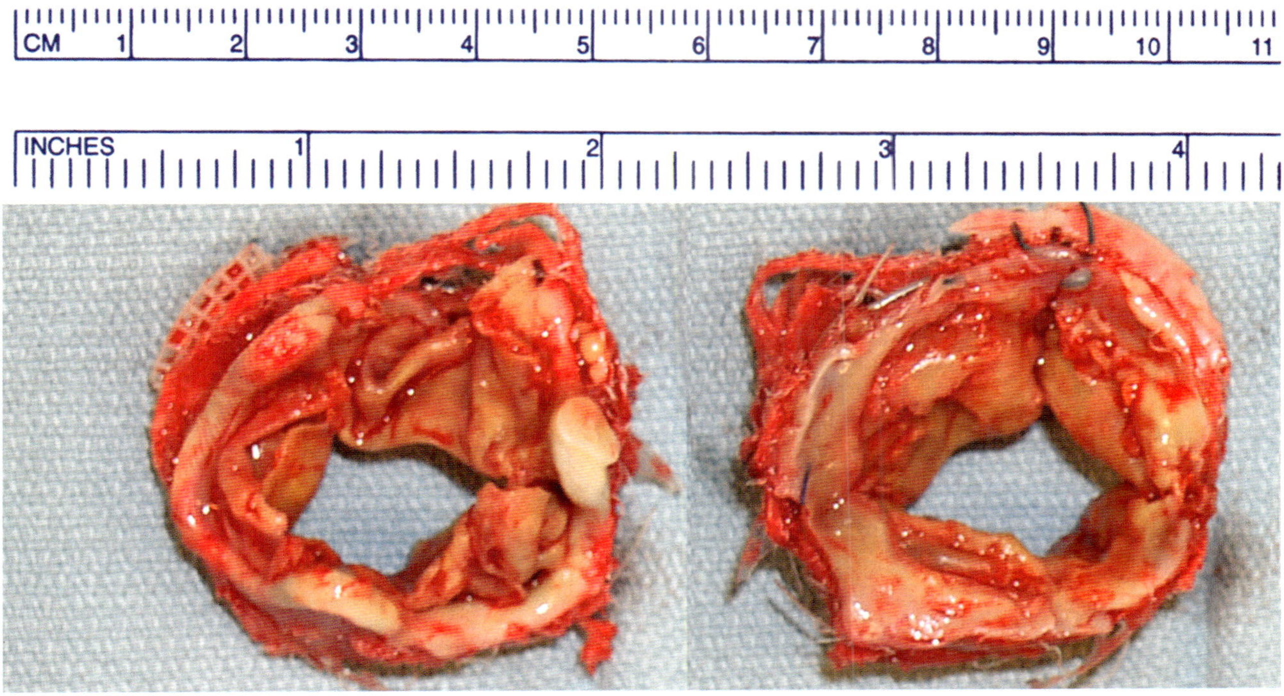

Fig 4.38 The explanted valve has been photographed from both the ventricular *(left)* and atrial *(right)* sides of the valve. Valve leaflet destruction by endocarditis is seen.

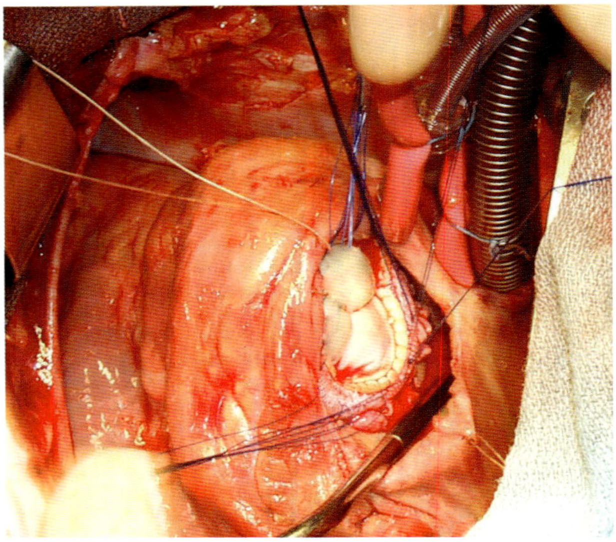

Fig 4.39 A new normal-appearing tricuspid valve prosthesis was sutured in the tricuspid annulus. The pacer and pacer leads were also explanted and replaced.

Comments

The diagnosis of prosthetic valve endocarditis is based on the same criteria as native valve endocarditis, with the caveat that visualization of valve vegetations is more difficult. With tissue prosthetic valves, infection may result in typical valvular vegetations, as in this case, although often transesophageal imaging is needed for identification. However, with mechanical valves, echocardiography may fail to detect infection because (1) infection is often limited to the sewing ring and annulus, and thus not evident on imaging, and (2) shadowing and reverberations from the metal sewing ring and valve occluders limit visualization of the valve or any adherent vegetations. Paravalvular abscess formation is common with prosthetic valve endocarditis, occurring in 60% to 70% of infected aortic prosthetic valves and in 20% to 25% of infected mitral prosthetic valves.

Suggested Reading

1. Hill EE, Herijgers P, Claus P, et al: Abscess in infective endocarditis. The value of transesophageal echocardiography and outcome: A 5-year study, Am Heart J 154:923–928, 2007.
2. Bruun NE, Habib G, Thuny F, et al: Cardiac imaging in infectious endocarditis, Eur Heart J 35(10):624–632, 2014.

CASE 4-9
Mechanical Mitral Valve Endocarditis

This 67-year-old woman had undergone mitral valve replacement 5 years ago. Over the past 5 years, she had a complicated clinical course with persistent heart failure, chronic atrial fibrillation, and severe pulmonary hypertension. About 2 weeks prior to the current admission she presented with a 2-week history of fatigue, vague neurologic symptoms, and the sudden onset of severe substernal chest pressure associated with ECG changes of acute anterior myocardial infarction. Emergent coronary angiography revealed a proximal left anterior descending artery occlusion. She subsequently became febrile and TEE showed a large mitral valve vegetation. She was then transferred to our medical center for surgical intervention.

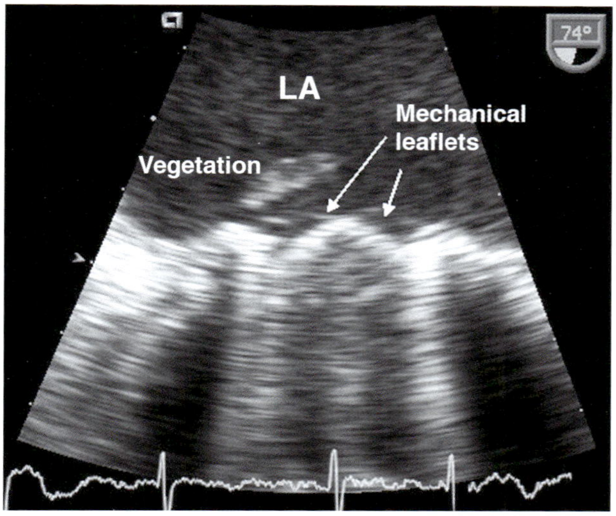

Fig 4.40 In a magnified image of the mitral valve in the four-chamber view, the closed bileaflet mechanical valve with shadowing and reverberations obscuring the LV is seen. In addition, a large, mobile mass of echoes, with motion independent of the valve leaflet motion, is seen on the left atrial side of the valve, consistent with a vegetation. In real time, vegetations are seen obstructing mitral inflow during diastole.

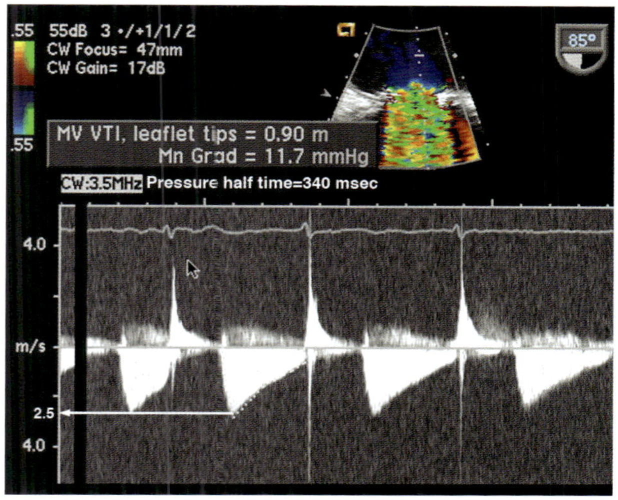

Fig 4.41 Continuous wave Doppler interrogation of the antegrade transmitral flow shows a peak velocity of 2.5 m/s, a mean gradient of 12 mm Hg and a pressure half-time of 340 ms. Using an empiric constant of 220, estimated mitral valve area is 0.65 cm^2.

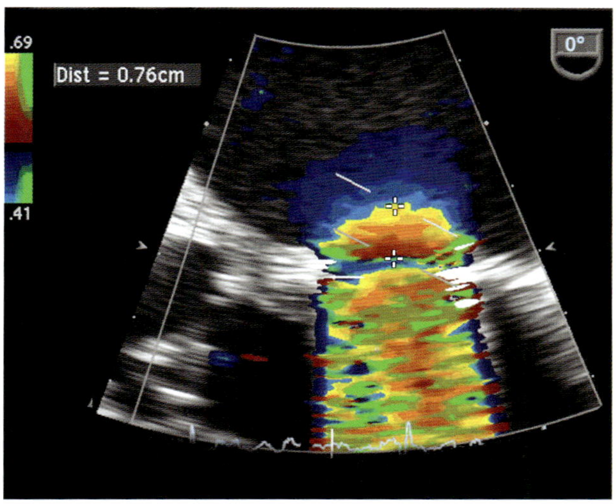

Fig 4.42 Color flow imaging shows the acceleration of flow proximal to the mitral orifice. The instantaneous transmitral flow rate is calculated as the surface area of the aliasing hemisphere ($2 \pi r^2$) × the aliasing velocity in the direction of mitral inflow. The calculation then becomes: [2 × π × (0.76 cm)^2] × 41 cm/sec, resulting in a transmitral flow rate of 149 ml/sec. Dividing this value by the peak antegrade mitral inflow velocity (2.5 m/sec from Fig 4.41) yields an estimated mitral valve orifice area of 0.6 cm^2.

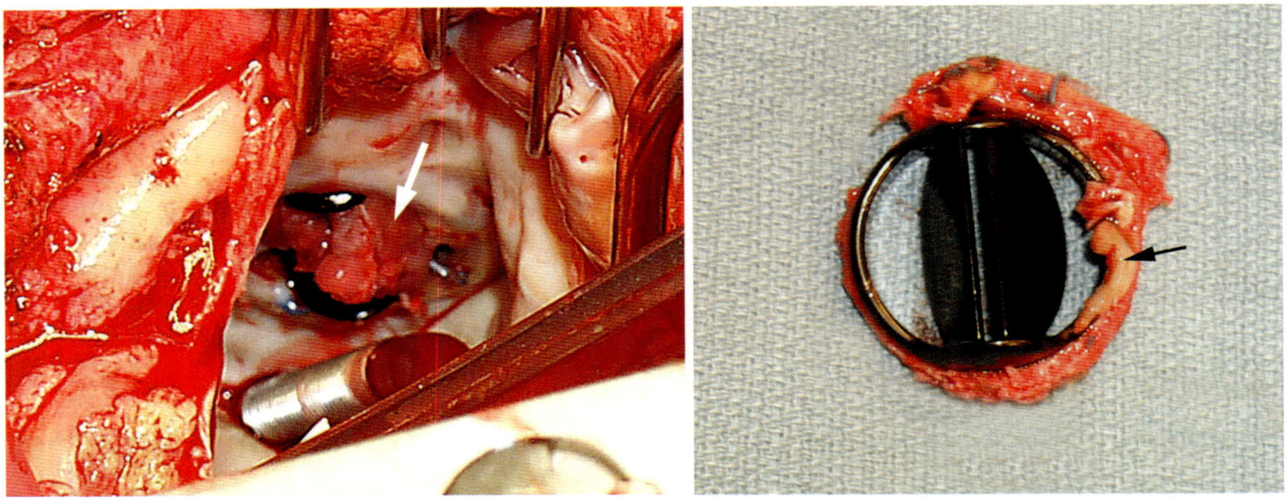

Fig 4.43 At surgery, a large vegetation was present on the atrial side of the valve, partially occluding the mitral orifice *(arrow, left)*. The resected valve shows that the mechanical valve itself is normal *(right)*. The site of attachment of the vegetation to the annulus is indicated by the arrow. Blood cultures and the resected vegetation grew coagulase-negative staphylococcus. The patient expired 10 days postoperatively with multiorgan system failure.

Comments

Endocarditis typically leads to valve regurgitation resulting from leaflet destruction. However, a large vegetation, as in this case, or infection involving the hinge points of a mechanical valve, can result in functional valve stenosis. Evaluation of the hemodynamic severity of valve obstruction follows the same principles as for any stenotic valve.

In addition to cerebral ischemic events or systemic emboli, fragments of valvular vegetations may embolize to the coronary arteries, resulting in acute myocardial infarction, as in this case. When the coronary angiogram suggests an embolic occlusion in a patient with a valve prosthesis, evaluation for infection or thrombus formation on the valve is needed.

Suggested Reading

1. Habib G, Badano L, Tribouilloy C, et al: Recommendations for the practice of echocardiography in infective endocarditis, Eur J Echocardiogr 11:202–219, 2010.
2. Prendergast BD, Tornos P: Surgery for infective endocarditis: Who and when? Circulation 121(9):1141–1152, 2010.

CASE 4-10
Mechanical Aortic Valve Endocarditis

This 35-year-old man had a history of aortic valve bacterial endocarditis complicated by an aortic root abscess that was treated with surgical excision of the valve and bileaflet mechanical prosthetic valve replacement. One month later he was admitted with signs and symptoms of heart failure, and was found to have a large paravalvular leak. He was taken to the OR and the mechanical valve was excised and replaced with a homograft.

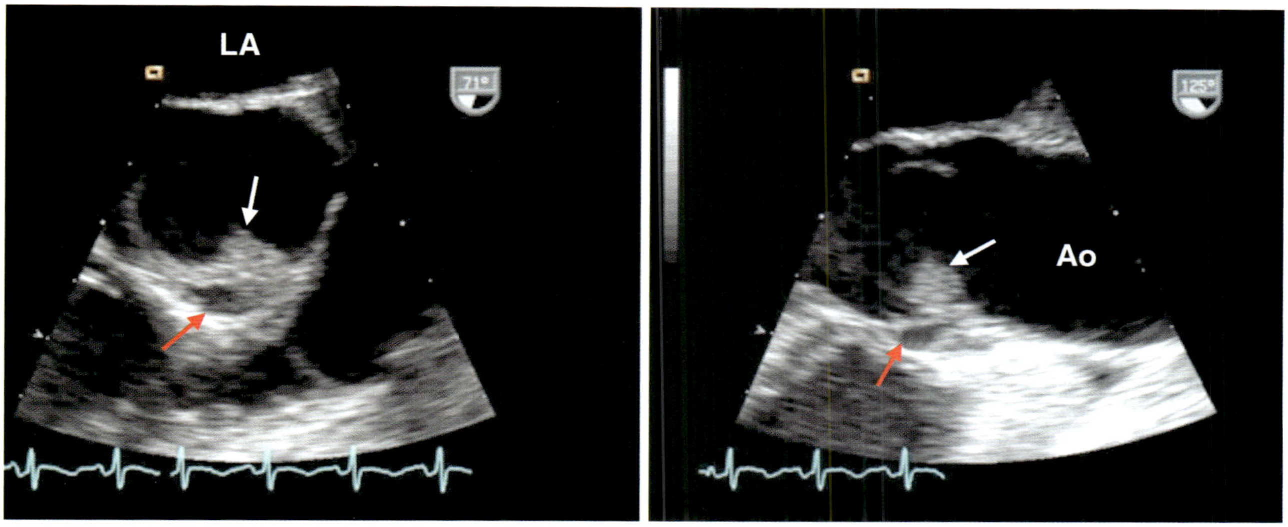

Fig 4.44 At his first operation, his native aortic valve was found to have an abscess anteriorly. In the left panel, a midesophageal short-axis view shows the vegetation *(white arrow)* with abscess formation *(red arrow)*. In the right panel, a midesophageal long-axis view also demonstrates the vegetation *(white arrow)* with abscess formation *(red arrow)*.

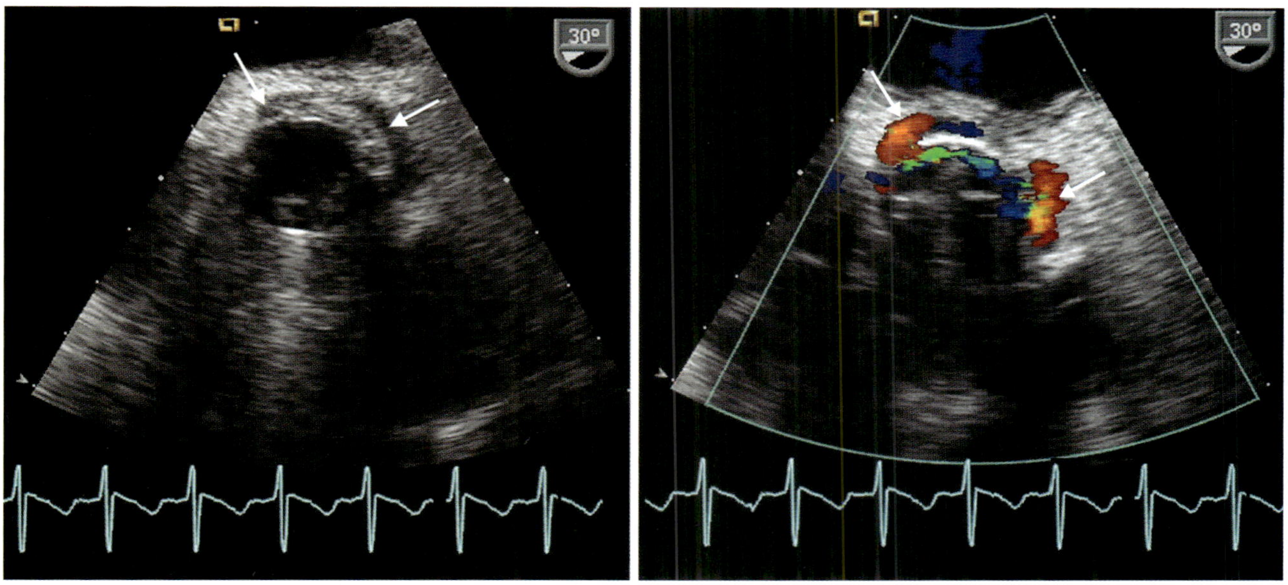

Fig 4.45 At reoperation, a midesophageal short-axis view of the aortic valve prosthesis shows echolucent areas external to the valve sewing ring, consistent with abscess or areas of valve dehiscence *(left panel, arrows)*. Color Doppler demonstrates regurgitation in these areas *(right panel, arrows)*.

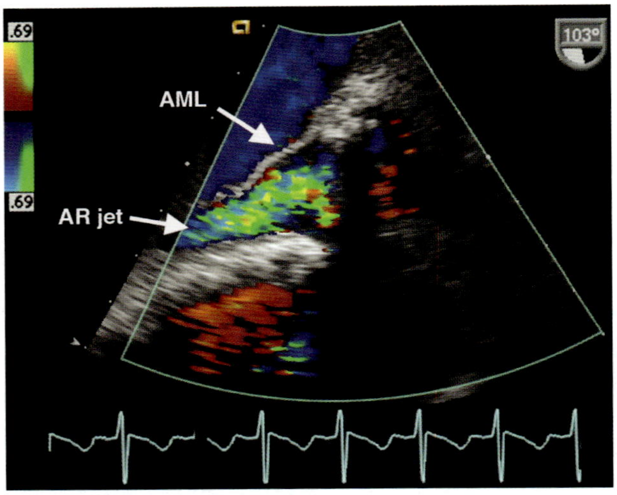

Fig 4.46 A midesophageal long-axis view shows a broad jet of aortic regurgitation that nearly fills the LV outflow tract.

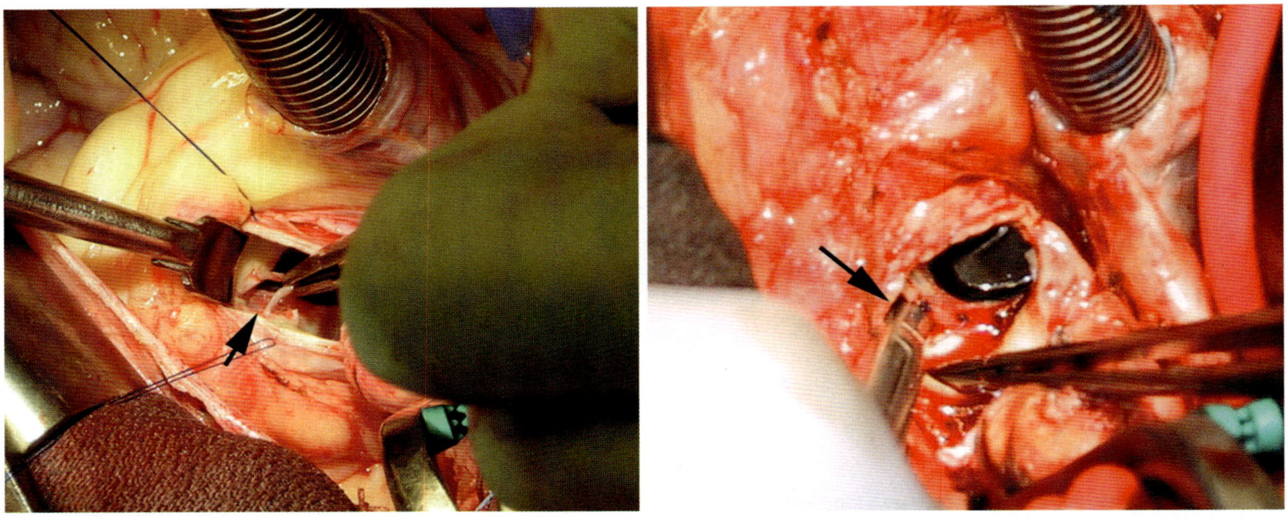

Fig 4.47 In the left panel, the native valve has been explanted in the first operation, and the black arrow indicates the subannular abscess. In the right panel, at the start of the second operation, the surgeon demonstrates an area of dehiscence to be in the same location of the previous abscess *(black arrow)*.

Comments

A small amount of paravalvular regurgitation is seen in up to 10% of mechanical valve replacements, even in the absence of endocarditis. However, new or worsening paravalvular regurgitation suggests infection of the sewing ring.

The severity of prosthetic valve regurgitation in patients with prosthetic valve endocarditis is evaluated using the same approaches as for evaluation of native valves. However, often only a semiquantitative measure of severity is needed because the decision about timing of surgical intervention is typically based on clinical events and the presence of valve dysfunction, rather than a specific measure of regurgitant severity.

For aortic regurgitation, the most useful quick methods to evaluate regurgitant severity are (1) the intensity and diastolic slope of the continuous wave (CW) Doppler curve and (2) the presence of holodiastolic flow reversal in the proximal abdominal aorta. Color Doppler is more helpful for defining the site and mechanism of regurgitation than for quantitation of hemodynamics in this situation.

Suggested Reading

1. Davila-Roman VG, Waggoner AD, Kennard ED, et al: Prevalence and severity of paravalvular regurgitation in the Artificial Valve Endocarditis Reduction Trial (AVERT) echocardiography study, J Am Coll Cardiol 44(7):1467–1472, 2004.

5 Surgical Prosthetic Valves

Prosthetic Valves

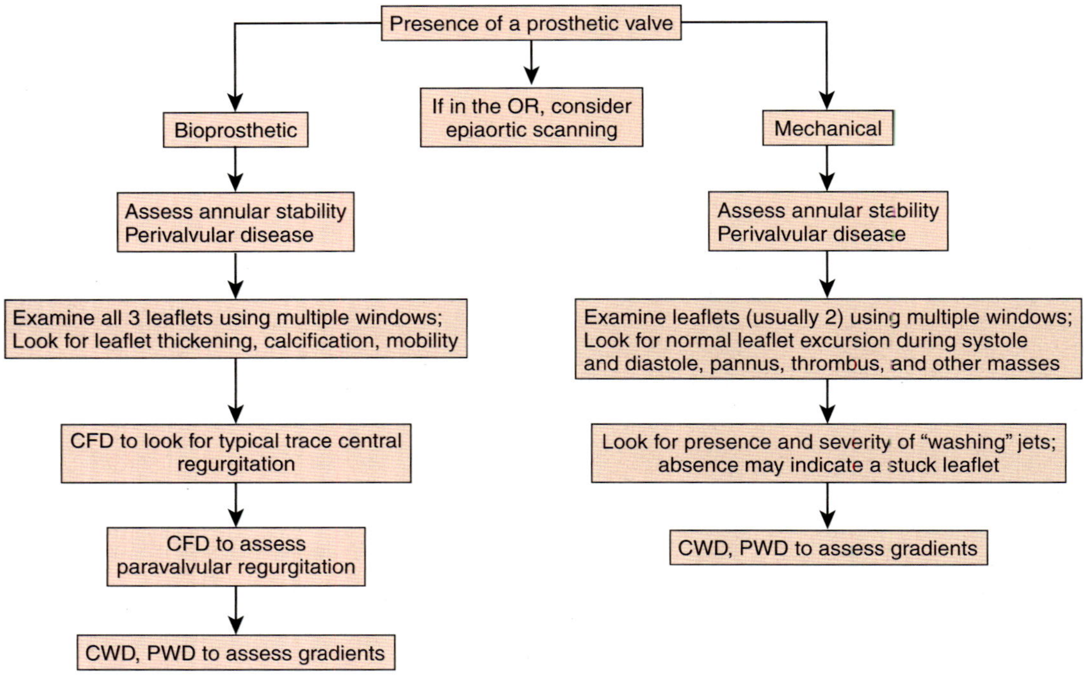

Fig 5.1 Flow chart of perioperative assessment of prosthetic valves. CFD, color flow Doppler; PWD, pulsed wave Doppler. (From Oxorn D, Intraoperative Echocardiography, Elsevier, 2012; p. 97, fig. 5-1.)

Normal Valves

CASE 5-1
Bioprosthetic Aortic Valve

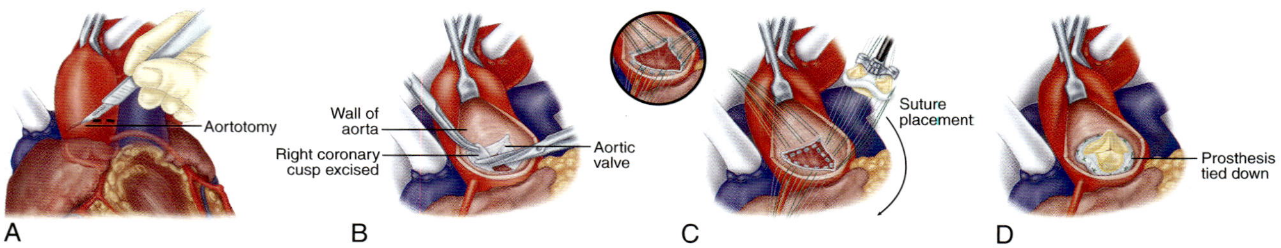

Fig 5.2 Example of insertion of normal stented bioprosthetic valve in aortic position. (From Sellke, Rule. Atlas of Cardiac Surgical Techniques, Saunders Elsevier, 2010.)

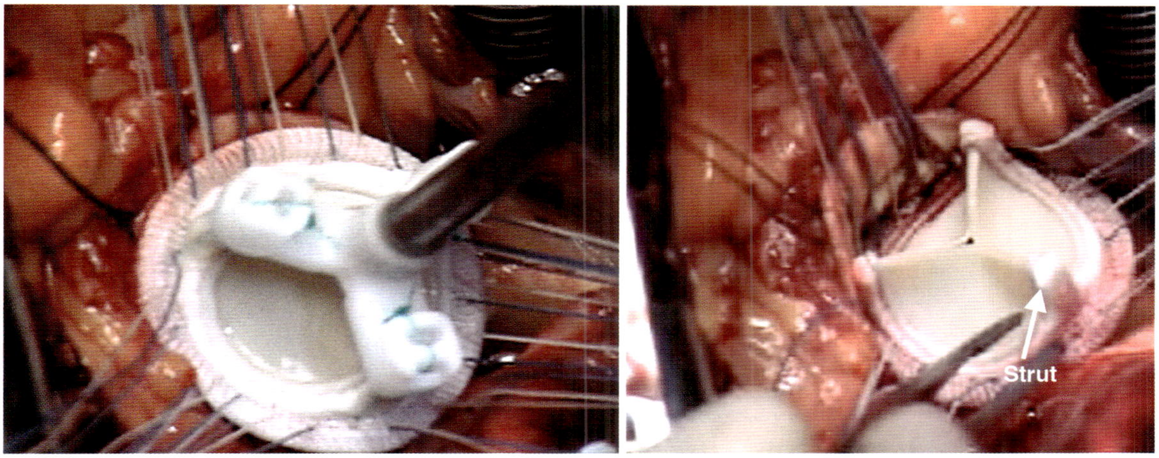

Fig 5.3 Sutures have been placed at equidistant intervals in sewing ring and aortic annulus *(left panel)*. Valve is lowered into position before the sutures are tied. (Perimount bovine pericardial valve, Edwards Lifesciences, Irvine, California.) With the valve-holding device removed, three struts (also known as posts or stents) at commissures of valve are easily visible *(right panel)*. Note that height of struts parallels normal anatomy of native aortic valve, with valve commissures more cephalad than valve sewing ring, resulting in typical curvature of valve leaflets. Normal overlap between leaflets in closed position is greatest adjacent to commissures and least in center of valve.

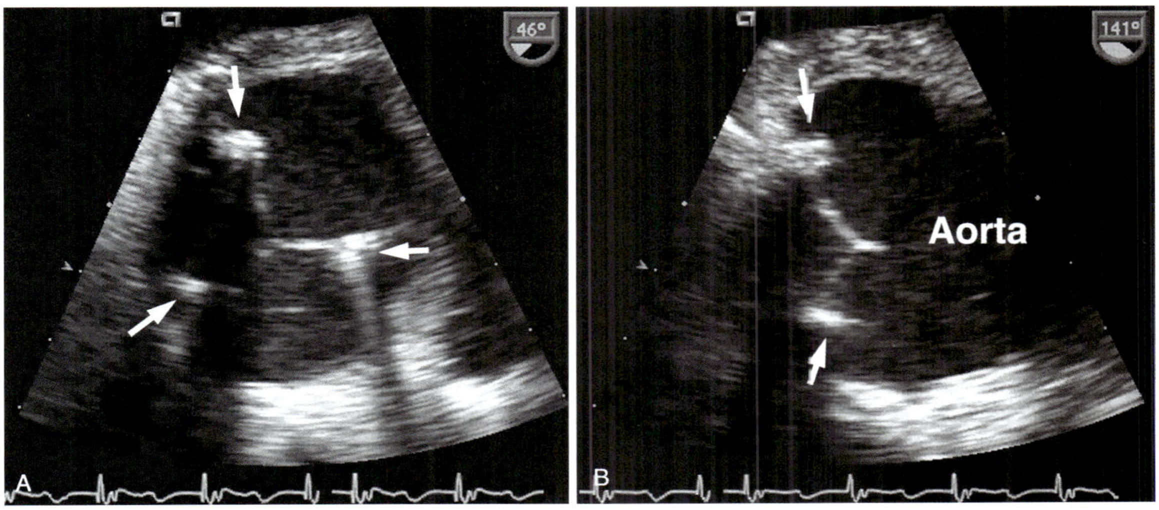

Fig 5.4 Short-axis (**A**) and long-axis (**B**) TEE views of aortic bioprosthesis show three struts in short axis and two struts in long axis *(arrows)* with thin leaflets in closed position in diastole.

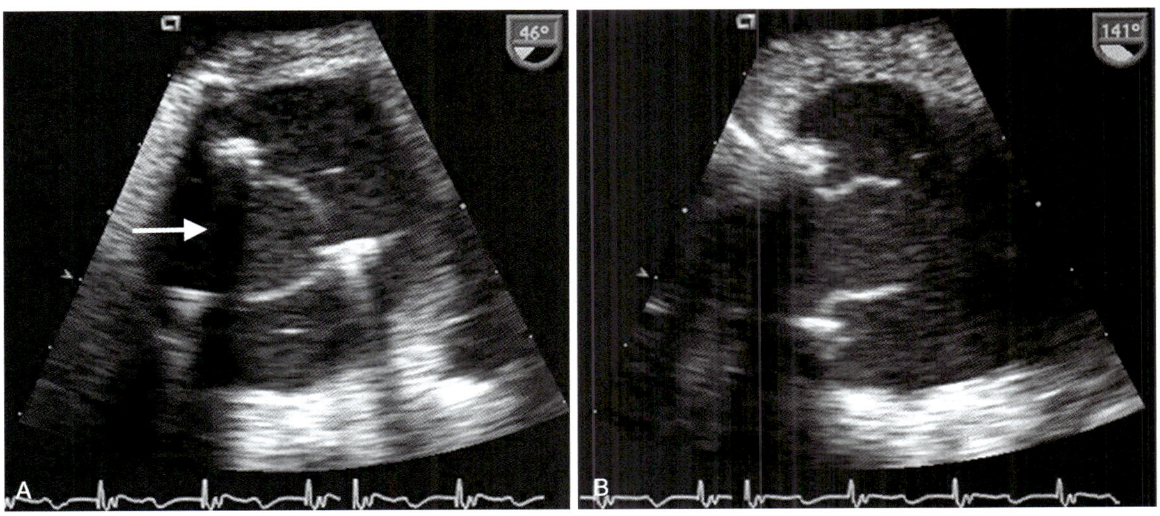

Fig 5.5 In systole, short-axis (**A**) and long-axis (**B**) TEE views show open leaflets during ventricular ejection. Acoustic shadowing from the strut prevents visualization of the noncoronary leaflet in short axis *(arrow)*.

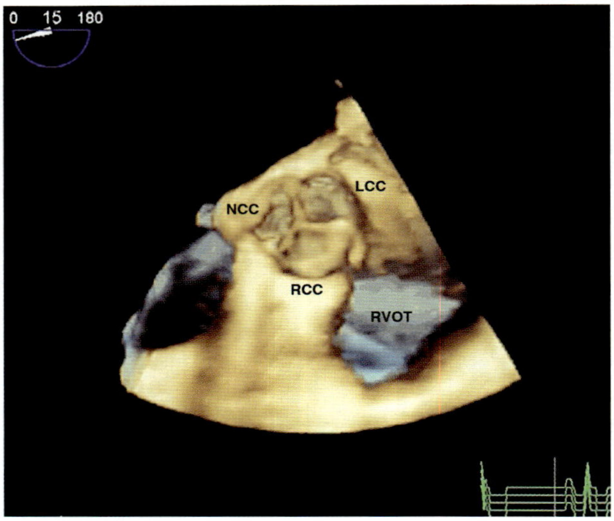

Fig 5.6 In another patient with similar prosthesis, 3D TEE from ascending aortic perspective shows cusps named according to position of native valve.

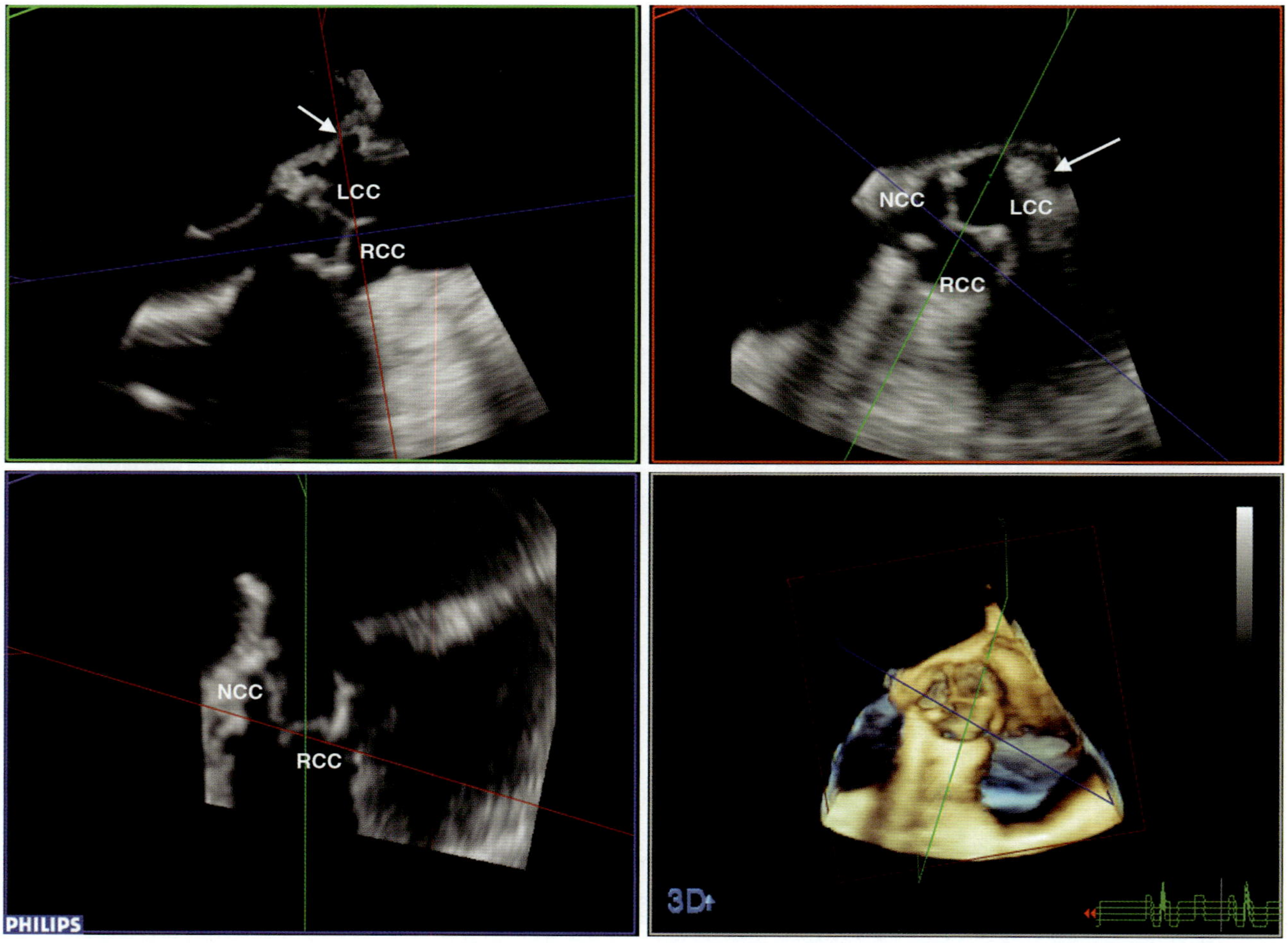

Fig 5.7 In this 3D multiplanar reconstruction of valve in Fig 5.6, upper right frame shows green and blue planes intersecting LCC/RCC and NCC/RCC. These are seen in long axis in upper left and lower left frames, respectively. The arrow indicates the position of the LMCA.

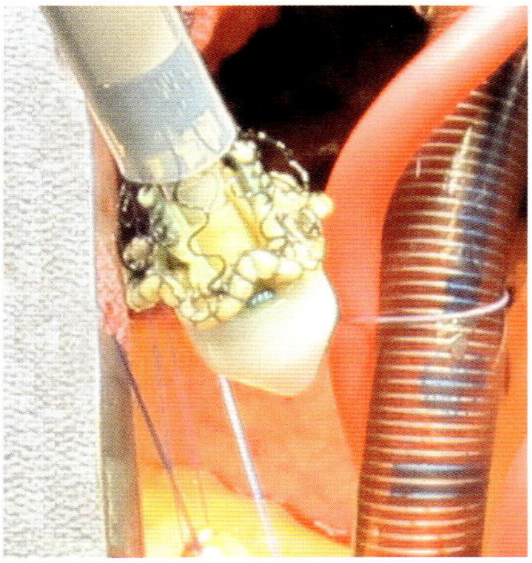

Fig 5.8 Self-expandable Perceval© valve (Sorin Group, Milan, Italy), unlike transcatheter aortic valve implantation (TAVR), is placed operatively via aortotomy. Ratio of effective orifice area to diameter of sewing ring is larger relative to other tissue prostheses. Image is of collapsed valve just before implantation.

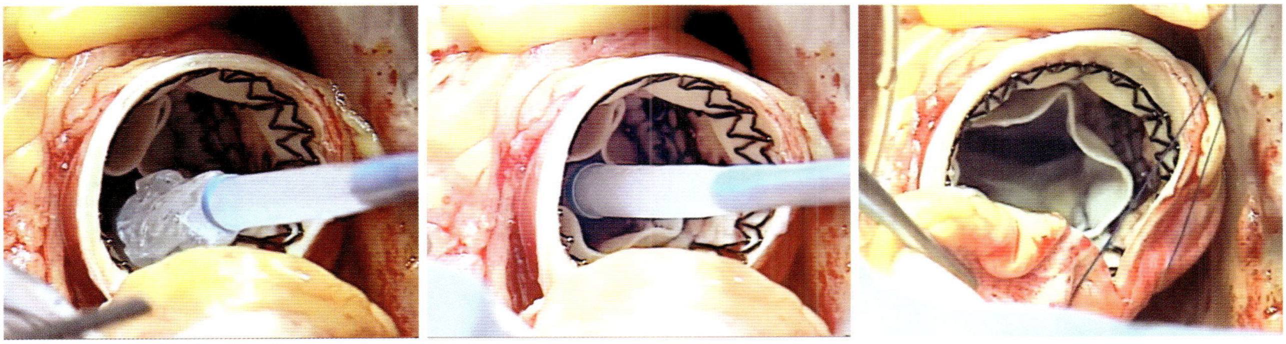

Fig 5.9 In left panel, initial valve deployment has been accomplished, and inflatable balloon placed to facilitate expansion of annular ring. Right panel shows valve fully deployed.

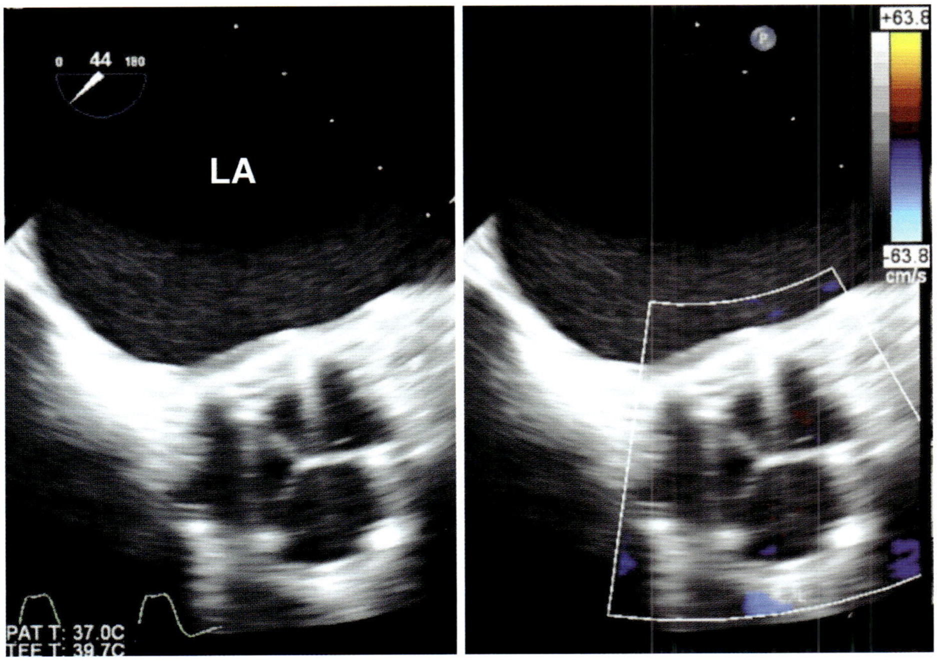

Fig 5.10 ▶ Midesophageal short-axis view of valve in diastole. No aortic regurgitation is visible.

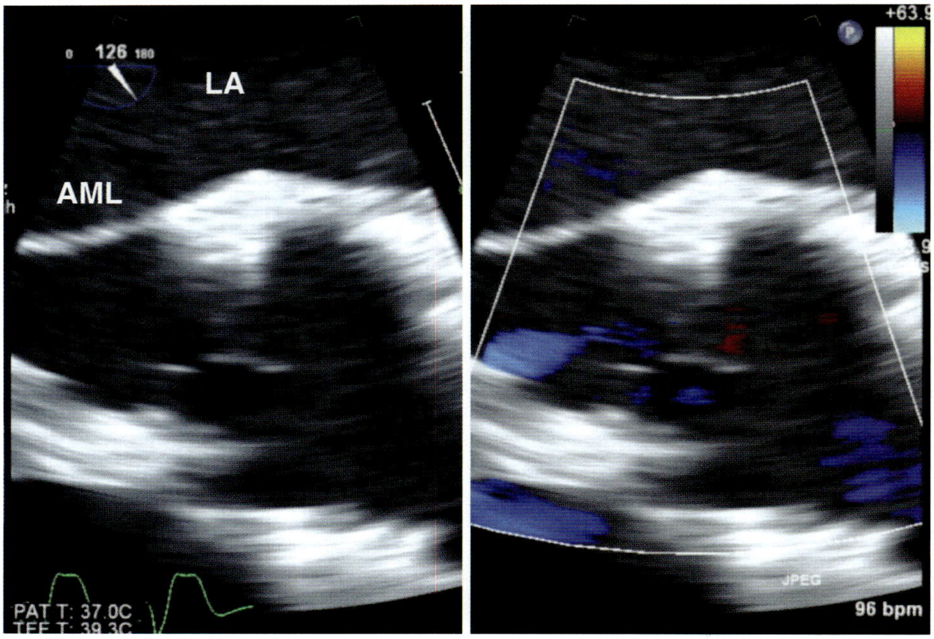

Fig 5.11 Corresponding mid-esophageal long-axis images.

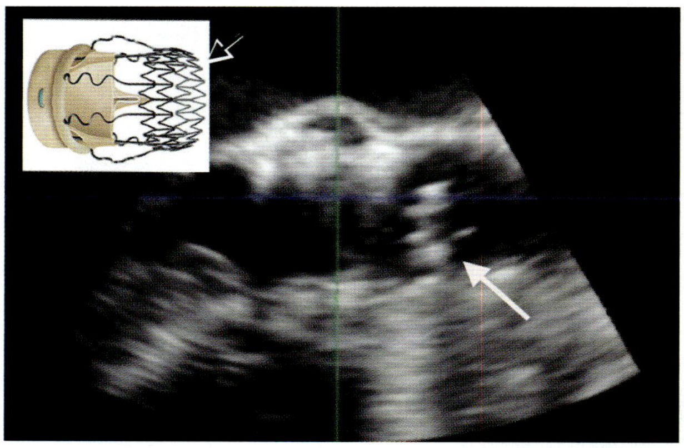

Fig 5.12 From midesophageal short-axis view of valve, with slight probe rotation, upper end of deployment apparatus is visible *(white arrow; black arrow in inset).*

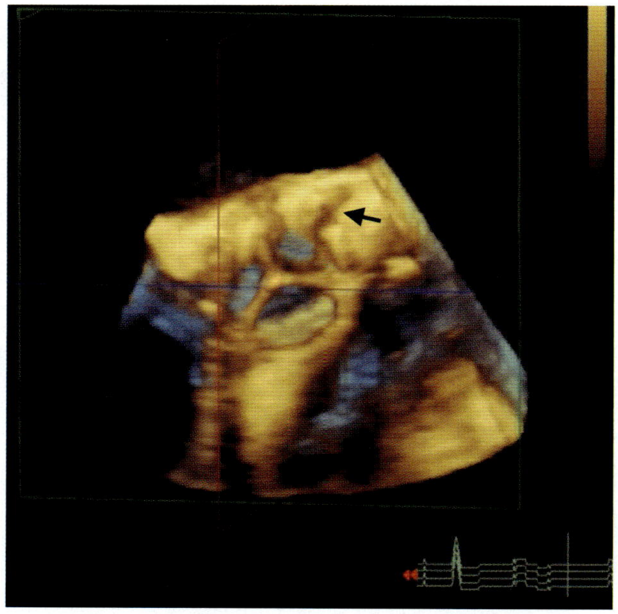

Fig 5.13 Valve on midesophageal 3D TEE from aortic perspective. The black arrow indicates the LMCA.

Comments

The two major categories of prosthetic valves are tissue valves and mechanical valves. Bioprosthetic (or tissue) valve leaflets are fashioned from bovine pericardium or a porcine aortic valve. The leaflets are supported by a rigid ring around the annulus with metal or polymer stents that support the commissures of the valve leaflets or by the cylindrical stent of the self-expandable valve. Implantation of these "stented" bioprostheses involves sewing an appropriately sized valve into the annulus, with the valve height and symmetry ensured by the annular ring and struts. In contrast, stentless tissue valves are supported only by a cylinder of flexible fabric or tissue. Implantation of stentless valves involves placement and suturing both at the annulus, and at the top of the commissures at the appropriate height.

Tissue valves open with a central circular orifice with a valve opening and closing motion similar to a native trileaflet aortic valve. However, the antegrade velocities (and pressure gradient) are higher than expected for a native valve because the sewing ring reduces the effective orifice area. At smaller valve sizes, the degree of functional stenosis can be significant, with a smaller effective orifice area than a similar-size mechanical valve. Thus the optimal valve choice in each patient depends on the size of valve that can be implanted, in addition to considerations of valve durability and long-term anticoagulation. If the implanted valve is too small for the patient size, patient-prosthesis mismatch (defined as an indexed effective valve area <0.85 cm^2/m^2) is associated with increased short-term mortality and suboptimal long-term outcomes.

Echocardiographic evaluation of the prosthetic valve after implantation should follow a standard format as shown in Fig 5.1

Suggested Reading

1. Yoganathan AP, Raghav V. Fluid dynamics of prosthetic valves. In Otto CM, editor: The practice of clinical echocardiography, ed 5, Philadelphia, 2016, Elsevier.
2. Maslow AD, Bert AA: Echocardiographic evaluation of prosthetic valves. In Oxorn D, editor: Intraoperative echocardiography. Practical echocardiography series, Philadelphia, 2012, Elsevier, pp 95–130.

CASE 5-2
Bioprosthetic Mitral Valve

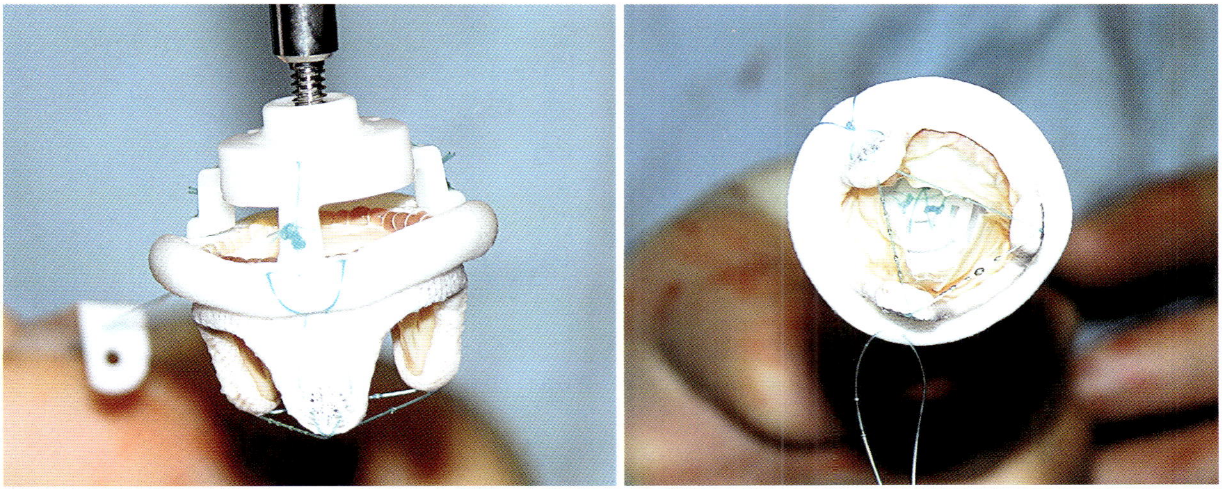

Fig 5.14 Stented mitral bioprosthesis (Medtronic Mosaic Mitral Prosthesis, Minneapolis, Minnesota), attached to holder, is seen from lateral view *(left)* and from ventricular aspect of valve *(right)* with leaflets in open position. Blue sutures maintain shape of prosthesis and provide orientation but are removed at time of implantation.

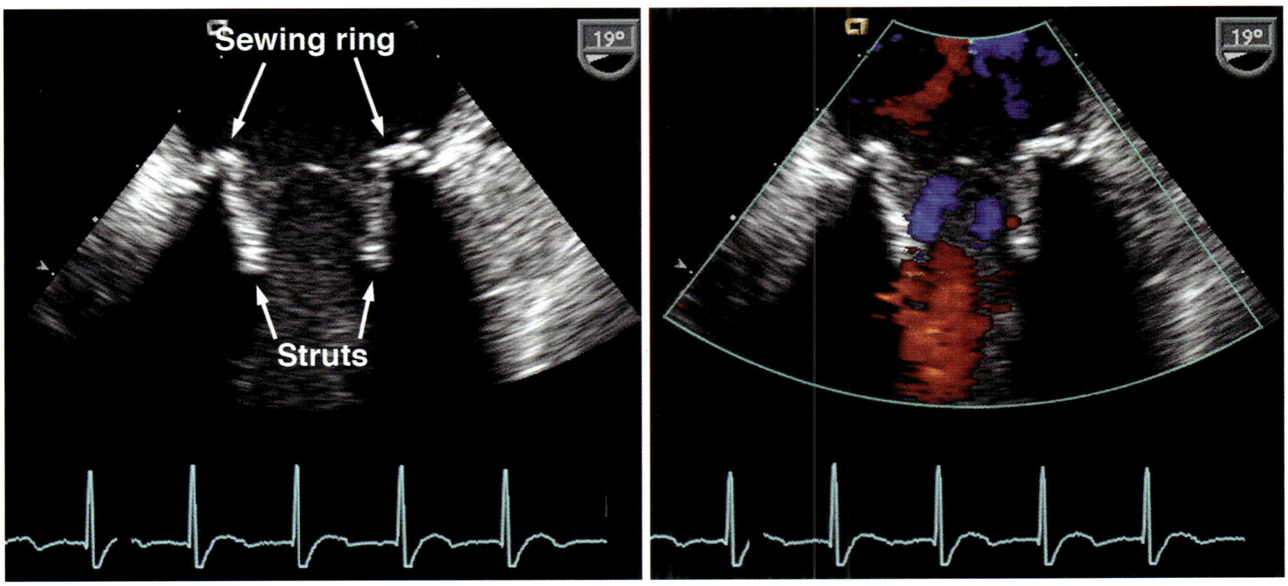

Fig 5.15 ▶ With valve implanted, four-chamber TEE view shows sewing ring, struts, and valve leaflets in systole. There are prominent acoustic shadows from sewing ring on 2D image *(left)*. Color Doppler *(right)* shows no mitral regurgitation.

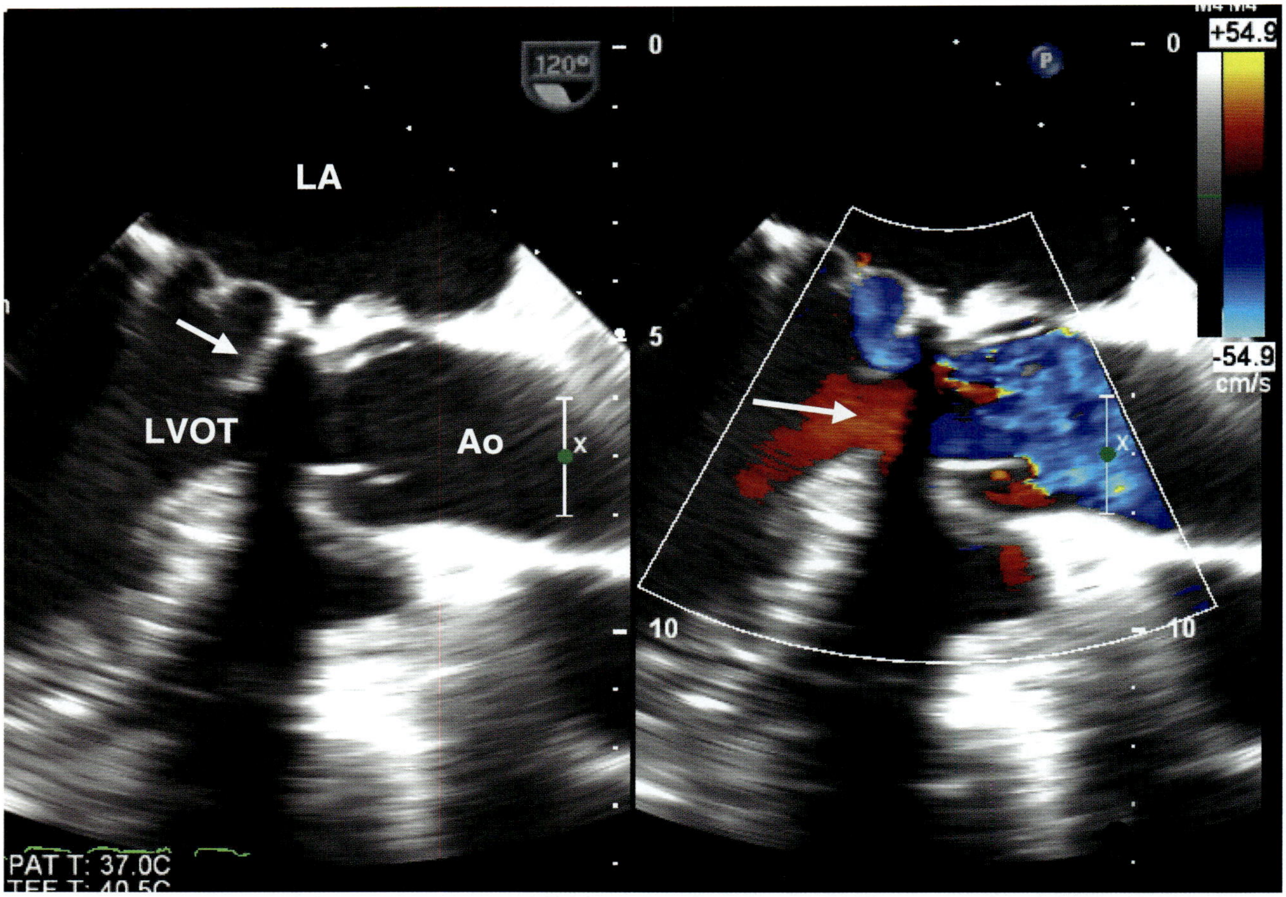

Fig 5.16 TEE midesophageal long-axis view shows one of the mitral struts protruding into the LVOT *(arrow)*. On the right, color Doppler shows no evidence of systolic signal aliasing, implying laminar, unobstructed flow *(arrow)*. Although this 2D image suggests LVOT obstruction, in most instances, there is enough room around the strut to allow unobstructed flow.

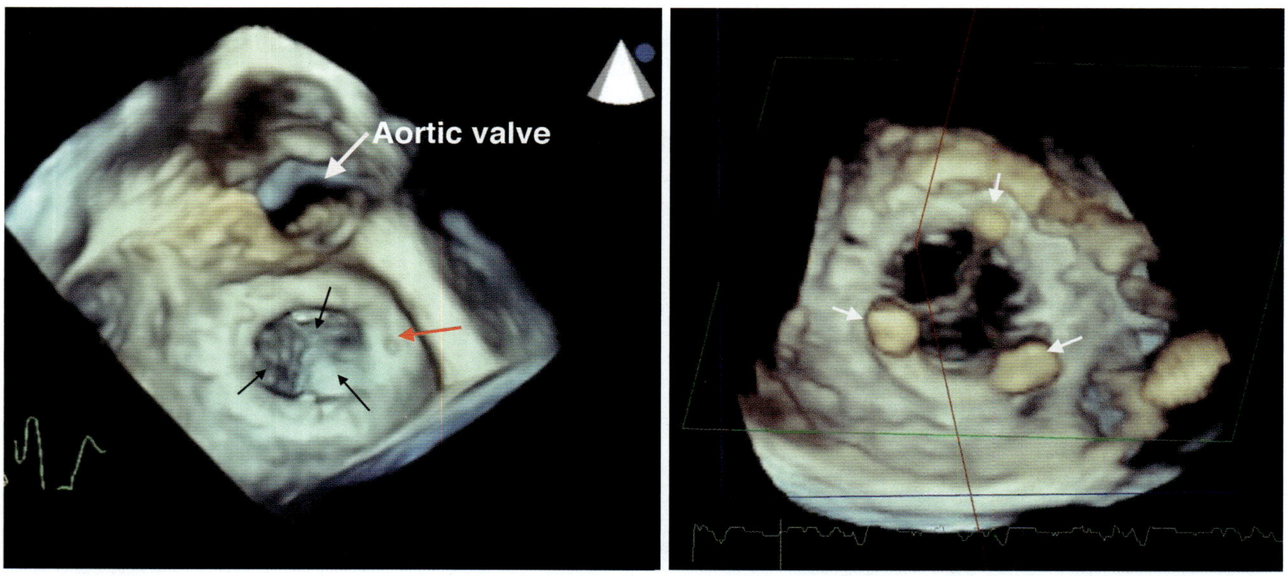

Fig 5.17 This image from different patient is 3D image from LA perspective. Black arrows indicate three leaflets, and red arrow, sewing ring *(left frame)*. In right frame, valve is now seen from LV perspective, with visualization of three struts *(white arrows)*. Each strut supports edge of two of three leaflets.

Comments

In the mitral position, mechanical valves are often used, as many of these patients are on chronic anticoagulation for atrial fibrillation. When bioprosthetic valves are used, stented valves are needed, rather than stentless valves, given the anatomy of the mitral annulus and left ventricle. The appearance of the valve in the mitral position is similar to a native aortic valve, with the stents protruding into the LV outflow tract. In the absence of a small and hypertrophied left ventricle, the stents rarely produce outflow tract obstruction (Fig 5.16). The flow through the mitral prosthesis is similar to a normal mitral valve, with an early diastolic peak (E-velocity), normal deceleration time and an atrial velocity peak (A-velocity) if the patient is in sinus rhythm. Velocities are only slightly higher than for a native valve, due to the large effective valve area and low left atrial to left ventricular pressure gradient in diastole.

Suggested Reading

1. O'Gara PT: Prosthetic heart valves. In Otto CM, Bonow RO, editors: Valvular heart disease, ed 4, Philadelphia, 2014, Elsevier, pp 420–438.

CASE 5-3
Bioprosthetic Tricuspid and Pulmonic Valves

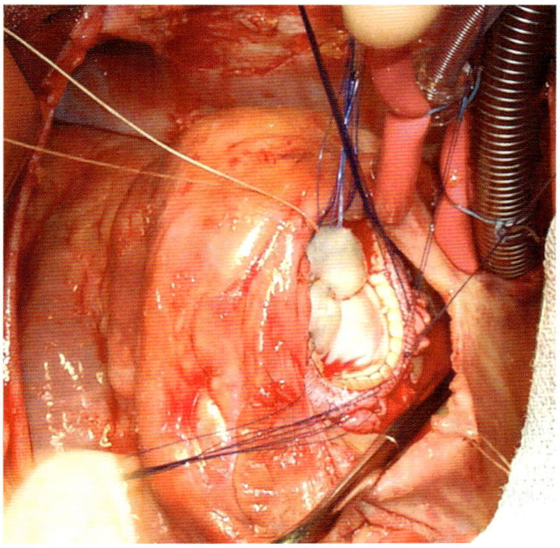

Fig 5.18 Surgical view of tricuspid valve bioprosthesis from right atrial side.

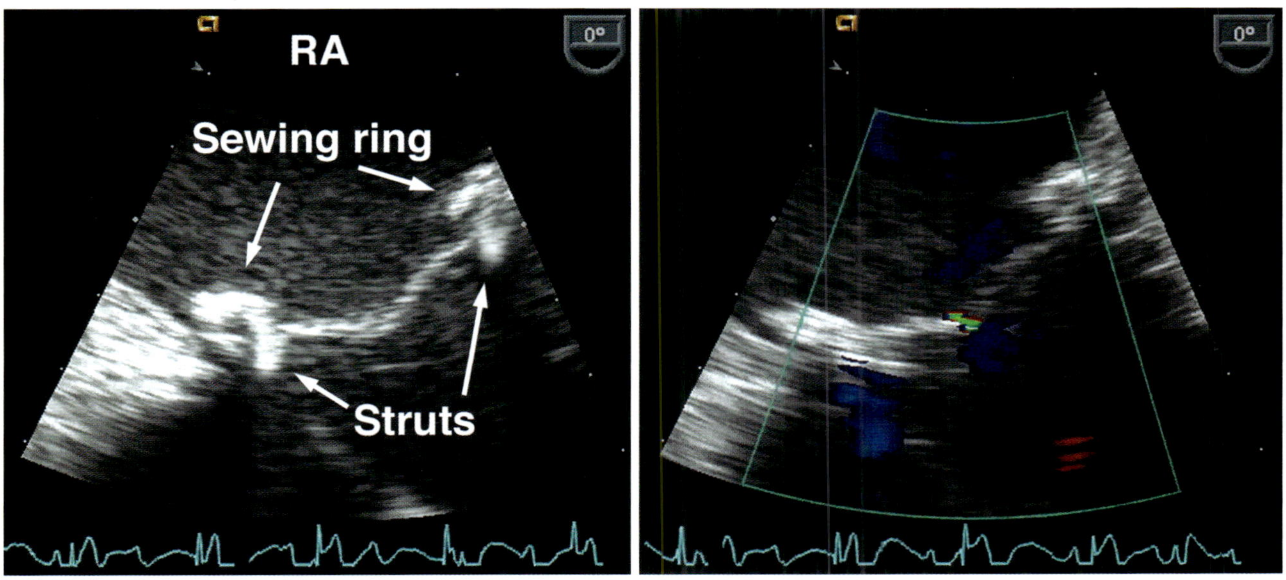

Fig 5.19 In four-chamber orientation at 0-degree rotation, tricuspid bioprosthetic sewing ring and struts are seen. Valve leaflets close at slight angle in systole *(left)* with no detectable regurgitation on color Doppler *(right)*.

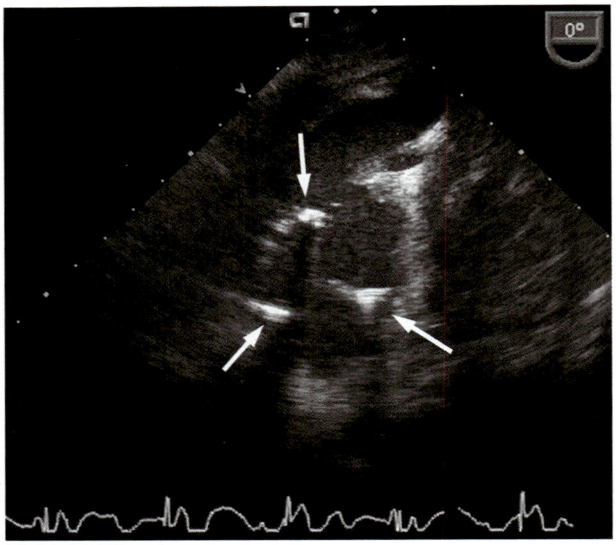

Fig 5.20 Transgastric short-axis view of tricuspid bioprosthesis shows three struts *(arrows)* and closed leaflets in systole.

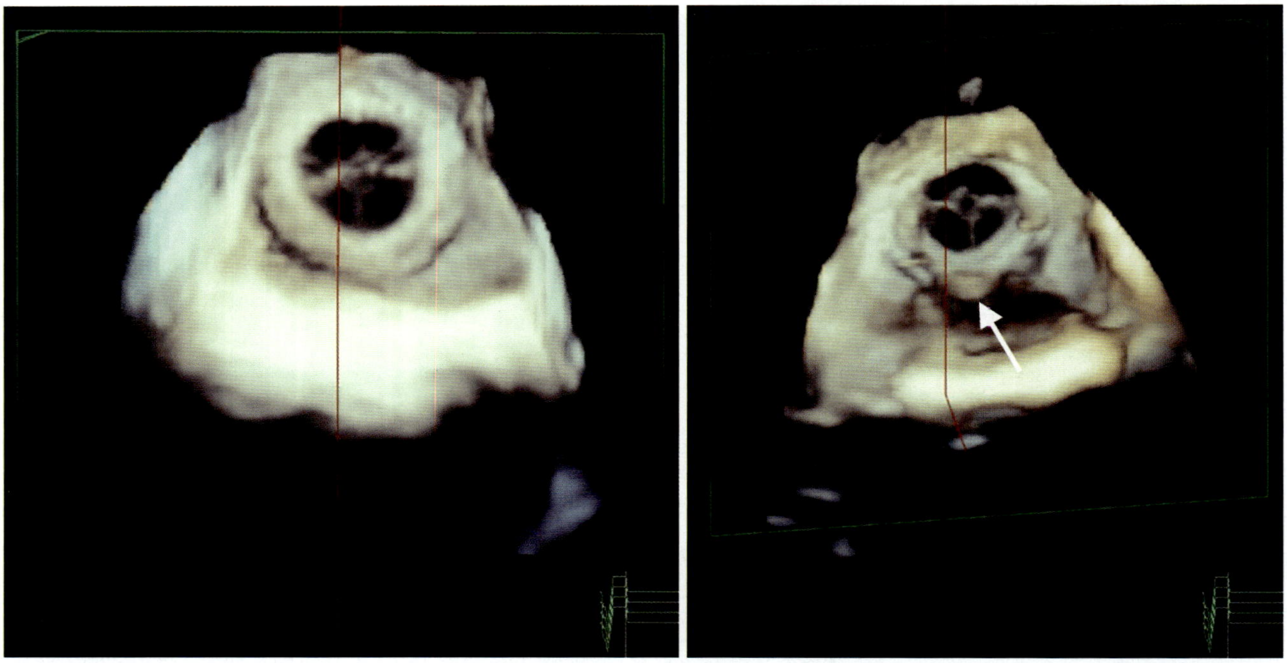

Fig 5.21 3D TEE of tricuspid valve from RA perspective *(left)* and from RV perspective *(right)*. White arrow indicates a strut.

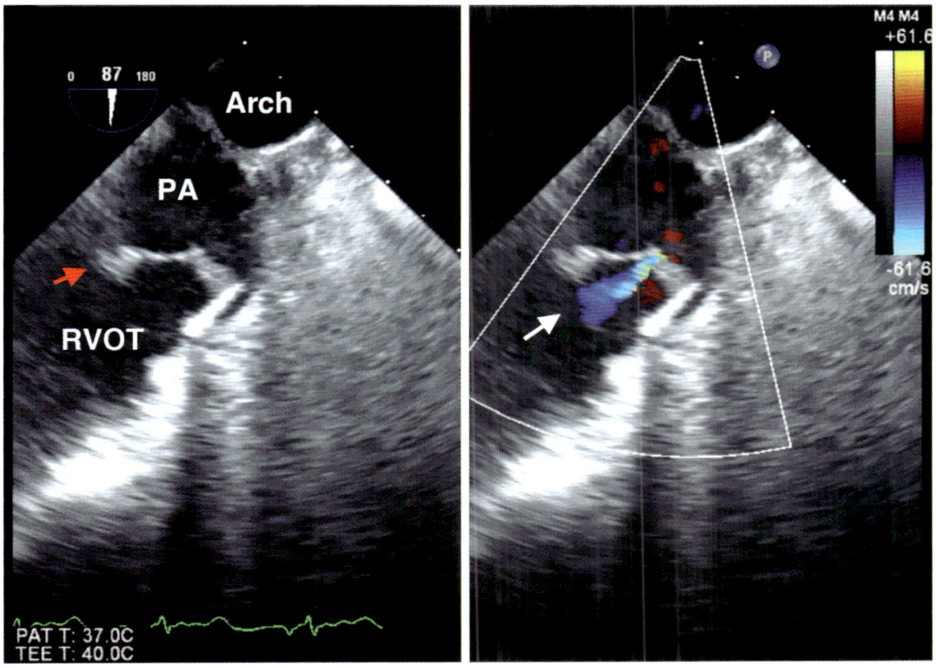

Fig 5.22 In a different patient, from high esophageal window, prosthetic pulmonic valve is seen; red arrow indicates one of valve struts. White arrow indicates small jet of pulmonic regurgitation.

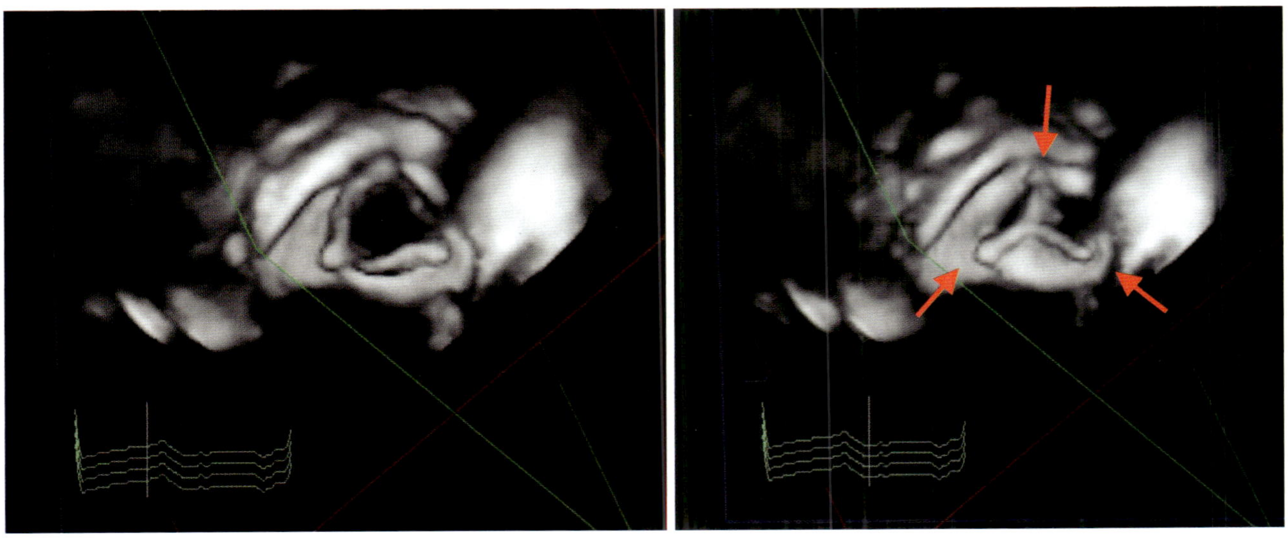

Fig 5.23 In a 3D TEE image corresponding to Fig 5.22, pulmonic prosthesis is seen from aspect of main pulmonary artery in systole *(left)*, and in diastole *(right)*. Three struts *(red arrows)* are more clearly visible.

Comments

Replacement of right-sided valves is less common than left-sided valves in adults. Mechanical valves in the tricuspid position have a high rate of valve thrombosis, whereas tissue valves have rapid valve deterioration. Thus tricuspid valve repair is preferred whenever possible. Bioprosthetic tricuspid valves have an appearance and flow dynamics similar to a mitral bioprosthesis. A small degree of central regurgitation is normal with bioprosthetic valves in any position, although not seen in this case.

Suggested Reading

1. Lin G, Bruce CJ, Connolly HM: Diseases of the tricuspid and pulmonic valves. In Otto CM, Bonow RO, editors: Valvular heart disease, ed 4, Philadelphia, 2014, Elsevier, pp 375–395.

CASE 5-4
Bileaflet Mechanical Mitral Valve

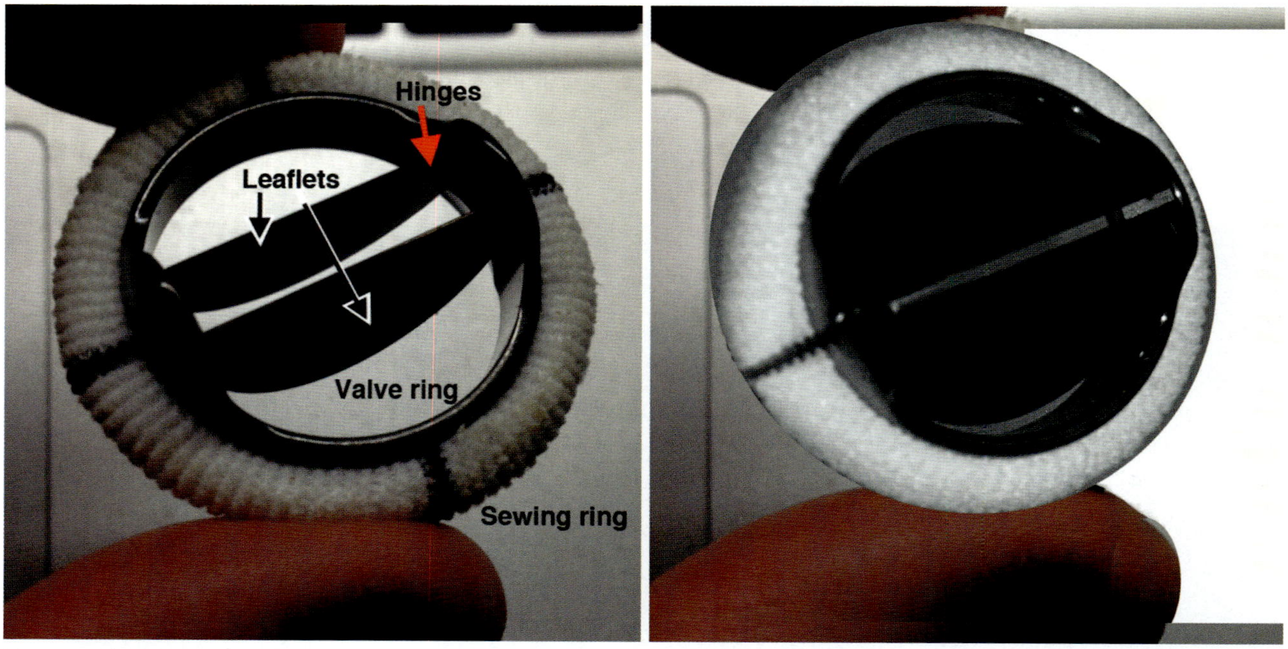

Fig 5.24 Bileaflet mechanical mitral valve as it would appear from left atrial side of valve. In left panel, valve is in diastolic position with leaflets open. Two semicircular occluders (or leaflets) are free at edges, with attachment only at small "hinges" near center of valve ring. Sewing ring is covered with cloth to allow attachment of sutures. In right panel, valve is almost completely closed; full closure would occur in systole.

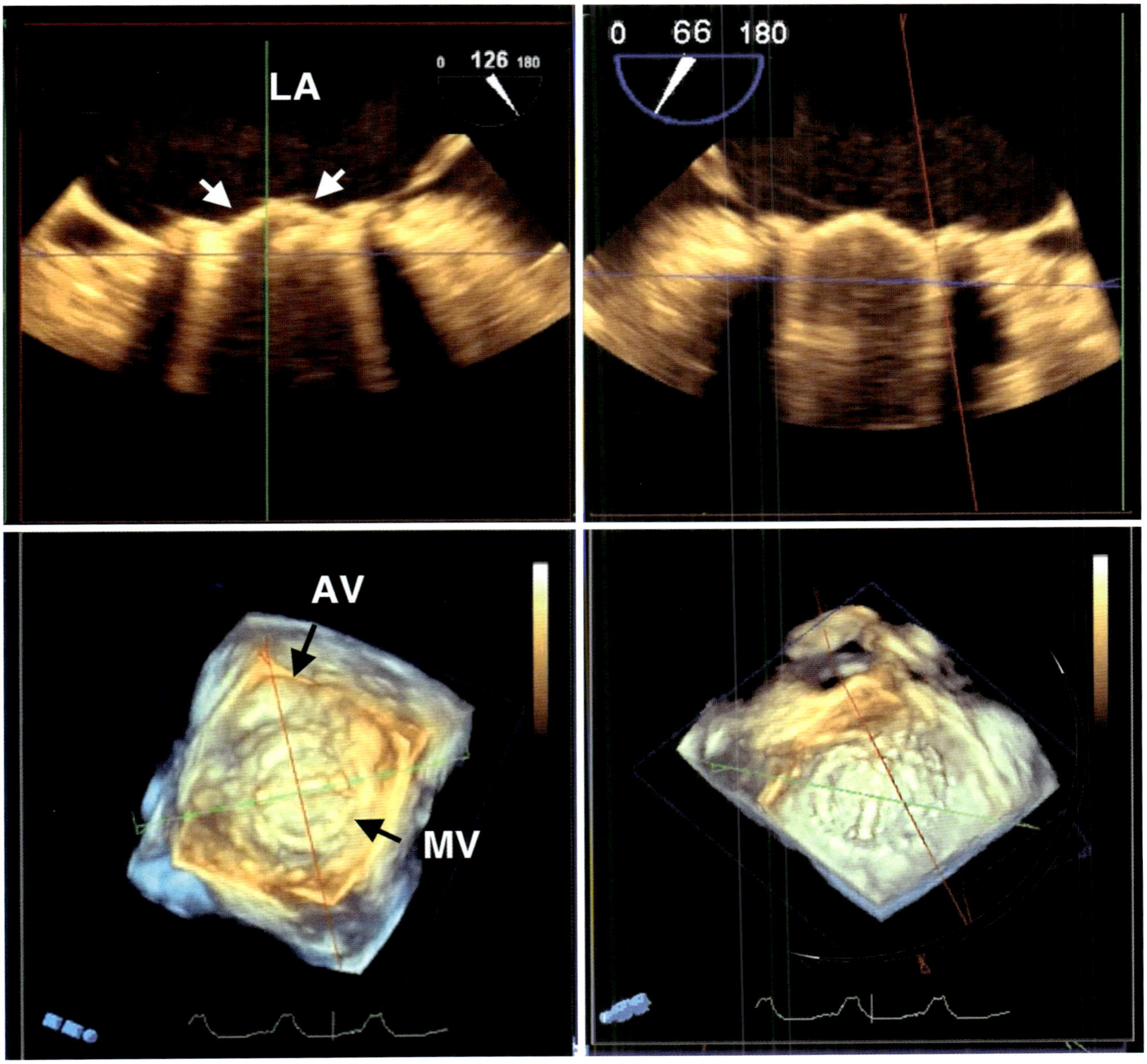

Fig 5.25 In patient at left, mitral valve has been implanted in "anatomic" position, with location of two prosthetic valve occluders matching normal positions of native anterior and posterior mitral valve leaflets. Bottom left panel shows "surgeons view"—view surgeon would have from right side of operating table with left atrium open—with red line intersecting valve, resulting in reconstructed 2D midesophageal long-axis view seen in top left image. Leaflets close symmetrically and are indicated with white arrows. In patient on right, valve has been implanted in "antianatomic position" with prosthetic valve occluders oriented at about 90 degrees from positions of native valve leaflets. In 3D image *(lower right)*, green line now intersects valve symmetrically, resulting in a similar reconstructed 2D image *(top right)*. In the videos, examples of how the valve looks at different transducer angles is shown.

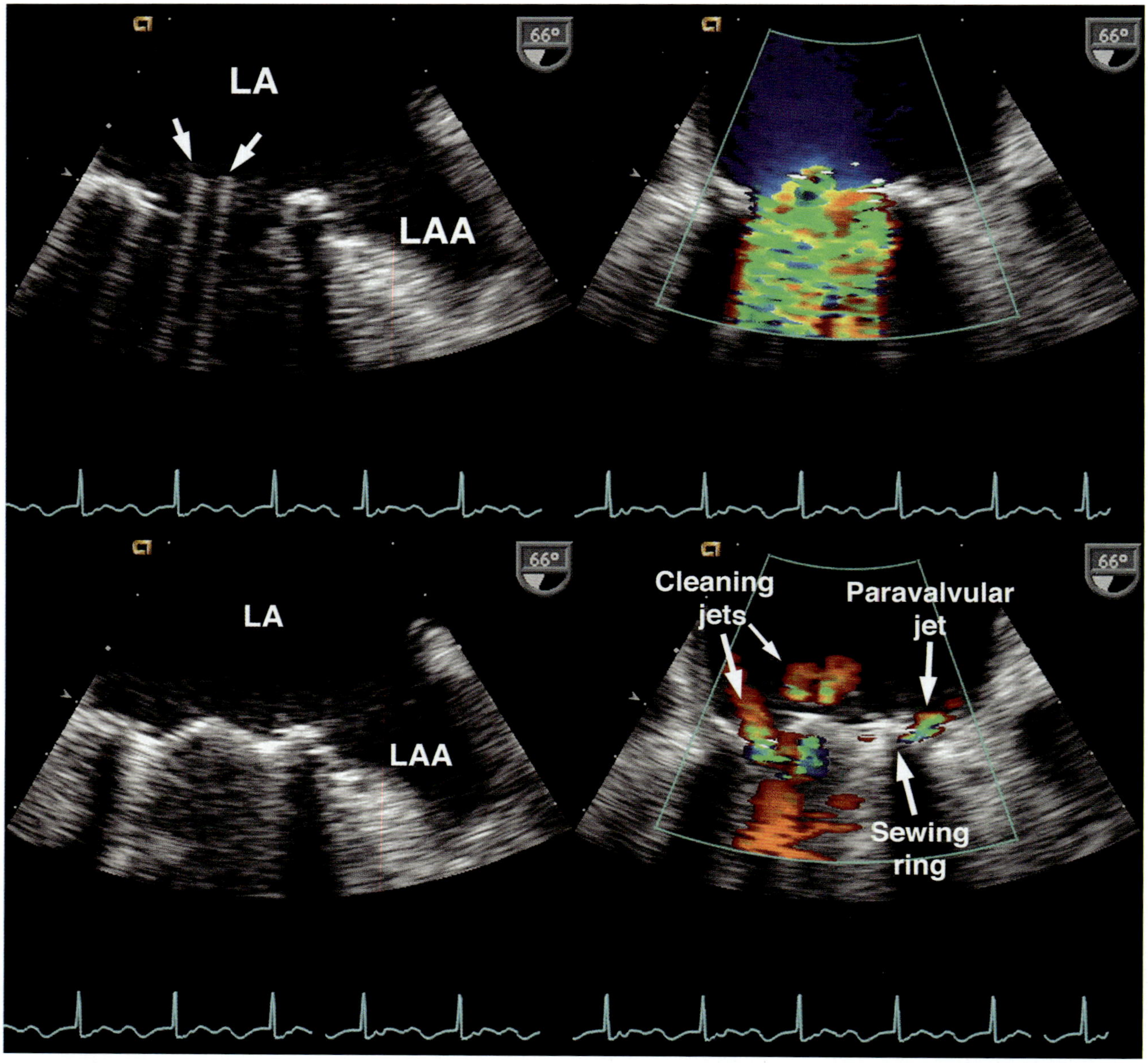

Fig 5.26 In two-chamber view, standard 2D *(left)* and color Doppler (*right*) images of valve shows parallel alignment of open leaflets *(arrows)* in diastole *(top)*. In systole *(bottom),* closed leaflets are at slight angle to each other. Note shadows cast by sewing ring and reverberations due to disk occluders that obscure left ventricle in this view. Color Doppler *(right)* shows normal antegrade flow through narrow central orifice and larger lateral orifices in diastole *(top)* with typical small eccentric jets due to closure of leaflets ("cleaning" jets) in systole *(bottom)*. Small paravalvular jet outside sewing ring is also seen—this closed spontaneously, shortly after separating from cardiopulmonary bypass.

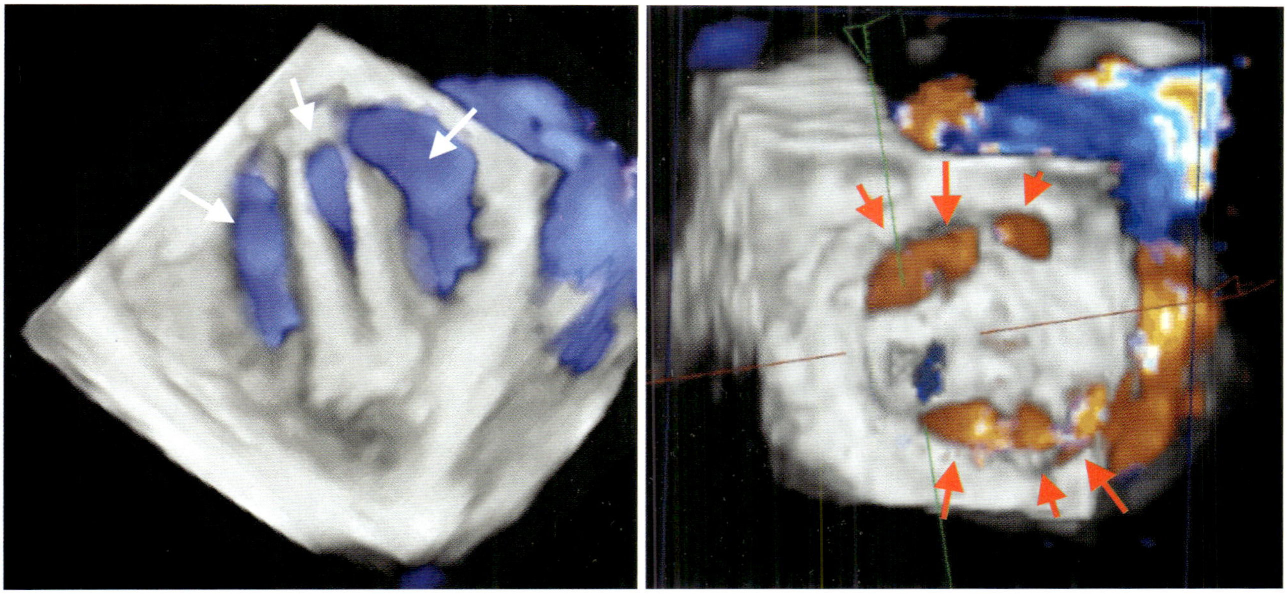

Fig 5.27 3D color Doppler of mitral valve from left atrial perspective shows three jets of inflow in diastole *(left, white arrows)* and multiple washing jets during systole *(right, red arrows)*.

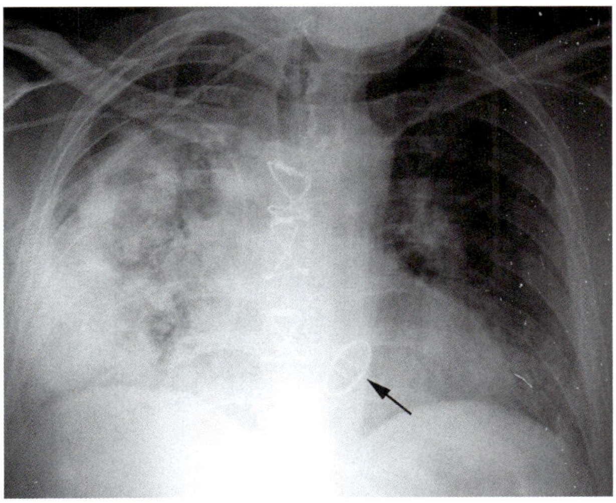

Fig 5.28 Portable AP chest radiograph shows open bileaflet mechanical valve in mitral position.

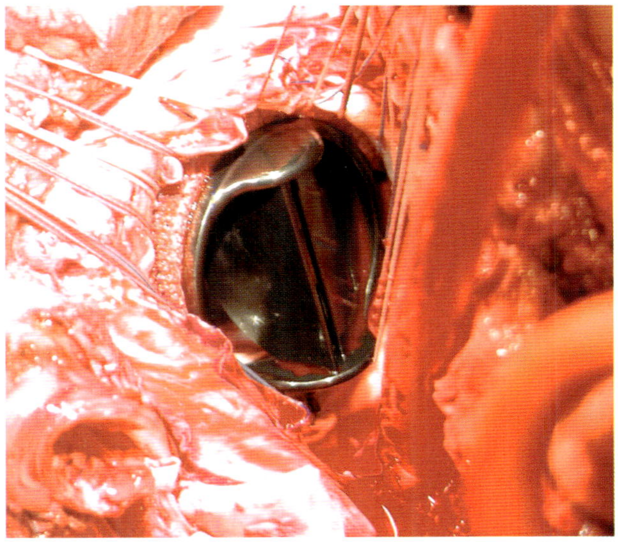

Fig 5.29 Bileaflet valve after insertion, viewed via open left atrium.

Comment

The most common type of mechanical valve is a bileaflet valve with two semicircular leaflet occluders or a tilting disk valve with a single circular occluder that pivots on hinges or a central strut. Older mechanical valve types, such as ball-in-cage valves now are rarely seen. The normal fluid dynamics of bileaflet mechanical valve prosthesis are characterized by a small amount of regurgitation due to the closure of the valve occluders. With a bileaflet valve, there are typically two converging jets from the pivot points, a small central jet, and a variable number of peripheral jets, with little signal aliasing. In addition, these normal regurgitant jets are small in size, originating from within the sewing ring.

In contrast, pathologic regurgitation occurs in unexpected locations, often paravalvular, and is usually associated with larger, more eccentric jets. Prosthetic valve regurgitation is evaluated using the same approaches as for native valves, including measurement of the vena contracta width, evaluation of the intensity and shape of the continuous wave Doppler curve, and calculation of regurgitant volume and orifice area. However, evaluation of prosthetic valves, particularly in the mitral position, requires transesophageal imaging because shadowing and reverberations from the prosthesis preclude evaluation from the transthoracic approach. Detection of the proximal isovelocity surface area (PISA) on the ventricular side of the valve is helpful for identification of the origin of the regurgitant jet, but measurements are often difficult due to PISA asymmetry and poor image quality.

Suggested Reading

1. Pibarot P: Prosthetic valve dysfunction: echocardiographic recognition and quantitation (including paravalvular regurgitation and closure) In Otto CM, editor: The practice of clinical echocardiography, ed 5, Philadelphia, 2016, Elsevier.
2. Beigel R, Siegel RJ: Evaluation of prosthetic valve dysfunction with the use of echocardiography, Rev Cardiovasc Med 15(4): 332–350, 2014.
3. Hahn RT: Mitral prosthetic valve assessment by echocardiographic guidelines, Cardiol Clin 31(2):287–309, 2013.

CASE 5-5
Bileaflet Mechanical Aortic Valve

Example of a normal bileaflet mechanical aortic valve replacement. Compared with the bileaflet valve in the mitral position, the valve in the aortic position is flipped on its vertical axis.

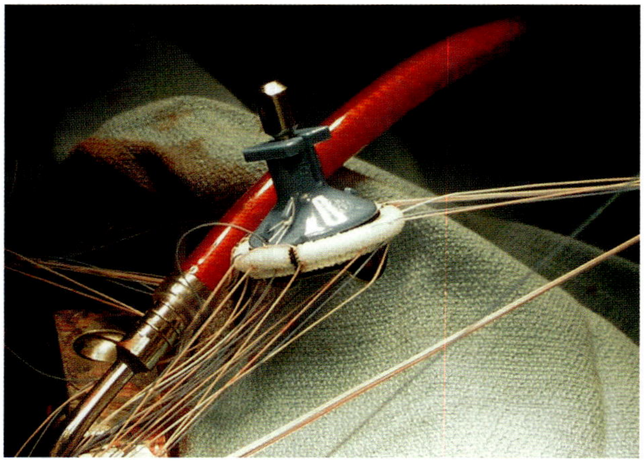

Fig 5.30 Mechanical valve is positioned in holder, with only sewing ring of valve visible. Sutures have been placed equidistant around sewing ring for attaching prosthesis to aortic annulus.

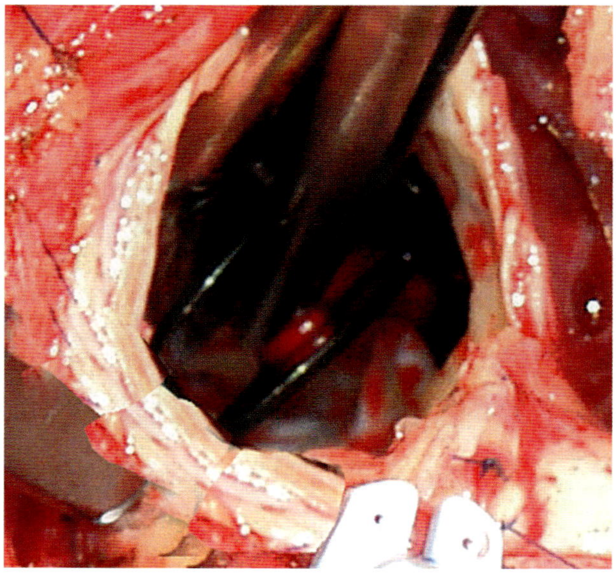

Fig 5.31 Bileaflet valve in aortic position with forceps opening two leaflets. Note narrow slit-like central orifice and two larger semicircular orifices.

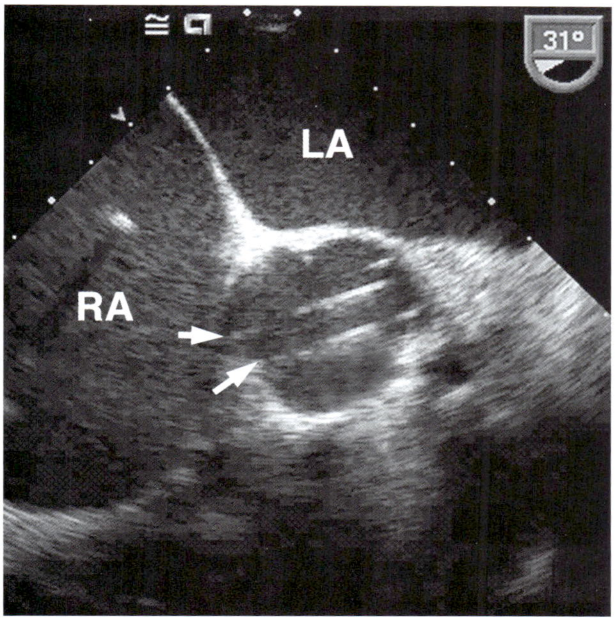

Fig 5.32 In view similar to surgical view, this echocardiographic short-axis view of aortic valve at 31-degree rotation shows two leaflets open in systole *(arrows)* with central slit-like orifice and two larger semicircular orifices anteriorly and posteriorly.

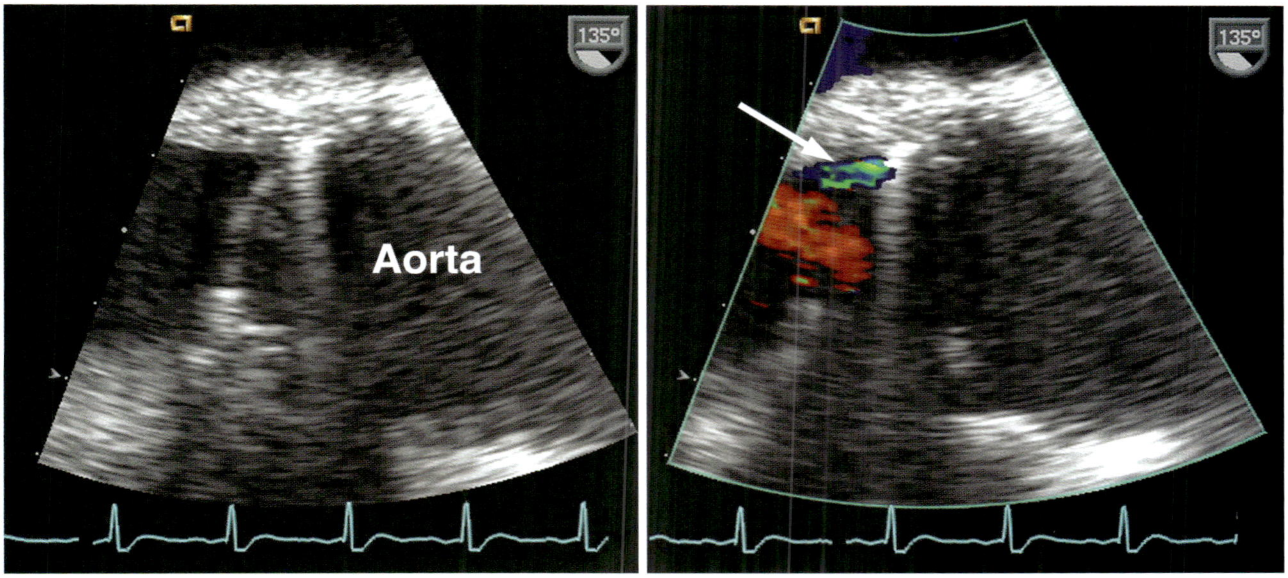

Fig 5.33 Long-axis view at 135 degrees. In real time, normal leaflet motion is seen with some shadowing and reverberations by proximal aspect of valve. Color Doppler *(right)* shows small amount of regurgitation *(arrow)*, as expected for this valve type.

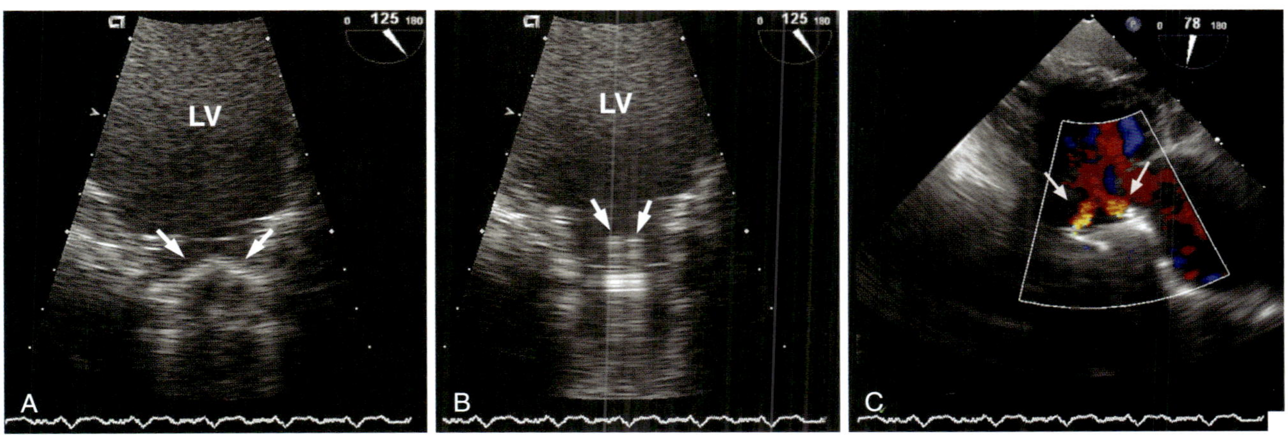

Fig 5.34 Transgastric apical view of left ventricle (LV) and ascending aorta in long-axis view shows bileaflet valve in aortic position in diastole **(A)** and systole **(B)**. Note that in normal closed position, leaflets *(arrow, left)* are at slight angle to each other whereas open leaflets *(arrow, right)* assume parallel orientation. Color Doppler **(C)** shows two normal "washing jets" *(arrows)*.

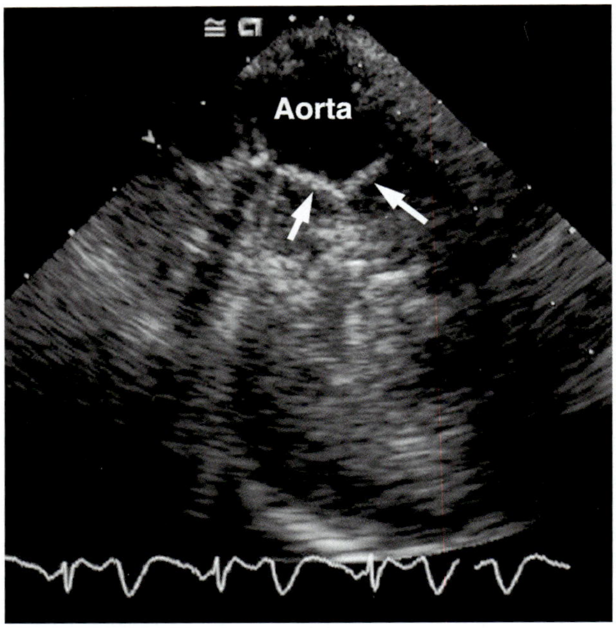

Fig 5.35 With sterile transducer placed epicardially during surgery on ascending aorta, this view of aortic prosthesis was obtained. Closed leaflets *(arrows)* are at slight angle, as seen in apical view.

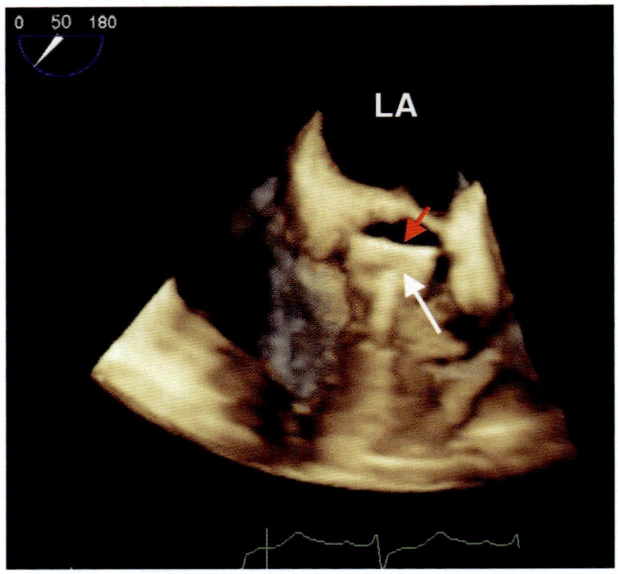

Fig 5.36 This 3D TEE midesophageal from left atrial perspective illustrates two problems when imaging mechanical valve from midesophageal position-lots of artifacts *(white arrow)* arising from mechanical leaflet *(red arrow)*, and inability to assess leaflet motion, which may be more readily accomplished from transgastric position (Fig 5.34).

Comments

The bileaflet valve consists of two pyrolytic carbon disks attached to a rigid ring by two small hinges. This design results in a small central slit-like orifice and two larger lateral semicircular orifices when the valve is open. As for tissue valves, the hemodynamics of a normally functioning mechanical valve are inherently stenotic, compared with a normal native valve, with tables available listing the expected transvalvular velocities, pressure gradients, and expected orifice areas for each valve type and size. Even higher velocities may be recorded with normally functioning valves due to the fluid dynamics of the central slit-like orifice. Effective orifice areas can be calculated using the continuity equation, as for native valves. Because the velocity and pressure gradient across a prosthesis valve depend on transvalvular flow rate, as well as valve type and size, a baseline examination when valve function is clinically normal is useful for distinguishing valve stenosis from normal hemodynamics on serial examinations.

Suggested Reading

1. Blauwet LA, Miller FA Jr: Echocardiographic assessment of prosthetic heart valves, Prog Cardiovasc Dis 57(1):100–110, 2014.
2. Eleid MF, Thomas JD, Nishimura RA: Increased prosthetic valve gradients: abnormal prosthetic function or pressure recovery? Catheter Cardiovasc Interv 84(6):903–911, 2014.

CASE 5-6
Bileaflet Tricuspid and Pulmonic Valves

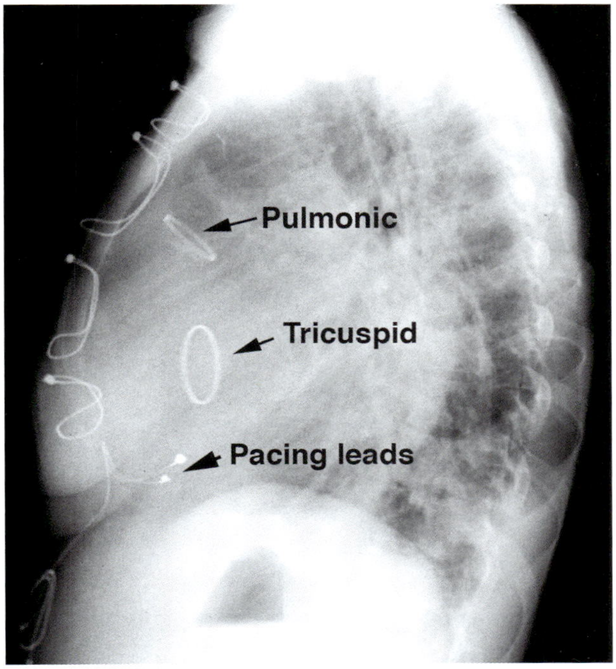

Fig 5.37 Lateral chest radiograph in this patient demonstrates sewing ring of both prosthetic pulmonic and prosthetic tricuspid valve. Epicardial pacing leads and sternal closure wires are also seen.

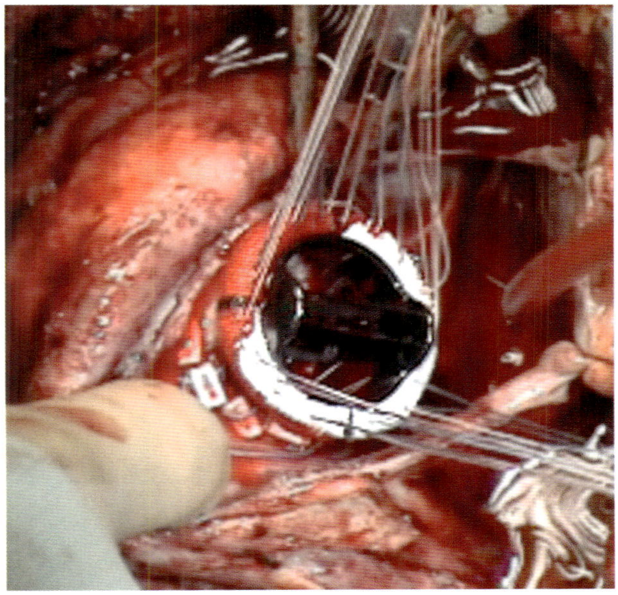

Fig 5.38 Intraoperative view from right atrium of mechanical valve being sutured into tricuspid annulus. Note that sutures are passed through small rectangular pledgets (near tip of surgeon's finger) to secure valve to annulus. These pledgets can sometimes be seen on echocardiography.

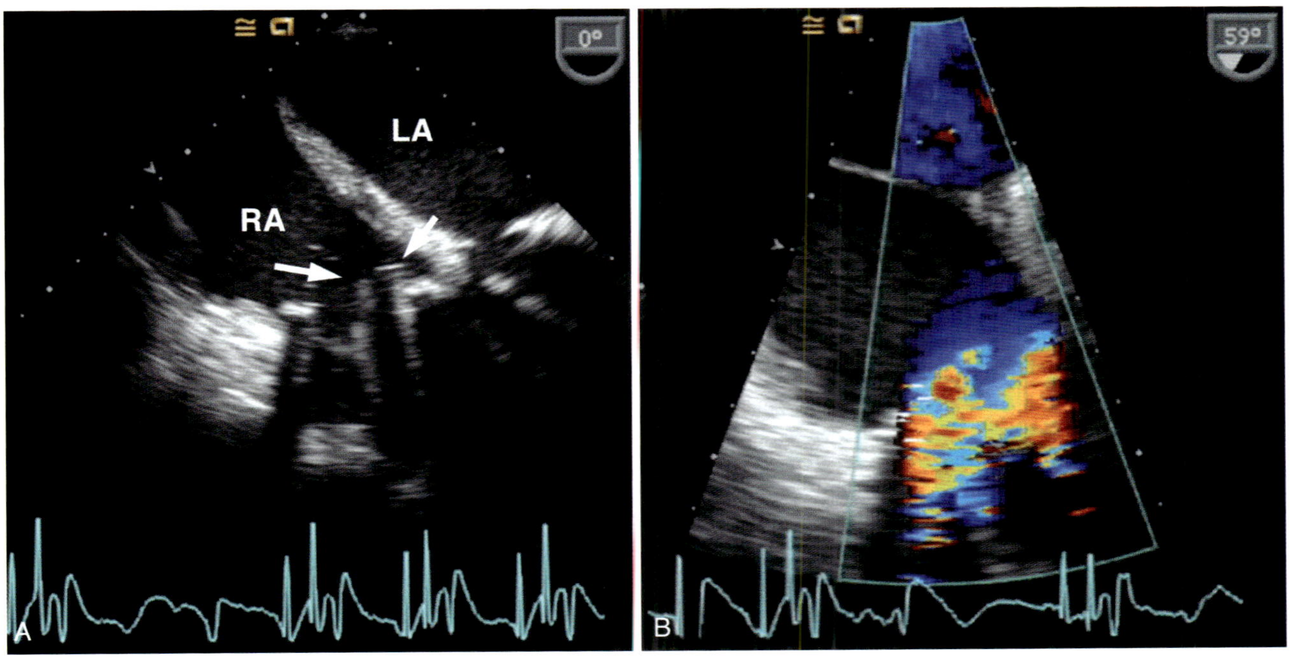

Fig 5.39 In **(A)**, midesophageal four-chamber view at 0 degrees demonstrates mechanical valve in tricuspid position in diastole with leaflets open *(arrows)*. In **(B)**, color Doppler in short-axis view at 59-degree rotation shows normal antegrade flow across valve.

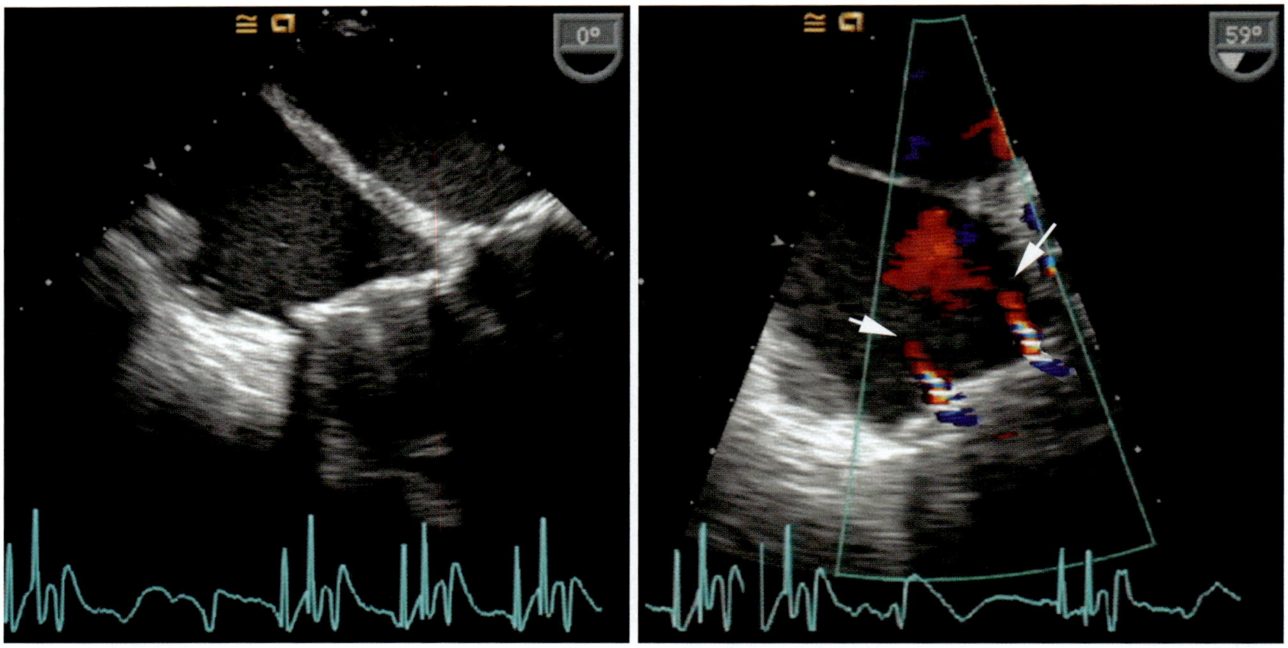

Fig 5.40 In same two views as in Fig 5.39, closed valve leaflet and normal prosthetic regurgitation *(arrows)* are seen.

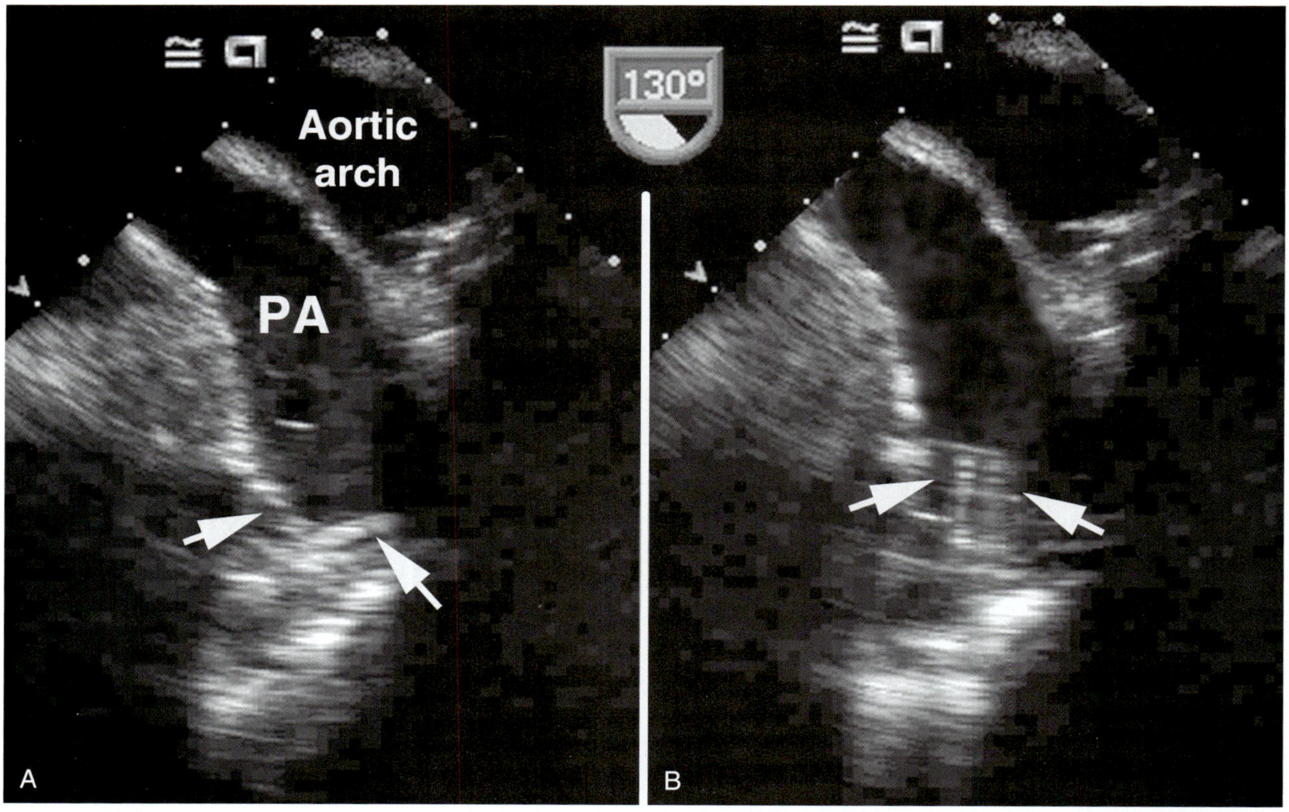

Fig 5.41 In high esophageal position at 130 degrees, bileaflet mechanical pulmonic valve is seen closed in diastole (**A**, *arrows*) and open in systole (**B**, *arrows*).

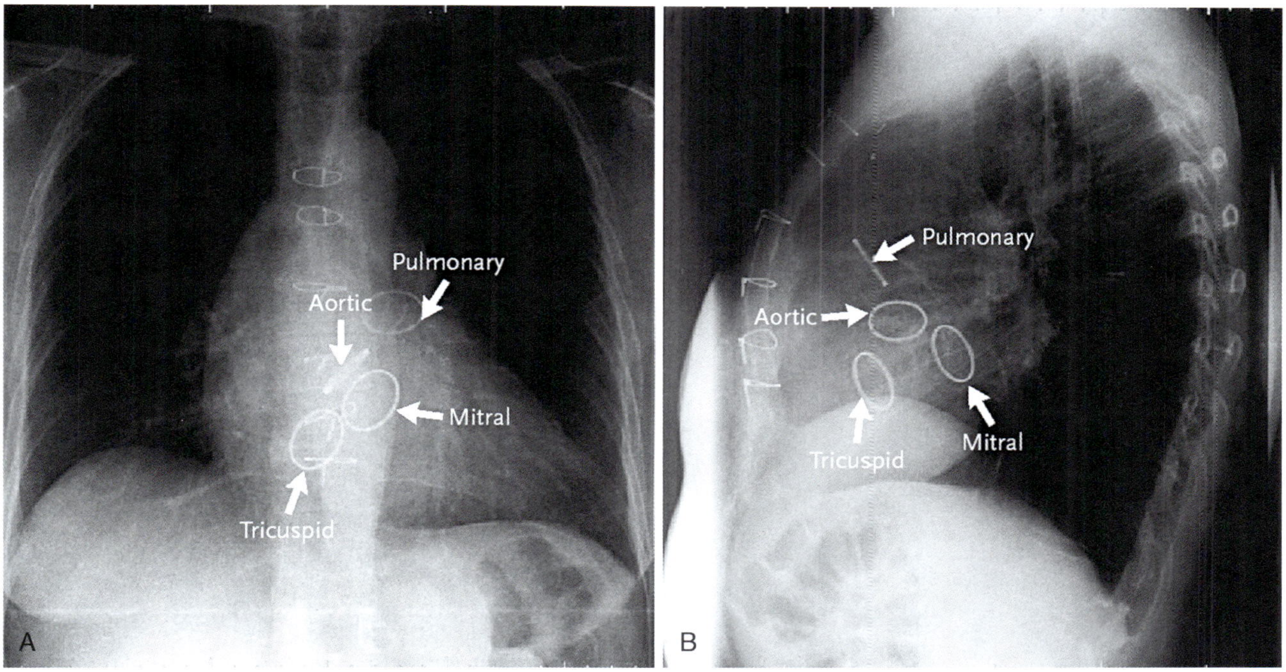

Fig 5.42 Normal positions of prosthetic valves in cardiac silhouette are demonstrated in this posterolateral and lateral chest x-ray. (Reproduced with permission from van den Brink B. Four artificial heart valves. N Engl J Med 2005; 353:712. ©Massachusetts Medical Society.)

Comments

Although the most straightforward way to determine the type and location of valve prostheses in a patient is to review the medical record or the valve card patients are given to carry with them. In some cases valve position and type must be inferred from physical examination or chest radiography. As shown in this example, a standard postero-anterior and lateral chest radiograph allows identification of valve position, based on the normal position of the valves within the cardiac silhouette (Figs 5.37, 5.42).

A valve prosthesis in the tricuspid position has an appearance and flow dynamics similar to the prosthetic mitral valve, although velocities and pressure gradients may be even lower because a larger prosthesis can be placed in the tricuspid annulus. In addition to the mean pressure gradient, evaluation of mechanical atrioventricular valves includes measurement of the pressure half-time. The empiric constant of 220, derived from studies of native mitral stenosis, can also be used for central orifice bioprosthetic valves and for mechanical valves to estimate valve area.

Suggested Reading

1. Otto CM: Prosthetic valves. In Otto CM, editor: Textbook of clinical echocardiography, ed 5, Philadelphia, 2013, Elsevier, pp 342–371.

Bioprosthetic Valves: Dysfunction

CASE 5-7
Bioprosthetic Aortic Valve Degeneration

This 56-year-old man, presented with signs and symptoms of congestive heart failure 11 years after the placement of a 27-mm pericardial bioprosthetic valve for endocarditis. The patient currently denies fevers, weight loss, fatigue, or other symptoms of endocarditis. Physical examination revealed a diastolic murmur and he was referred for echocardiography and then cardiac surgery.

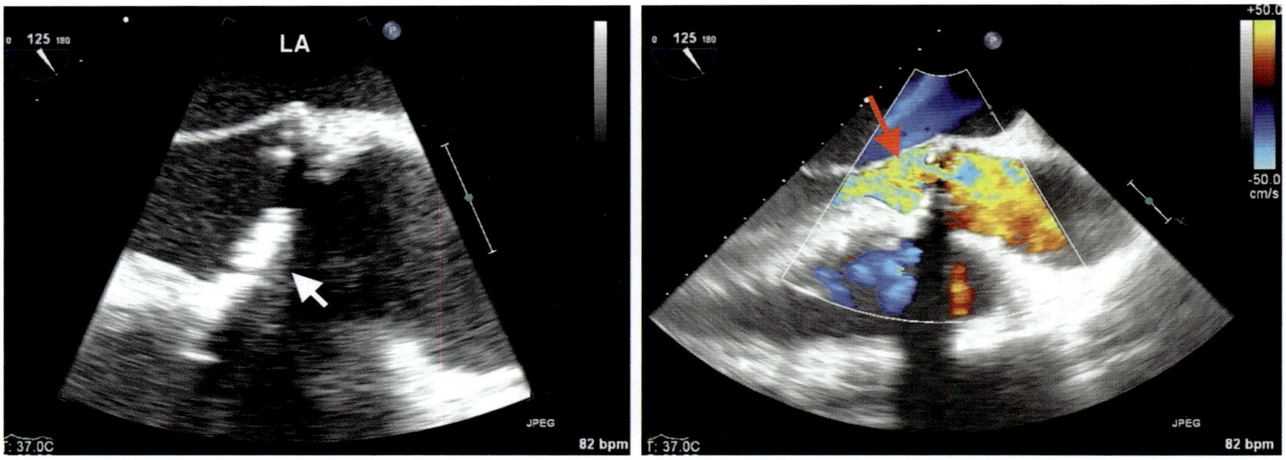

Fig 5.43 In left panel of this midesophageal long-axis image, right coronary cusp is heavily calcified *(white arrow)*. More posterior cusp is also calcified. In right panel, color Doppler shows jet of tricuspid regurgitation, which broadens to fill entire LV outflow tract. Vena contracta measurement is difficult due to shadowing by valve calcification but appearance suggests severe aortic regurgitation.

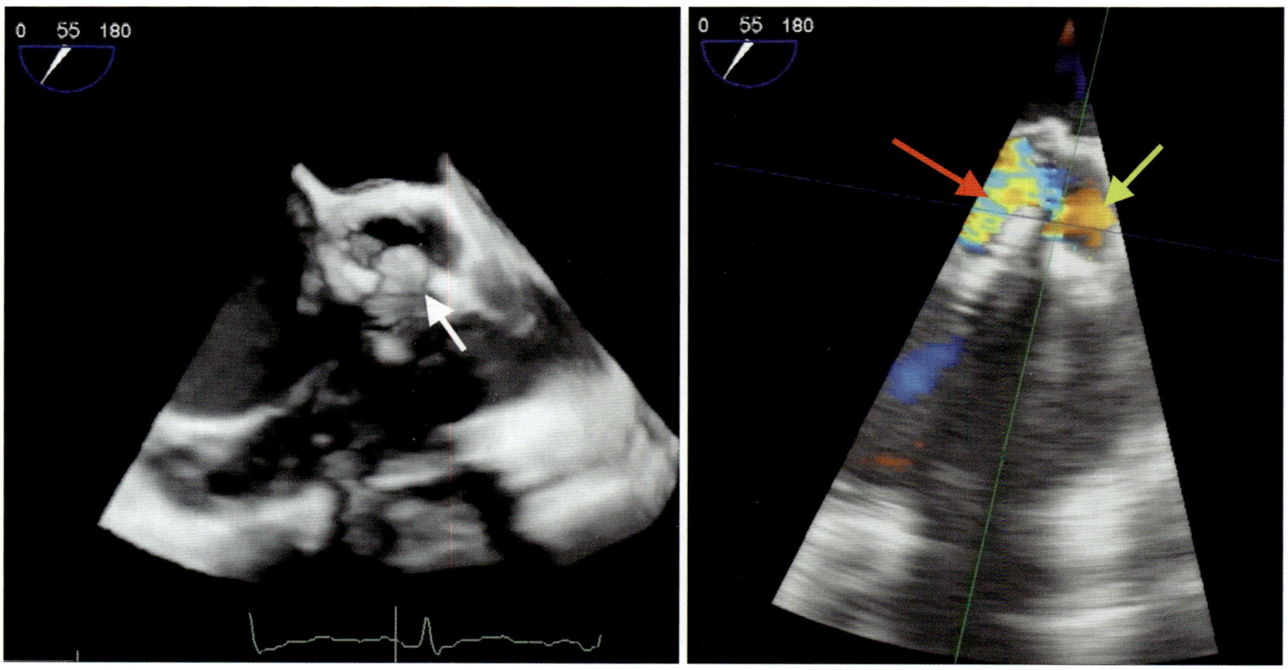

Fig 5.44 In left panel, 3D TEE image of aortic valve is seen from aspect of ascending aorta. At end diastole, thickened right coronary cusp is evident *(white arrow)*. Right panel is result of multiplanar reconstruction, showing aortic regurgitation primarily in vicinity of noncoronary cusp *(red arrow)*, but also left coronary cusp *(yellow arrow)*.

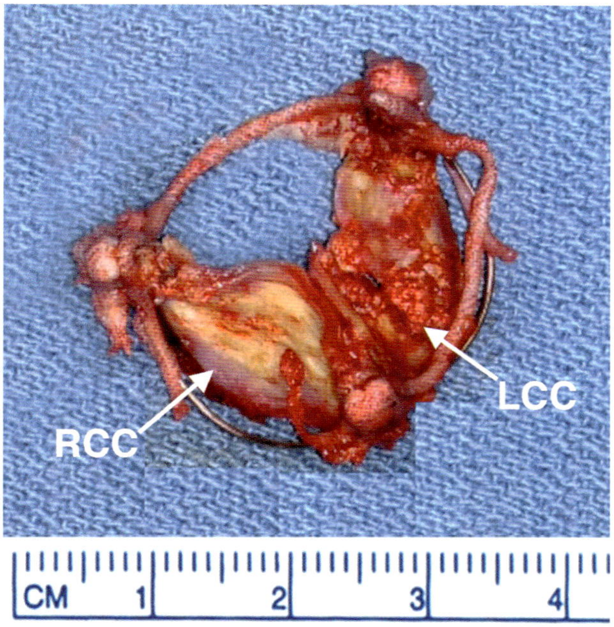

Fig 5.45 Valve was explanted, with surgeon noting severe calcification of right coronary leaflet, partial destruction of left coronary leaflet, and near total absence of noncoronary leaflet.

Comments

The major disadvantage of tissue valves is eventual structural deterioration. The prevalence of primary valve failure 15 years after valve implantation is about 20% for aortic bioprostheses and nearly 40% for mitral bioprostheses. Mechanisms of valve failure include (1) tissue deterioration, resulting in loss of leaflet integrity (as in this case) with consequent regurgitation, and (2) tissue calcification, resulting in valve stenosis or regurgitation.

In a patient with a bioprosthetic valve, the differential diagnosis of a mobile mass in or near the valve should always include a flail leaflet, as well as valve vegetation or thrombosis. Transesophageal imaging is often needed to fully define the mechanism of valve dysfunction.

Suggested Reading

1. Johnston DR, Soltesz EG, Vakil N, et al: Long-term durability of bioprosthetic aortic valves: implications from 12,569 implants, Ann Thorac Surg 99(4):1239–1247, 2015.
2. Chiang YP, Chikwe J, Moskowitz AJ, et al: Survival and long-term outcomes following bioprosthetic vs mechanical aortic valve replacement in patients aged 50 to 69 years, JAMA 312(13):1323–1329, 2014.

CASE 5-8
Bioprosthetic Aortic Valve Stenosis

This 68-year-old male was seen for increasing shortness of breath and fatigue. Nine years previously he had undergone a valve replacement with a 27-mm Carpentier-Edwards pericardial prosthesis because of aortic valve endocarditis.

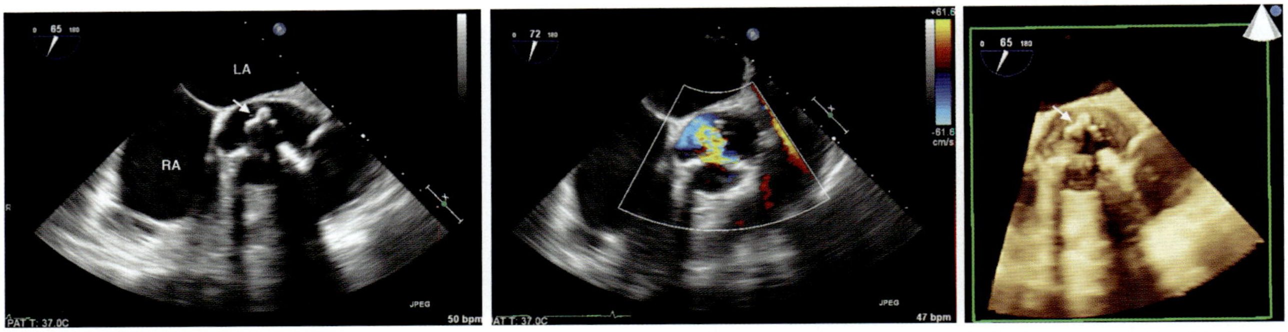

Fig 5.46 Three panels are all taken in systole. In midesophageal short-axis view of aortic valve *(left)*, there is restricted leaflet mobility (more clearly seen in accompanying video clip) and calcification *(arrow)*. Color Doppler imaging shows flow through narrowed systolic orifice *(center)*. 3D images *(right)* from aortic perspective demonstrates leaflet thickening and calcification *(arrow)* adjacent to one of valve struts.

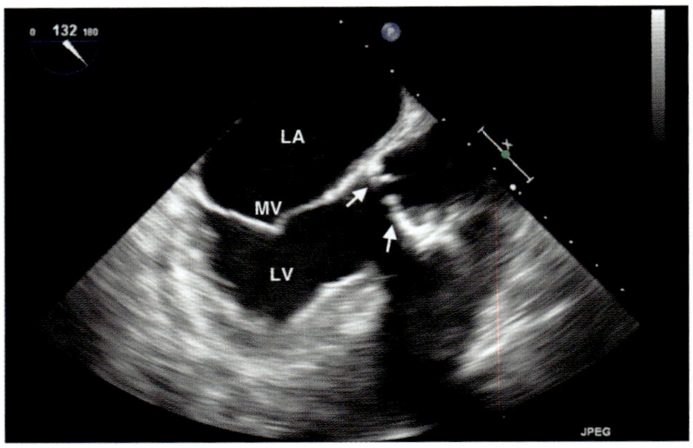

Fig 5.47 Midesophageal long-axis view of aortic valve again demonstrate prosthetic valve leaflet calcification *(arrows)* and, in the accompanying video, restricted leaflet motion. AAo = Ascending aorta.

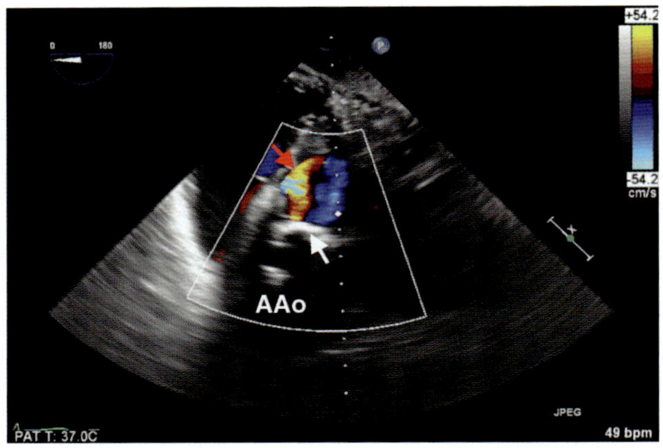

Fig 5.48 In this apical transgastric diastolic image, jet of aortic regurgitation is appreciated *(red arrow)*. Prosthetic calcification is again seen *(white arrow)*.

Comments

The durability of bioprosthetic valves is inversely related to patient age at the time of implantation. In older adults, bioprosthetic valve dysfunction is uncommon for the first 10 years, followed by progressive leaflet fibrosis and calcification, which results in valve stenosis in some patients. Diagnosis of prosthetic valve stenosis should take into consideration the baseline postoperative valve hemodynamics. Compared with a normal native valve, a bioprosthetic valve has a higher antegrade velocity and mean pressure gradient and a lower valve area with the specific hemodynamics in an individual patient dependent on valve size, flow rates, and other clinical factors. A baseline echocardiographic study 3 to 6 months after valve implantation is recommended for comparison with future studies. The diagnosis of prosthetic valve stenosis is most secure when there has been a progressive increase in gradient and decrease in valve area over time and when the valve leaflets are calcified with reduced systolic motion. Hemodynamics suggesting stenosis in the absence of leaflet changes or without evidence of progressive disease may be due to patient-prosthesis mismatch, not valve stenosis.

Suggested Reading

1. Zoghbi WA, Chambers JB, Dumesnil JG, et al: Recommendations for evaluation of prosthetic valves with echocardiography and Doppler ultrasound: a report from the American Society of Echocardiography's Guidelines and Standards Committee and the Task Force on Prosthetic Valves, J Am Soc Echocardiogr 22(9):975–1014; quiz 1082–1084, 2009.

CASE 5-9
Rocking Aortic Valve Prosthesis

This 69-year-old male presented with a 2-week history of increasing shortness of breath, and generalized swelling. He denied any fevers, chills, or night sweats. He had undergone aortic valve replacement and interposition aortic graft because of an ascending aortic aneurysm and dilated aortic annulus with severe aortic regurgitation 2 years before the current admission. There was no evidence of active infection at that time.

At surgery, the valve was found to be dehisced anteriorly. After the valve was removed, inflammation of the native annulus was evident, and this was confirmed on pathological examination.

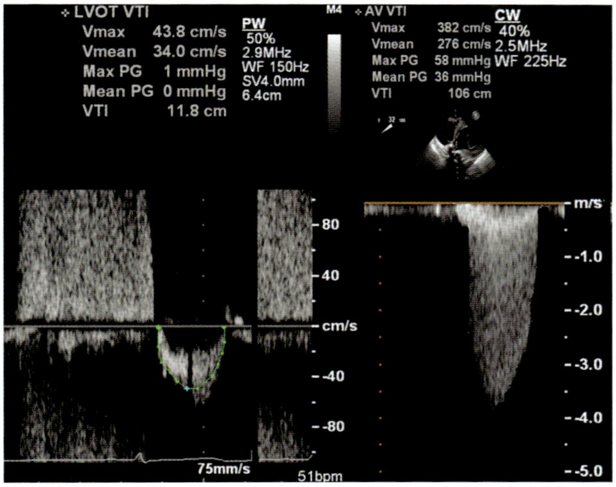

Fig 5.49 Pulsed wave Doppler of LV outflow tract *(left)* suggests low cardiac output with velocity of only 0.44 m/sec. Continuous-wave Doppler of transaortic flow *(right)* shows velocity of 3.8 m/sec and mean gradient of 36 mm Hg. Although gradient is only moderately elevated, functional valve area (with outflow tract diameter of 2.2 cm) is only 0.5 cm^2. These findings are consistent with severe prosthetic stenosis, with low stroke volume.

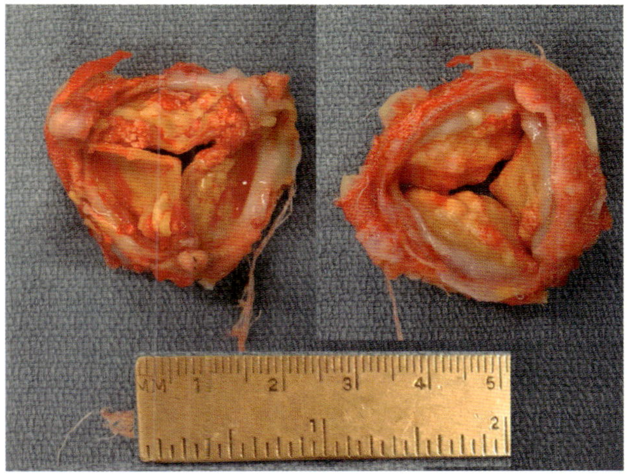

Fig 5.50 Explanted prosthetic valve is seen from aortic *(left panel)* as well as ventricular *(right panel)* aspects. There is thickening and nodularity in all three cusps.

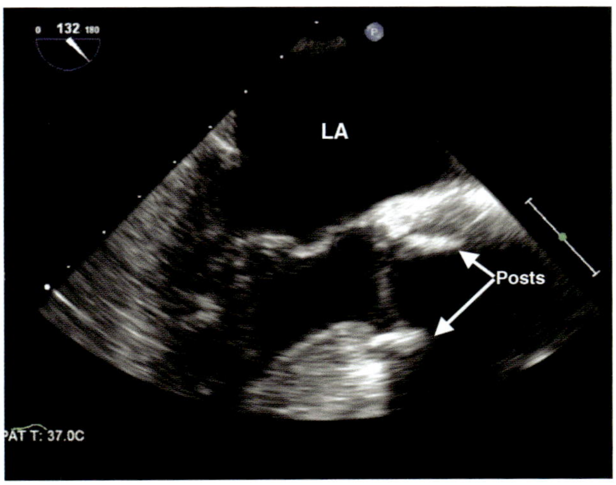

Fig 5.51 This midesophageal long-axis image was taken after placement of original aortic tissue prosthesis. It is well seated, and there was no color Doppler evidence of aortic regurgitation.

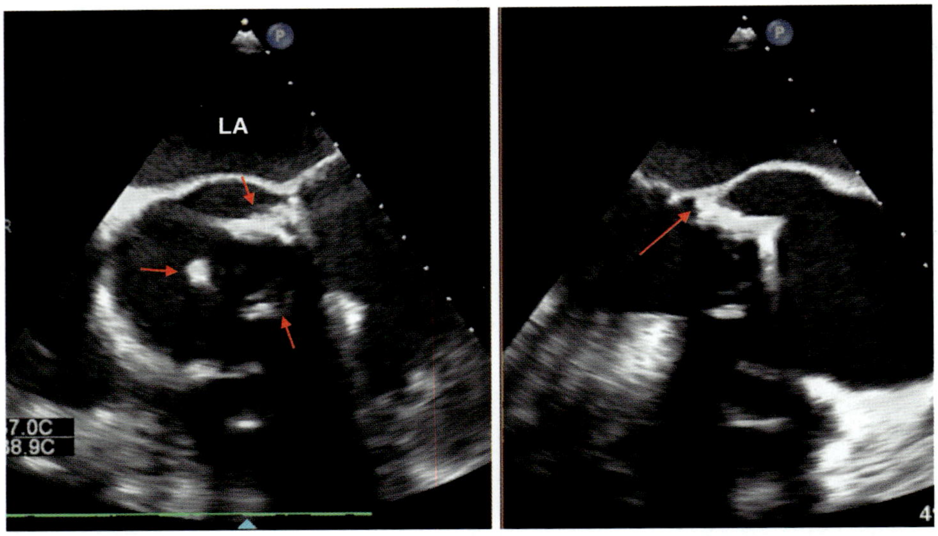

Fig 5.52 This biplane TEE image was obtained after induction of anesthesia for second operation. In left panel, midesophageal short-axis image shows large area of valvular dehiscence. Red arrows indicate valve posts. In right panel, red arrow indicates area where rocking motion is seen in real time.

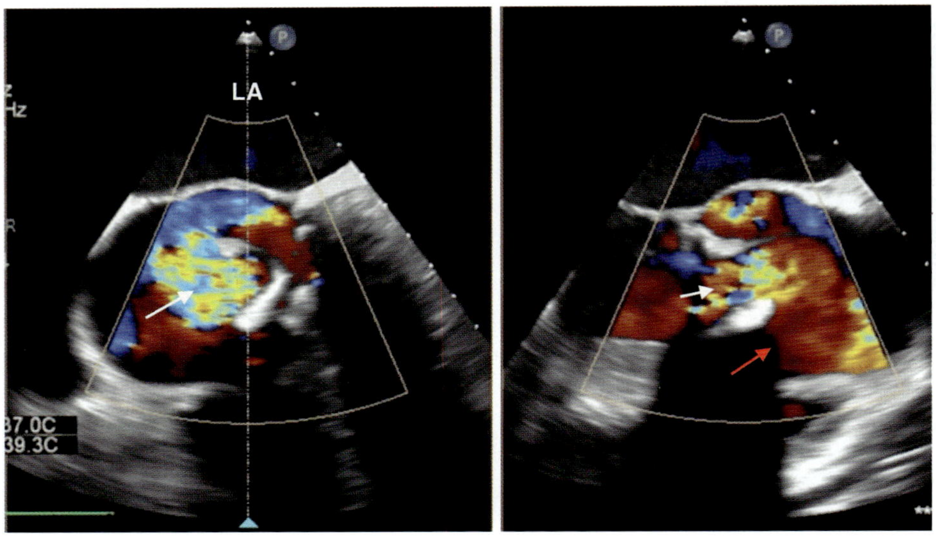

Fig 5.53 Color Doppler is applied to Fig 5.52, and in systole there is flow through the valve *(white arrow)* as well anterior to the valve *(red arrow)* although this latter jet is affected by dropout. The valve leaflets remain competent, with only trace AR through the valve.

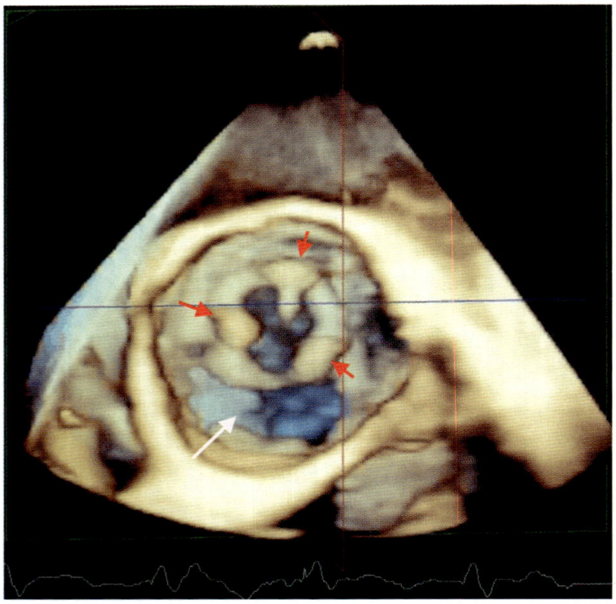

Fig 5.54 In this 3D image of aortic valve from ascending aortic perspective, valvular dehiscence is again appreciated. Red arrows again indicate three valve posts, whereas white arrow indicates broad area of dehiscence. Second video associated with this figure is taken with slight horizontal angulation so that rocking motion of valve may be fully appreciated.

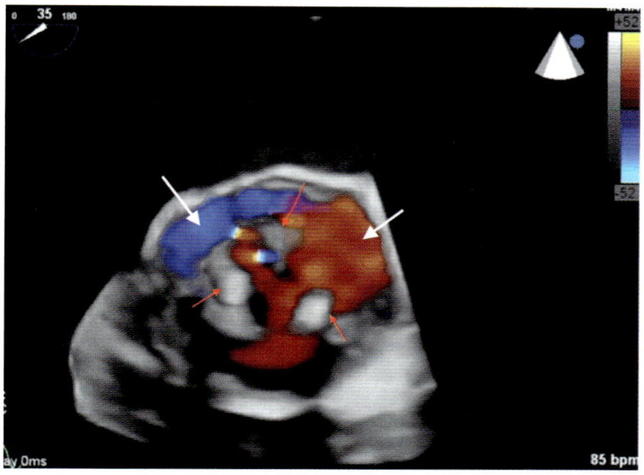

Fig 5.55 3D color Doppler is applied to previous image. Red arrows indicate valve posts, whereas white arrows indicate areas of paravalvular regurgitation.

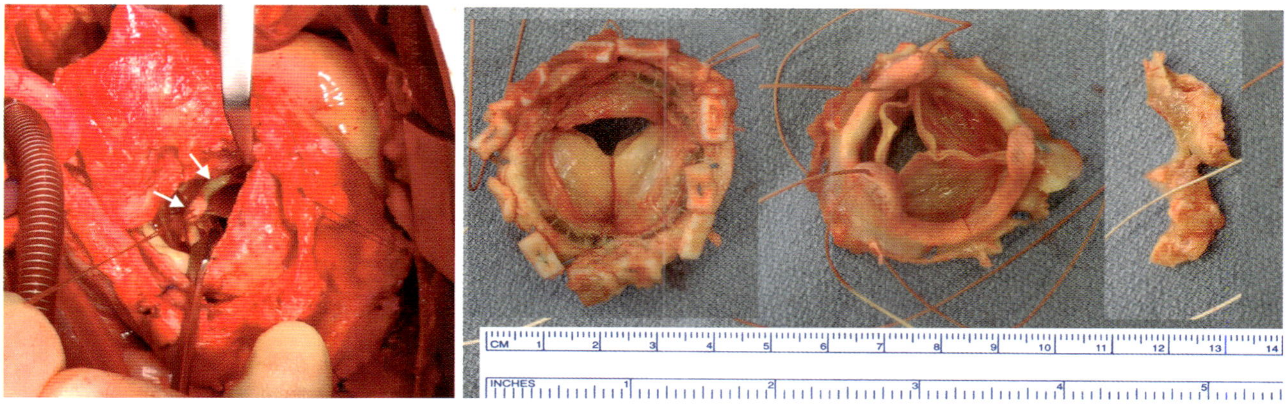

Fig 5.56 Following aortotomy, free edge of dehisced valve is seen *(left)*. The leaflets from the explanted valve *(right)* are neither thickened nor calcified.

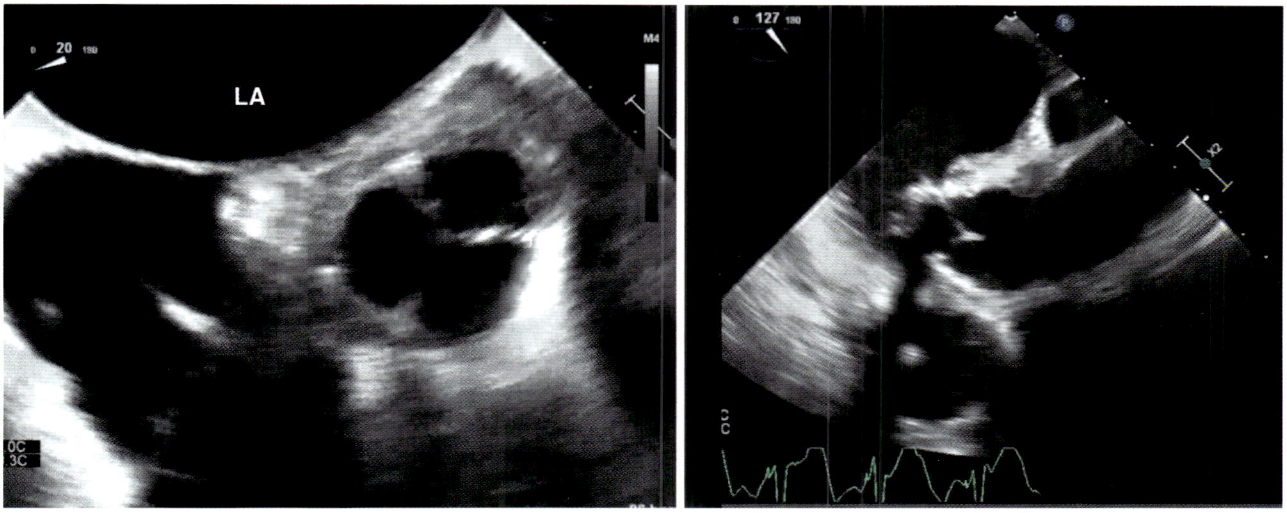

Fig 5.57 Valve within homograft, anchored well with normal leaflet motion (left midesophageal short axis, right midesophageal long axis).

Comments

In patients presenting with valve dehiscence and paravalvular regurgitation, the initial diagnostic evaluation should include blood cultures because endocarditis is a likely cause of new paravalvular regurgitation. Paravalvular regurgitation also can occur due to inadequate annular tissue structural integrity, for example with tissue destruction due to paravalvular abscess, or to annular fibrosis and calcification resulting in suture breakage due to excessive mechanical forces between the prosthetic material and native valve annulus. These complications may be seen early after valve replacement but also can occur late as in this case.

In addition to standard surgical criteria for intervention for valve regurgitation, other indications for intervention for paravalvular regurgitation include the concern that further valve dehiscence may occur abruptly. In addition, hemolytic anemia that is refractory to medical therapy may require intervention.

Although surgical repair remain the standard, in some patients, paravalvular leaks can be closed with percutaneously placed devices.

Suggested Reading

1. Mahjoub H, Pibarot P, Dumesnil JG: Echocardiographic evaluation of prosthetic heart valves, Curr Cardiol Rep 17(6):48, 2015.
2. Sorajja P, Bae R, Lesser JA, Pedersen WA: Percutaneous repair of paravalvular prosthetic regurgitation: patient selection, techniques and outcomes, Heart 101(9):665–673, 2015.

CASE 5-10
Bioprosthetic Mitral Valve Stenosis

A 34-year-old woman was referred from an outside hospital in cardiogenic shock, and acute respiratory failure 10 days after delivery of an infant. She had a bioprosthetic mitral valve, placed several years ago for bacterial endocarditis which now showed evidence for severe bioprosthetic stenosis and pulmonary hypertension. Her peripartum clinical course also was complicated by pulmonary embolism.

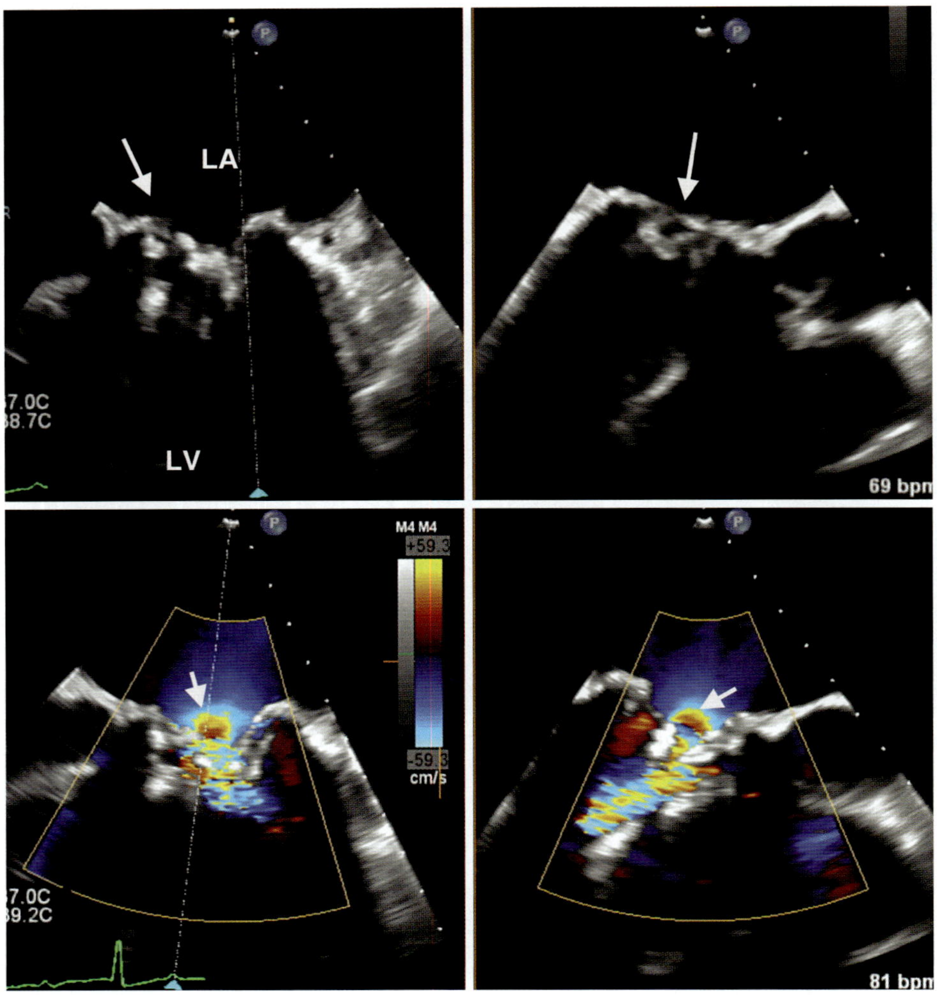

Fig 5.58 In two orthogonal midesophageal views *(top)* of mitral prosthesis *(arrow)*, there is extensive thickening and calcification of valve leaflets, as well as shadowing distal to valve. Left panels show four-chamber view and right panels show long-axis view. In real time, valve opens minimally during diastole. Color Doppler in same image planes *(bottom)* shows flow acceleration on left atrial side of valve and narrow flow stream through valve orifice.

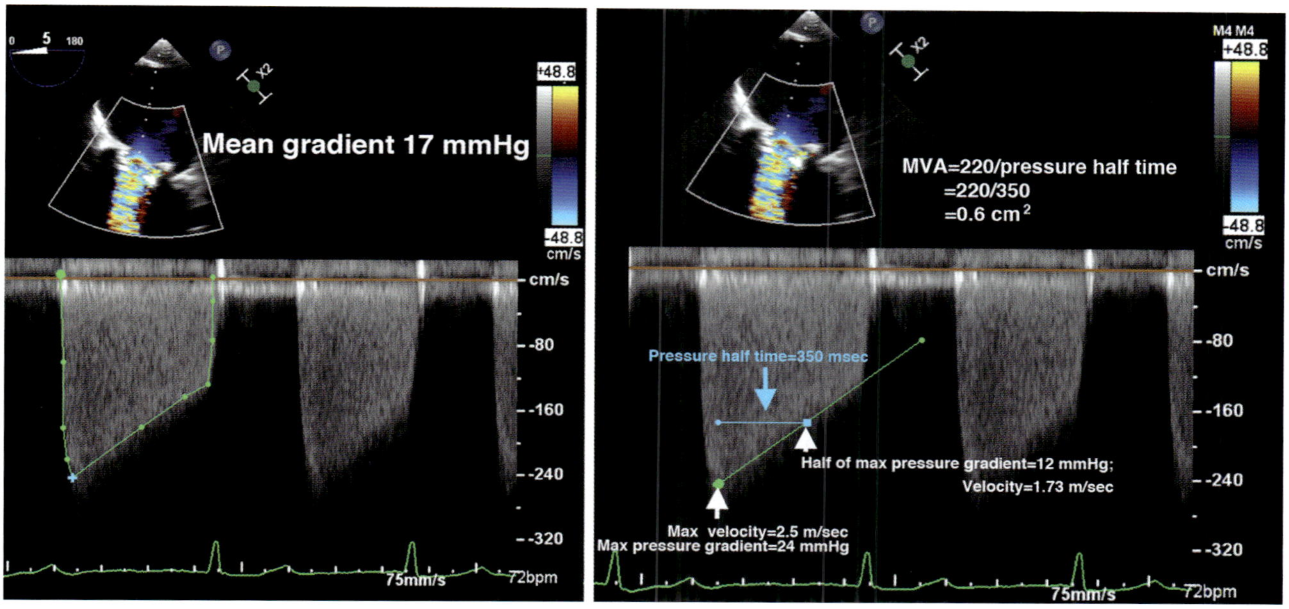

Fig 5.59 Continuous wave Doppler demonstrates mean gradient across mitral prosthesis of 17 mm Hg, and mitral valve area, calculated by pressure half time equation, of 0.6 cm^2. Both values are consistent with severe mitral stenosis. As patient is in atrial fibrillation, Doppler data were averaged over several beats.

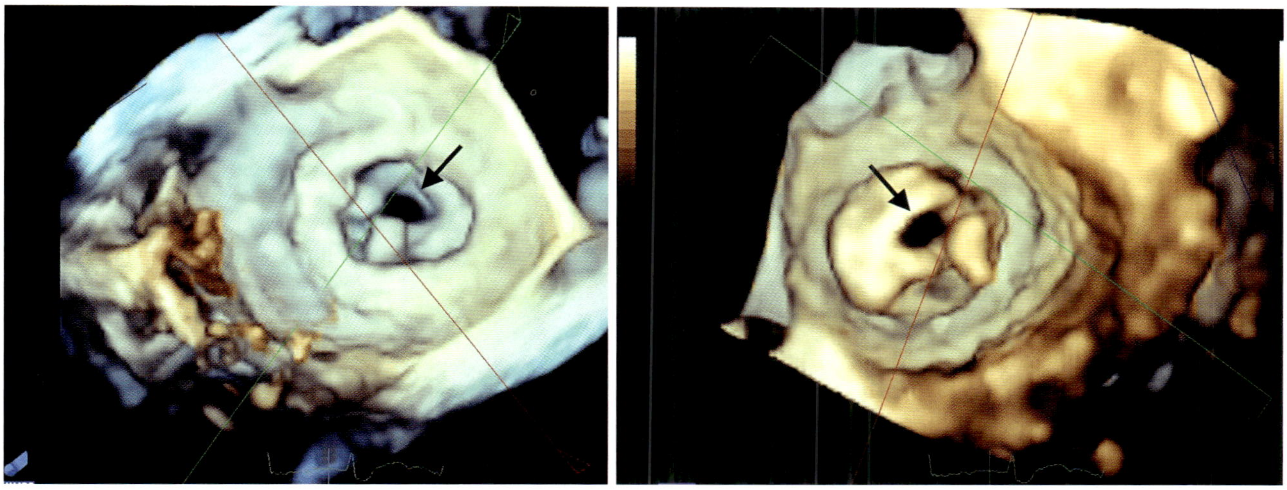

Fig 5.60 3D TEE during diastole of mitral bioprosthesis from LA perspective *(left)* and LV perspective *(right)*. Black arrows indicate maximal leaflet opening. Thickened leaflets are evident.

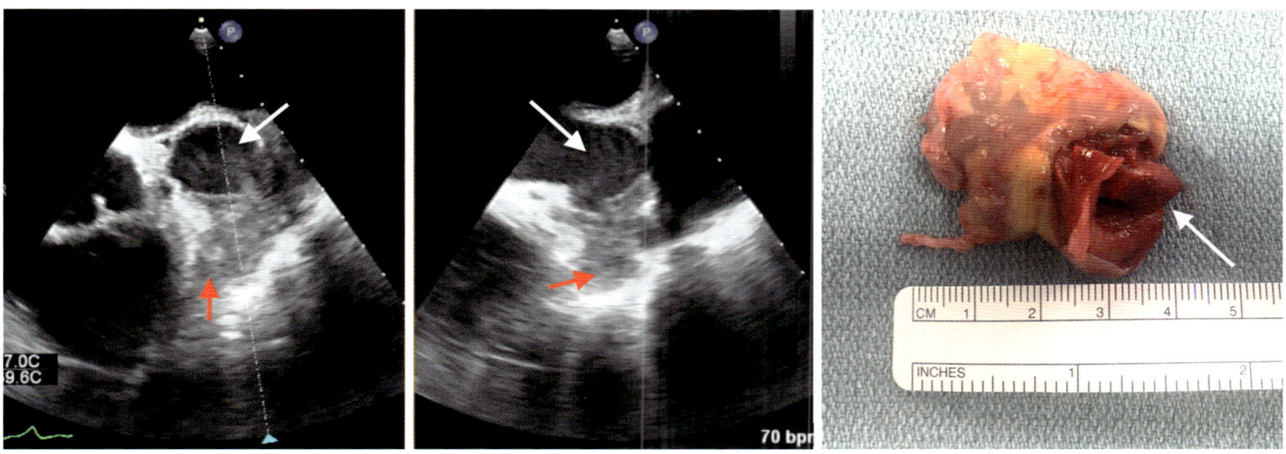

Fig 5.61 Biplane imaging of LA appendage *(left and center)* shows probable thrombus *(red arrows)* and spontaneous echo contrast, colloquially called "smoke" in LA appendage *(white arrows)*, which is more fully appreciated in real time. At surgery, resected left atrial appendage *(right)* was filled with thrombus *(white arrow)*.

Comments

Bioprosthetic valve stenosis usually presents with gradual onset of exertional symptoms or is diagnosed due to a new murmur on physical examination. In an asymptomatic patient with severe stenosis, the presentation may be acute in the setting of a superimposed hemodynamic load, such as pregnancy, fever, or anemia, as in this case. A bioprosthetic valve often is chosen in young women to avoid the risks of warfarin anticoagulation during pregnancy, despite the known shorter longevity of bioprosthetic valves in younger patients.

Suggested Reading

1. Silversides C, Siu S: Heart disease in pregnancy. In Otto CM, editor: The practice of clinical echocardiography, ed 5, Philadelphia, 2016, Elsevier.
2. Chikwe J, Chiang YP, Egorova NN, Itagaki S, Adams DH: Survival and outcomes following bioprosthetic vs mechanical mitral valve replacement in patients aged 50 to 69 years, JAMA 313(14):1435–1442, 2015.

CASE 5-11
Bioprosthetic Mitral Valve Thrombosis

This 28-year-old male had been operated on 3 days previously for rheumatic heart disease. His tricuspid valve was repaired, his 10-year-old, 23-mm aortic bioprosthesis replaced, and his regurgitant and stenotic mitral valve replaced with a bioprosthesis. Because of a long pump complicated by respiratory and cardiac failure, he was placed on ECMO (extracorporeal membrane oxygenation) for pulmonary and cardiac support.

Because of rising pulmonary artery pressures, a TTE was done.

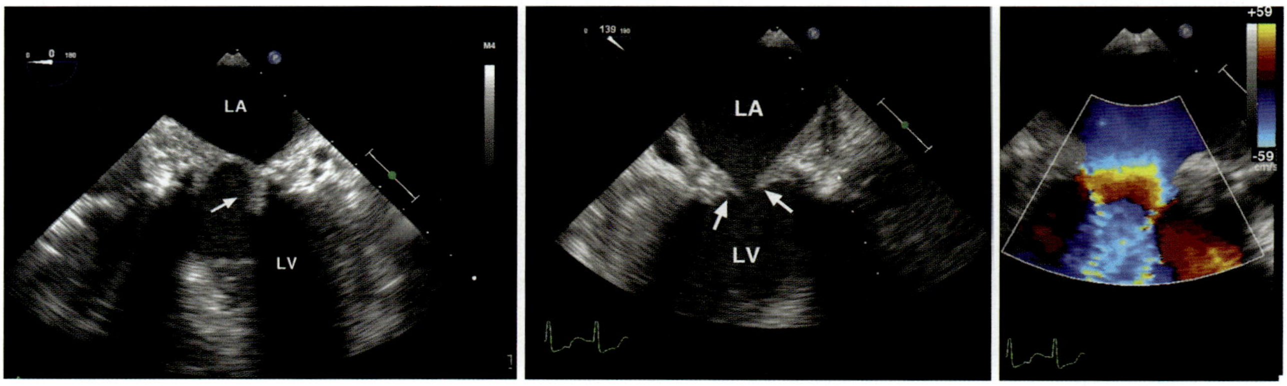

Fig 5.62 In left and middle frames, midesophageal views during diastole show mitral bioprosthetic leaflets to be extremely thickened with reduced diastolic excursion. In right frame, color Doppler shows large proximal flow convergence region *(blue to red transition)* even though velocity scale is set at relatively high Nyquist limit.

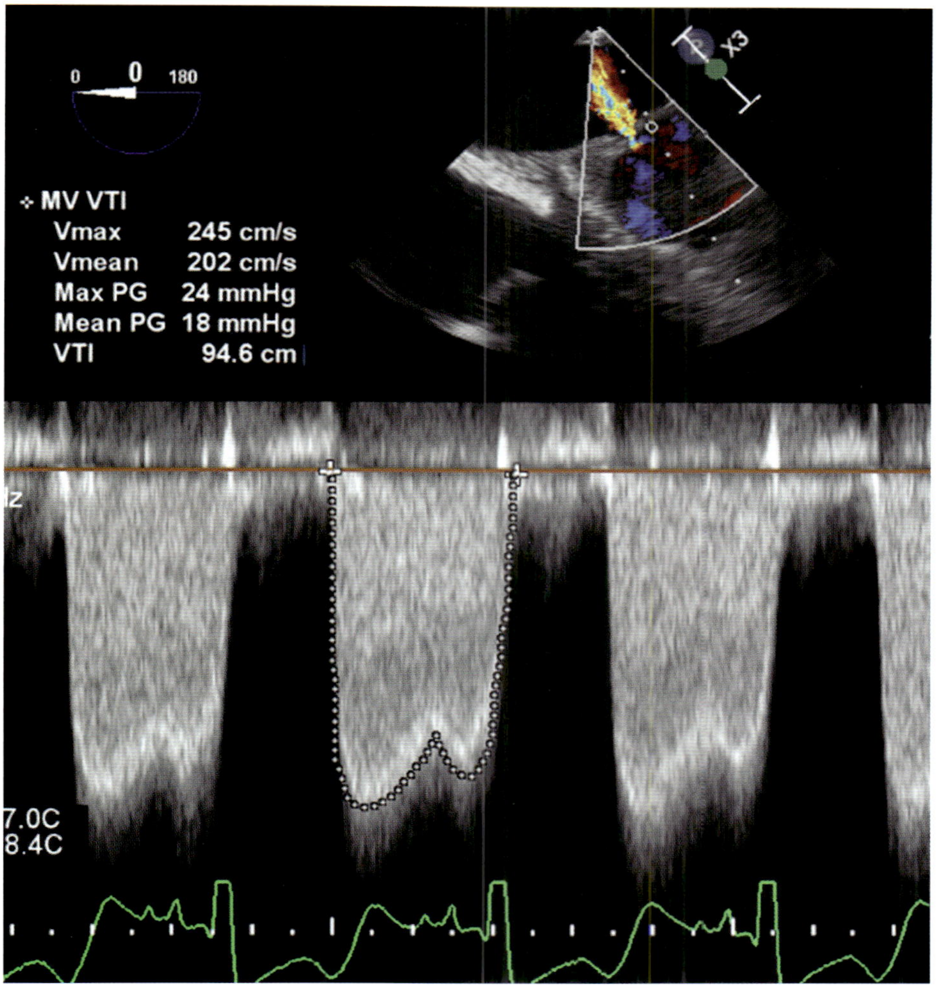

Fig 5.63 CW Doppler through mitral prosthesis shows markedly elevated mean diastolic gradient of 18 mm Hg.

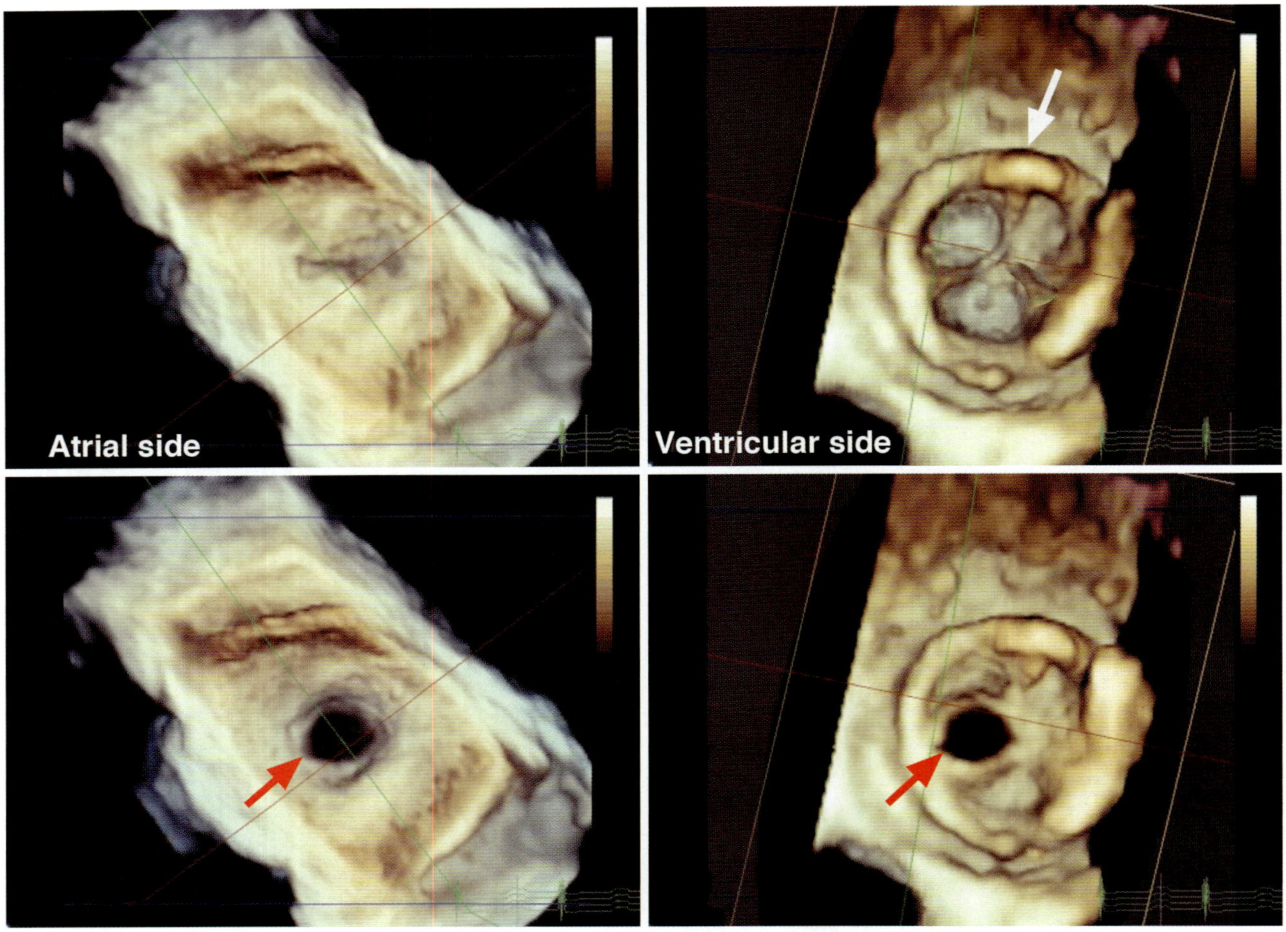

Fig 5.64 Image is 3D TEE of mitral bioprosthesis. Top two frames show valve in systole, bottom two frames in diastole. White arrow indicates one of valve posts. From atrial side, valve leaflets appear obscured in systole although they appear relatively normal in view from ventricular side. In lower two frames, there is extreme restriction of leaflet opening and in real time, two of three cusps do not move. Red arrows indicate valvular orifice.

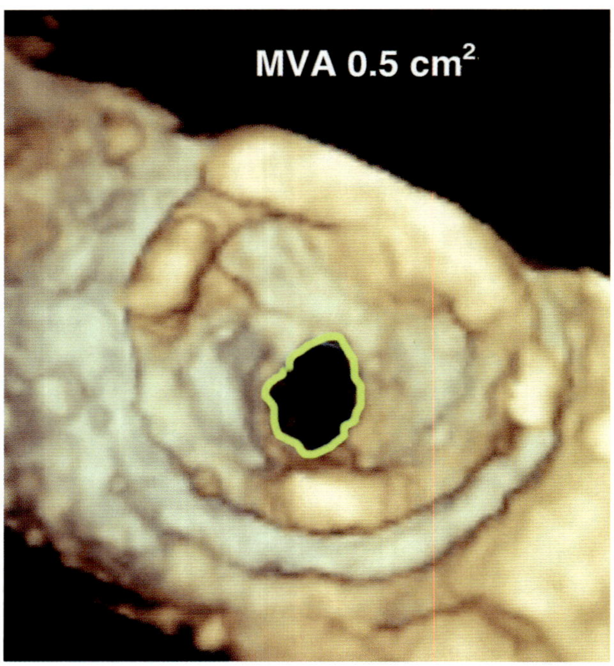

Fig 5.65 Using multiplanar reconstruction, orifice was identified and planimetry was used to measure mitral valve area (MVA) of 0.5 cm^2.

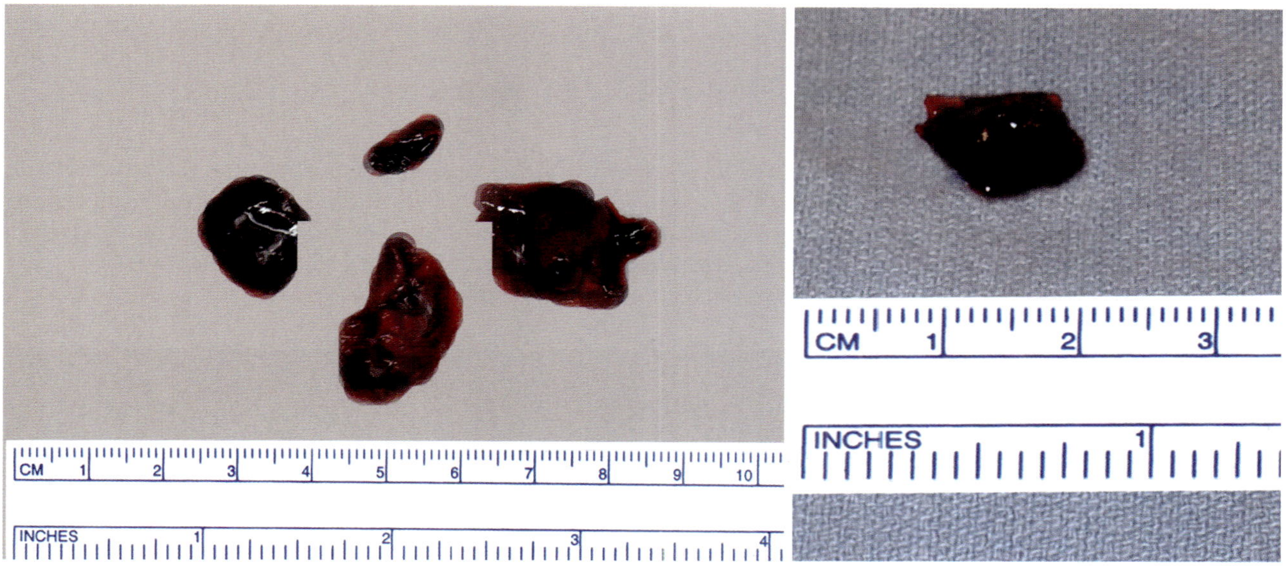

Fig 5.66 Illustrated are multiple thrombi removed from valve. Prosthesis was left in situ, and functioned well after separating from cardiopulmonary bypass.

Comments

Acute thrombosis of a bioprosthetic valve early after implantation is rare but does occur, possibly related to lack of endothelialization for bioprosthetic leaflets and sewing ring. In the current case, thrombosis was facilitated by the stagnation of blood in the left-sided chambers secondary to the use of ECMO. Thrombolysis is not indicated for left-sided valve thrombosis due to the risk of systemic embolism. Prompt diagnosis and surgical intervention in this patient led to a good clinical outcome without a systemic embolic event. Current guidelines indicate that anticoagulation with warfarin is reasonable for the first 3 months after bioprosthetic mitral valve replacement (Class IIa) and may be considered for the first 3 months after bioprosthetic aortic valve replacement (Class IIb)

Suggested Reading

1. Nishimura RA, Otto CM, Bonow RO, et al: American College of Cardiology/American Heart Association Task Force on Practice Guidelines: 2014 AHA/ACC guideline for the management of patients with valvular heart disease: executive summary: a report of the American College of Cardiology/American Heart Association Task Force on Practice Guidelines, J Am Coll Cardiol 63(22):2438–2488, 2014.
2. Griffin BP, Rodriguez R, Tan C, et al: Early bioprosthetic valve failure: mechanistic insights via correlation between echocardiographic and operative findings, J Am Soc Echocardiogr 28(10): 1131–1148, 2015.

CASE 5-12
Bioprosthetic Mitral Valve Regurgitation

This 40-year-old woman first underwent mitral valve replacement at age 23 years for rheumatic mitral valve disease, with a repeat mitral valve replacement at age 30 years with a stented bioprosthetic valve. At age 35 years, she developed heart failure symptoms after the birth of her son, followed by the new onset of atrial fibrillation. Her medical course has been complicated by diabetes, hypothyroidism, anemia, and sleep apnea. Echocardiography showed a flail prosthetic valve leaflet with severe mitral regurgitation. She was referred for repeat valve replacement.

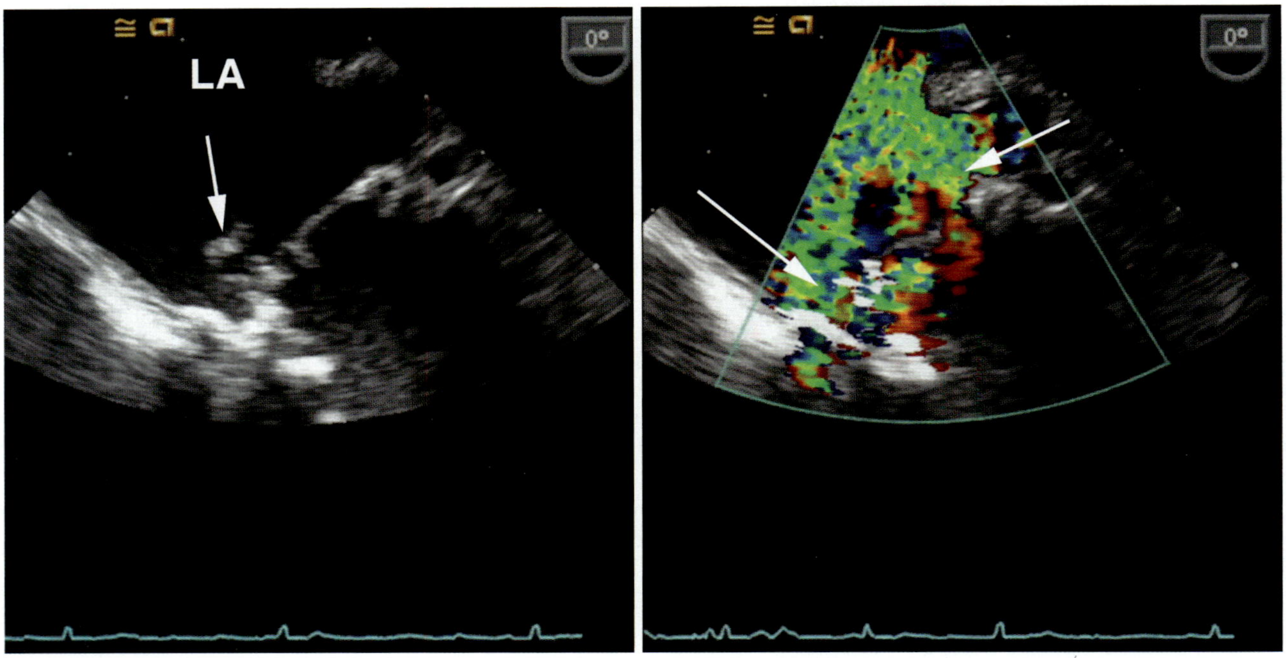

Fig 5.67 In TEE four-chamber view at 0 degrees, mass attached to mitral valve leaflet prolapses into left atrium in systole *(left)* with color Doppler *(right)* showing at least two regurgitant jets, one paravalvular medially and one through central area of valve leaflets *(arrows)*.

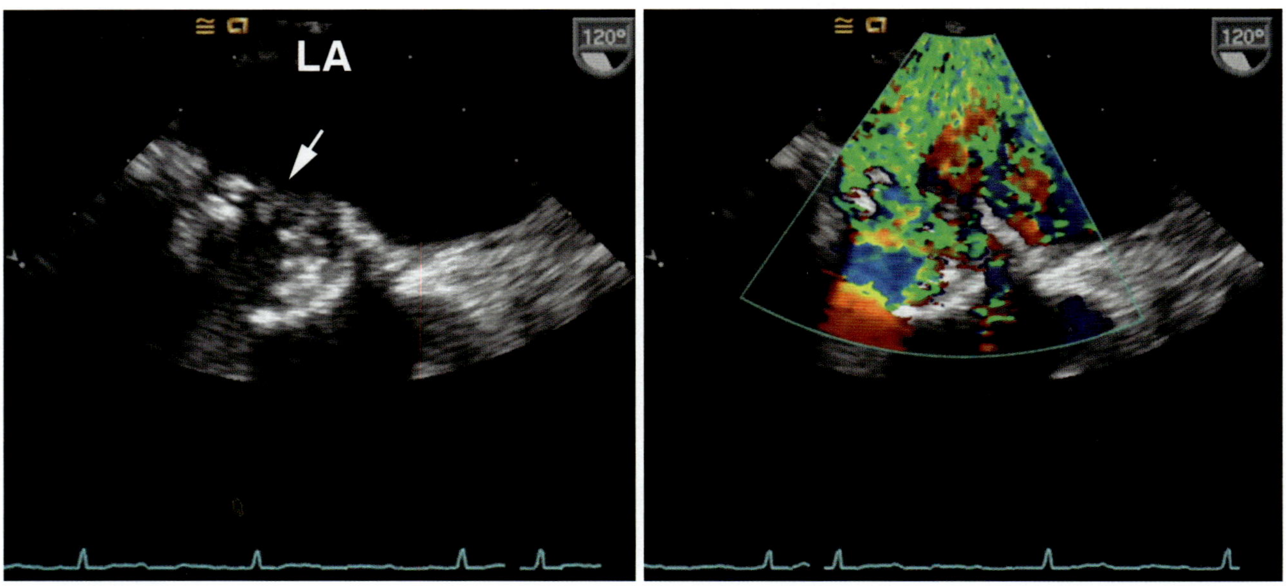

Fig 5.68 In long-axis view at 120 degrees, marked irregularity of leaflets of stented valve *(arrow)* and severe regurgitation are again seen.

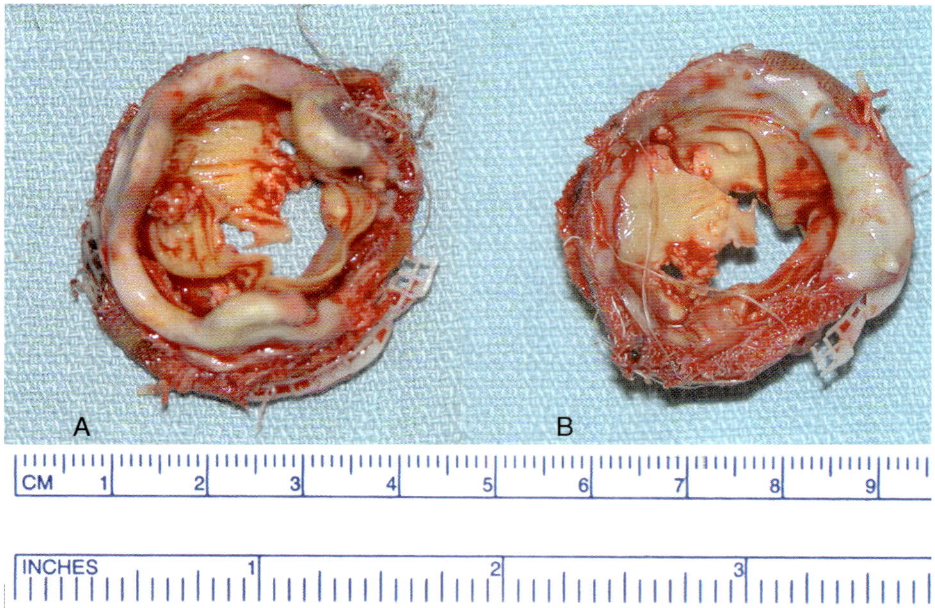

Fig 5.69 Explanted valve shows severe destruction of valve leaflets when viewed from left ventricular **(A)** or left atrial **(B)** side of valve.

Comments

This woman had structural failure of a mitral bioprosthesis only 10 years after valve replacement, with symptoms consistent with prosthetic valve dysfunction as early as 6 years after valve implantation. The longevity of older models of bioprosthetic valves was inversely related to patient age at the time of surgery. For example, the 10-year rate of freedom from structural deterioration in patients over age 70 years old was about 90% compared with only 10% in patients aged 16 to 39 years and 35% in patients aged 40 to 49 years. It remains controversial whether pregnancy accelerates the rate of bioprosthetic valve deterioration, but careful monitoring of bioprosthetic valve function during pregnancy is warranted given the rapid rate of structural deterioration in women in this age range. However, the optimal choice of valve in younger adults is in transition given the availability of transcatheter valve-in-valve implantation for structural deterioration of bioprosthetic valves.

Suggested Reading

1. Yun KL, Miller DC, Moore KA, et al: Durability of the Hancock MO bioprosthesis compared with standard aortic valve bioprostheses, Ann Thorac Surg 60(2 Suppl):S221–S228, 1995.
2. Johnston DR, Soltesz EG, Vakil N, et al: Long-term durability of bioprosthetic aortic valves: implications from 12,569 implants, Ann Thorac Surg 99(4):1239–1247, 2015.
3. Lawley CM, Lain SJ, Algert CS, et al: Prosthetic heart valves in pregnancy, outcomes for women and their babies: a systematic review and meta-analysis, BJOG 122(11):1446–1455, 2015.

CASE 5-13
Bioprosthetic Mitral Valve Endocarditis with Paravalvular Regurgitation

This 52-year-old male had undergone mitral valve replacement 15 years previously for endocarditis, with repeat mitral valve replacement 2 months ago for tissue degeneration of the prosthesis. His postoperative course was complicated by sternal wound infection, adult respiratory distress syndrome (ARDS), *Staph aureus* sepsis, and acute renal failure. At that time, both transthoracic and transesophageal echocardiography showed normal valve function with no evidence of infection. He was treated with IV antibiotics and sternal wound debridement but had progressive clinical deterioration. He is now transferred to our medical center in acute cardiogenic shock with severe mitral regurgitation, presumed due to prosthetic valve endocarditis.

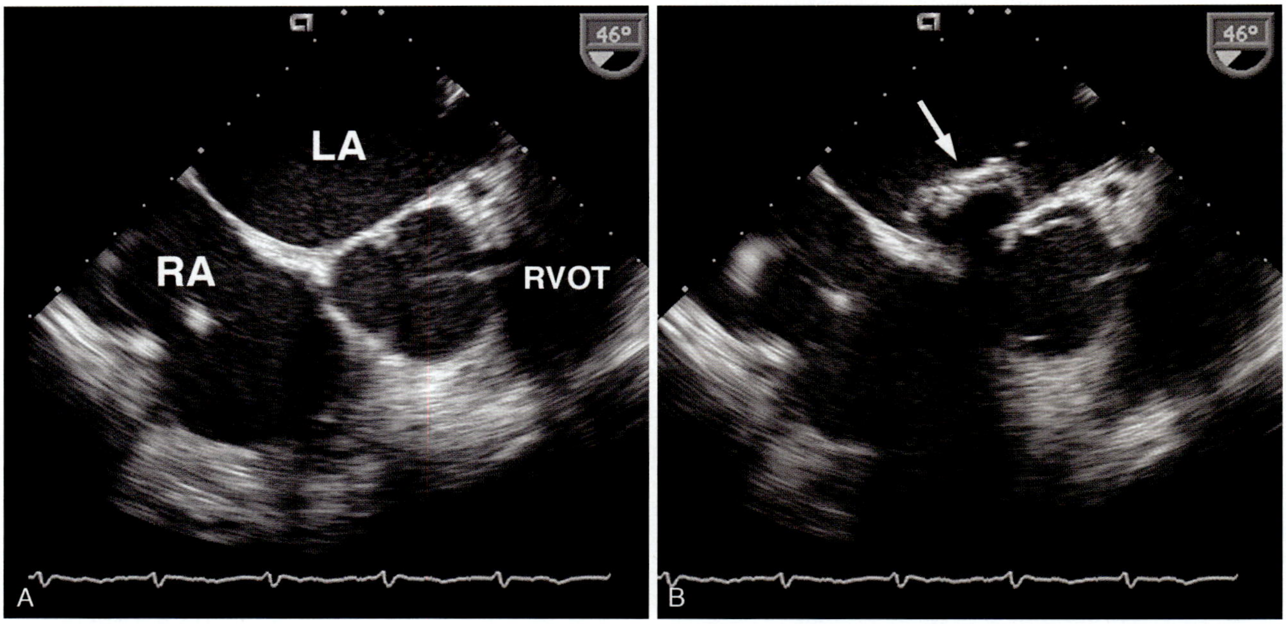

Fig 5.70 Short-axis view at level of aortic valve (at 46-degree rotation) in diastole **(A)** shows closed aortic valve and normal left atrium (LA). Catheter is present in right atrium (RA). In systole **(B)**, large echodense mass prolapses into LA *(arrow)*, presumably from mitral valve prosthesis.

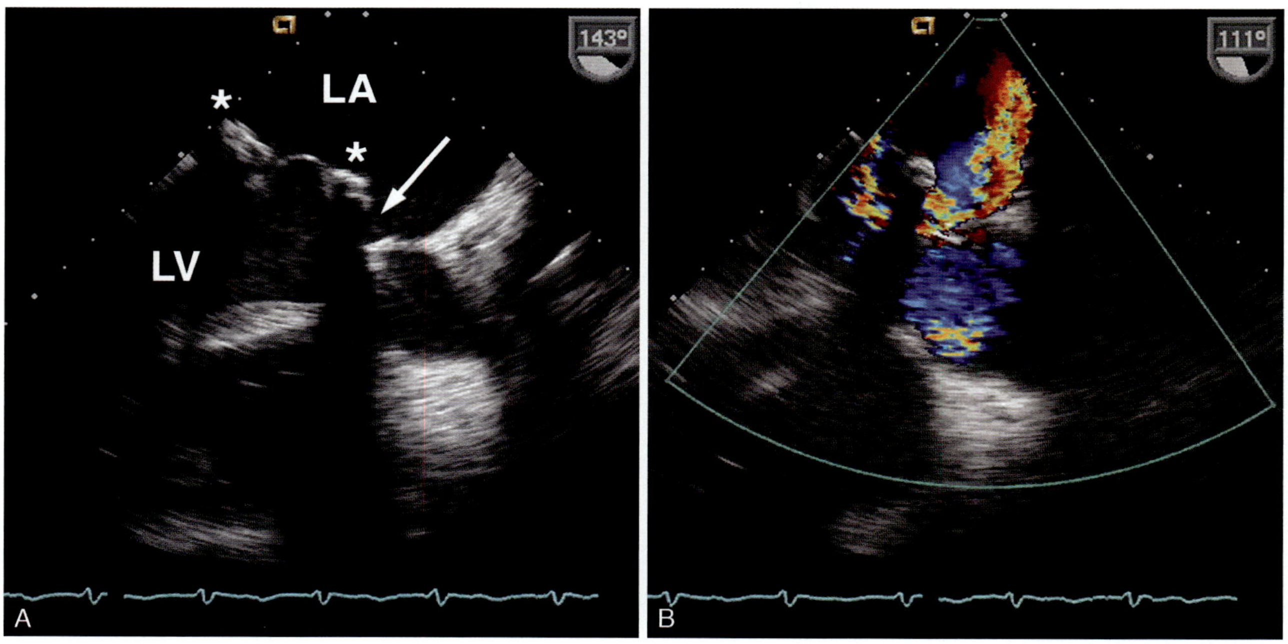

Fig 5.71 Long-axis view (at 143-degree rotation) confirms that prolapsing mass *(asterisks)* is attached to mitral leaflet. Arrow indicates where valve has become dehisced from annulus **(A)**. Color flow **(B)** demonstrates significant mitral regurgitation. At surgery, mitral valve prosthesis was encircled by vegetations and was dehisced from annulus, being held in place only by two remaining pledgets in posterior-lateral aspect of annulus. Pathologic examination demonstrated vegetations with gram-positive coccal bacterial forms. Cultures of valve tissue showed no growth. Although cultures of mediastinal tissue grew *Candida albicans*, there were no fungal forms seen in valve tissue.

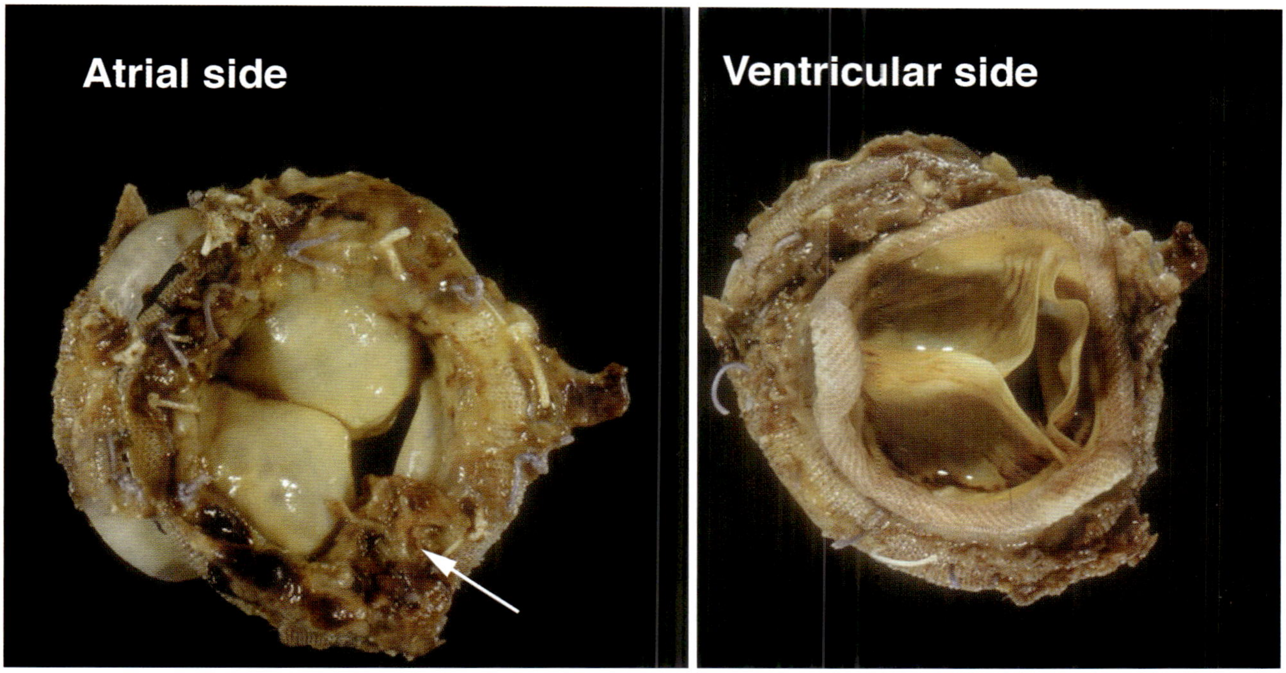

Fig 5.72 Pathologic examination of valve revealed inflammatory tissue circumferentially around metallic rim of valve, as well as lesion projecting over one of cusps *(arrow)*. Pathologic examination was consistent with bacterial vegetation. All three cusps were intact.

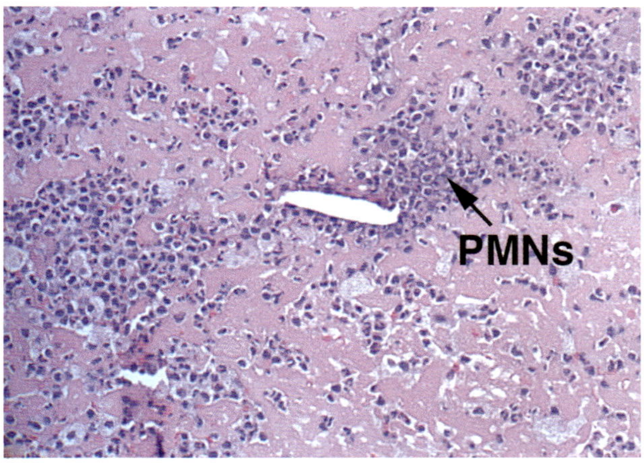

Fig 5.73 Microscopic examination of tissue around annulus revealed active inflammation with sheets of polymorphonuclear leukocytes (PMNs).

Comments

This patient has early prosthetic valve endocarditis with a large vegetation on the valve leaflet and infection of the sewing ring, resulting in valve dehiscence. Most cases of prosthetic valve endocarditis require removal of the prosthesis, in addition to prolonged antibiotic therapy. In this patient with fungal infection of the mediastinum and a large vegetation on the prosthetic valve, fungal endocarditis was suspected. However, the pathologic examination was most consistent with *Staph aureus* endocarditis, emphasizing that large vegetations may be seen with bacterial, as well as fungal, endocarditis. *Staph aureus* is a very virulent organism and there is a high prevalence of paravalvular abscess and poor outcomes in patients with *Staph aureus* endocarditis.

Suggested Reading

1. Cahill TJ, Prendergast BD: Infective endocarditis, Lancet 387(10021):882–893, 2016.
2. Kang DH: Timing of surgery in infective endocarditis, Heart 101(22):1786–1791, 2015.

CASE 5-14
Bioprosthetic Mitral Valve Stenosis with Leaflet Perforation

This 49-year-old male who over the past few months reported significant worsening of exercise tolerance with shortness of breath on minimal exertion. He underwent bioprosthetic aortic and mitral valve replacement for endocarditis 10 years prior, and then a redo bioprosthetic aortic valve replacement several years after his original surgery. Recent TTE demonstrates severe bioprosthetic mitral stenosis.

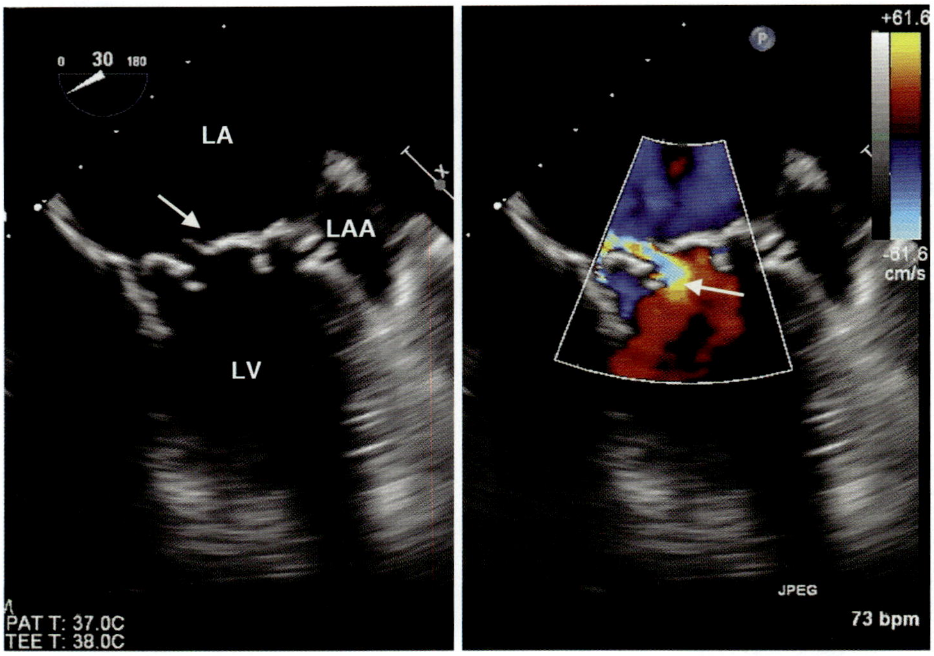

Fig 5.74 In midesophageal view at 30 degrees, leaflet or portion of leaflet is seen to prolapse *(left panel, white arrow).* In right panel, white arrow indicates eccentric jet of mitral regurgitation.

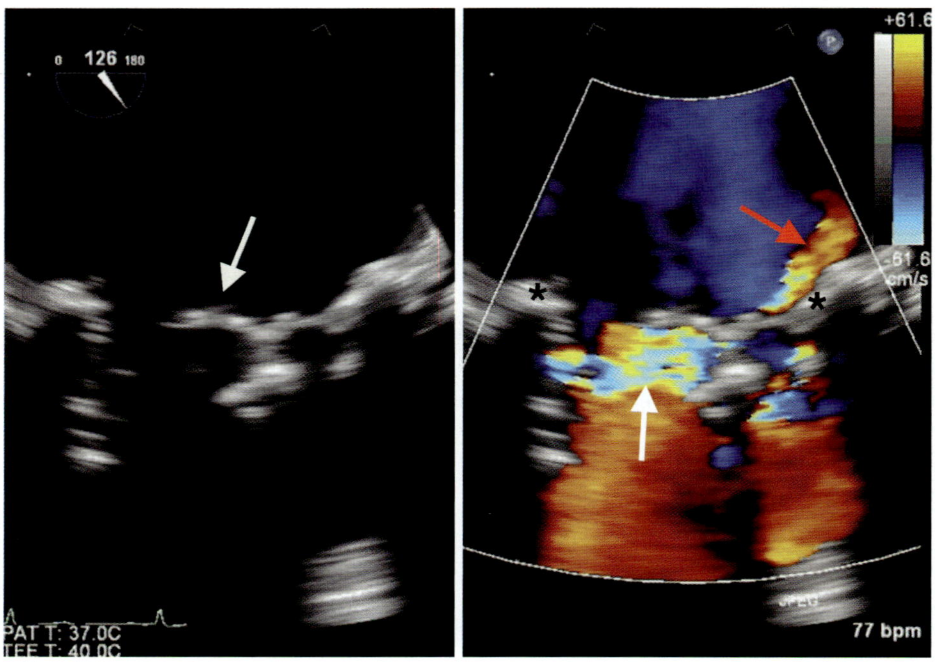

Fig 5.75 With transducer now rotated to angle of 126 degrees, left panel again demonstrates disruption of systolic coaptation *(white arrow).* Color Doppler demonstrates same central transvalvular jet as previous figure, but there is now evidence of smaller eccentrically directed jet as well that seems to originate within sewing ring *(red arrow).* Jet's eccentricity raises suspicion of leaflet perforation. Asterisks mark sewing ring of valve.

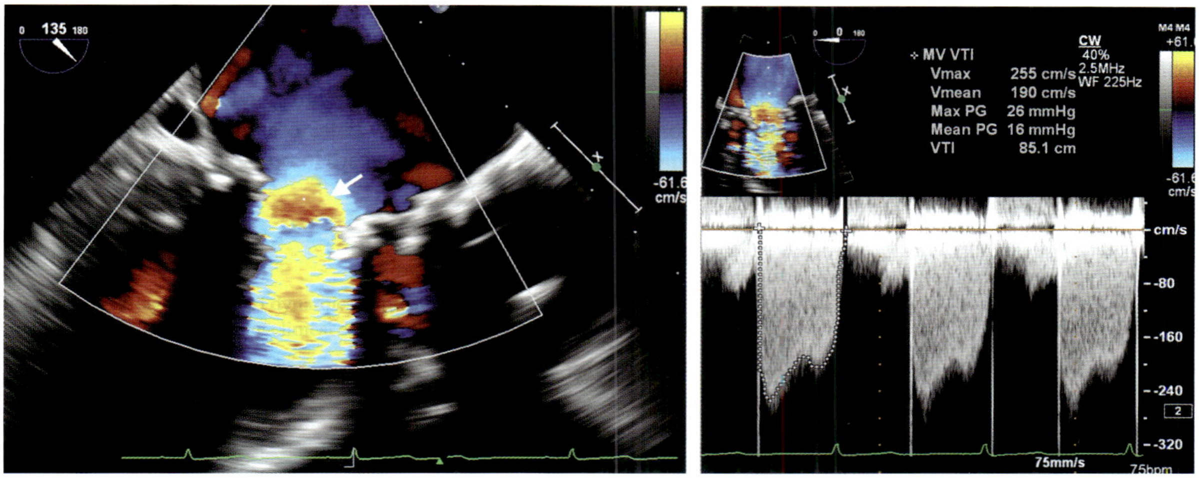

Fig 5.76 Left panel demonstrates flow acceleration *(arrow)* at mitral orifice. In right panel, CW Doppler shows mean gradient of 16 mm Hg, indicative of severe prosthetic valve stenosis.

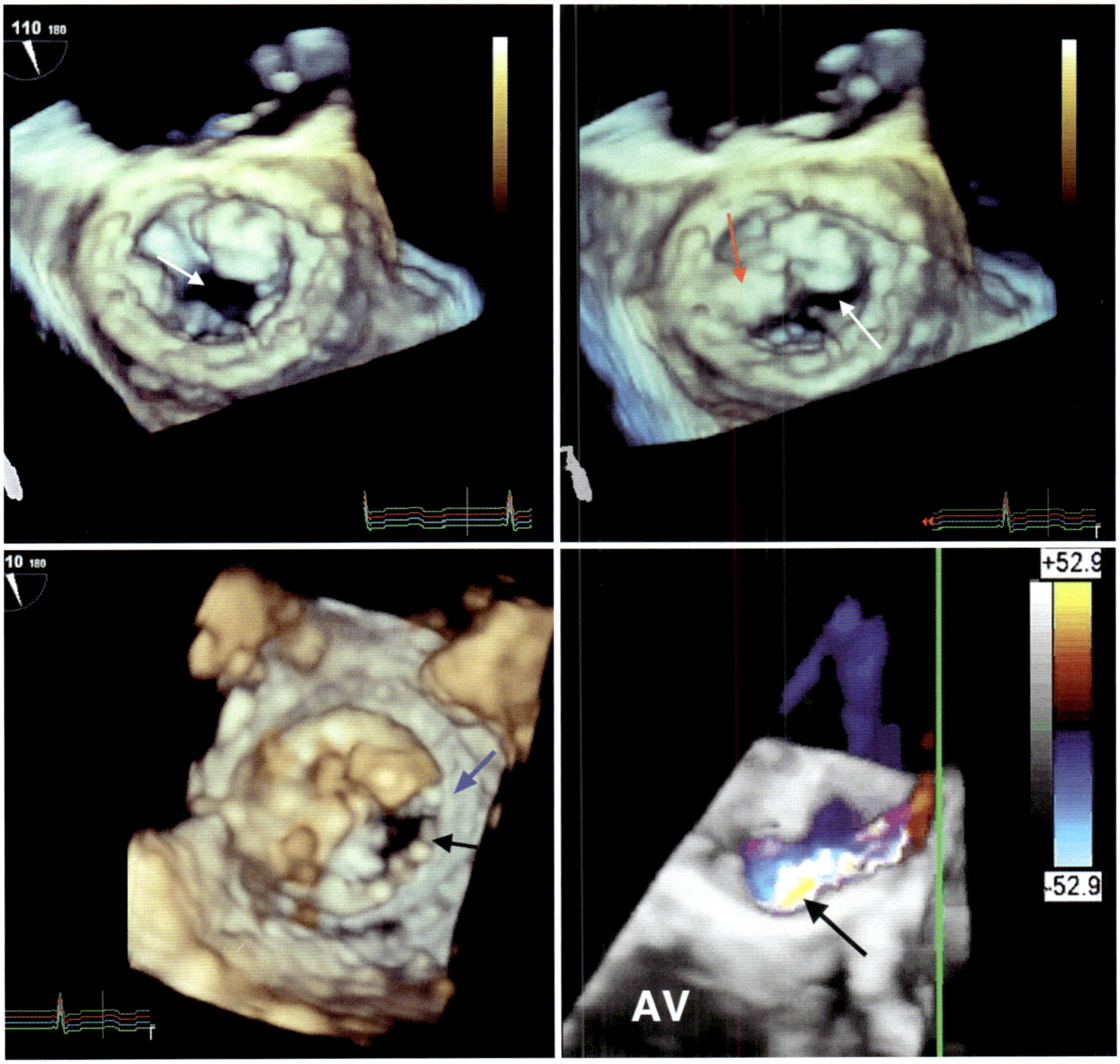

Fig 5.77 3D TEE from midesophageal position. Images are from LA perspective in upper left (diastole) and upper right (systole) panels, and LV perspective in lower left panel. Diastolic orifice is small *(white arrow)*, and during systole, there is incomplete coaptation *(white arrow)*. Calcified portion of one of leaflets *(red arrow)* is seen in real time to prolapse freely. From LV perspective black arrow points to defect that is most likely leaflet perforation; it is clearly inside valve sewing ring *(blue arrow)*. In lower right panel, 3D color Doppler shows that eccentric jet is directed anterolaterally.

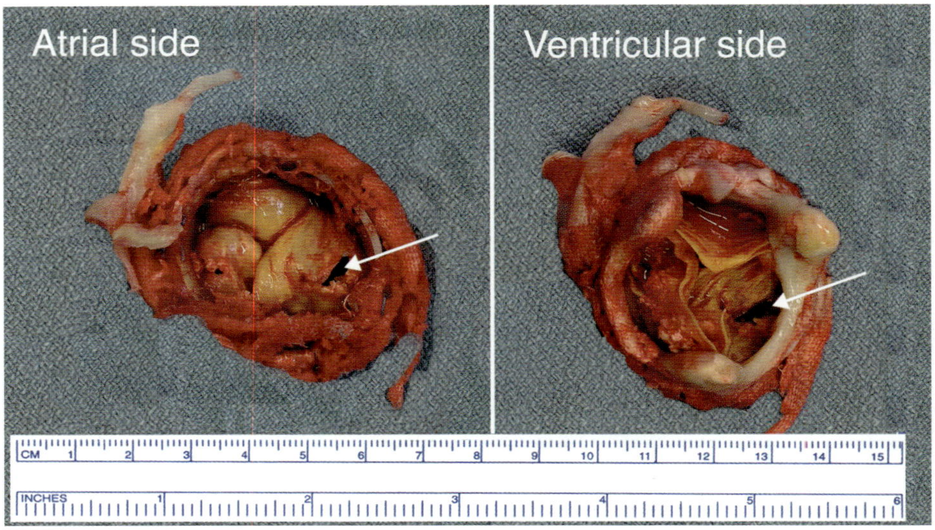

Fig 5.78 Explanted valve is seen from atrial and ventricular perspectives. There is generalized leaflet thickening, and leaflet perforation is seen.

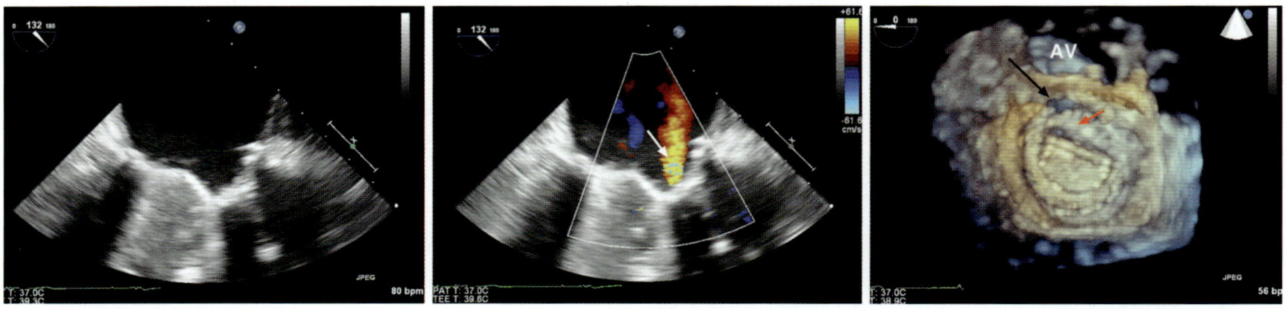

Fig 5.79 Bileaflet mechanical prosthesis was placed *(left panel)*, but upon weaning from cardiopulmonary bypass, anterolateral perivalvular regurgitant jet was noted *(white arrow, center panel)*. 3D TEE *(right panel)* shows where sewing ring *(red arrow)* has pulled away from native annulus, creating defect *(black arrow)*. Patient was returned to cardiopulmonary bypass and defect closed.

Comment

This case illustrates the use of 3D imaging to demonstrate a leaflet perforation of a degenerated bioprosthetic mitral valve. Although Doppler data suggested the leak was due to leaflet dysfunction, the diagnosis could not be established with 2D imaging. The distinction between transvalvular and paravalvular regurgitation is important because treatment options for a paravalvular leak include surgical repair (as in this case) or closure with a device by a transcatheter approach (see Chapter 14).

Suggested Reading

1. Lang R, Tsang W: 3D echocardiography: principles of image acquisition, display and analysis. In Otto CM, editor: The practice of clinical echocardiography, ed 5, Philadelphia, 2016, Elsevier.

CASE 5-15
Bioprosthetic Tricuspid Valve Regurgitation

The patient presented nearly 20 years before this hospitalization with motor vehicle trauma resulting in severe tricuspid regurgitation, requiring a bioprosthetic valve replacement. He now presents with increasing fatigue, severe tricuspid regurgitation with massive RA enlargement. On CT scan, the patient was found to have a very enlarged RV with several adhesions against the sternum. Because of this, a limited right thoracotomy approach was proposed with minimally invasive approach with groin cannulation.

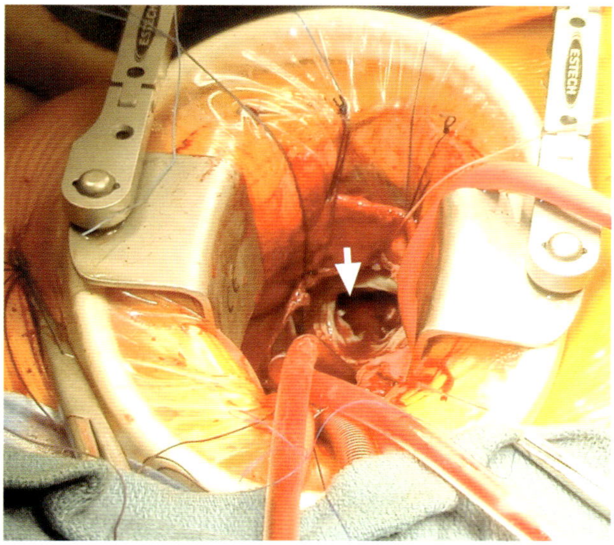

Fig 5.80 Through right thoracotomy, right atrium is incised and tricuspid valve is exposed *(arrow)*.

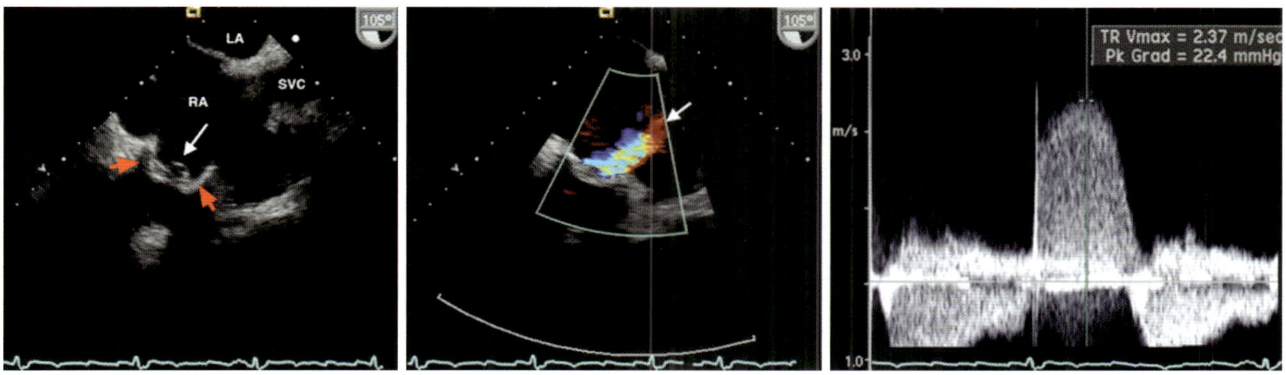

Fig 5.81 In this midesophageal bicaval view rotated slightly medially to include tricuspid valve, left panel illustrates flail portion of tricuspid bioprosthesis *(white arrow)*. Red arrows indicate two of three valve posts. In center panel, eccentric jet of TR is seen *(white arrow)*. Width of jet suggests at least moderate regurgitation. CW Doppler in right panel shows antegrade velocity of 2.37 m/sec.

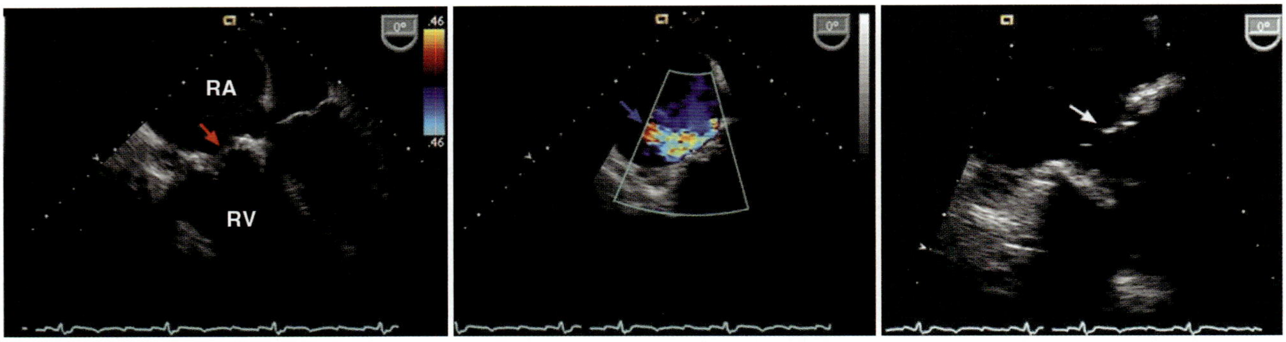

Fig 5.82 In left panel, midesophageal four-chamber view again shows tricuspid bioprosthesis with thickened leaflet tissue *(red arrow, left panel)*. In center frame, blue arrow indicates jet of TR. Right frame is zoom-mode image of tricuspid bioprosthesis; calcification is seen.

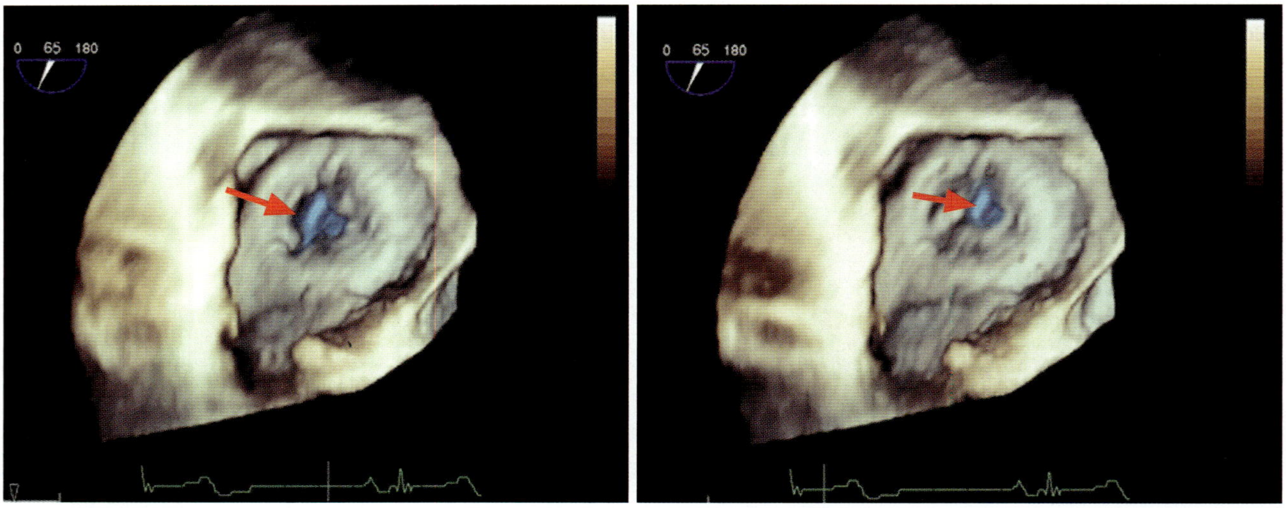

Fig 5.83 3D TEE of tricuspid prosthesis is seen from right atrial perspective in diastole *(left frame)* and systole *(right frame)*. Red arrows indicate valve orifice which appears smaller than sewing ring in diastole, consistent with mild stenosis. In addition, valve does not close completely in systolic with large regurgitant orifice.

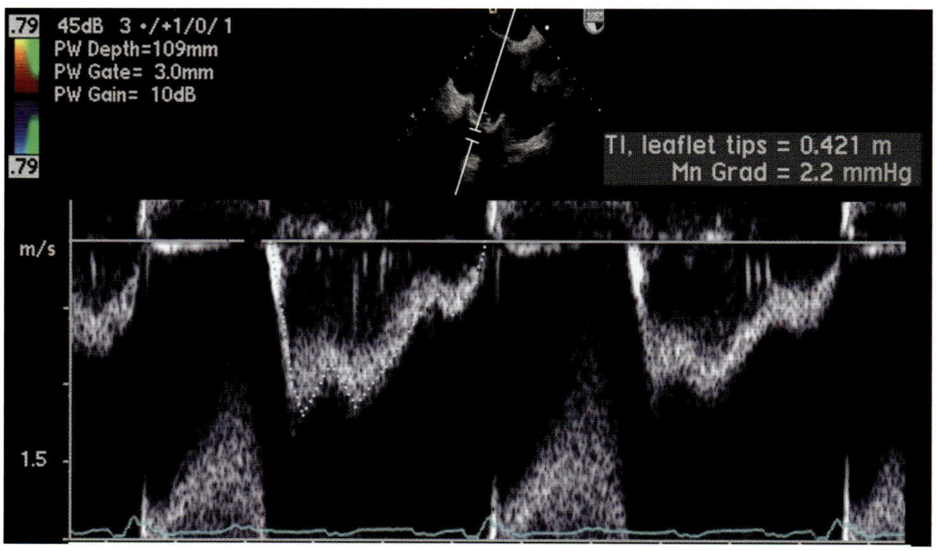

Fig 5.84 Mean tricuspid inflow gradient obtained from midesophageal four-chamber view was only 2.2 mm Hg, consistent with regurgitation being primary hemodynamic lesion in this patient.

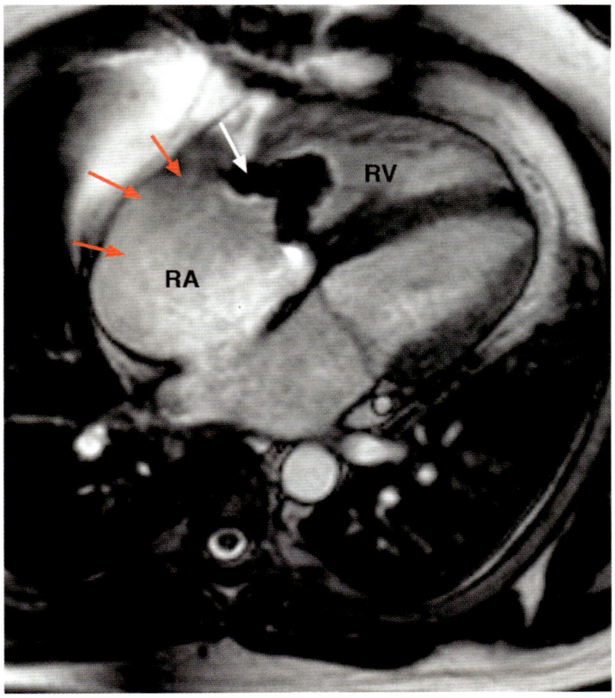

Fig 5.85 Cardiac MRI shows right-sided chamber dilation as well as tricuspid bioprosthesis *(white arrow)*. In real time, jet of TR can be appreciated in part of RA indicated by red arrows.

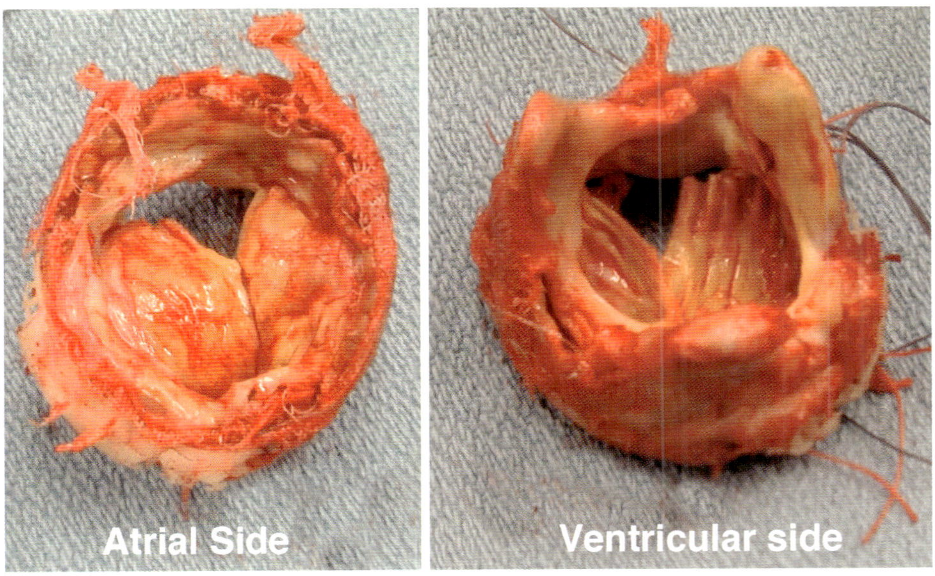

Fig 5.86 Explanted valve is seen from both atrial and ventricular perspectives. There is leaflet thickening, and one of three leaflets is retracted, accounting for large regurgitant orifice area.

Comments

Evaluation of a bioprosthetic tricuspid valve can be challenging because gradients may be low, even when severe stenosis is present, if flow rates are low. Severe tricuspid regurgitation may not be recognized because the low pressure gradient between the RV and RA results in relatively laminar to-and-fro flow across the large regurgitant orifice area, rather than a dramatic color Doppler jet as seen with a high-velocity mitral regurgitant jet. The pulsed Doppler recording of flow across the tricuspid valve in this case (Fig 5.84) also shows laminar retrograde flow in systole, which is aliased so that it appears at the bottom of the velocity scale.

Suggested Reading

1. Lee SH, Kim SA, Jo SH, et al: Combined traumatic tricuspid regurgitation and acute myocardial infarction after fist blows to the chest, Circulation 129(20):e496–e498, 2014.
2. Avegliano G, Corneli M, Conde D, Ronderos R: Traumatic rupture of the tricuspid valve and multi-modality imaging, Cardiovasc Diagn Ther 4(5):401–405, 2014.

Mechanical Prosthetic Valves: Dysfunction

CASE 5-16
Paravalvular Aortic Regurgitation

This 55-year-old man had undergone aortic valve replacement 6 months earlier with a bileaflet mechanical valve. He now presented with a new diastolic murmur and an echocardiogram showing severe aortic regurgitation. He was referred for surgical treatment.

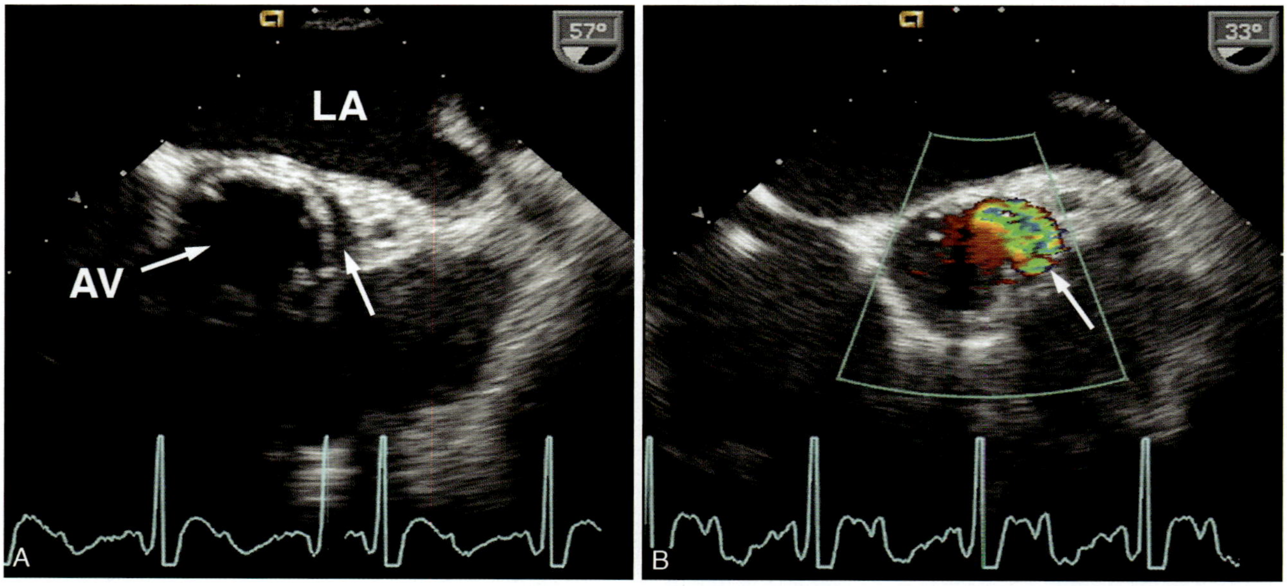

Fig 5.87 Short-axis TEE view **(A)** at 57 degrees shows crescent-shaped echolucent area *(arrow)* around left coronary cusp aspect of sewing ring. Color Doppler **(B)** shows diastolic flow in this region consistent with aortic regurgitation *(arrow)*. This represents vena contracta in short axis at level of valve.

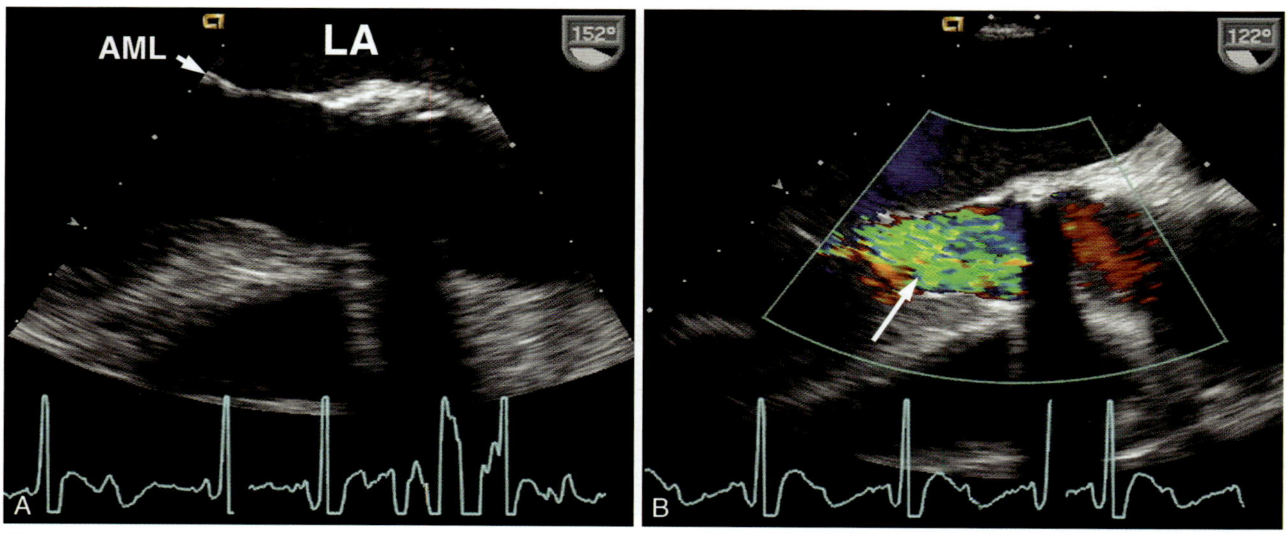

Fig 5.88 In TEE long-axis view **(A)** at 152 degrees, there is shadowing from mechanical valve, but color Doppler **(B)** shows broad jet *(arrow)* of aortic regurgitation that fills LVOT.

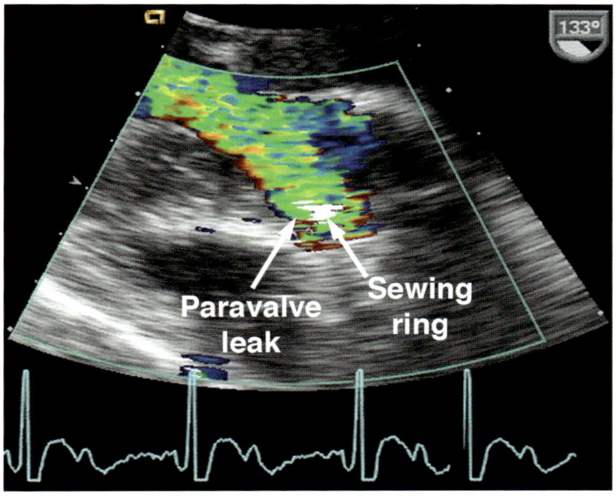

Fig 5.89 Transgastric long-axis view was obtained starting in transgastric short-axis view at 0 degrees and then rotating image plane to 133 degrees and turning transducer medially. Color Doppler shows broad aortic regurgitant jet. This view is helpful with prosthetic aortic valves, as valve does not shadow outflow tract from this angle.

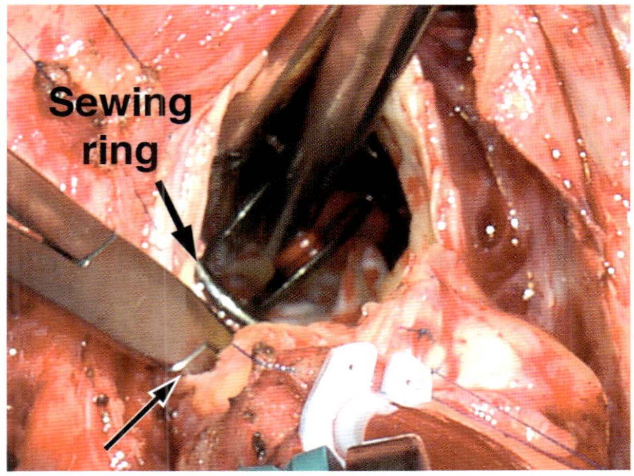

Fig 5.90 At surgery, valve appeared intact. However, on very close inspection there was an area of dehiscence (*arrow*, instrument in dehisced area) extending from just under left main coronary artery laterally to junction of left and right native commissure. Given fact that there was no evidence of infection, this was thought to be mechanical failure and amenable to repair.

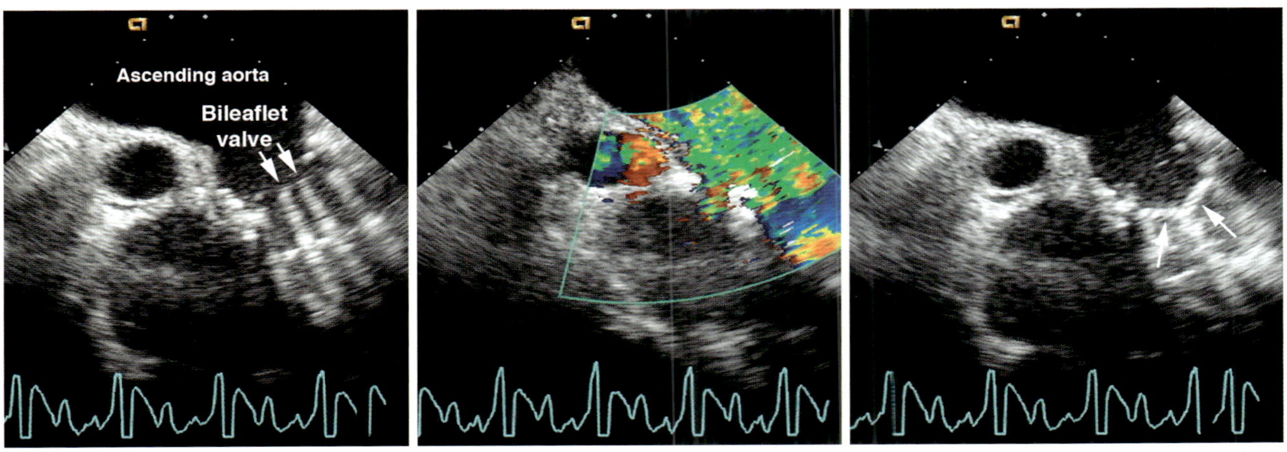

Fig 5.91 Epiaortic scanning after correction in systole shows full excursion of mechanical leaflets *(left panel)* and normal antegrade flow *(center panel)*. Right panel in diastole shows normal slightly obtuse closure angle of leaflets (not 180 degrees) *(arrows)*.

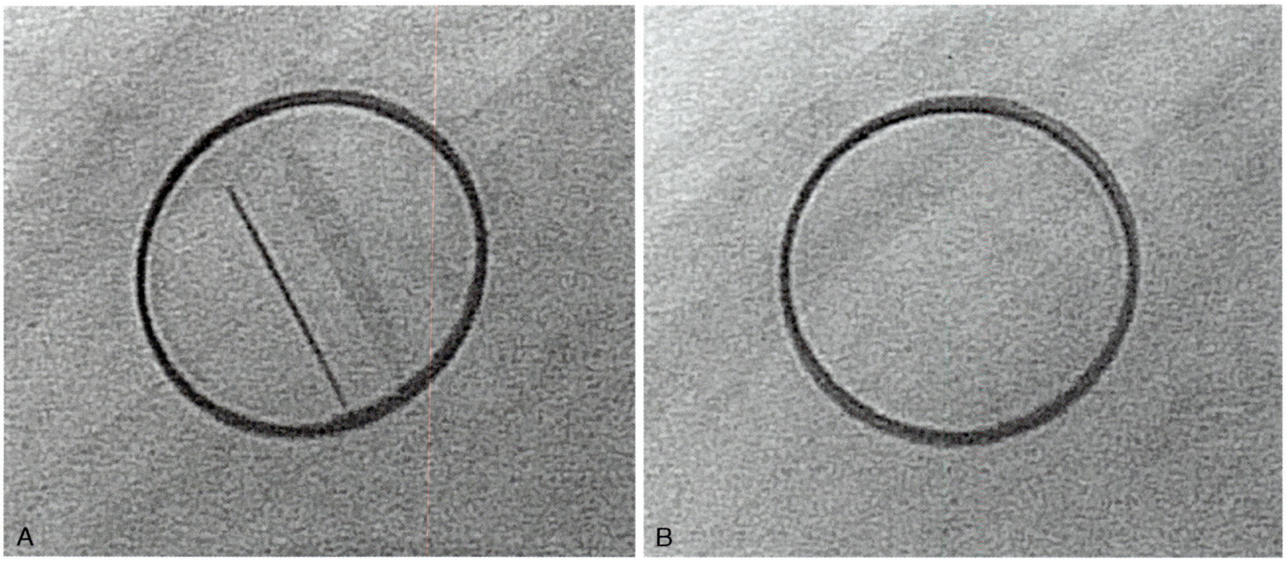

Fig 5.92 Postoperative fluoroscopy shows leaflets fully opened in systole **(A)** and not visible during diastole **(B)** due to relative angle of valve leaflets and x-ray source.

Comments

Mechanical valves have a very low rate of primary structural deterioration, with the interface between the valve sewing ring and the native annular tissue being the most vulnerable location for dysfunction. In this patient, the sutures attaching the valve to the aortic annulus were disrupted. Early after surgery, suture disruption may occur due to friction if there is any movement of the valve ring or if the annulus is fibrotic or calcified, which is the most likely explanation in this case. Later after surgery, mechanical disruption of the sutures is less likely due to tissue growth onto the sewing ring. The most common cause of late paravalvular regurgitation is infection, with paravalvular abscess formation.

Regurgitation of a mechanical aortic valve is often best evaluated from a transthoracic approach because the valve is well seen from this position and the outflow tract is not shadowed by the valve. With transesophageal imaging for prosthetic aortic valves, care is needed to demonstrate aortic regurgitation. As in this case, transgastric views may be helpful for color Doppler demonstration of regurgitation. Continuous wave Doppler examination can also be diagnostic.

The epiaortic imaging and fluoroscopy of the valve demonstrate the normal opening and closing of this bileaflet valve.

Suggested Reading

1. Konoske R, Whitener G, Nicoara A: Intraoperative evaluation of paravalvular regurgitation by transesophageal echocardiography, Anesth Analg 121(2):329–336, 2015.

CASE 5-17
Paravalvular Mitral Regurgitation

This 55-year-old man had a complex cardiac history with three previous mitral valve surgical procedures. He was admitted for hemolytic anemia with symptoms of lightheadedness and one episode of syncope. Transthoracic echocardiography showed paravalvular mitral regurgitation and he was referred for surgical consideration.

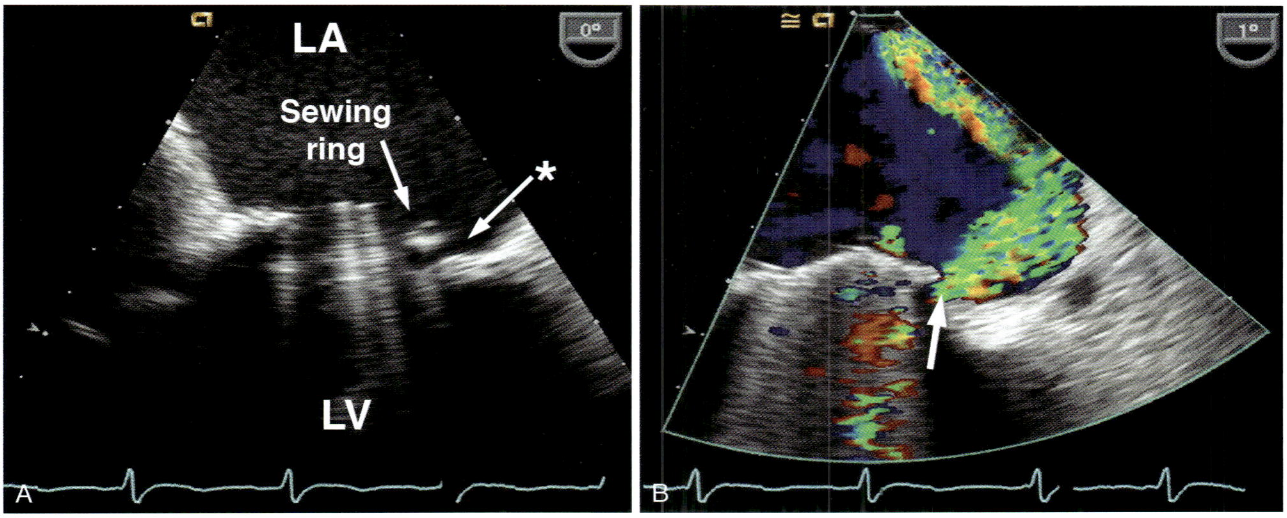

Fig 5.93 Four-chamber TEE view at 0 degrees shows bileaflet mitral valve open in diastole (**A**) with area of apparent discontinuity *(arrow)* at lateral sewing ring. Color Doppler during systole (**B**, *arrow*) shows large jet of paravalvular mitral regurgitation originating at this site that is eccentric in direction and extends along lateral wall of left atrium. Vena contracta width of 5 mm *(arrow)* is consistent with at least moderate regurgitation.

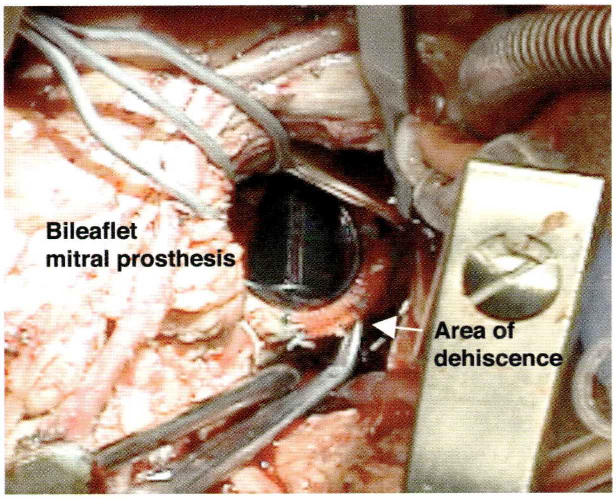

Fig 5.94 At surgery, view from left atrial side of valve showed area of paravalvular dehiscence.

Comments

This patient had recurrent paravalvular regurgitation due to a calcified and fibrotic annulus, resulting in disruption of the sutures, without evidence of infection. Regurgitation of mechanical prosthetic valves in the mitral position is best evaluated by transesophageal imaging. In this case it is obvious that regurgitation is pathologic because it originates outside the sewing ring, the vena contracta is wide and the jet is eccentric and turbulent. Compare the pathologic regurgitant jet in this example with the normal regurgitant jet seen in Case 5-4.

Hemolytic anemia is most common with paravalvular regurgitation of the mechanical valve in the mitral position, as in this case. The severity of regurgitation is often only mild to moderate, as in this case, with symptoms due to anemia, not regurgitation. Some cases of hemolytic anemia can be treated conservatively with folate and iron replacement and occasional transfusion, but more severe anemia, refractory to medical therapy, requires surgical intervention.

Suggested Reading

1. Mahjoub H, Pibarot P, Dumesnil JG: Echocardiographic evaluation of prosthetic heart valves, Curr Cardiol Rep 17(6):48, 2015.

CASE 5-18
Impaired Occluder Motion, Mitral Position

This 69-year-old male had 10 years previously undergone a mitral valve repair for myxomatous mitral valve disease, with P2 resection and ring annuloplasty. Over the 3 to 4 months before this admission, he had noted an increase in shortness of breath and dramatic decrease in exercise tolerance. A TTE showed severe aortic regurgitation, and an anteriorly directed eccentric jet at the previous mitral repair. He was scheduled for aortic and mitral valve replacements.

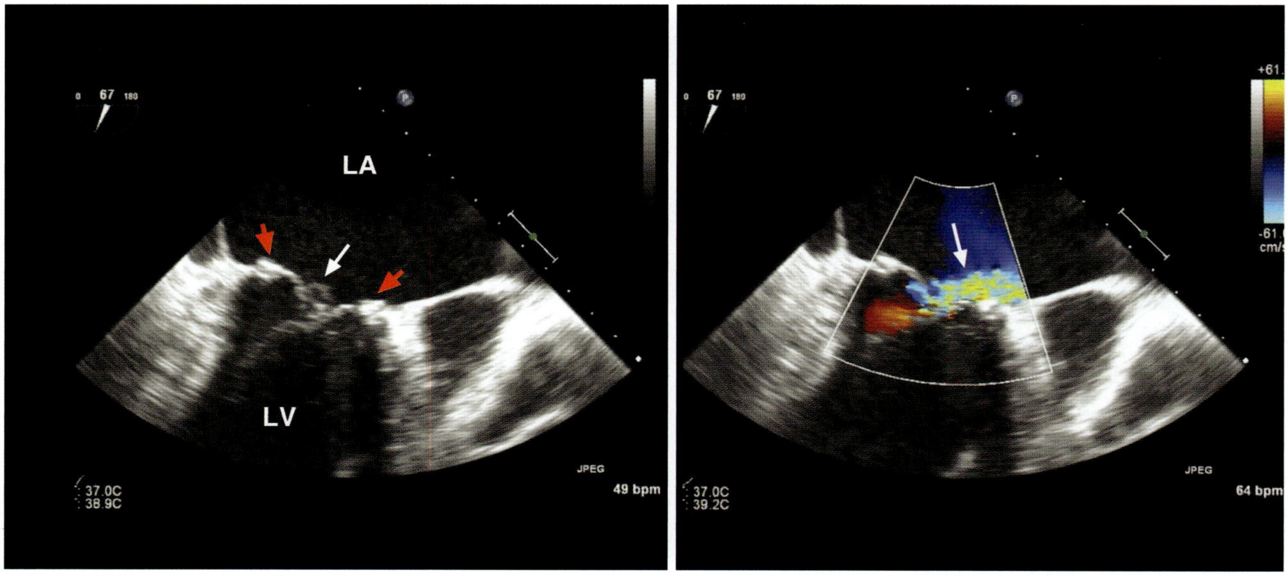

Fig 5.95 In this midesophageal view, left panel illustrates previously placed annuloplasty ring in mitral position *(red arrows)*. White arrow indicates prolapsed valvular tissue. In right panel, white arrow indicates eccentric jet of mitral regurgitation.

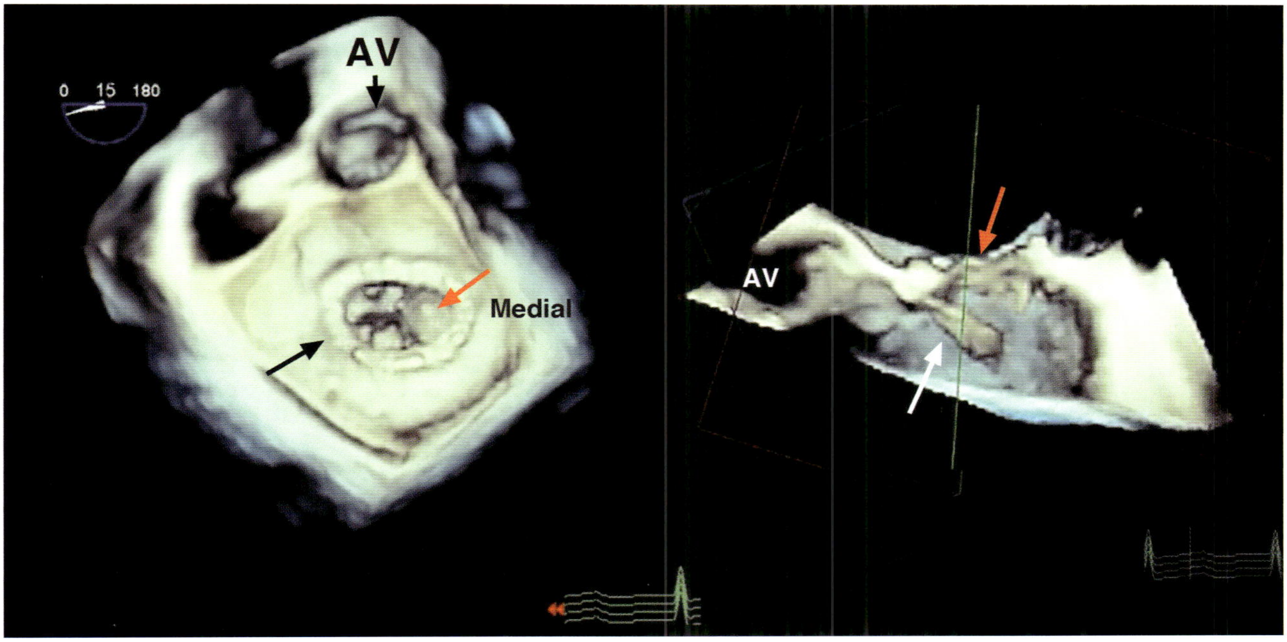

Fig 5.96 Left panel is 3D TEE midesophageal view of mitral valve from left atrium. Annuloplasty ring is seen *(black arrow)* as is prolapsing leaflet tissue *(red arrow)*. Right panel shows valve cropped from medial aspect. Prolapsing portion comes from posterior leaflet.

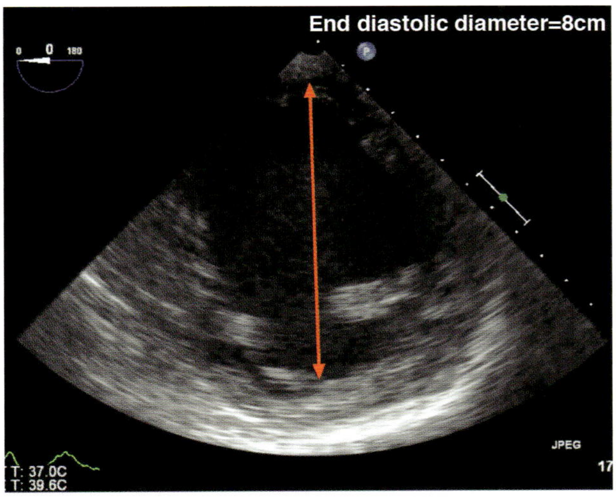

Fig 5.97 In this diastolic frame of transgastric short-axis image of left ventricle, end diastolic diameter is elevated at 8 cm. In real time, overall systolic function is reduced.

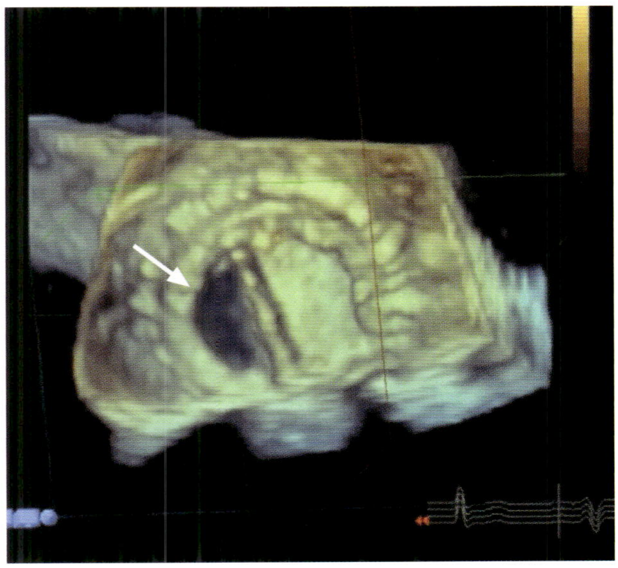

Fig 5.98 Mechanical bileaflet prosthesis was placed in mitral position; however, only one of the leaflets opens normally in diastole showing dark hemi-circular diastolic orifice *(white arrow)*. Other leaflet remains closed in diastole.

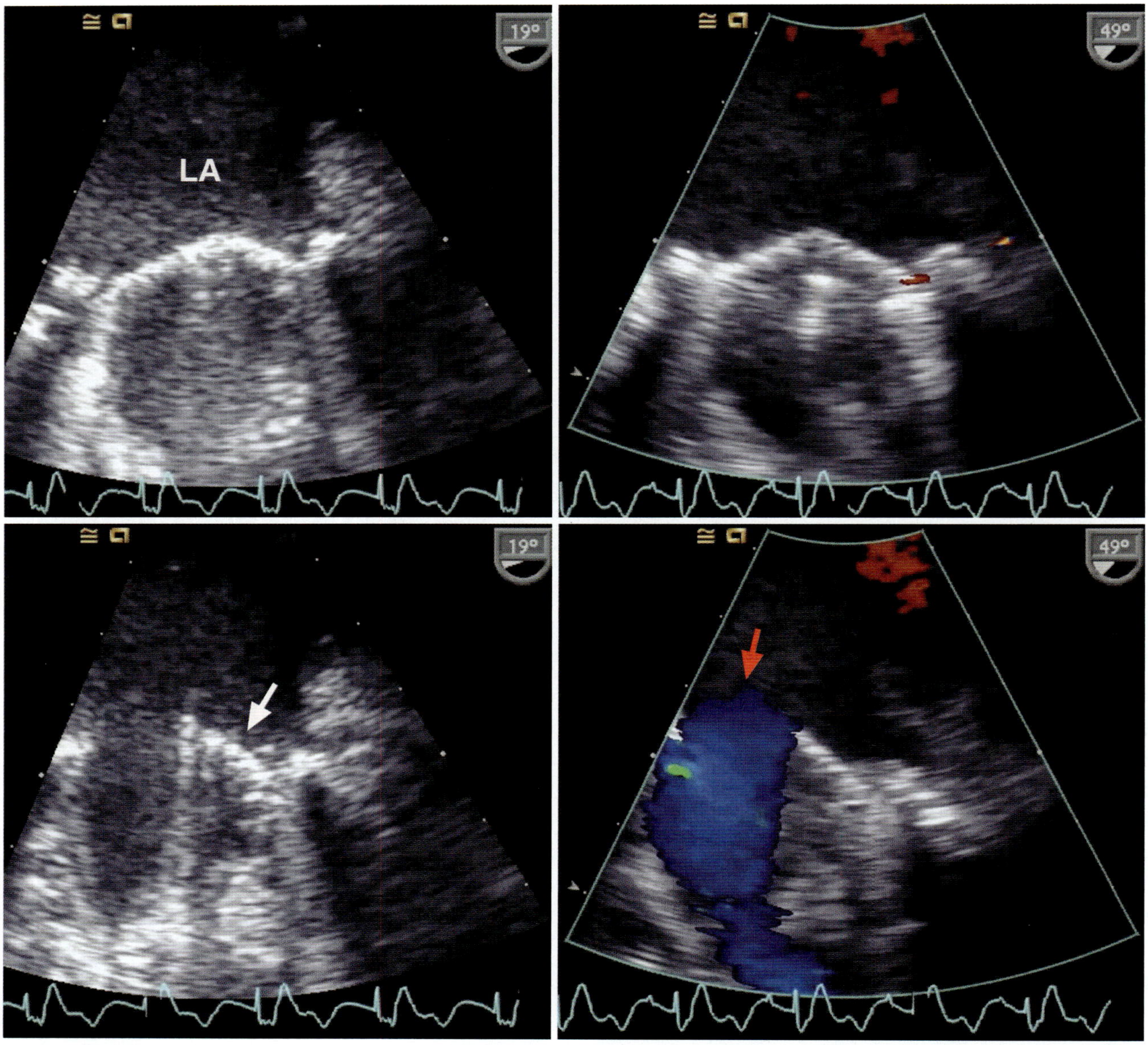

Fig 5.99 In patient with similar clinical presentation midesophageal view of bileaflet prosthesis demonstrates adequate closure during systole *(top panels)* without regurgitation, but stuck leaflet during diastole *(bottom panels, white arrow)* with color Doppler confirmation of unilateral mitral inflow *(red arrow)*.

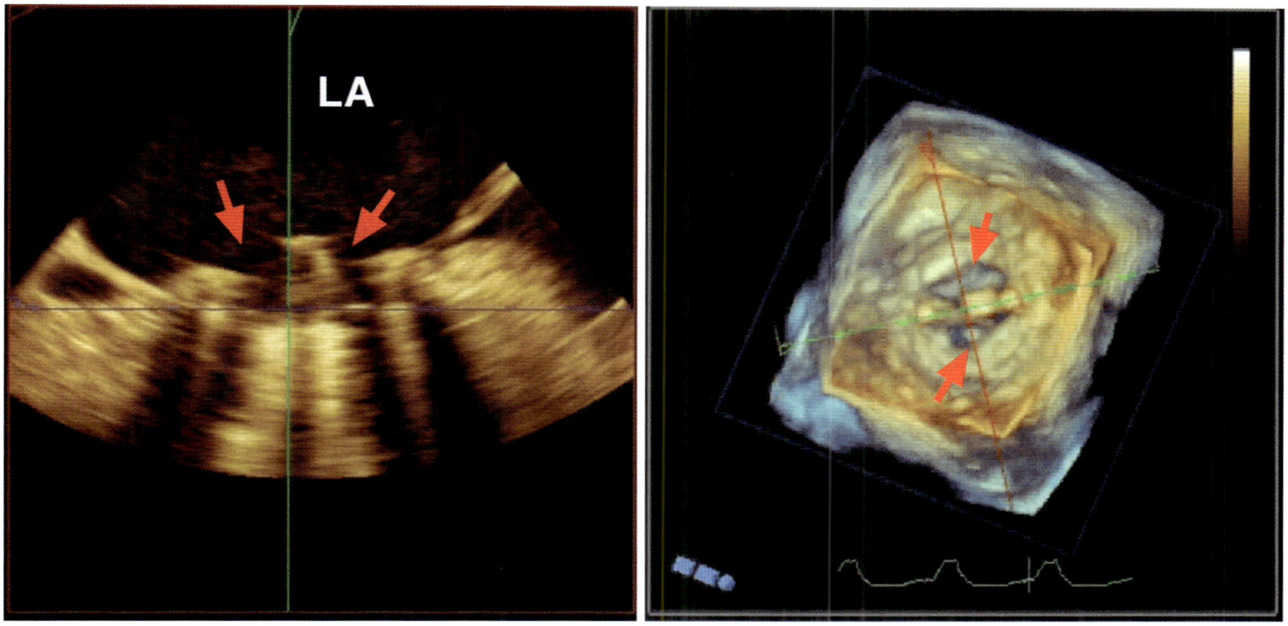

Fig 5.100 Patient was returned to cardiopulmonary bypass, and valve rotated to anatomic position; subsequently, both leaflets moved freely and allowed more complete inflow orifice *(red arrows)*.

Comments

The most common mechanisms of mechanical valve dysfunction are infection and thrombosis. Valve thrombosis may be acute, for example thrombus in the hinges of a bileaflet valve limiting disk excursion, or chronic, with a slowly enlarging thrombus leading to impairment of disk motion. In addition, tissue ingrowth (or pannus) around the annulus on the upstream side of the valve, as seen in this case, can prevent normal disk opening and/or closing. The risk factors for pannus ingrowth have not been studied. In some cases, pannus ingrowth seems to be associated with suboptimal long-term anticoagulation suggesting a pattern of repetitive thrombosis and tissue ingrowth. However, other cases do not appear to be related to adequacy of anticoagulation. Pathologic examination of the tissue is nonspecific, showing fibrous tissue.

Suggested Reading

1. Bouzas-Mosquera A, Álvarez-García N: Orientation of bileaflet mechanical aortic valve prostheses for optimal evaluation by transthoracic echocardiography, J Thorac Cardiovasc Surg 150(2):428–430, 2015.

CASE 5-19
Impaired Occluder Motion, Tricuspid Position

This 28-year-old woman with complex congenital heart disease is status posttricuspid valve replacement and classic Glenn shunt for Ebstein's anomaly as a child. She has a history of several right lung arterial-venous vascular malformations with cyanosis, complete heart block with a transvenous atrial lead and an epicardial ventricular lead, and significant LV systolic dysfunction. She has been treated for congestive heart failure with an improvement in her ejection fraction from 15% to 45%. However, she continues to have persistent symptoms and signs of right-sided heart failure and is wheelchair bound due to exertional limitations. Transthoracic echocardiography shows a mean gradient of about 12 mm Hg across the mechanical tricuspid valve and severe tricuspid regurgitation. She is referred to surgery for formation of a bidirectional Glenn shunt, insertion of new atrial and ventricular pacer leads, and consideration of repeat tricuspid valve replacement.

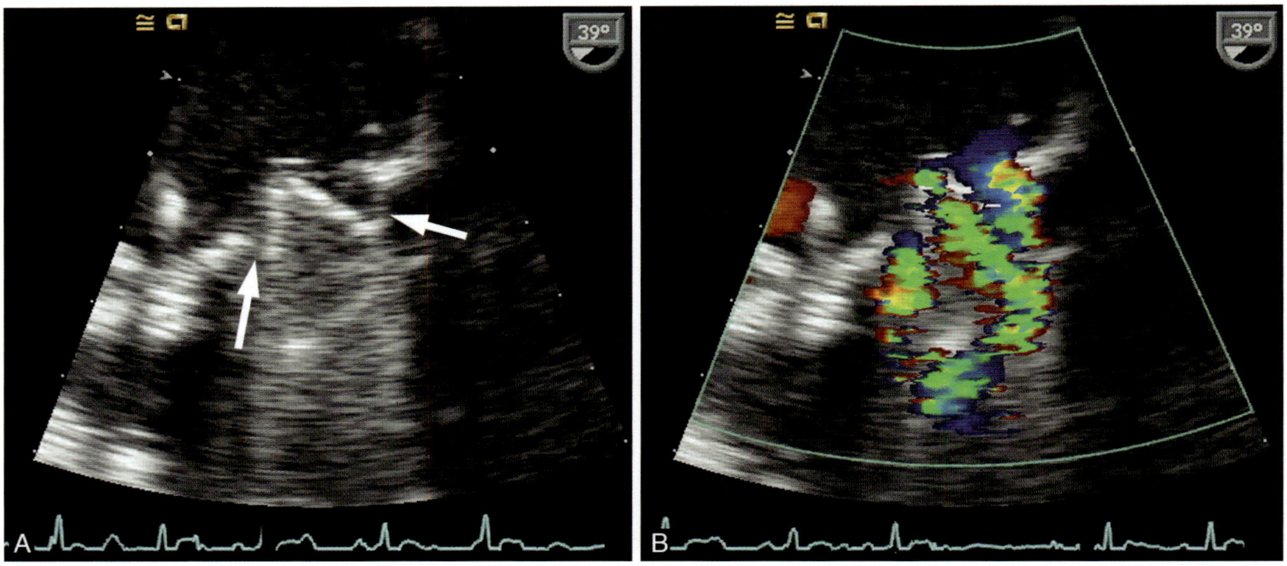

Fig 5.101 View of tricuspid prosthesis at 39-degree rotation shows reduction in maximum opening of leaflets in diastole (**A**, *arrows*). Instead of parallel alignment, leaflets only partly open at acute angle. Color Doppler (**B**) of antegrade flow shows three narrow jets, instead of normal pattern of antegrade flow across bileaflet valve.

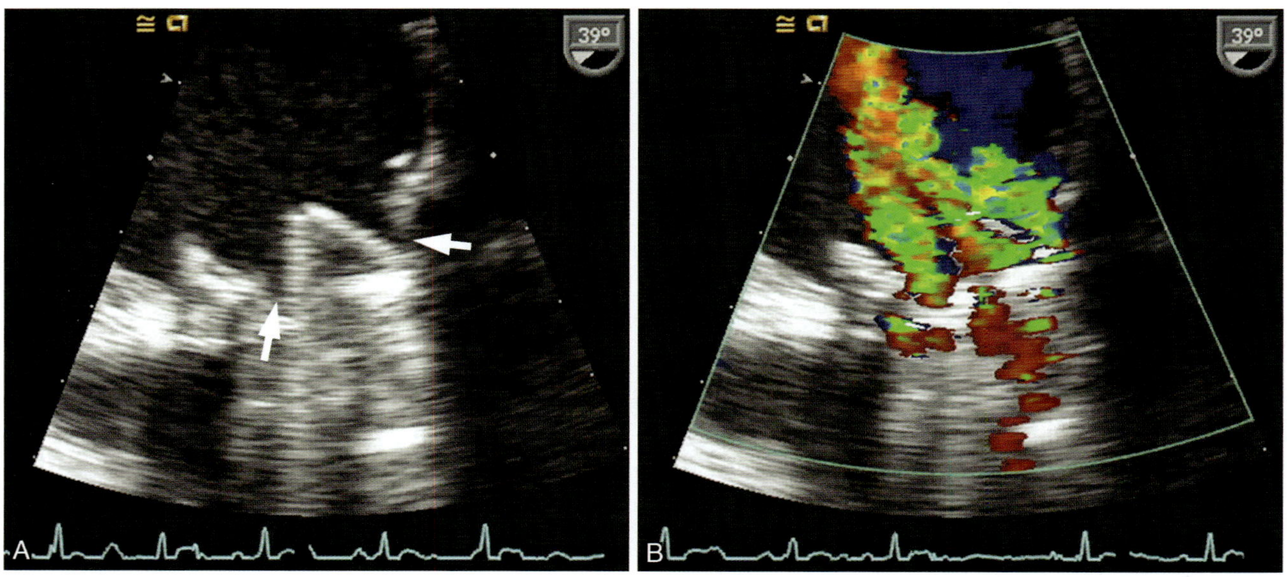

Fig 5.102 In same orientation, valve leaflets fail to close in systole (**A**, *arrows*) with color Doppler (**B**) showing severe tricuspid regurgitation.

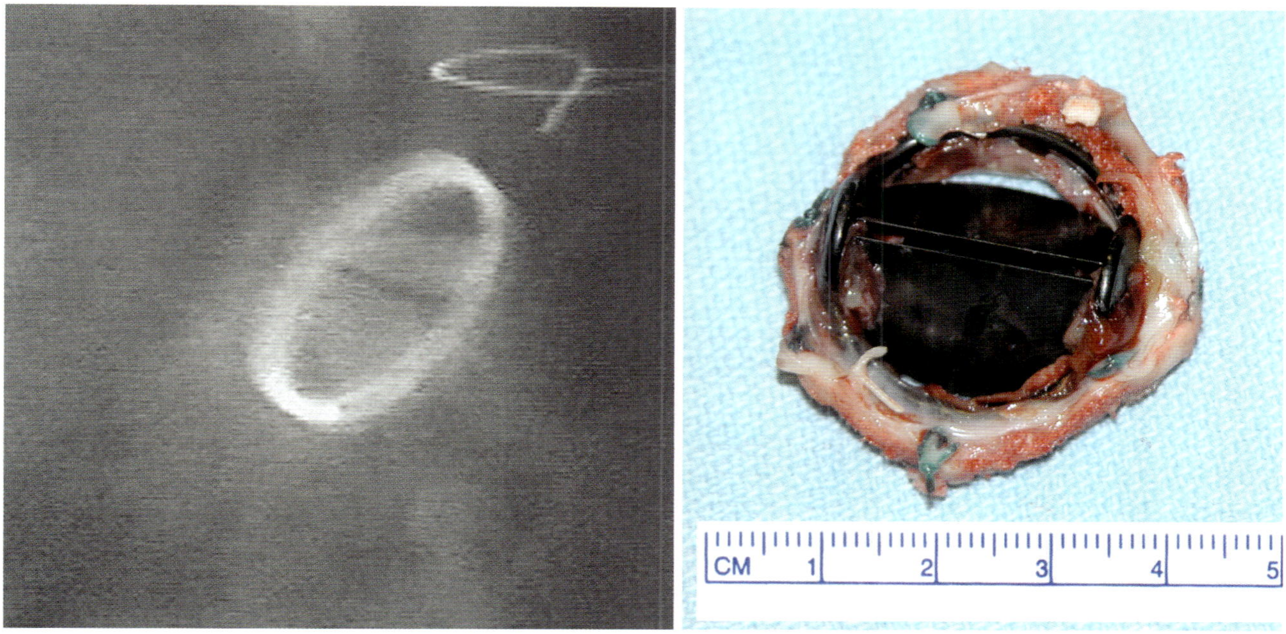

Fig 5.103 Fluoroscopy of valve shows position of leaflets; in real time, leaflets fail to move during cardiac cycle. In right panel, resected valve demonstrates pannus, particularly in region of leaflet "hinges," with resultant restriction of leaflet motion. Valve was replaced with 27-mm pericardial tissue prosthesis. The patient had dramatic clinical improvement after surgery, with substantial improvement in exercise tolerance.

Comments

In this patient with complex cyanotic congenital heart disease, it was difficult to differentiate whether symptoms were due to tricuspid valve dysfunction or inadequate pulmonary blood flow. At surgery, she had both repeat tricuspid valve surgery and restoration of the connection between the right and left pulmonary arteries so that flow from the Glenn shunt now supplies both lungs. The resected tricuspid valve was clearly dysfunctional, so it is likely that her clinical improvement was due, at least in part, to improvement in the function of the tricuspid valve. Because of the risk of tissue degeneration of valves in the tricuspid position, she will need periodic echocardiographic evaluation of tricuspid valve function.

Suggested Reading

1. Quevedo HC, Samson R, Li Z, et al: Role of four-dimensional transesophageal echocardiography in diagnosis of mechanical tricuspid valve obstruction due to thrombus, Echocardiography 32(8):1307–1310, 2015.

CASE 5-20
Systolic Anterior Leaflet Motion after Mechanical Mitral Valve Replacement

This 29-year-old male had a bileaflet mechanical prosthesis with preservation of the anterior mitral leaflet performed 12 years previously, and now presents with increasing dyspnea on exertion and fatigue. A transthoracic echocardiogram revealed a depressed ejection fraction of 40% with an 82 mmHg peak gradient in the left ventricular outflow tract.

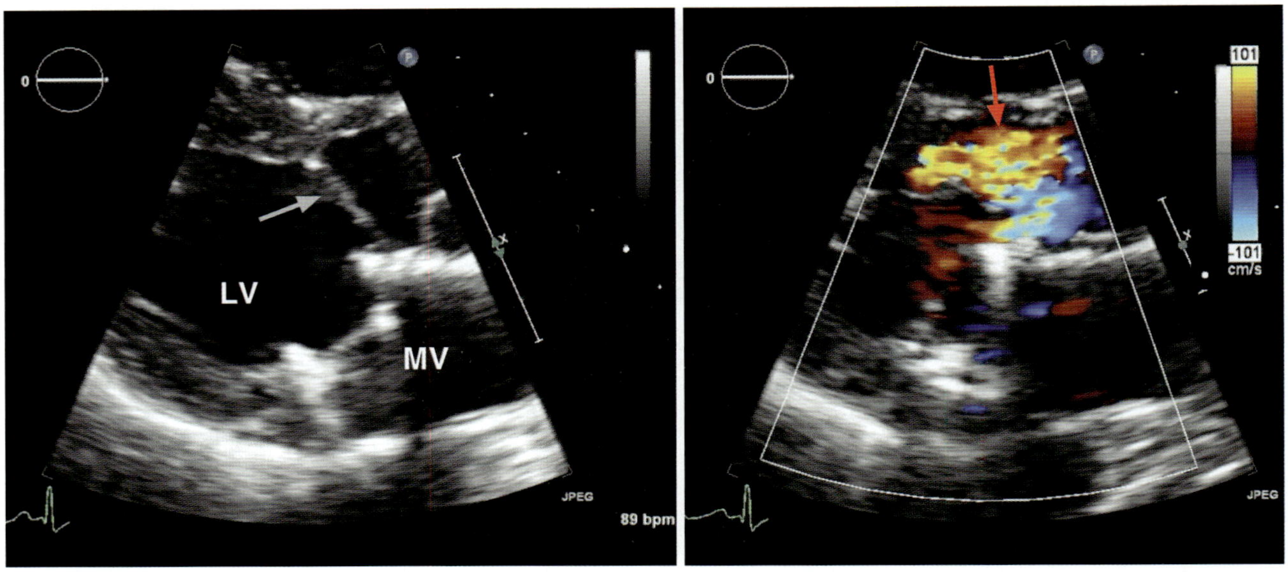

Fig 5.104 In left panel, transthoracic parasternal long-axis image shows mitral prosthesis, as well as obstruction of LVOT by residual native anterior mitral leaflet *(arrow)*. In right frame, there is flow acceleration in LVOT *(red arrow)*, even at aliasing velocity of 101 cm/sec.

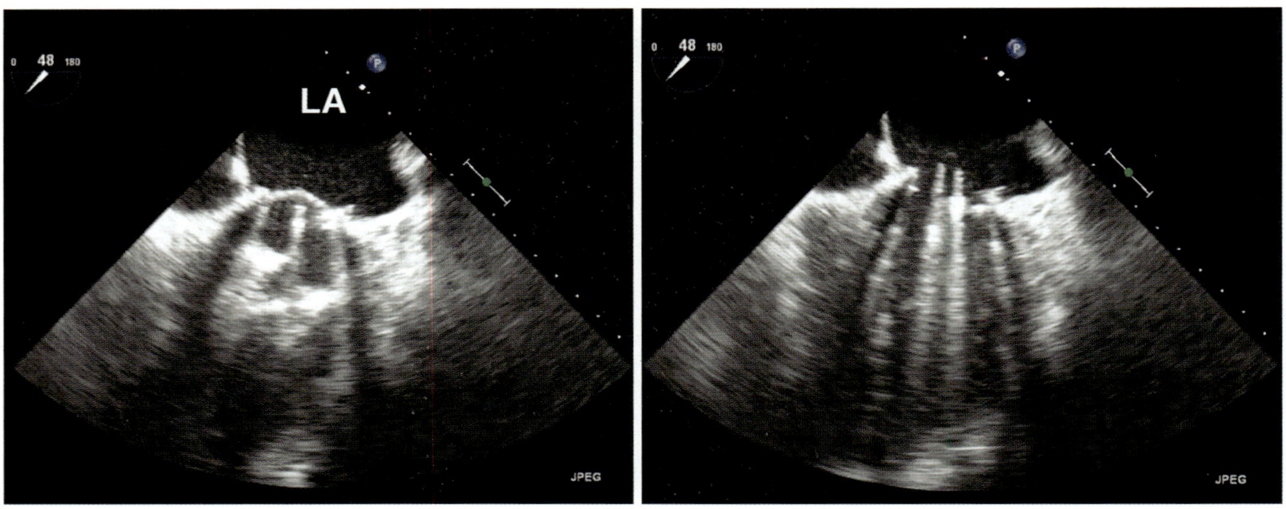

Fig 5.105 Midesophageal TEE shows normally functioning mitral prosthesis in systole *(left panel)* and diastole *(right panel)*.

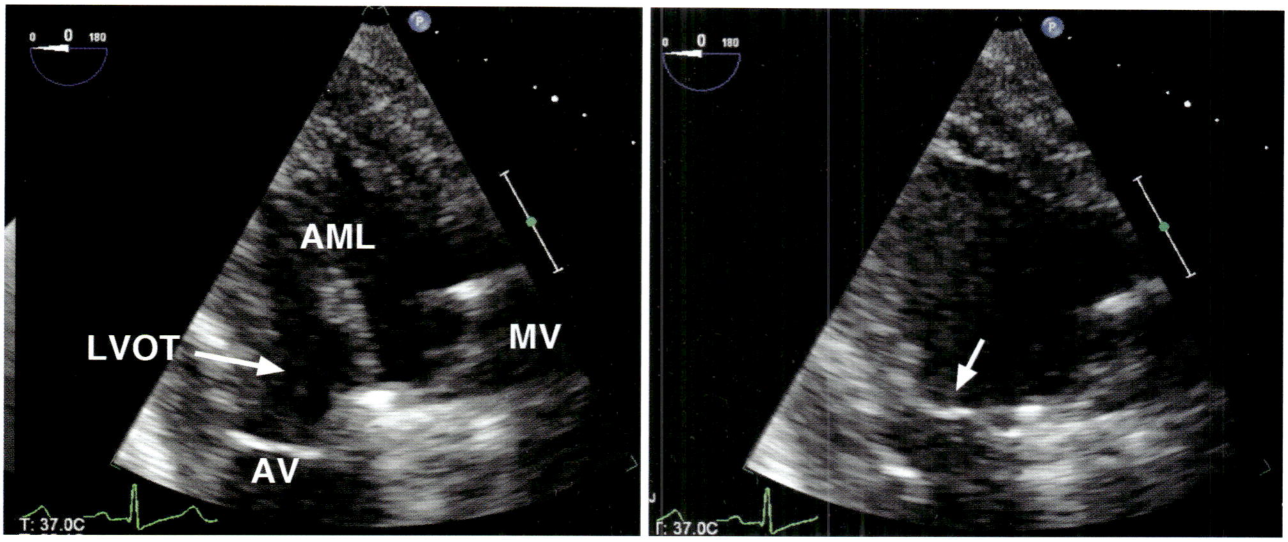

Fig 5.106 In this deep transgastric view, residual native AML is seen during diastole *(left panel),* which is displaced anteriorly during systole *(right panel)* causing LVOT obstruction. In real time, aortic valve is seen "fluttering" consistent with LVOT obstruction.

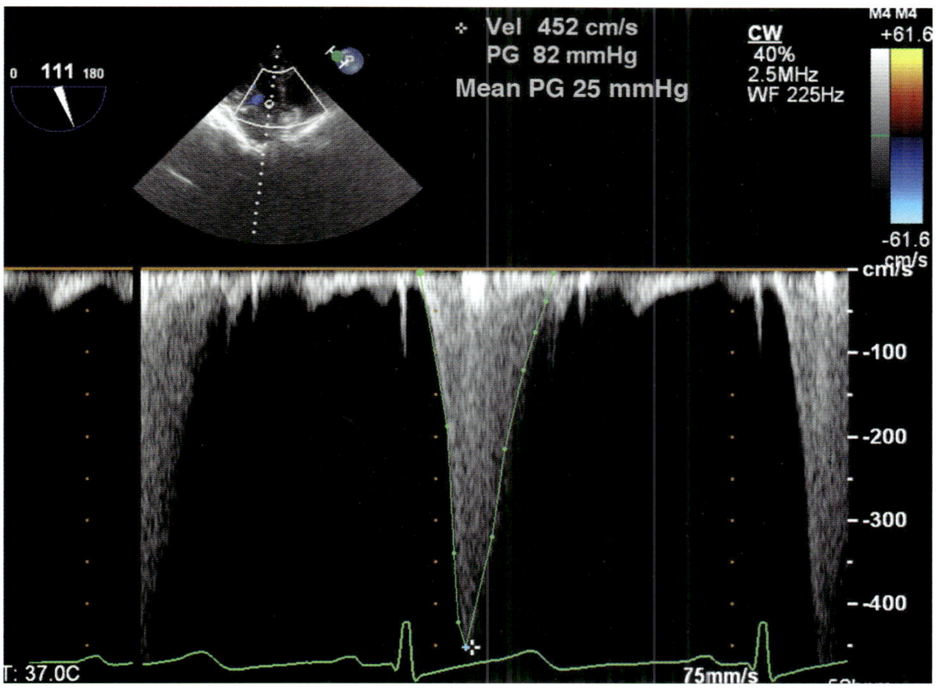

Fig 5.107 CW Doppler from deep transgastric window reveals typical "icepick pattern" of dynamic LVOT obstruction, with elevated peak and mean pressure gradients.

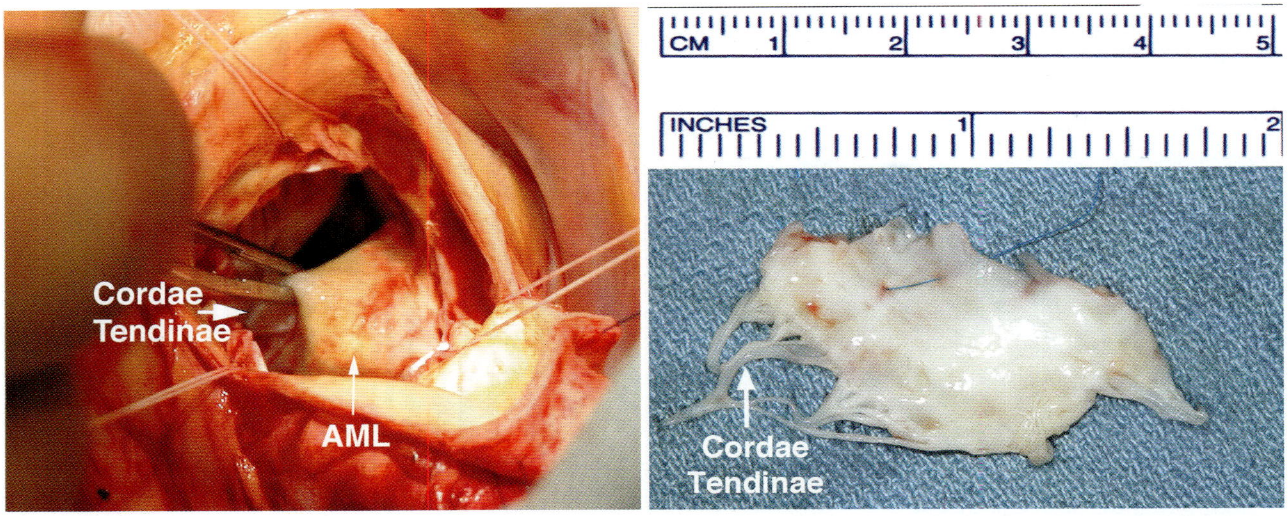

Fig 5.108 Mitral valve anatomy and surgical approach is illustrated in different patient undergoing aortic valve replacement. In this surgical view, native aortic valve has been excised, exposing anterior mitral leaflet (AML) *(left)*. In patient presented here, ascending aortotomy was performed, aortic leaflets spread open, and residual anterior mitral leaflet excised *(right)*. This avoided more complicated approach via left atrium.

Comments

Preservation of the continuity between the mitral annulus and papillary muscles helps maintain normal left ventricular systolic function after mitral valve surgery. When a valve repair is not possible, it is still preferable to preserve the native valve leaflets at the time of valve replacement. The posterior leaflet is easily retained, with a low likelihood of interference with mitral valve function. The anterior leaflet is often divided, with the two segments positioned so that they do not interfere with mechanical valve function. In this case it is likely that the preserved native anterior leaflet was not obstructing the LV outflow tract initially but that the leaflet became more redundant over time, resulting in systolic anterior motion and subaortic obstruction. More typically, this complication presents at the time of the initial surgery with postoperative hypotension and difficulty weaning from cardiopulmonary bypass. This complication is recognized on echocardiography by the presence of an increased velocity in the subaortic region as illustrated here.

Suggested Reading

1. Matsuno Y, Mori Y, Umeda Y, Takiya H: Bioprosthetic mitral valve dysfunction due to native valve preserving procedure, Asian Cardiovasc Thorac Ann 24(3):276–279, 2016.

6 Right-Sided Valve Disease

TABLE 6-1
Best Views for Assessing Tricuspid Valve

ME four-chamber view	With probe anteflexed, septal leaflet will be seen adjacent to interventricular septum, and anterior leaflet adjacent to right ventricular free wall. Retroflexion will allow visualization of posterior leaflet adjacent to free wall.
ME RV inflow–outflow view	With transducer angle rotated to about 50–80 degrees, anterior leaflet and posterior leaflet are seen.
TG views	Transgastric short-axis view of tricuspid valve with all three leaflets can be seen with transducer angle rotated to approximately 0–30 degrees. Transgastric long-axis view at 90–120 degrees with probe rotated to patient's right shows anterior and posterior leaflets. Advancing and flexing probe allows visualization pulmonic in addition to tricuspid valves.
3D echocardiography	Obtain view of tricuspid valve from 0–30 degrees midesophageal, four-chamber view tilted so that the valve is centered in imaging plane, or transgastric view with anteflexion. Acquire using narrow-angle, single-beat mode. Guidelines indicate that TTE may be preferable to TEE for 3D of tricuspid valve.

TABLE 6-2
Best Views for Assessing Pulmonic Valve

ME RV inflow–outflow view	With transducer angle rotated to about 50–80 degrees from midesophageal four-chamber view, two leaflets of pulmonic valve are seen anterior to aortic valve.
High esophageal views	Image descending aorta in midesophageal longitudinal plane (approximately 70–110 degrees). Withdraw probe to level of aortic arch. Rotate probe clockwise to image pulmonic valve and RVOT. Rotating transducer position back to approximately 0 degrees, and adjustment of transducer depth and flexion allows pulmonary valve, main PA, and its bifurcation to be seen.
TG views	Transgastric long-axis view at 90–120 degrees with probe rotated to patient's right shows anterior and posterior leaflets of tricuspid valve. Advancing and flexing probe allows visualization of pulmonic in addition to tricuspid valves.
3D echocardiography	Obtain view of pulmonic valve from either 90-degree, high-esophageal, or 120-degree, midesophageal three-chamber view rotated to center pulmonic valve. Acquire using narrow-angle, single-beat mode. Guidelines indicate that TTE may be preferable to TEE for 3D of pulmonic valve.

Normal Tricuspid and Pulmonic Valves

CASE 6-1
Normal Tricuspid and Pulmonic Valves

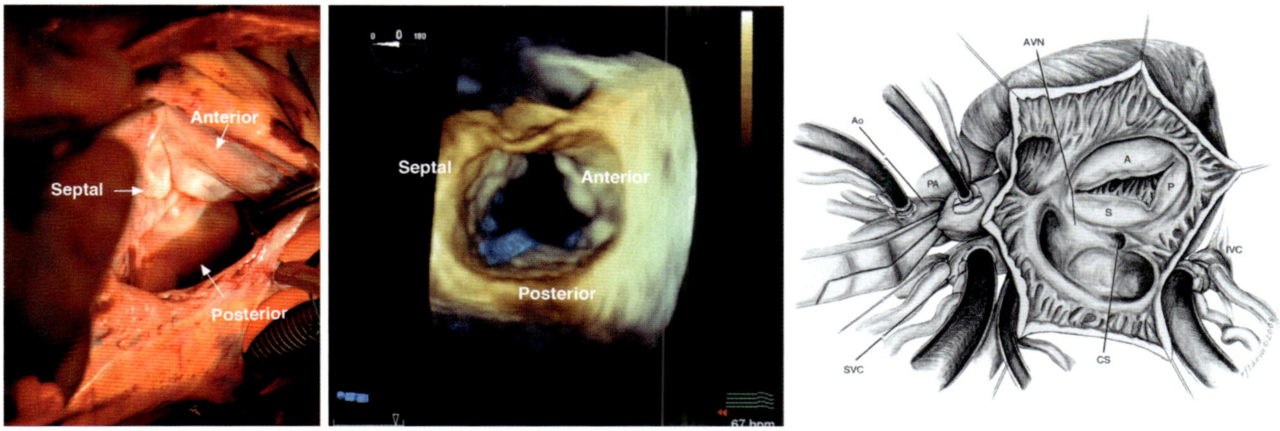

Fig 6.1 Left panel shows three leaflets of tricuspid valve at time of surgery, with normal leaflets appearing thin, smooth, and with complete coaptation in systole. In the center panel, the corresponding 3D TEE image is seen from right atrial aspect. Video clip shows both right atrial *(left)* and right ventricular *(right)* aspects of valve. Right panel shows exposure of tricuspid valve after right atriotomy. Approximate position of AVN is displayed. It is susceptible to injury during procedures on tricuspid valve. (Reproduced with permission from Elsevier Limited, Kidlington, Oxford, UK.) Ao = aorta; CS = coronary sinus; IVC = inferior vena cava; PA = pulmonary artery; AVN = atrio-ventricular node; S, A, P = septal, anterior, and posterior leaflets of tricuspid valve; SVC = superior vena cava. (Right panel used with permission of Elsevier.)

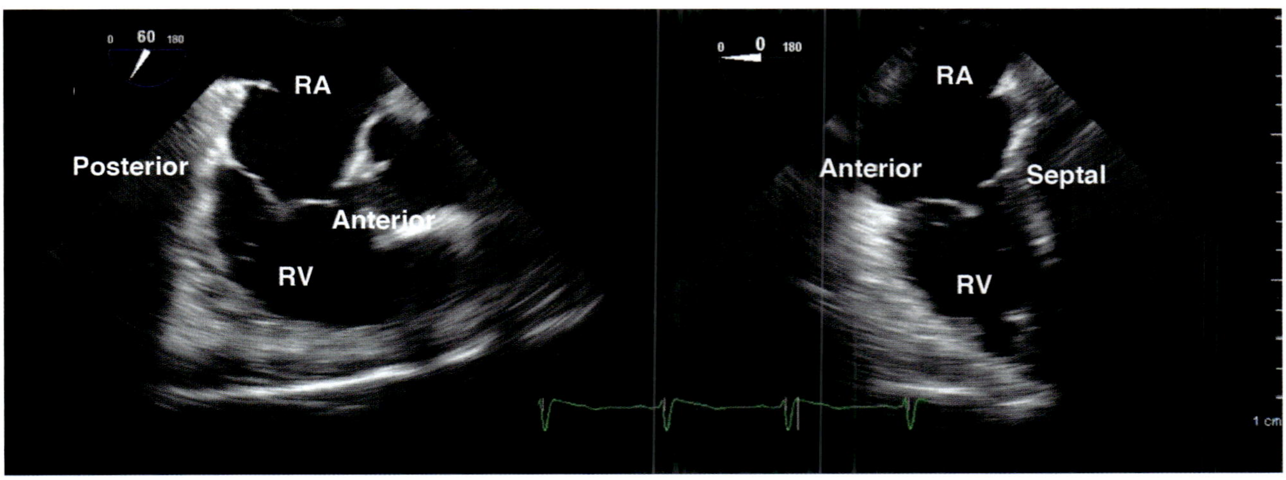

Fig 6.2 With probe in midesophageal position and anteflexed, four-chamber view *(right panel)* shows anterior and septal leaflets. At 60 degrees, anterior and posterior leaflets are seen.

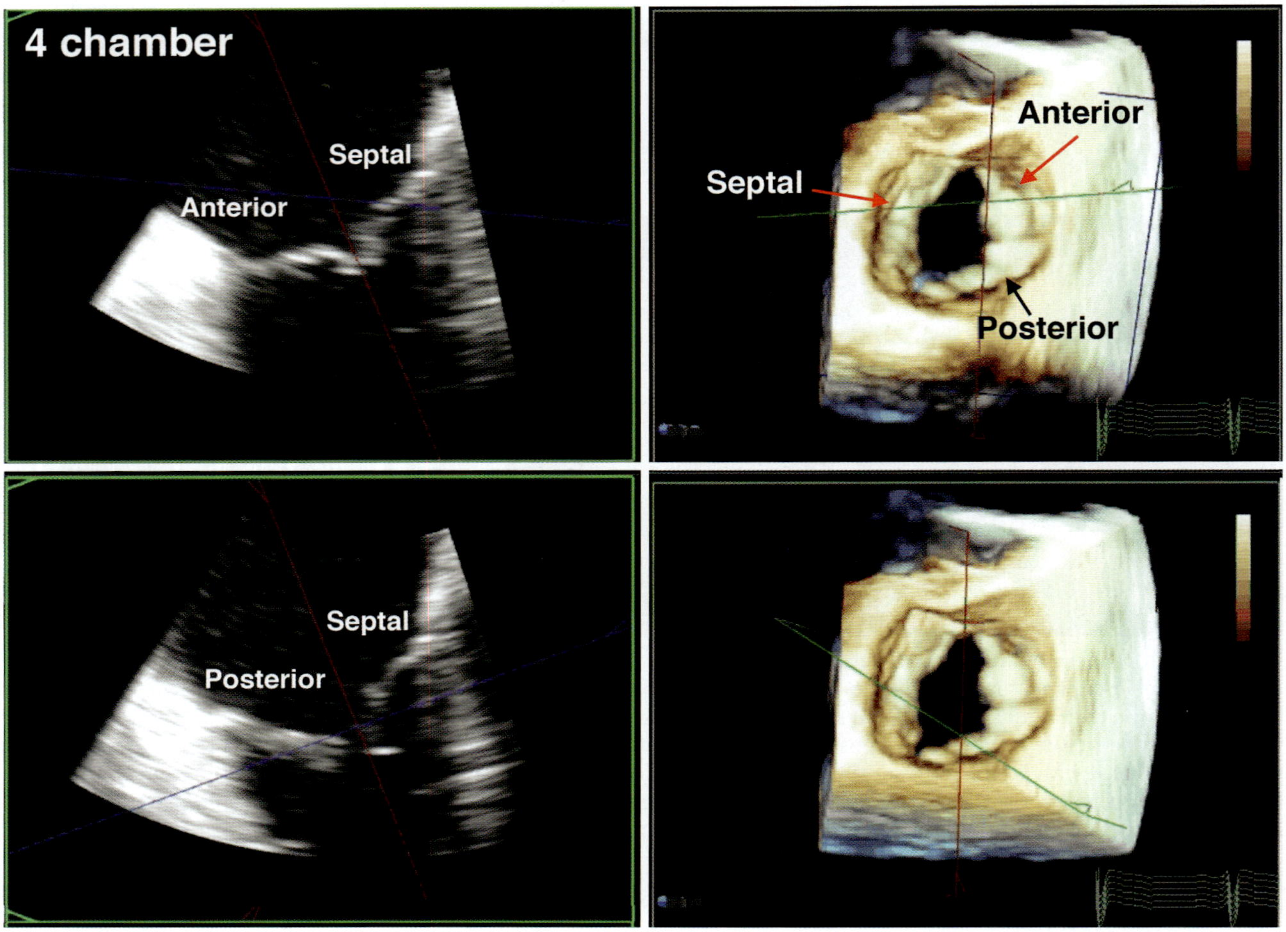

Fig 6.3 The use of 3D echocardiography allows definitive identification of the tricuspid leaflets. In two top panels, with probe anteflexed, green plane is seen to intersect anterior and septal leaflets; in bottom two panels, with probe retroflexed, green plane is seen to intersect posterior and septal leaflets.

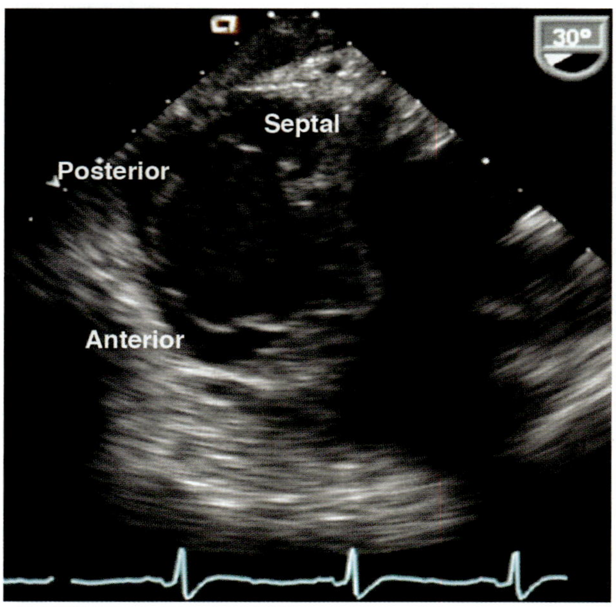

Fig 6.4 From transgastric position, tricuspid valve is imaged in short axis at 30 degrees, demonstrating all three leaflets.

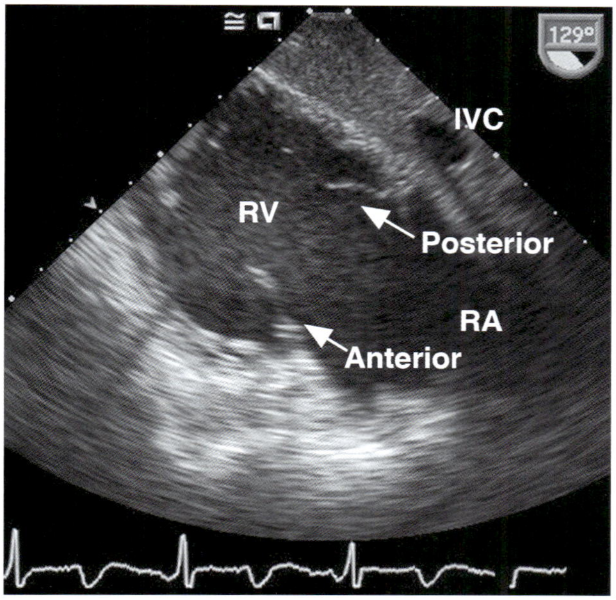

Fig 6.5 From transgastric view, right ventricular inflow view is obtained by starting in short-axis view of left ventricle, rotating image plane to about 120 degrees, and turning transducer slightly to patient's right. Posterior and anterior tricuspid valve leaflets are seen. Proximal outflow tract is also frequently seen and slight advancement of probe may allow imaging and Doppler interrogation of pulmonic valve.

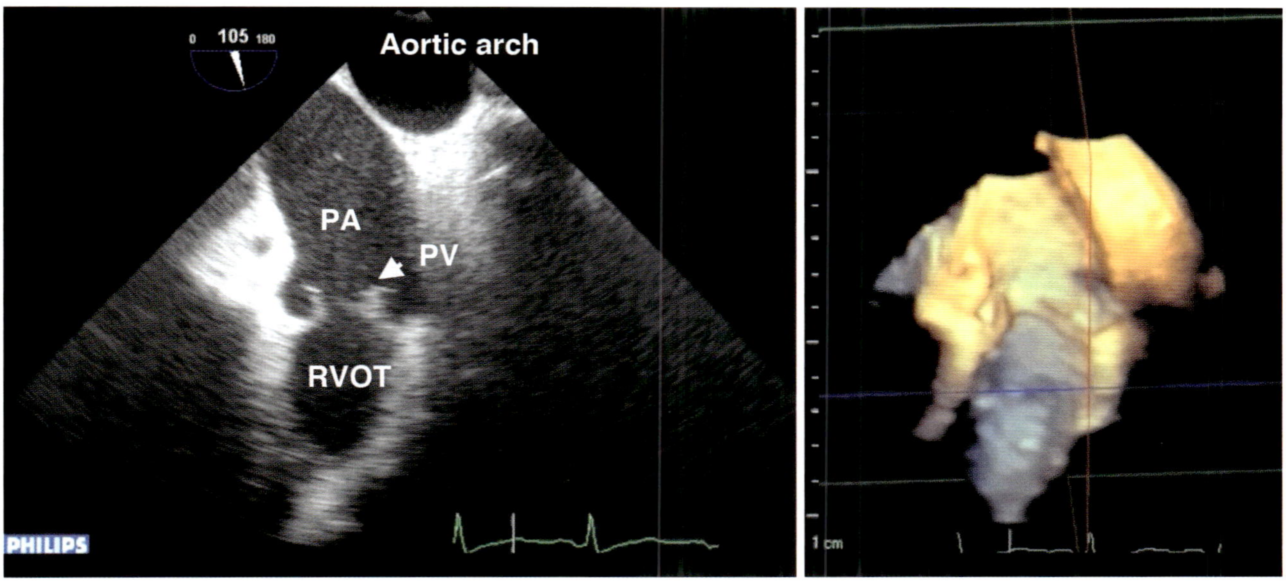

Fig 6.6 This view of pulmonic valve and right ventricular outflow tract *(left panel)* was acquired from very high esophageal position. In right panel, comparable 3D image is seen.

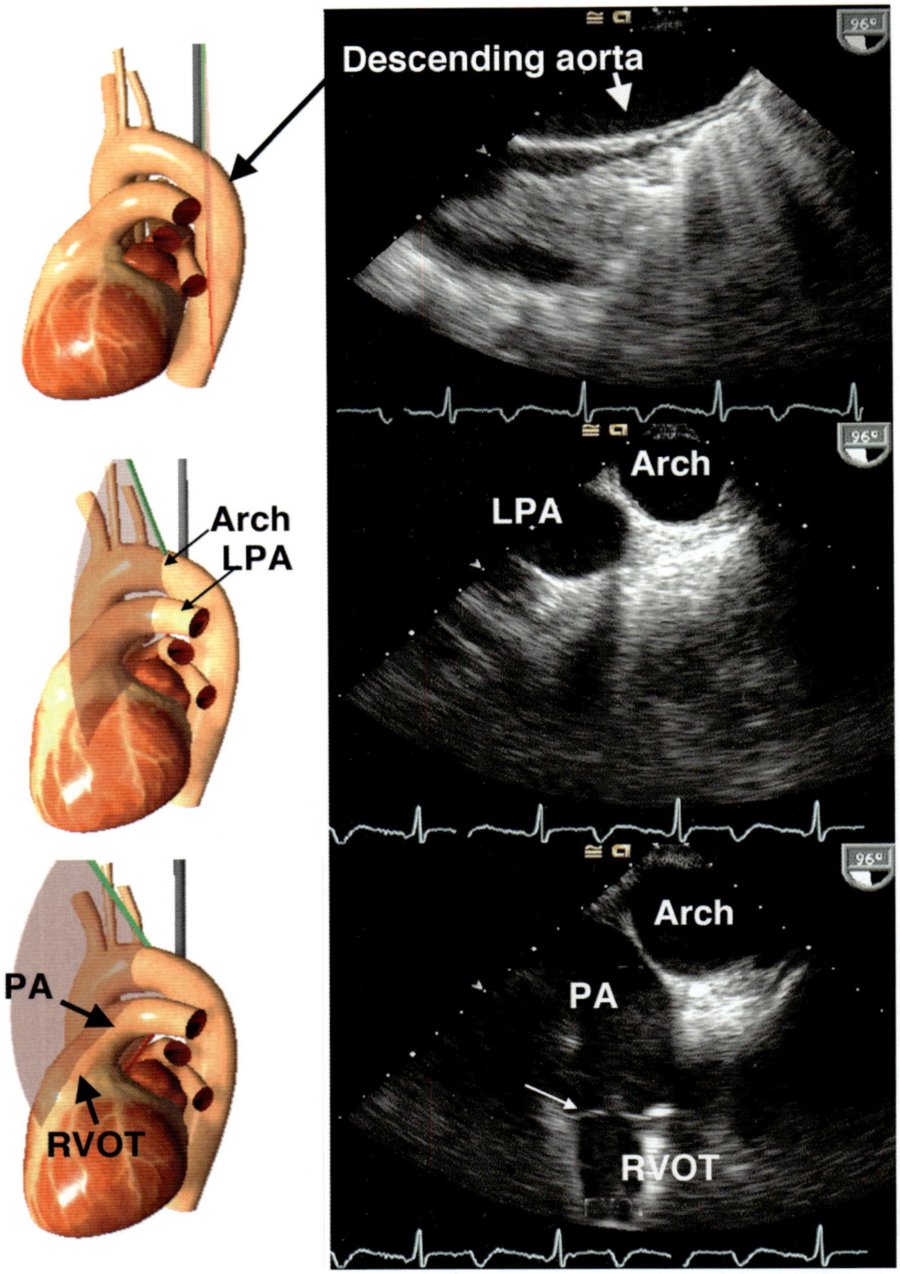

Fig 6.7 Steps to image pulmonic valve and RV outflow tract from high esophageal position. *1.* Image descending aorta in long axis, then slowly withdraw probe making small rotational adjustments to keep aorta centered. *2.* As arch is approached it will be imaged in short axis. Begin rotating probe to patient's right. Left pulmonary artery will come into view. *3.* Continue rotating probe until main pulmonary artery, pulmonic valve *(arrow),* and RV outflow tract come into view. (3D animation was reproduced with permission from TEE Simulation on Virtual TEE website at http://pie.med.utoronto.ca/TEE.)

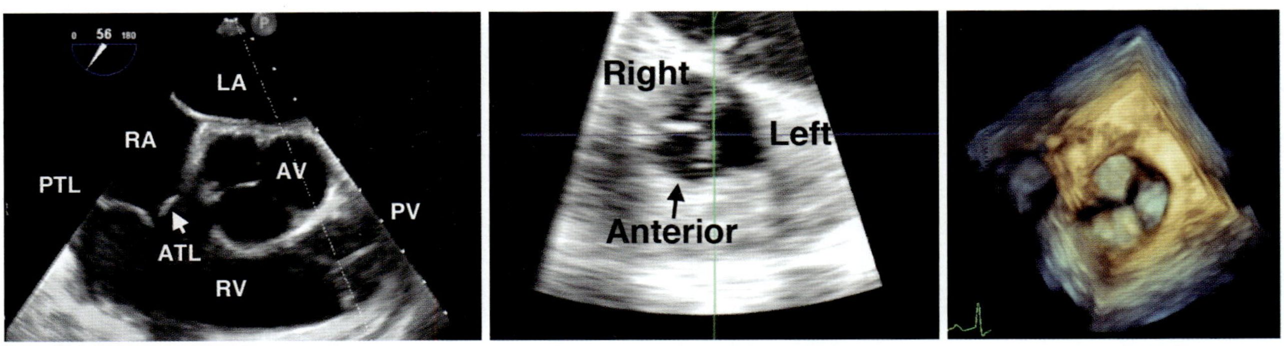

Fig 6.8 In left panel at midesophageal position, image plane is rotated to about 50 to 80 degrees from four-chamber view to obtain "inflow–outflow" view of RV. Orthogonal view of pulmonic valve in middle panel shows three leaflets of pulmonic valve. Right panel shows comparable 3D image.

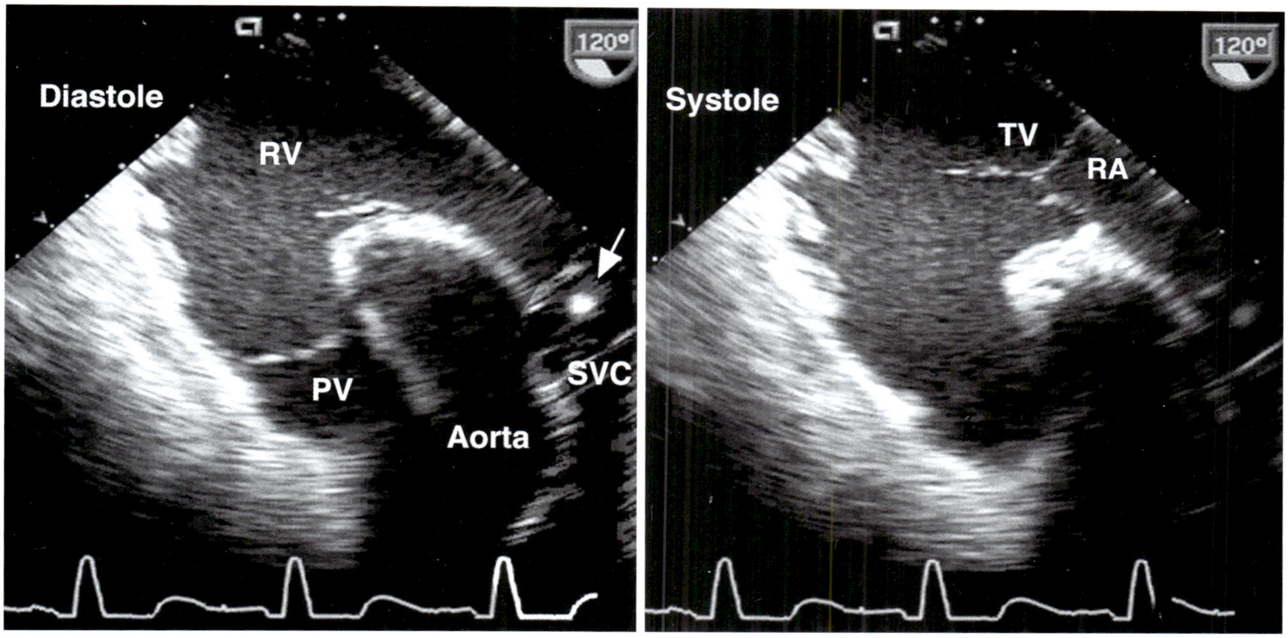

Fig 6.9 By moving transducer to position just on gastric side of gastroesophageal junction, view of both tricuspid and pulmonic valves (shown in diastole on *left* and in systole on *right*) can be obtained. Note that this image plane is same as shown in Fig 6.8, rotated 90 degrees counterclockwise, due to different position of transducer in transgastric compared with midesophageal position. Arrow points to central venous catheter in superior vena cava.

Comments

The tricuspid valve is routinely evaluated on TEE in at least two views. Most often the four-chamber view and short-axis ("inflow–outflow") view are used, with 2D imaging of leaflet thickness and mobility and annulus size with color Doppler evaluation of regurgitation. When regurgitation is present, severity is evaluated based on the vena contracta width. In addition, velocity is recorded using continuous wave Doppler, although velocity may be underestimated, as it is not always possible to obtain parallel intercept angle between the ultrasound beam and direction of the tricuspid regurgitant jet on TEE examination. Additional views of the tricuspid valve are typically obtained only if initial images are abnormal or if there is clinical concern for tricuspid valve involvement, such as a patient with suspected endocarditis. 3D imaging, either on TEE or TTE imaging, may be helpful in assuring correct identification of the three valve leaflets (Fig 6.3).

The pulmonic valve is routinely evaluated in long-axis view from the midesophageal inflow–outflow view (Fig 6.8). When indicated, the pulmonic valve and RV outflow tract may be imaged from the high esophageal position (Fig 6.7) or the transgastric position (Fig 6.9).

Rheumatic Heart Disease

CASE 6-2
Rheumatic Mixed Tricuspid Disease Associated with Mitral Stenosis

This 36-year-old woman had long history of valvular heart disease secondary to rheumatic fever. She had suffered a stroke 15 years before admission, thought to be embolic in nature, and was started on warfarin. She now presented with increasing fatigue and shortness of breath, and clinical evidence of congestive heart failure.

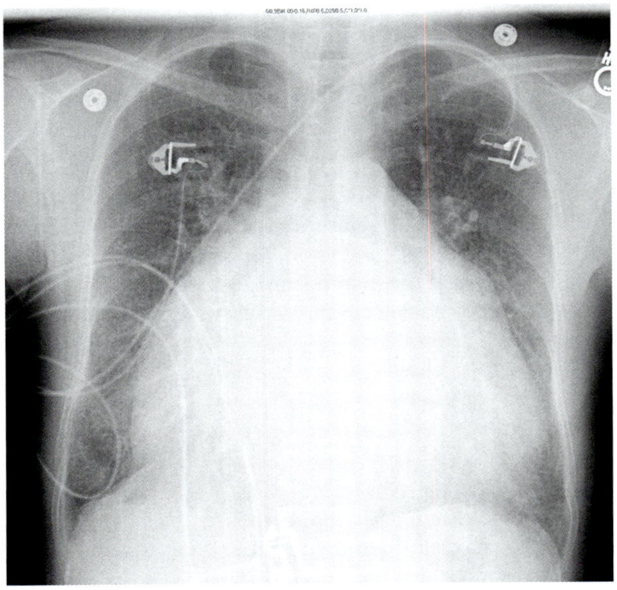

Fig 6.10 Chest radiography revealed global cardiomegaly and central pulmonary congestion.

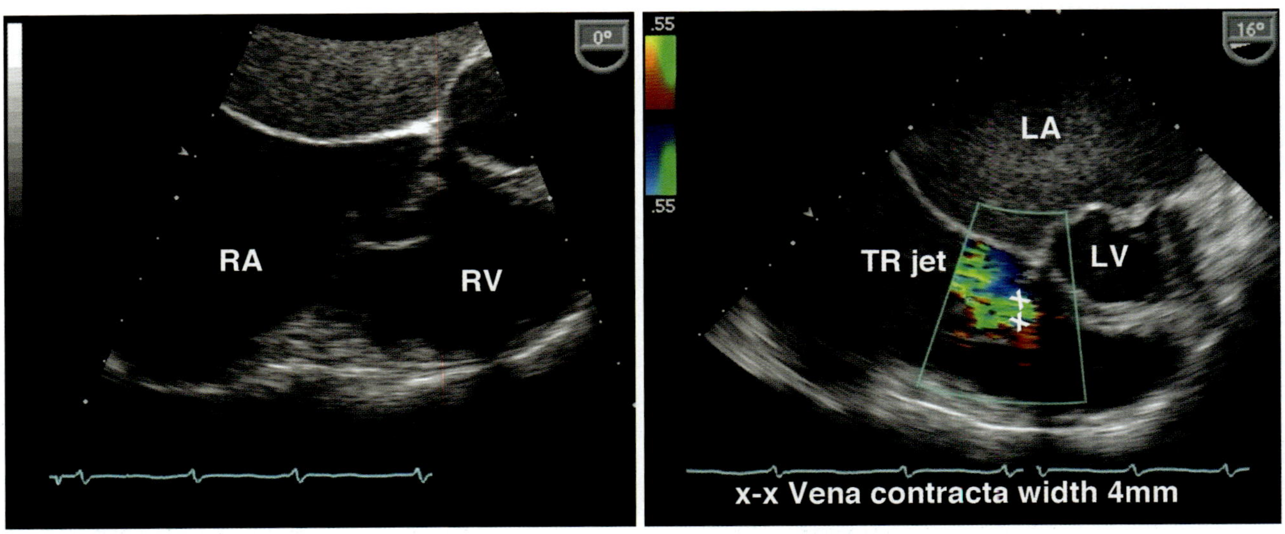

Fig 6.11 In TEE four-chamber plane at 0-degree rotation, zoom image of tricuspid valve in systole reveals significant leaflet thickening. Color Doppler flow imaging demonstrates moderate tricuspid regurgitation with vena contracta width of 4 mm. There is coexistent mitral stenosis, with spontaneous contrast visible in enlarged left atrium.

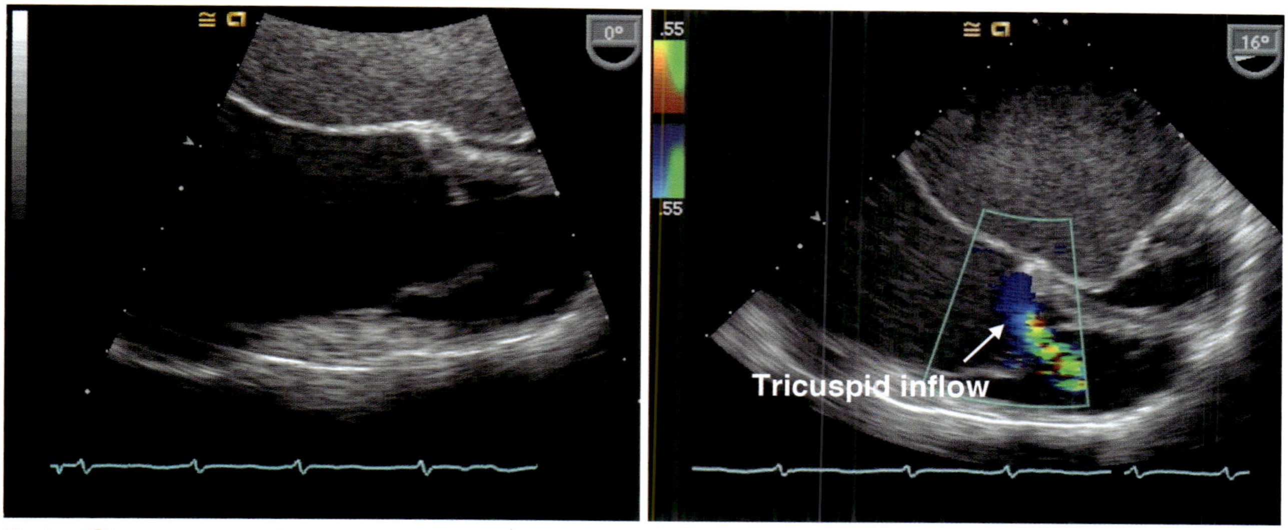

Fig 6.12 In same image plane as Fig 6.11, diastolic image shows doming of tricuspid leaflets, consistent with rheumatic disease, with narrow antegrade flow stream suggesting tricuspid stenosis.

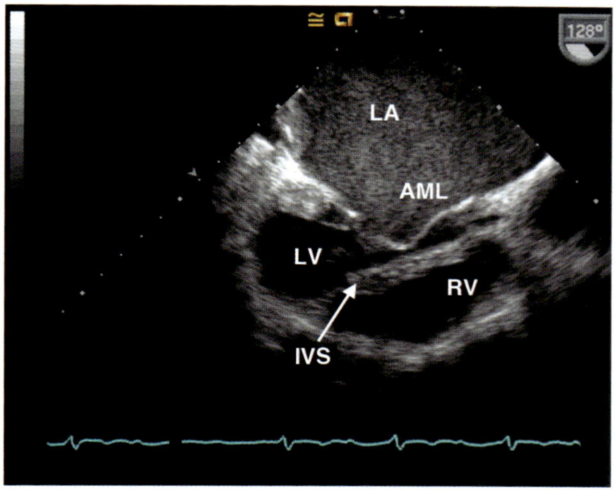

Fig 6.13 With probe now rotated to 120 degrees, diastolic doming (sometimes called "hockey stick shape") of anterior mitral leaflet is typical for rheumatic valve disease. Interventricular septum bows toward LV during systole and diastole so that LV appears "D"-shaped in short-axis view (see video), characteristic of RV pressure overload.

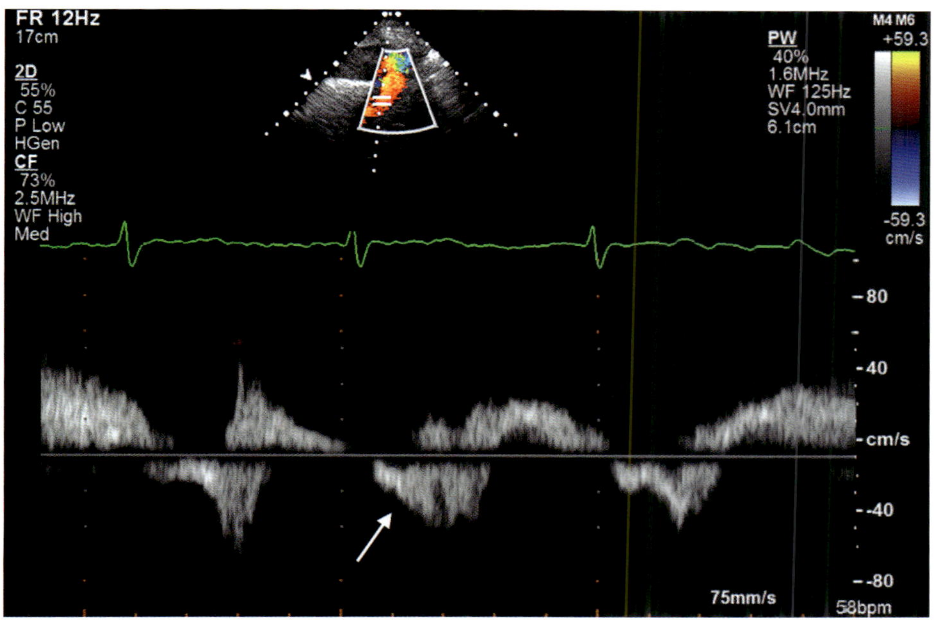

Fig 6.14 With probe now advanced to transgastric position and rotated to 70 degrees, pulsed wave Doppler of hepatic vein demonstrates systolic flow reversal *(arrow)*, which is typical of severe tricuspid regurgitation. However, this finding is only specific for severe tricuspid regurgitation when normal sinus rhythm is present. In this patient, there is no P wave on ECG or a-velocity on Doppler because patient is in atrial fibrillation. Thus this finding is consistent with other findings suggesting moderate tricuspid regurgitation.

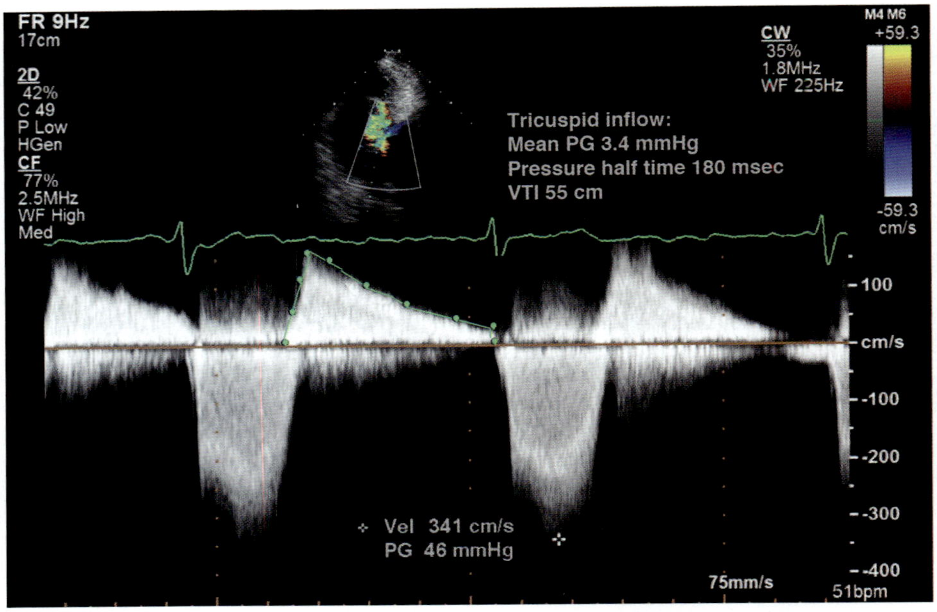

Fig 6.15 From apical transgastric transducer position, continuous-wave Doppler of tricuspid inflow demonstrates mean gradient of 3.4 mm Hg, and pressure half-time of 180 msec, consistent with mild tricuspid stenosis. Density of systolic signal of tricuspid regurgitation is less dense than antegrade flow, consistent with moderate tricuspid regurgitation. Velocity of tricuspid regurgitation jet is 3.4 m/sec, consistent with RV to RA peak systolic gradient of 46 mm Hg. Added to central venous pressure of 15 mm Hg yields estimated RV systolic pressure of 61 mm Hg.

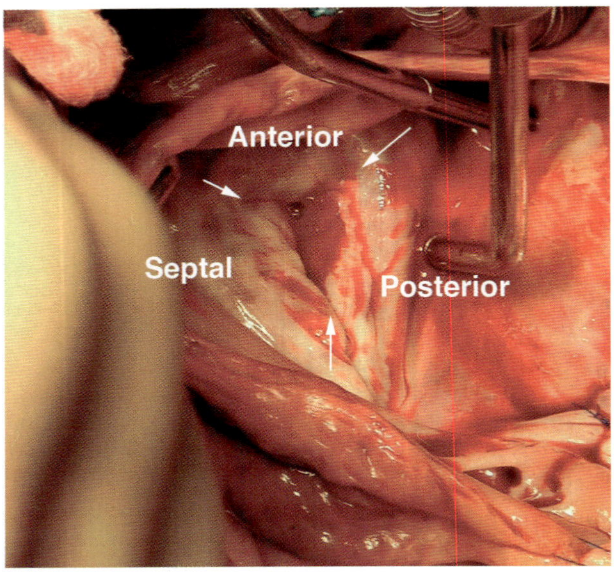

Fig 6.16 At surgery, three leaflets of tricuspid valve are seen; they are all severely thickened, with fusion of all three commissures *(arrows)*, which is pathognomonic for rheumatic valve disease.

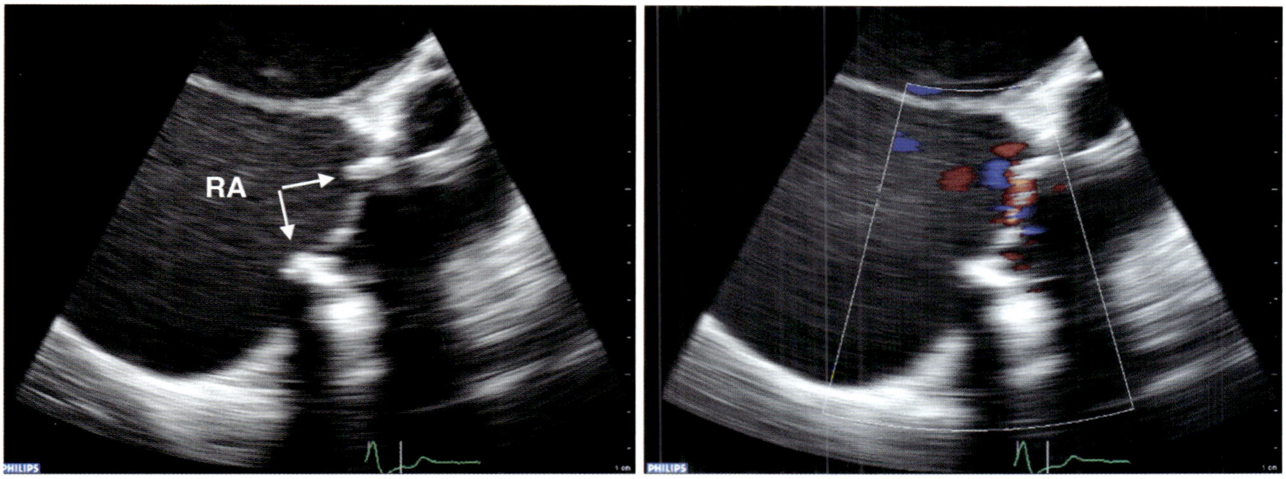

Fig 6.17 Postoperatively in four-chamber view, two posts of prosthetic tricuspid valve are seen *(arrows)*. In right frame, color Doppler shows only mild tricuspid regurgitation.

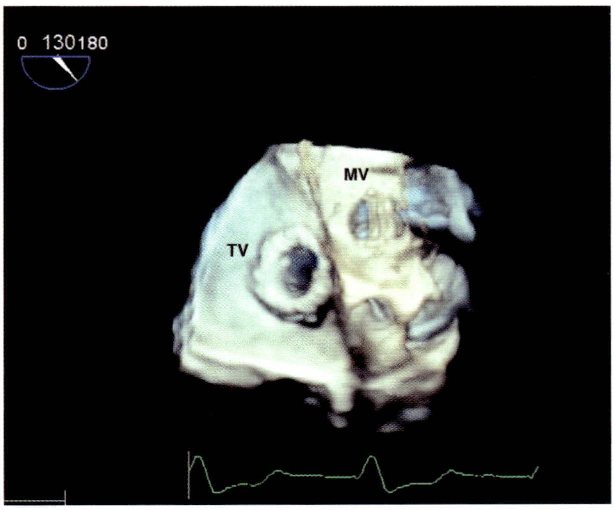

Fig 6.18 From the atrial perspective, 3D TEE allows enface visualization of tissue tricuspid prosthesis, as well as bileaflet mechanical prosthesis in mitral position.

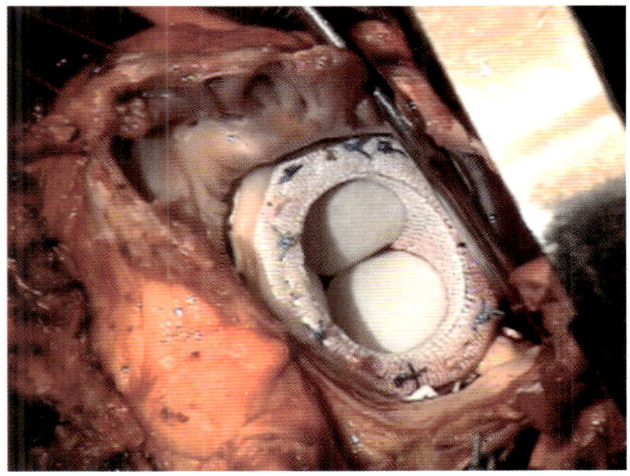

Fig 6.19 Surgical view with right atrium still open shows trileaflet tissue prosthesis in tricuspid valve position.

Comments

The tricuspid valve is affected by the rheumatic process in about 5% to 10% of patients with rheumatic mitral valve disease. Rheumatic involvement of the tricuspid valve results in leaflet thickening, commissural fusion, and fusion and shortening of the chords, although findings are often subtle compared with the mitral valve. Rheumatic involvement of the tricuspid valve can cause stenosis, due to commissural fusion, or regurgitation, due to chordal shortening and fusion, but severe stenosis is uncommon. Most often, there is a combination of stenosis and regurgitation, which may result in symptoms even when either lesion, in isolation, might not be considered severe. With left-sided rheumatic mitral valve disease, intervention for tricuspid involvement or severe annular dilation is recommended with any degree of valve dysfunction because progressive tricuspid disease often occurs late after surgery for rheumatic mitral valve disease.

Suggested Reading

1. Lin G, Bruce CJ, Connolly HM: Diseases of the tricuspid and pulmonic valves. In Otto CM, Bonow RO, editors: Valvular heart disease, ed 4, Philadelphia, 2014, Elsevier, pp 375–395.

CASE 6-3
Rheumatic Tricuspid Regurgitation in Patient with Bioprosthetic Aortic Valve

A 28-year-old man presented with 2-month history of increasing dyspnea on exertion and leg edema. Past medical history was notable for bioprosthetic aortic valve replacement 10 years previously for severe symptomatic aortic regurgitation. Echocardiography revealed prosthetic aortic valve stenosis and regurgitation, as well as anatomic changes consistent with rheumatic mitral and tricuspid valve disease with mixed stenosis/regurgitation of both atrioventricular valves. There was severe LV dilation with normal systolic function.

Right heart catheterization revealed an RA mean pressure 8 mm Hg, RV pressure of 46/6 mm Hg, PA pressure of 46/23 mm Hg with mean of 30 mm Hg, wedge pressure of 17 mm Hg, transpulmonary gradient of 13 mm Hg, pulmonary vascular resistance (Fick) of 4.5 wood units, and systemic vascular resistance (Fick) of 1384 dsc-5.

Surgical intervention was recommended for symptomatic prosthetic valve dysfunction and concurrent rheumatic mitral valve disease. After mitral and aortic valve replacements were performed, attention was turned to the tricuspid valve. An attempt at valve repair was unsuccessful so the tricuspid valve was replaced with bioprosthetic valve.

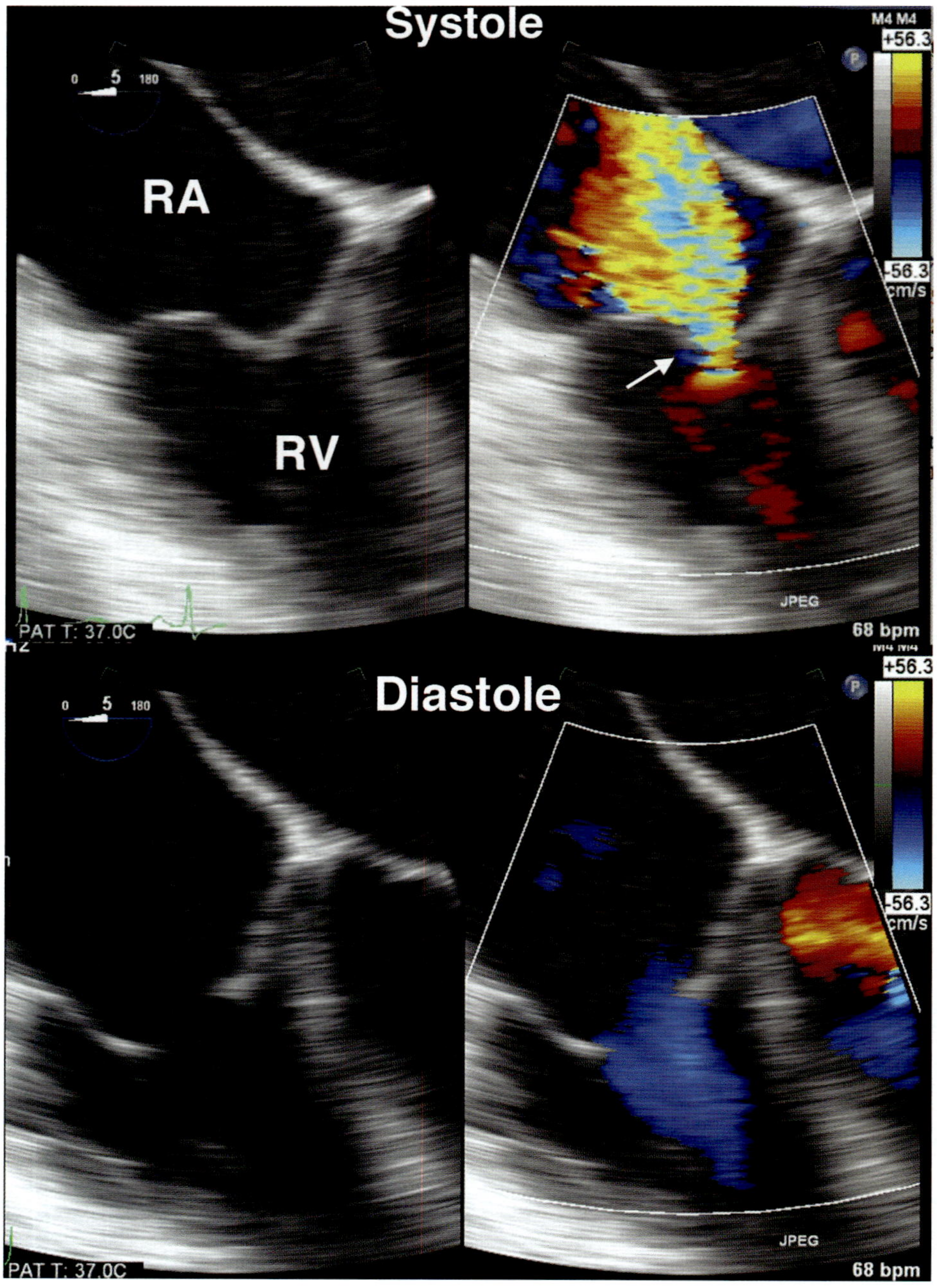

Fig 6.20 In midesophageal four-chamber view, two leaflets most likely visualized are septal and anterior, as probe is anteflexed. During systole jet of tricuspid regurgitation *(arrow)* is seen with vena contract width of 8 mm. During diastole, restricted leaflet motion with diastolic doming and relatively immobility of septal leaflet is seen.

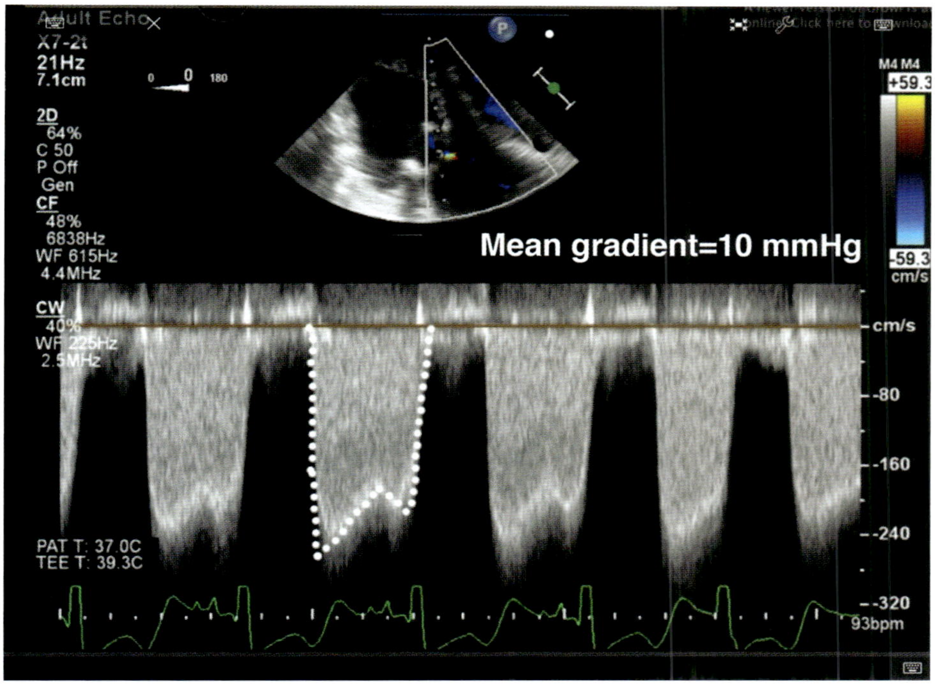

Fig 6.21 Continuous-wave Doppler shows diastolic mean gradient of 10 mm Hg, consistent with high transvalvular flow rate, most likely due to tricuspid regurgitation. Measurement of pressure half-time is challenging in this patient because short diastolic filling period (rapid heart rate) and superimposed atrial velocity obscure early diastolic deceleration slope. However, slope appears consistent with only mild to moderate tricuspid stenosis.

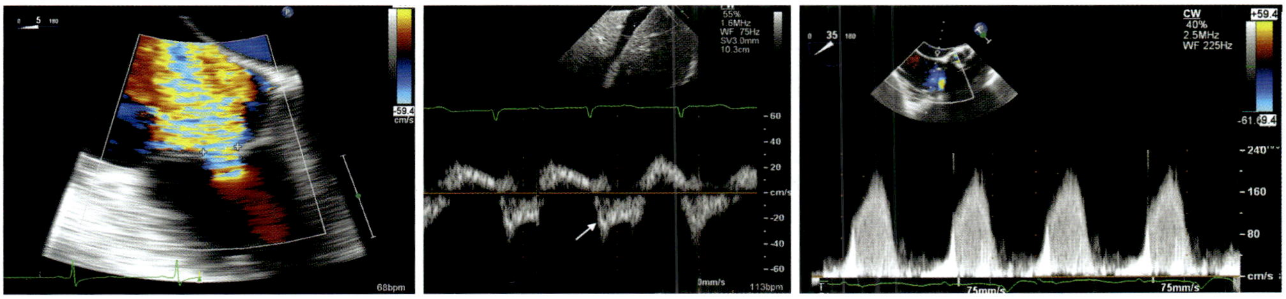

Fig 6.22 Vena contracta of tricuspid regurgitant jet is measured at 8 mm using zoom mode to show narrow neck between region of flow acceleration on RV size of valve and turbulence jet in RA. Holo-systolic flow reversal is present in hepatic vein *(arrow)*. Both vena contracta width >7 mm and systolic flow reversal in hepatic veins (with patient in sinus rhythm) are specific for severe TR. Continuous-wave Doppler of tricuspid regurgitant jet *(right)* shows dense, early peaking jet, also consistent with severe tricuspid regurgitation.

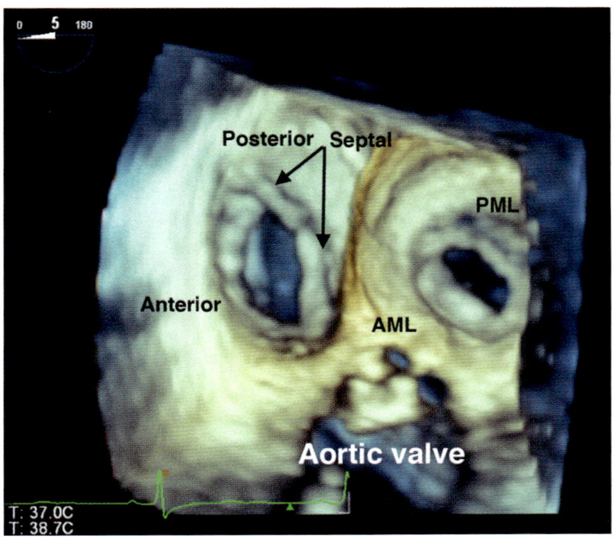

Fig 6.23 3D echocardiography from atrial perspective reveals typically appearing rheumatic mitral valve with thickening of both leaflets. Tricuspid valve leaflets are also thickened, and valve appears bileaflet due to fusion of septal and posterior leaflets. In real time, there is incomplete coaptation of tricuspid leaflets.

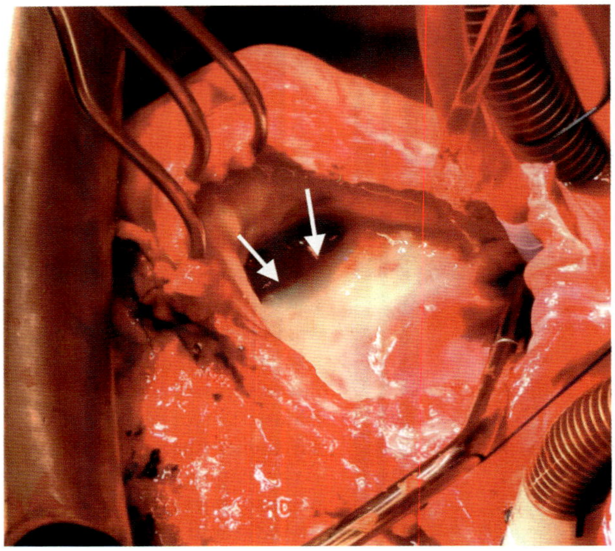

Fig 6.24 At time of right atriotomy, there is severe thickening of tricuspid apparatus. Arrows indicate fused posterior and septal leaflets.

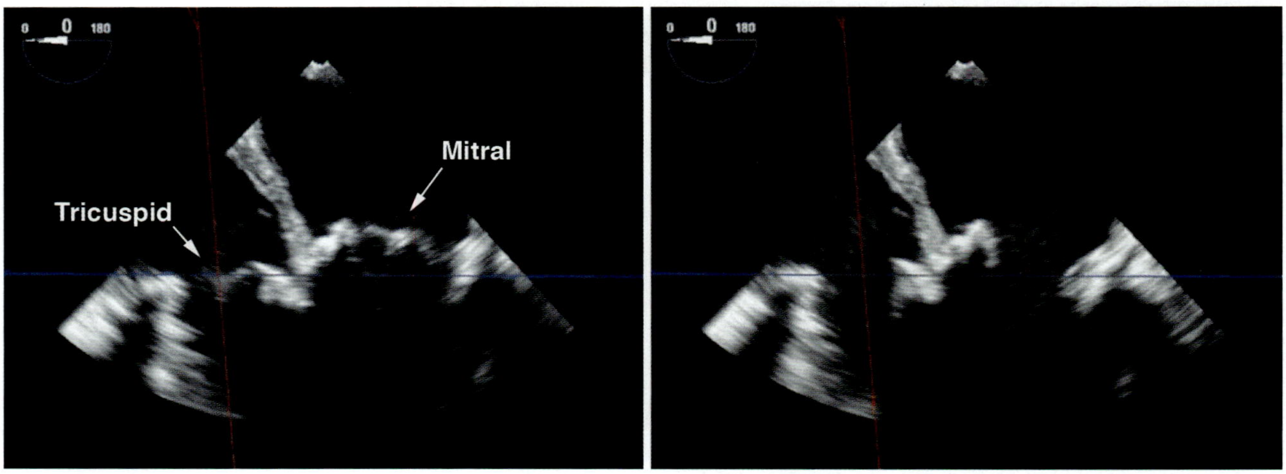

Fig 6.25 Postoperatively, tissue prostheses were placed in both tricuspid and mitral positions. In this four-chamber image, tissue valves are seen in systole *(left panel)* and diastole *(right panel).*

Comments

Most patients with rheumatic mitral stenosis have significant tricuspid regurgitation. The cause of tricuspid regurgitation may be rheumatic involvement of the tricuspid valve leaflets and chords but often the tricuspid leaflets are unaffected by rheumatic disease. Functional tricuspid regurgitation is present in about 80% of patients with rheumatic mitral stenosis and about 40% of those with severe rheumatic mitral regurgitation.

In these patients, chronic pulmonary hypertension secondary to mitral stenosis results in right ventricular and tricuspid annular dilation. With severe annular dilation, the normal tricuspid leaflets cannot completely close in systole, leading to tricuspid regurgitation. It is postulated that the additional right ventricular volume overload from tricuspid regurgitation leads to further right ventricular enlargement and progressive tricuspid regurgitation. In addition, there may be subtle rheumatic involvement of the tricuspid leaflets that may be better evaluated by 3D echocardiography.

Suggested Reading

1. Bruce CJ, Connolly HM: Right-sided valve disease in adults. In Otto CM, editor: The practice of clinical echocardiography, ed 5, Philadelphia, 2016, Elsevier.

Tricuspid Annuloplasty

CASE 6-4
Tricuspid Annuloplasty for Secondary Tricuspid Regurgitation

This 49-year-old man with prior mitral commissurotomy for rheumatic mitral valve disease presented with right-sided heart failure, atrial fibrillation, recurrent mitral stenosis, and severe tricuspid regurgitation. He was referred for mitral valve replacement, tricuspid annuloplasty, and radiofrequency ablation of atrial fibrillation.

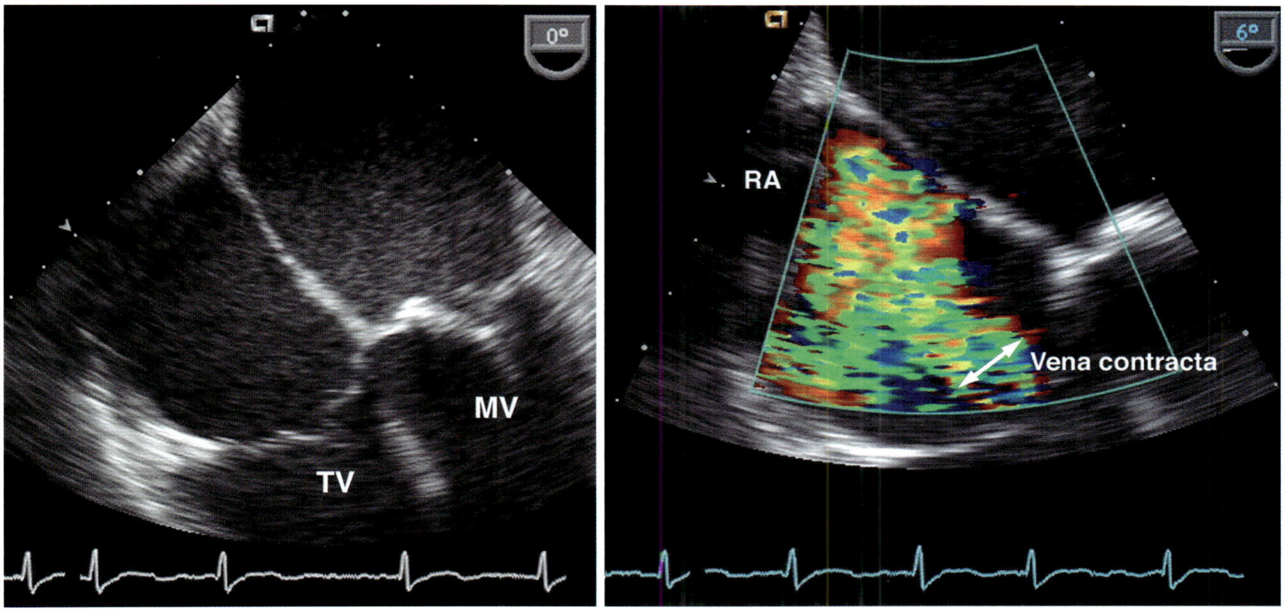

Fig 6.26 In four-chamber view, rheumatic mitral valve disease is seen but tricuspid leaflets appear thin with normal mobility. Tricuspid annulus is severely dilated. Central tricuspid regurgitation is demonstrated by color Doppler imaging.

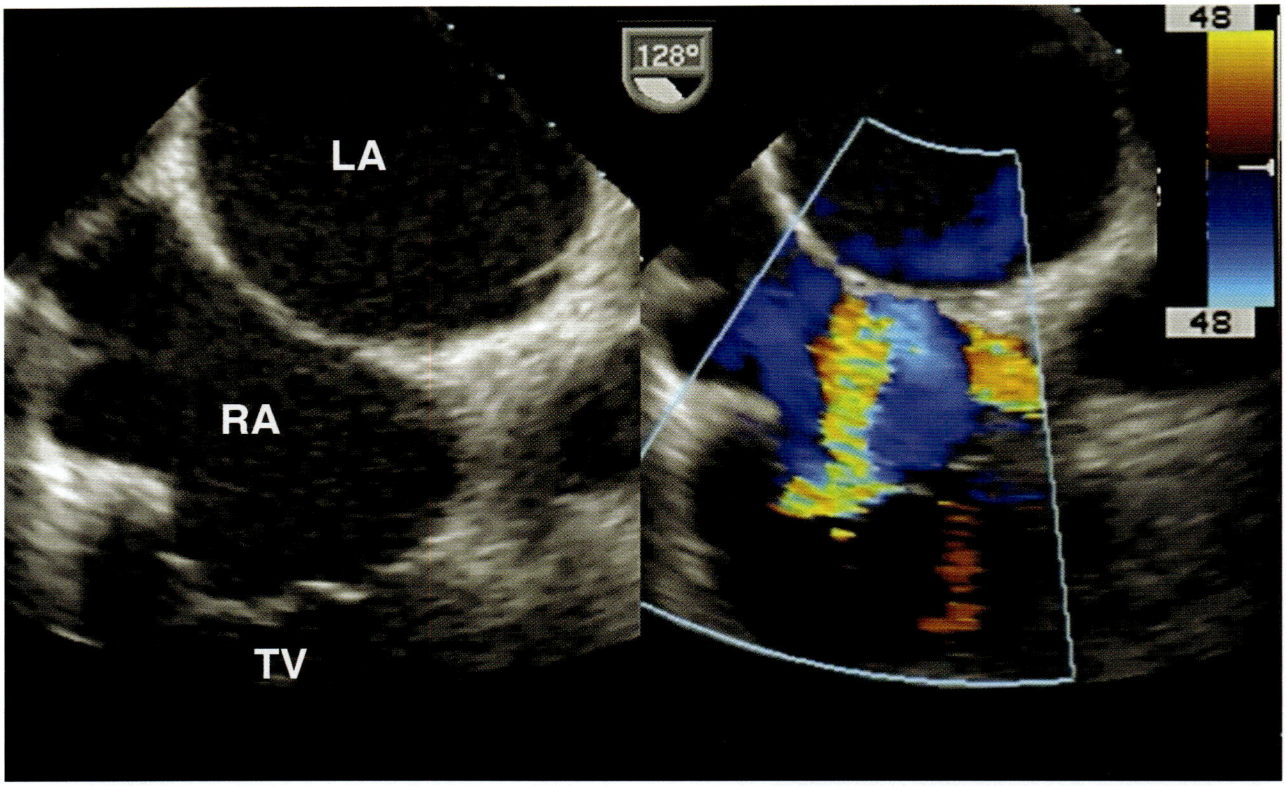

Fig 6.27 From bicaval view probe was rotated to patient's left, and color Doppler showed moderate jet of TR. RVSP was estimated at 51 mm Hg.

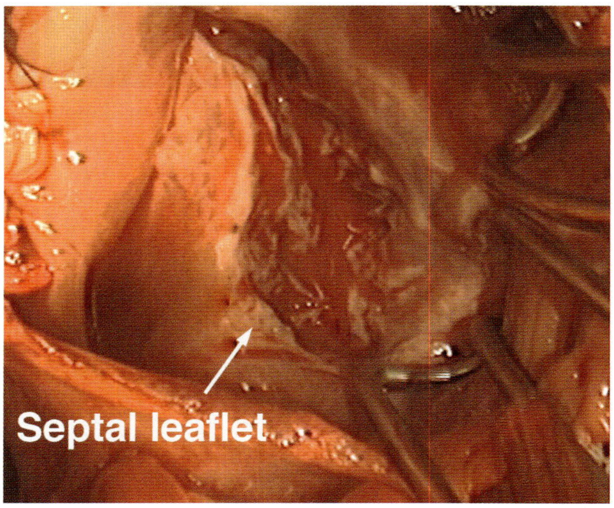

Fig 6.28 On direct inspection, tricuspid leaflets were normal in thickness, with no evidence of commissural fusion. However, annulus was dilated to 40 mm.

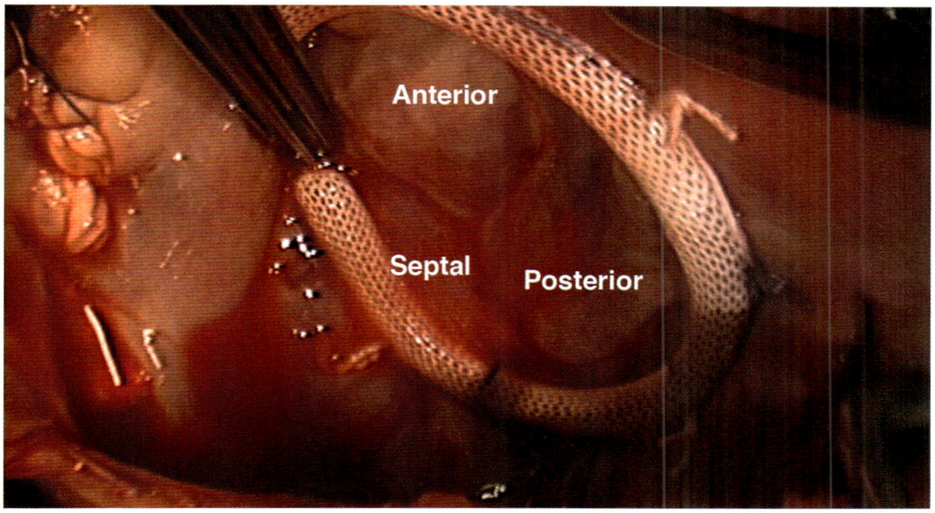

Fig 6.29 After replacing mitral valve, 32-mm tricuspid valve ring was placed. "C"-shaped ring is placed in such fashion to avoid suturing into A-V node.

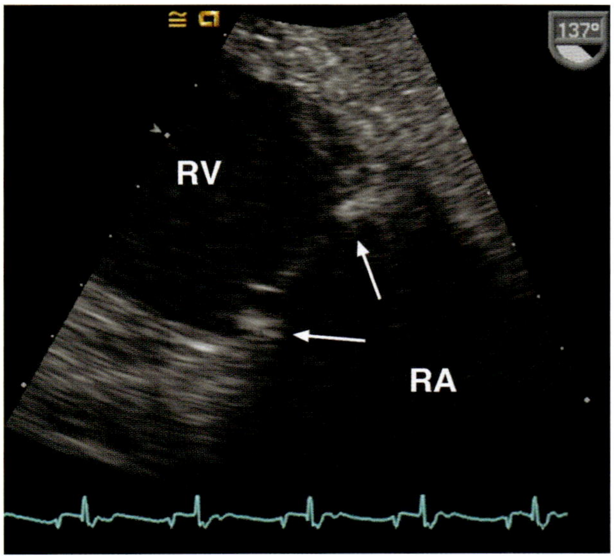

Fig 6.30 From transgastric long axis of TV, leaflets and annuloplasty ring *(arrows)* are seen.

Comments

Tricuspid valve repair or replacement is recommended in patients with severe symptomatic tricuspid regurgitation due to disease of the valve leaflets. In patients undergoing left-sided valve surgery, tricuspid valve surgery is recommended for both symptomatic and asymptomatic patients with severe functional tricuspid regurgitation. Even with only mild to moderate rheumatic tricuspid regurgitation, tricuspid valve repair is recommended at the time of left-sided valve surgery if there is significant tricuspid annular dilation (>40 mm on TTE or >70 mm on direct surgical inspection) or if there is significant pulmonary hypertension.

When tricuspid valve surgical intervention is necessary, tricuspid valve repair is preferable to valve replacement whenever possible. Tricuspid valve repair often includes placement of an annular ring to reduce the size of the annulus, which is particularly effective for treatment of functional tricuspid regurgitation when pulmonary hypertension and annular dilation are present. When valve replacement is needed, bioprosthetic valve is often chosen because of higher risk of thrombosis with right-sided mechanical valve prostheses.

Suggested Reading

1. Nishimura RA, Otto CM, Bonow RO, et al: ACC/AHA Task Force Members: 2014 AHA/ACC guideline for the management of patients with valvular heart disease: A report of the American College of Cardiology/American Heart Association Task Force on Practice Guidelines, Circulation 129(23):e521–e643, 2014.
2. Dreyfus GD, Martin RP, Chan KM, Dulguerov F, Alexandrescu C: Functional tricuspid regurgitation: A need to revise our understanding, JACC 65(21):2331–2336, 2015.

Ebstein's Anomaly

CASE 6-5
Ebstein's Anomaly

This 40-year-old female with Ebstein's anomaly of the tricuspid valve was referred for surgical intervention because of increasing shortness of breath in association with increasing tricuspid regurgitation.

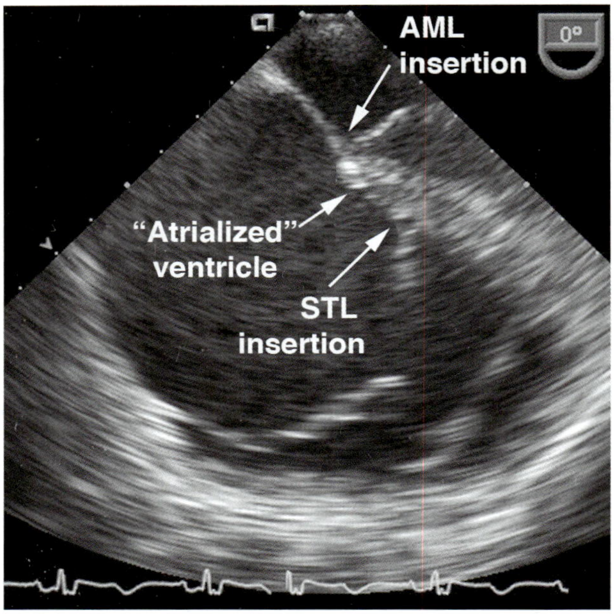

Fig 6.31 Four-chamber view shows apical displacement of septal leaflet of tricuspid valve (STL) compared with insertion point of anterior mitral valve leaflet (AML). Normal distance between mitral and tricuspid insertion points is less than 1 cm. Greater distance, as in this case, suggests Ebstein's anomaly. Right atrial and ventricular enlargement can also be appreciated in this view. Segment of right ventricular myocardium on atrial side of displaced tricuspid valve is considered "atrialized" because it exhibits ventricular electrical activity but is exposed to atrial pressures.

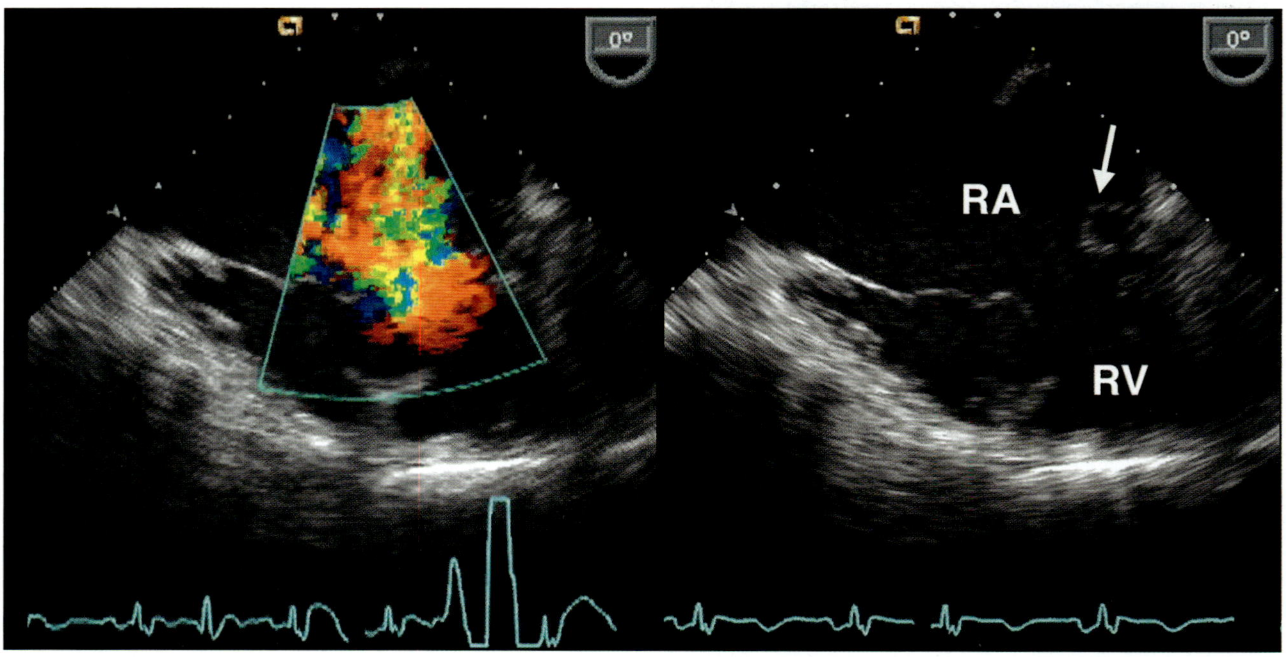

Fig 6.32 With probe advanced in esophagus and turned toward right, color flow Doppler shows severe tricuspid regurgitation with broad vena contracta, measuring 18 mm. The arrow indicates the septal leaflet.

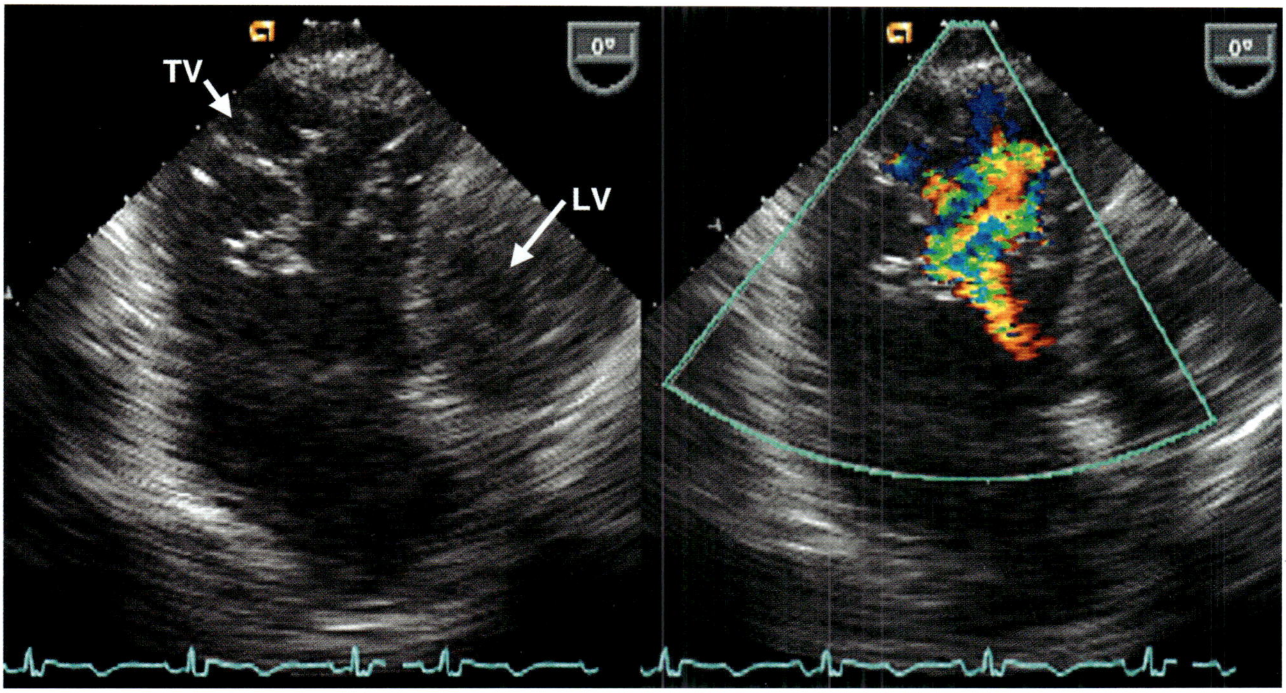

Fig 6.33 Transgastric short-axis view of tricuspid valve shows severe right-sided chamber enlargement in comparison to normal size of left ventricle. Color flow demonstrates severe central tricuspid regurgitation.

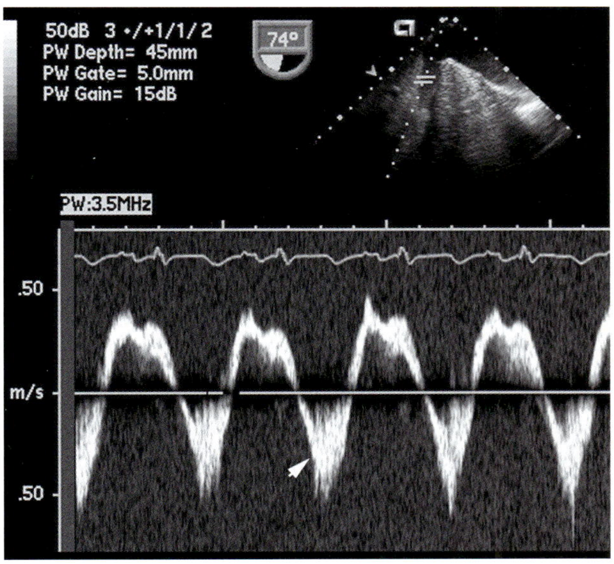

Fig 6.34 Hepatic vein is imaged from transgastric position. Pulsed Doppler shows normal flow into right atrium in diastole (greater than baseline), with reversed flow in systole *(arrowhead)*. This finding is consistent with severe tricuspid regurgitation. However, correlation with other measures of regurgitant severity is needed because systolic flow reversal can be seen in absence of severe tricuspid regurgitation in patients with severely elevated venous pressures or with atrial fibrillation.

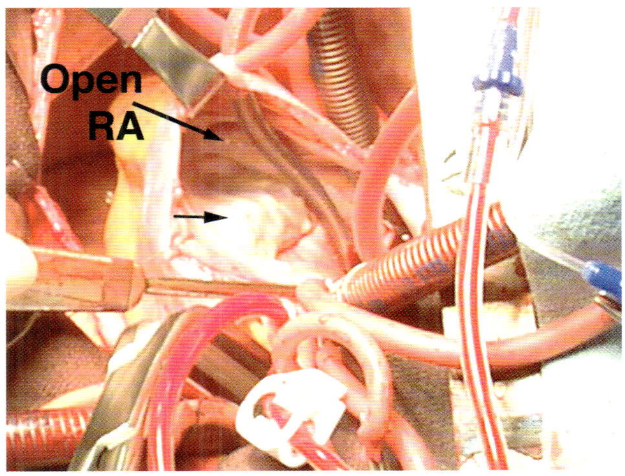

Fig 6.35 Intraoperative inspection of valve demonstrates apically displaced, elongated tricuspid valve leaflets *(arrow)*. Valve repair was not successful in this patient, so she underwent tricuspid valve replacement.

Comments

Some patients with Ebstein's anomaly who reach adulthood without previous surgical procedure remain asymptomatic, without clinical evidence of right heart failure, despite moderate to severe tricuspid regurgitation. In some cases, regurgitant severity increases or chronic right-sided volume overload leads to right heart failure symptoms, prompting surgical intervention.

Ebstein's anomaly may be associated with atrial septal defects in about one-third of patients, and patent foramen ovale is common in those without an atrial septal defect. Elevated right atrial pressures due to tricuspid regurgitation may lead to right-to-left shunting at the atrial level with systemic arterial oxygen desaturation and cyanosis. Ebstein's anomaly is also associated with ventricular preexcitation (e.g., Wolff–Parkinson–White syndrome).

Patients with Ebstein's anomaly are unlikely to have pulmonary hypertension. However, the apparent tricuspid regurgitant jet signal is often difficult to interpret due to the effect of motion of the large, displaced tricuspid valve and there may be erroneous overestimation of pulmonary pressures by Doppler. When pulmonary hypertension is suspected in patients with Ebstein's anomaly, right heart catheterization should be performed for direct measurement of pulmonary pressures.

Suggested Reading

1. Booker OJ, Nanda NC: Echocardiographic assessment of Ebstein's anomaly, Echocardiography 32(Suppl 2):S177–S188, 2015.
2. Bruce CJ, Connolly HM: Right-sided valve disease in adults. In Otto CM, editor: The practice of clinical echocardiography, ed 5, Philadelphia, 2016, Elsevier.

CASE 6-6
Ebstein's Anomaly and Patent Foramen Ovale

This 55-year-old man with Ebstein's anomaly of the tricuspid valve and no prior heart surgery presented with progressive right heart failure symptoms, atrial fibrillation, worsening hypoxia (oxygen saturation 85%), and severe peripheral edema. Echocardiography demonstrated patent foramen ovale with right-to-left shunting, Ebstein's anomaly with severe RA and RV enlargement and moderately reduced right ventricular systolic function. At right heart catheterization, pulmonary pressures were 22/9 (mean 15) mm Hg. After careful discussion, he was referred for surgical intervention.

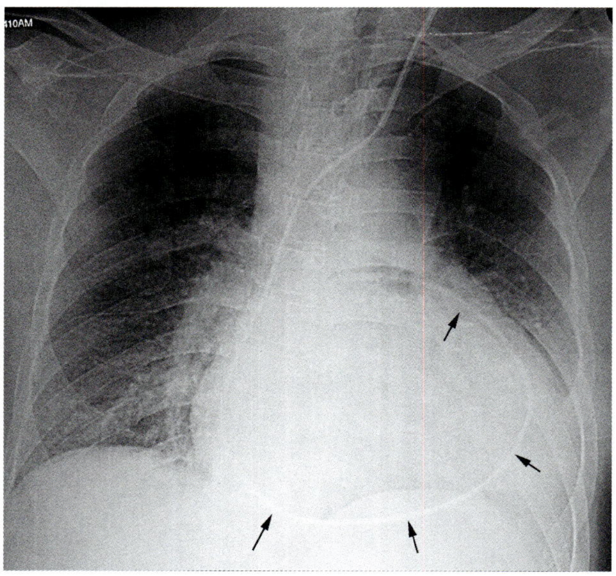

Fig 6.36 Preoperative chest radiograph shows pulmonary artery catheter *(arrows)* in severely enlarged right heart.

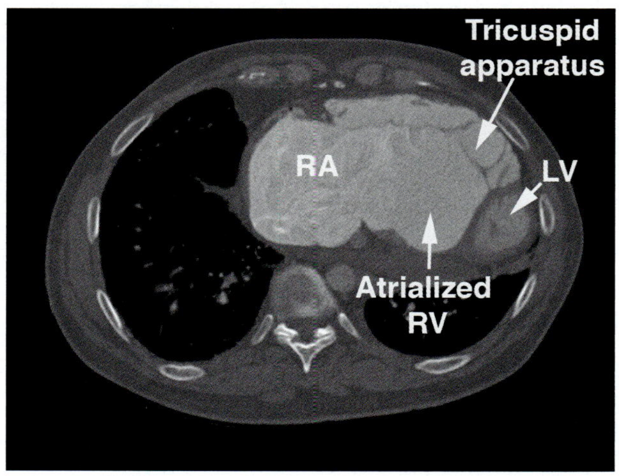

Fig 6.37 Chest CT demonstrated enlarged right atrium (RA), apically displaced tricuspid valve apparatus, and atrialized segment of right ventricle (RV). For comparison, note size of left ventricle (LV).

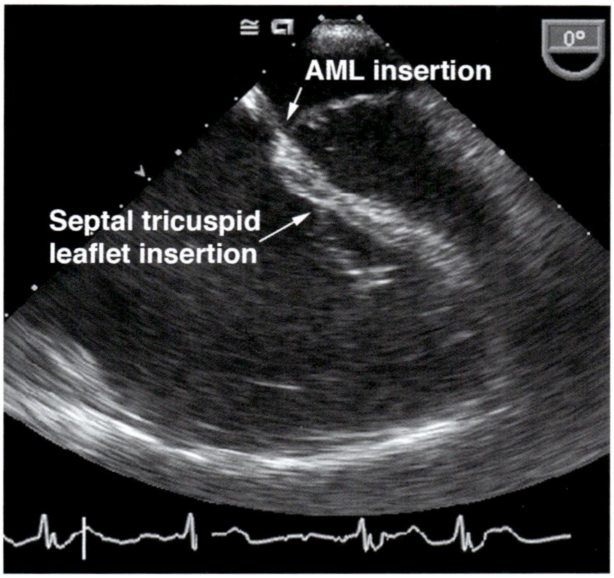

Fig 6.38 TEE imaging in four-chamber view shows severe right heart enlargement with apical displacement of septal leaflet of tricuspid valve, compared with anterior mitral leaflet (AML).

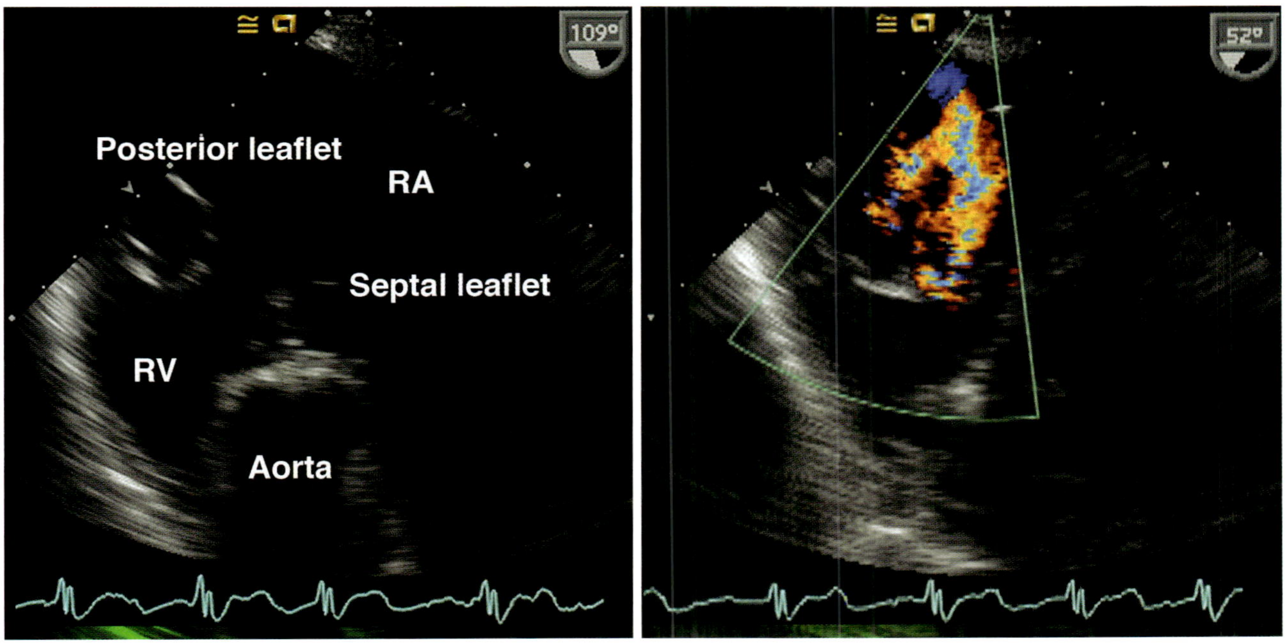

Fig 6.39 From transgastric view, long-axis view of right heart shows apically displaced tricuspid valve leaflets, with color flow indicating at least moderate tricuspid regurgitation.

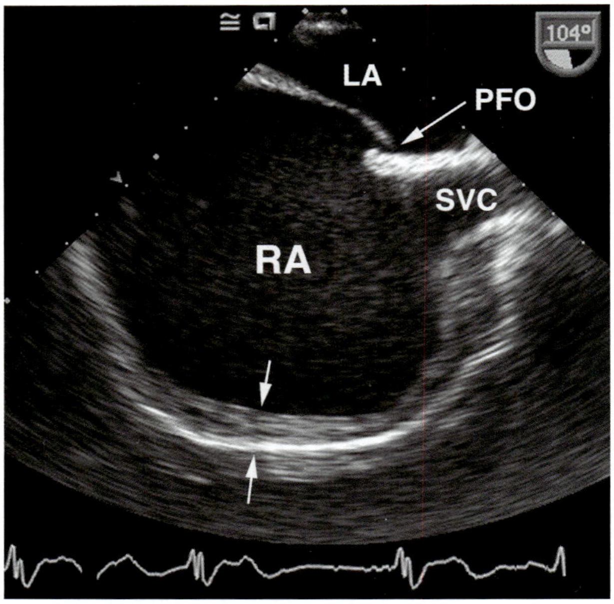

Fig 6.40 TEE right atrial view shows increased thickness of right atrial wall (*arrows*) and patent foramen ovale (PFO) in atrial septum.

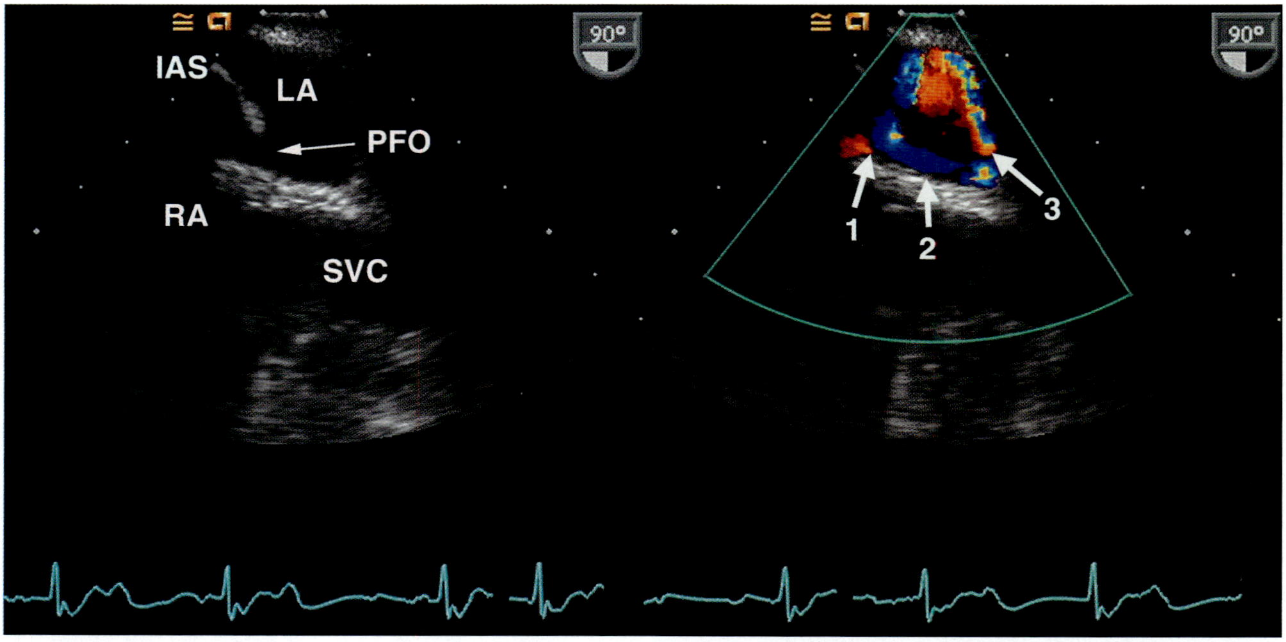

Fig 6.41 Color flow through PFO is demonstrated. Arrow 1 indicates flow going from right atrium through defect and into left atrium; arrow 2 indicates flow hugging left atrial side of interatrial septum (IAS); arrow 3 indicates flow heading toward dome of left atrium.

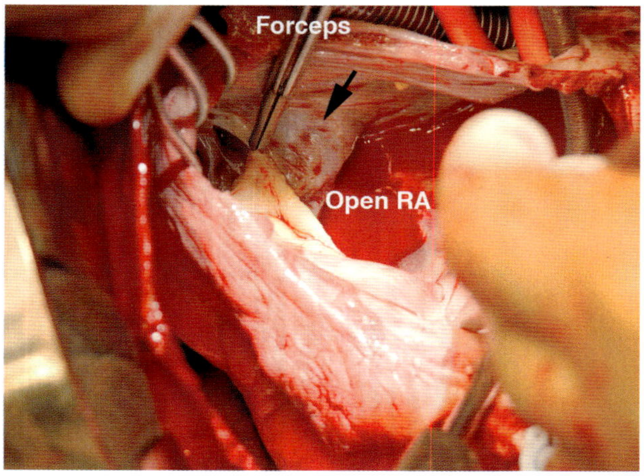

Fig 6.42 At surgery, atrialized segment of right ventricle is seen *(arrow)* with ventricular trabeculation on atrial side of tricuspid valve. Forceps are seen grasping tricuspid leaflet.

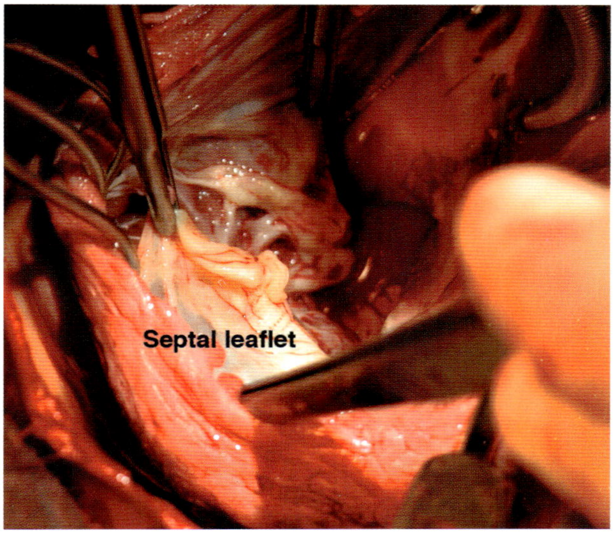

Fig 6.43 Elongated, apically displaced septal leaflet of tricuspid valve. The leaflet edge, lifted by the forceps, is thickened.

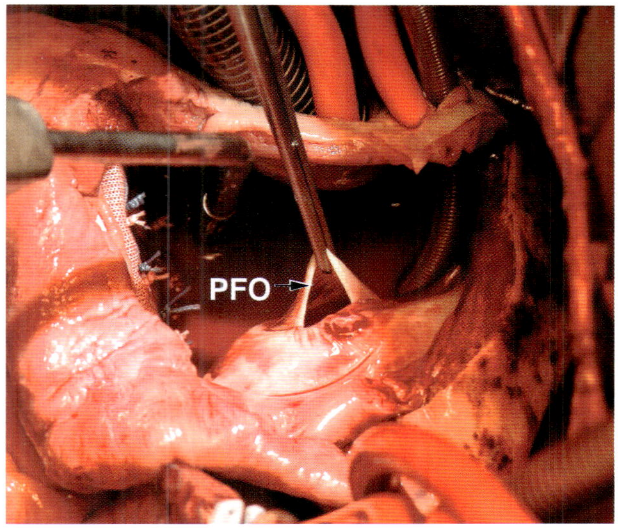

Fig 6.44 Patent foramen ovale can be stretched easily, as shown.

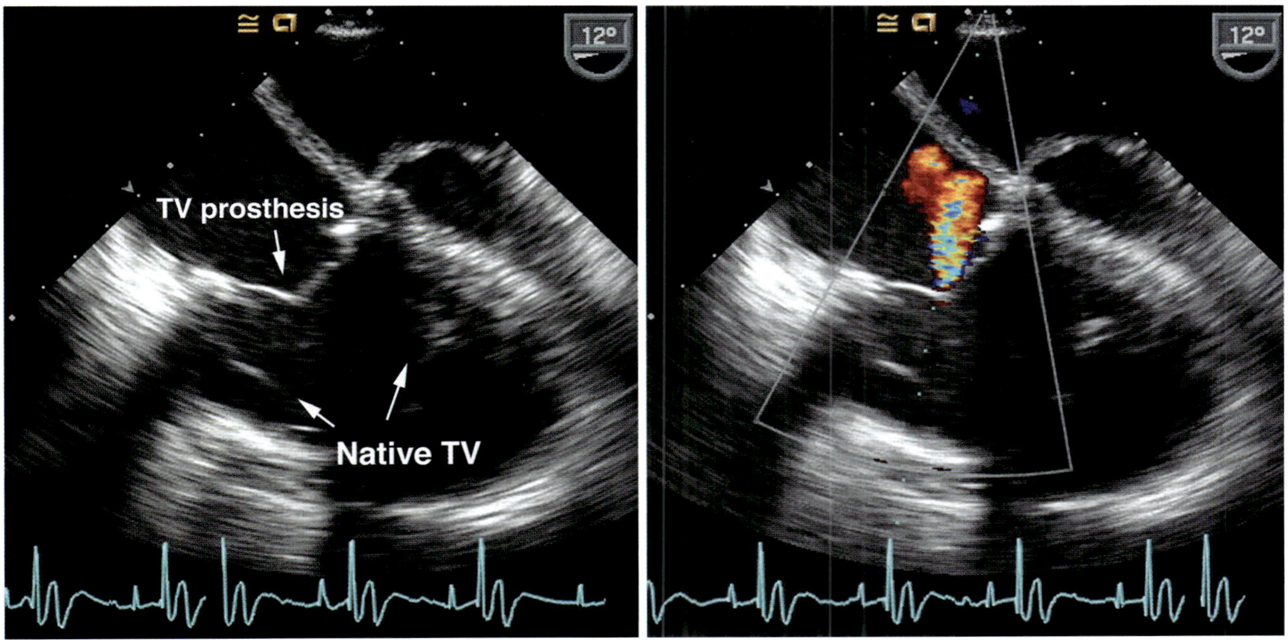

Fig 6.45 After tricuspid valve replacement and PFO closure, prosthesis is seen at annulus level with residual native valve leaflets apically *(left)*. Color Doppler demonstrates small amount of central regurgitation *(right)*. There is no flow across interatrial septum.

Comments

This patient tolerated severe tricuspid regurgitation due to Ebstein's anomaly for many years, without symptoms of heart failure. Eventually, volume overload resulted in RA enlargement with stretching of the patent foramen ovale. RA pressure exceeded LA pressure (due to the tricuspid regurgitation), with consequent right-to-left shunting across the patent foramen ovale and arterial oxygen desaturation.

Although repair of the tricuspid valve is often possible in pediatric patients, repair is less likely to be successful in adult patients due to fibrosis of the valve structures and adherence of the apically displaced leaflets to the underlying ventricular wall.

Suggested Reading

1. Davies RR, Pasquali SK, Jacobs ML, et al: Current spectrum of surgical procedures performed for Ebstein's malformation: an analysis of the Society of Thoracic Surgeons Congenital Heart Surgery Database, Ann Thorac Surg 96(5):1703–1709, 2013.

Tricuspid Valve Prolapse/Flail

CASE 6-7
Traumatic Tricuspid Regurgitation

The patient is a 25-year-old male who was previously in good health until approximately 1 month before the current admission when he was involved in a high-speed motor vehicle accident where he was passenger in car that struck a telephone pole, deploying the airbags. He was admitted to our level I trauma center where he was found to have fractures of right ribs 3 and 4 and left ribs 6 through 10, as well as sternal fracture, splenic laceration, bilateral pneumothoraxes, and pleural effusions that were treated with tube thoracostomies. On echocardiogram, he was found to have severe tricuspid regurgitation with wide vena contracta and systolic flow reversal in the hepatic veins. His RV was dilated with normal systolic function.

Currently, the patient complains of some sternal and rib pain. He denies any shortness of breath, dyspnea on exertion, orthopnea, or lower extremity edema.

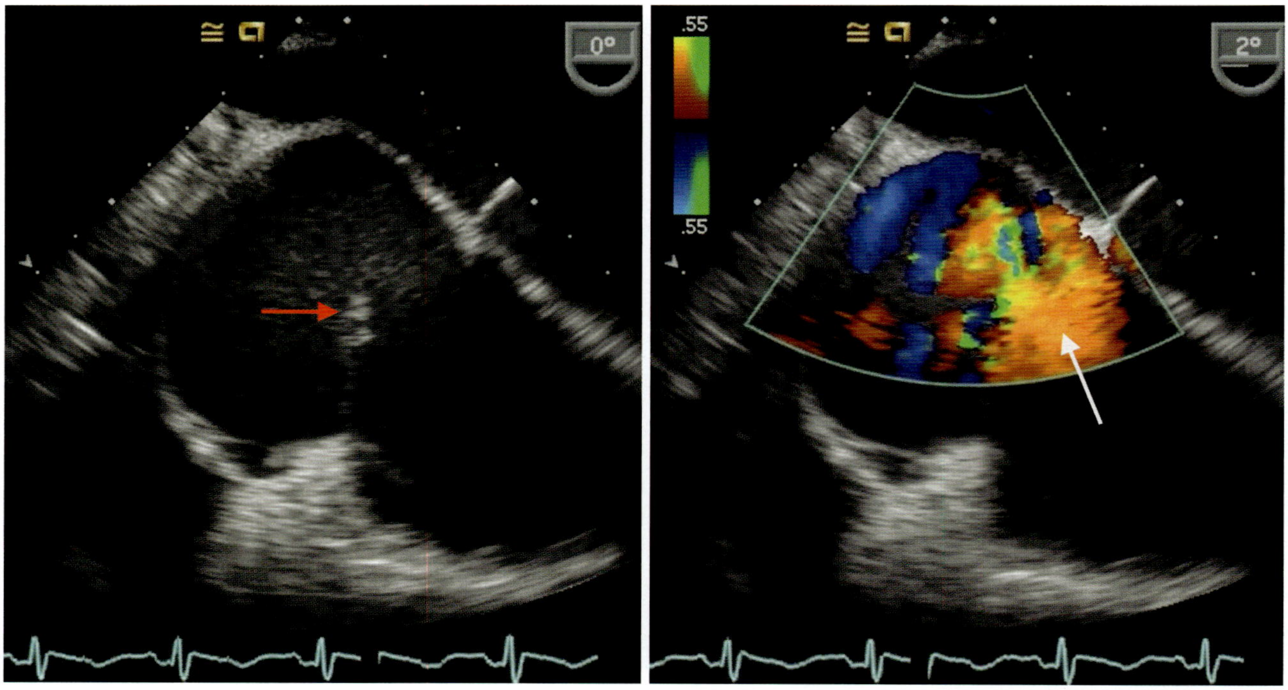

Fig 6.46 In this four-chamber view, systolic frame shows flail tricuspid leaflet, most likely anterior leaflet *(red arrow)*. There is mass at tip, which most likely is portion of ruptured papillary muscle. Both RA and RV are dilated. In right panel, white arrow indicates broad jet of tricuspid regurgitation, with to-and-fro low-velocity flow backward and forward across valve.

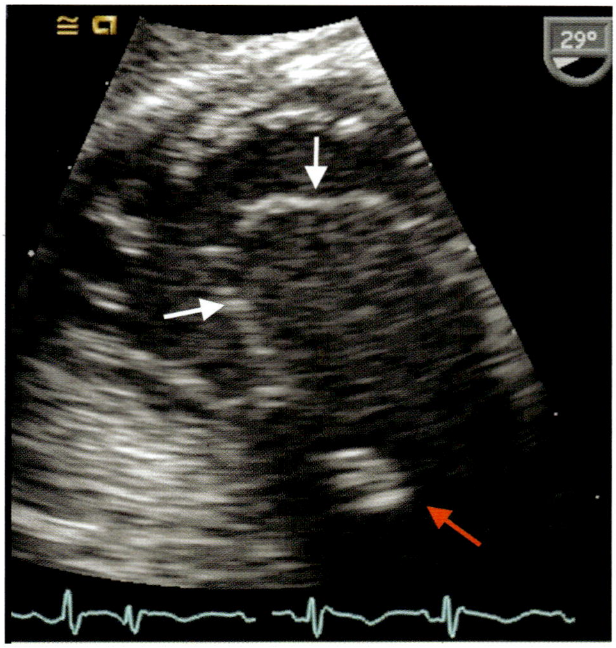

Fig 6.47 In this transgastric image of tricuspid valve, white arrows indicate leaflet edges during diastole, and red arrow indicates what is likely injured papillary muscle attached to anterior leaflet.

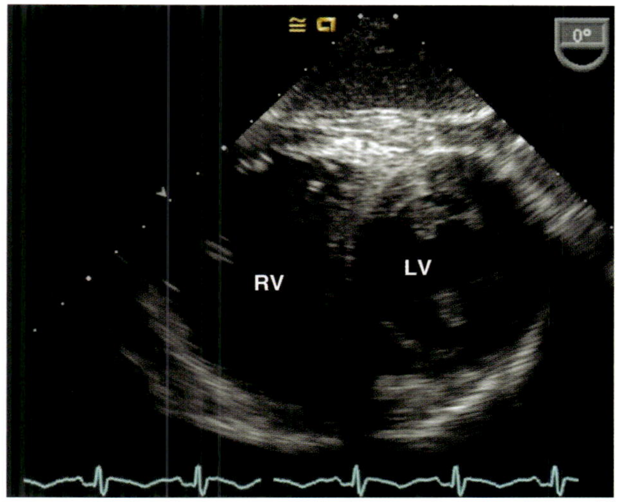

Fig 6.48 In this transgastric short axis of right and left ventricles, right ventricle is significantly dilated with paradoxical motion of interventricular septum, consistent with volume overload of right ventricle.

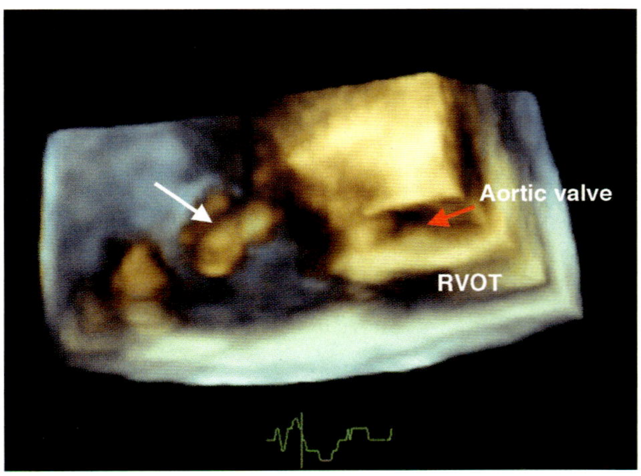

Fig 6.49 This 3D image shows flail anterior leaflet *(arrow)*.

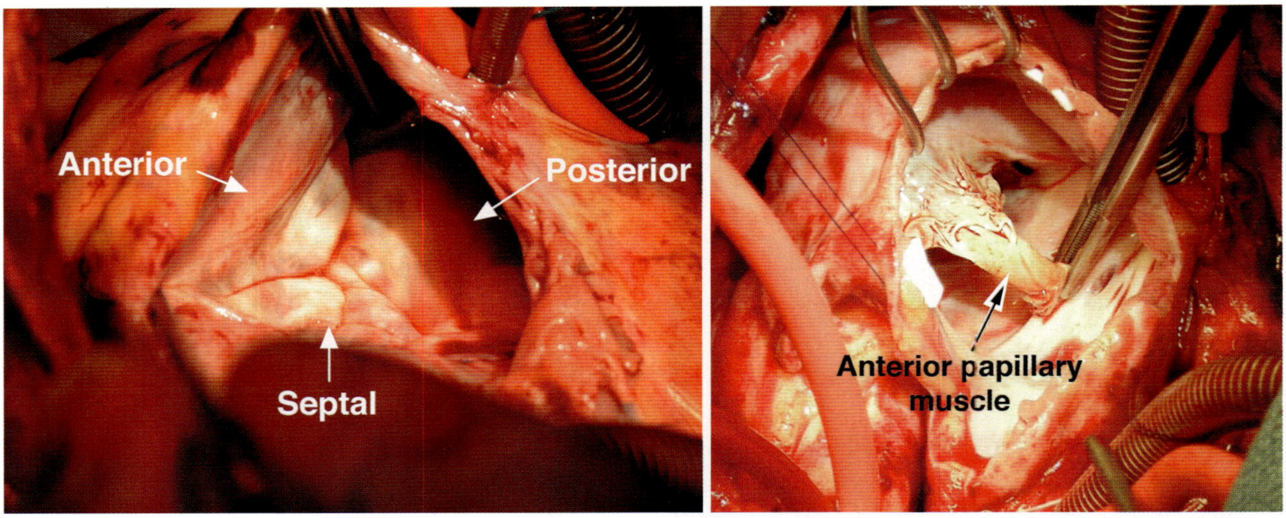

Fig 6.50 At surgery, with right atrium opened, ruptured papillary muscle to anterior leaflet is shown. Surgeon is grasping end with pair of forceps. The left panel shows normal tricuspid valve for comparison.

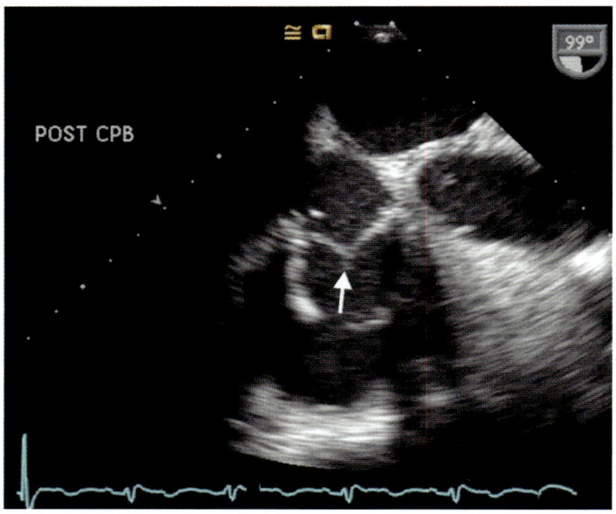

Fig 6.51 After weaning from cardiopulmonary bypass (CPB) after bioprosthetic tricuspid valve replacement, this view at 99 degrees, with probe rotated toward patient's right, shows two leaflets of bioprosthetic valve coapting normally in systole *(white arrow)*. There was no tricuspid regurgitation identified.

Comments

Blunt chest wall trauma can result in severe tricuspid regurgitation due to chordal or papillary muscle rupture, as in this case. Some patients tolerate tricuspid regurgitation and may present years later with progressive RV dilation and systolic dysfunction. Others present more acutely with signs of right heart failure and reduced forward cardiac output. Tricuspid regurgitation also may result from iatrogenic leaflet or chordal damage at the time of catheter-based cardiac procedures. Permanent pacer leads also are associated with tricuspid regurgitation due to the lead impairing normal leaflet motion or due to fibrous adhesions developing over time.

Suggested Reading

1. Lee SH, Kim SA, Jo SH, et al: Combined traumatic tricuspid regurgitation and acute myocardial infarction after fist blows to the chest, Circulation 129(20):e496–e498, 2014.
2. Looi JL, Lee AP, Wong RH, Yu CM: 3D echocardiography for traumatic tricuspid regurgitation, JACC Cardiovasc Imaging 5(12):1285–1287, 2012.
3. Frizzell JD, West MB, Snider RL: Severe tricuspid regurgitation with giant C-v waves after pacer implantation, Circulation 130(4):e23–e25, 2014.

CASE 6-8
Tricuspid Valve Prolapse

This 33-year-old man with myxomatous mitral valve disease and partial flail posterior leaflet with severe mitral regurgitation was referred for mitral valve repair. The tricuspid valve was evaluated intraoperatively because of the concern for myxomatous involvement of the tricuspid valve.

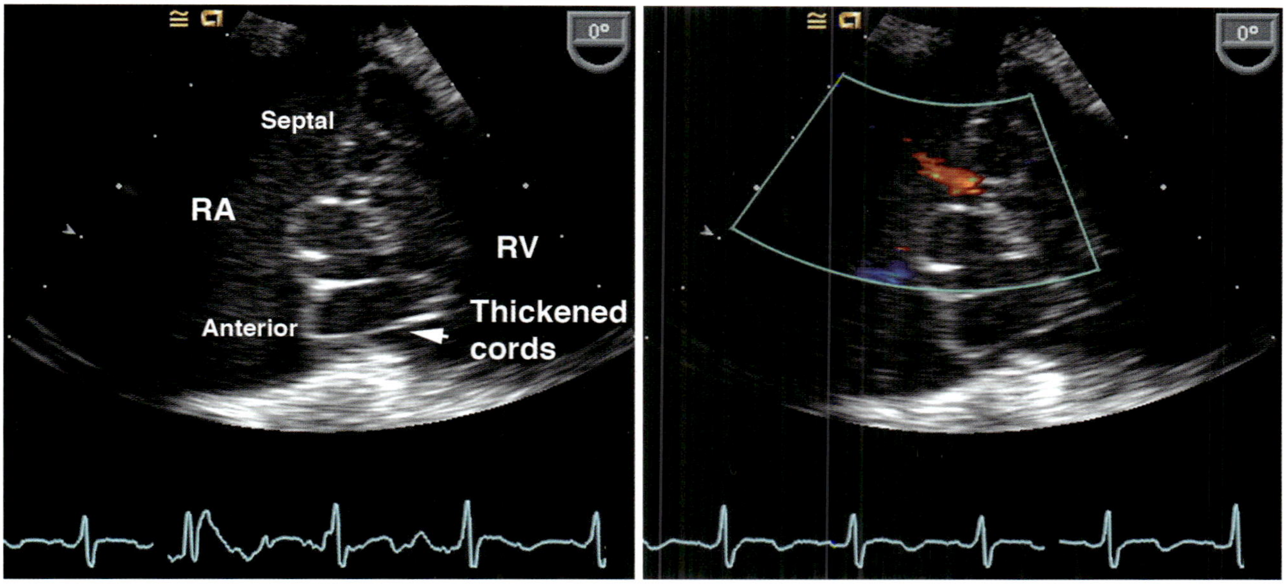

Fig 6.52 Low TEE view of tricuspid valve in four-chamber orientation shows mildly thickened, redundant leaflets with prolapse of anterior and septal leaflets and prominent thickened chords. Color Doppler *(right)* demonstrates only small jet of regurgitation.

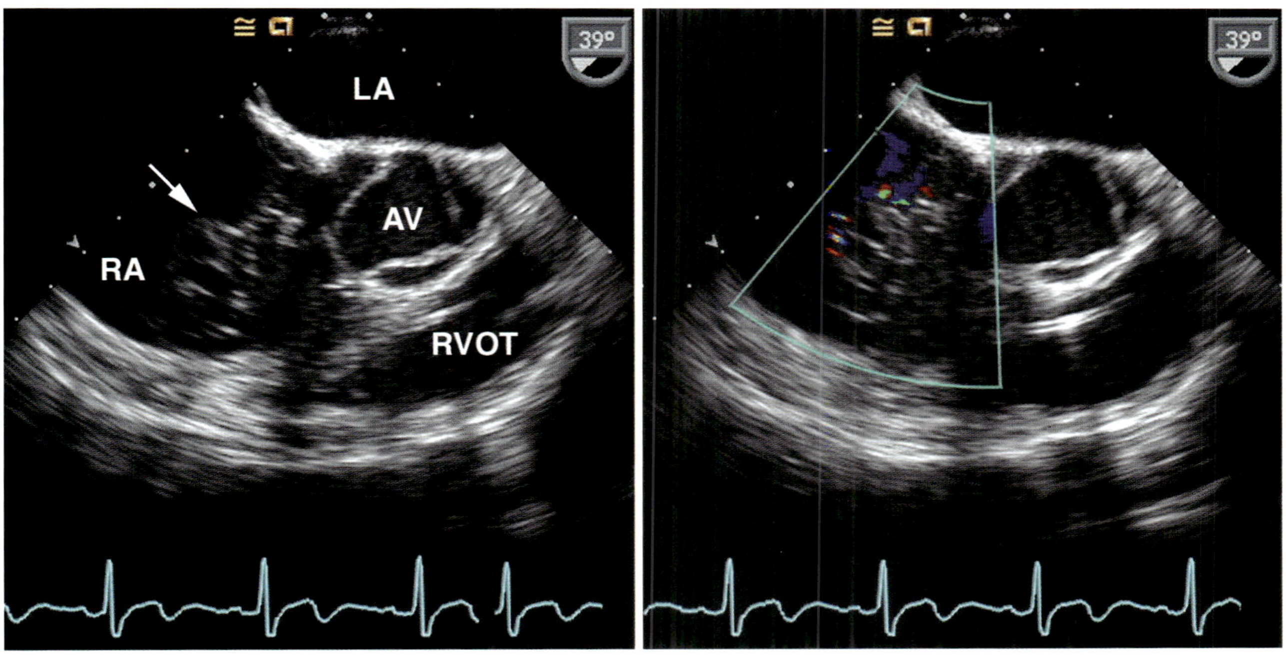

Fig 6.53 With image plane rotated to 39 degrees, redundant tricuspid valve leaflets are seen *(arrow)* in orientation similar to transthoracic short-axis view at aortic valve level. Again, only mild regurgitation is demonstrated.

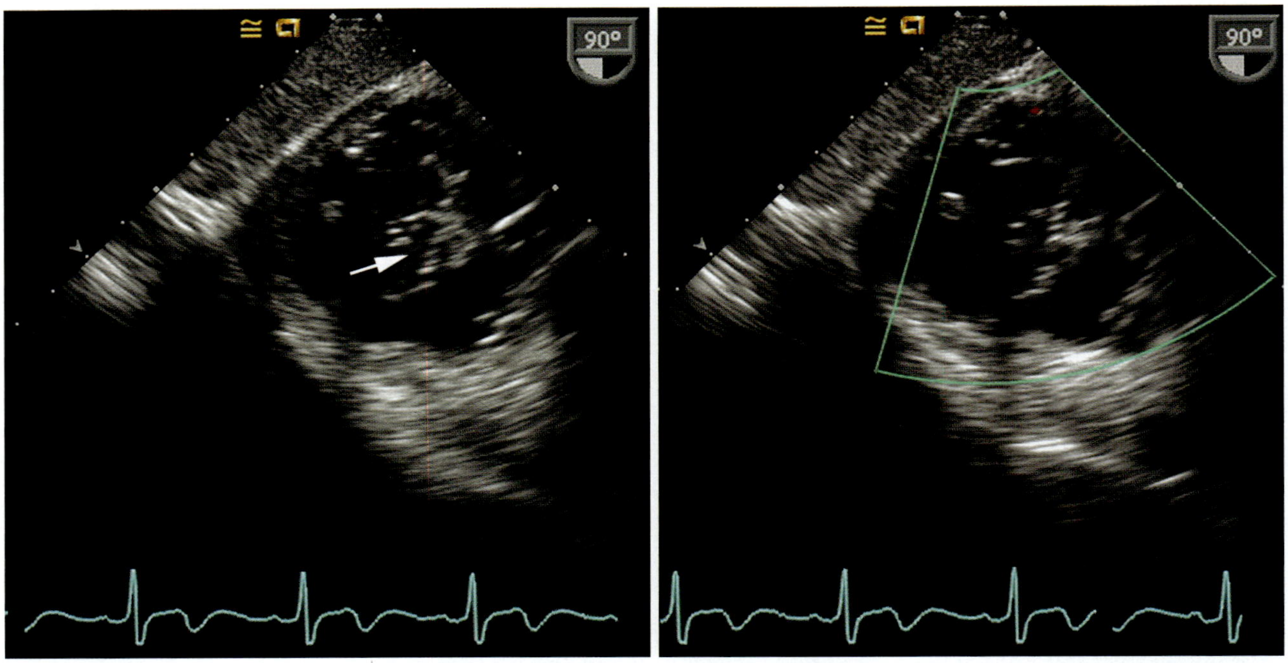

Fig 6.54 ▶ Transgastric short-axis view of tricuspid leaflets *(arrow)* again shows their redundancy.

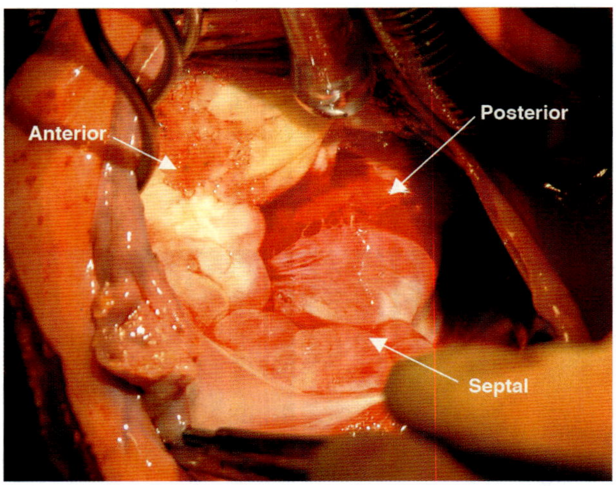

Fig 6.55 ▶ Intraoperative inspection of valve demonstrates myxomatous appearance of valve leaflets with redundancy and prolapse of all three leaflets.

Comments

Myxomatous valve disease most often affects the mitral valve, but other valves can also be affected. In patients with mitral valve prolapse, about one-third have tricuspid valve prolapse, although valve dysfunction is often only mild. The pulmonic valve can also occasionally be affected in patients with mitral valve prolapse.

Suggested Reading

1. Elsayed M, Thind M, Nanda NC: Two- and three-dimensional transthoracic echocardiographic assessment of tricuspid valve prolapse with mid-to-late systolic tricuspid regurgitation, Echocardiography 32(6):1022–1025, 2015.
2. Haake RM, Maqsood MA, et al: Tricuspid regurgitation of varying severity: leaflet prolapse or pacemaker lead–induced obstruction? J Cardiothorac Vasc Anesth 25(4):753–754, 2011.

Carcinoid Valve Disease

CASE 6-9
Carcinoid Valve Disease

This 71-year-old man presented with progressive signs and symptoms of right heart failure over the past 5 months. Ten years before this admission, the patient had colon resection for carcinoid tumor. He was subsequently noted to have chronic flushing and diarrhea, and at that time underwent two abdominal explorations for excision of liver metastases after which he was asymptomatic until the current symptoms developed.

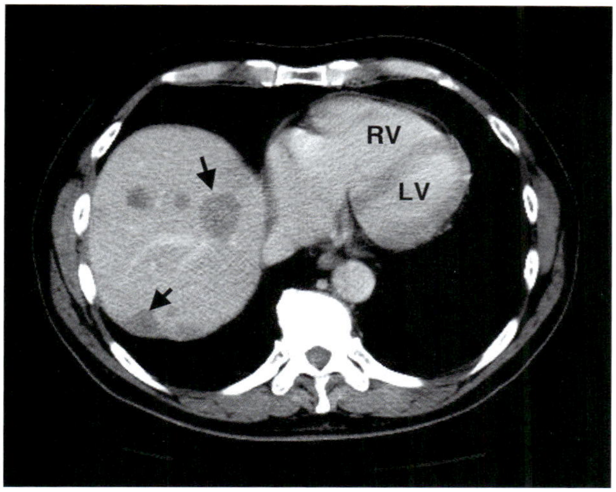

Fig 6.56 Abdominal CT scan reveals numerous liver metastases *(arrows)* from previous intestinal carcinoid; this is almost always seen when carcinoid syndrome is present.

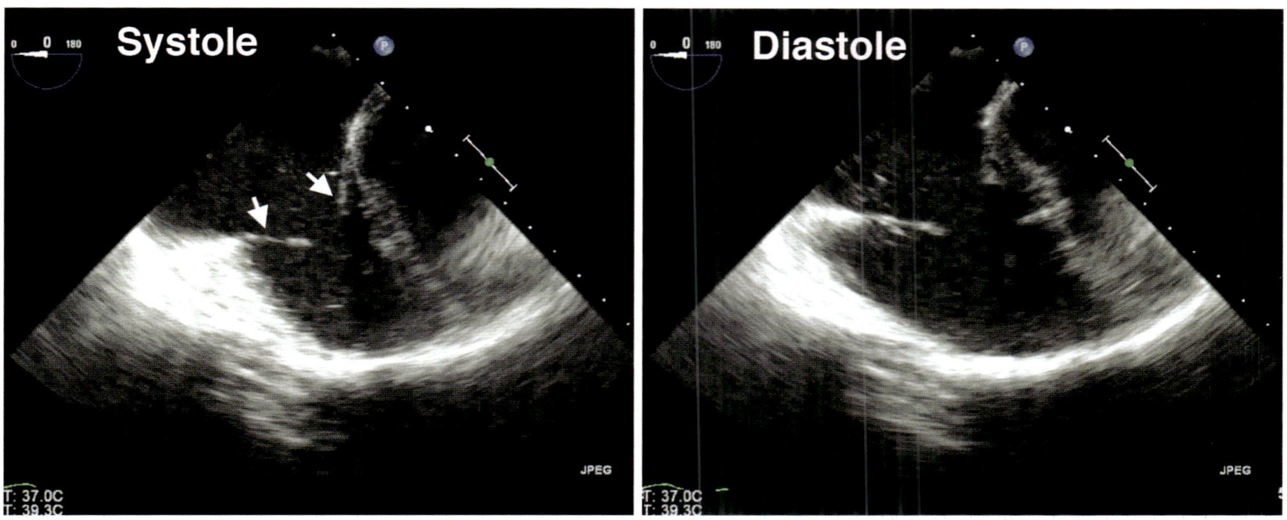

Fig 6.57 In this four-chamber view, tricuspid valve leaflets are rigid and fixed *(arrows)* during both phases of cardiac cycle, as is typical in carcinoid heart disease This often results in tricuspid regurgitation and stenosis. RA and RV are dilated. In real time, there is paradoxical movement of interventricular septum, consistent with right ventricular volume overload.

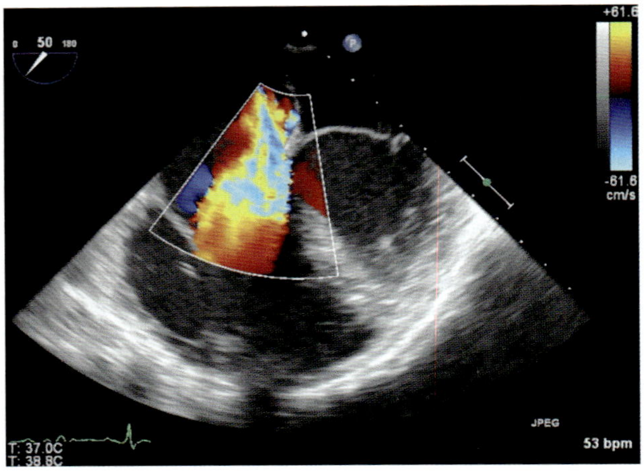

Fig 6.58 Color Doppler shows severe tricuspid regurgitation with low velocity reflecting normal RV and pulmonary systolic pressures.

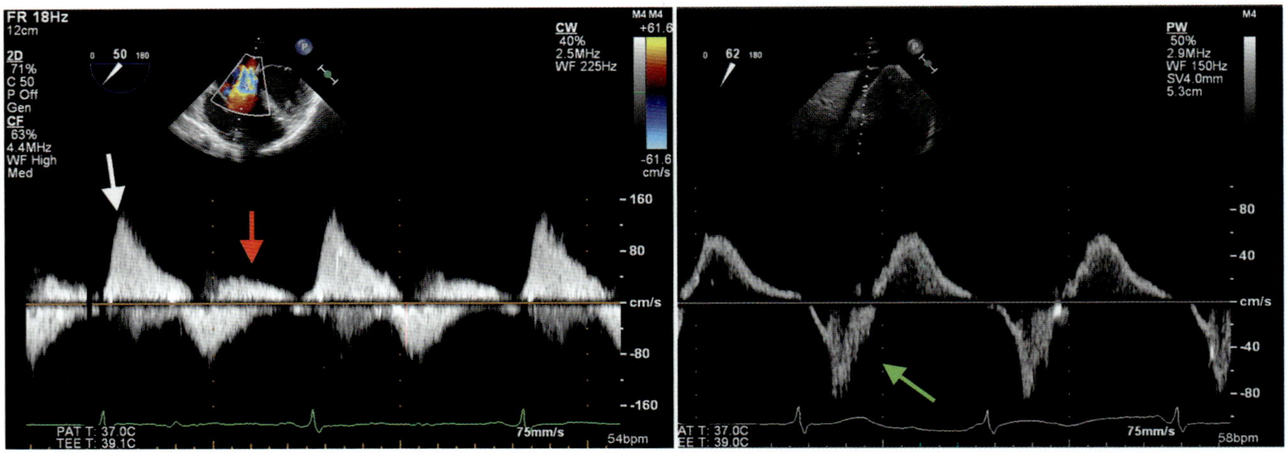

Fig 6.59 Continuous- and pulse-wave Doppler of tricuspid valve and hepatic vein, respectively, speak to severity of tricuspid regurgitation. Tricuspid regurgitation jet peaks early in systole *(white arrow)*, and it is dense and triangular shaped. The red arrow shows presence of diastolic regurgitation. In hepatic vein, there is systolic reversal *(green arrow)*.

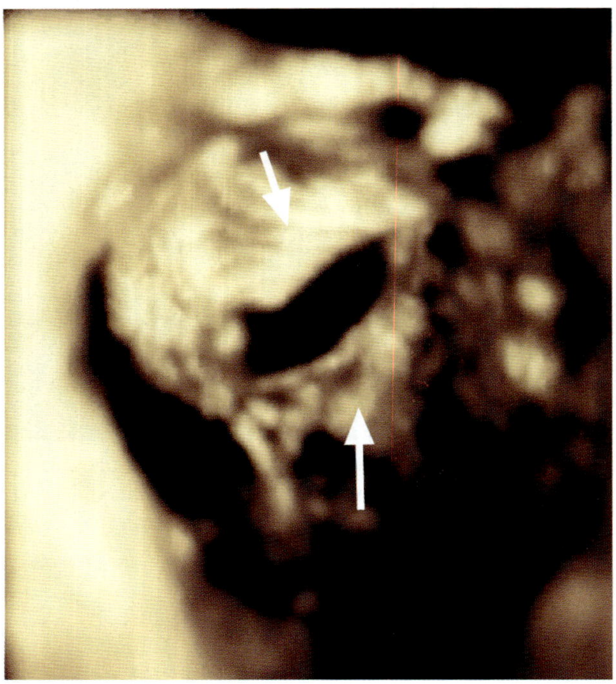

Fig 6.60 3D imaging from ventricular aspect of tricuspid valve *(arrows)* during systole show incomplete coaptation.

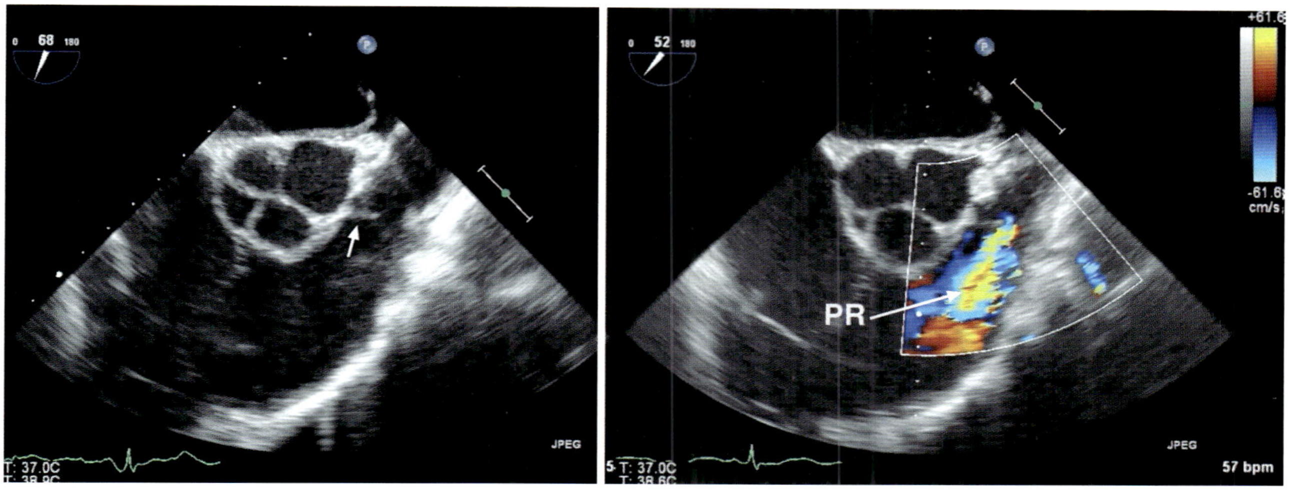

Fig 6.61 In this right ventricular inflow–outflow view, one leaflet of pulmonic valve is seen *(arrow)*. Leaflet is thickened, and there is severe pulmonic regurgitation.

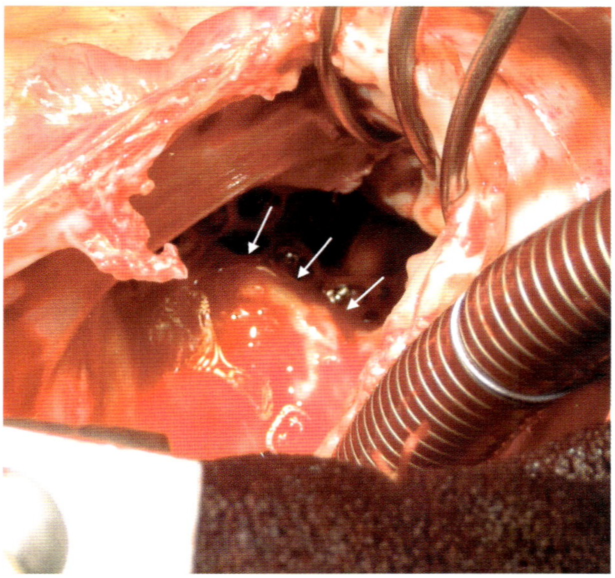

Fig 6.62 At surgery, after incising right atrial wall, thickened tricuspid valve is seen. Arrows indicate grossly abnormal edge of one of leaflets.

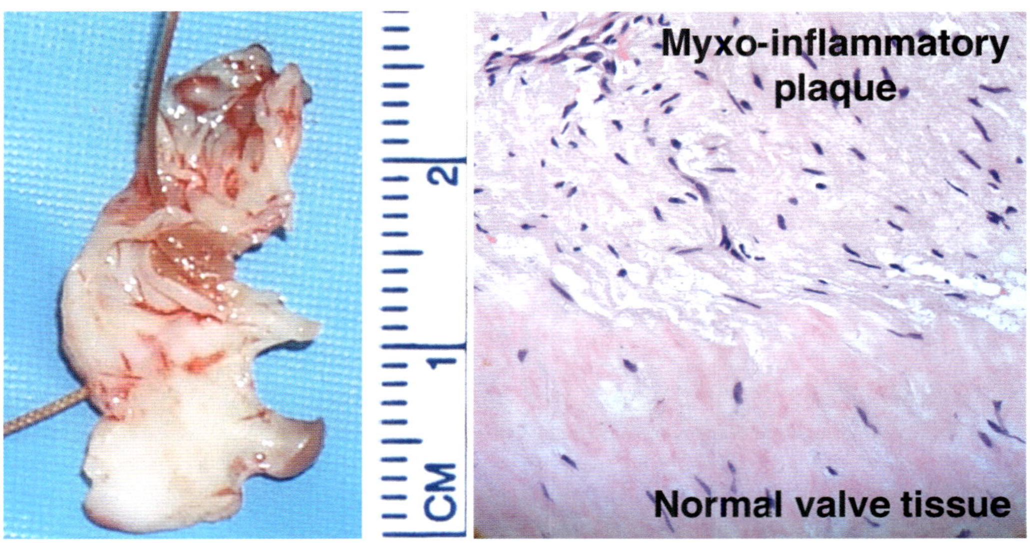

Fig 6.63 In another case with similar presentation, explanted tricuspid valve shows diffuse thickening and shortening of leaflets. Histologic section in right panel demonstrates normal tricuspid valve tissue with superficial plaques of myxo-inflammatory material consistent with carcinoid heart disease.

Comments

Carcinoid valve disease is rare, but has pathognomonic appearance on echocardiography with thickening, shortening, and retraction of the tricuspid valve leaflets. Carcinoid valve disease is seen in patients with carcinoid tumor metastatic to the liver and is thought to be due to elevated levels of vasoactive substances such as serotonin (5-hydroxytryptamine), 5-hydroxytryptophan, histamine, bradykinin, tachykinins, and prostaglandin. The clinical presentation typically includes vasomotor changes (flushing or blood pressure instability), although right heart failure may be present with end-stage disease. With cardiac involvement, over 90% have severe tricuspid regurgitation and most also have pulmonic valve involvement with combined stenosis and regurgitation. Left-sided involvement is unusual and is typically associated with patent foramen ovale or lung metastases, as otherwise the vasoactive agents are inactivated in the lungs.

Suggested Reading

1. Miles LF, Leong T, McCall P, Weinberg L: Carcinoid heart disease: correlation of echocardiographic and histopathological findings, BMJ Case Rep November 24, 2014.
2. Patel C, Mathur M, Escarcega RO, Bove AA: Carcinoid heart disease: current understanding and future directions, Am Heart J 167(6):789–795, 2014.

Pulmonic Valve

CASE 6-10
Severe Pulmonic Regurgitation

This 26-year-old man had undergone surgical repair for tetralogy of Fallot as a child, with closure of ventricular septal defect and pulmonary valvotomy. He presents now with increasing shortness of breath and atrial flutter. Echocardiography showed severe pulmonic regurgitation with severe RV enlargement but only mildly reduced RV systolic function. Estimated pulmonary systolic pressure was normal by echocardiography, which was confirmed at catheterization, with no evidence of branch pulmonary stenosis. He was referred for pulmonary valve replacement.

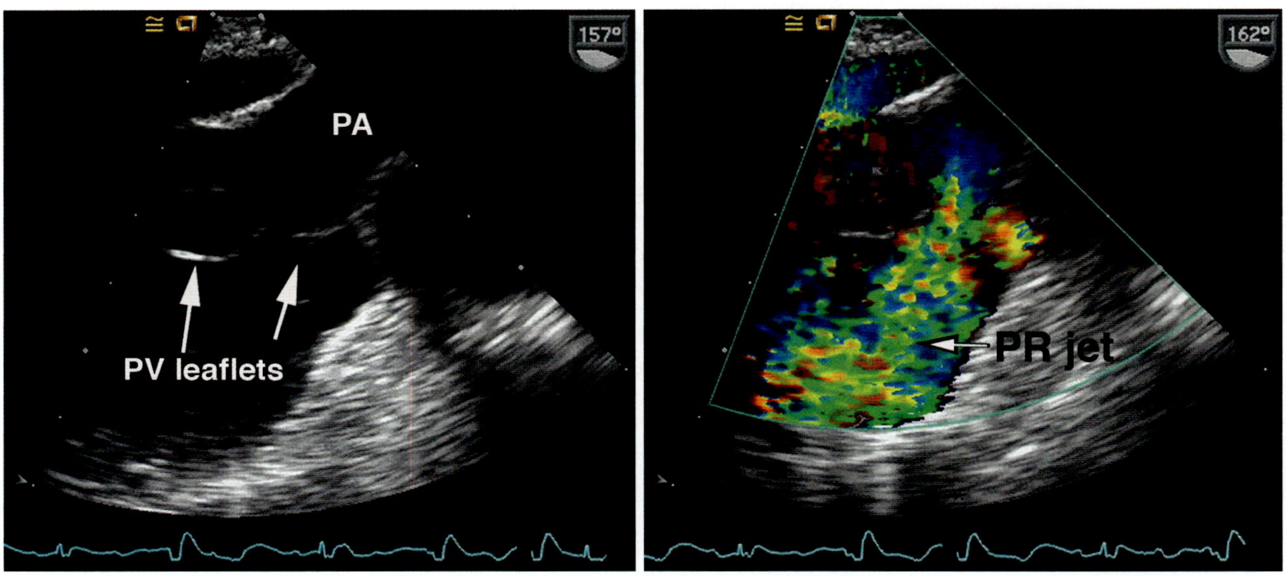

Fig 6.64 High TEE view of pulmonic valve in long axis with image plane rotated to 157 degrees shows pulmonic valve (PV) leaflets with severe thinning and prolapse of one leaflet *(left)*. Color flow shows severe pulmonic regurgitation with regurgitant jet nearly filling RVOT.

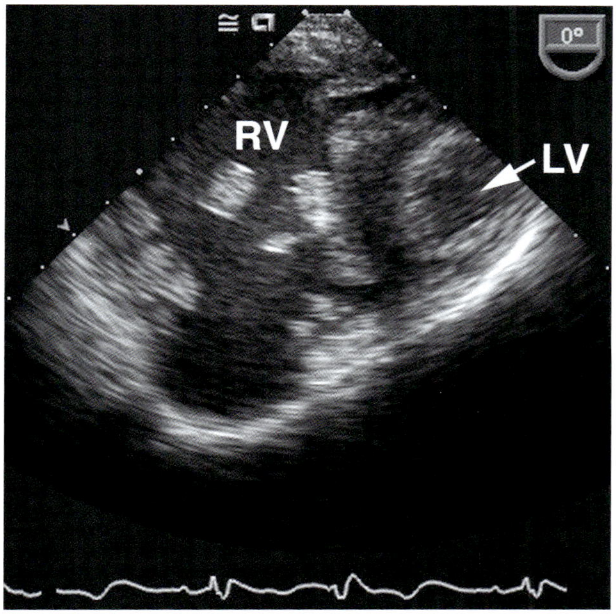

Fig 6.65 Transgastric view demonstrated severe right ventricular dilation. Although pulmonary pressures were normal, right ventricular wall appears hypertrophied. Note relatively much smaller left ventricle. In real time, there is paradoxical septal motion and septal diastolic flattening consistent with right ventricular overload.

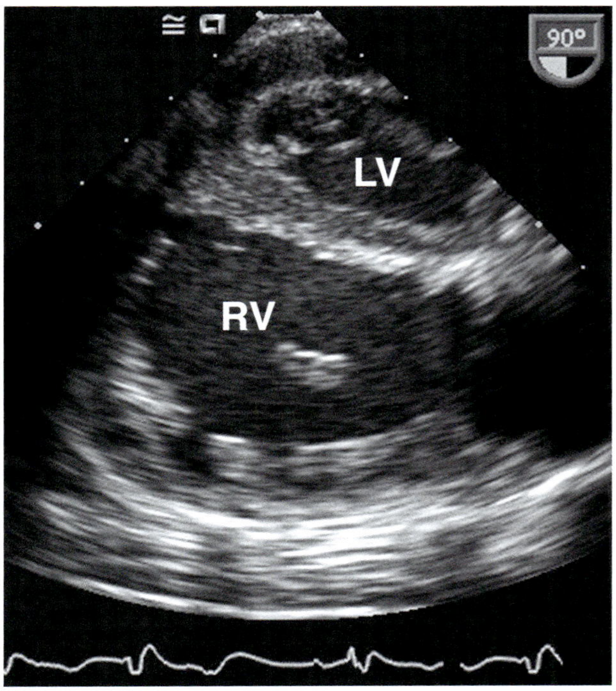

Fig 6.66 This 90-degree basal transgastric image looks more like 0 degrees because of abnormal orientation of heart; this latter phenomenon is related to mismatch in right and left chamber sizes. Right ventricular hypertrophy is again noted. In real time, paradoxical motion of interventricular septum and septal diastolic flattening related to right ventricular volume overload are seen.

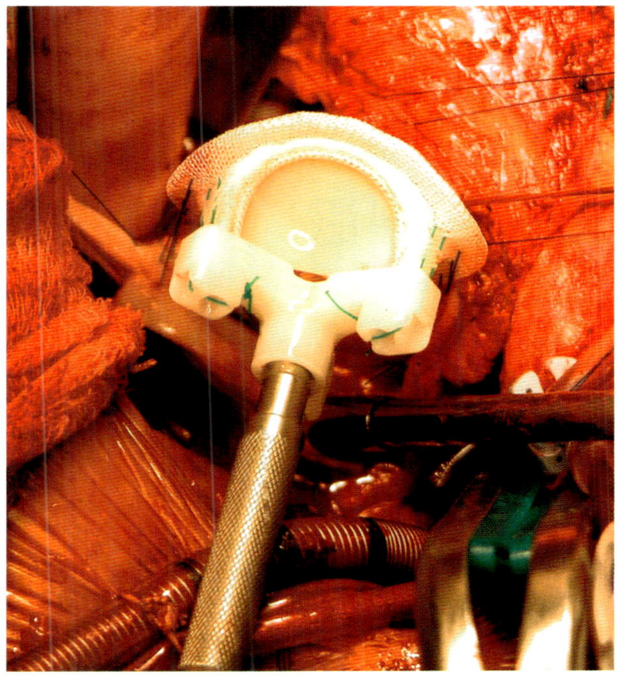

Fig 6.67 Stented tissue prosthetic valve is prepared for implantation.

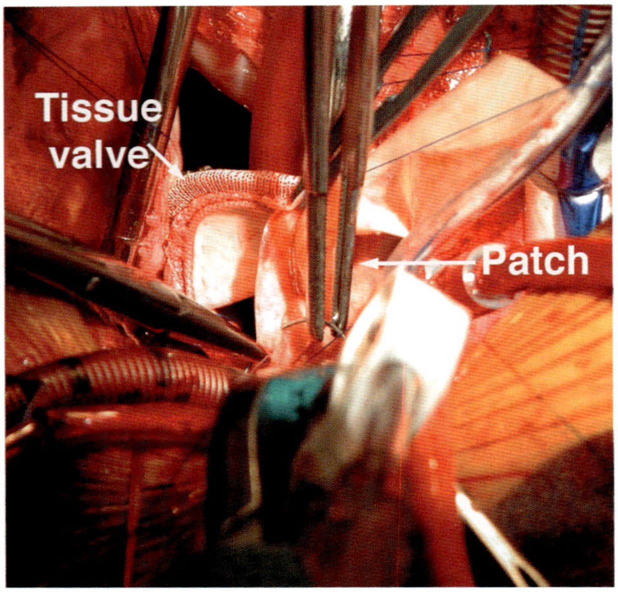

Fig 6.68 With valve in position, patch is used to enlarge pulmonic annulus.

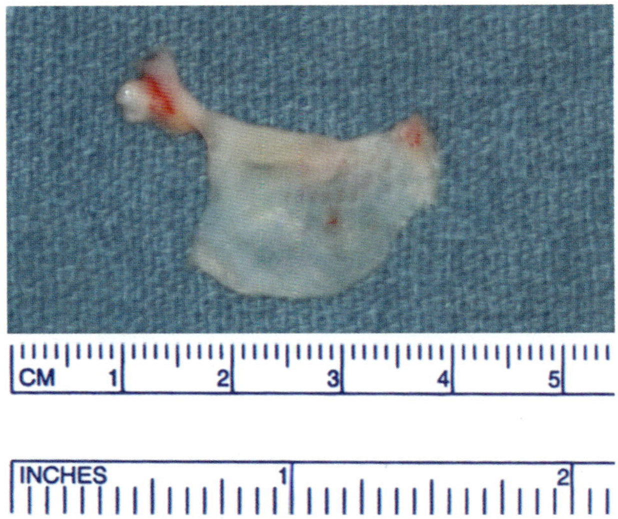

Fig 6.69 Excised valve leaflet is dysmorphic and thin. Only one leaflet was identified. Of other two leaflets, only blighted remnants were seen.

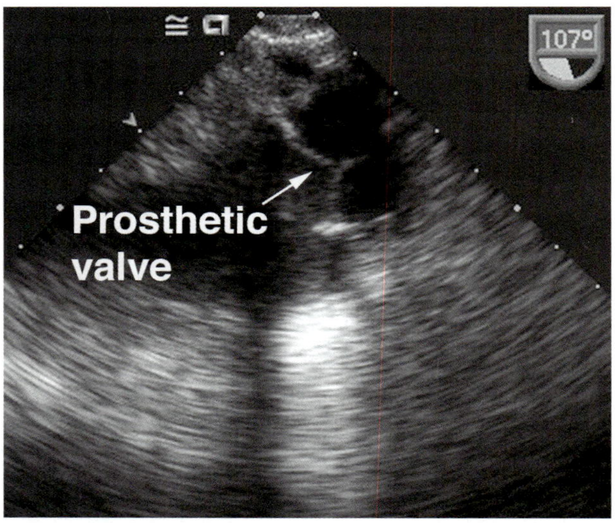

Fig 6.70 Tissue prosthetic valve on TEE images after procedure shows thin leaflets with normal motion. There was no regurgitation.

Comments

Pulmonic regurgitation late after repair of tetralogy of Fallot is common, with moderate-to-severe regurgitation in up to 50% of patients. The consequent right ventricular volume overload results in progressive RV enlargement and eventual systolic dysfunction. However, evaluation of the severity of pulmonic regurgitation can be problematic. The width of the diastolic flow stream by color Doppler is helpful, with narrow jet consistent with mild regurgitation and jet that fill the RVOT consistent with severe regurgitation. Because the velocity of pulmonic regurgitation is low, when pulmonary pressures are normal, regurgitation may be missed by color Doppler unless the examiner is aware of this possibility. Other helpful parameters are the intensity of the continuous wave Doppler regurgitant signal, relative to antegrade flow, and the slope (or pressure half-time) of the diastolic signal. Holodiastolic flow reversal in the main pulmonary artery, due to severe pulmonic regurgitation, should be distinguished from diastolic flow due to patent ductus arteriosus.

Suggested Reading

1. Cuypers JA, Menting ME, Konings EE, et al: Unnatural history of tetralogy of Fallot: prospective follow-up of 40 years after surgical correction, Circulation 130(22):1944–1953, 2014.
2. Swamy P, Bharadwaj A, Varadarajan P, Pai RG: Echocardiographic evaluation of tetralogy of Fallot, Echocardiography 32(Suppl 2): S148–S156, 2015.

CASE 6-11
Pulmonary Homograft Regurgitation/Stenosis after Ross Procedure

This 29-year-old woman with history of rheumatic valvular disease had Ross procedure and mitral valve replacement 8 years previously. She has had recent history of increased shortness of breath, cardiac cachexia, and right-sided congestive heart failure with ascites, and was found to have severe tricuspid regurgitation, and severe pulmonic valve and insufficiency. Her aortic autograft and prosthetic mitral valve were functioning well.

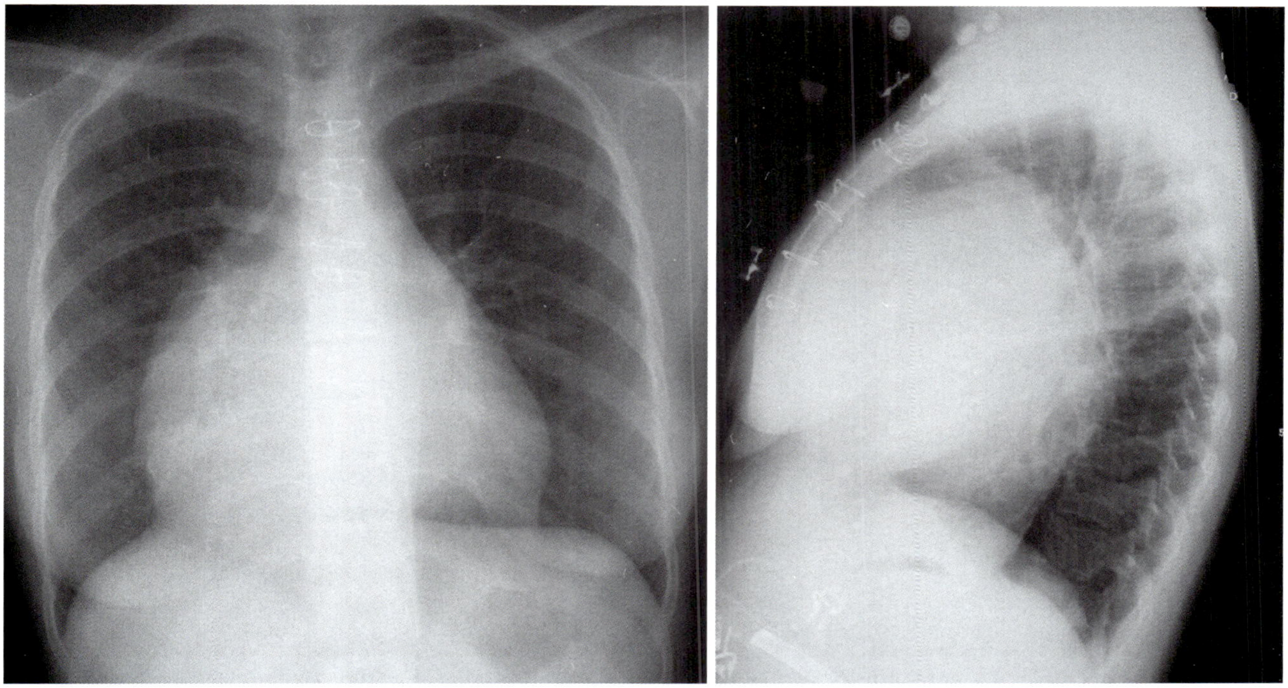

Fig 6.71 PA and lateral chest x-rays show generalized enlargement of right-sided chambers.

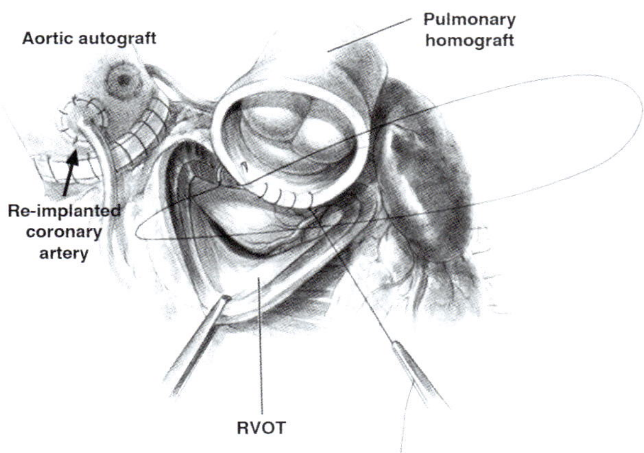

Fig 6.72 In this illustration, native aortic valve has been excised, and native pulmonary root has been resected just proximal to its bifurcation into right and left pulmonary arteries and transplanted to aorta. Coronary arteries have been reimplanted into aortic autograft. Pulmonary homograft is being sutured into place. (Reproduced with permission from Elsevier Limited, Kidlington, Oxford, UK.)

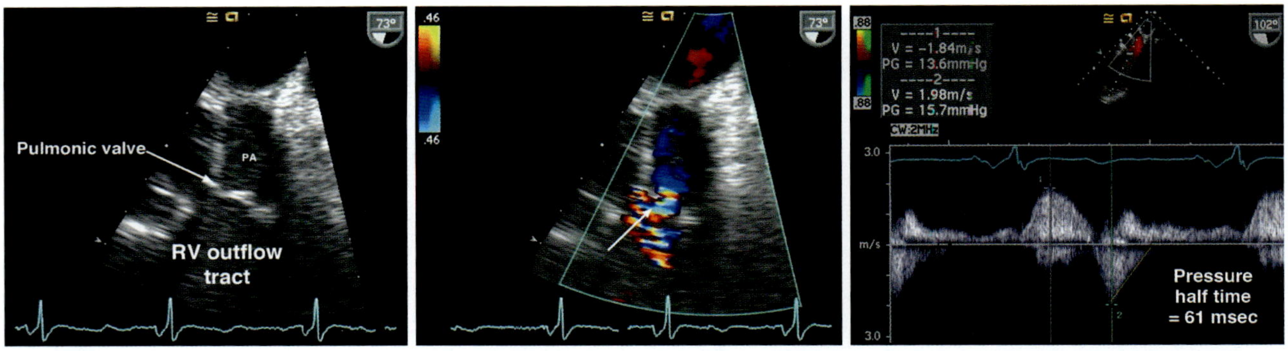

Fig 6.73 In high esophageal position, pulmonic regurgitation is seen *(arrow, middle frame)*. CW Doppler is seen in right panel. Antegrade velocity is approximately 2 m/sec, whereas pressure half-time of regurgitant jet is 61 msec, consistent with severe pulmonic regurgitation.

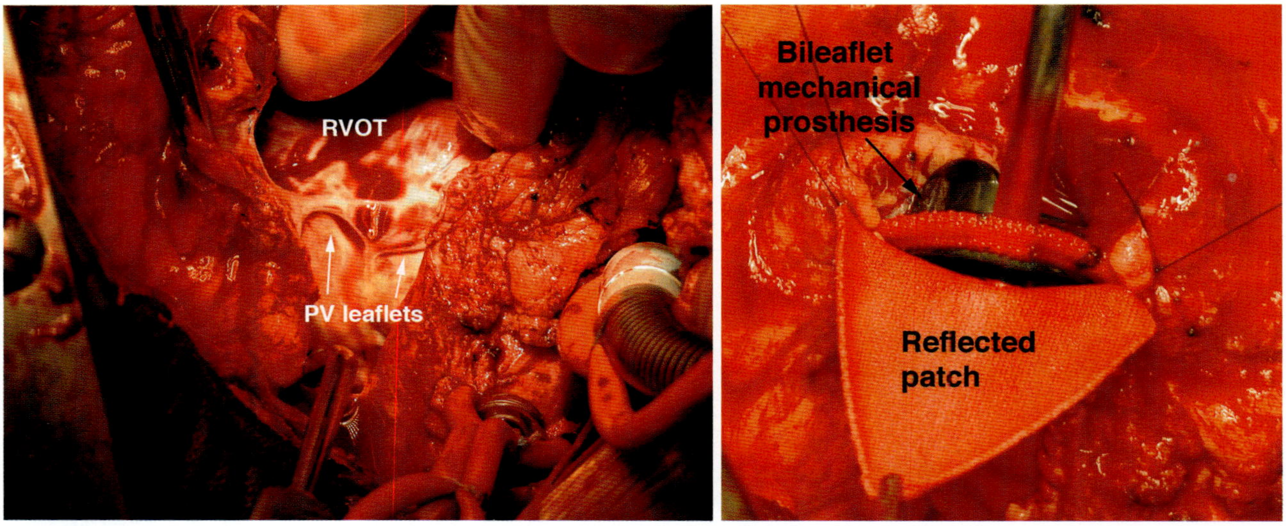

Fig 6.74 After incision of RV outflow tract, thickened leaflets of pulmonary homograft are seen. On right, leaflets have been excised, bileaflet mechanical valve placed, and outflow tract closed with pericardial patch.

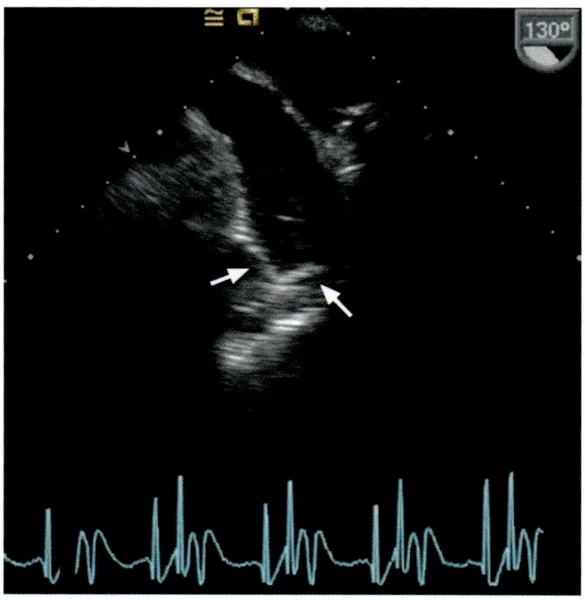

Fig 6.75 Postoperative high esophageal imaging shows bileaflet mechanical prosthesis in diastole, with leaflets closed *(arrows)*.

Suggested Reading

1. Oury J, Maxwell M: An appraisal of the Ross procedure: goals and technical guidelines, Oper Tech Thorac Cardiovasc Surg 2(4):289–301, 1997.

7 Adult Congenital Heart Disease

Atrial Septal Defects

CASE 7-1
Anatomy and Imaging of the Atrial Septum

The atrial septum is close to the TEE transducer position and is well visualized, as the normal orientation is perpendicular to the ultrasound beam. From a single high TEE probe position, the entire atrial septum can be examined by starting in a four-chamber view and then incrementally rotating the image plane to the bicaval view at approximately 90 to 120 degrees rotation. 3D imaging is especially helpful for visualization of the entire atrial septum and positioning of transcatheter closure devices.

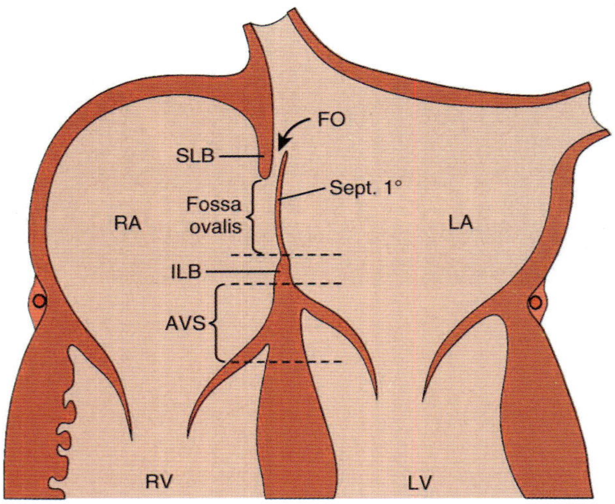

Fig 7.1 Diagram of atrial septal components showing foramen ovale (FO), septum primum (Sept 1°), left atrium (LA), left ventricle (LV), fossa ovalis, superior limbic bands (SLB) and inferior limbic bands (ILB), atrioventricular septum (AVS), right atrium (RA), right ventricle (RV). (Adapted from Keane JF, Lock JE, Fyler DC (eds.): Nadas Pediatric Cardiology, 2e, Philadelphia, 2006, Elsevier/Saunders.)

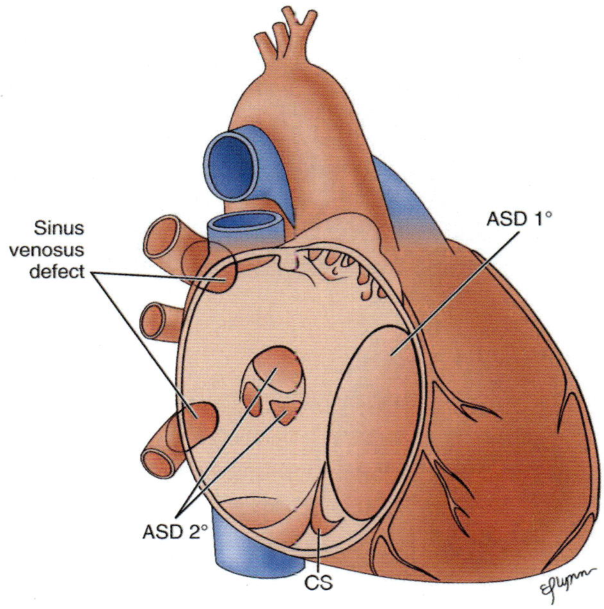

Fig 7.2 Diagram of atrial septum showing several types of atrial septal defects. (Adapted from Keane JF, Lock JE, Fyler DC (eds.): Nadas Pediatric Cardiology, 2e, Philadelphia, 2006, Elsevier/Saunders.)

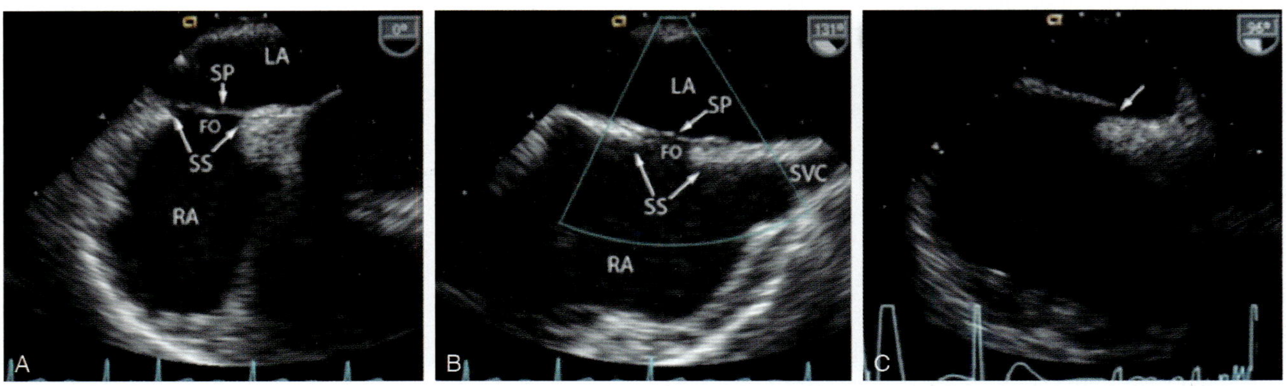

Fig 7.3 From high TEE position, fossa ovalis (FO) is seen in both four-chamber **(A)** and bicaval **(B)** views. At rotation angle between 60 and 90 degrees, opening between septum primum and septum secundum *(arrow)* or patent foramen ovale is seen. LA = left atrium, RA = right atrium, SP = septum primum, SS = septum secundum, FO = fossa ovalis.

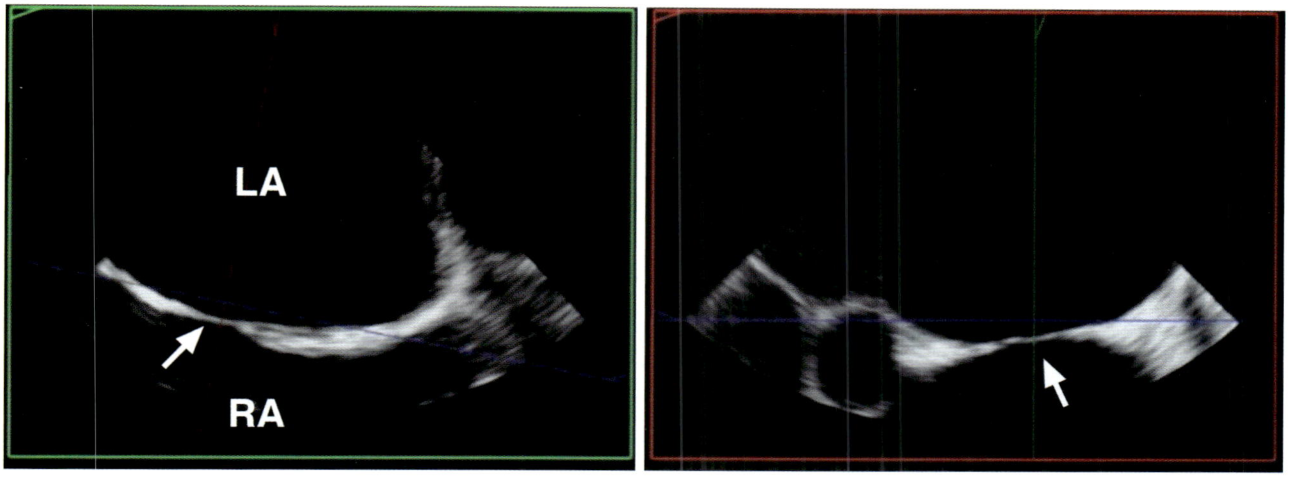

Fig 7.4 In midesophageal position, orthogonal views at 110 degrees *(left)* and 20 degrees *(right)* will be used to construct 3D image. Pyramidal truncated data set (3D Zoom, QLAB; Philips, Medical Systems) includes entire atrial septum (see Fig 7.5).

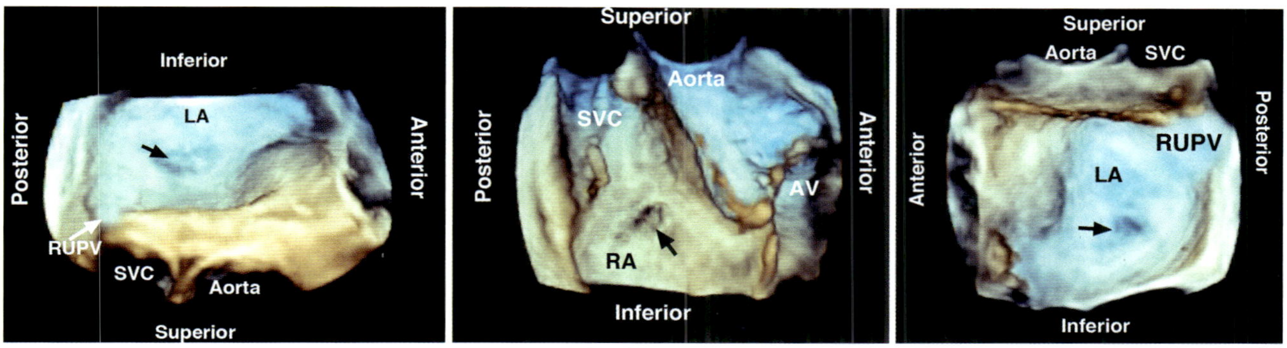

Fig 7.5 Using multiplanar reconstruction modality base (QLAB; Philips, Medical Systems), initial 3D image *(left frame)* shows atrial septum from left atrial perspective. Rotating image along its horizontal axis *(middle frame)* allows imaging of atrial septum from right atrial perspective; proximity of ascending aorta can be appreciated, crucial concept in periprocedural septal puncture. Subsequent rotation of image along its vertical axis allows better appreciation of atrial septum from left atrial perspective. In all three frames, black arrow indicates fossa ovalis.

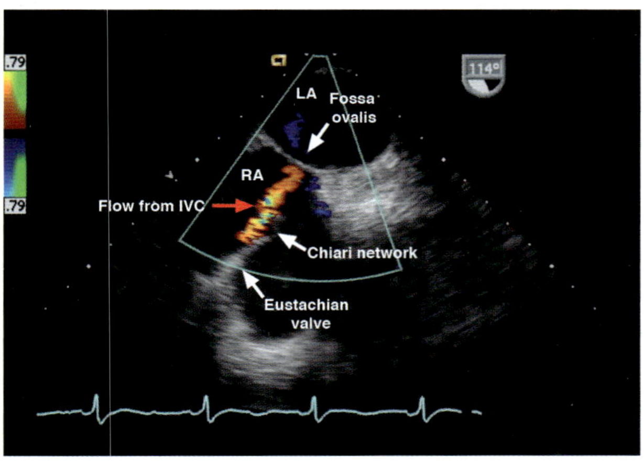

Fig 7.6 In this midesophageal view at 114 degrees, there is persistence of fetal remnants; Eustachian Valve and Chiari network. Red arrow indicates flow into right atrium from IVC. As can be seen, color Doppler signal *(red arrow)* is directed by these structures to fossa ovalis. In utero, this allows oxygenated blood returning from placenta to cross through patent foramen ovale to left atrium.

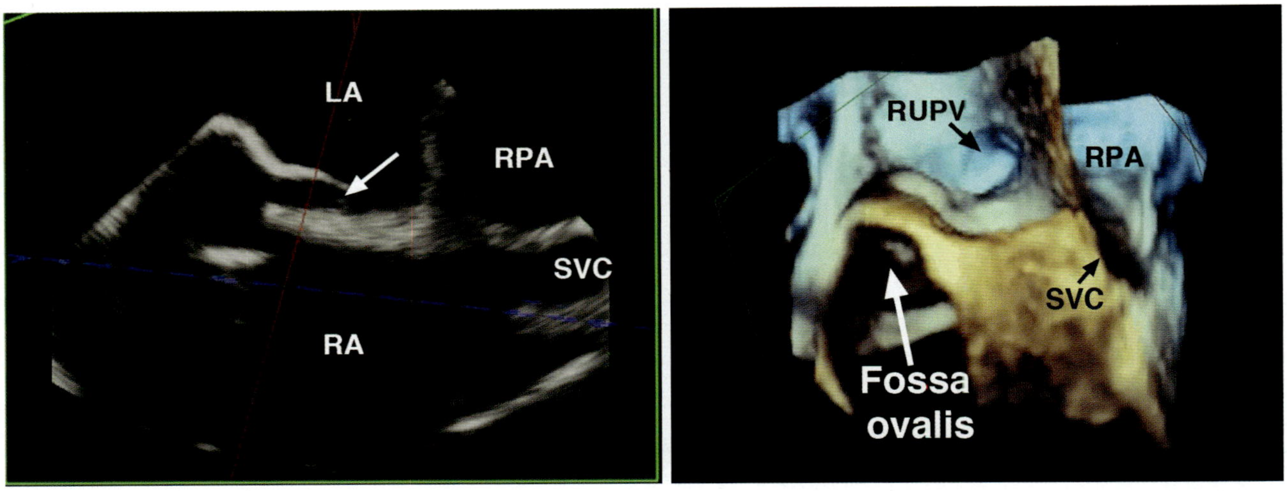

Fig 7.7 In left panel, midesophageal view at approximately 110 degrees shows PFO *(arrow)*. Right panel is corresponding 3D image. In the video, bubbles are seen passing from the RA to LA indicative of a shunt through the PFO.

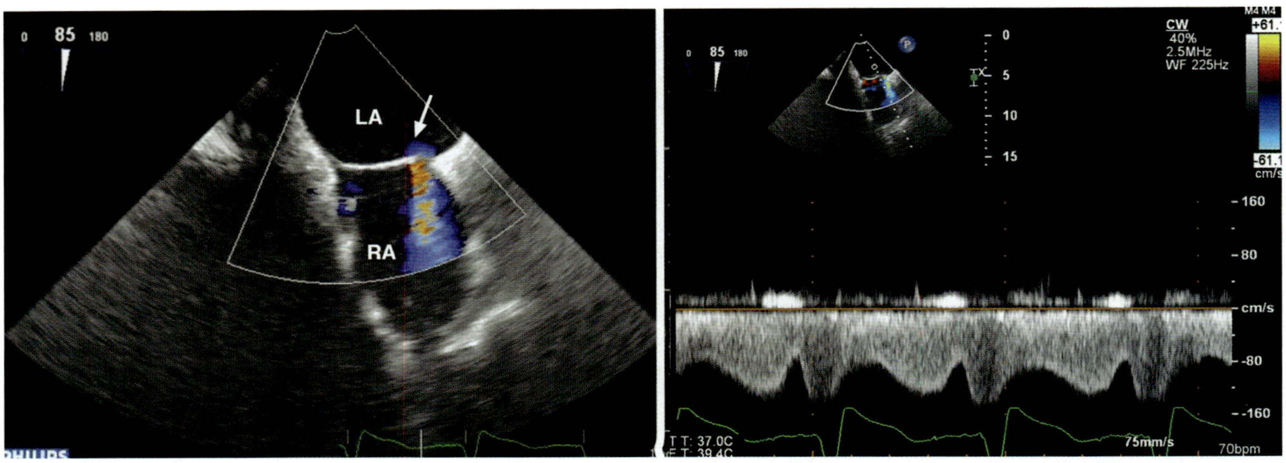

Fig 7.8 At left, color Doppler shows flow through PFO. Arrow indicates flow convergence on left atrial side; both color and spectral Doppler *(right)* indicate that flow is from left atrium to right atrium.

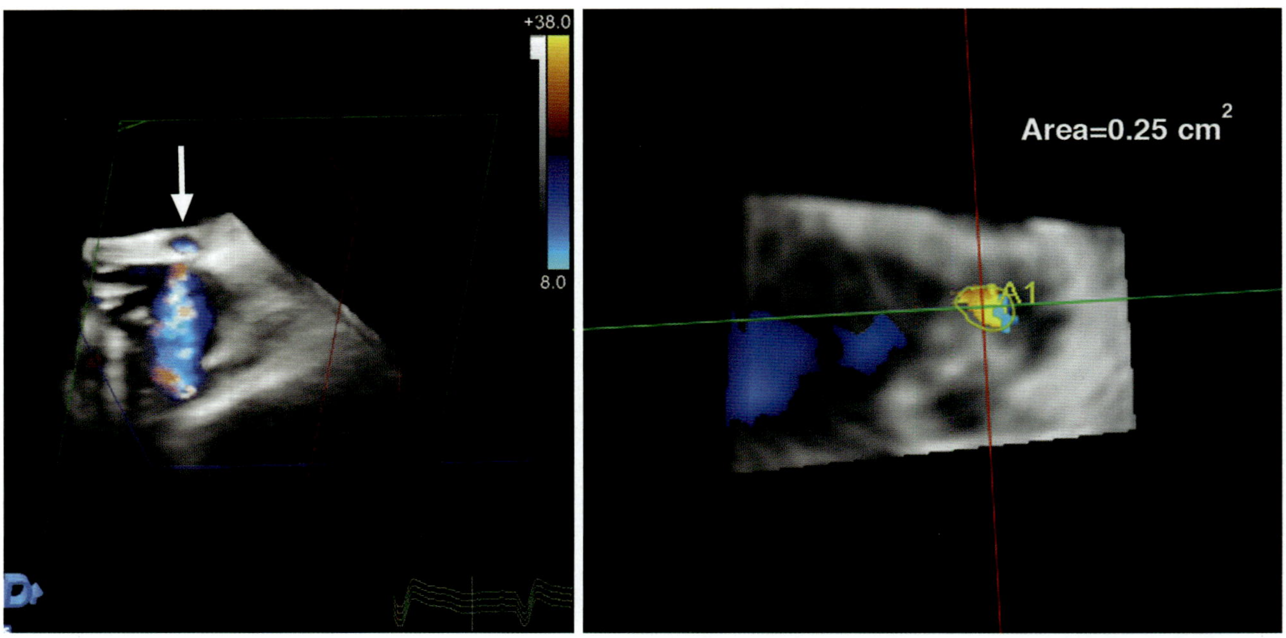

Fig 7.9 3D color Doppler shows hemispherical shape of flow acceleration *(arrow)*. On right, multiplanar reconstruction is used to calculate dimension of PFO.

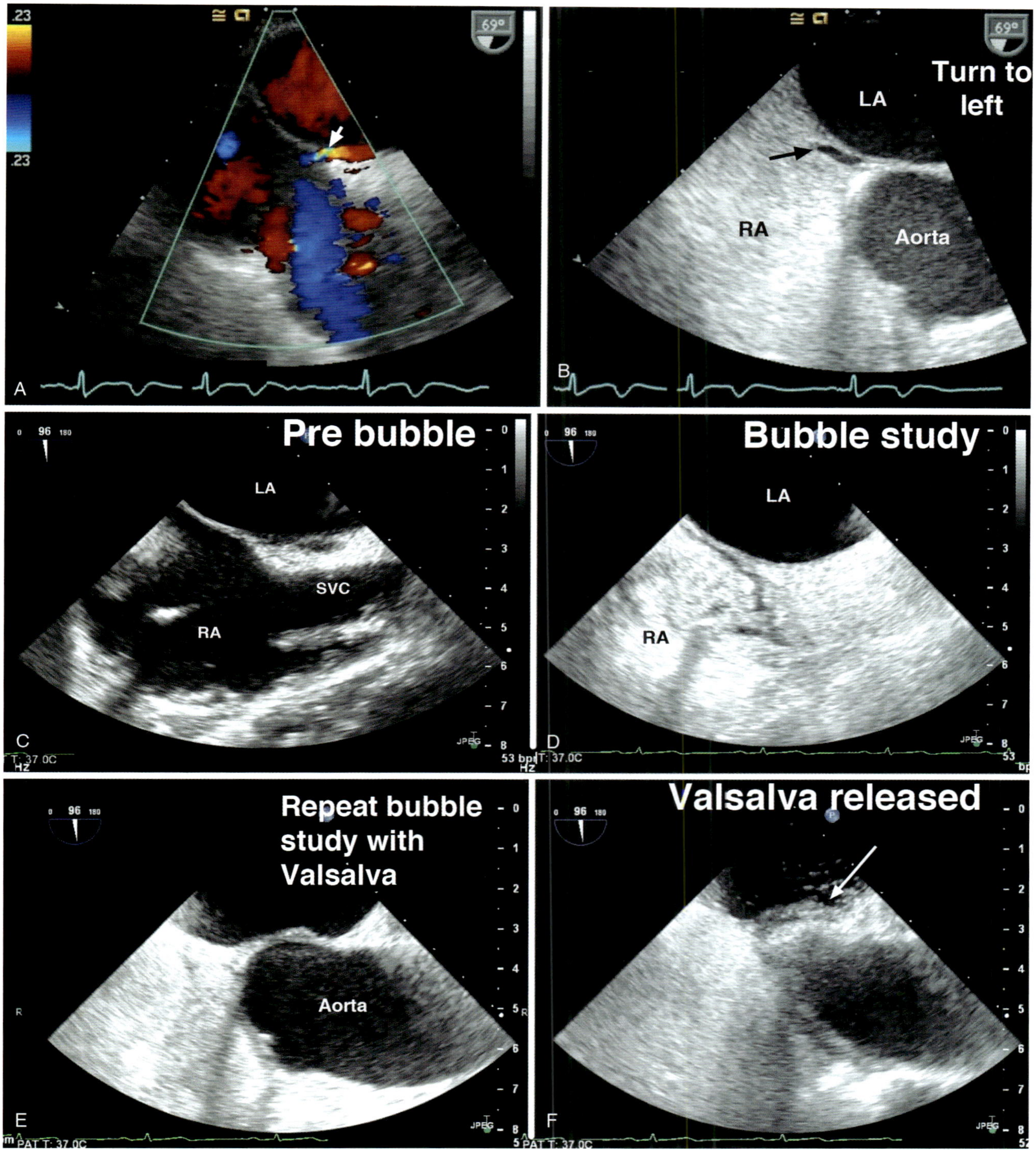

Fig 7.10 In patients in whom PFO is suspected but saline contrast study is negative, there are several diagnostic strategies. In panels **A** and **B**, probe is in midesophageal position with slight turning to patient's left; color Doppler evidence of left-to-right shunt is confirmed by presence of "negative contrast" *(black arrow)* in right atrium. In panels **C** through **F**, first saline contrast study is unequivocally negative; however, injection of contrast with Valsalva maneuver is followed quickly by release of Valsalva, subsequent increase in right atrial pressure, and appearance of microbubbles in left atrium; red arrow in video indicates negative contrast from IVC flow.

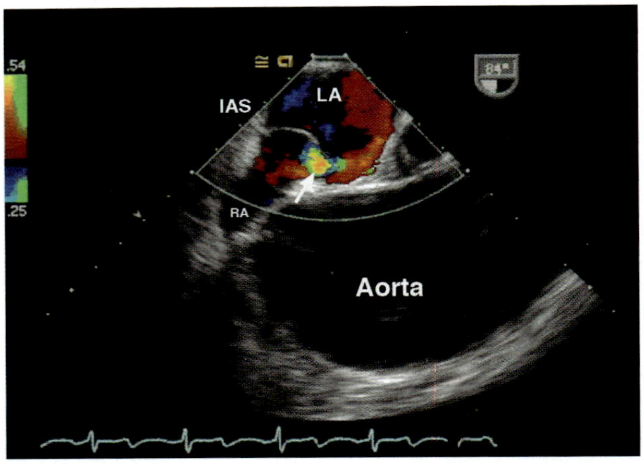

Fig 7.11 In another patient with elevated right atrial pressure secondary to pulmonary hypertension, color Doppler is indicative of right atrial to left atrial flow.

CASE 7-2
Patent Foramen Ovale

Intraoperative transesophageal echocardiography (TEE) in a patient undergoing coronary artery bypass grafting demonstrated a patent foramen ovale (PFO).

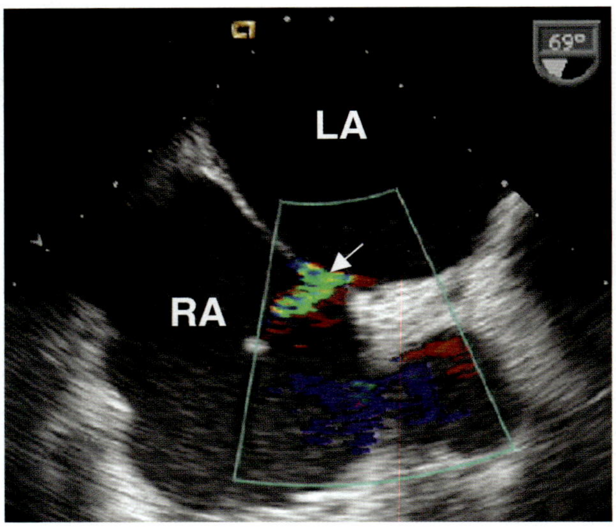

Fig 7.12 View of left atrium (LA) and right atrium (RA) from high esophageal position at 69 degrees rotation demonstrates PFO at limbus of fossa ovalis with color Doppler showing small jet of flow from left to right *(arrow)*.

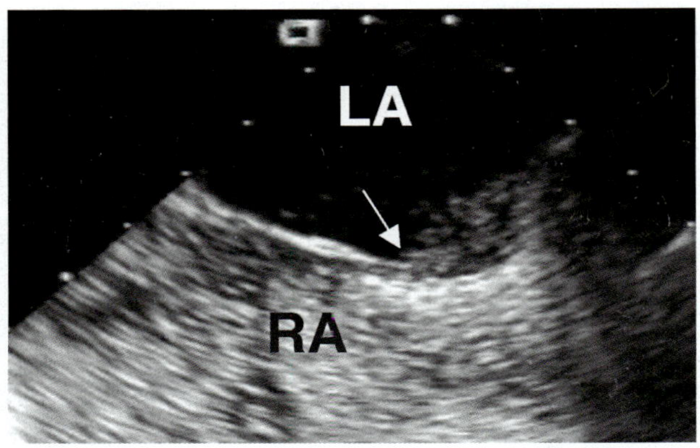

Fig 7.13 Injection of agitated saline in peripheral vein opacifies right heart due to effect of microbubbles. Microbubbles in hand-agitated saline do not pass through pulmonary capillaries, leaving left heart unopacified in absence of intracardiac shunt. In this case, magnified image at about 70 degrees rotation shows passage of contrast from right to left across patent foramen ovale *(arrow)*.

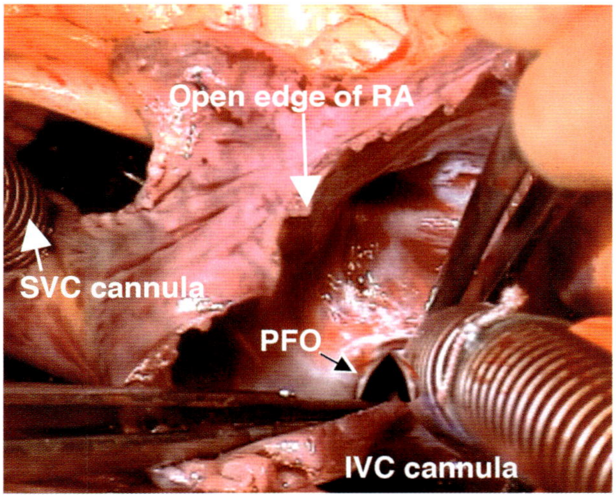

Fig 7.14 Intraoperative view, with right atrium (RA) opened, demonstrates PFO in interatrial septum.

Comments

A PFO can be demonstrated on TEE in 20% to 25% of adults. The PFO typically is best seen from a high esophageal view of the atrial septum, with the transducer rotated between 60 and 90 degrees. The PFO is seen at the junction of the secundum septum (covering the fossa ovalis) and the primum septum. In most patients the PFO is small and functions as a "flap valve," with no flow across the septum when atrial pressures are low and left atrial pressure is slightly higher than right atrial pressure. With a transient elevation in right atrial pressure, for example with Valsalva maneuver, the flap valve opens and blood can flow from right to left. With chronic elevation in atrial pressure, the PFO may become stretched with a defect between the right and left atrium allowing flow, even at rest. A small PFO is typically a benign incidental finding without associated clinical symptoms or signs. However, there is an association between the presence of a PFO and cryptogenic stroke, with studies in progress testing the hypothesis that closing the PFO will decrease the risk of recurrent stroke.

Suggested Reading

1. Asrress KN, Marciniak M, Marciniak A, Rajani R, Clapp B: Patent foramen ovale: the current state of play, Heart 101(23): 1916–1925, 2015.
2. Gupta SK, Shetkar SS, Ramakrishnan S, Kothari SS: Saline contrast echocardiography in the era of multimodality imaging—importance of "bubbling it right". Echocardiography 32(11): 1707–1719, 2015.

CASE 7-3
Atrial Septal Aneurysm

This 48-year-old woman with recurrent neurologic events was found to have an atrial septal aneurysm with evidence of right-to-left shunting on intracardiac echocardiography with agitated saline used for right heart contrast.

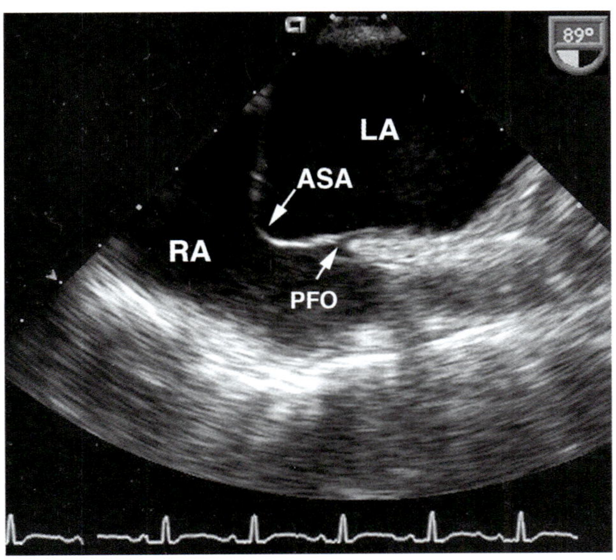

Fig 7.15 In high TEE view at about 90 degree of rotation bulging of atrial septum into RA is seen. Curvature of atrial septum exceeds 1.5 cm and persists in both systole and diastole, consistent with diagnosis of atrial septal aneurysm (ASA). See also small patent foramen ovale.

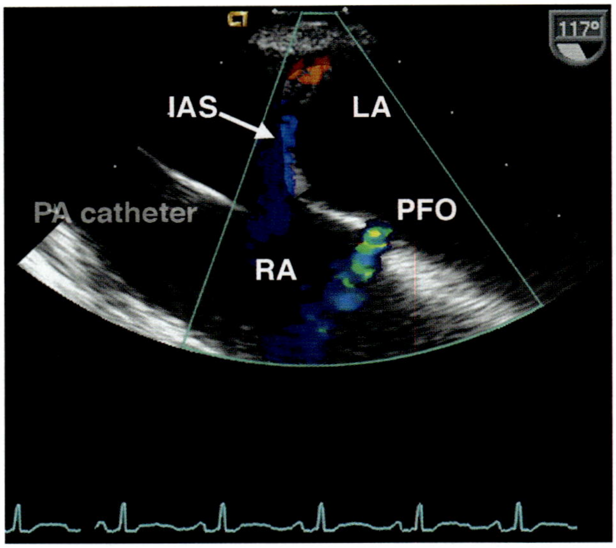

Fig 7.16 Color Doppler demonstrates left-to-right flow across PFO.

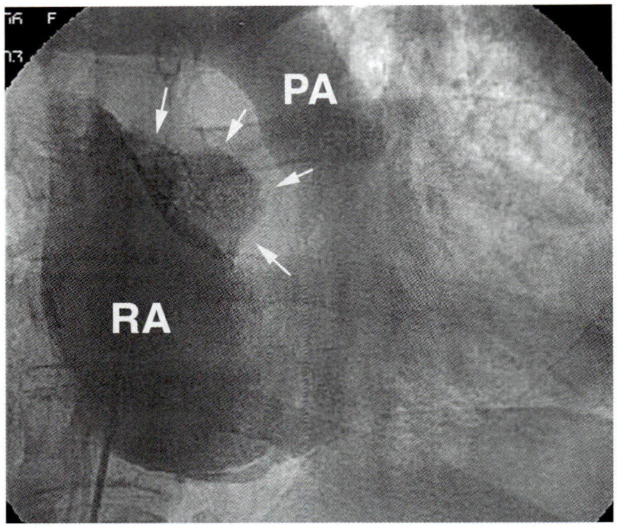

Fig 7.17 Right atrial angiography shows opacified right atrium with septum bulging into left atrium. With elevation of right atrial pressure during angiogram, septal curvature reverses *(arrows)* (see Fig 7.15).

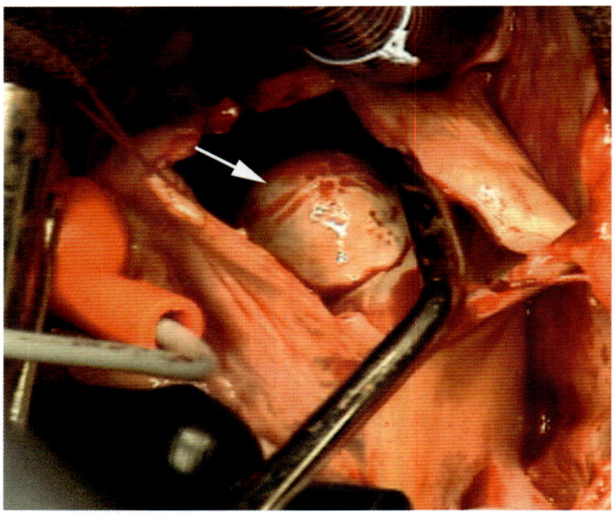

Fig 7.18 Intraoperative view from opened right atrium shows central septum *(arrow)* bulging into right atrium.

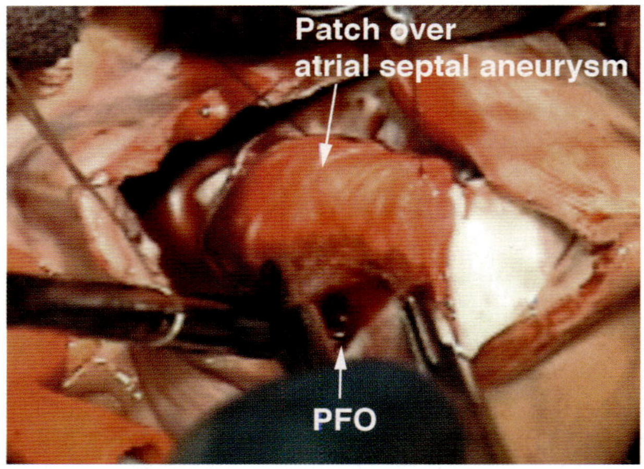

Fig 7.19 At surgery, with right atrium open, large atrial septal aneurysm and small atrial septal defect were plicated and closed using pericardial patch.

Comments

In addition to a PFO, this patient has an atrial septal aneurysm, defined as transient bulging of the fossa ovalis region greater than 1.5 cm in the absence of chronically elevated left or right atrial pressures. The presence of an atrial septal aneurysm is associated with a higher risk of embolic stroke than a PFO alone, most likely related to the high (>90%) prevalence of fenestrations of the septum in patients with a septal aneurysm. In patients with recurrent neurologic events despite adequate medical therapy, PFO closure may be considered, either surgically or using a percutaneously inserted closure device.

Suggested Reading

1. McGrath ER, Paikin JS, Motlagh B, et al: Transesophageal echocardiography in patients with cryptogenic ischemic stroke: a systematic review, Am Heart J 168(5):706–712, 2014.

CASE 7-4
Secundum Atrial Septal Defect

This 50-year-old man presented with increasing shortness of breath on exertion. After a negative pulmonary evaluation, he underwent echocardiography that demonstrated a secundum atrial septal defect (ASD).

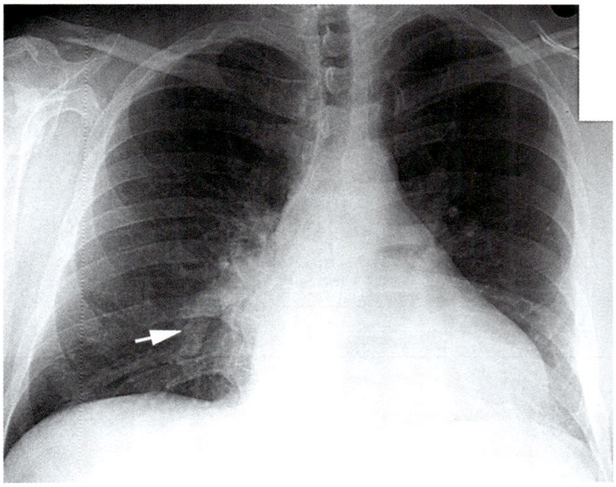

Fig 7.20 PA chest radiograph shows cardiomegaly with prominent right atrial border and enlarged right pulmonary artery *(arrow)*.

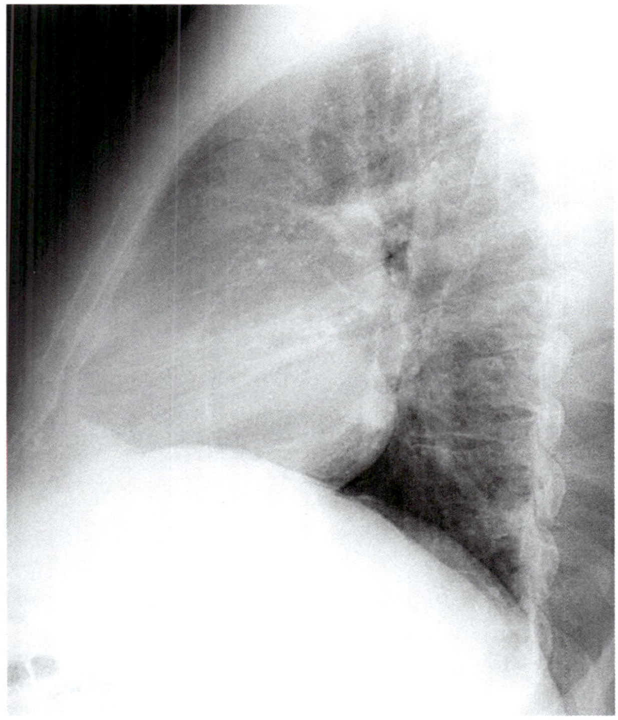

Fig 7.21 On lateral chest radiograph, right ventricular enlargement is evident with opacification of retrosternal space by enlarged right ventricle.

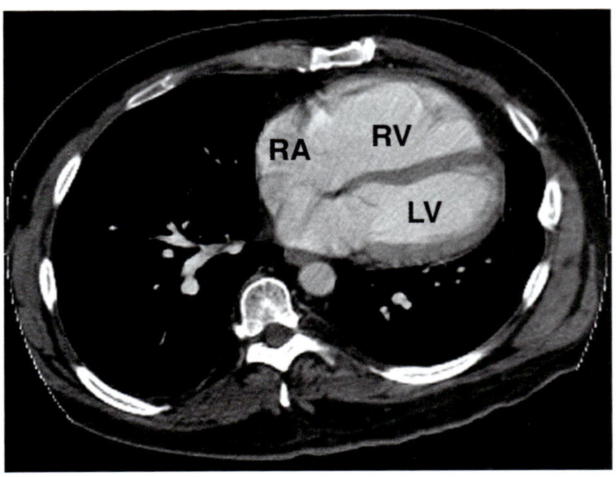

Fig 7.22 Chest CT demonstrates severe right ventricular and right atrial enlargement.

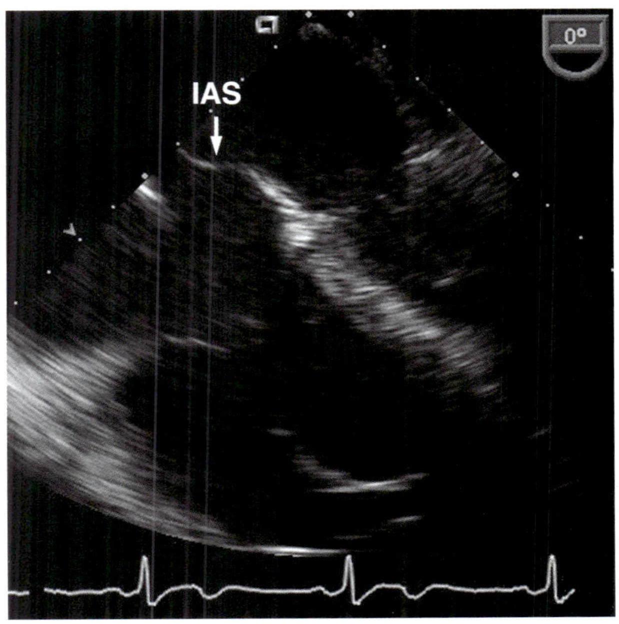

Fig 7.23 TEE four-chamber view shows enlarged right ventricle and atrium, although atrial septum appears intact in this image plane.

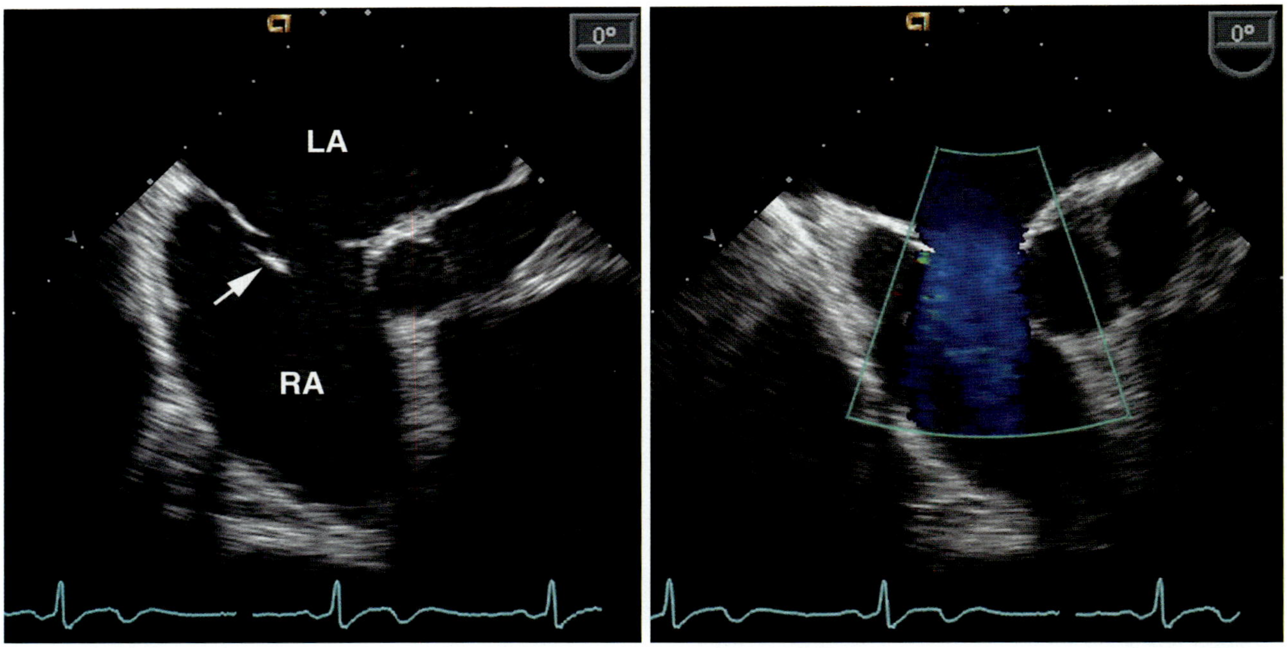

Fig 7.24 Slight anteflexion of probe, with image plane now including aortic valve, demonstrates ASD with left-to-right flow and defect diameter of 18 mm. Arrow indicates pulmonary artery catheter in right atrium.

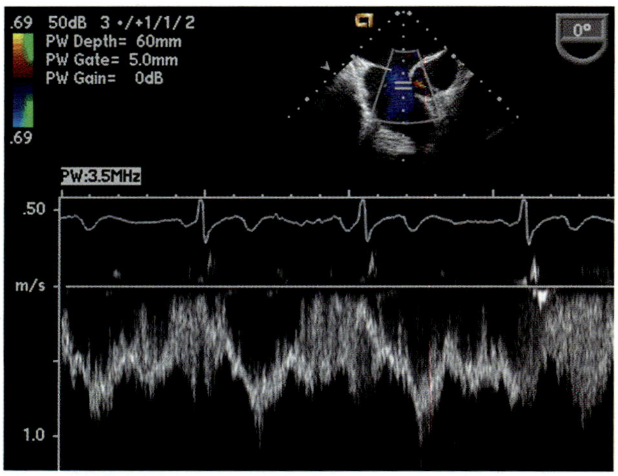

Fig 7.25 Pulsed Doppler confirms left-to-right flow in both systole and diastole.

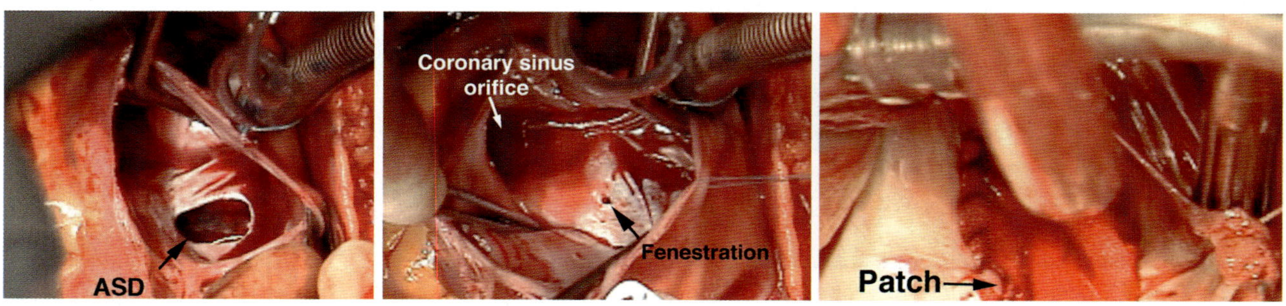

Fig 7.26 After sternotomy, right atrial appendage was noted to be redder than usual, consistent with shunting of oxygenated left atrial blood. Through open right atrium, 2 × 1 cm ASD was identified *(left frame)*. In addition, smaller but separate defect was noted adjacent to tendon of Todaro (at origin of coronary sinus) *(center)*. Both defects were closed with single pericardial patch, with postoperative image demonstrating patch across defect *(right frame)*. Patient had atrial flutter 5 days postoperatively and was easily cardioverted back into sinus rhythm. However, he subsequently had recurrent atrial flutter that was treated with radiofrequency catheter ablation of caval tricuspid isthmus.

Comments

The most common type of atrial septal defect (ASD) is a secundum ASD, with the defect located centrally in the septum typically measuring ≥1 cm diameter. Although most ASDs are diagnosed and treated in childhood, a substantial number are not recognized until young adulthood, with a few diagnosed only later in life, as in this case.

The TEE features of an atrial septal defect are the consequence of right-sided volume overload. Blood flows left to right across the atrial defect so that the right heart pumps a larger stroke volume than the left heart. The severity of shunting is measured as the pulmonary flow (Qp) to systemic flow (Qs) ratio, where 1 is normal. A Qp:Qs ratio >1.5:1 is associated with progressive right atrial and right ventricular enlargement. In addition, ventricular septal curvature is reversed with "paradoxical" septal motion. Pulmonary hypertension is unusual with a secundum ASD. TTE may demonstrate the atrial defect itself with color Doppler showing left-to-right flow. A contrast study can be performed when right heart enlargement is present and images of the atrial septum are suboptimal.

TEE provides better images of the interatrial septum and is helpful when percutaneous closure is planned, to measure the size of the defect and evaluate the rim of tissue that will anchor the device.

Suggested Reading

1. Brickner ME, Hillis LD, Lange RA: Congenital heart disease in adults. First of two parts, N Engl J Med 342:256–263, 2000.
2. Brickner ME, Hillis LD, Lange RA: Congenital heart disease in adults. Second of two parts, N Engl J Med 342:334–342, 2000.
3. Faletra FF, Pedrazzini G, Pasotti E, et al: 3D TEE during catheter-based interventions, JACC Cardiovasc Imaging 7(3):292–308, 2014.

CASE 7-5
Primum Atrial Septal Defect

This 34-year-old asymptomatic woman was incidentally noted to have a murmur, which prompted echocardiography. This study revealed a large primum ASD with left-to-right flow and a Qp:Qs of 2.5:1. In addition, a cleft anterior leaflet of the mitral valve with moderate mitral regurgitation was demonstrated.

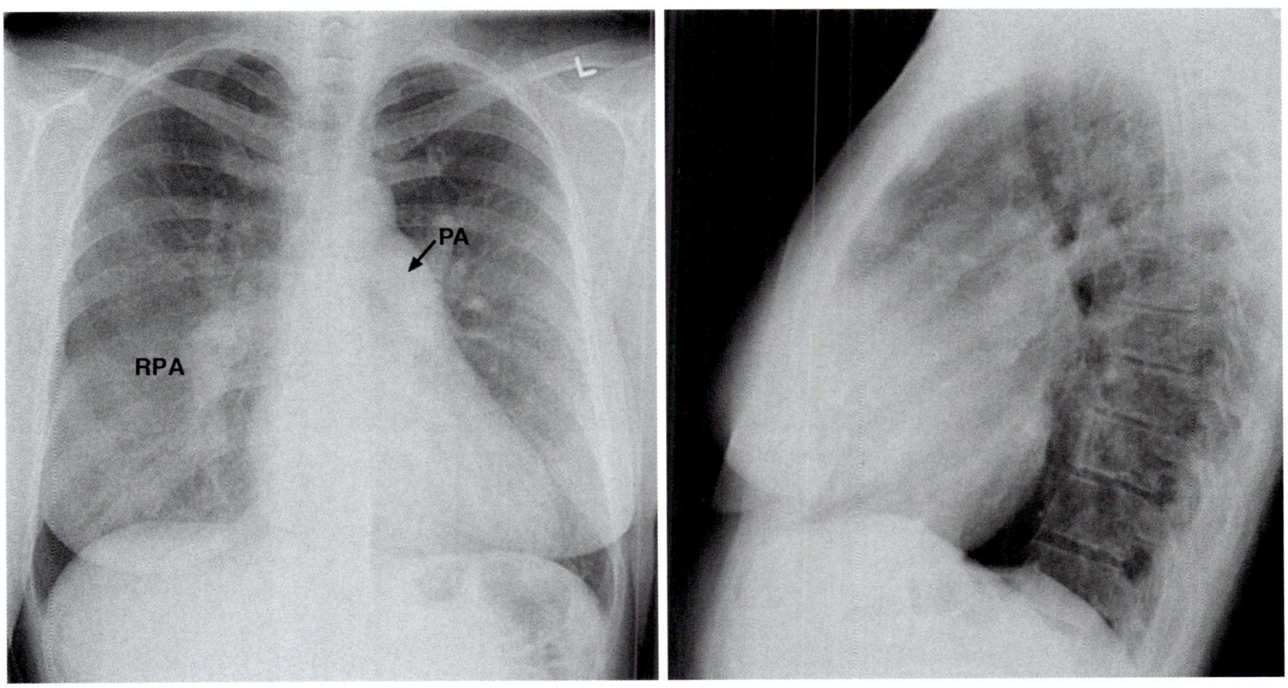

Fig 7.27 Chest radiography shows enlargement of right and left atrium, right ventricle, and pulmonary artery, with increased pulmonary blood flow.

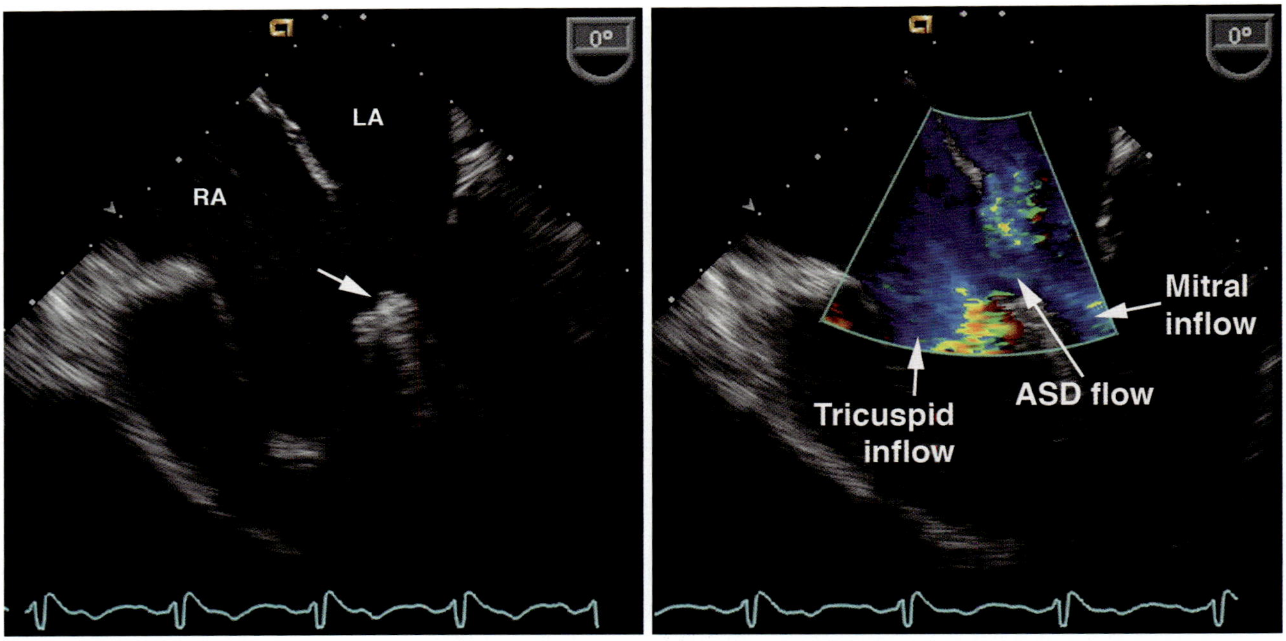

Fig 7.28 In four-chamber view in diastole on 2D *(left)* and color *(right)* crest of ventricle septum is seen *(arrow)* with open tricuspid and mitral valve on either side. With mitral and tricuspid valves open and large atrial defect, all four cardiac chambers have equal pressures in diastole.

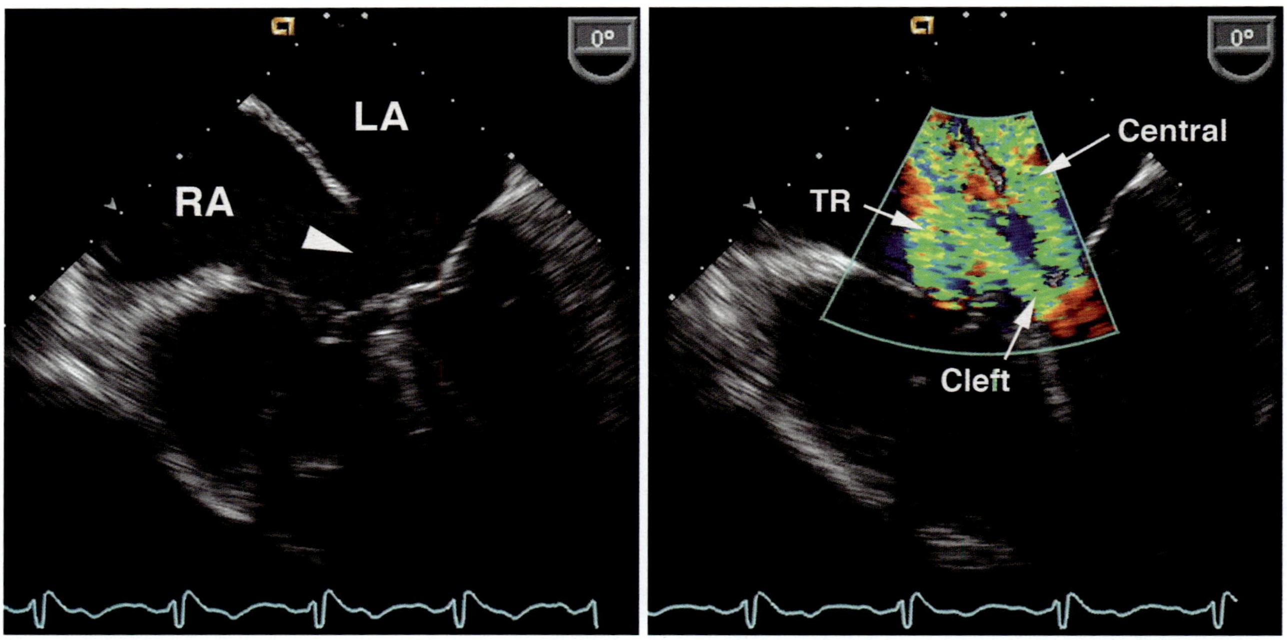

Fig 7.29 In same view in systole, tricuspid and mitral valve are closed. Arrowhead indicates ASD. Moderate-to-severe mitral regurgitation is seen, in part due to cleft anterior mitral valve leaflet.

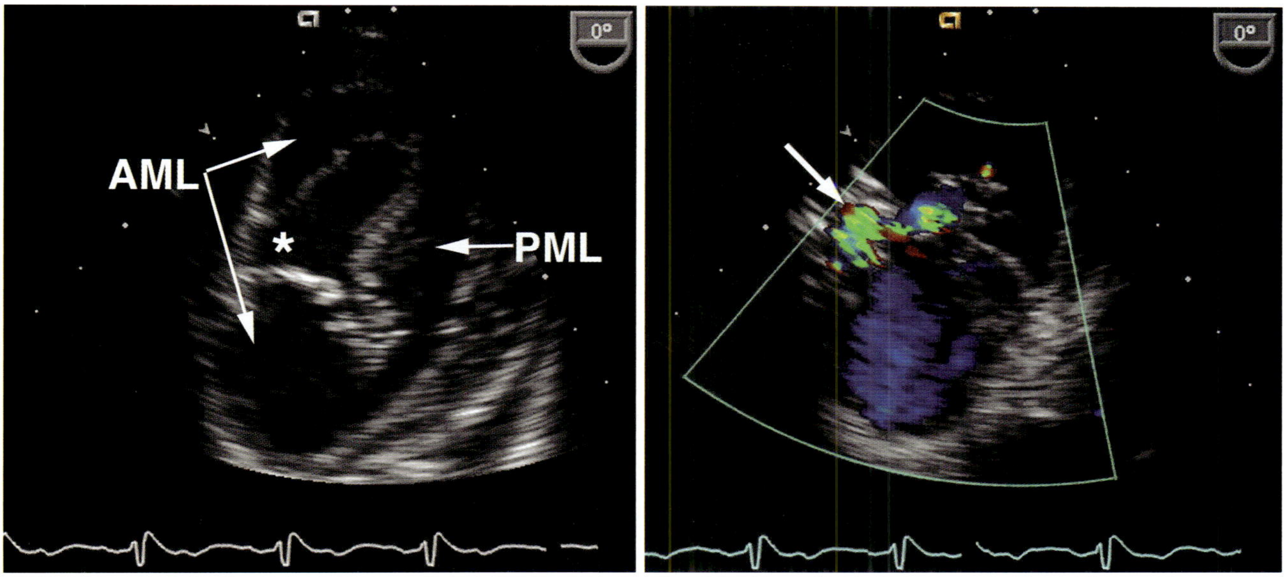

Fig 7.30 Short-axis view of mitral valve obtained with probe retroflexed just distal to gastroesophageal junction, demonstrates cleft *(asterisk)* in anterior mitral leaflet (AML). On right, regurgitant flow is seen through cleft *(arrow)*.

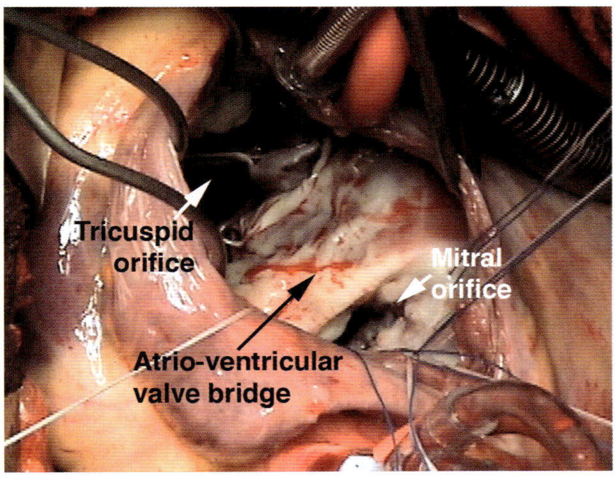

Fig 7.31 At surgery, opening right atrium reveals absence of primum septum, and two atrioventricular valves.

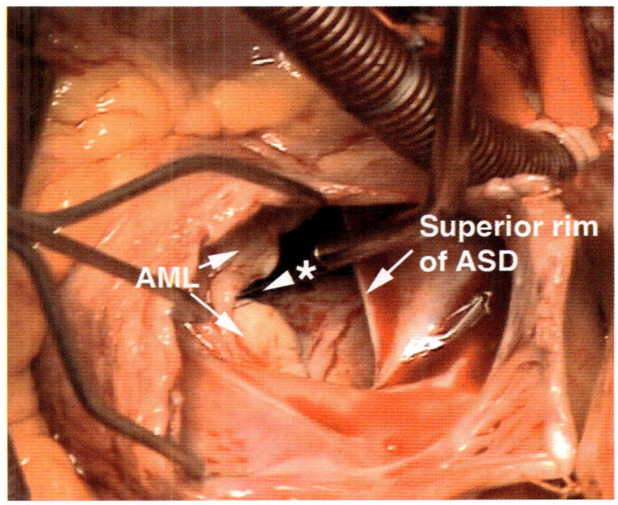

Fig 7.32 Cleft in anterior mitral leaflet is demonstrated *(asterisk)*.

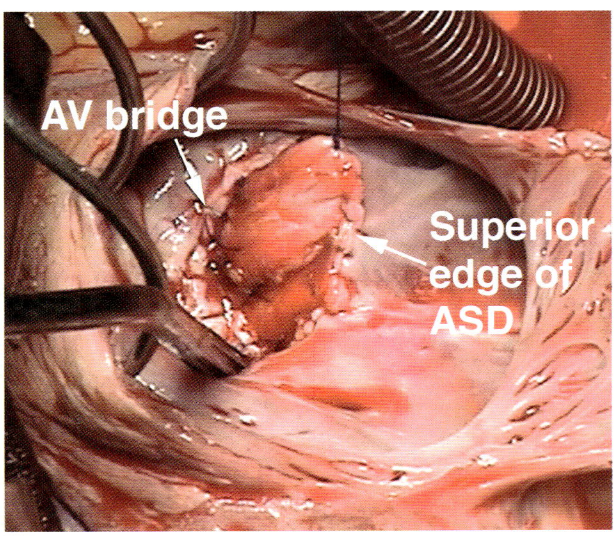

Fig 7.33 At surgery, ostium primum defect was closed with pericardial patch.

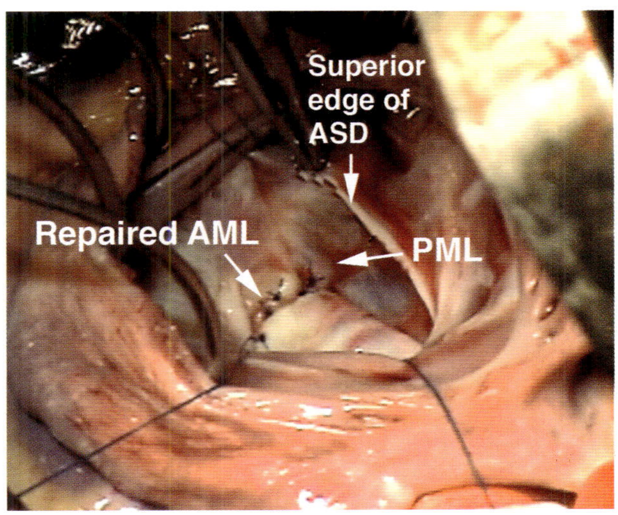

Fig 7.34 Anterior mitral leaflet (AML) was repaired by suturing cleft leaflet and placing 30-mm annuloplasty ring.

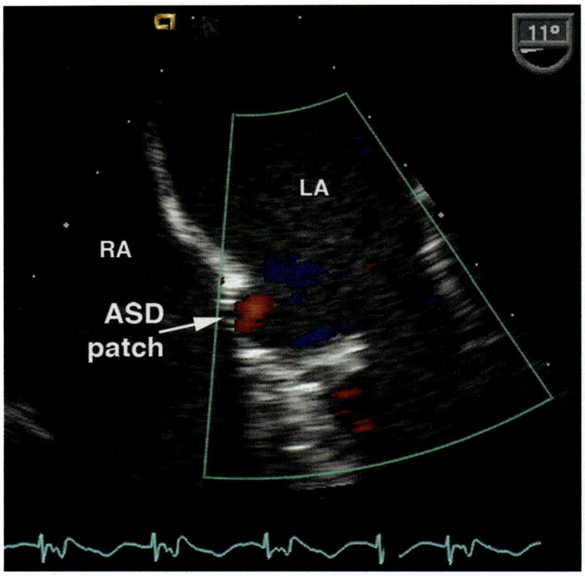

Fig 7.35 Postprocedure four-chamber view shows ASD patch with no residual flow.

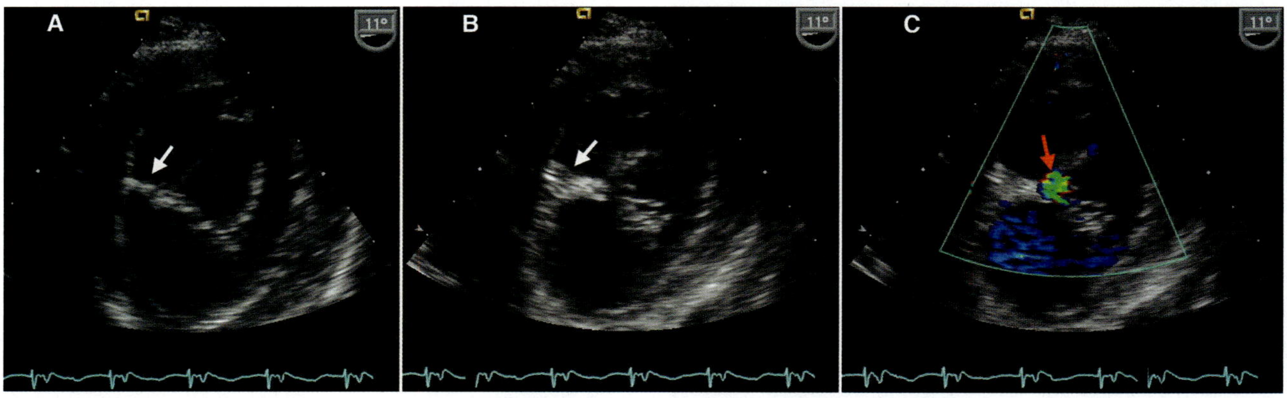

Fig 7.36 Postprocedure short-axis view of mitral valve in diastole **(A)**, and in the same orientation as Fig 7.30, shows repair of cleft leaflet *(white arrow)*. In systole **(B)**, the repair of cleft leaflet *(white arrow)* is again seen, with some residual central mitral regurgitation seen on color Doppler (**C**, *red arrow*).

Comments

A primum ASD is seen in the base of the septum, adjacent to the atrioventricular valve plane and, in effect, is a partial atrioventricular canal defect. The defect is best seen in a four-chamber view, both on 2D imaging and with color Doppler. These defects are large, typically requiring surgical closure with placement of a patch. Many patients have associated abnormalities of the atrioventricular valve, most commonly a cleft anterior mitral valve leaflet. Some cleft leaflets can be repaired by approximation of the two segments, but others require replacement if the valve is deformed or if there is excessive tension when the segments are sutured together. The echocardiographer should also carefully evaluate for a ventricular septal defect (VSD) in patients with a primum ASD.

Suggested Reading

1. Mahmood F: Perioperative transesophageal echocardiography: Current status and future direction, Heart 102:1159–1167, 2016.
2. Randolph GR, Hagler DJ, Connolly HM, et al: Intraoperative transesophageal echocardiography during surgery for congenital heart defects, J Thorac Cardiovasc Surg 124:1176–1182, 2002.

CASE 7-6
Primum Atrial Septal Defect with Previous Atrioventricular Canal Defect Repair

The patient, a 29-year-old woman, who had an atrioventricular canal defect repaired as a child, presents with increasing shortness of breath, and on TTE was found to have a residual left-to-right shunt at the atrial level, most likely from a residual atrial septal defect. Mitral regurgitation and a persistent left superior vena cava were also present.

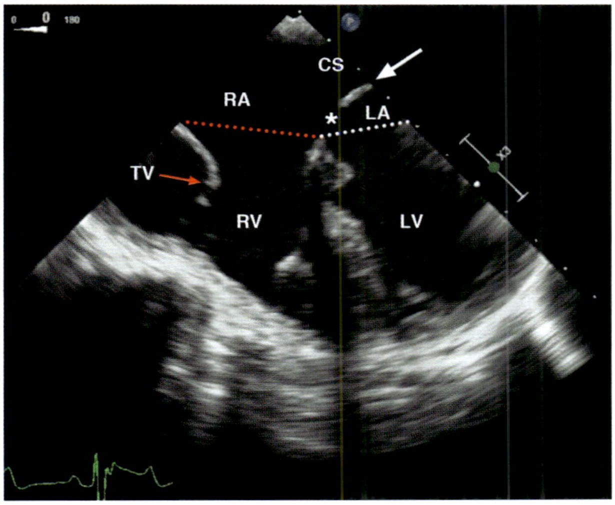

Fig 7.37 Complex anatomy is demonstrated in this diastolic midesophageal four-chamber view. Red dotted line indicates tricuspid annulus, whereas white dotted line indicates mitral annulus. White arrow indicates interatrial septum, and asterisk, primum ASD. Large coronary sinus (CS) can be seen emptying into right atrium, just above tricuspid valve.

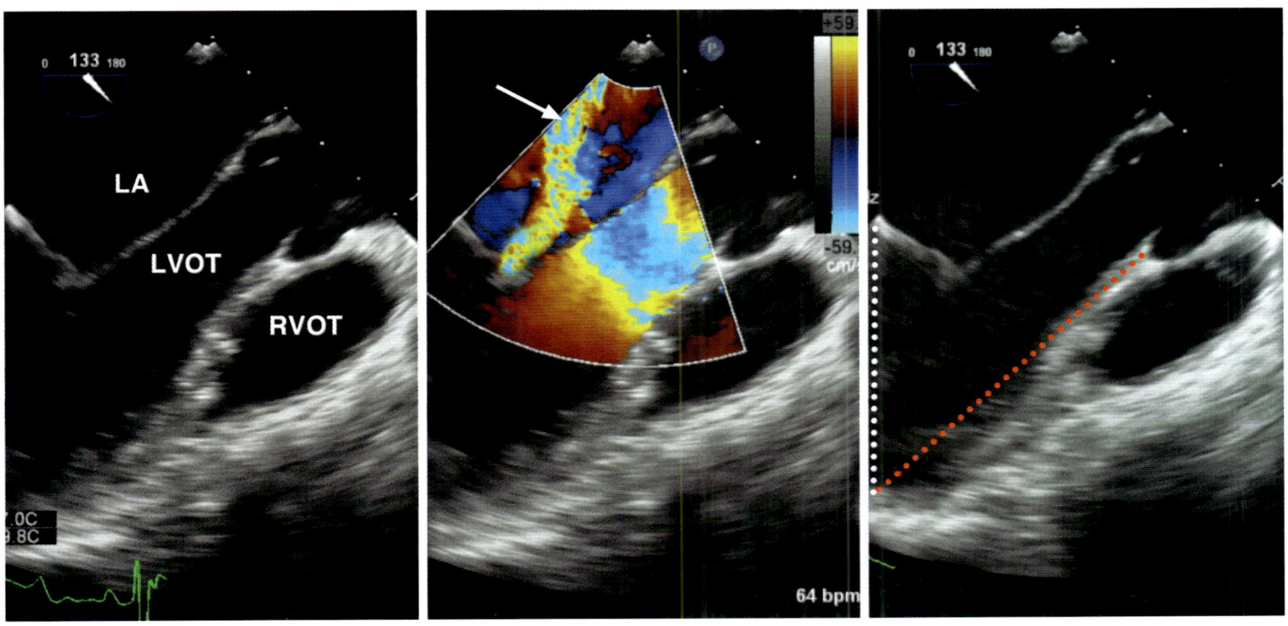

Fig 7.38 In this midesophageal long-axis view during systole, left and center panels show central jet of mitral regurgitation *(arrow)*, and flow in left ventricular outflow tract. Right panel demonstrates so-called "goose-neck" deformity in which distance from left ventricular apex to posterior mitral annulus *(white dotted line)* is 20% to 25% shorter than distance from left ventricular apex to aortic annulus *(red dotted line)*.

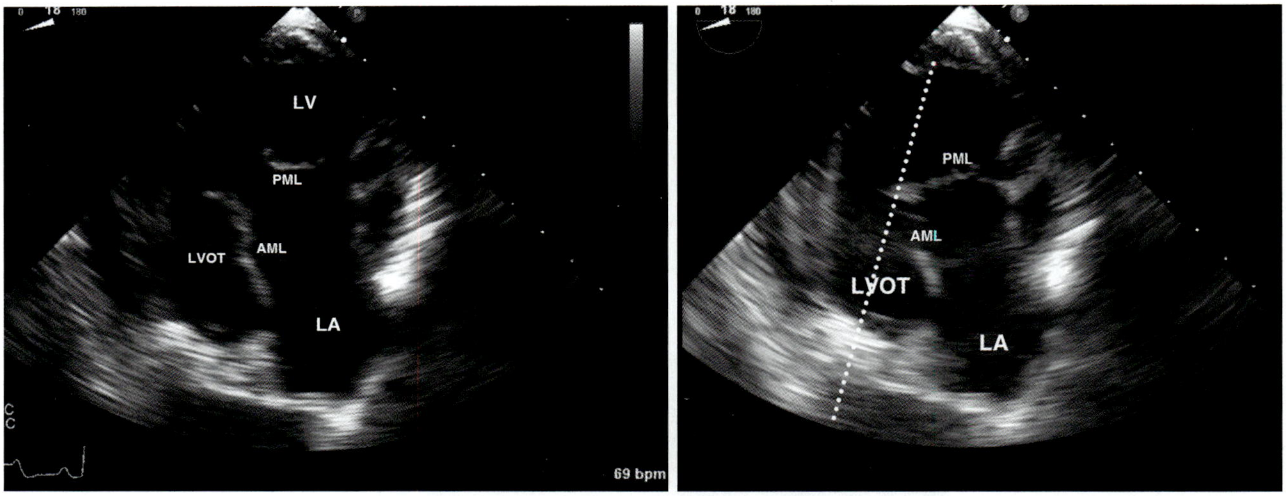

Fig 7.39 In this deep transgastric image, left frame is in diastole. In systolic frame on right, dashed line indicates that continuous wave Doppler can be aligned reasonably parallel to flow to measure gradient in left ventricular outflow tract (LVOT).

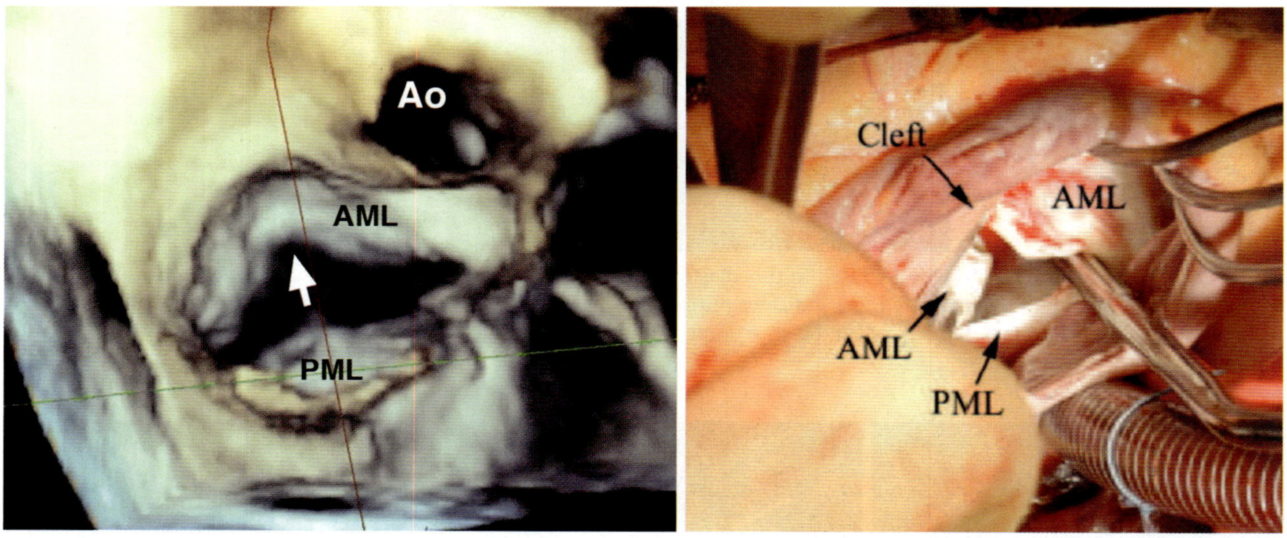

Fig 7.40 On left is 3D TEE of mitral valve from left atrial perspective, in which partial cleft in anterior leaflet of mitral valve is noted *(arrow)*. On right is valve as seen in surgical field.

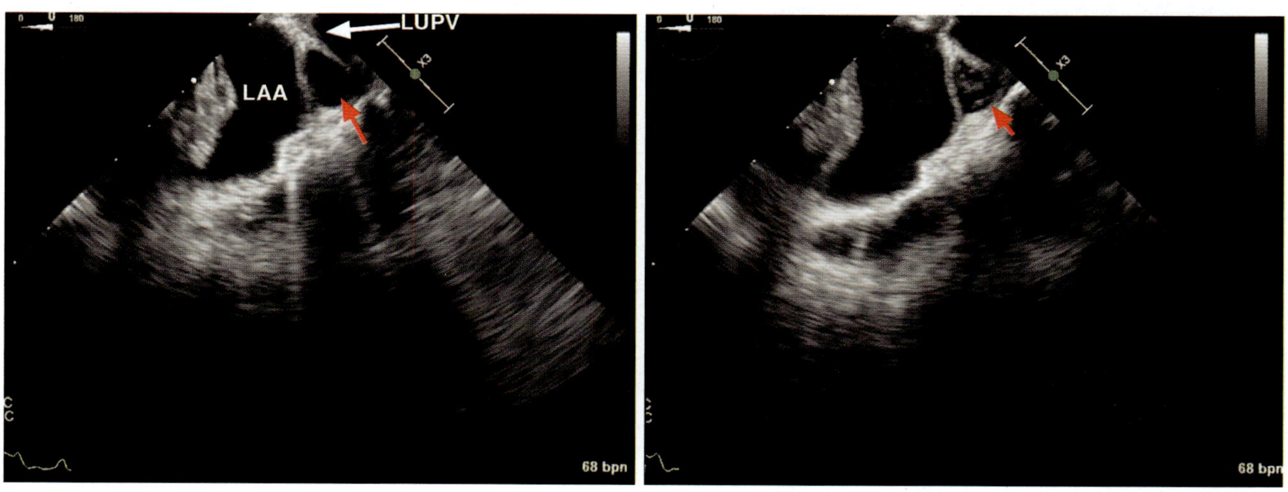

Fig 7.41 In this midesophageal image rotated to patient's left, left atrial appendage, left upper pulmonary vein (LUPV), and persistent left superior vena cava *(red arrow)* are seen. On right, agitated saline is seen in persistent left superior vena cava after injection of saline in left antecubital vein.

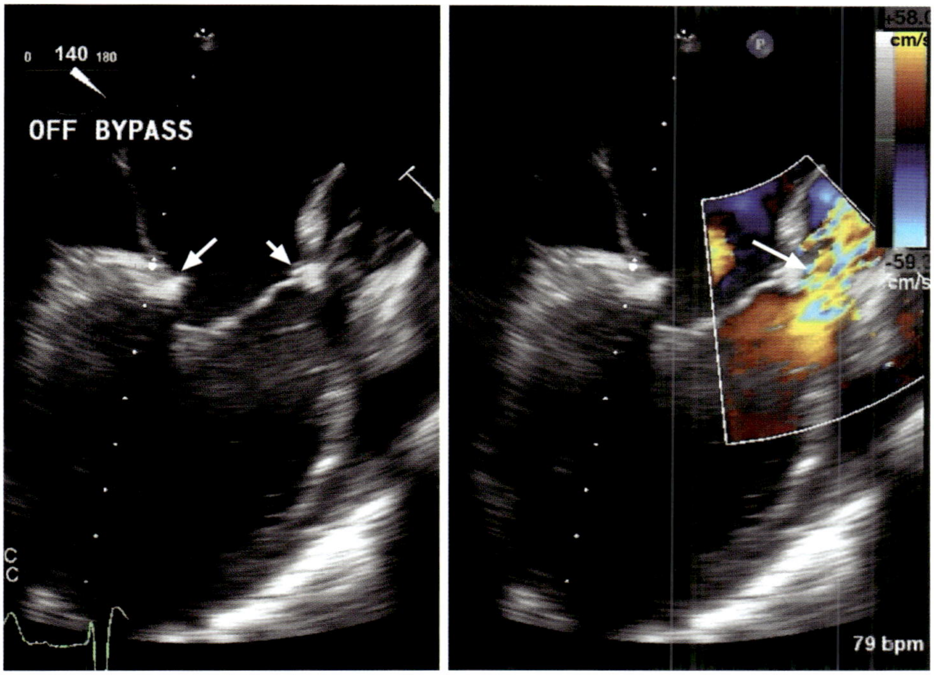

Fig 7.42 Intraoperatively, atrial septal defect was closed successfully with pericardial patch, cleft in anterior mitral leaflet repaired, and mitral ring annuloplasty placed. However, as seen in this midesophageal long-axis view, ring annuloplasty *(white arrows)* is displaced anteriorly, producing narrowing and turbulence in left ventricular outflow tract.

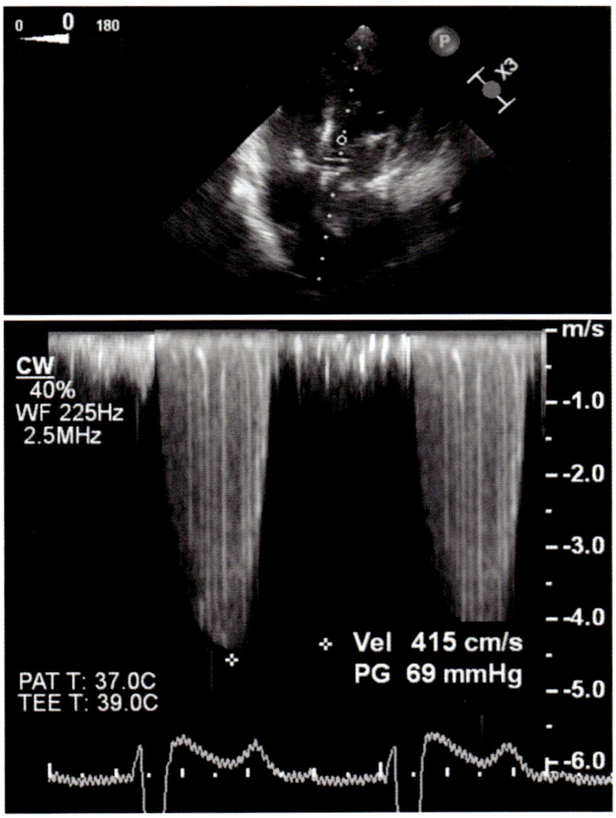

Fig 7.43 From deep transgastric view, late-peaking systolic left ventricular outflow tract velocity of 4.2 m/s, corresponding to peak gradient of 69 mm Hg, was measured.

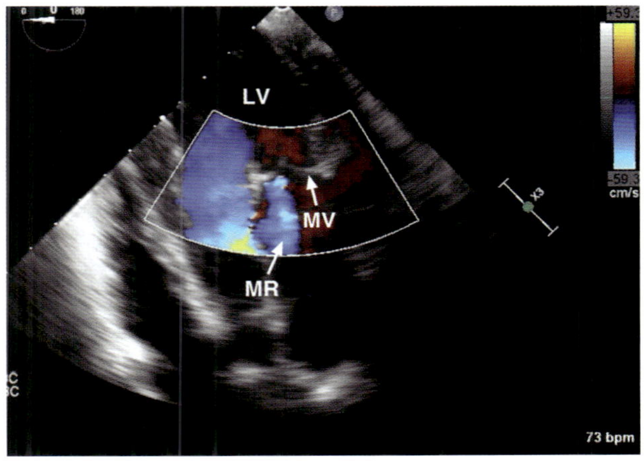

Fig 7.44 Patient was returned to cardiopulmonary bypass. Because of outflow tract gradient, annuloplasty ring was removed. After second separation from cardiopulmonary bypass, there was no longer any evidence for obstruction in outflow tract with normal blue laminar flow seen in this transgastric apical view. Only mild to moderate amount of mitral regurgitation (MR) remained.

Comments

This case illustrates the utility of intraoperative TEE guidance during surgery for complex congenital heart disease. Recognition of subaortic obstruction due to the annuloplasty ring impinging on the narrow LV outflow tract in this patient with a history of an AV canal defect resulting in prompt correction at the same surgical procedure.

Suggested Reading

1. De Mey N, Couture P, Denault AY, et al: Subaortic stenosis after atrioventricular septal defect repair, Anesth Analg 113:236–238, 2011.
2. Kutty S, Smallhorn JF: Evaluation of atrioventricular septal defects by three-dimensional echocardiography: benefits of navigating the third dimension, J Am Soc Echocardiogr 25(9): 932–944, 2012.

CASE 7-7
Sinus Venosus Atrial Septal Defect

This 34-year-old man presented with increasing fatigue, shortness of breath, and palpitations. After an episode of atrial fibrillation, he underwent echocardiography, which showed a probable ASD with moderate right ventricular and right atrial enlargement. TEE demonstrated the anatomy of the sinus venosus defect, with a maximum diameter of 2.4 cm. Right heart catheterization showed normal right heart pressures with a Qp:Qs ratio of 2.5:1.

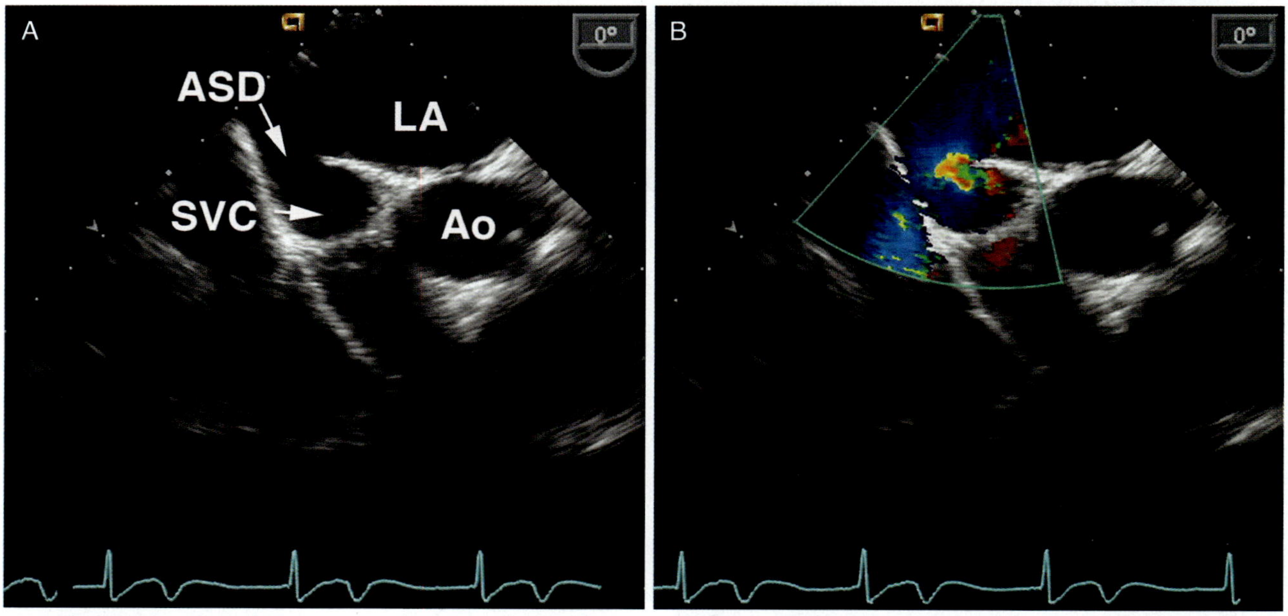

Fig 7.45 From high TEE position at 0 degrees, communication (*arrow*, ASD) between superior vena cava (SVC) and left atrium (LA) is seen (**A**). Color flow demonstrates low-velocity flow through this region (**B**).

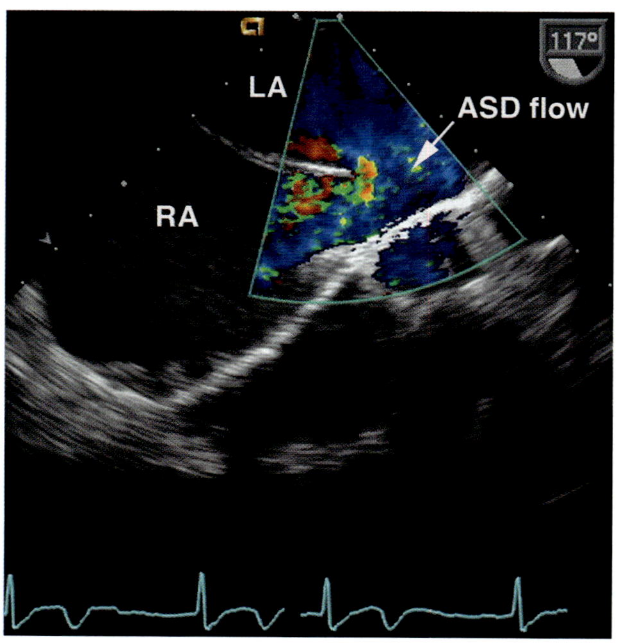

Fig 7.46 Color flow demonstrates flow between two atria at superior aspect of atrial septum.

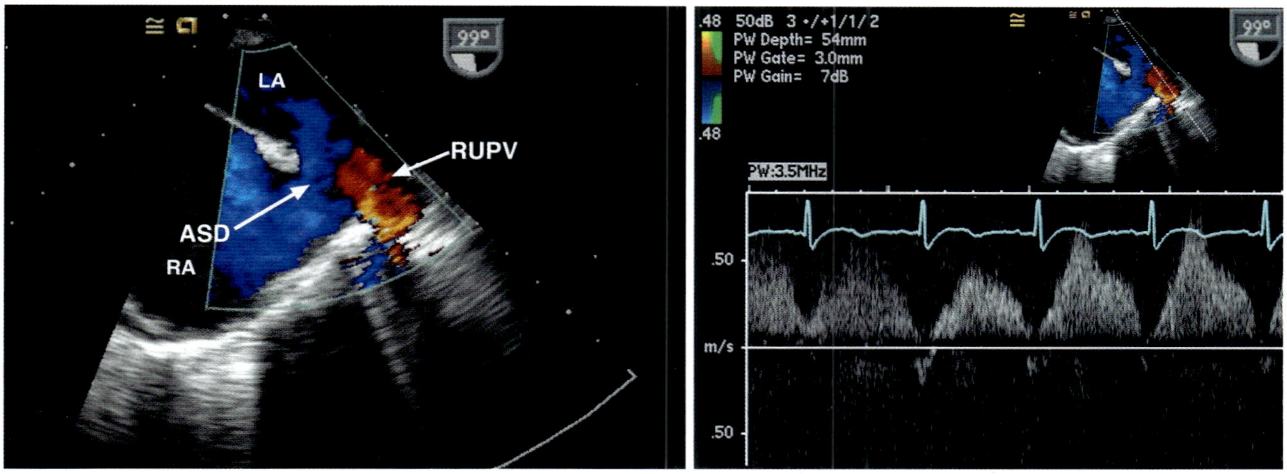

Fig 7.47 With probe further rotated to patient's right, right upper pulmonary venous flow as well as atrial septal defect flow is seen. Pulsed wave Doppler reveals characteristic pulmonary venous tracing.

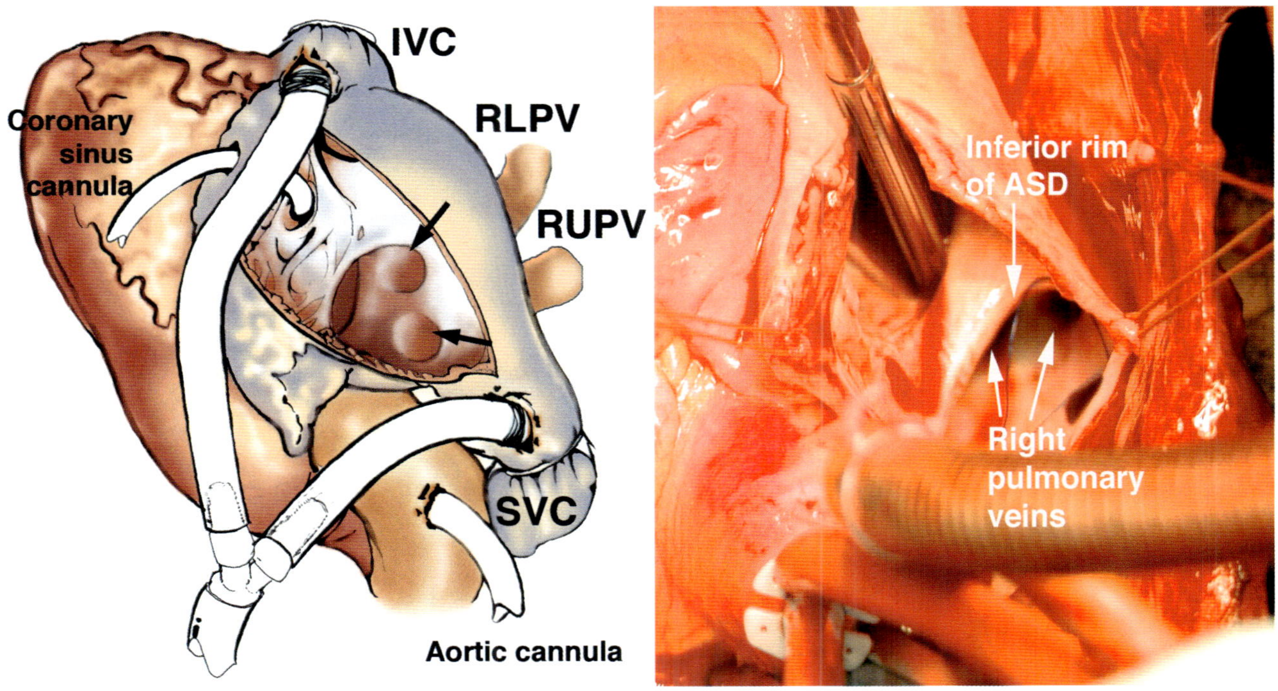

Fig 7.48 Schematic drawing of surgical findings with ASD straddling right upper and lower pulmonary veins *(arrows)*. Cannulas are present in superior and inferior vena cava and in ascending aorta for cardiopulmonary bypass. On right is corresponding intraoperative photograph. (Courtesy of Starr Kaplan.)

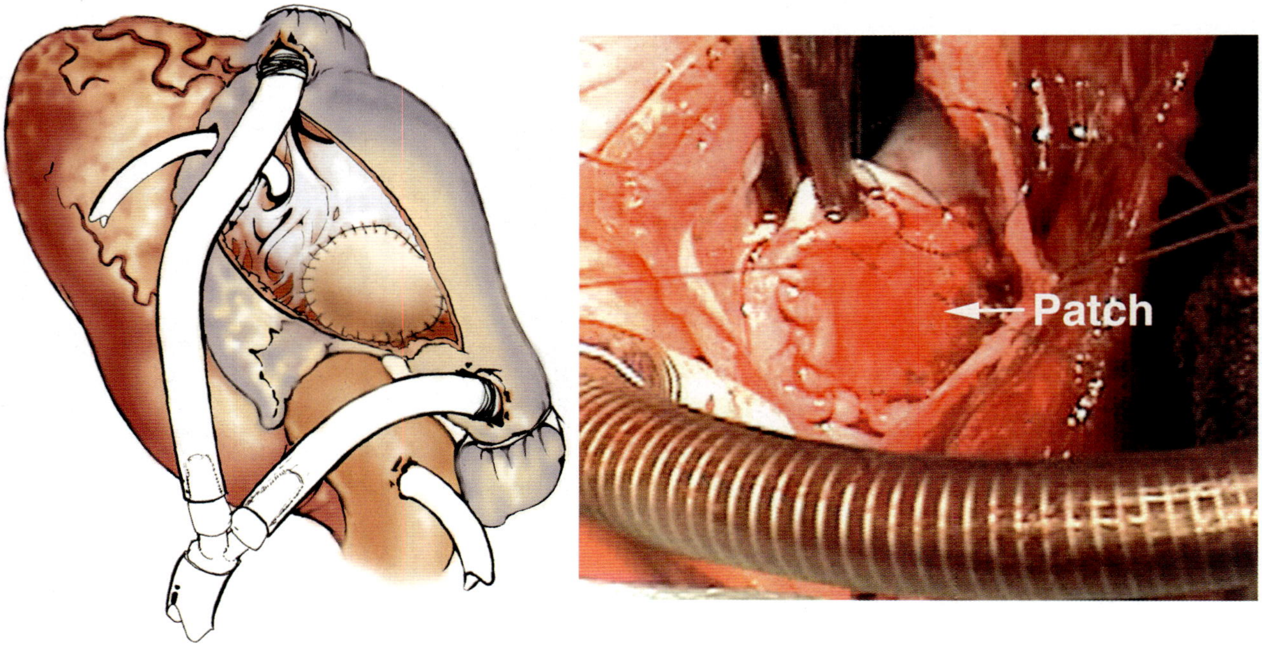

Fig 7.49 As shown in this schematic, defect was closed using double-patch repair technique, including repositioning pulmonary venous drainage to left side of septum. On right is corresponding intraoperative photograph. (Drawing courtesy of Starr Kaplan.)

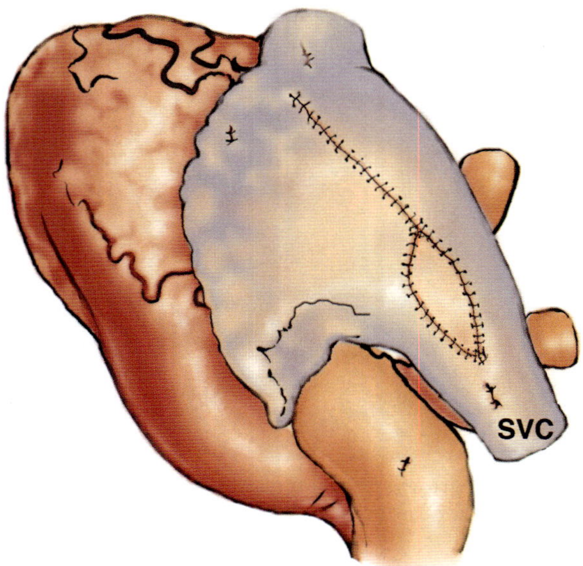

Fig 7.50 Heart is decannulated. Closure of right atrium extends to include distal part of superior vena cava (SVC). (Courtesy of Starr Kaplan.)

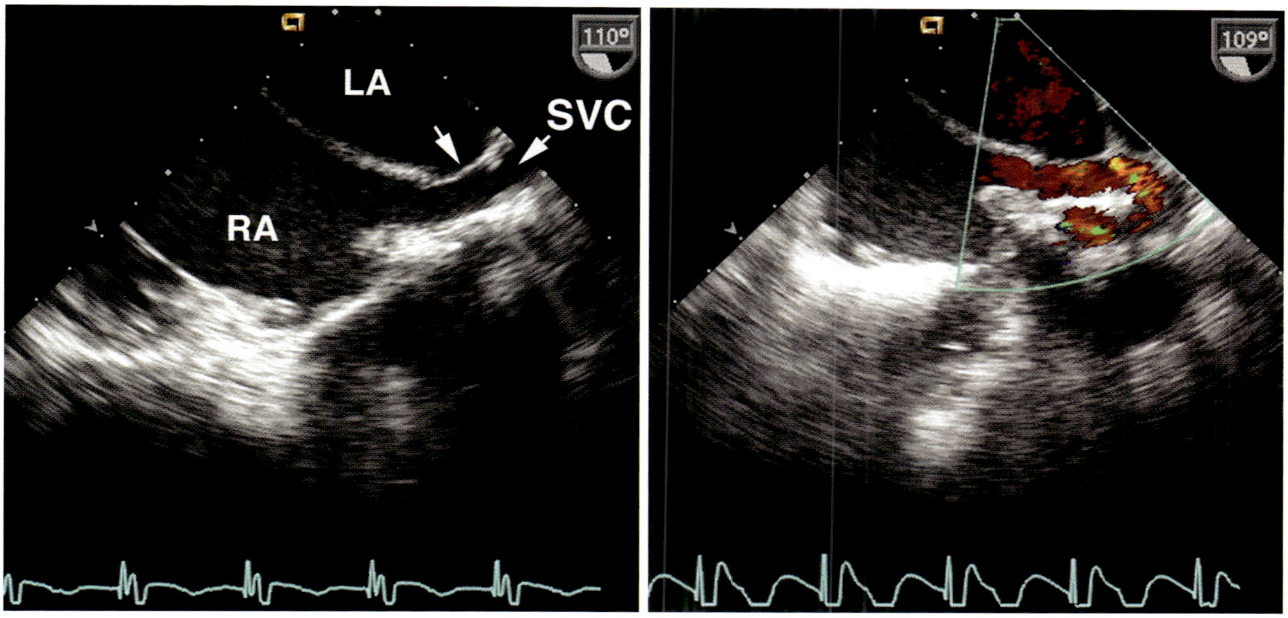

Fig 7.51 Postoperative TEE image at 110 degrees shows patch repair of defect *(arrow)* with no residual interatrial flow *(right)* on color Doppler.

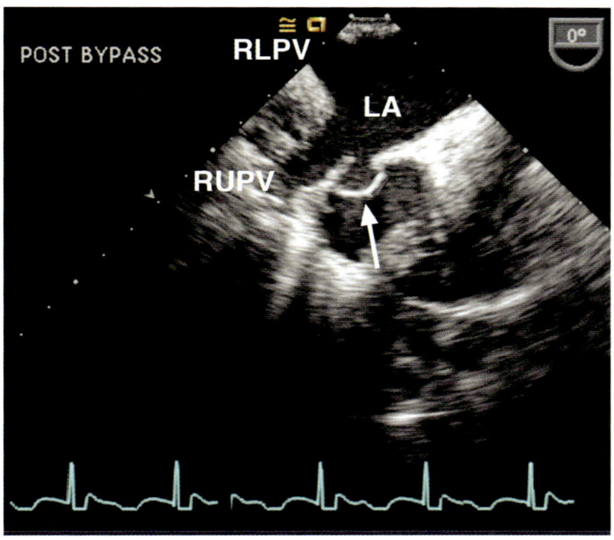

Fig 7.52 Postoperative TEE image at 0 degrees shows patch repair of defect *(arrow)*. Both right-sided pulmonary veins drain into left atrium.

Comments

Sinus venosus defects are most often located at the superior aspect of the atrial septum near the junction with the superior vena cava, although some are found near the junction of the inferior vena cava and right atrium. Diagnosis can be difficult on transthoracic echocardiography (TEE) because the atrial septum appears intact in most views. Often the diagnosis is suspected based on the presence of right heart enlargement and a positive contrast study, with the defect itself only visualized on TEE. Even with TEE imaging, these defects can be missed unless care is taken to examine the entire atrial septum, including the segments at the entrance of the superior and inferior vena cava. Sinus venous defects may be associated with anomalous entry of one or more pulmonary veins into the right atrium, as in this case. On TEE, the examiner should take time to identify all four pulmonary veins and the atria to which they drain.

Suggested Reading

1. Martin SS, Shapiro EP, Mukherjee M: Atrial septal defects—clinical manifestations, echo assessment, and intervention, Clin Med Insights Cardiol 8(Suppl 1):93–98, 2015.

CASE 7-8
Coronary Sinus Atrial Septal Defect

A 35-year-old man presented with increasing shortness of breath, and episodes of paroxysmal atrial fibrillation. On transthoracic echocardiography a bubble study was positive with no obvious PFO nor secundum atrial septal defect. Further investigations showed a markedly enlarged coronary sinus, an unroofed coronary sinus atrial septal defect, and the absence of a left superior vena cava. Calculation of his pulmonary to systemic blood flow ratio was estimated at 1.9:1. There was RA and RV enlargement.

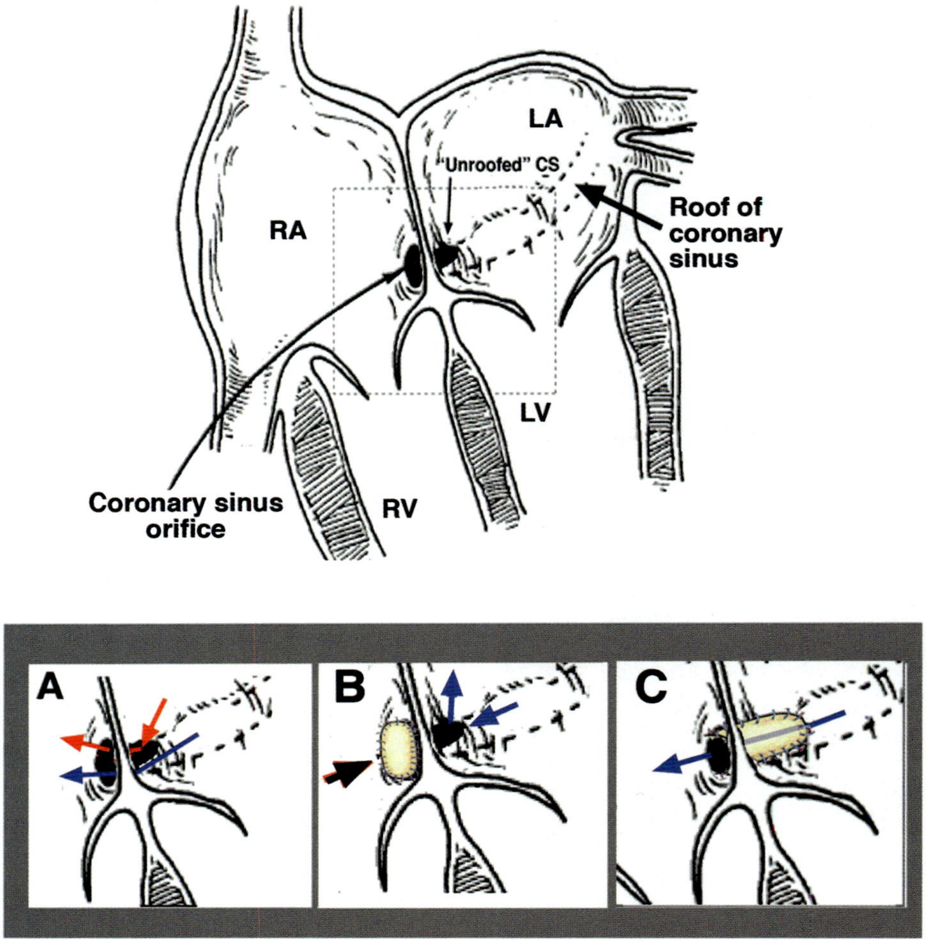

Fig 7.53 In this illustration, fenestration or "unroofing" of portion of coronary sinus is demonstrated. In left inset, left and right atria can communicate through unroofed portion of coronary sinus and coronary sinus ostium *(red arrow).* Blue arrows represent coronary sinus flow that drains normally though coronary sinus ostium and into right atrium. In middle inset, patch covers coronary sinus ostium, so that coronary sinus blood shunts through unroofed portion into left atrium; if there is persistent left superior vena cava, this option is contraindicated because of large shunt that would result. In right inset, pericardial baffle covers unroofed portion of coronary sinus, and by suturing baffle to coronary sinus ostium directs all coronary sinus blood into right atrium while preventing any interatrial shunt. This option is indicated with persistence of left superior vena cava. (From Quaegebeur J, Kirklin JW, Pacifico AD, Bargeron Jr LM: Surgical experience with unroofed coronary sinus. Ann Thor Surg 27:418–425, 1979. Used with permission.)

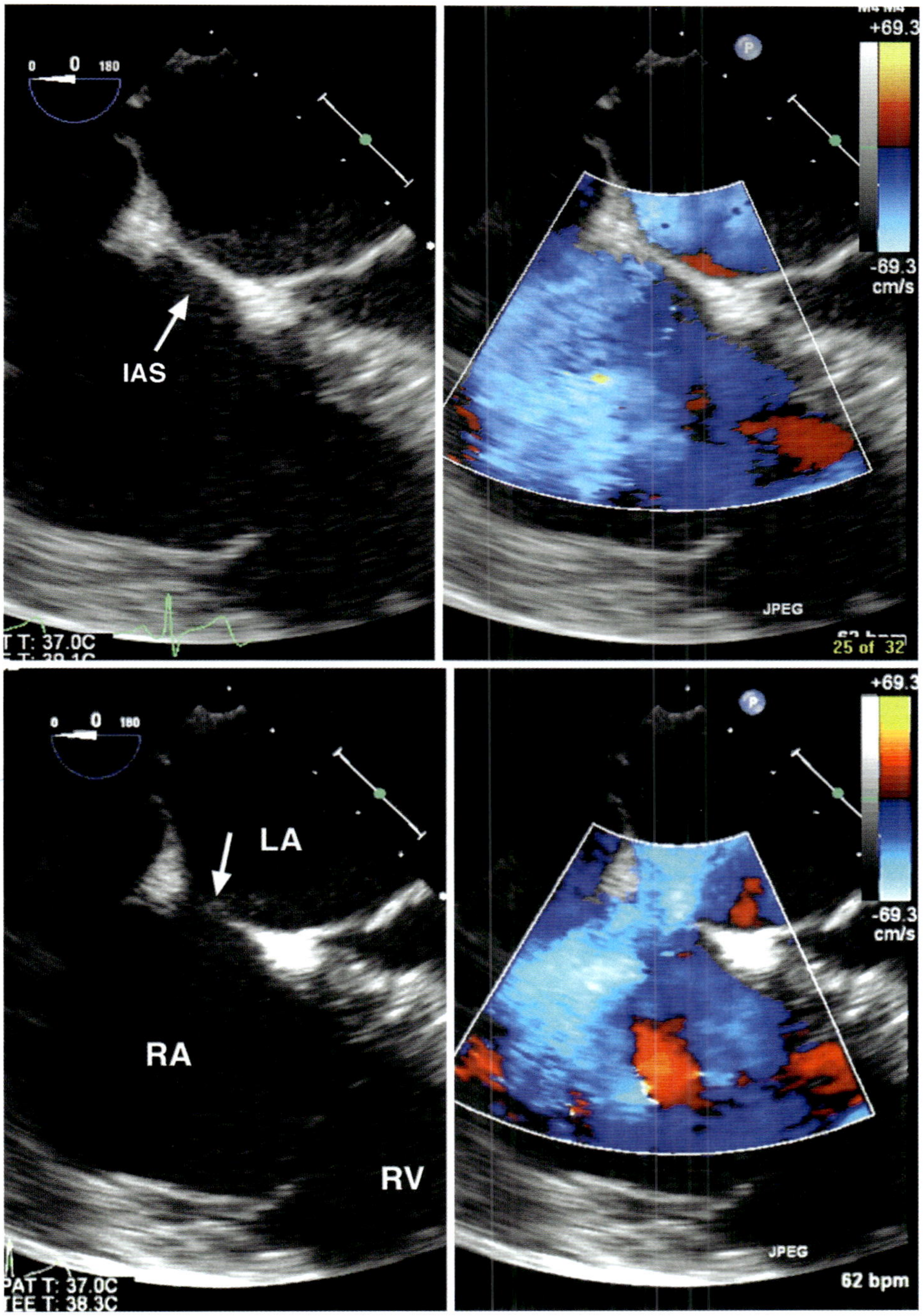

Fig 7.54 In upper two panels, midesophageal four-chamber view shows intact interatrial septum; however, when probe is retroflexed *(lower two panels)*, large coronary sinus is demonstrated *(arrow)*, suggesting either persistent left superior vena cava, unroofed coronary sinus, or both.

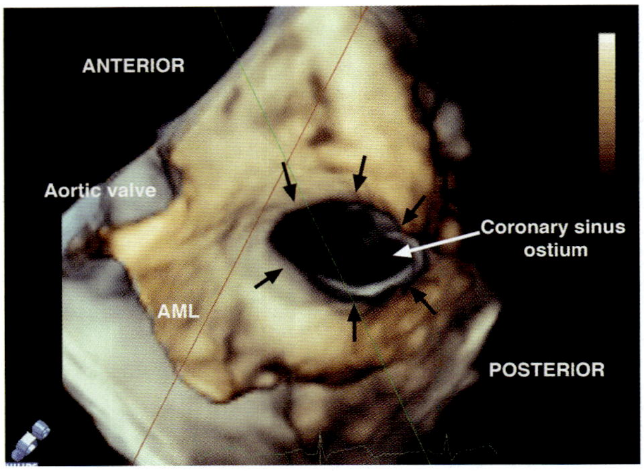

Fig 7.55 In this 3D TEE from left atrial perspective, left atrium has been cropped down to unroofed portion *(black arrows)*, which communicates directly with coronary sinus.

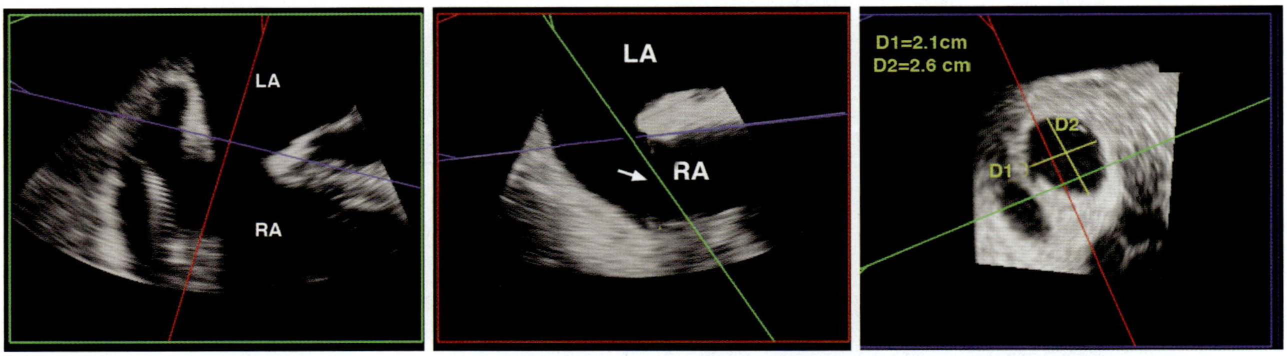

Fig 7.56 Using multiplanar reconstruction, blue planes in left and center panels define diameters of unroofed portion of coronary sinus. In right plane, cross-sectional representation of this area is shown.

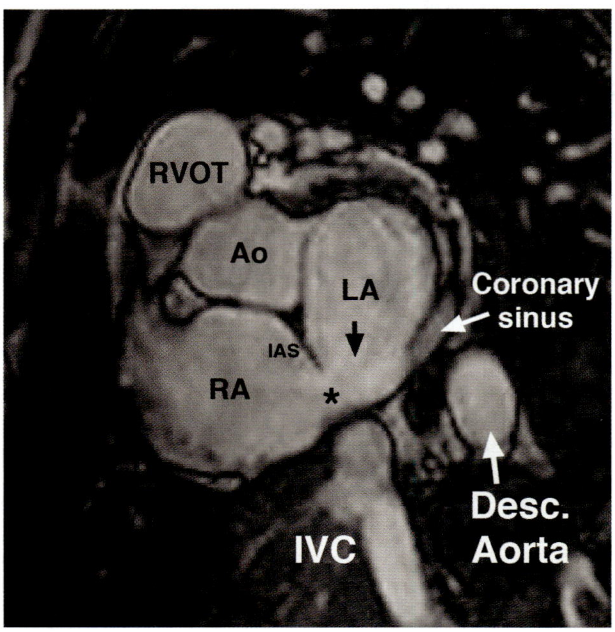

Fig 7.57 MRI shows unroofing of coronary sinus *(arrow)* and coronary sinus ostium *(asterisk)*.

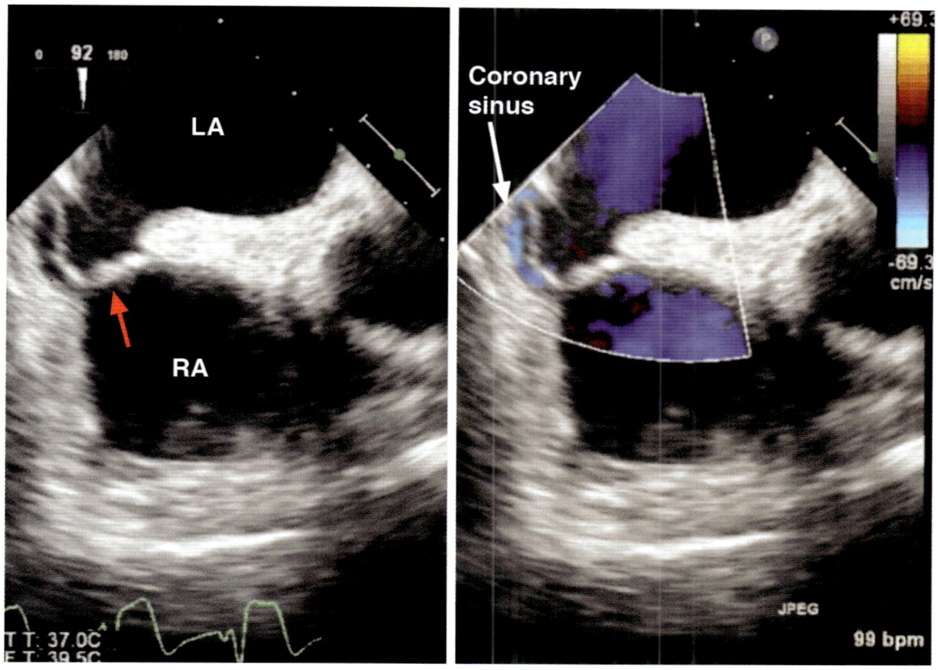

Fig 7.58 Baffle *(red arrow)* closes interatrial communication, and directs all coronary sinus flow into right atrium.

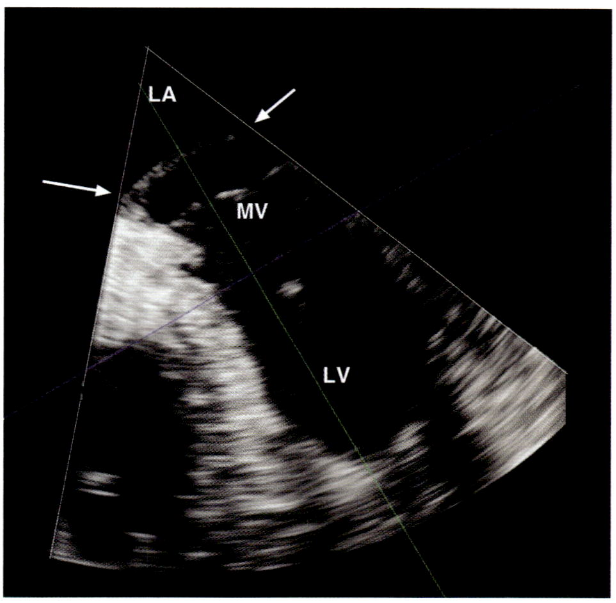

Fig 7.59 In this midesophageal four-chamber view with the probe retroflexed, baffle can be seen in left atrium *(arrows)*.

Comments

An atrial septal defect due to an "unroofed" coronary sinus is very uncommon but was recognized in this case by imaging to show the interatrial communication on both 2D imaging and with color Doppler.

Suggested Reading

1. Joffe DC, Oxorn DC, Rivo J: Coronary sinus atrial septal defect, Anesth Analg 107:1163–1165, 2008.

Ventricular Septal Defects

CASE 7-9
Anatomy and Imaging of the Ventricular Septum

In planning for procedures involving the ventricular septum, there a number of important views, both 2D and 3D. The septal segments are named according to the AHA guidelines. (See Standardized myocardial segmentation and nomenclature for tomographic imaging of the heart: A statement for healthcare professionals from the Cardiac Imaging Committee of the Council on Clinical Cardiology of the American Heart Association. Circulation 2002; 105:539–542.)

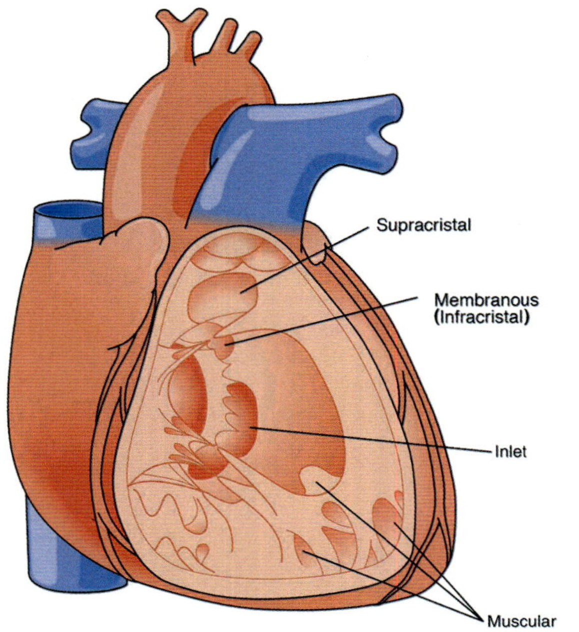

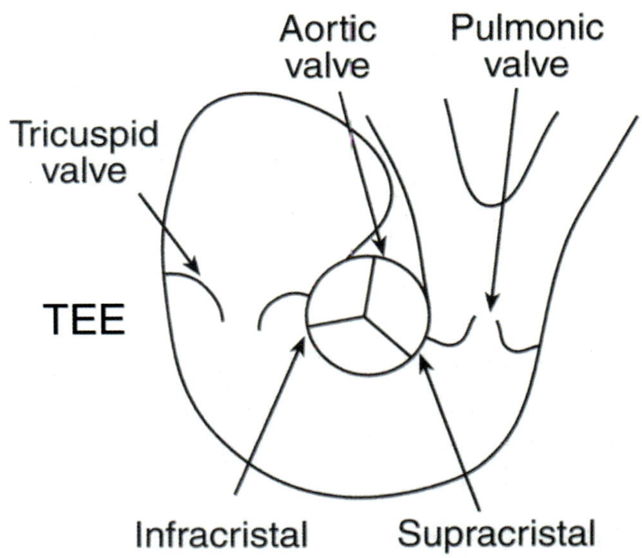

Fig 7.60 At left, diagram of types of VSDs as viewed on TEE from right ventricle. (Adapted from Fyler DC (ed.): Nadas Pediatric Cardiology, 2e, Philadelphia: 1992, Hanley & Belfus.) On right, position of different VSDs as seen on TEE. (Reproduced with permission from Linker D: Practical Echocardiography of Congenital Heart Disease, Philadelphia: 2000, Churchill Livingstone. Elsevier Inc.)

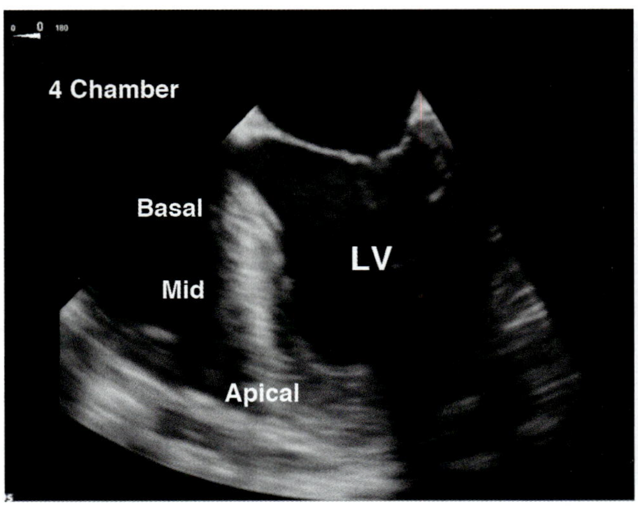

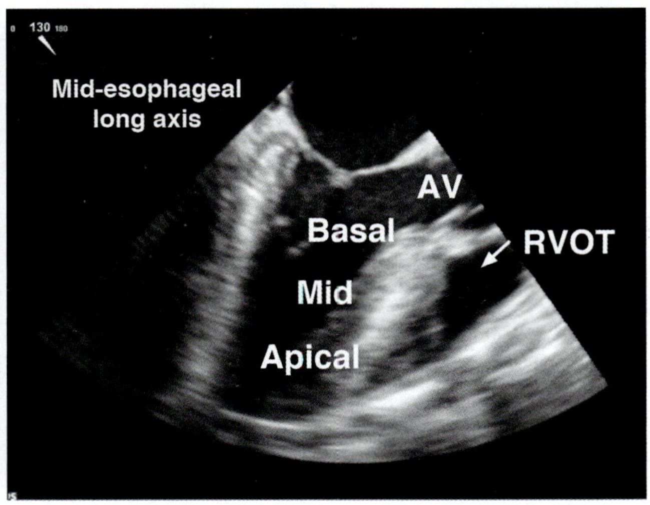

Fig 7.61 Ventricular septum is imaged in midesophageal four-chamber and long-axis views. In four-chamber view, inferior septum is seen with portion of anterior septum seen if image plane is angulated anteriorly to include aortic valve. In long-axis view, anterior septum is seen.

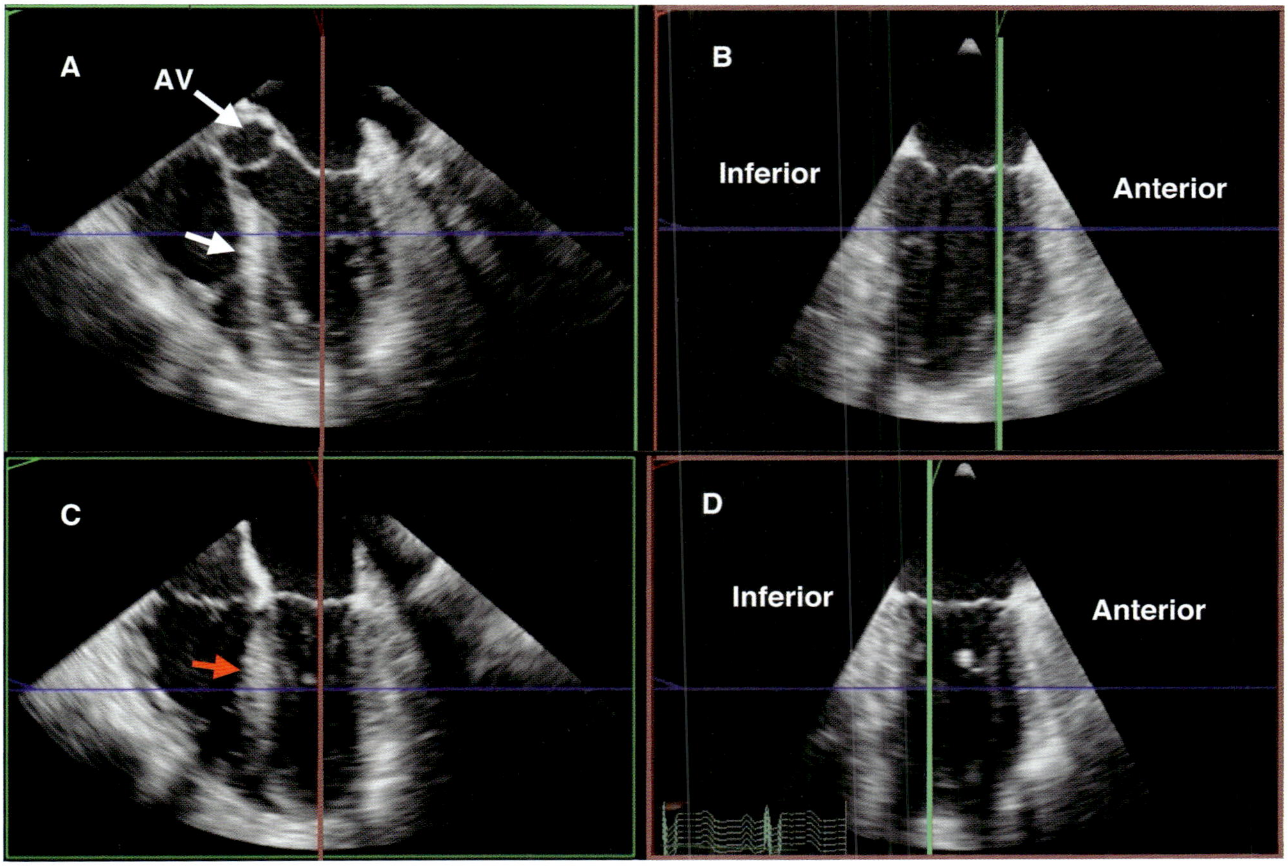

Fig 7.62 With use of multiplanar reconstruction, midesophageal anteriorly angulated four-chamber view is in upper left quadrant, and midesophageal two-chamber view in upper right quadrant. Movement of green plane toward anterior wall (**B**) allows one to conclude that septum seen in (**A**), *(white arrow)* is indeed anterior. Subsequent movement of green plane toward inferior wall (**D**) would allow one to conclude that septum seen in (**C**), *(red arrow)* is indeed inferior.

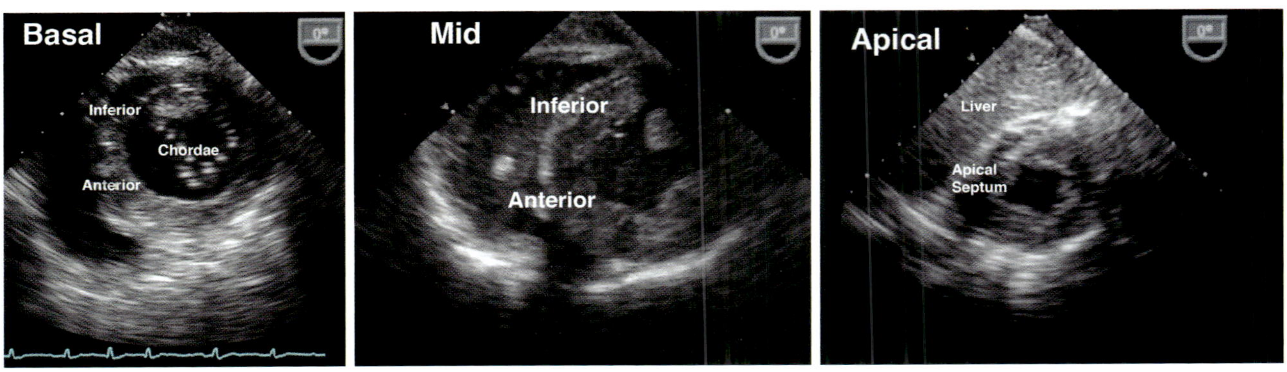

Fig 7.63 Transgastric short-axis views allow imaging of all components of ventricular septum. After imaging at base, probe is progressively advanced and retroflexed to obtain midpapillary and apical views.

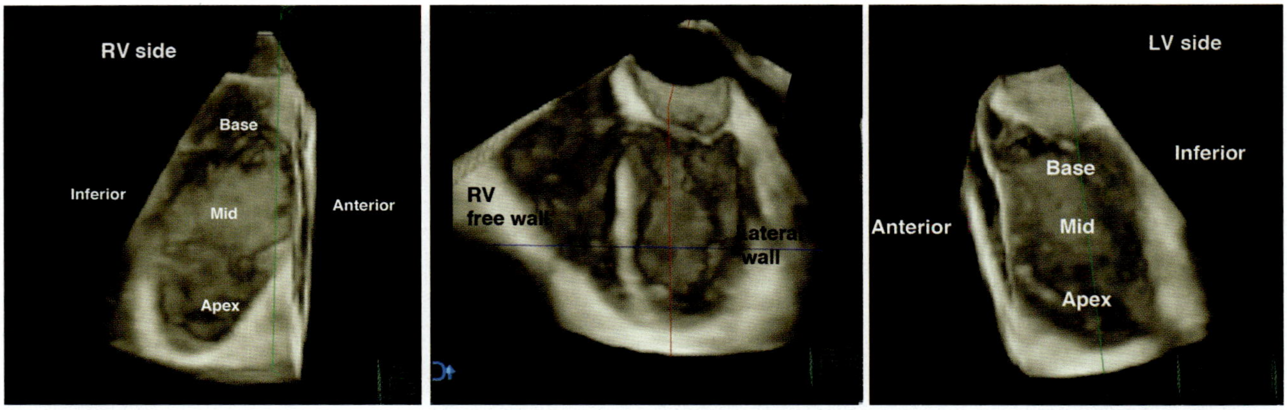

Fig 7.64 3D acquisition techniques can be used to image ventricular septum. We have chosen to use full-volume mode. Center image shows both ventricles, with anterior part of heart cropped away in coronal plane. Rotating this image in counterclockwise direction along its vertical axis, cropping away free wall of RV, and restoring anterior portion of heart that was initially cropped allows full visualization of right ventricular side of septum *(left)*. Similarly, rotating center image in clockwise direction along its vertical axis, cropping away lateral wall of LV, and restoring anterior portion of heart that was initially cropped allows full visualization of left ventricular side of septum.

Comments

Narrow-section live 3D imaging can be used in the initial evaluation of a ventricular septal defect but better images are obtained by cropping a full-volume 3D acquisition as illustrated by this case. The approach to transcatheter closure of a ventricular septal defect depends on the location and size of the defect so that imaging is critical in the success of this procedure. It is also important to ensure that additional ventricular septal defects are not present.

Suggested Reading

1. Cossor W, Cui VW, Roberson DA: Three-dimensional echocardiographic en face views of ventricular septal defects: Feasibility, accuracy, imaging protocols and reference image collection, J Am Soc Echocardiogr 28:1020–1029, 2015.

CASE 7-10
Membranous VSD

This 41-year-old man with diabetes and hypertension had a known small VSD since childhood. After a scrape on his ankle became infected, he developed *Staphylococcus aureus* endocarditis with vegetations involving the right side of the VSD. His clinical course was complicated by septic shock, septic pulmonary emboli, adult respiratory distress syndrome, and acute ST-elevation myocardial injury, with a normal coronary angiogram. He fully recovered and was referred for closure of the VSD.

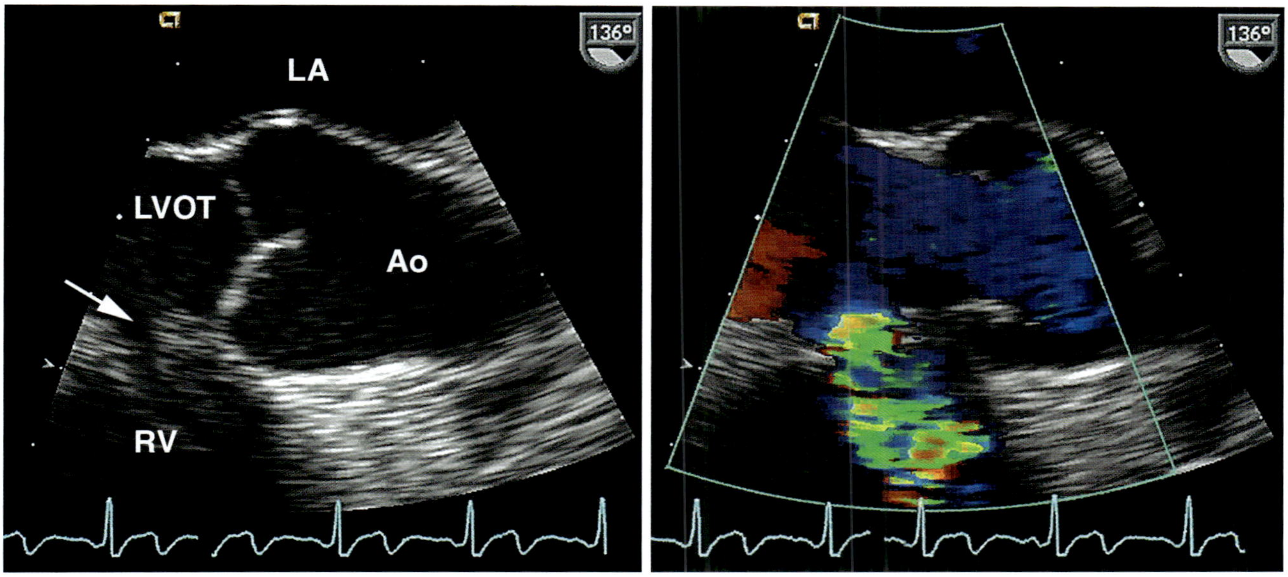

Fig 7.65 In long-axis view (at 135 degrees) of left ventricular outflow tract (LVOT), apparent loss of continuity is seen in region of membranous ventricular septum *(arrow)*. There is mobile sock-like aneurysm on right ventricular side.

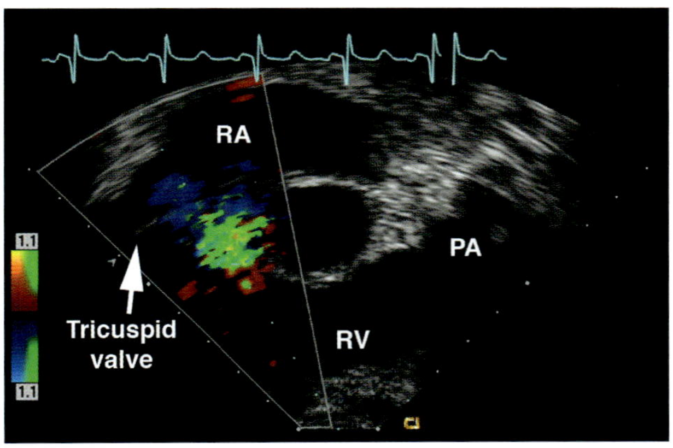

Fig 7.66 In transthoracic study, reoriented to simulate TEE orientation, VSD flow is seen to enter RV adjacent to tricuspid valve.

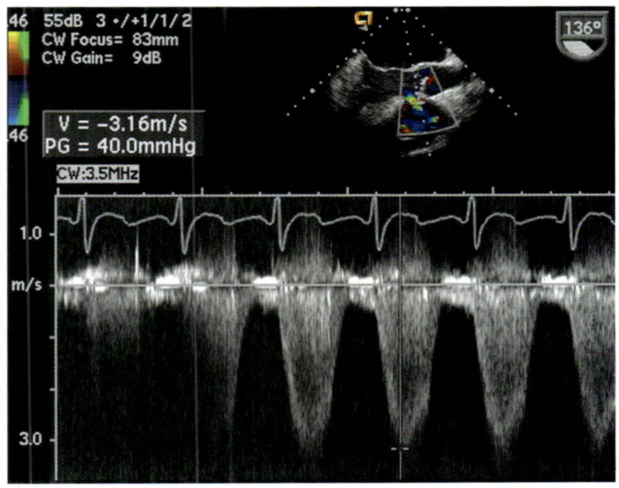

Fig 7.67 Continuous wave Doppler of this flow indicates systolic ejection-type velocity of at least 3.2 m/s. This is consistent with flow from left to right ventricle (estimated pressure difference by Doppler of 40 mm Hg), although pressure difference may be underestimated due to nonparallel intercept angle between ultrasound beam and direction of blood flow.

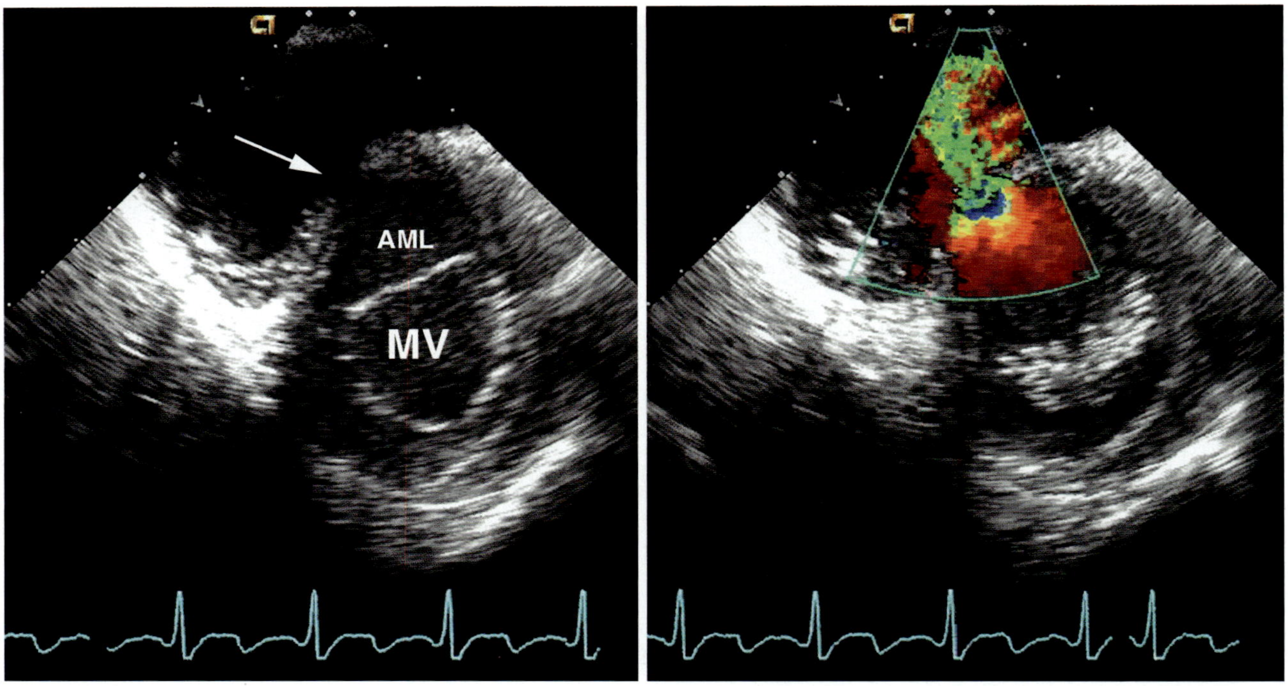

Fig 7.68 Epicardial images were acquired by surgeon, with ultrasound transducer in sterile sleeve, for further evaluation of anatomy of defect. There is discontinuity *(arrow)* in septum just apical to aortic valve (note anterior mitral leaflet in this view) and color flow demonstrates left-to-right flow across this defect.

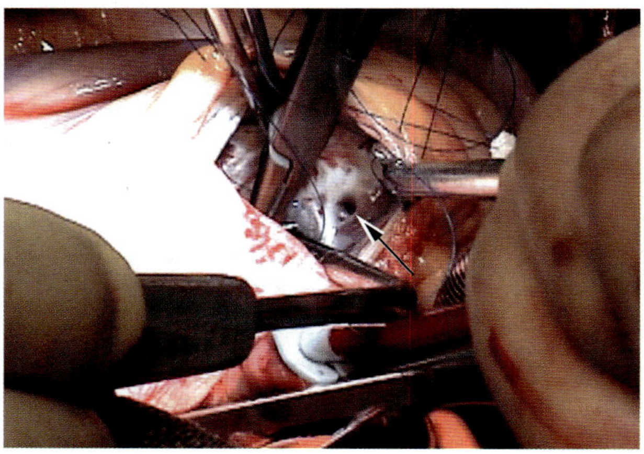

Fig 7.69 VSD *(arrow)* was inspected first via incision in pulmonary artery. Defect was 8 mm in diameter, with no evidence of active infection.

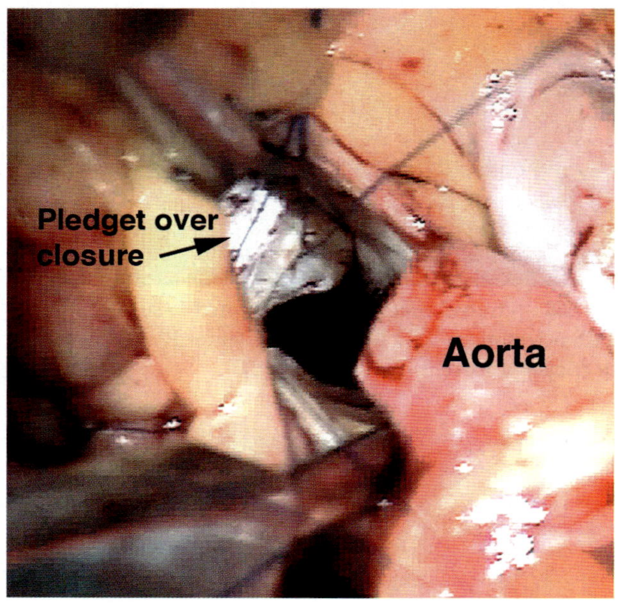

Fig 7.70 Next, aortotomy was performed and defect was visualized from left side of septum. Again, there was no evidence of active infection. Because of small size of defect, it was repaired with primary closure.

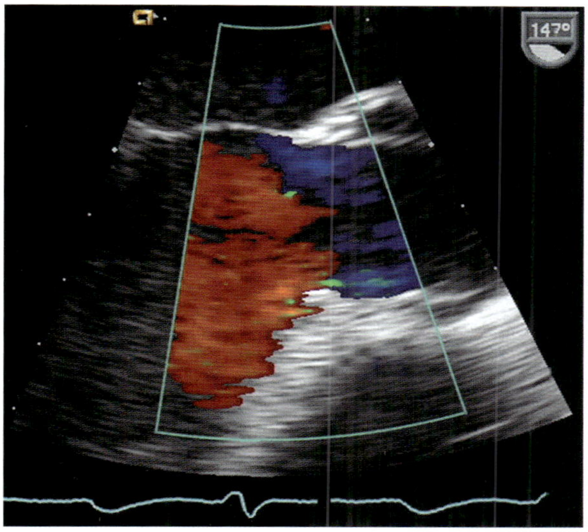

Fig 7.71 Postprocedure echocardiographic images showed no residual defect.

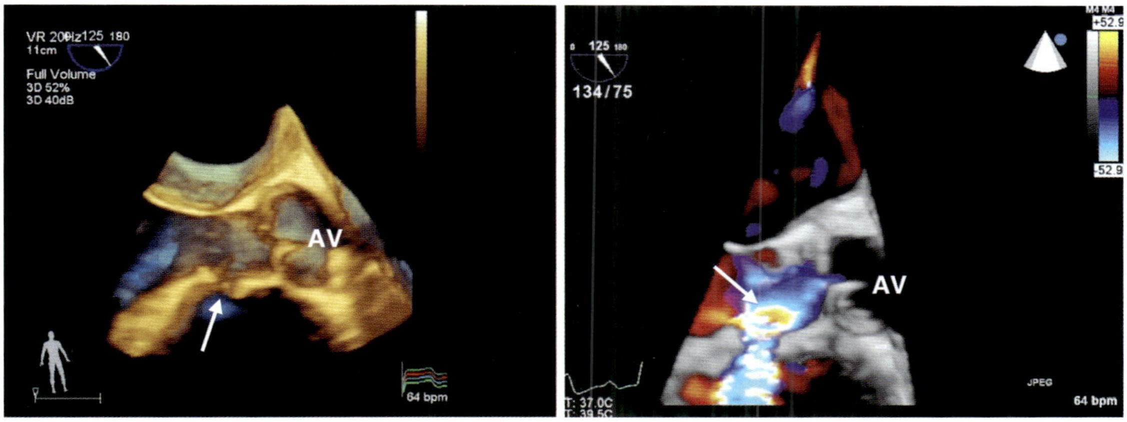

Fig 7.72 In another patient with similar clinical presentation, 3D TEE *(left)* clearly demonstrates membranous ventricular defect *(arrow)*. On the right, during isovolumic contraction, the increase in LV pressure initiates flow through the VSD; the arrow indicates the area of flow convergence.

Comments

In adults, a small membranous VSD is typically asymptomatic. Diagnosis is based on the presence of a loud systolic murmur, with echocardiographic confirmation of the diagnosis. Many membranous defects are partially closed by thin tissue, possibly related to the tricuspid valve apparatus, with an echocardiographic appearance described as a ventricular septal "aneurysm," even though this tissue is normal. Most small membranous VSDs are not closed, as these defects are well tolerated hemodynamically with no data to suggest adverse cardiovascular outcomes. However, patients with a VSD are at increased risk of endocarditis and should receive antibiotic prophylaxis. When endocarditis occurs, vegetations are typically located in the area of jet turbulence, on the right ventricular side of the defect and the tricuspid valve. Once endocarditis occurs, closure of the defect is often recommended to prevent recurrent infection.

Suggested Reading

1. Walpot J, Peerenboom P, van Wylick A, et al: Aneurysm of the membranous septum with ventricular septal defect and infective endocarditis, Eur J Echocardiogr 5:391–393, 2004.
2. Charakida M, Pushparajah K, Anderson D, Simpson JM: Insights gained from three-dimensional imaging modalities for closure of ventricular septal defects, Circ Cardiovasc Imaging 7(6): 954–961, 2014.

CASE 7-11
Muscular VSD

This 32-week premature infant was noted to have a systolic murmur.

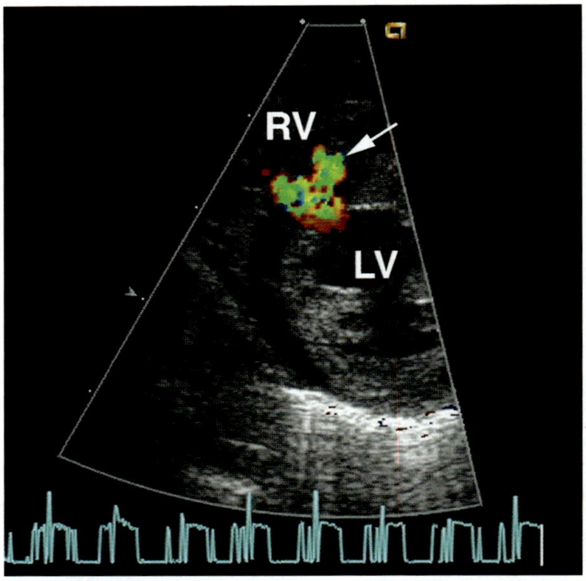

Fig 7.73 Transthoracic short-axis view demonstrates small VSD in midsegment of septum with left-to-right flow in systole *(arrow)*.

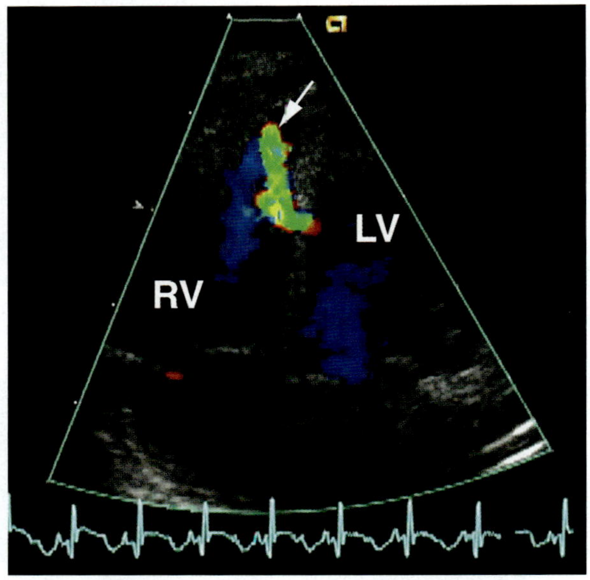

Fig 7.74 In four-chamber transthoracic view, VSD is again seen, with localized area of left-to-right flow *(arrow)*.

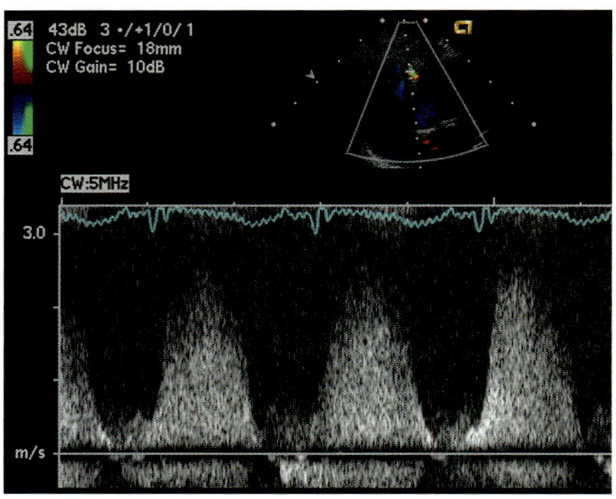

Fig 7.75 Continuous wave Doppler shows high-velocity signal, although maximum velocity is probably underestimated due to nonparallel intercept angle.

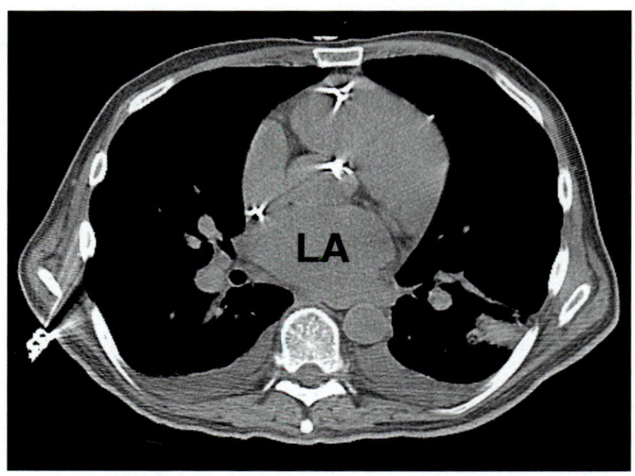

Fig 7.76 In different patient, undergoing surgery for aortic stenosis, preoperative CT showed large left atrium.

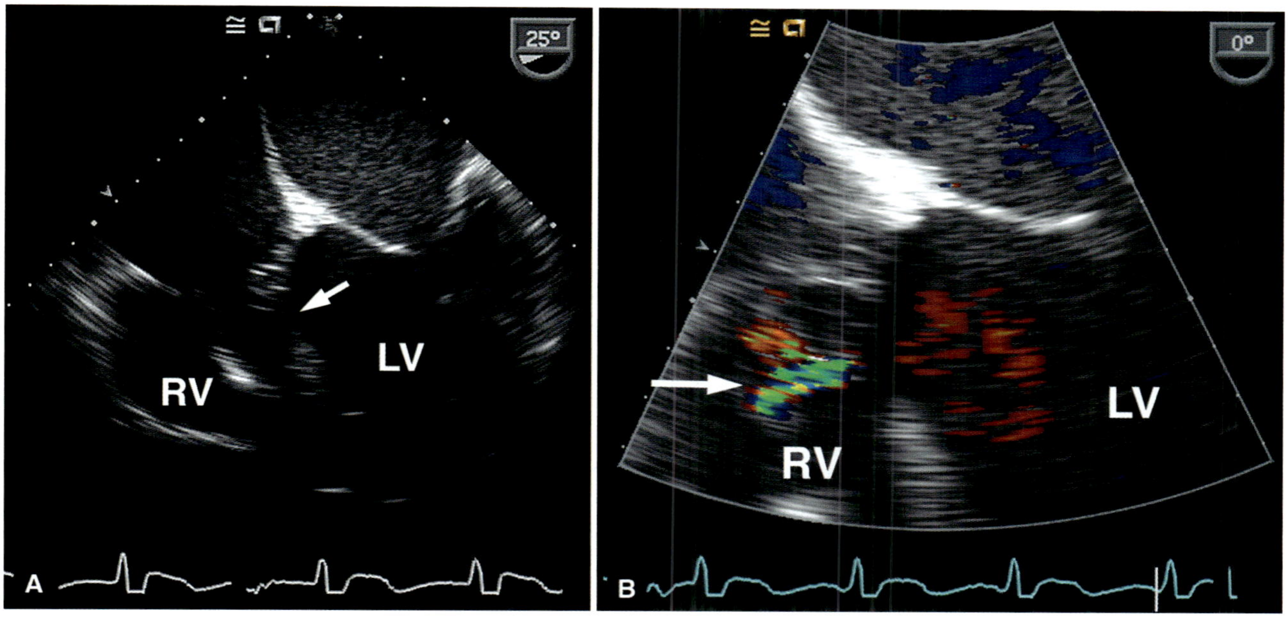

Fig 7.77 In this patient, small muscular VSD was found on 2D imaging (**A**, *arrow*), confirmed by color Doppler (**B**, *arrow*), and closed through aortic root at time of aortic valve replacement.

Comments

Most muscular VSDs are small and many close spontaneously in childhood. In this infant, the murmur resolved by 18 months of age. Occasionally, a small congenital muscular VSD is seen in an adult. However, most defects of the muscular septum in adults are acquired as a result of endocarditis or ventricular septal rupture after myocardial infarction. (See Chapter 1.)

Suggested Reading

1. Zhang J, Ko JM, Guileyardo JM, Roberts WC: A review of spontaneous closure of ventricular septal defect, Proc (Bayl Univ Med Cent) 28(4):516–520, 2015.
2. Anderson RH, Brown NA, Mohun TJ: Insights regarding the normal and abnormal formation of the atrial and ventricular septal structures, Clin Anat 29(3):290–304, 2016.

CASE 7-12
Supracristal VSD

This 51-year-old man with a VSD and enlargement of the sinuses of Valsalva was referred for repair of the VSD and aortic root replacement.

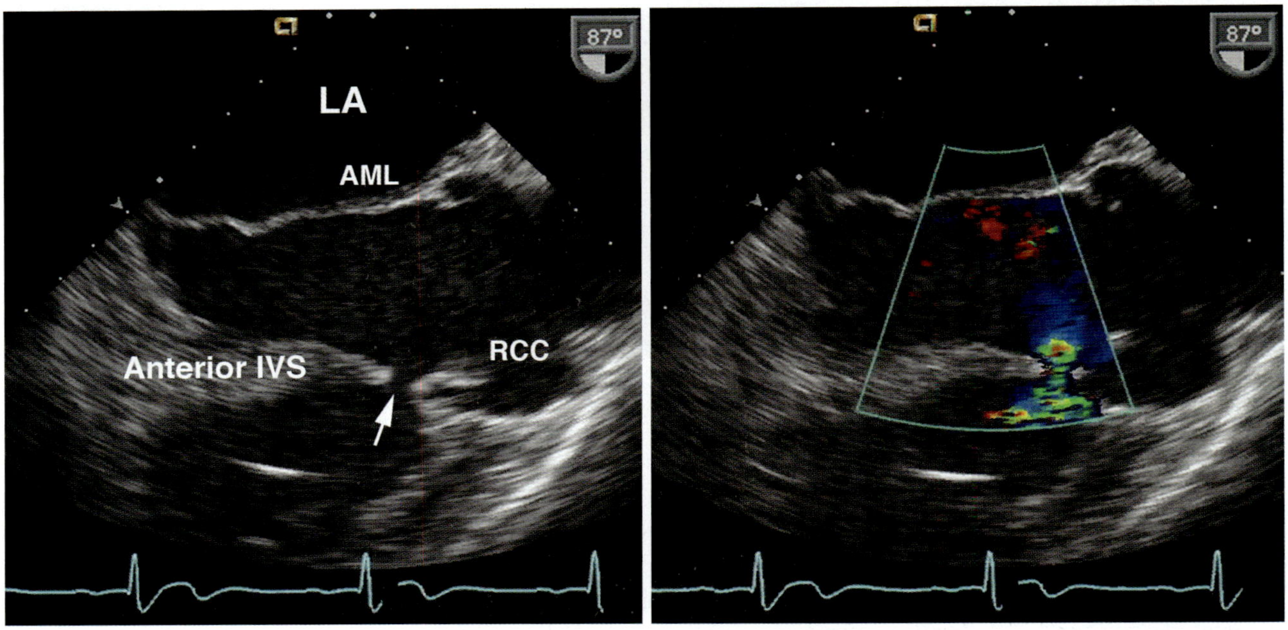

Fig 7.78 In long-axis view of aortic valve, small defect in anterior interventricular septum (IVS) is seen immediately adjacent to right coronary cusp (RCC) of aortic valve, with color Doppler *(right)* demonstrating left-to-right flow through this region. Compare this image with Fig 7.65 and note position of defect relative to aortic valve. Sinuses of Valsalva diameter is 53 mm in this view.

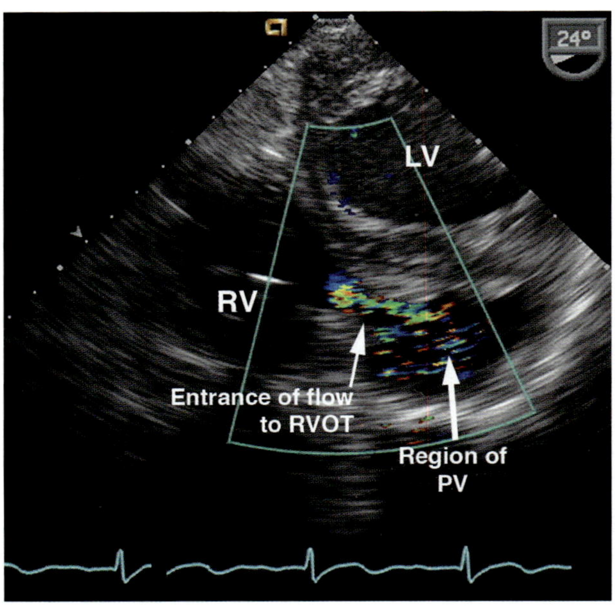

Fig 7.79 In transgastric view of RVOT, entrance of VSD flow just proximal to pulmonic valve is seen.

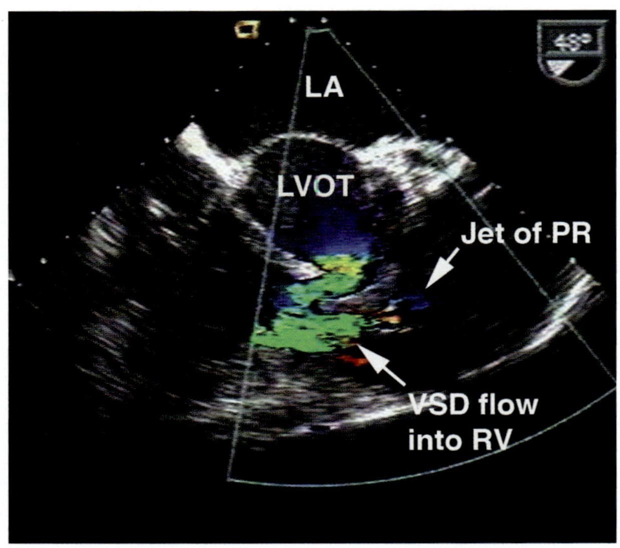

Fig 7.80 In short-axis view, VSD is seen to empty into right ventricle just below pulmonic valve.

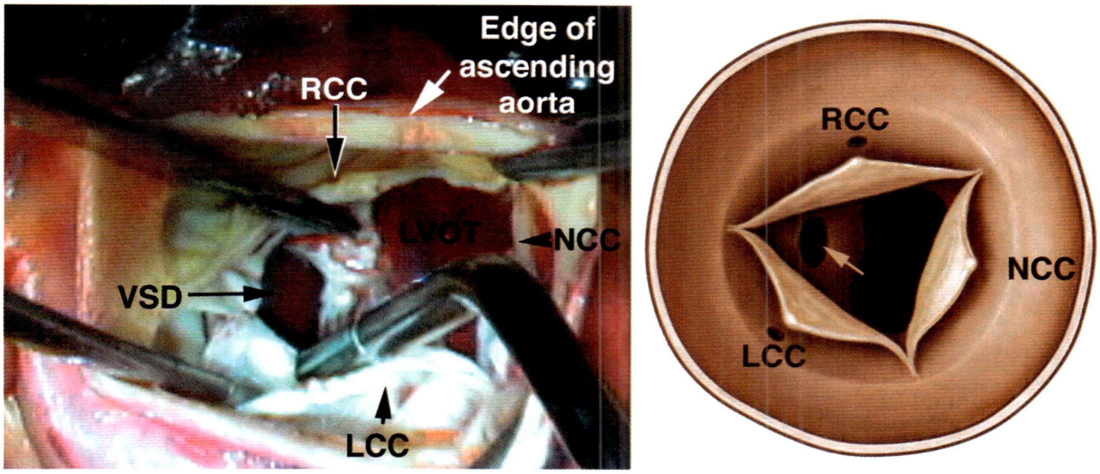

Fig 7.81 At surgery and in corresponding drawing *(arrow)*, VSD is seen via aortotomy incision immediately adjacent to aortic valve.

Comments

Supracristal VSDs are uncommon compared with membranous VSDs in adults. A supracristal VSD is located just inferior to the pulmonic valve and, as in this case, is often associated with abnormal anatomy of the aortic sinuses and/or dysfunction of the aortic valve due to lack of support of the aortic annulus.

A short-axis view of the aortic valve is very helpful in differentiating the types of VSDs. In the short-axis view, a membranous VSD is seen immediately adjacent to the right coronary cusp (near the tricuspid valve). In contrast, a supracristal VSD is closer to the left coronary cusp, adjacent to the pulmonic valve (see Fig 7.60).

Suggested Reading

1. Hartlage GR, Consolini MA, Pernetz MA, et al: Intraoperative transesophageal echocardiography for paediatric cardiac surgery—an audit of 200 cases, Anaesth Intensive Care 27:591–595, 1999.
2. Hartlage GR, Consolini MA, Pernetz MA, et al: Bad company: Supracristal VSD presenting with ruptured sinus of valsalva aneurysm. A case presentation with echocardiographic depiction and an analysis of contemporary literature, Echocardiography 32(3):575–583, 2015.

Abnormalities of the Great Vessels

CASE 7-13
Aortic Coarctation

This 29-year-old man, with a history of coarctation repair at age 5 years, presented with hypertension and was found to have a recurrent coarctation.

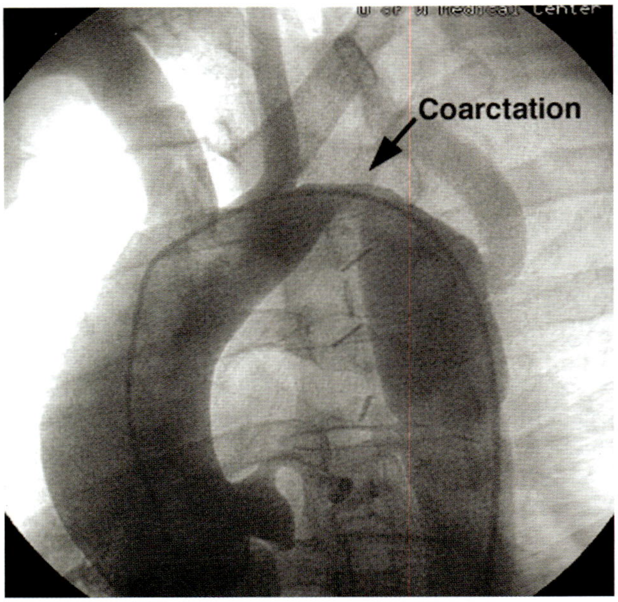

Fig 7.82 Contrast aortogram shows severe coarctation of aorta in distal arch.

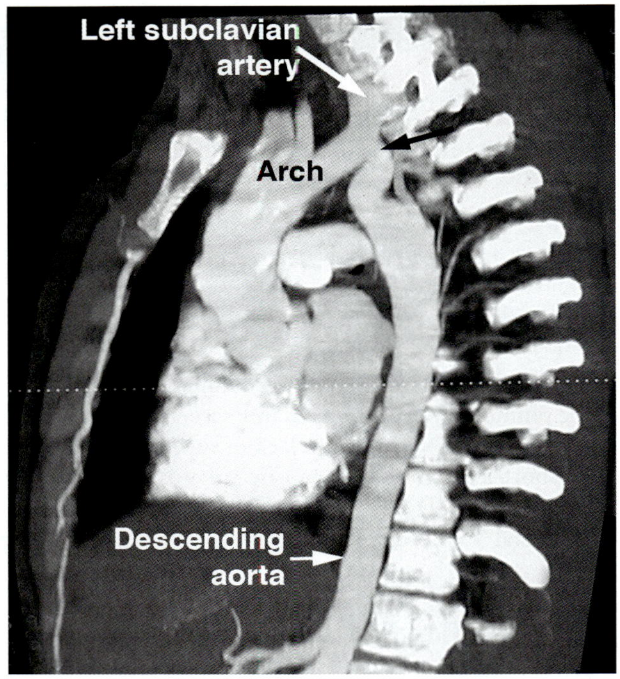

Fig 7.83 Sagittal CT image shows coarctation *(arrow)* just distal to left subclavian artery.

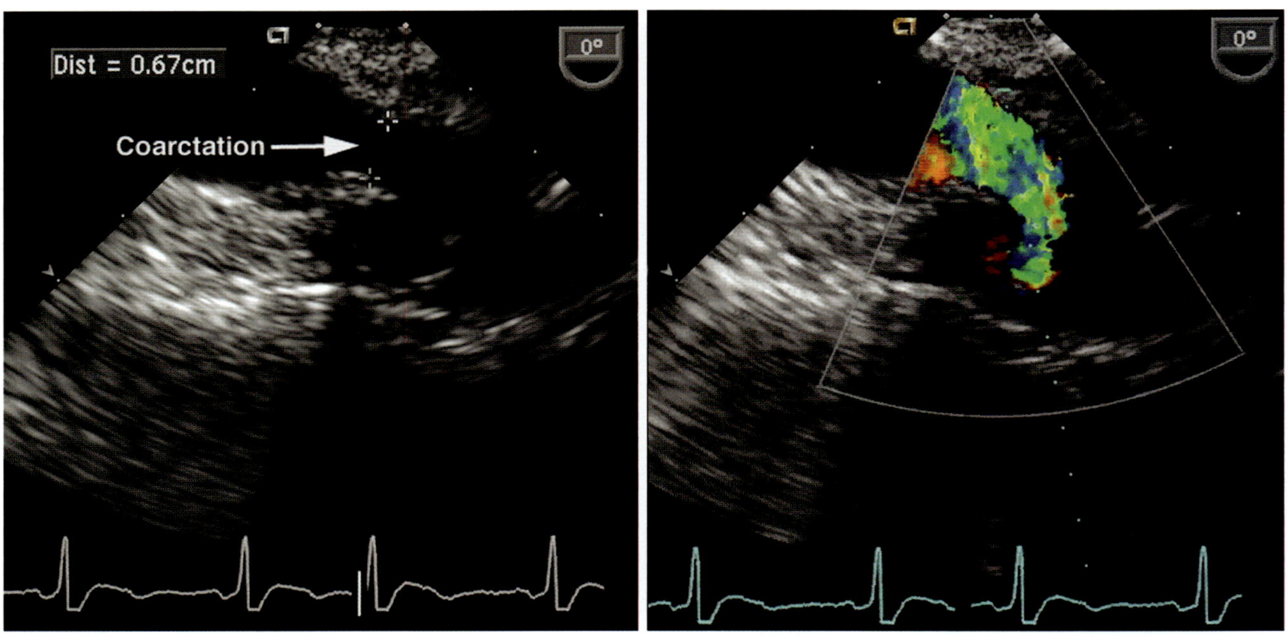

Fig 7.84 On intraoperative TEE, view of distal aortic arch from very high esophageal position shows narrowing *(left)* and increased flow velocity *(right)* at coarctation site.

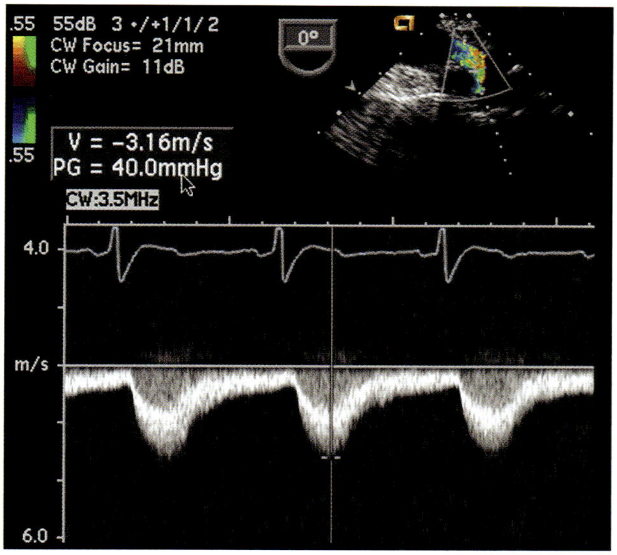

Fig 7.85 Continuous wave Doppler of this region shows high-velocity signal with persistent decrescendo velocity pattern in diastole, consistent with severe coarctation. Antegrade velocity peak likely is underestimated.

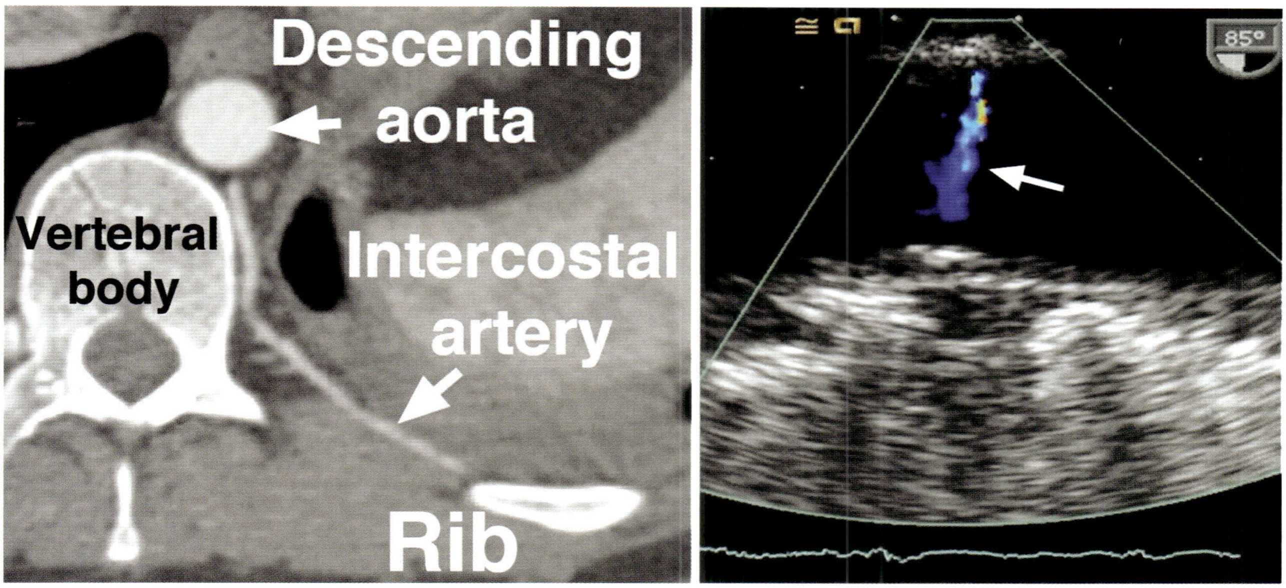

Fig 7.86 In this CT scan, intercostal artery can be seen entering aorta. In midesophageal long-axis view of descending thoracic aorta, collateral flow from intercostal artery is seen entering aorta *(arrow)*.

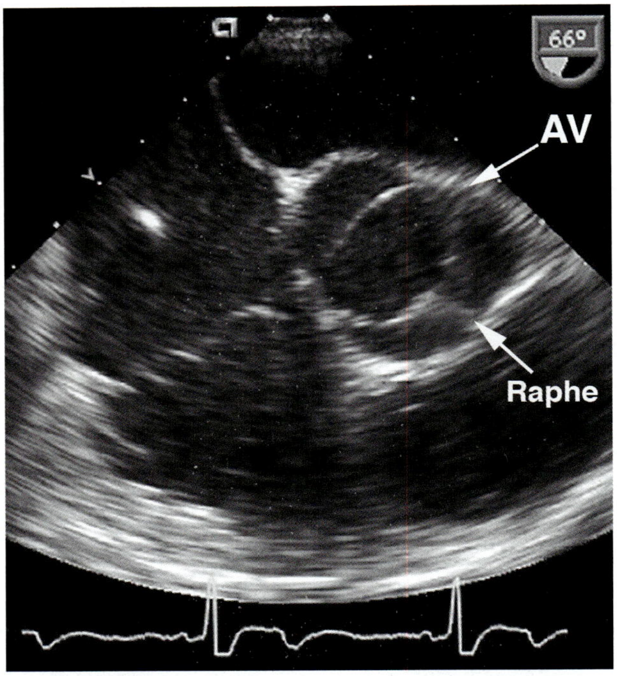

Fig 7.87 Short-axis image of aortic valve demonstrates bicuspid valve with anterior-posterior orientation of leaflets and raphe in larger leaflet (corresponding to fusion of right and left coronary cusps).

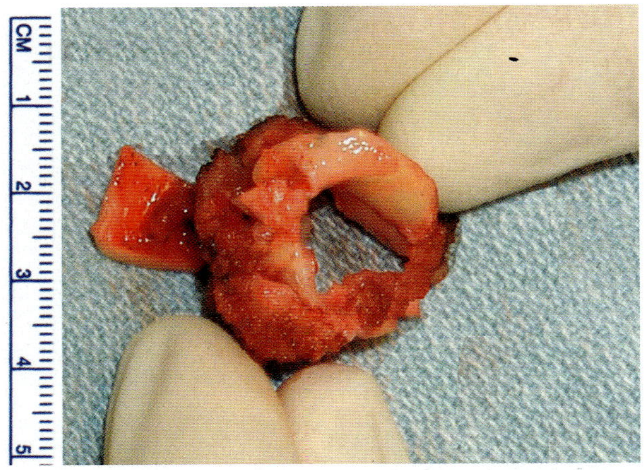

Fig 7.88 At surgery, narrowed segment of aorta was resected and aorta was reconstructed with Dacron tube graft.

Comments

In patients with an aortic coarctation, 50% have a bicuspid aortic valve. Conversely, about 10% of patients with a bicuspid aortic valve also have an aortic coarctation. In patients with Turner's syndrome, there is a high prevalence of both bicuspid aortic valve and aortic coarctation. Although the exact mechanism of this association is not known, because both conditions are inherited, it is assumed that this phenotype represents an underlying developmental disorder of the aortic valve and aorta. Similar to other patients with a bicuspid aortic valve, those with an associated aortic coarctation are also at risk for progressive dilation of the aorta. The clinical implication of this association is that aortic valve anatomy should be assessed in patients with an aortic coarctation. In addition, echocardiographic examination in patients with a bicuspid aortic valve should include recording of the velocity signal in the descending thoracic aorta, as well as measurement of upper- and lower-extremity blood pressures.

Suggested Reading

1. Aboulhosn J, Child JS: Echocardiographic evaluation of congenital left ventricular outflow obstruction, Echocardiography 32(Suppl 2):S140–S147, 2015.

CASE 7-14
Persistent Left Superior Vena Cava

This 49-year-old woman was referred for evaluation of hypertension and a cardiac murmur. A blood pressure difference of 40 mm Hg was noted between the arm and leg, and transthoracic echocardiography showed an aortic coarctation. At surgery, the coarctation was located between the left carotid and left subclavian arteries. The coarctation was repaired using a patch repair. Incidentally, a persistent left superior vena cava was noted.

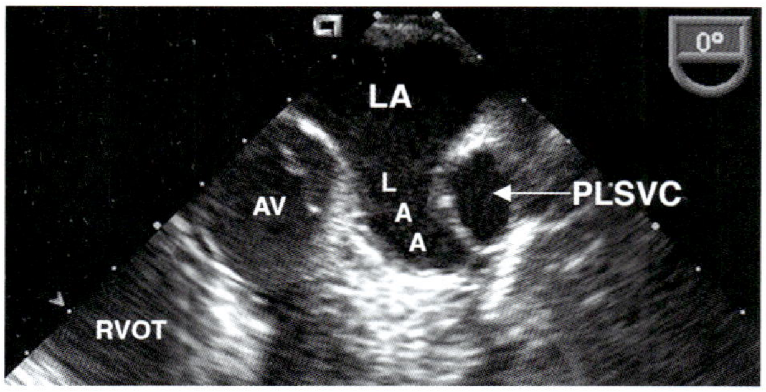

Fig 7.89 High esophageal view at 0 degrees shows echo-free circular structure, persistent left superior vena cava (PLSVC) lateral to left atrial appendage (LAA).

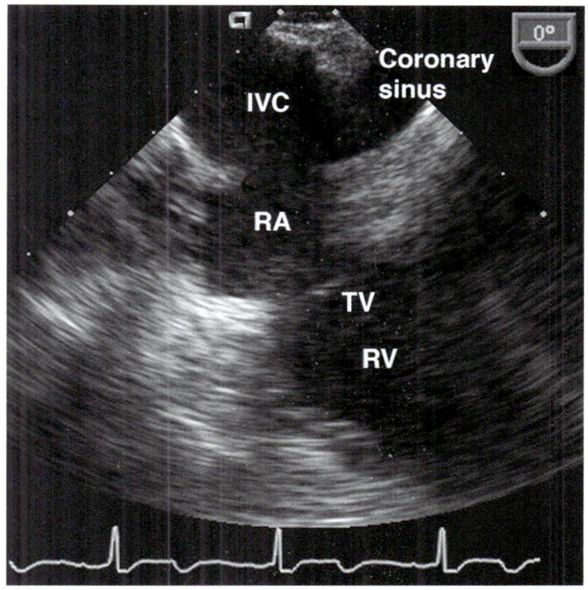

Fig 7.90 Low esophageal view shows entrance of enlarged coronary sinus into right atrium.

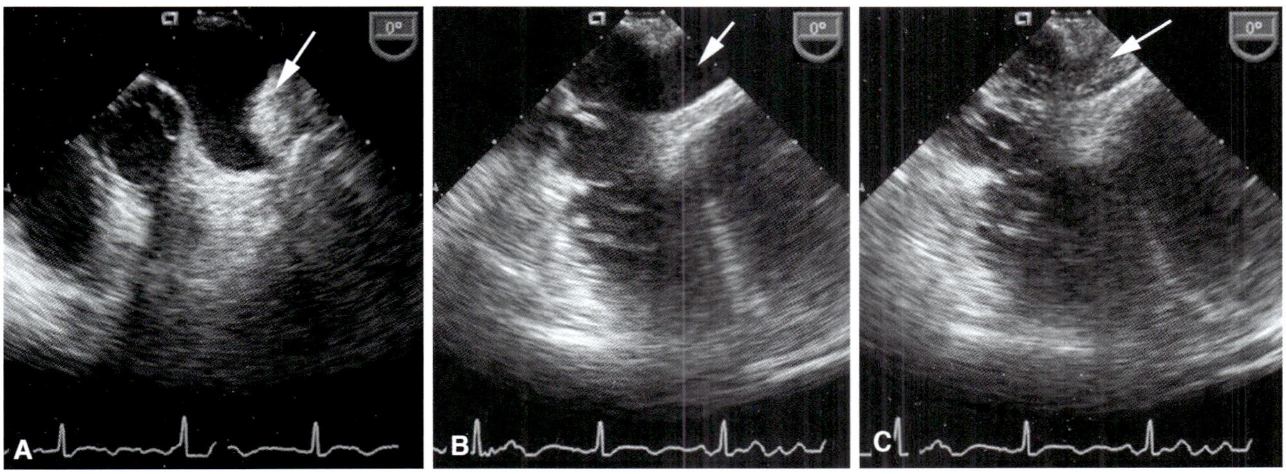

Fig 7.91 Injection of contrast via left arm shows appearance of contrast in structure *(arrow)* lateral to left atrial appendage **(A)** and contrast entering right atrium via coronary sinus *(arrows)* (**B** and **C**). These findings are consistent with persistent left superior vena cava.

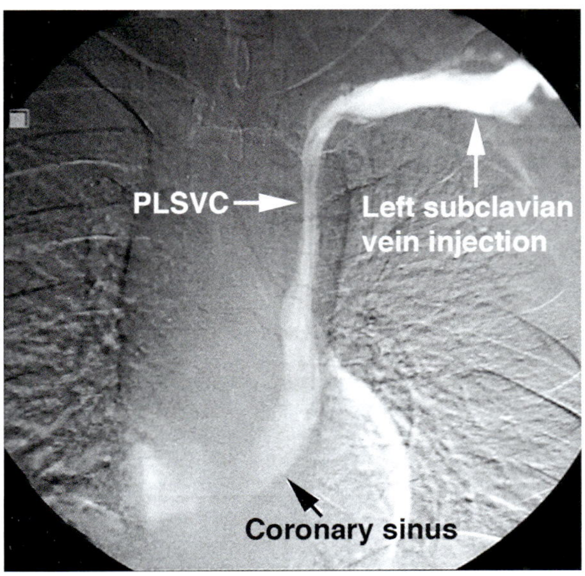

Fig 7.92 Venogram with injection of contrast into left subclavian vein shows left-sided superior vena cava entering coronary sinus.

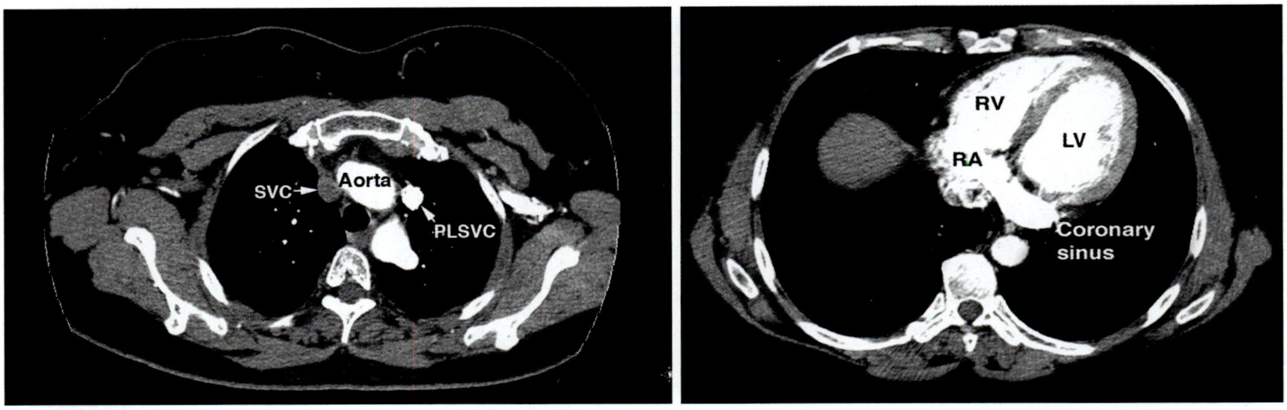

Fig 7.93 On left, CT scan with contrast at level of ascending aorta shows opacification of left SVC but not right SVC, as contrast was injected via left arm. On right, CT scan at heart level shows dilated coronary sinus.

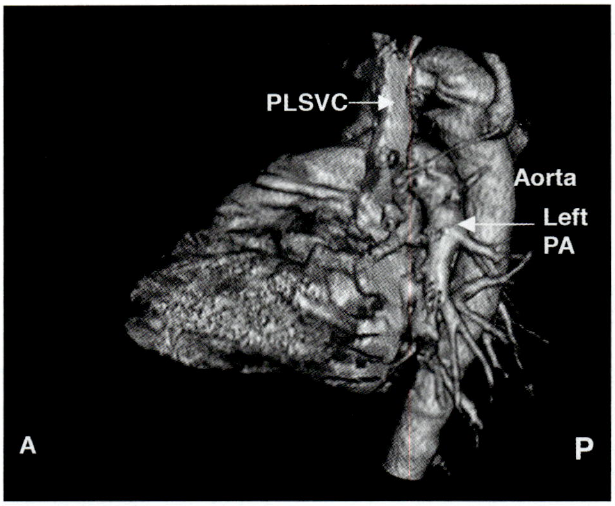

Fig 7.94 3D reconstruction of CT images with heart rotated to left shows PLSVC.

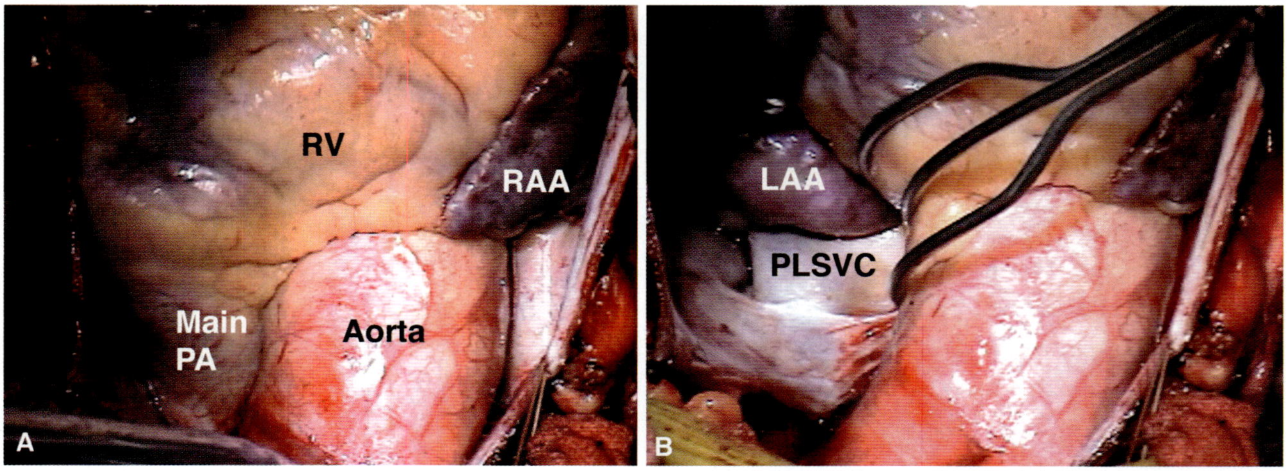

Fig 7.95 Intraoperative findings show normal position of aorta and pulmonary artery **(A)**. When great arteries are retracted gently, PLSVC and LAA can be seen **(B)**.

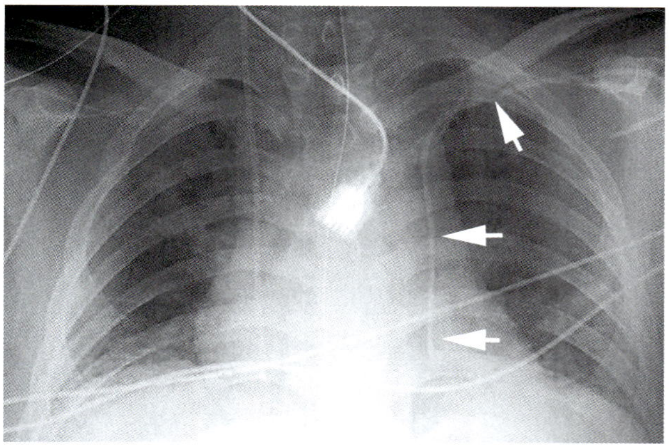

Fig 7.96 Chest radiograph showing central venous catheter in PLSVC *(arrows)*.

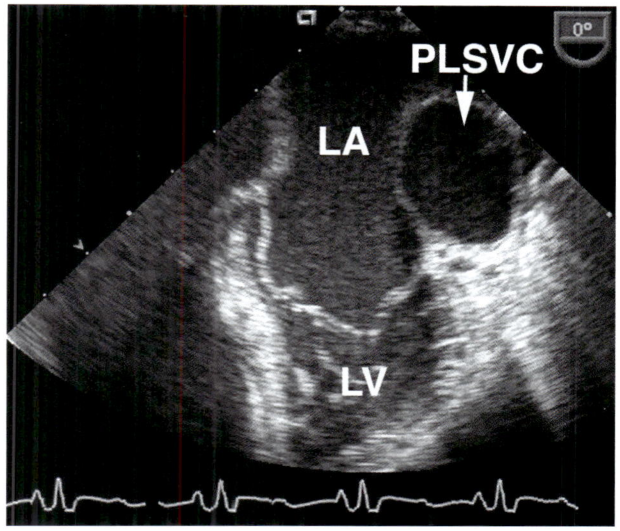

Fig 7.97 This 22-year-old woman had previously undergone repair of tetralogy of Fallot as a child, and now presented for tricuspid and pulmonic valve replacements for valvular regurgitation. This midesophageal four-chamber view shows large PLSVC lateral to LA.

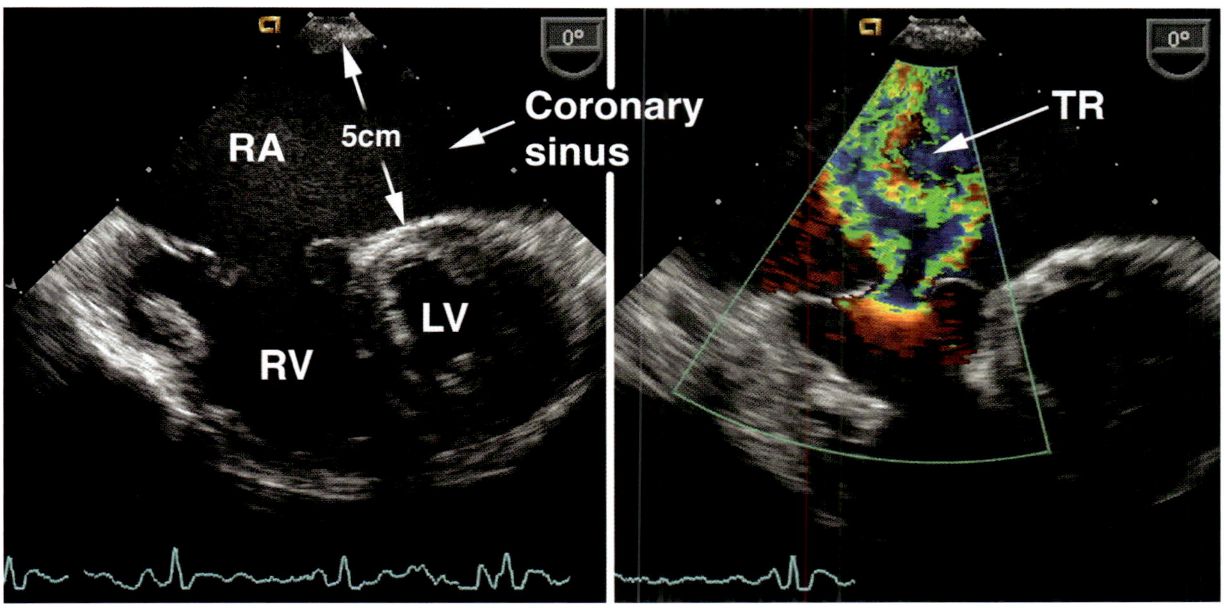

Fig 7.98 In this low esophageal view, there is non-coaptation of tricuspid leaflets, resulting in severe TR. Coronary sinus measures 5 cm in diameter.

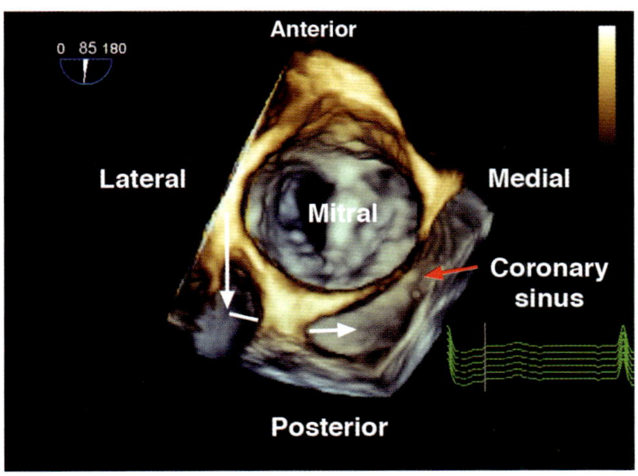

Fig 7.99 In another patient with persistent left SVC, white arrows indicate path of injection of agitated saline into left antecubital vein; descending from left SVC into enlarged coronary sinus. In real time, movement of "bubbles" can be seen more clearly.

Comments

About 0.5% of adults have both a normal superior vena cava entering the right atrium from the right side of the mediastinum, as well as a persistent left-sided superior vena cava. This PLSVC typically drains into the coronary sinus and, from there, into the right atrium. Because the pattern of blood flow is normal, there are no clinical symptoms or signs associated with a PLSVC. Most of these patients are diagnosed when they become ill, if echocardiography is performed or if a central venous catheter enters the right atrium from a left mediastinal position.

On echocardiography, a PLSVC is recognized based on the finding of an enlarged coronary sinus. The coronary sinus is seen in short axis in a left ventricular long-axis view. From the standard four-chamber view, the transducer can be advanced in the esophagus and retro-flexed to visualize the coronary sinus along its long axis. This view shows the entrance of the coronary sinus into the right atrium. Typically, the size of the dilated coronary sinus is 1 to 2 cm. The massive enlargement of the coronary sinus in the second case is most likely due as well to the severely elevated right atrial pressure.

If the diagnosis of a PLSVC is in doubt, a contrast injection in a left arm vein will demonstrate contrast in the coronary sinus before contrast is seen in the right atrium. Chest CT or MR also can be used to define the caval anatomy in more detail.

During open heart surgery, the presence of a PLSVC with coronary sinus enlargement will negate the effectiveness of retrograde cardioplegia.

Suggested Reading

1. Goyal SK, Punnam SR, Verma G, Ruberg FL: Persistent left superior vena cava: A case report and review of literature, Cardiovasc Ultrasound 6:50, 2008.
2. Gonzalez-Juanatey C, Testa A, Vidan J, et al: Persistent left superior vena cava draining into the coronary sinus: report of 10 cases and literature review, Clin Cardiol 27:515–518, 2004.

CASE 7-15
Right Pulmonary Artery Stenosis

This 59-year-old man with complex congenital heart disease had a history of tetralogy of Fallot with several prior surgeries, most recently a bileaflet mechanical aortic valve prosthesis 10 years ago. About 7 months before the present admission he suffered a witnessed cardiac arrest, for which a pacemaker-defibrillator was placed. However, after placement of the AICD, he continued to complain of fatigue and shortness of breath with mild exertion. Right heart catheterization and pulmonary angiography revealed elevated right-sided pressures, significant ostial stenosis of the right pulmonary artery, and a hypoplastic left lung circulation with severe distal pruning of vessels. Echocardiography revealed biventricular dysfunction, severe pulmonic regurgitation, and tricuspid regurgitation. He was scheduled for surgery.

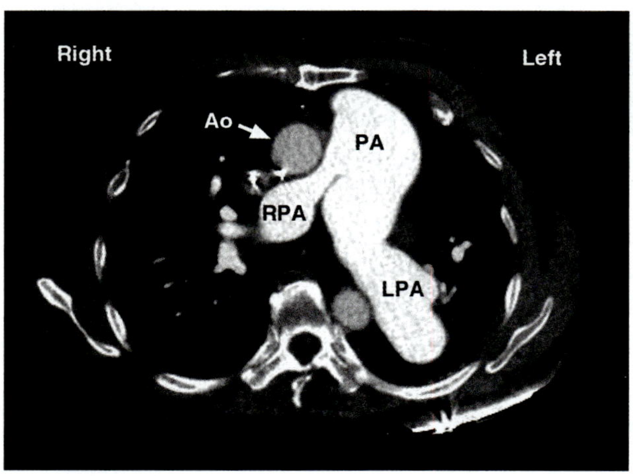

Fig 7.100 CT scan showed dilated main and left pulmonary arteries, and stenotic origin of right pulmonary artery. Left lung is much smaller than right lung.

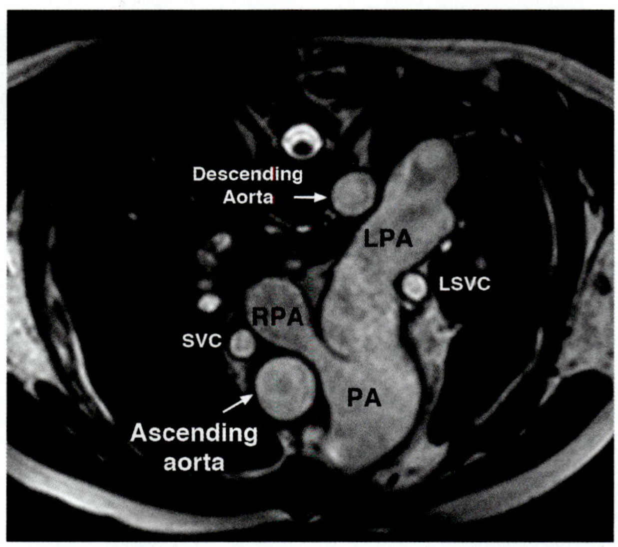

Fig 7.101 MRI has been rotated to match image seen with TEE. In addition to findings on CT scan, both right and left superior vena cavae are seen.

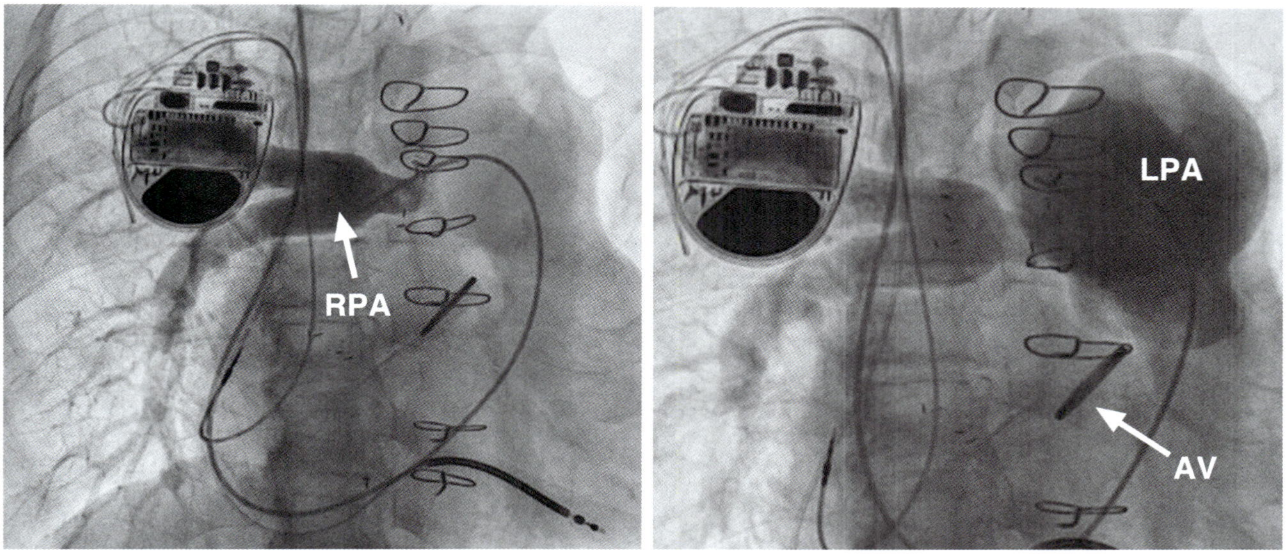

Fig 7.102 Pulmonary angiography shows marked discrepancy in size of pulmonary artery branches. Prosthetic aortic valve is also visualized.

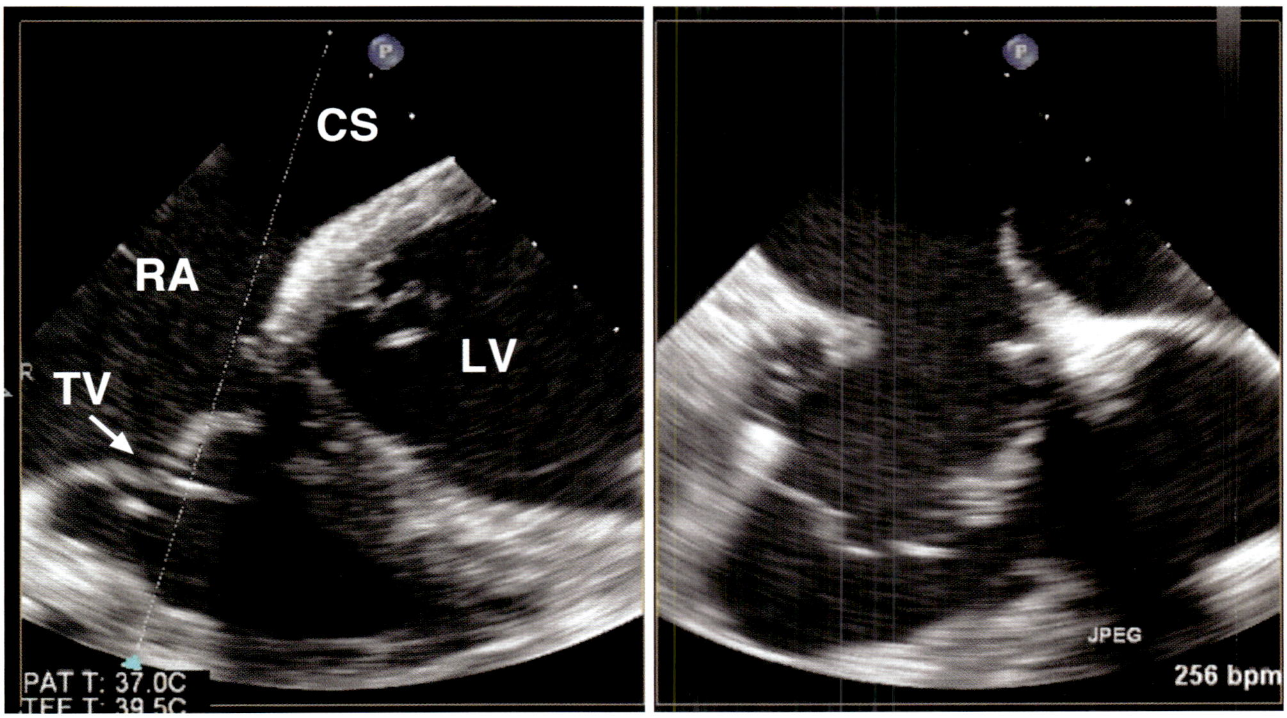

Fig 7.103 Enlarged coronary sinus, consistent with left-sided SVC is seen.

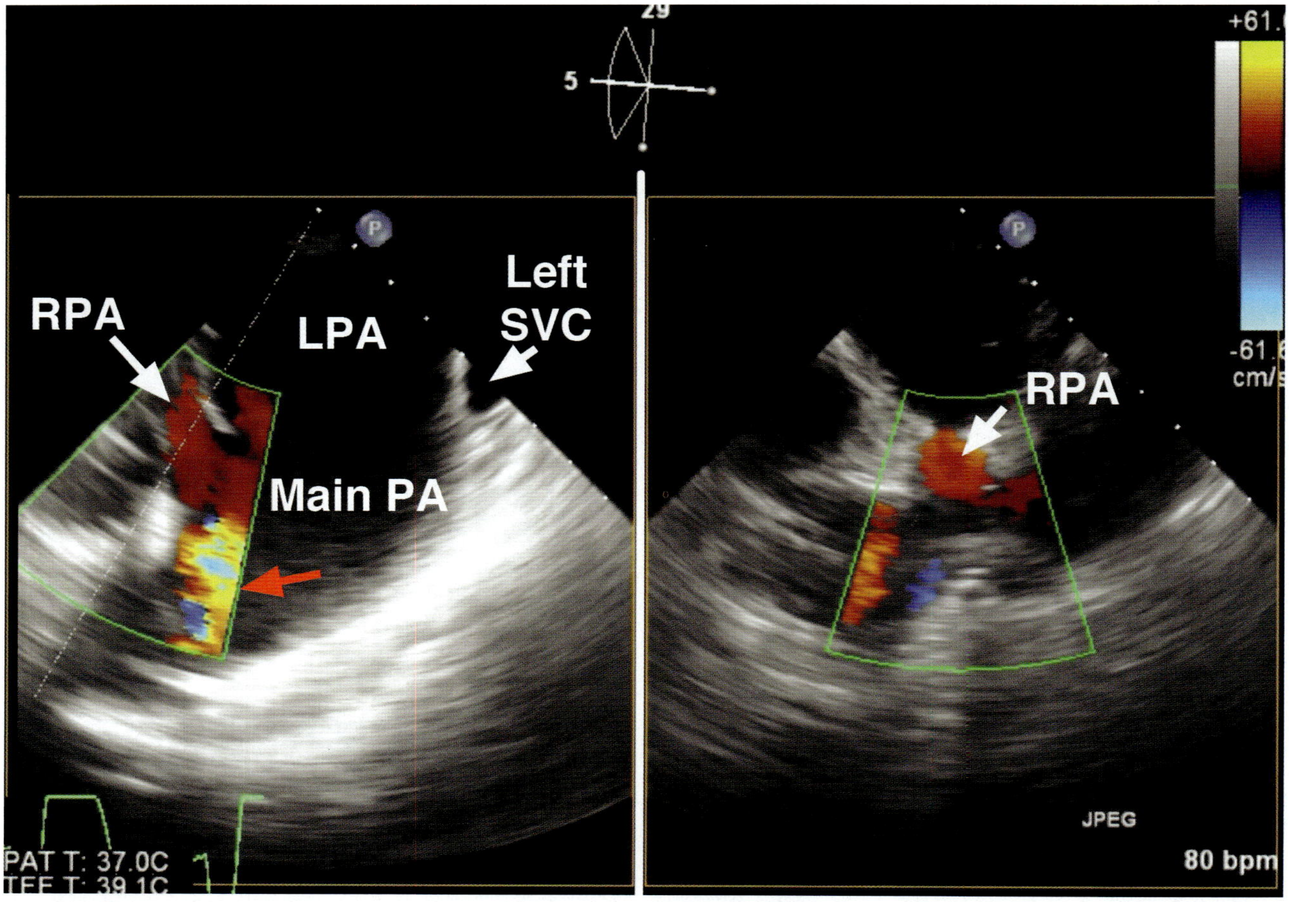

Fig 7.104 In this high esophageal TEE, abnormal pulmonary artery bifurcation is seen.

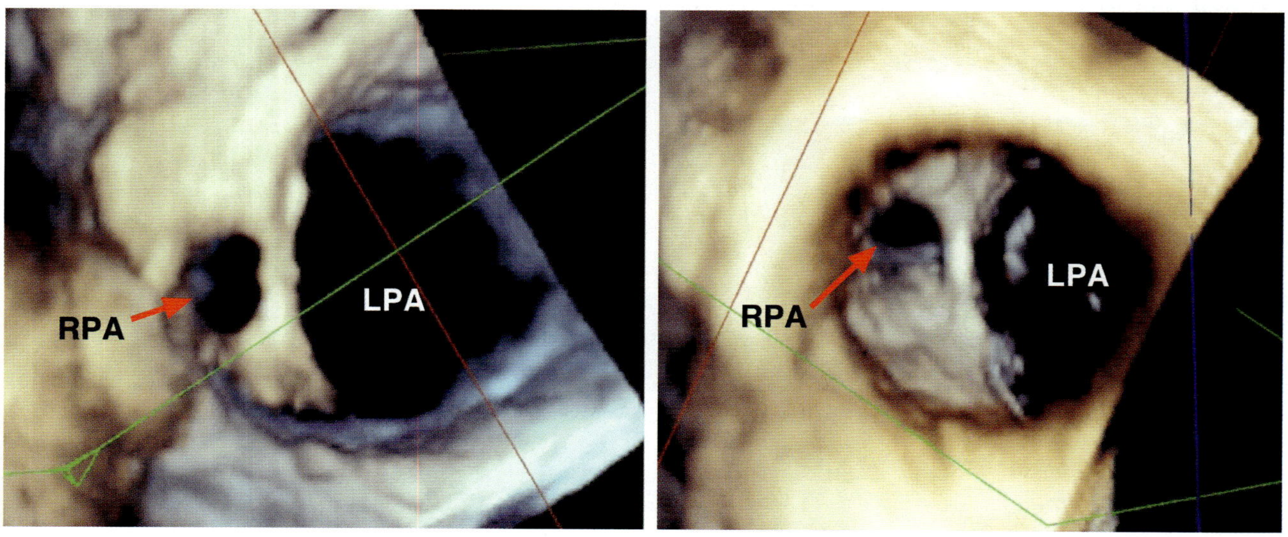

Fig 7.105 On left, pulmonary artery bifurcation is seen from superior perspective, and on right, bifurcating is seen from right ventricular outflow tract perspective.

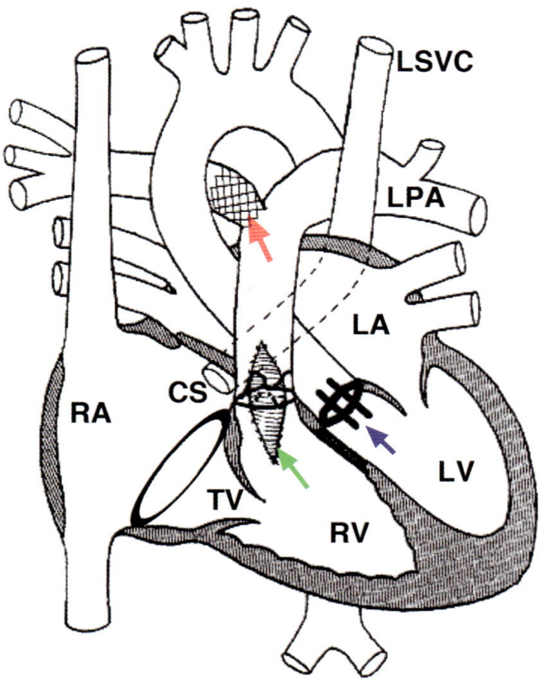

Fig 7.106 Schematic shows components of procedure: incision of RVOT and pulmonic valve replacement *(green arrow)*, introduction of stent *(red arrow)* into right pulmonary artery via RVOT incision, and tricuspid ring annuloplasty. Preexisting bileaflet mechanical aortic valve prosthesis is indicated by blue arrow.

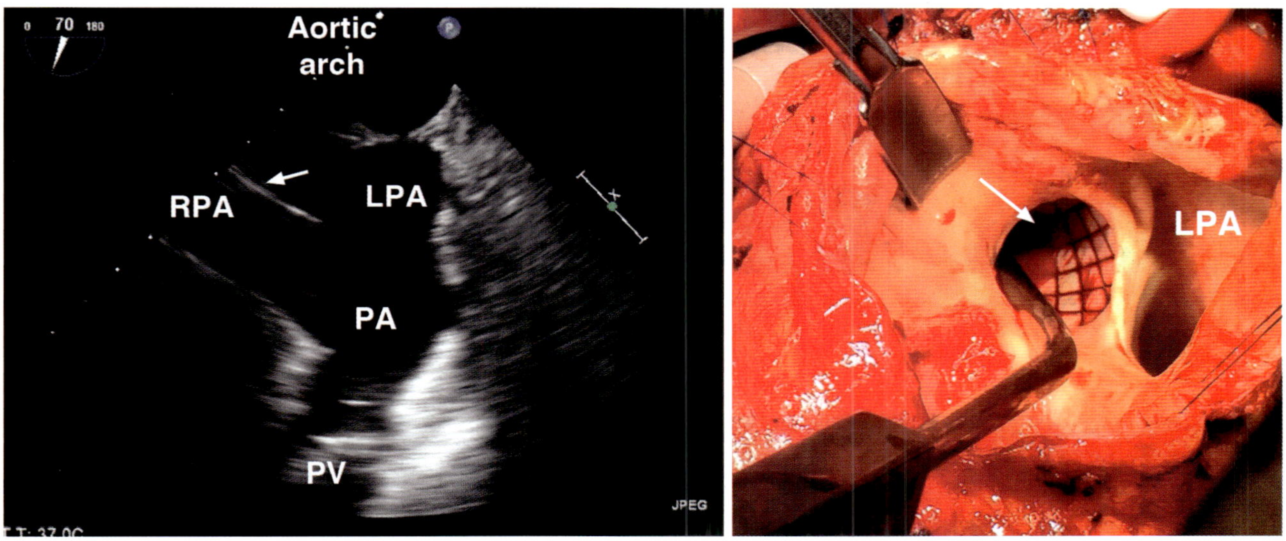

Fig 7.107 In this high esophageal TEE, stent *(arrow)* is seen bridging right pulmonary artery orifice. On right is in vivo image showing stent in right pulmonary artery.

Comments

Branch pulmonary artery stenosis often accompanies tetralogy of Fallot and can lead to clinical symptoms as in this case. TTE diagnosis can be challenging because of limited visualization of the pulmonary artery branches but may be suspected with an unexplained high velocity systolic Doppler flow signal is found. This case illustrates the utility of TEE for visualization of the branch pulmonary arteries and for guiding placement of the stent to relieve stenosis.

Suggested Reading

1. Maskatia SA, Spinner JA, Morris SA, et al: Effect of branch pulmonary artery stenosis on right ventricular volume overload in patients with tetralogy of Fallot after initial surgical repair, Am J Cardiol 111(9):1355–1360, 2013.
2. Narayan HK, Glatz AC, Rome JJ: Bifurcating stents in the pulmonary arteries: A novel technique to relieve bilateral branch pulmonary artery obstruction, Catheter Cardiovasc Interv 86(4):714–718, 2015.
4. Wilder TJ, Van Arsdell GS, Pham-Hung E, et al: Aggressive patch augmentation may reduce growth potential of hypoplastic branch pulmonary arteries after tetralogy of Fallot repair, Ann Thorac Surg 101(3):996–1004, 2016.

Complex Congenital Heart Disease

CASE 7-16
Subaortic Membrane

This 25-year-old woman presented during pregnancy with increasing exertional dyspnea. Examination revealed a 4/6 systolic murmur at the base radiating to the carotids. Transthoracic echocardiography demonstrated a subaortic membrane with an antegrade velocity of 5.4 m/s.

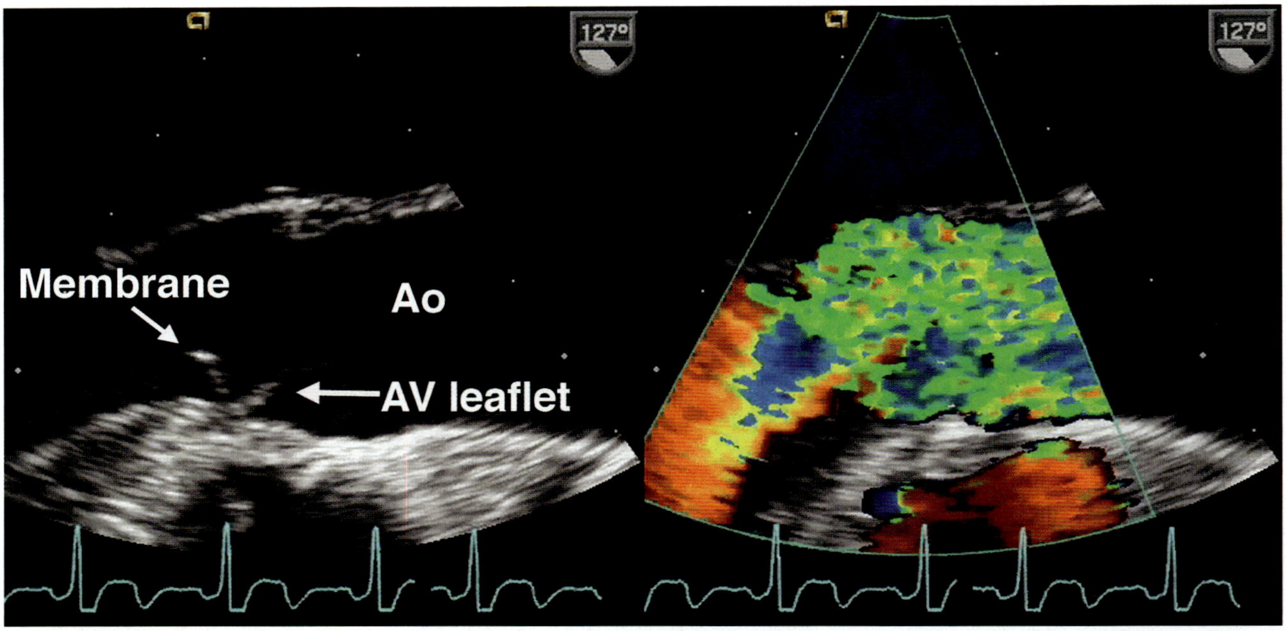

Fig 7.108 In long-axis TEE view at 127 degrees, linear echo consistent with subaortic membrane is seen adjacent to right coronary cusp of aortic valve. Color Doppler *(right)* shows aliasing at level of membrane, suggesting increased velocity due to obstruction to blood flow. In real time, small amount of aortic regurgitation is appreciated.

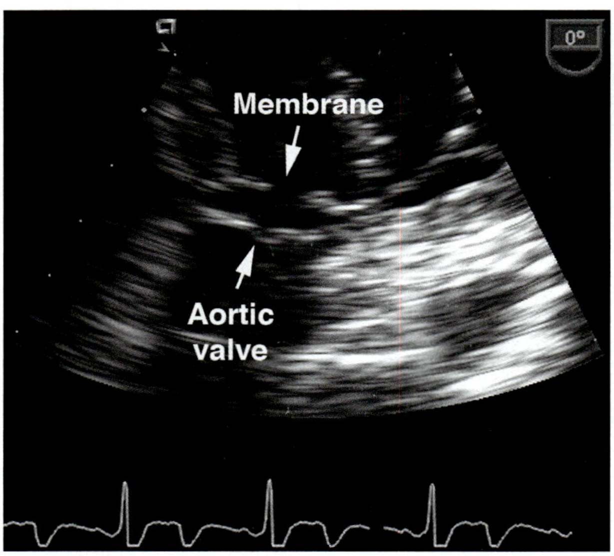

Fig 7.109 In transgastric apical view angled anteriorly to image aortic valve, linear membrane is seen about 0.5 cm proximal to aortic valve plane. In real time, a transgastric long-axis view shows proximal flow convergence at the level of the membrane.

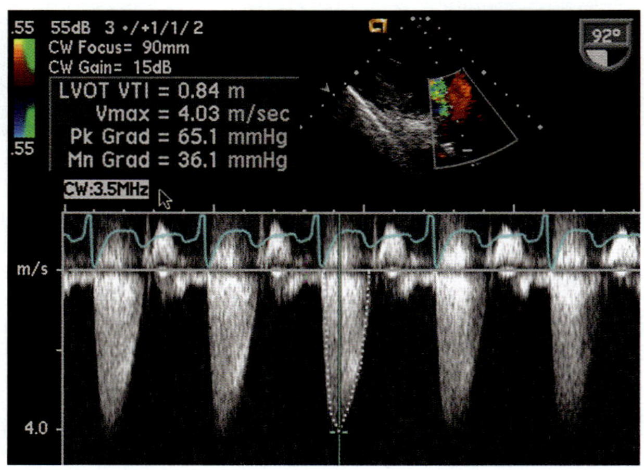

Fig 7.110 Continuous wave Doppler interrogation of aortic valve from transgastric long-axis view yields maximum velocity of at least 4.0 m/s, with mean gradient of 36 mm Hg.

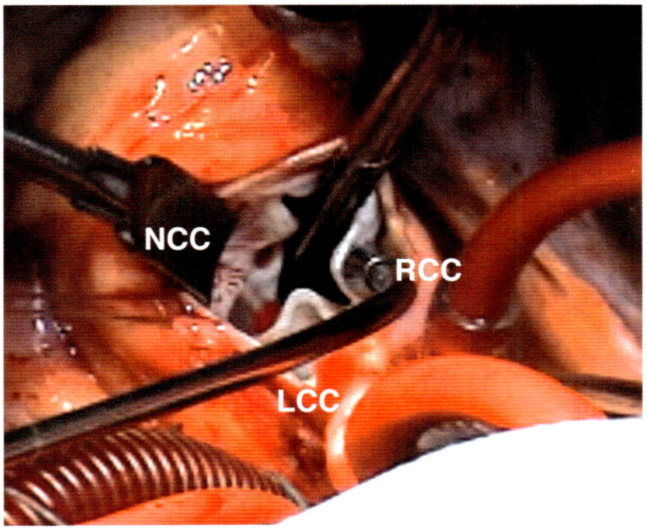

Fig 7.111 Intraoperative photograph of aortic valve with non (NCC), right (RCC), and left coronary cusps (LCC).

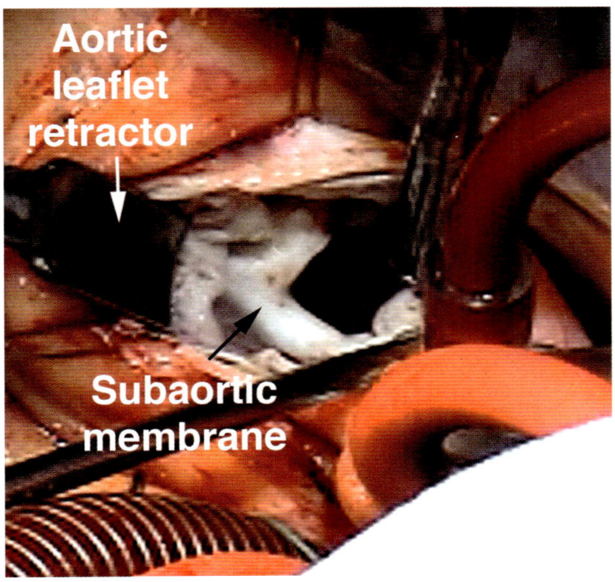

Fig 7.112 With aortic leaflets retracted, white subaortic membrane is seen. Membrane was uneventfully resected.

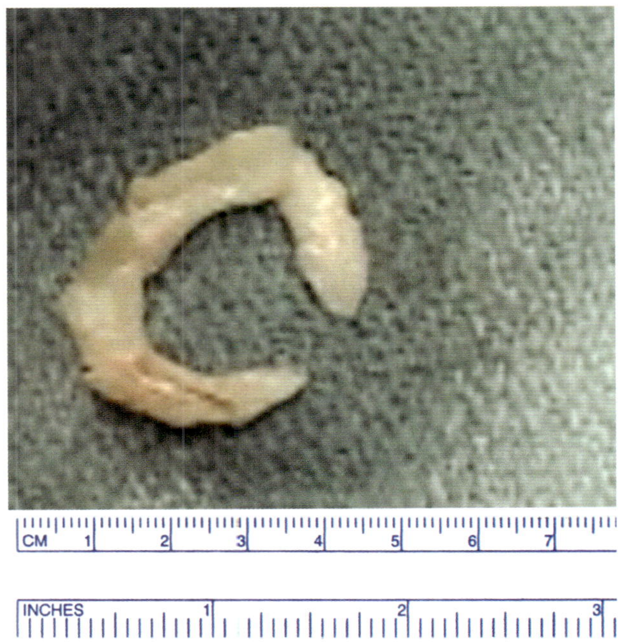

Fig 7.113 Resected membrane showing C-shaped membrane that nearly encircled outflow tract. Echocardiography 1 month after surgery showed only small area of increased echogenicity along ventricular septum in subaortic region with no evidence for significant obstruction to flow.

Comments

The symptoms and physical examination findings of subaortic membranes are similar to valvular aortic stenosis, and this diagnosis should be considered in younger patients with evidence of left ventricular outflow obstruction. The membrane itself may be difficult to visualize on transthoracic imaging. However, color and pulsed Doppler evidence for acceleration of flow proximal to the aortic valve suggests this possibility. Aortic regurgitation may be present if turbulence from the subaortic stenosis has damaged the valve leaflets. TEE imaging both confirms the diagnosis and allows delineation of the anatomy of the membrane. Aspects important in surgical planning are the type of subaortic obstruction (muscular versus membranous), the distance between the membrane and the aortic valve, the presence of severity of aortic regurgitation and any evidence for attachments between the membrane and the valve leaflets. When aortic valve function is normal, the subaortic membrane typically can be resected with preservation of the aortic valve, as in this case.

Suggested Reading

1. Mancuso AJ, Clark J, Mahmood F: Left ventricular outflow tract obstruction: Is it the valve or something else? J Cardiothorac Vasc Anesth 28(3):848–849, 2014.
2. Anderson MJ, Arruda-Olson A, Gersh B, Geske J: Subaortic membrane mimicking hypertrophic cardiomyopathy, BMJ Case Rep 2015.
3. Pickard SS, Geva A, Gauvreau K, et al: Long-term outcomes and risk factors for aortic regurgitation after discrete subvalvular aortic stenosis resection in children, Heart 101(19):1547–1553, 2015.

CASE 7-17
Corrected Transposition of the Great Arteries (Ventricular Inversion)

This 19-year-old woman with congenitally corrected transposition of the great vessels was referred for systemic atrioventricular valve replacement for severe regurgitation with worsening systemic ventricular function and progressive heart failure symptoms. Physical examination showed a blood pressure of 103/55mm Hg, regular heart rate at 118 bpm, weight of 106 lb, a hyperdynamic precordium, and a 3/6 holosystolic murmur heard throughout the precordium.

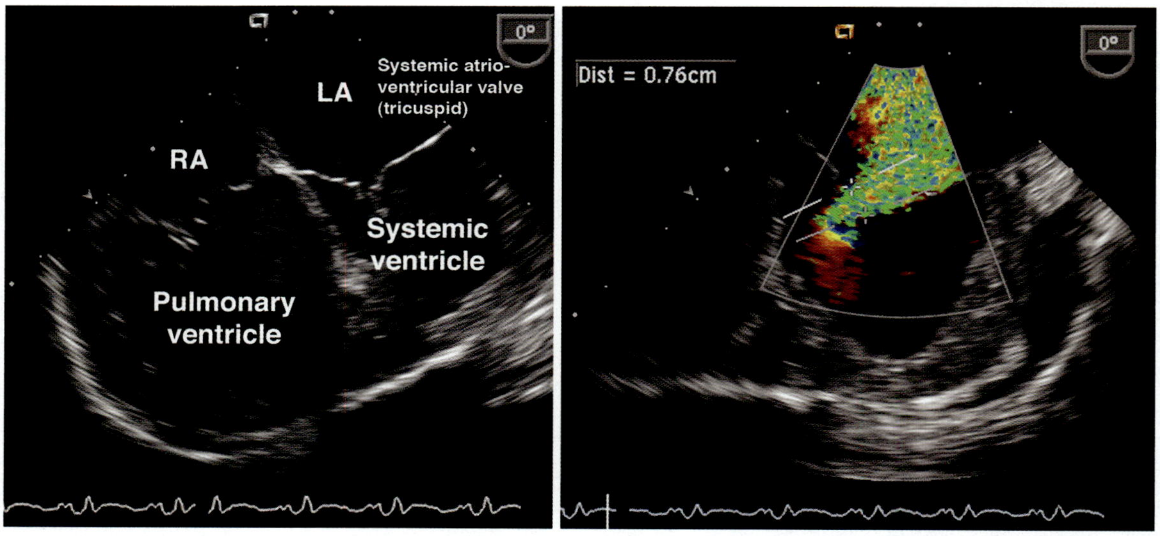

Fig 7.114 TEE four-chamber view *(left)* demonstrates dilated systemic and pulmonary ventricles. Systemic ventricle is anatomic right ventricle that ejects into aorta. Pulmonary ventricle is anatomic left ventricle that ejects into pulmonary artery. Pulmonary ventricle is severely dilated, with severely reduced systolic function. Systemic ventricle is mildly dilated, with moderate global hypokinesis. Color Doppler *(right)* demonstrates severe regurgitation of systemic atrioventricular valve (anatomic tricuspid valve) with vena contracta width of 0.8 cm.

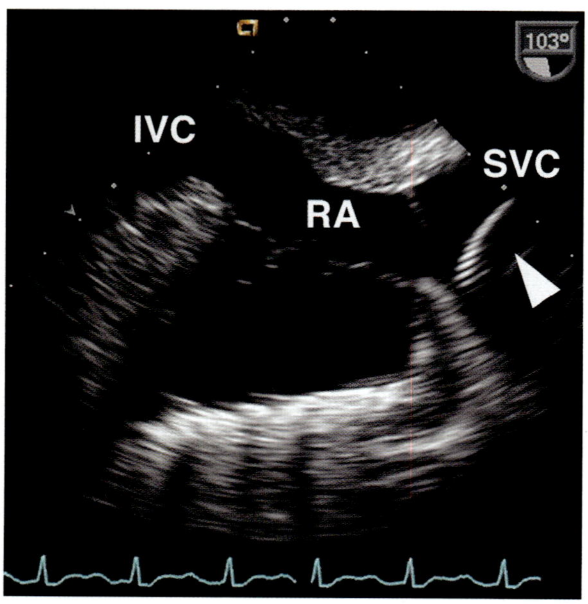

Fig 7.115 Bicaval view shows superior vena cava and inferior vena cava (SVC, IVC) entering right atrium (RA). Venous drainage cannula *(arrowhead)* is seen in SVC.

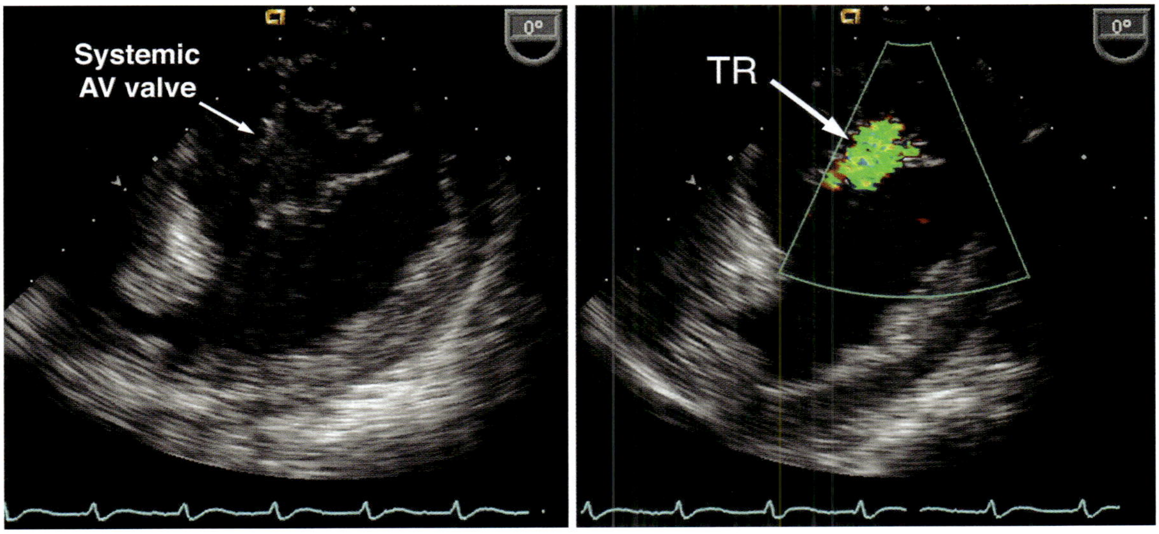

Fig 7.116 Transgastric short-axis view in diastole *(left)* demonstrates tricuspid valve in systemic ventricle. In systole *(right)*, central regurgitant jet is appreciated.

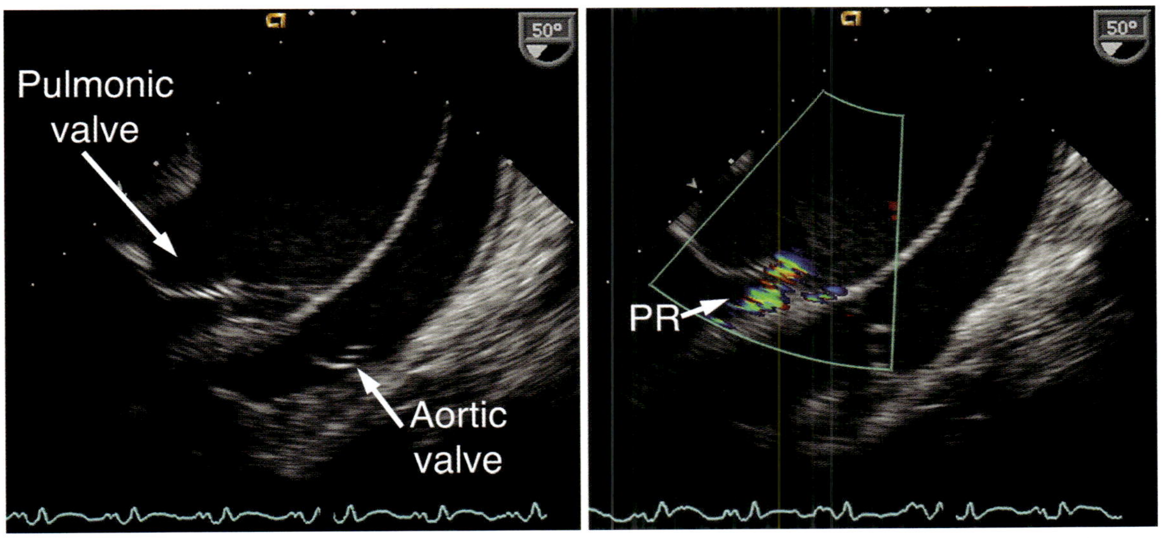

Fig 7.117 Long-axis view of aorta shows that aortic and pulmonic valves are seen in long axis in same image plane and great vessels are parallel to each other. Pulmonary artery is markedly dilated compared with smaller aorta. Color Doppler (*right*) shows mild pulmonic regurgitation (PR).

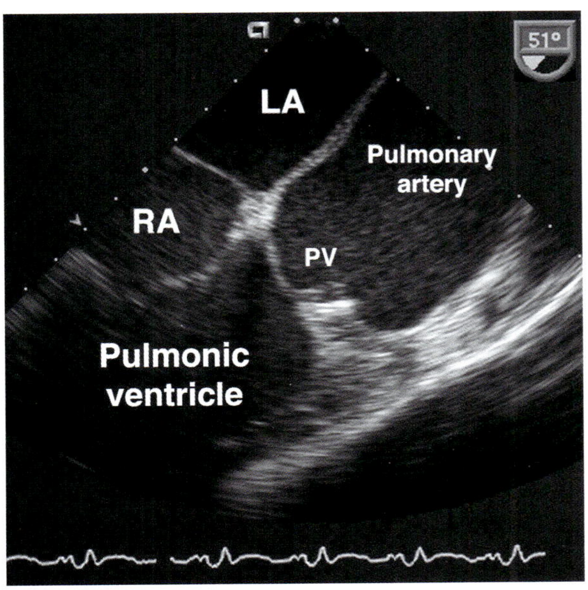

Fig 7.118 Changing angle of interrogation to 51 degrees, with slight rightward turning of probe, gives view of right atrium (RA), pulmonic ventricle, pulmonic valve (PV), and pulmonary artery, similar to long-axis view.

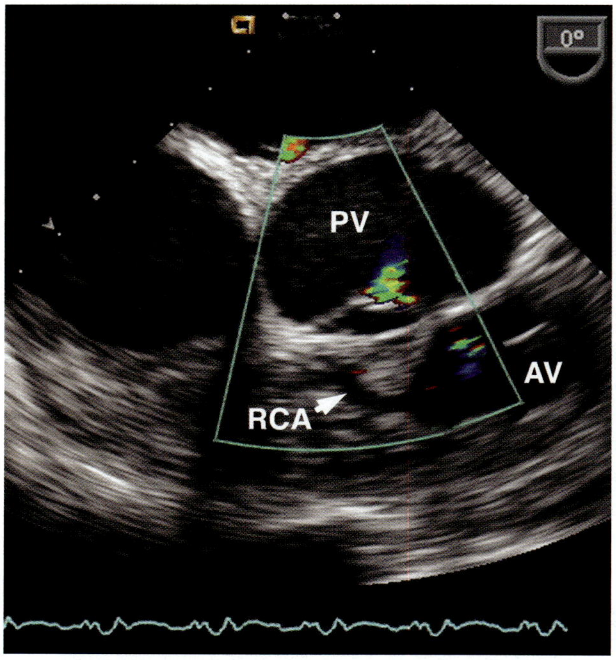

Fig 7.119 Short-axis view shows aortic and pulmonic valves in same image plane. Origin of right coronary artery (RCA) is also seen.

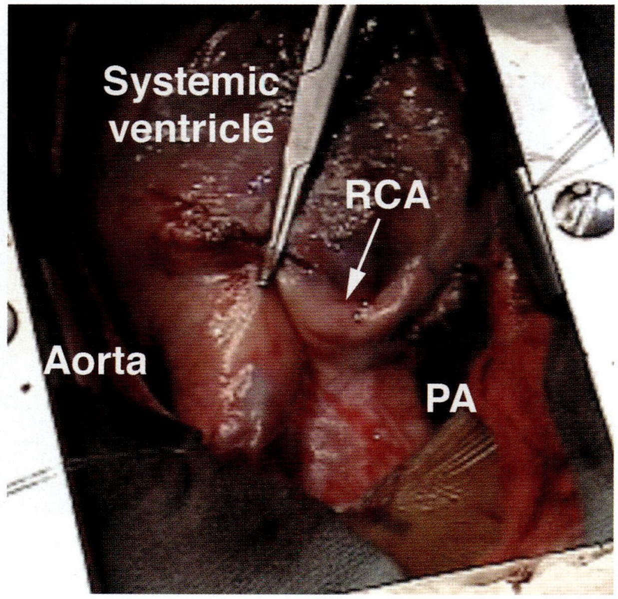

Fig 7.120 Intraoperative photograph shows side-by-side great vessels with anterior aorta (note right coronary artery arising from aorta).

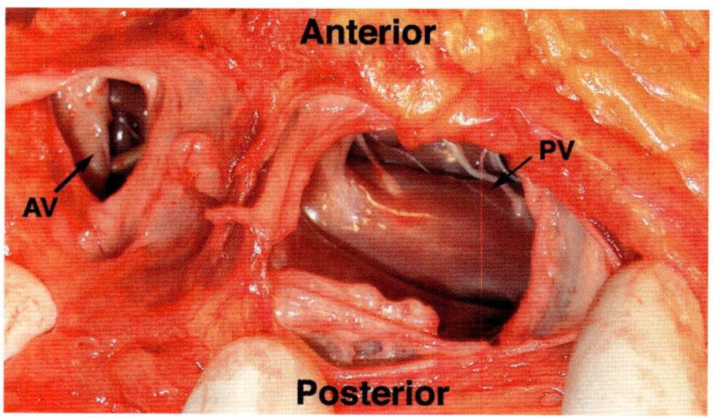

Fig 7.121 In another patient with similar anatomy who underwent heart transplantation, photograph of explanted heart with great vessels removed shows side-by-side pulmonic and aortic valves.

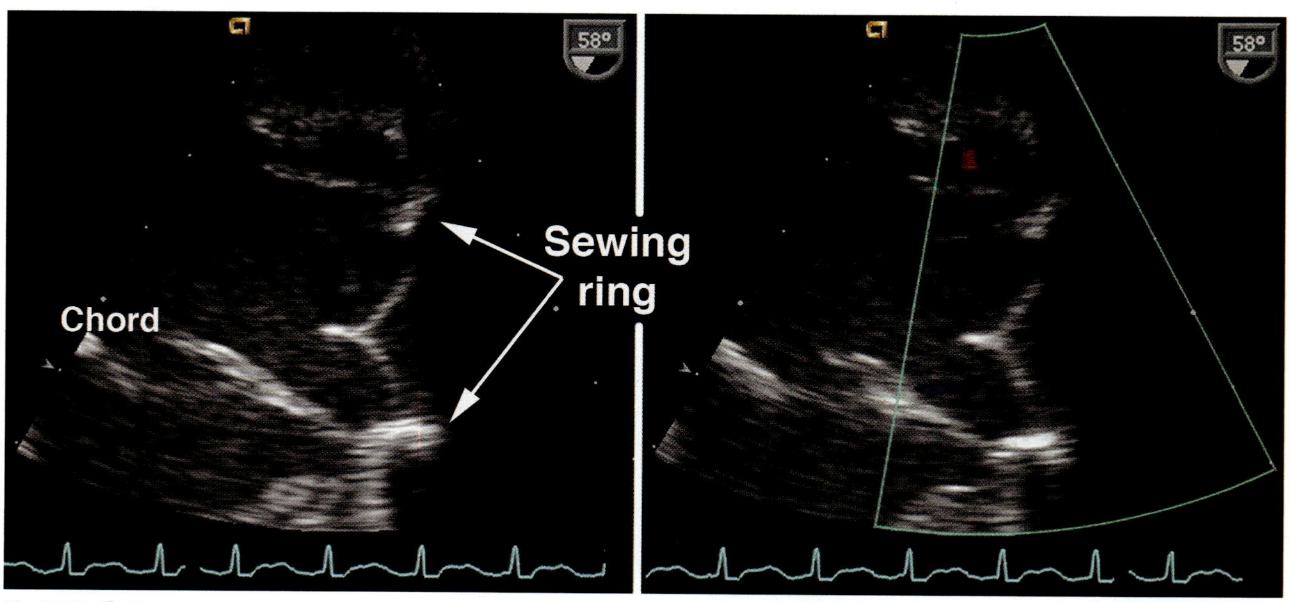

Fig 7.122 Tissue prosthesis in systemic atrioventricular position is seen in transgastric two-chamber view in systole. Some of valve chords were retained to help preserve ventricular function. Color Doppler *(right)* demonstrated no regurgitation.

Comments

With complex congenital heart disease, the echocardiographer should seek to define the pathway of blood flow and identify each cardiac chamber and valve. With congenitally corrected transposition of the great vessels, systemic venous blood returns to the right atrium, flows through the mitral valve into the left ventricle and is then ejected into the pulmonary artery, across the pulmonic valve. The pulmonary veins drain into the left atrium, oxygenated blood crosses the tricuspid valve into the right ventricle and is then ejected across the aortic valve into the aorta. Thus the movement of oxygenated blood is normal, only the ventricles are reversed; therefore, this condition is sometimes called "ventricular inversion." These patients typically come to medical attention because of associated defects such as tricuspid (systemic atrioventricular valve) regurgitation, VSD, pulmonic stenosis, and heart block.

The identification of the right atrium is based on the entrance of the IVC and SVC into this chamber. The pulmonary veins usually drain into the left atrium.

Shape and wall thickness cannot be used to distinguish the right and left ventricles when there is transposition of the great vessels, as dilation and hypertrophy alter the geometry of both ventricles. However, the atrioventricular valves stay with the corresponding ventricular chamber, so that the mitral valve identifies the anatomic left ventricle and the tricuspid valve the anatomic right ventricle, although it is important to distinguish a cleft mitral valve from a trileaflet tricuspid valve. Other features that identify the anatomic right ventricle include:

- The annular plane of the tricuspid valve is slightly more apical than the mitral annulus (see Fig 7.114).
- The right ventricle has a moderator band and more prominent trabeculation.

Great vessel anatomy is determined by following the vessels distally. The pulmonary artery is identified based on bifurcation into branches that supply the pulmonary vasculature. The aorta is identified by the arch and head and neck vessels. The semilunar valves are positioned in the corresponding great vessel: for example, aortic valve in the aorta and pulmonic valve in the pulmonary artery. Unlike the normal perpendicular orientation of aortic and pulmonic valve planes, both valves are in the same plane with transposition of the great vessels. The aorta and pulmonary artery are side by side (with the aorta anterior) unlike the normal crisscross relationship with the pulmonary artery anteriorly.

Suggested Reading

1. Placci A, Lovato L, Bonvicini M: Congenitally corrected transposition of the great arteries in an 83-year-old asymptomatic patient: Description and literature review, BMJ Case Rep 2014.
2. Mah K, Friedberg MK: Congenitally corrected transposition of the great arteries: Situs solitus or inversus, Circ Cardiovasc Imaging 7(5):849–851, 2014.

CASE 7-18
Tricuspid Atresia with Fontan Physiology

This 42-year-old man with tricuspid atresia underwent surgical palliation as a child with connection of the right atrium to the pulmonary artery. Thus all the systemic venous return was directed to the pulmonary artery without an intervening ventricle (e.g., Fontan physiology). The pulmonary artery was oversewn just distal to the pulmonic valve so that the entire ventricular output was directed to the systemic vasculature. He did well for many years, leading an active life, including bicycling. He was able to complete a college education followed by a full-time professional career.

His major cardiac limitation was due to recurrent atrial arrhythmias, which were treated with medication, a pacemaker, and several ablation procedures. However, progressive right atrial enlargement was associated with worsening arrhythmias, symptoms and signs of right heart failure, and evidence of a protein-losing enteropathy. He was referred for right atrial reduction with surgical revision of the Fontan conduit.

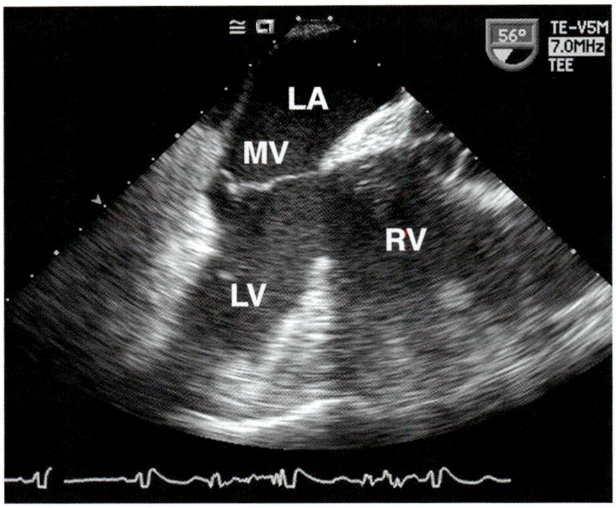

Fig 7.123 TEE view at 56 degrees demonstrates left atrium, mitral valve, and left ventricle. Large ventricular septal defect is present so that left and right ventricles function as common chamber.

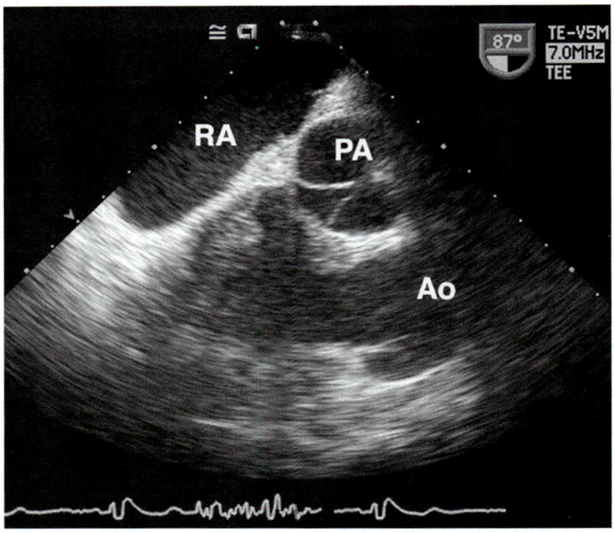

Fig 7.124 With image plane rotated further to 87 degrees, pulmonary artery (PA) and aorta (Ao) are seen. In this patient, pulmonary artery had been oversewn just distal to pulmonic valve. Although there is some motion of bicuspid pulmonic valve, there is no significant antegrade flow. Both pulmonic and aortic valve arise from common ventricular chamber.

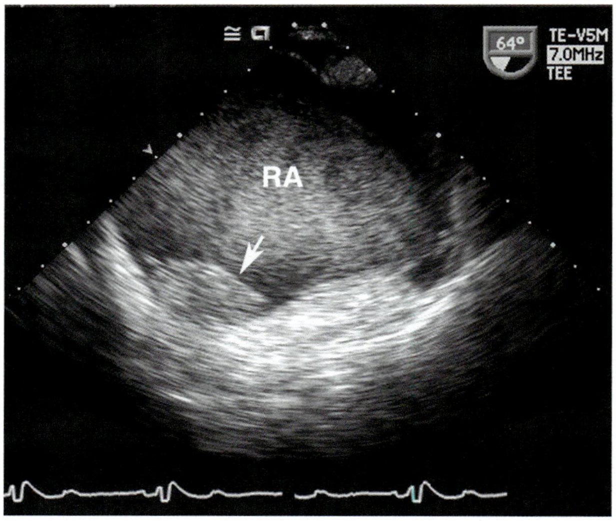

Fig 7.125 With transducer turned toward patient's right side at image plane of 64 degrees, severe enlarged right atrium (RA) with marked spontaneous contrast and mural thrombus *(arrow)* is seen.

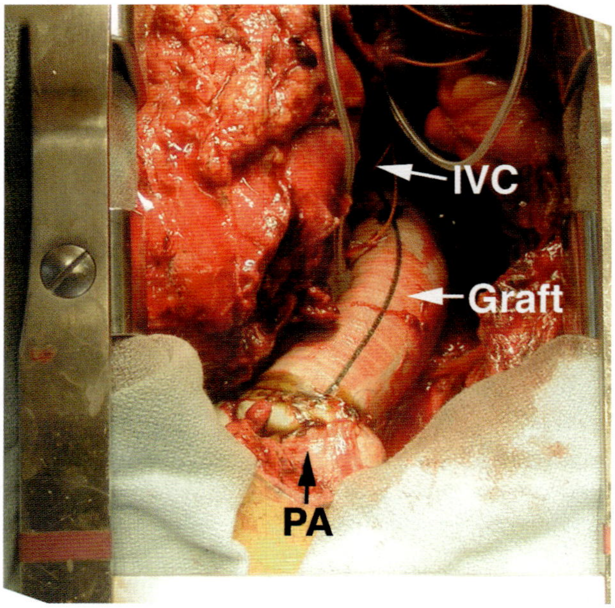

Fig 7.126 At surgery, right atrial size was reduced and common atrium formed with right and left chambers. Dacron nonvalved conduit was placed from IVC to main PA, as seen in this photograph. SVC was connected directly to right PA.

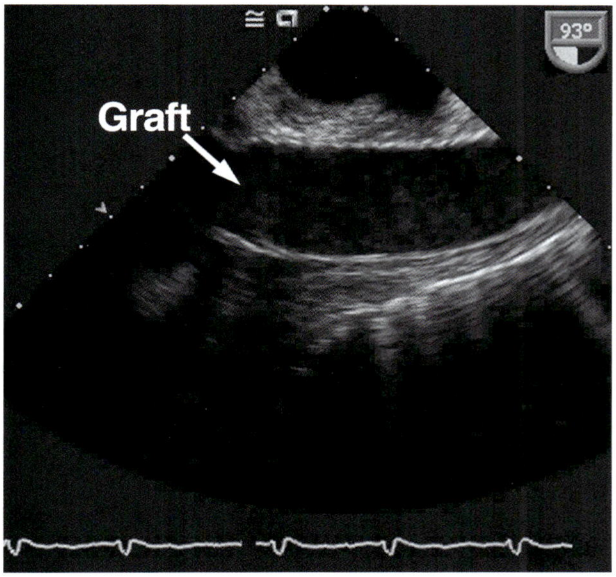

Fig 7.127 Graft is visualized on TEE using 93-degree image plane with transducer turned toward patient's right side.

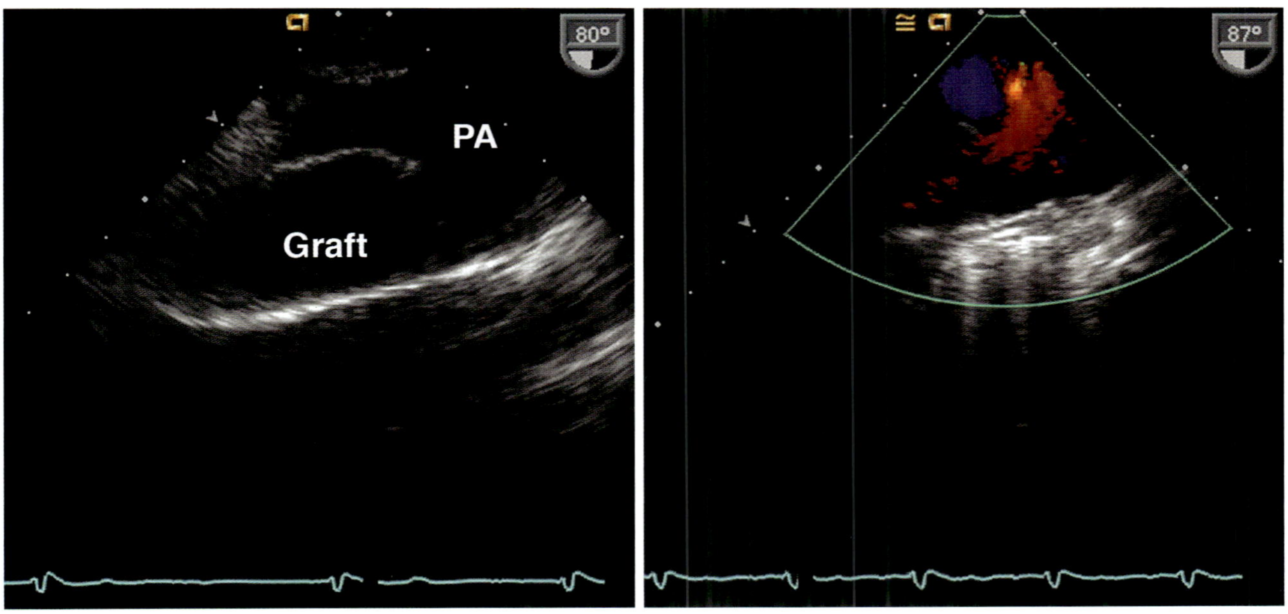

Fig 7.128 Transducer is moved cephalad to image more superior segments of graft and connection to PA. Color Doppler shows no obstruction to flow at distal anastomosis of graft.

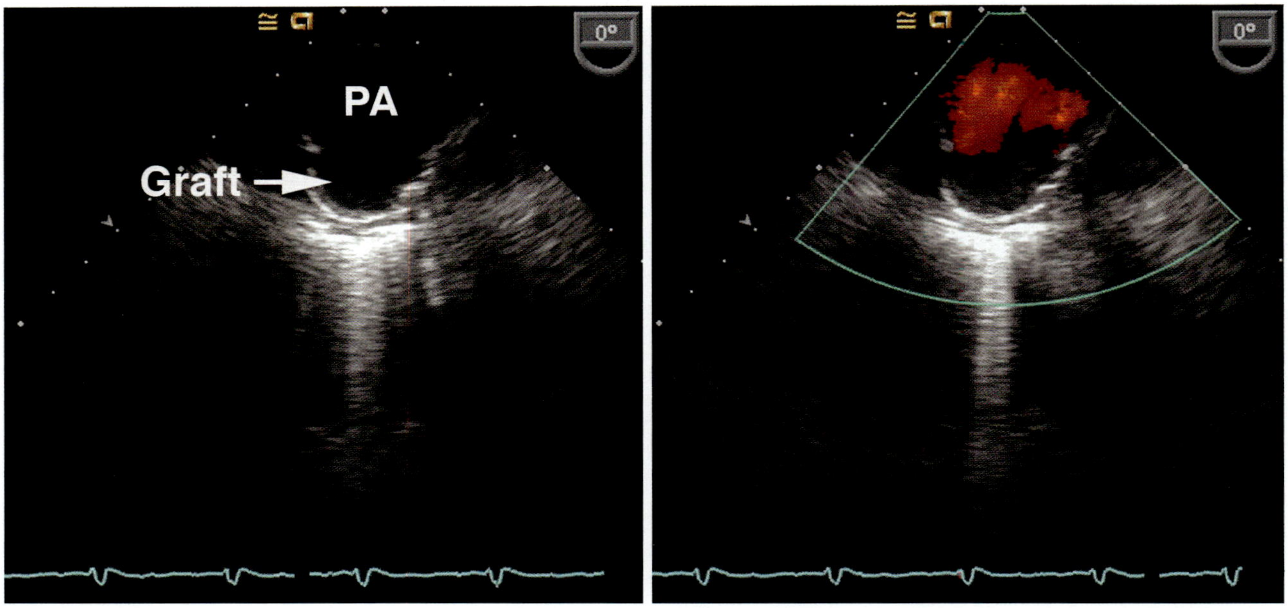

Fig 7.129 Rotation of image plane to 0 degrees provides short-axis view of graft at entrance into PA.

Comments

In complex congenital heart disease with only one functional ventricle, as in this patient with tricuspid atresia, one surgical option is to direct the systemic venous return into the pulmonary vasculature without an intervening ventricle. Thus pulmonary blood flow is not pulsatile, and adequate forward flow depends on systemic venous pressure being higher than left atrial pressure, a pattern of pulmonary flow often termed Fontan physiology. Early in the history of this procedure, the vena caval connections were left intact and the right atrium was connected to the pulmonary artery. However, as these patients grew to adulthood, the right atrium progressively enlarged, leading to refractory atrial arrhythmias, elevated systemic venous pressures, and compression of the pulmonary veins. The current surgical approach is to connect the SVC and IVC more directly to the pulmonary artery, to avoid progressive right atrial enlargement. In patients with the earlier procedure, as in this patient, revision of the Fontan procedure to eliminate the right atrium may be considered when arrhythmias are refractory or for progressive right heart failure symptoms.

Suggested Reading

1. Kutty S, Rathod RH, Danford DA, Celermajer DS: Role of imaging in the evaluation of single ventricle with the Fontan palliation, Heart 102(3):174–183, 2016.
2. Zaragoza-Macias E, Schwaegler RG, Stout KK: Echocardiographic evaluation of univentricular physiology and cavopulmonary shunts, Echocardiography 32(Suppl 2):S166–S176, 2015.

CASE 7-19
Severe Pulmonic Regurgitation after Remote Pulmonary Valvotomy

This 53-year-old woman with a history of a pulmonary valvotomy at the age of 5 for congenital pulmonary stenosis was referred because of a 6-month history of increasing shortness of breath, syncope, fluid retention, and generalized fatigue. Prior to the last 6 months she had done well, with little limitation. TTE showed increasing tricuspid and pulmonic regurgitation, as well as right ventricular enlargement.

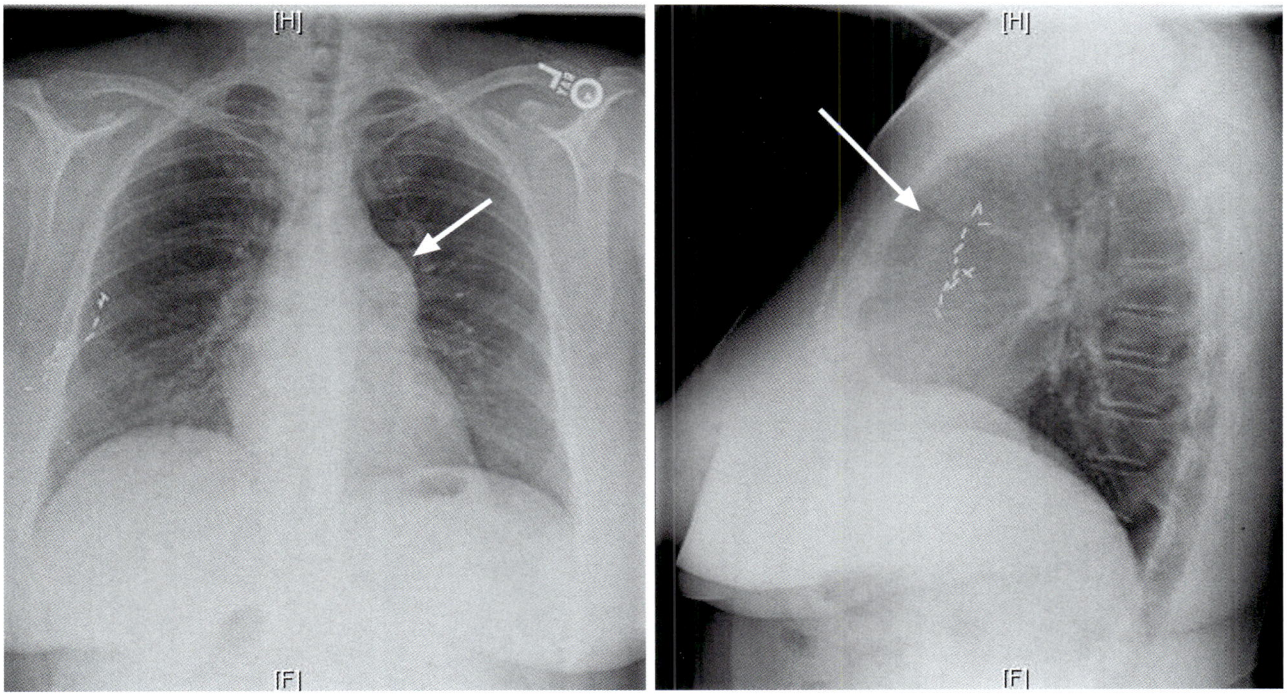

Fig 7.130 Preoperative chest x-ray showed enlarged main pulmonary artery *(left, arrow)*, and diminished retrosternal airspace, suggestive of right ventricular enlargement *(right, arrow)*.

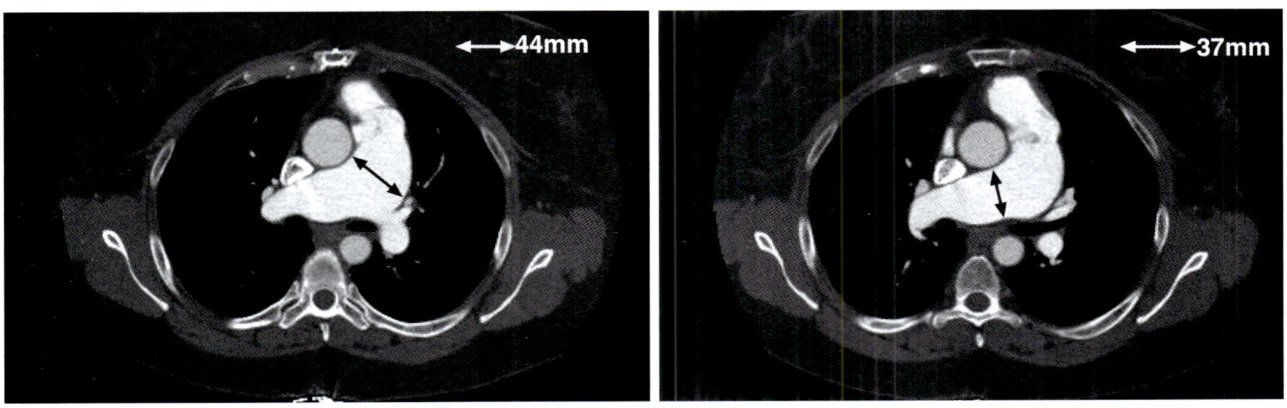

Fig 7.131 CT scan showed enlargement of main pulmonary artery *(left)* and right pulmonary artery *(right)*.

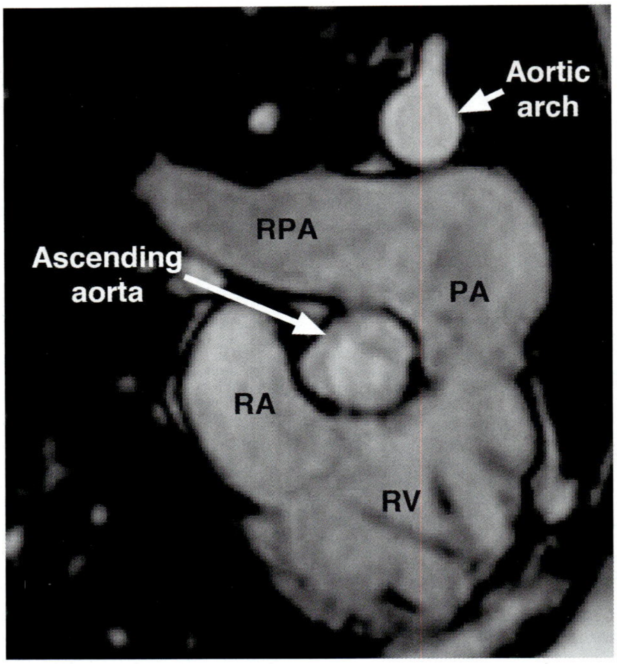

Fig 7.132 Preoperative MRI showed enlargement of all right-sided cardiac structures.

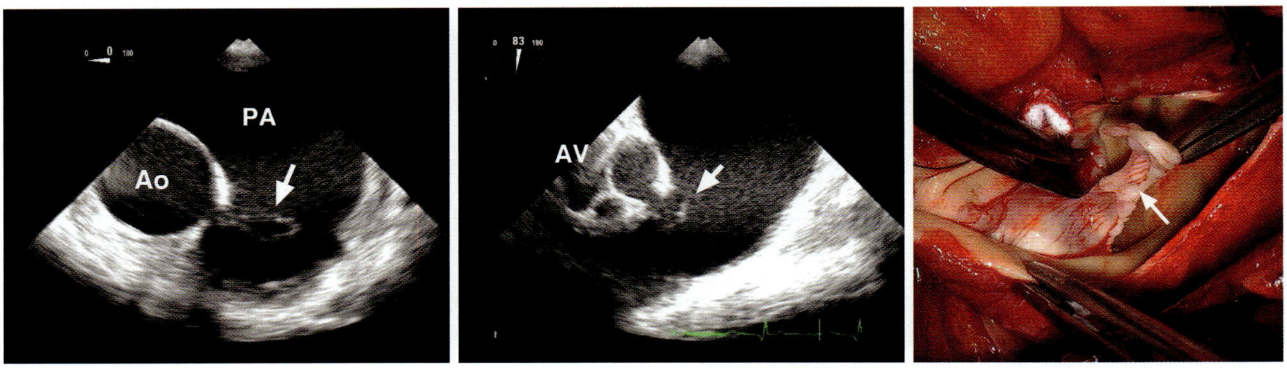

Fig 7.133 Form high esophageal window, orthogonal views of pulmonary artery are seen. In both, there is no functional valvular tissue identified; there are just remnants of pulmonic valve. On right, intraoperative image shows surgeon retracting pulmonic valvular tissue, just before resecting it.

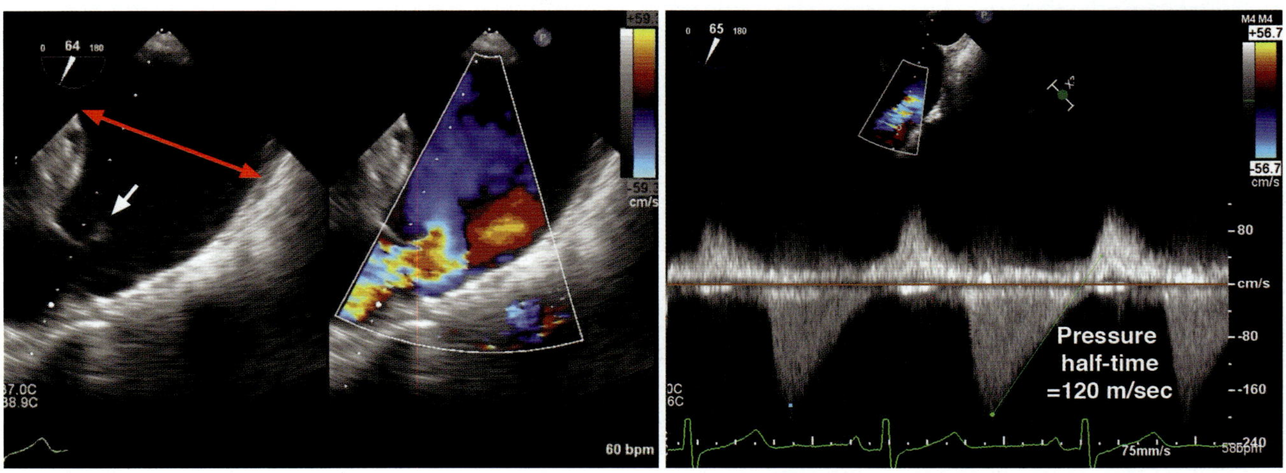

Fig 7.134 Simultaneous 2D and color Doppler imaging again reveals remnants of pulmonic valvular tissue, as well as broad jet of pulmonic regurgitation. Diameter of main pulmonary artery is measured at 44 mm *(red arrow)*. On right, continuous wave Doppler shows pulmonic regurgitation and jet shows steep deceleration slope with pressure half-time of 120 msec, consistent with severe pulmonic regurgitation.

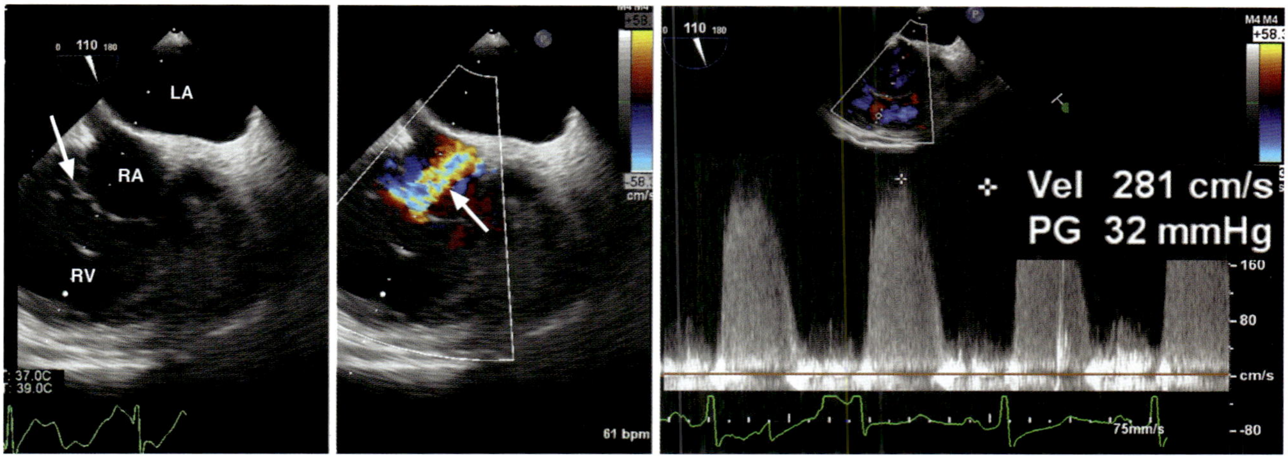

Fig 7.135 From midesophageal bicaval view with rotation to patient's left, jet of TR is seen. Tricuspid annular diameter had been measured at 48 mm. Continuous wave Doppler showed right atrial to right ventricular systolic gradient of 32 mm Hg; added to CVP of 15 yields RVSP of 47 mm Hg.

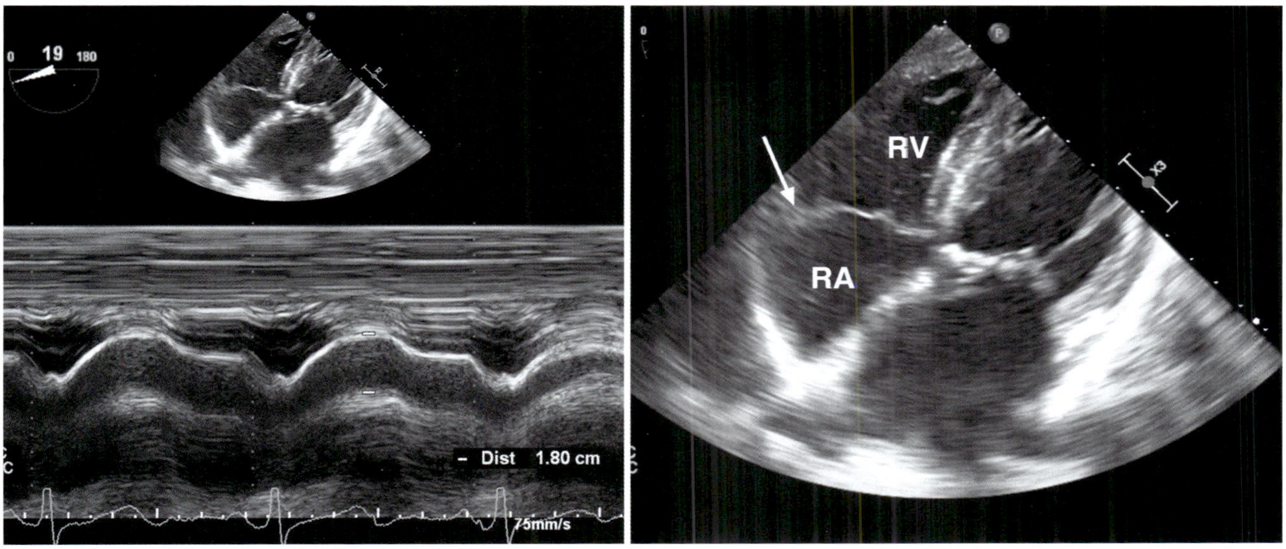

Fig 7.136 Although right ventricle was dilated, right ventricular systolic function was normal, as indicated by TAPSE of 1.8 cm. As seen in example in right frame, measurement can be made with TEE from deep transgastric position with probe turned to patient's right. Lateral tricuspid annulus is indicated by arrow.

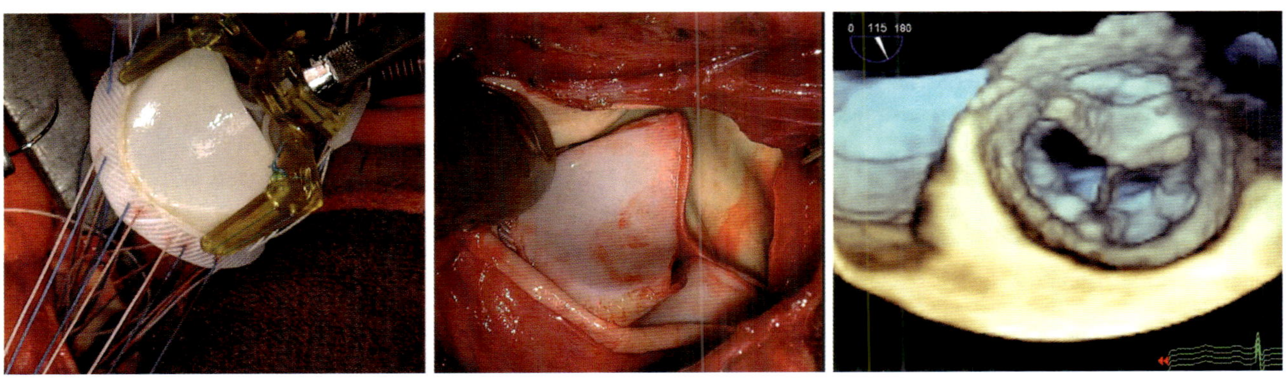

Fig 7.137 In left frame, trileaflet prosthetic tissue prosthesis is seen in its holder. In middle frame valve prosthesis is seen in its final position. On right is 3D TEE of tissue prosthesis in diastole.

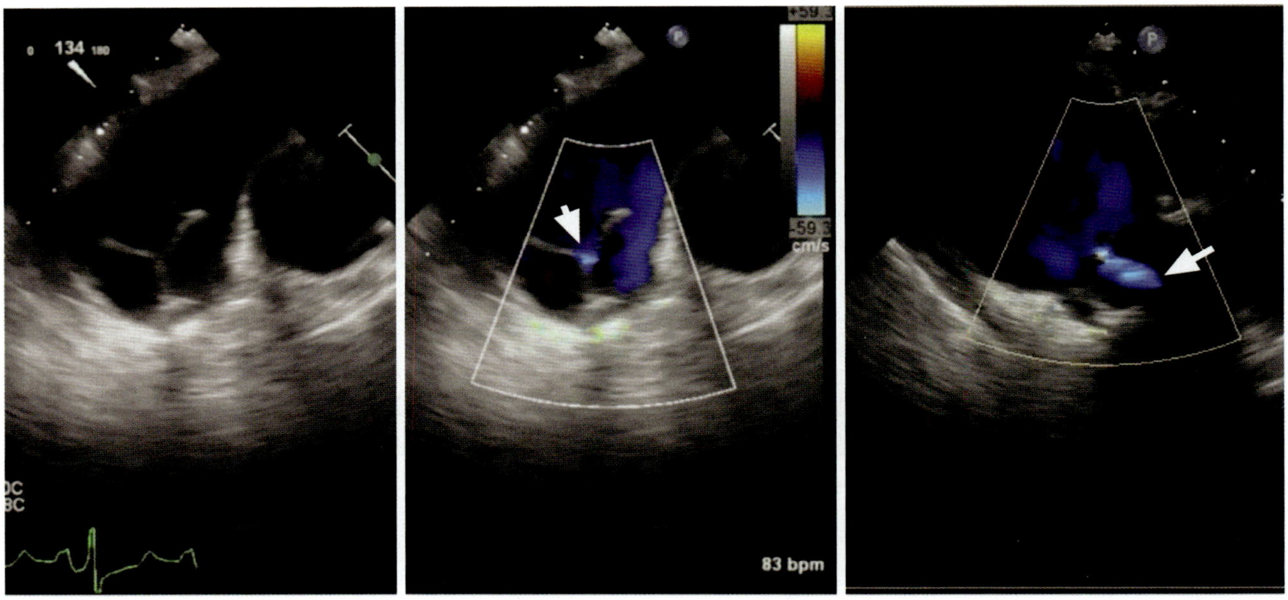

Fig 7.138 2D TEE after pulmonic valve implantation shows mild central pulmonic regurgitation (*arrows*) in short-axis (*center*) and long-axis (*right*) images.

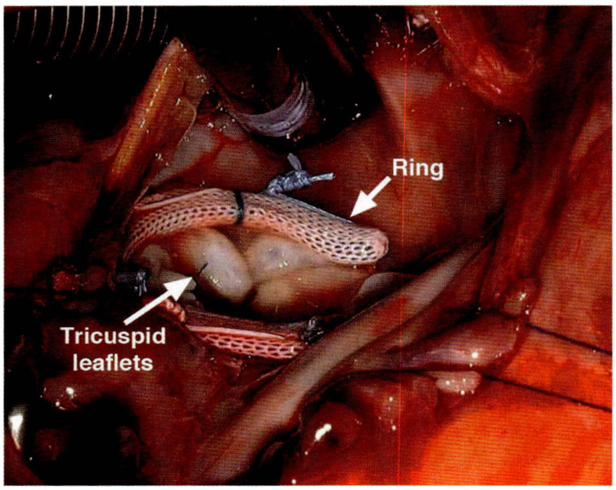

Fig 7.139 Tricuspid annuloplasty was performed with "C"-shaped ring, with only mild residual tricuspid regurgitation seen on 2D TEE.

Comments

Pulmonic regurgitation is the most common long-term complication after valvotomy for isolated pulmonic stenosis or after tetralogy of Fallot repair. Long-term follow-up of right ventricular size and systolic function is essential to optimize the timing of repeat intervention with a goal of performing pulmonic valve replacement before the onset of irreversible RV systolic function. The role of tricuspid valve annuloplasty at the time of pulmonic valve replacement remains controversial because tricuspid valve regurgitation may decrease after pulmonic valve replacement due to remodeling of the previously volume overloaded RV.

Suggested Reading

1. Zdradzinski MJ, Qureshi AM, Stewart R, et al: Comparison of long-term postoperative sequelae in patients with tetralogy of Fallot versus isolated pulmonic stenosis, Am J Cardiol 114(2): 300–304, 2014.
2. Bashore TM: Adult congenital heart disease: Right ventricular outflow tract lesions, Circulation 115:1933–1947, 2007.
3. Jassal DS, Thakrar A, Schaffer SA, et al: Percutaneous balloon valvuloplasty for pulmonic stenosis: The role of multimodality imaging, Echocardiography 25:231–235, 2008.
4. Kogon B, Patel M, Leong M, McConnell M: Book management of moderate functional tricuspid valve regurgitation at the time of pulmonary valve replacement: Is concomitant tricuspid valve repair necessary? Pediatr Cardiol 31:843–848, 2010.
5. Stephane David J, Tousignant C, Bowry R: Tricuspid annular velocity in patients undergoing cardiac operation using trans-esophageal echocardiography, J Am Soc Echocardiogr 19:329–334, 2006.

8 Hypertrophic Cardiomyopathy

CASE 8-1
Transplant for Hypertrophic Cardiomyopathy

This 26-year-old woman with hypertrophic cardiomyopathy and prolonged QT syndrome was referred for heart transplantation for low-output heart failure with clinical symptoms of fatigue and marked exercise intolerance with New York Heart Association (NYHA) class III symptoms despite maximal medical therapy. Right heart catheterization documented a pulmonary artery pressure of 24/9 mm Hg with a pulmonary wedge pressure of 10 mm Hg. Cardiac output was 5.8 L/min, with a cardiac index of 2.9 L/min.

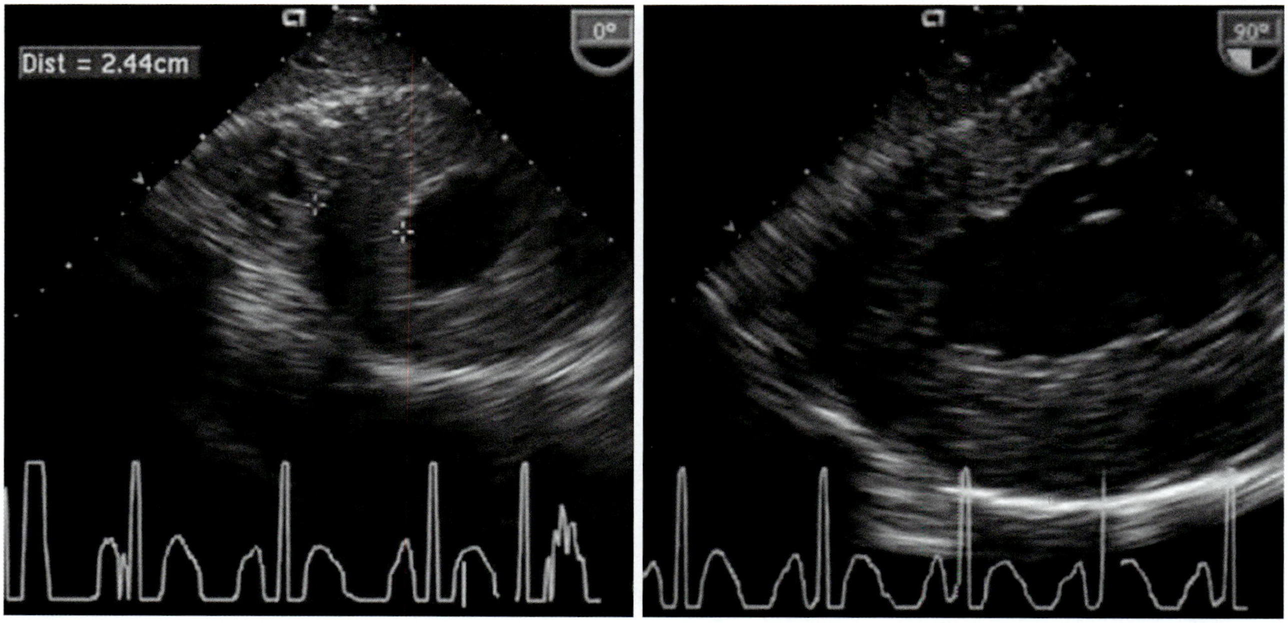

Fig 8.1 Transgastric short-axis view shows severe hypertrophy of left ventricle with septal thickness of 2.4 cm *(left)*. Transgastric long-axis view *(right)* also shows severe hypertrophy of left ventricle.

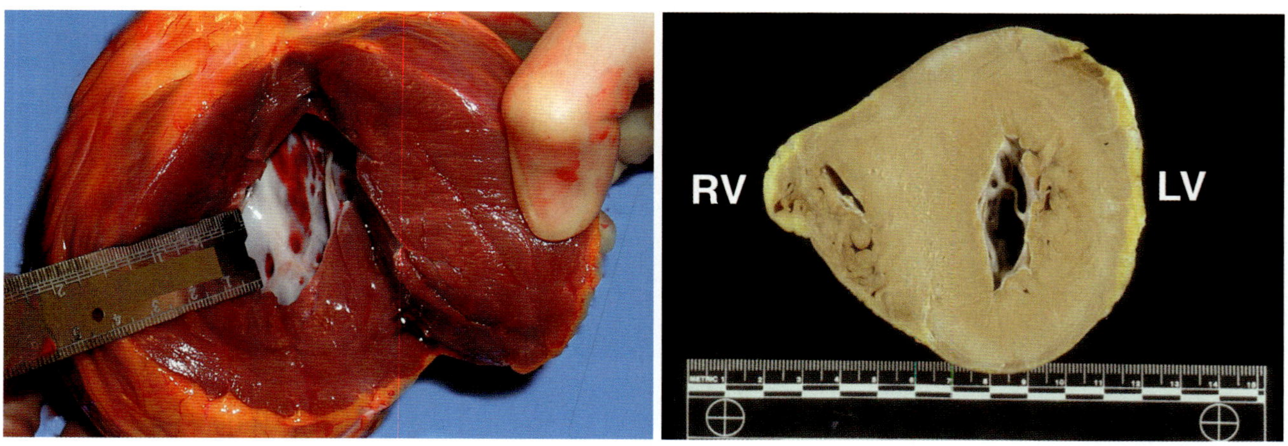

Fig 8.2 A section through apex of freshly explanted heart *(left)* demonstrates severe hypertrophy of ventricular myocardium. At pathologic examination *(right)*, heart was severely hypertrophied (cardiac mass = 655 g), with pattern typical for hypertrophic cardiomyopathy; left ventricular cavity was extremely small.

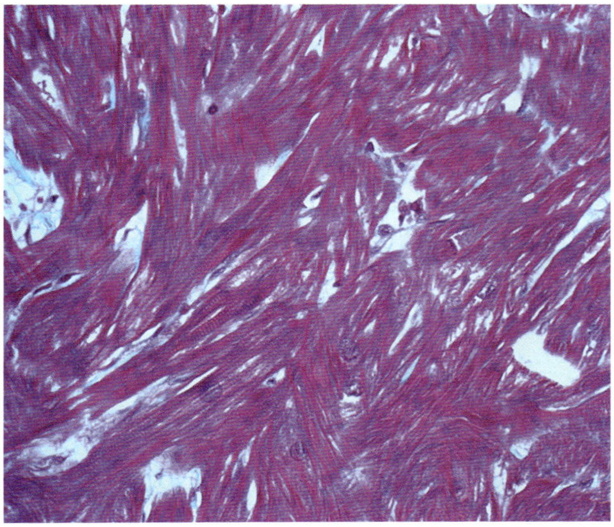

Fig 8.3 Histologic examination revealed severe cardiomyocyte disarray, with mild-to-moderate interstitial fibrosis.

CASE 8-2
Myomectomy for Dynamic Left Ventricular Outflow Tract Obstruction

This 64-year-old man was referred for surgical intervention for hypertrophic cardiomyopathy with severe dynamic subaortic obstruction. He had an 8-month history of increasing exertional dyspnea, chest pain, and syncope. Echocardiography showed hypertrophic cardiomyopathy with severe outflow obstruction and severe mitral regurgitation. Coronary angiography showed no significant epicardial coronary artery disease.

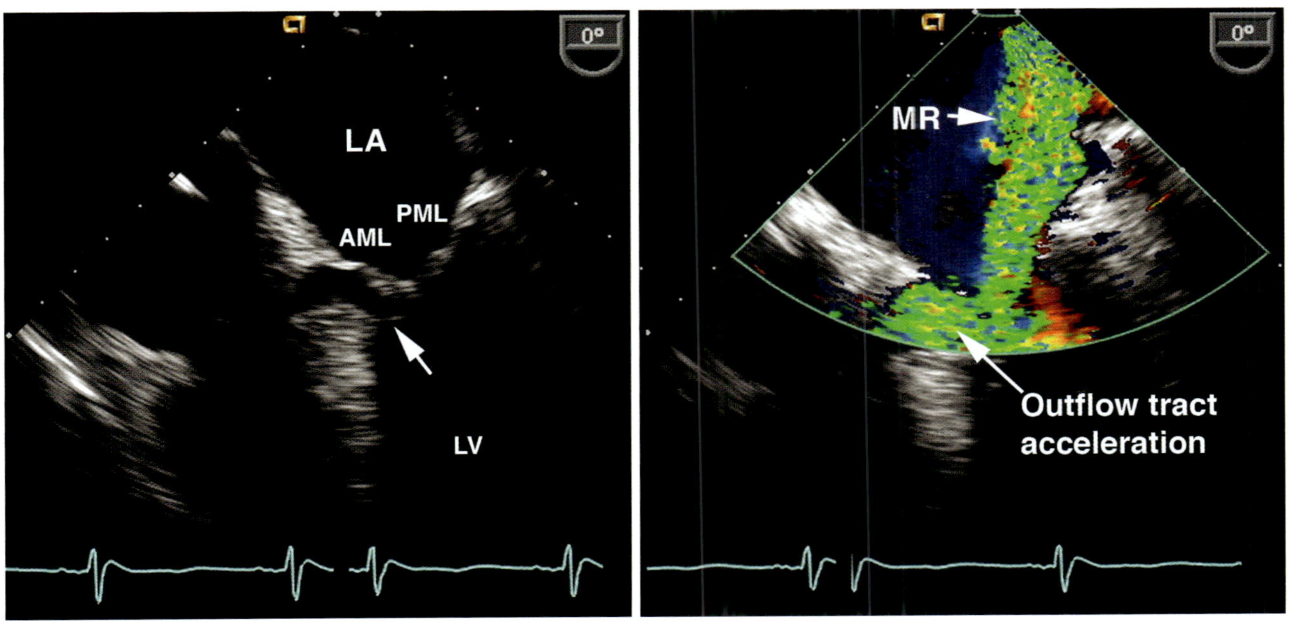

Fig 8.4 Four-chamber TEE view *(left)* demonstrates systolic anterior motion of mitral valve leaflet *(arrow)*. Color Doppler *(right)* shows both increased outflow tract velocity (*green* indicates variance due to high flow velocity with signal aliasing) and severe mitral regurgitation (MR).

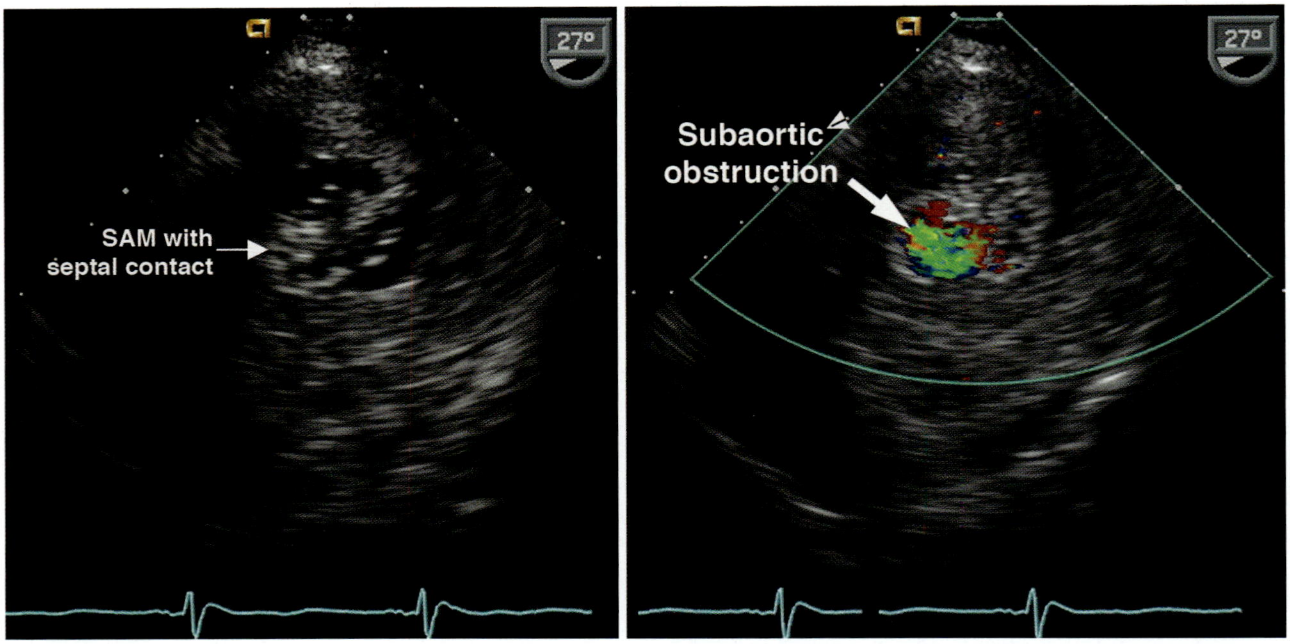

Fig 8.5 Transgastric short-axis view at mitral valve level shows severely hypertrophied left ventricle; there is systolic anterior motion (SAM) of anterior mitral leaflet with interventricular septal contact *(left)* and color flow *(right)* demonstrating subaortic obstruction.

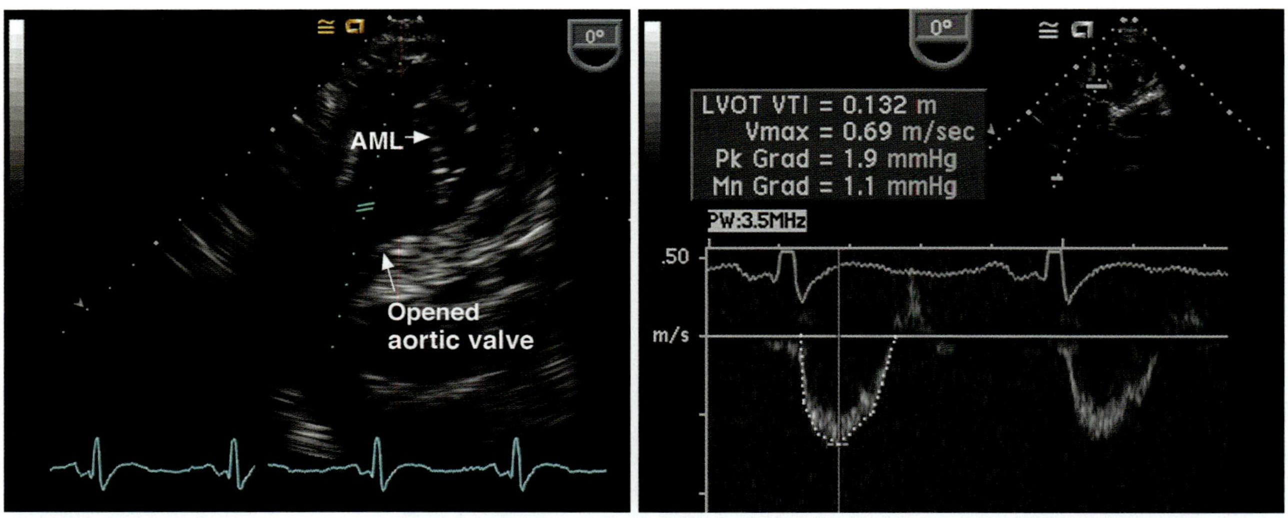

Fig 8.6 In different patient without hypertrophic cardiomyopathy, example of using transgastric apical view for evaluation of left ventricular outflow is shown. Image plane is angulated anteriorly from deep transgastric four-chamber view to show aortic valve *(left)*. Then, pulsed or continuous-wave Doppler examination of flow is recorded, in this case showing normal velocity of 0.7 m/s *(right)*. Maximal velocity may be underestimated by this approach, as it is not always possible to obtain parallel intercept angle between ultrasound beam and direction of blood flow. However, actual velocity is at least as high as recorded velocity.

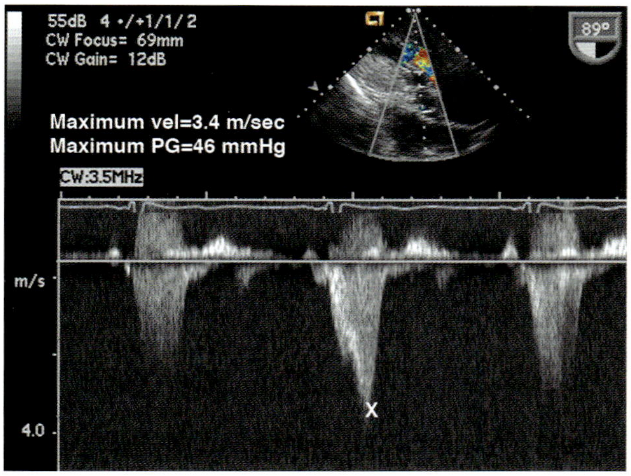

Fig 8.7 In this patient with hypertrophic cardiomyopathy, continuous-wave Doppler from transgastric long-axis view demonstrates late-peaking, high-velocity systolic signal with maximum velocity of 3.4 m/s, corresponding to maximum pressure gradient (PG) of 46 mm Hg. PG may be even higher when patient is awake and active.

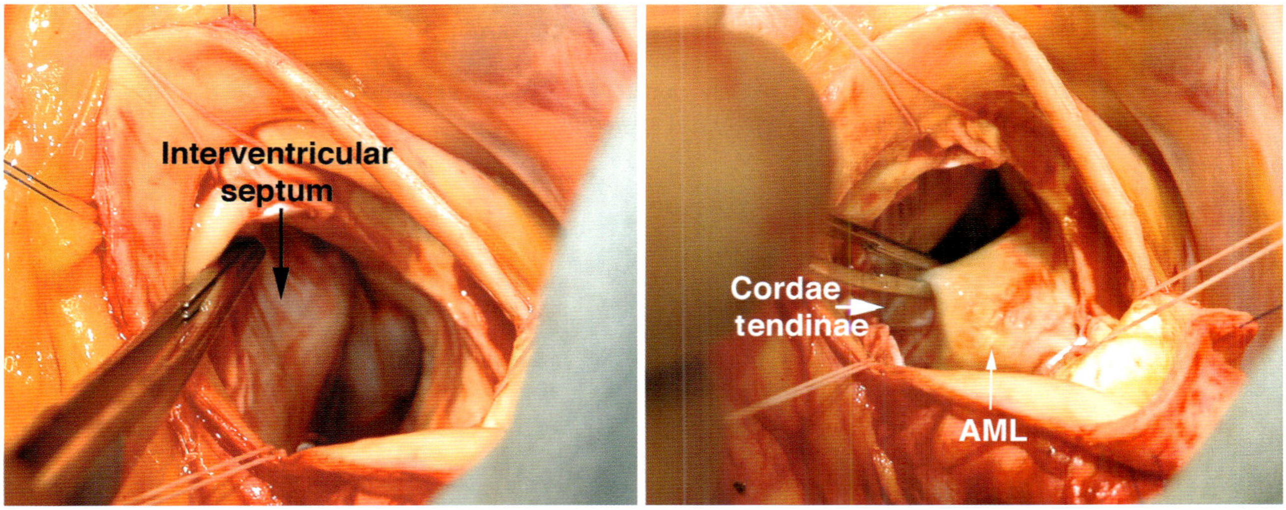

Fig 8.8 At surgery, left ventricular outflow tract is approached via ascending aorta, and through passively opened aortic valve. In normal example in which aortic valve has been removed, structures visible in LVOT include interventricular septum *(left)* anteriorly and AML *(right)* posteriorly.

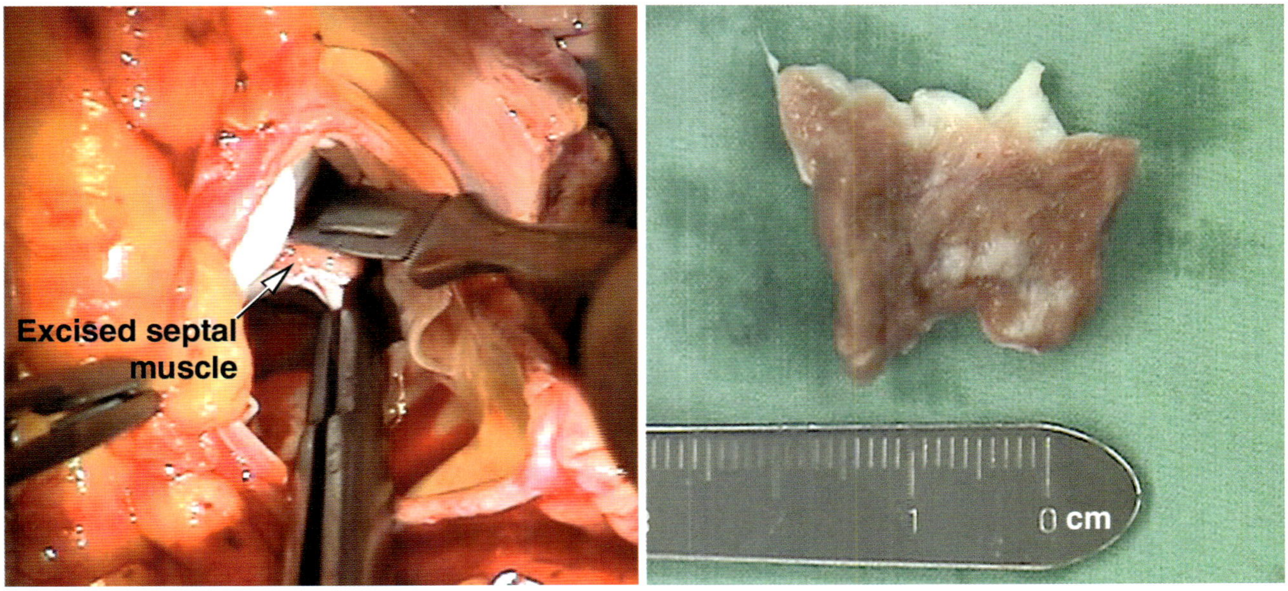

Fig 8.9 ▶ In this patient with hypertrophic cardiomyopathy, trough of septal myocardium was removed anteriorly with depth and length of approximately 1 cm, taking care to avoid creating VSD. Because of severe subaortic obstruction with systolic anterior motion of AML, mitral valve was replaced with low-profile mechanical valve. Both anterior and posterior chords were preserved, but anterior leaflet was partly excised, with remnants of AML incorporated into medial and lateral suture lines.

Comments

Hypertrophic cardiomyopathy is an autosomal dominant inherited disease that is characterized by asymmetric hypertrophy of the left ventricle, diastolic dysfunction, and, in a subset of patients, dynamic subaortic obstruction. There are several different patterns of left ventricular hypertrophy but all have in common relative sparing the basal segment of the inferior–posterior left ventricular wall. In some cases, symptoms are predominantly a result of diastolic dysfunction, as in the first Case 8-1. Typically, relaxation is decreased early in the disease, with decreased compliance occurring late in the disease. Diastolic dysfunction is associated with elevated filling pressures and a reduced forward cardiac output, resulting in symptoms of exertional fatigue and dyspnea.

The dynamic outflow obstruction that occurs in some patients is related to systolic anterior motion of the mitral leaflets and an anatomically abnormal mitral valve. There is often coexisting mitral regurgitation due to malcoaptation of the leaflets at the site of systolic anterior motion. Symptoms of angina, dyspnea, and syncope occur in some, but not all, patients with outflow obstruction. Outflow obstruction is dynamic in that it varies during the ejection period, with the maximal obstruction in late systole. In addition, the degree of outflow obstruction varies with loading conditions: typically, it increases with a decrease in ventricular volume (e.g., hypovolemia), a decrease in systemic vascular resistance (e.g., with vasodilators), or an increase in contractility (e.g., with exercise).

Treatment options include medical therapy, percutaneous ablation of the septal myocardium in selected patients, and surgical myomectomy, sometimes with concurrent mitral valve replacement.

Suggested Reading

1. Woo A: Hypertrophic cardiomyopathy: echocardiography in diagnosis and management of patients (including stress testing). In Otto CM, editor: The Practice of Clinical Echocardiography, ed 5, Philadelphia, 2016, Elsevier.
2. Gersh BJ, Maron BJ, Bonow RO, et al: 2011 ACCF/AHA guideline for the diagnosis and treatment of hypertrophic cardiomyopathy: executive summary: a report of the American College of Cardiology Foundation/American Heart Association Task Force on Practice Guidelines, Circulation 124(24):2761, 2011.
3. Caselli S, Maron MS, Urbano-Moral JA, et al: Differentiating left ventricular hypertrophy in athletes from that in patients with hypertrophic cardiomyopathy, Am J Cardiol 114(9):1383–1389, 2014.
4. Hensley N, Dietrich J, Nyhan D, et al: Hypertrophic Cardiomyopathy: A Review, Anesthesia Analgesia 120:554–559, 2015.

CASE 8-3
Myomectomy for Dynamic Left Ventricular Outflow Tract Obstruction with 3D TEE Imaging

This 52-year-old woman was diagnosed with hypertrophic cardiomyopathy at age 35 years. She was medically managed with disopyramide, which was initially successful, but over time the dose had to be steadily increased. She reached a point where her dose was maximal, but she still complained of increasing shortness of breath on exertion to the point of only being to walk 50 ft before stopping. She was referred for a surgical opinion. A surgical myotomy-myectomy was planned for relief of symptoms. At surgery, a total of 3 cm^3 of septal myocardial tissue was removed, as measured by displacement of saline in a sterile graduated cylinder. In addition, there was a short, thick cord from the anterior leaflet of the mitral valve and two smaller accessory chordae, directly connected to the interventricular septum, that were divided to relieve outflow obstruction.

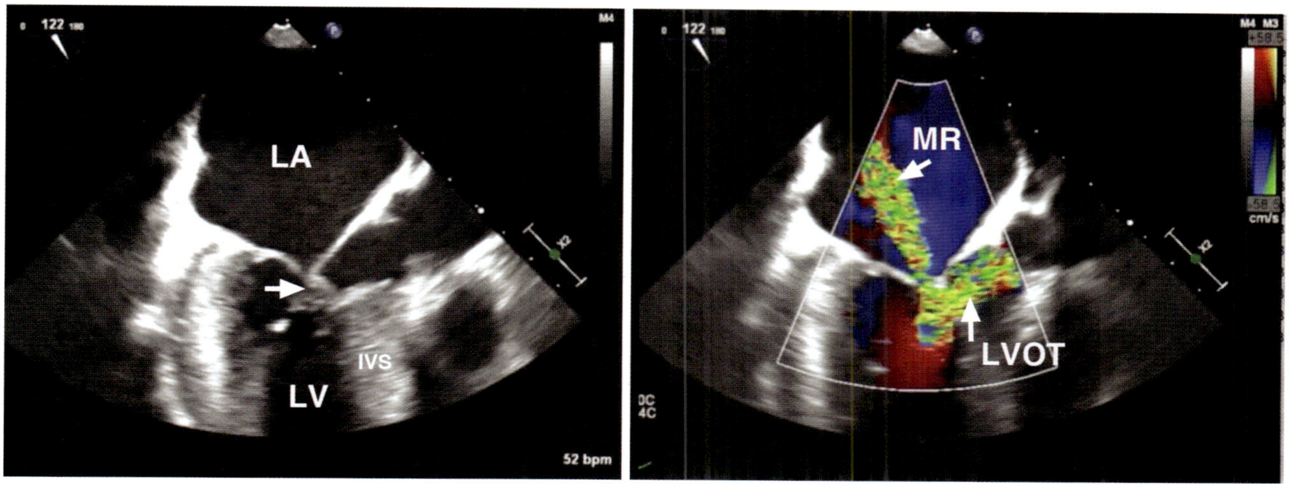

Fig 8.10 In this midesophageal long-axis view, there is systolic anterior motion of mitral coaptation point *(arrow)* that contacts interventricular septum (IVS). At right, see color flow acceleration in left ventricular outflow tract (LVOT) as well as mitral regurgitation (MR).

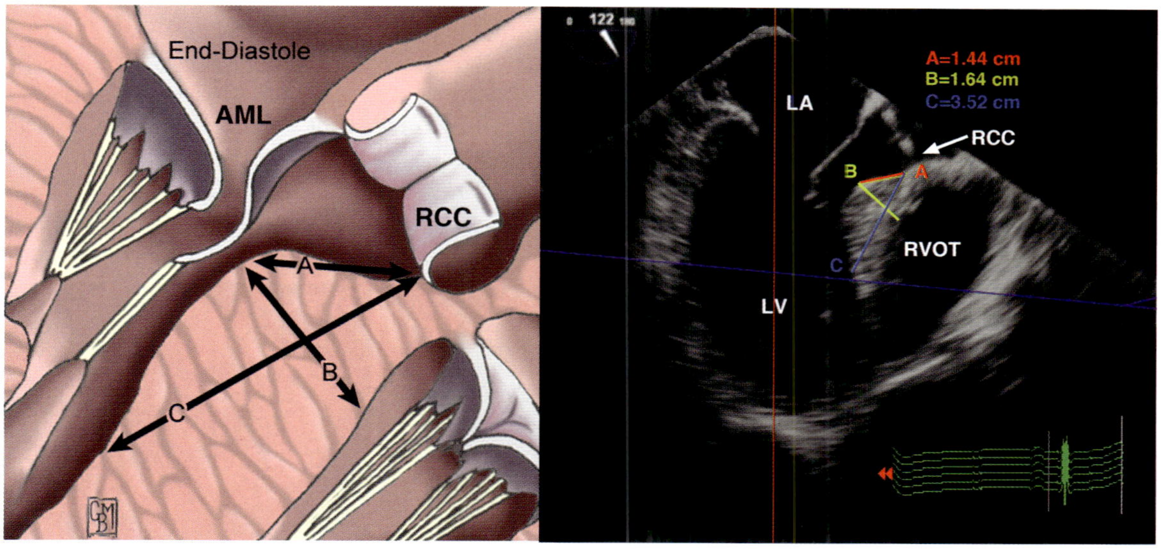

Fig 8.11 In left frame, artistic rendition corresponding to midesophageal long-axis view is seen. Several measurements are made that may help surgeon determine extent of septal resection; **(A)** is distance from base of right coronary cusp to septal contact point, **(B)** maximal septal width, and **(C)** distance from base of right coronary cusp to distal point of septal thickening. In right frame, representative midesophageal long-axis view with measurements is shown. All measurements are made at end-diastole. (Drawing courtesy of Annette Vegas, MD.)

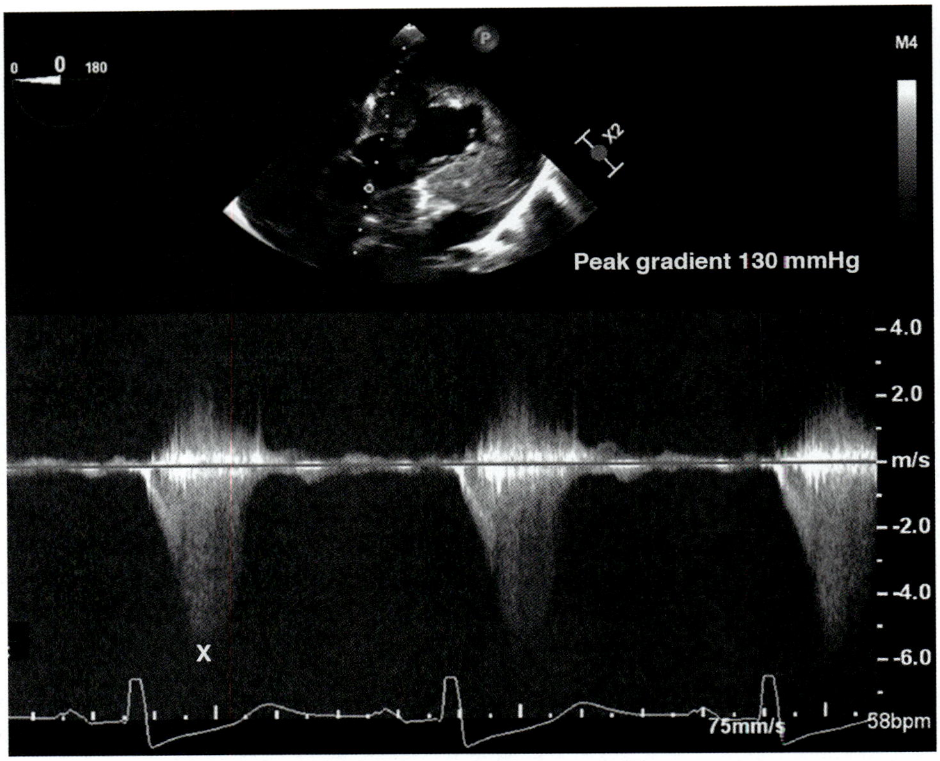

Fig 8.12 Deep transgastric imaging and continuous-wave Doppler allow velocity measurement across left ventricular outflow tract. Late-peaking, high-velocity, systolic signal appearance typical of dynamic outflow tract obstruction is seen. Peak gradient is 130 mm Hg.

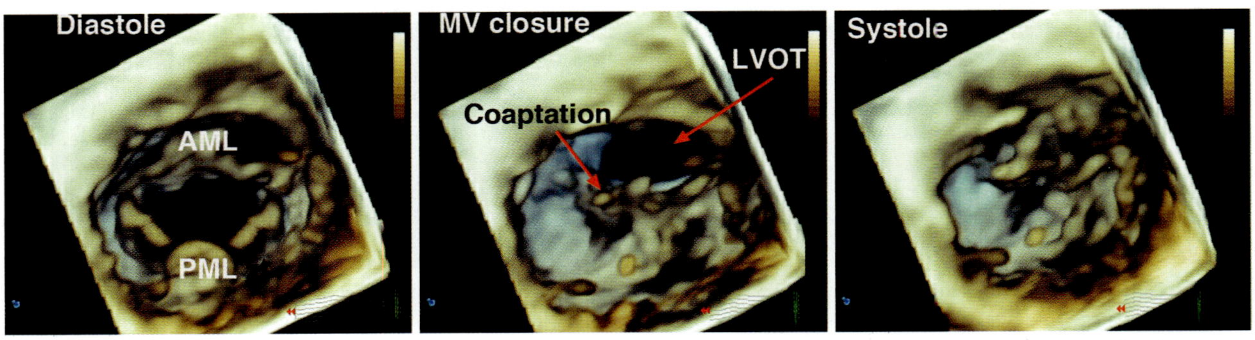

Fig 8.13 3D TEE views of mitral valve viewed from left ventricular side are shown. At left, anterior mitral leaflet (AML) and posterior mitral leaflet (PML) are open during diastole. In the middle panel, LV outflow tract is the dark area anterior to mitral valve, with mitral closure and normal coaptation during early systole. In late systole *(right)*, coaptation point has moved anteriorly toward interventricular septum, resulting in contact of mitral leaflets with septum, obstructing ejection of blood out of LV across aortic valve. Dynamics are especially obvious on real-time video.

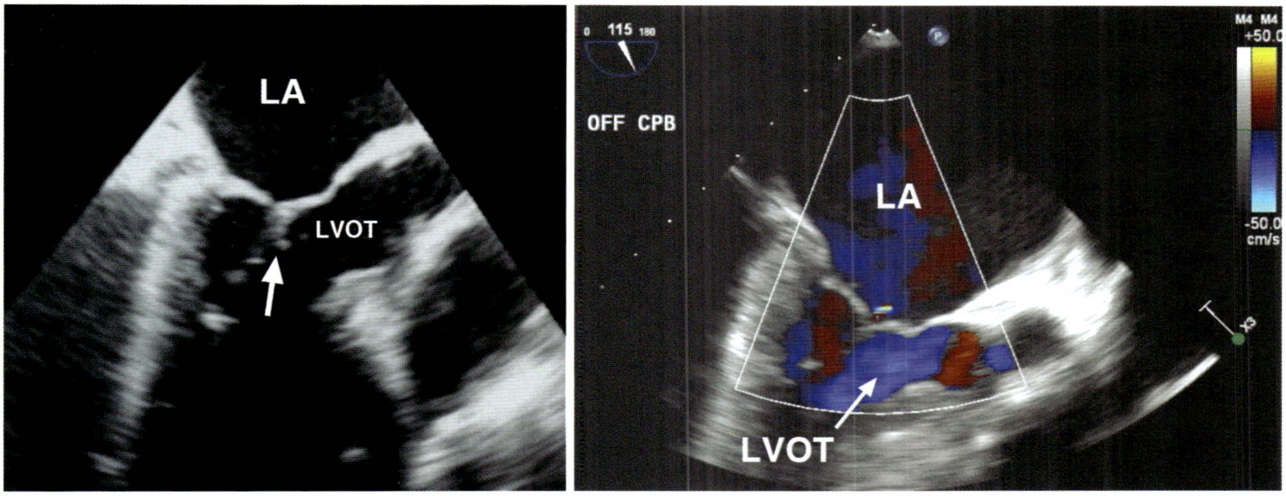

Fig 8.14 This midesophageal long-axis view was taken after myomectomy and separation from cardiopulmonary bypass. At left, mitral coaptation point has not moved toward interventricular septum, and at right, neither flow acceleration in left ventricular outflow tract nor mitral regurgitation are seen.

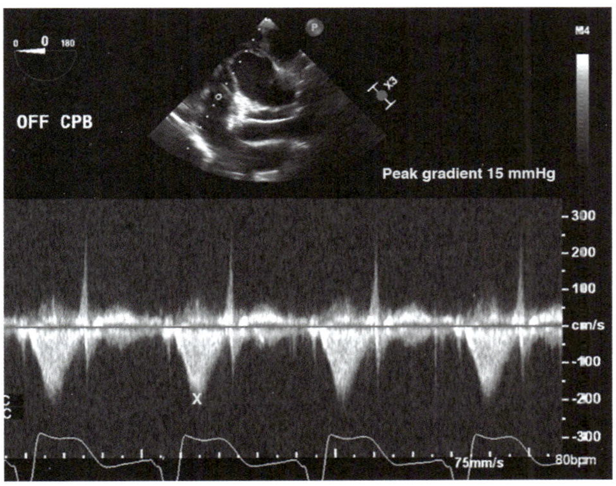

Fig 8.15 Postoperative deep transgastric imaging and continuous-wave Doppler velocity measurement across left ventricular outflow tract show much reduced peak gradient of 15 mm Hg.

CASE 8-4
Postmyomectomy Ventricular Septal Defect

The patient is a 71-year-old man who has been noticing increasing shortness of breath and dyspnea on exertion. He also complained of mild exertional chest pain as well as episodes of near syncope. Cardiac catheterization showed minimal nonobstructive coronary disease. A stress echocardiogram showed no aortic stenosis, an outflow tract gradient of 12 mm Hg, which increased to 120 mm Hg with exercise. Prominent basal septal hypertrophy was seen. He was scheduled for surgical myomectomy.

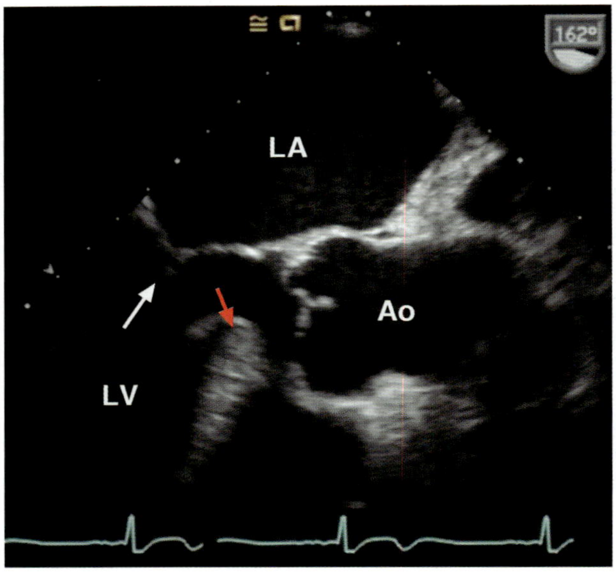

Fig 8.16 Preoperative TEE showed normal aortic valve function in midesophageal long-axis view. Coaptation point has moved close to top of interventricular septum, but does not contact it *(white arrow)*. There is prominent basal septal hypertrophy *(red arrow)*.

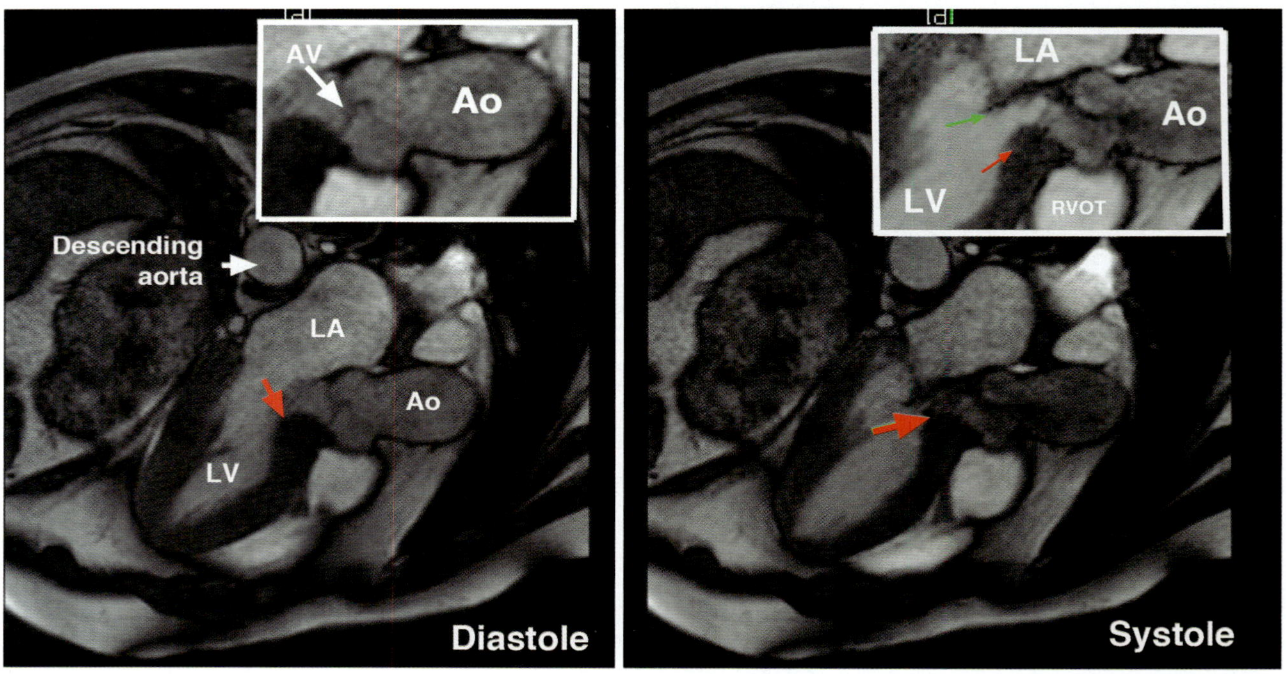

Fig 8.17 An MRI (reoriented to same position as midesophageal long-axis TEE) shows prominent basal septal hypertrophy in diastole *(red arrow)*. Inset shows aortic valve more clearly. Left ventricular outflow tract is narrowed during systole *(green arrow)*, seen more clearly in real time.

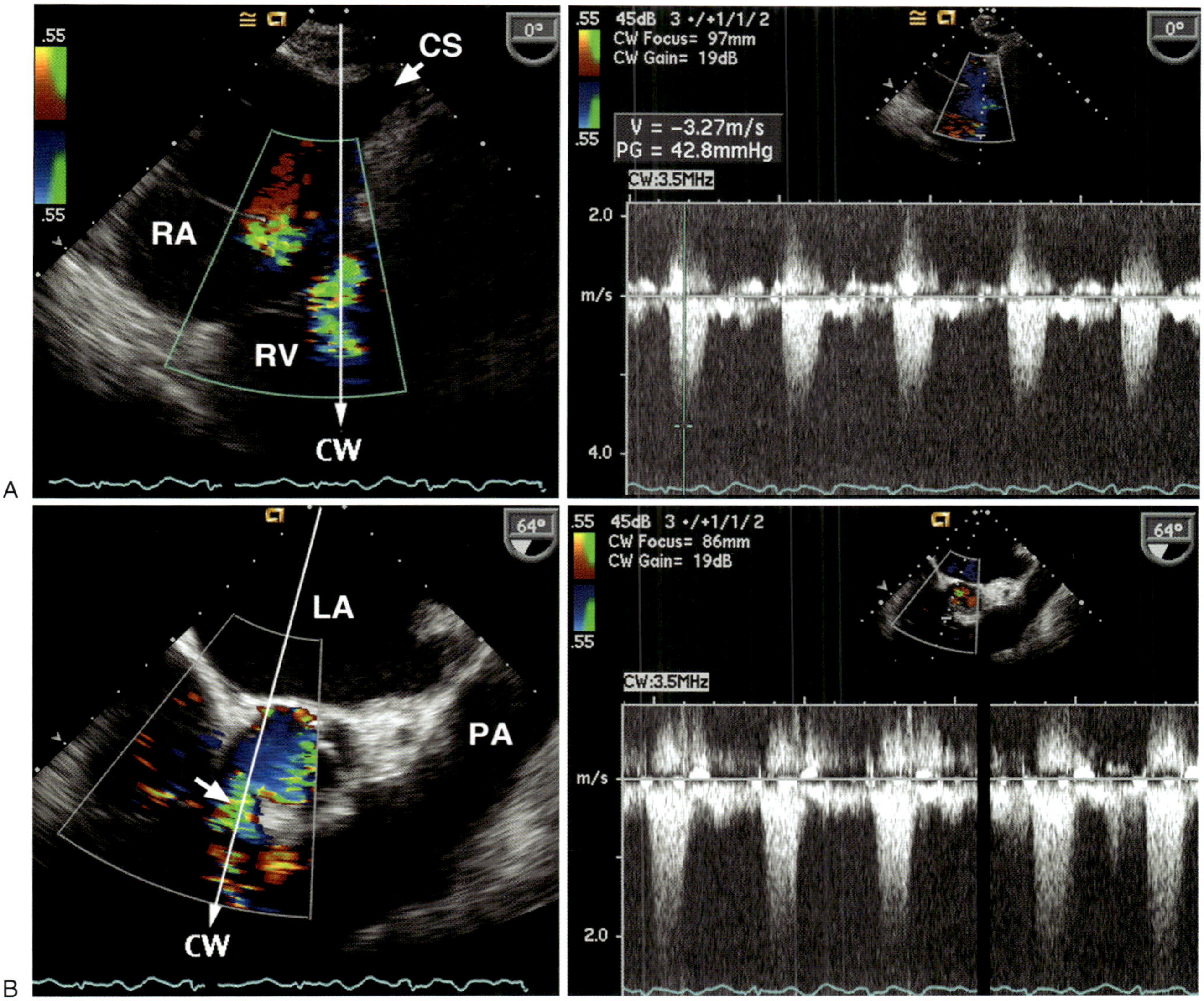

Fig 8.18 (**A**) After septal myomectomy, color Doppler from midesophageal position with probe retroflexion *(left)* showed color jet in systole on RV side of tricuspid valve. CW Doppler *(right)* showed high-velocity jet that was moving away from probe. (**B**) Color Doppler after slight withdrawal and ante-flexion of probe showed color Doppler flow disturbance consistent with ventricular septal defect in basal septum with flow into RV, adjacent to tricuspid valve *(white arrow)*. CW Doppler shows high-velocity signal with timing and shape similar to CW Doppler recording from midesophageal position. This finding is consistent with postmyectomy ventricular septal defect, although peak velocity likely is underestimated on both tracings due to nonparallel intercept angle.

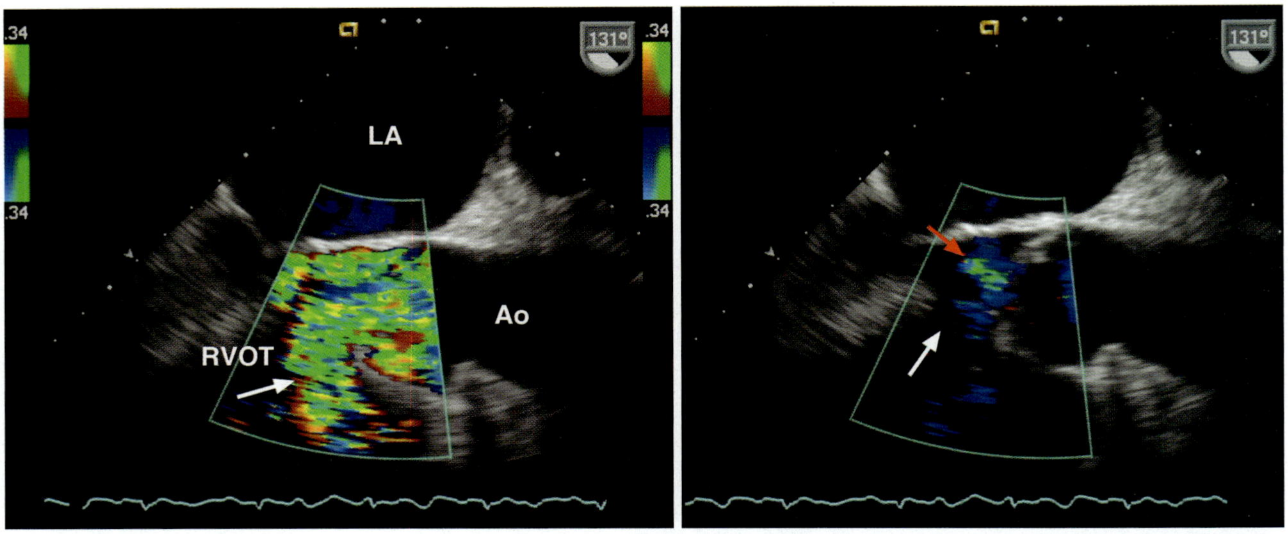

Fig 8.19 Midesophageal long-axis imaging during systole again showed VSD *(white arrow)*. On right, during diastole, defect is seen *(white arrow)*, as is small amount of aortic regurgitation *(red arrow)*.

Comments

Exercise testing is recommended in patients with hypertrophic cardiomyopathy and exertional symptoms but no obstruction at rest, as in this case. Abnormal findings seen on stress testing in patients with hypertrophic cardiomyopathy include symptoms of chest pain or presyncope, a provable subaortic gradient, a blunted or decreased blood pressure, arrhythmias, ST changes on ECG and an increase in mitral regurgitant severity.

At surgery, adequate removal of septal tissue is needed for relief of dynamic subaortic obstruction in patients with hypertrophic cardiomyopathy. However, depending on septal thickness and curvature, it can be a fine line between relieving obstruction and inadvertently creating a ventricular septal defect. On the baseline intraoperative TEE, it is important to define the spatial extent and thickness of septal hypertrophy, as well as the curvature of the septum, because the septum typically is viewed by looking down through the aortic valve. After the procedure, it is important to carefully search for a ventricular septal defect, residual outflow obstruction, and any changes to aortic valve function.

Suggested Reading

1. Lafitte S, Reant P, Touche C, et al: Paradoxical response to exercise in asymptomatic hypertrophic cardiomyopathy: a new description of outflow tract obstruction dynamics, J Am Coll Cardiol 62(9):842–850, 2013.
2. Shah JS, Esteban MT, Thaman R, et al: Prevalence of exercise-induced left ventricular outflow tract obstruction in symptomatic patients with nonobstructive hypertrophic cardiomyopathy, Heart 94(10):1288–1294, 2008.
3. Peteiro J, Bouzas-Mosquera A, Fernandez X, et al: Prognostic value of exercise echocardiography in patients with hypertrophic cardiomyopathy, J Am Soc Echocardiogr 25(2):182–189, 2012.

9 Pericardial Disease

CASE 9-1
Pericardial Effusion

Examples of pericardial effusions seen on intraoperative TEE in several different patients are shown.

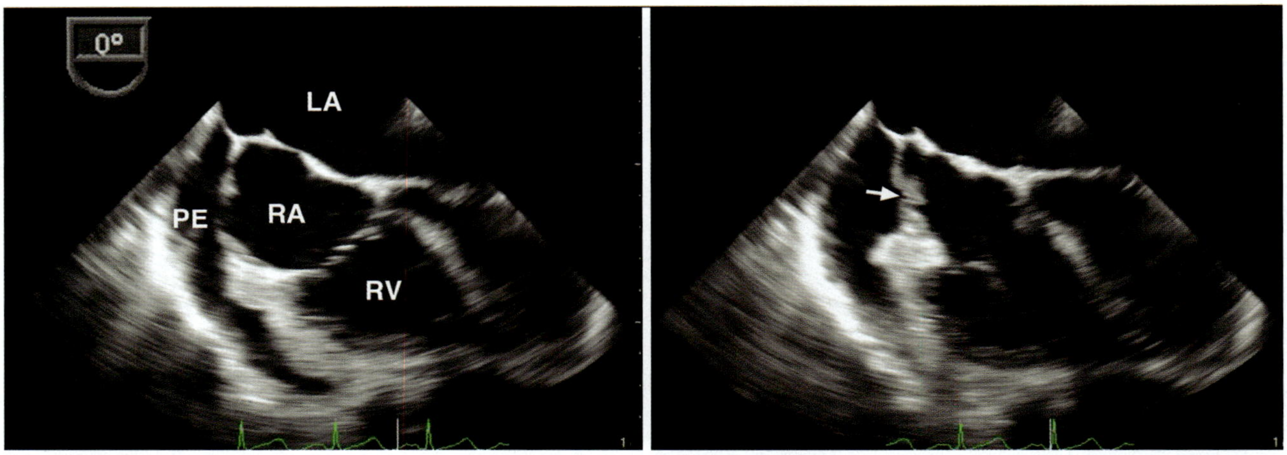

Fig 9.1 From high transesophageal position, echo-free space is seen adjacent to right atrium in four-chamber view. Patient is in diastole; right atrial free wall *(left)* shows normal convex contour. In early ventricular systole *(right)*, right atrial "collapse" is present with concave appearance of RA free wall because pericardial pressure is higher than RA pressure during atrial diastole.

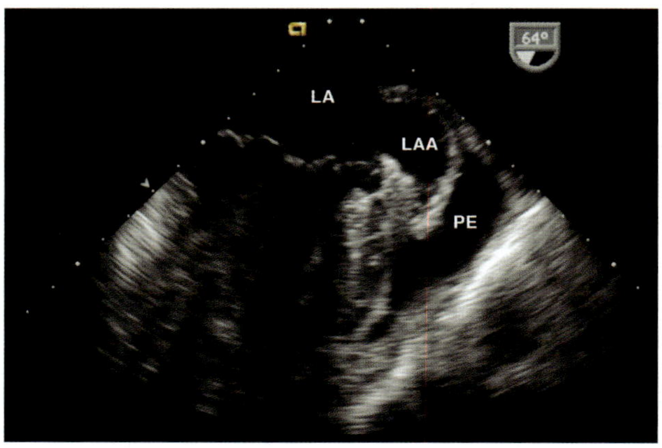

Fig 9.2 In midesophageal commissural view, left atrial appendage (LAA) is surrounded by pericardial effusion within transverse pericardial sinus.

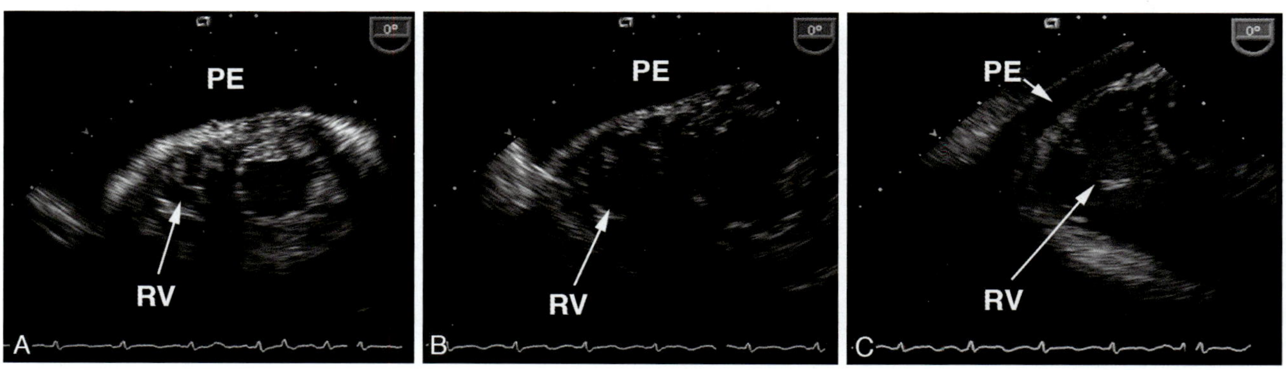

Fig 9.3 This series of transgastric images in short-axis view from left to right shows pericardial effusion (PE) of diminishing size as fluid is removed by percutaneous needle pericardiocentesis. Note that size of left and right ventricles increases as pericardial fluid is removed, suggesting that high intrapericardial pressures prevented normal diastolic ventricular filling, such as in pericardial tamponade physiology.

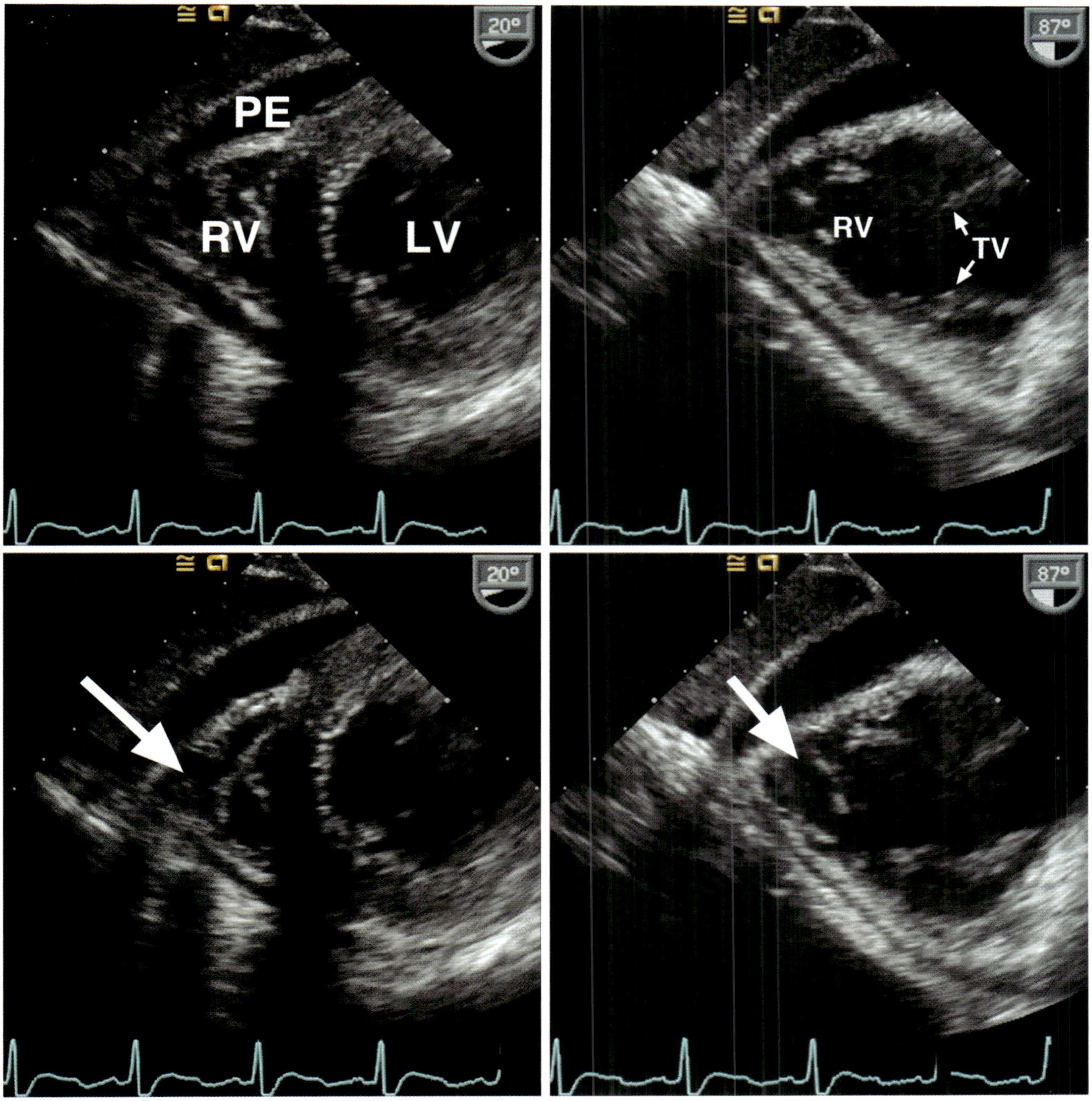

Fig 9.4 This patient presented with ascending aortic dissection, and signs of pericardial tamponade. In transgastric short-axis views *(top left)* and long-axis view *(top right)*, pericardial effusion is present. Although effusion is only small to moderate in size, pericardial pressure may be high due to rapid accumulation of pericardial fluid. Tamponade physiology is confirmed in two bottom frames, which show right ventricular diastolic "collapse" due to pericardial pressure higher than RV diastolic pressure. This phenomenon is better appreciated in the video. Compression of RV results in low forward stroke volume and hypotension.

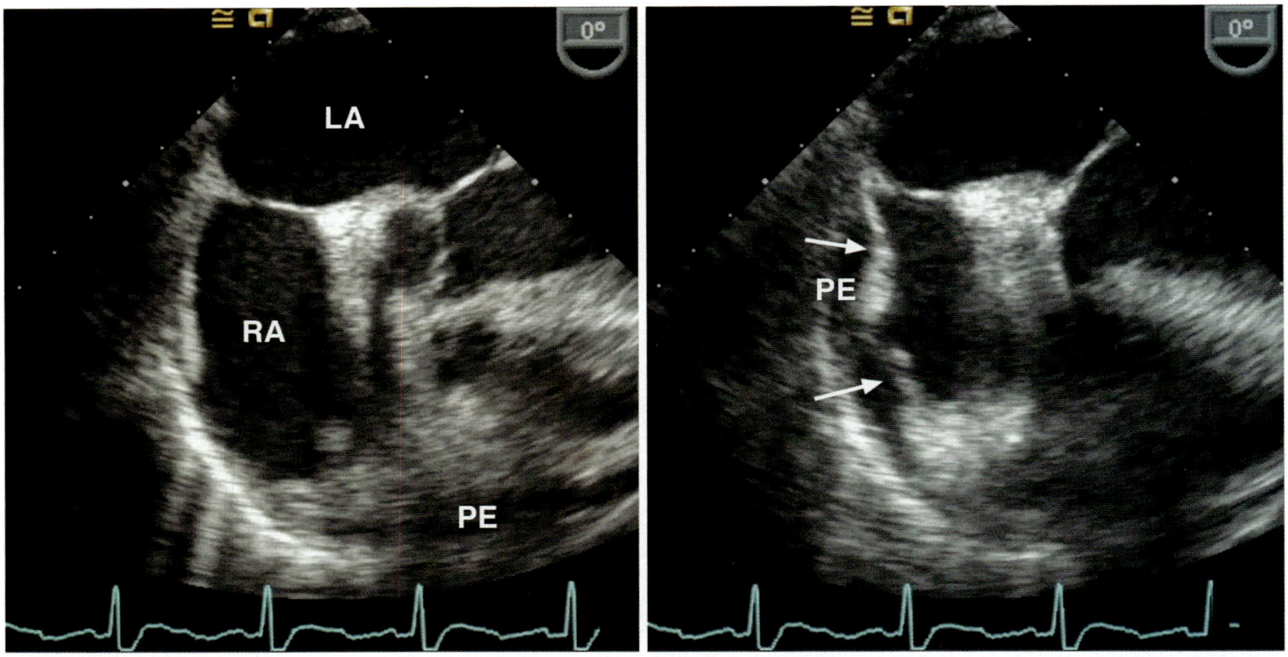

Fig 9.5 In same patient as Fig 9.1d, right atrial collapse is seen in right image *(arrows)*.

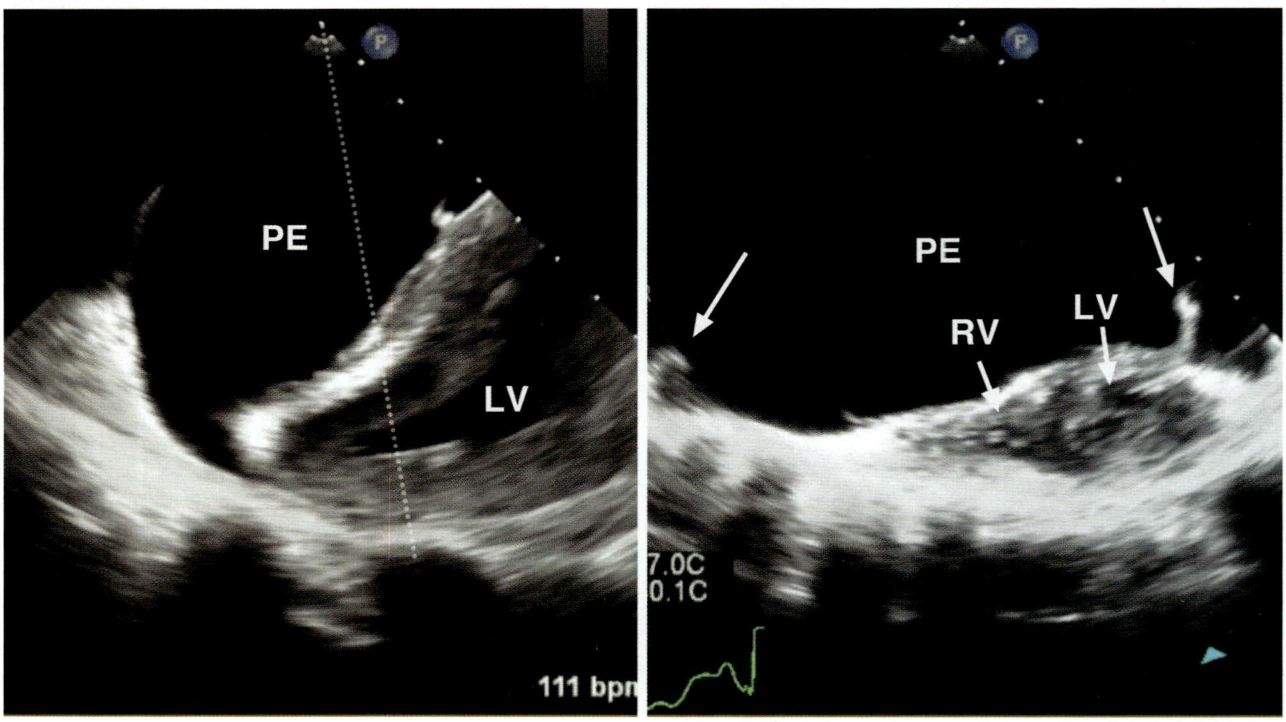

Fig 9.6 Next five images are from patient in whom heart transplant had been performed three weeks earlier. Pericardial effusion had been detected on TTE follow-up. Two attempts at subxiphoid drainage had been attempted with unsatisfactory results. In order to avoid redo sternotomy, left-sided, video-assisted thoracic surgical approach to draining effusion was planned. Biplane TEE from transgastric position revealed massive pericardial effusion; on left, long-axis view shows extremely small LV cavity, and on right, small ventricles are seen at level of apex. Fibrinous strands are seen within effusion *(arrow)*.

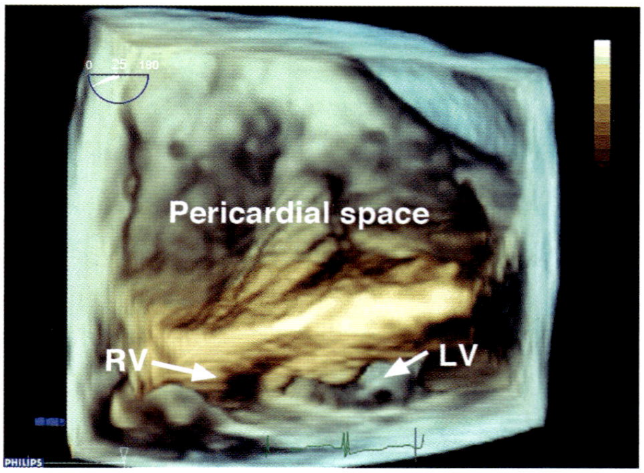

Fig 9.7 Same view as Fig 9.6, with use of 3D imaging. Large posterior pericardial effusion is appreciated.

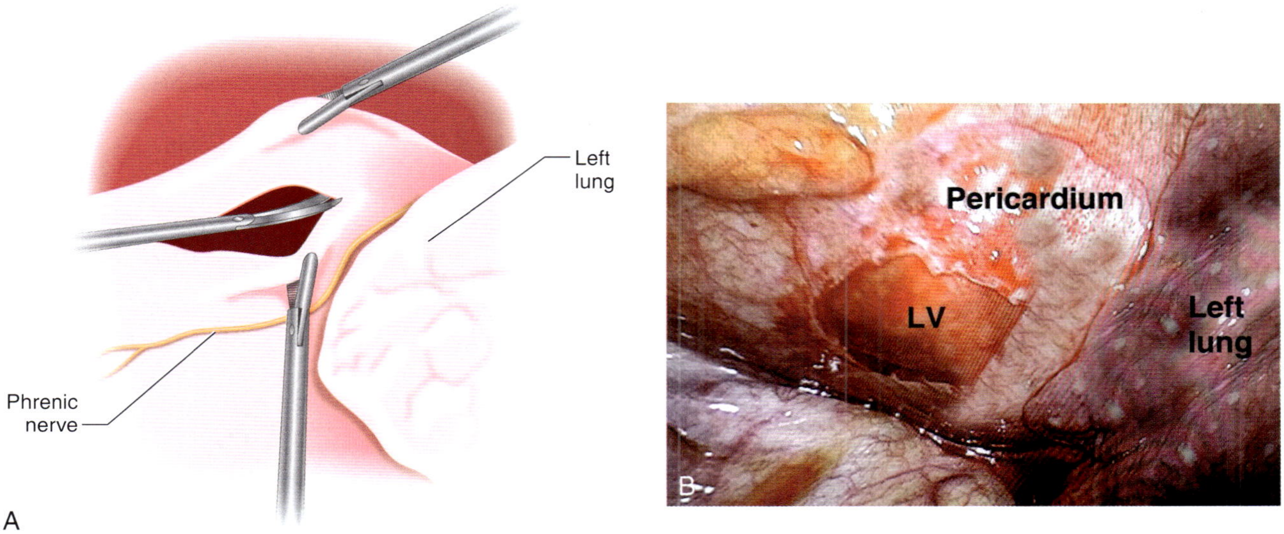

Fig 9.8 On the left is a drawing of typical view from thoracoscope showing grasper, which is placed through same thoracoscope incision at 6 o'clock on this picture, and additional grasper placed through third intercostal incision port at 1 o'clock. These two graspers are used to elevate and separate pericardium, which is divided using standard dissecting scissors placed through more anterior fifth intercostal incision. Care is taken to avoid left phrenic nerve during this dissection. On the right is the surgeon's view with the thoracoscope. (From Oper Techniques Thorac Cardiovasc Surg 2001; 6:132–139. With permission.)

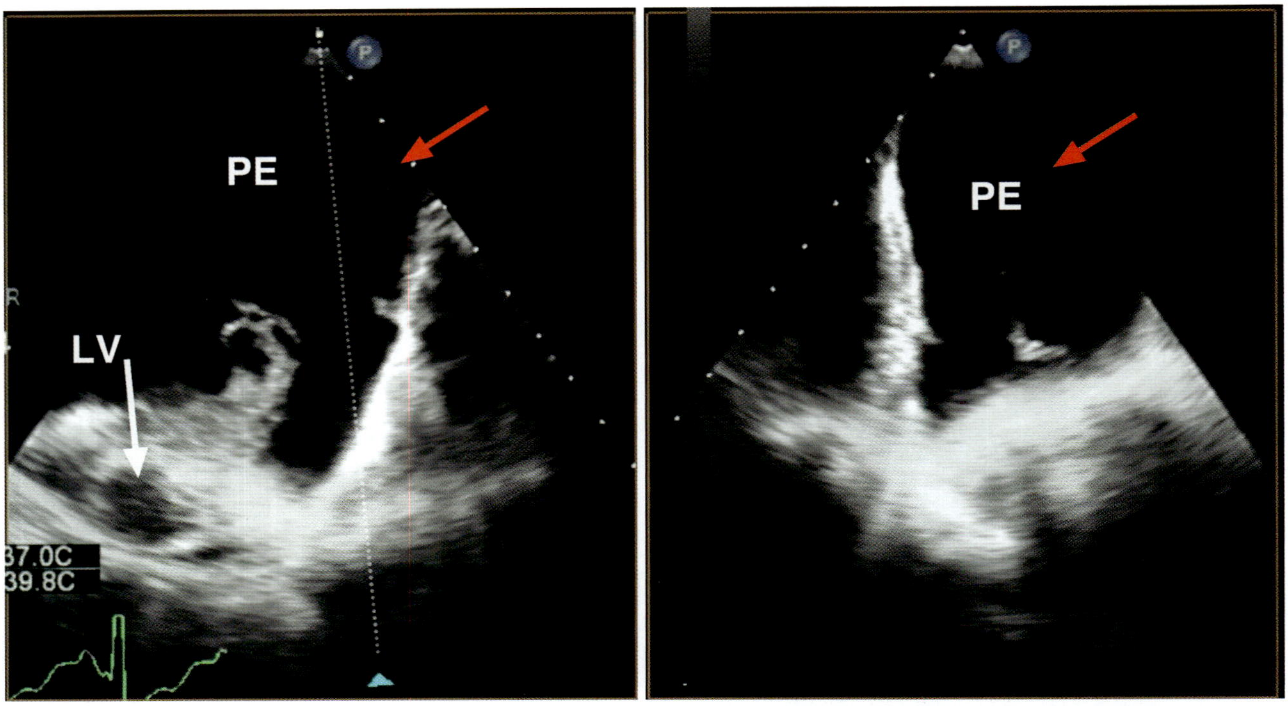

Fig 9.9 Biplane transgastric imaging, short-axis on left. Surgeon manually indented pericardial sac at level of red arrows, confirming direct approach to effusion; he then incised pericardium and drained over 1 L of pericardial fluid.

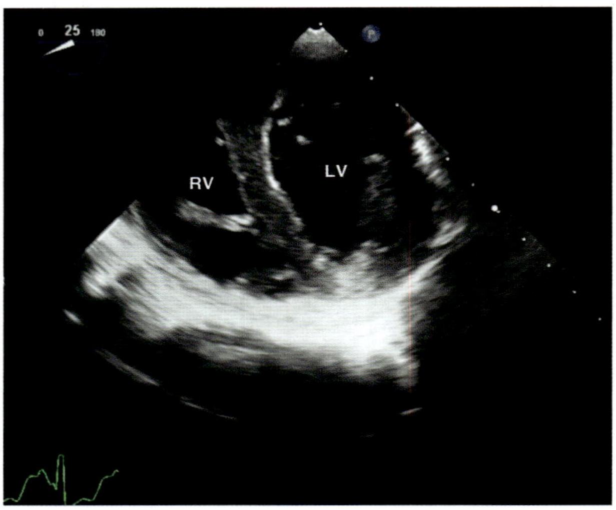

Fig 9.10 Postdrainage, right and left ventricular volumes are restored, with no evidence of RV compression. Patient's hemodynamics responded appropriately with increase in cardiac output and blood pressure. These changes are not reliable in patients receiving positive pressure ventilation.

Comments

A pericardial effusion is diagnosed based on the echocardiographic finding of an echo-lucent area around the heart. Pericardial effusions are usually circumferential, with fluid filling the entire pericardial space around the right and left ventricles, although pericardial effusions may also be asymmetric due to adhesions resulting in areas of loculated fluid, especially in patients with prior cardiac surgical procedures.

The pericardial space extends to the origin of the great vessels, with the narrow transverse sinus of the pericardium extending posterior to the aorta and pulmonary artery, and adjacent to the left atrial appendage. Fluid in the transverse sinus is uncommon but may be seen on TEE as in the example here. The pericardial space also encloses the right atrium, with pericardial reflections at the junctions of the SVC and IVC with the right atrium, so that fluid adjacent to the right atrium is commonly seen. A small pocket of pericardial fluid also may be seen posterior to the left atrium, where the oblique sinus of the pericardium extends into the region between the four pulmonary veins.

A pericardial effusion is distinguished from a pleural effusion by its location. Pericardial fluid is seen posterior to the left ventricle and left atrium but anterior to the descending thoracic aorta, whereas pleural fluid extends posterior to the descending aorta. Fluid adjacent to the right atrium may be either pleural or pericardial, with the latter inferred from the presence of a pericardial effusion in other views. The presence of a compressed lung in the echo-lucent space helps confirm a diagnosis of pleural effusion.

Pericardial fluid may be well tolerated if the pressure within the pericardial space is low, for example with a chronic effusion that has accumulated slowly. Even very large chronic effusions may be associated with normal hemodynamics. However, if the pressure in the pericardial space exceeds the diastolic pressure in the cardiac chambers, hemodynamic changes are seen. When pericardial pressure exceeds right atrial pressure, the free wall of the right atrium inverts or "collapses" and right atrial filling volumes are reduced. Similarly, the left atrium and right ventricle can be compressed when pericardial pressure exceeds the pressure in that cardiac chamber. Tamponade physiology can even occur with loculated effusions if there is compression of one of the cardiac chambers. The diagnosis of tamponade due to a loculated effusion can be challenging. In addition, chamber collapse may not be seen, even when pericardial pressures are high, if the wall of the chamber is thickened or fibrotic.

Along with chamber collapse, a high pericardial pressure restricts the total cardiac volume. Thus, as the right-sided chambers increase in size with inspiration, due to negative intrathoracic pressures and increased venous return, the left-sided chambers are compressed with a reduction in forward cardiac output. These reciprocal inspiratory changes in right and left ventricular diastolic filling result in the drop in blood pressure seen with inspiration, or pulsus paradoxus. These changes are not reliable in patients receiving positive pressure ventilation.

Suggested Reading

1. Welch T: Pericardial disease. In Otto CM, editor: The practice of clinical echocardiography, ed 5, Philadelphia, 2016, Elsevier.
2. Klein AL, Abbara S, Agler DA, et al: American Society of Echocardiography clinical recommendations for multimodality cardiovascular imaging of patients with pericardial disease: endorsed by the Society for Cardiovascular Magnetic Resonance and Society of Cardiovascular Computed Tomography, J Am Soc Echocardiogr 26(9):965–1012, e15, 2013.
3. Silbiger JJ, Garg V, Moss N, et al: Protruding fat from the posterior atrioventricular groove: a novel echocardiographic finding useful in distinguishing pericardial effusions from left pleural effusions, J Am Soc Echocardiogr 28(1):116–117, 2015.

CASE 9-2
Pericardial Constriction

This 57-year-old man was referred for coronary artery bypass grafting surgery and pericardiectomy for pericardial constriction. About 4 years ago, he presented with exertional dyspnea and lower extremity edema. Echocardiography showed a thickened pericardium with increased central venous pressure and evidence for reciprocal respiratory changes in right and left ventricular diastolic filling. Left and right ventricular size and systolic function were normal, and estimated pulmonary systolic pressure was 30 mm Hg. Cardiac catheterization confirmed equalization of right and left ventricular diastolic pressures, with a square-root sign (√) in the ventricular diastolic pressure curve. There was no etiology identified for his pericardial disease. Specifically, there was no history of pericarditis, chest surgery or trauma, radiation therapy, or rheumatologic disease. He denied a history of tuberculosis and a PPD was negative.

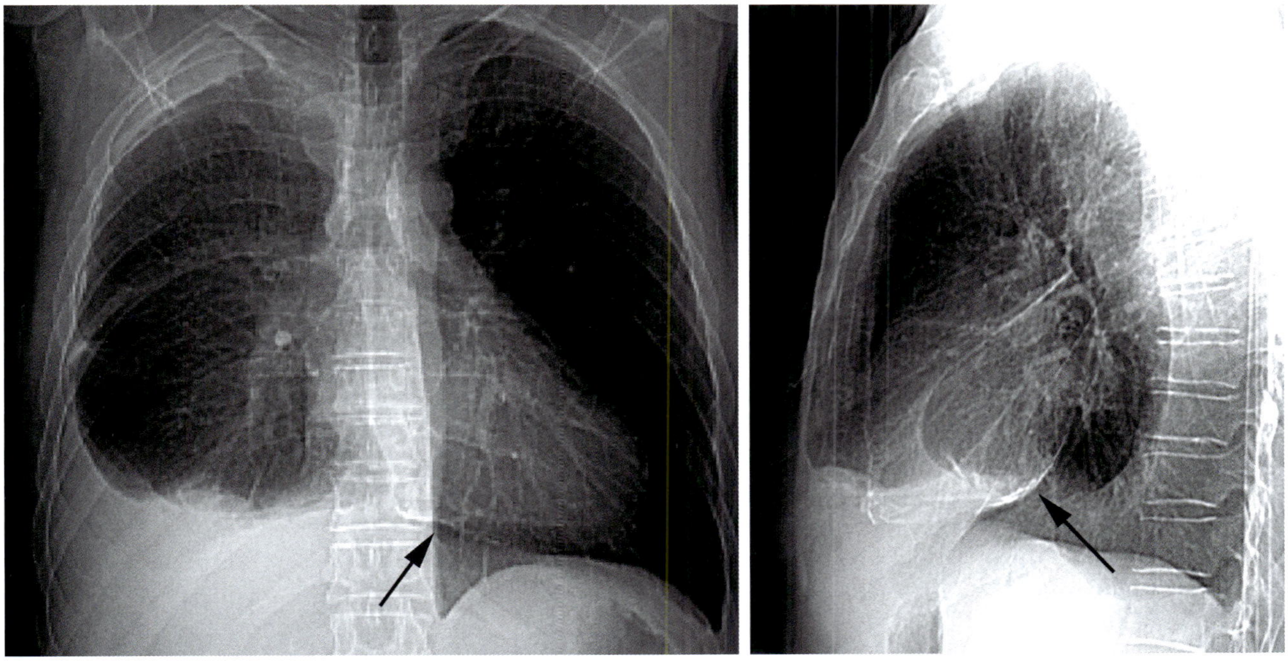

Fig 9.11 PA chest radiograph *(left)* shows right pleural effusion and very faint line of calcification *(arrow)* at inferior aspect of left ventricle. Lateral chest radiograph *(right)* shows area of dense pericardial calcification *(arrow)* along posterior aspect of left ventricle.

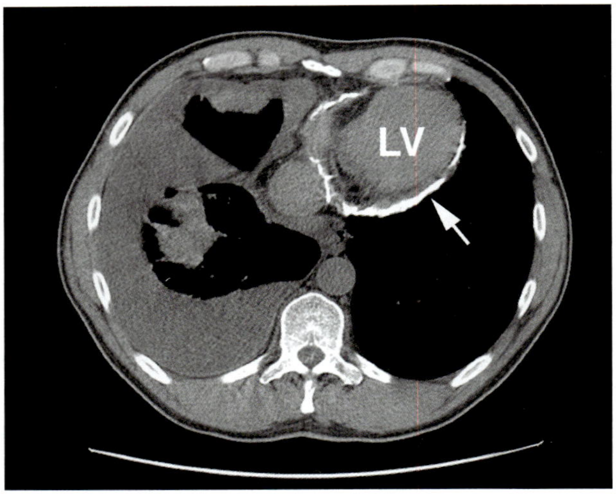

Fig 9.12 Chest CT scan shows marked thickening and increased density of pericardium, consistent with pericardial thickening and calcification. There is moderately sized right pleural effusion and some compressive right lower lobe atelectasis. Man's CT findings also included liver cirrhosis and splenomegaly, suggesting portal hypertension, probably related to his constrictive pericarditis.

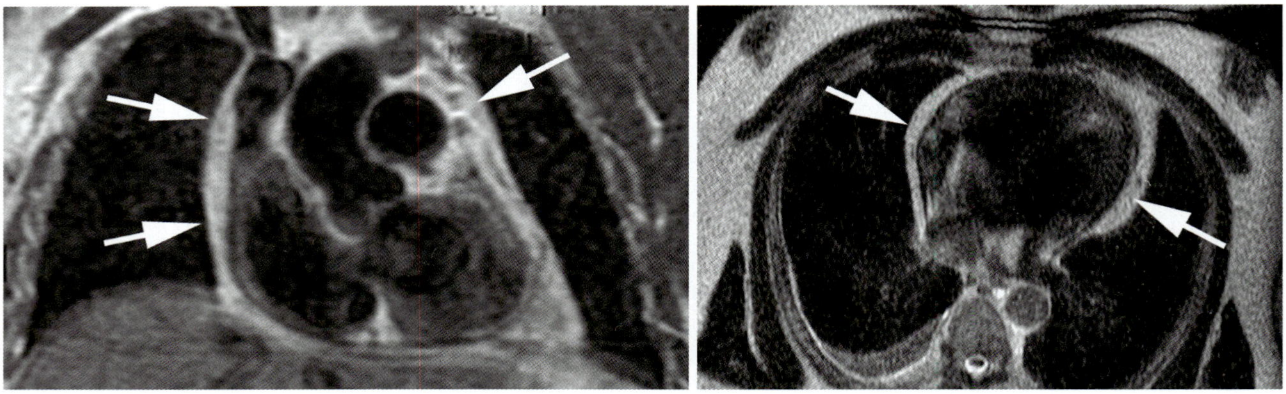

Fig 9.13 MRI demonstrates thickened pericardium *(arrows)* in both coronal *(left)* and axial *(right)* views.

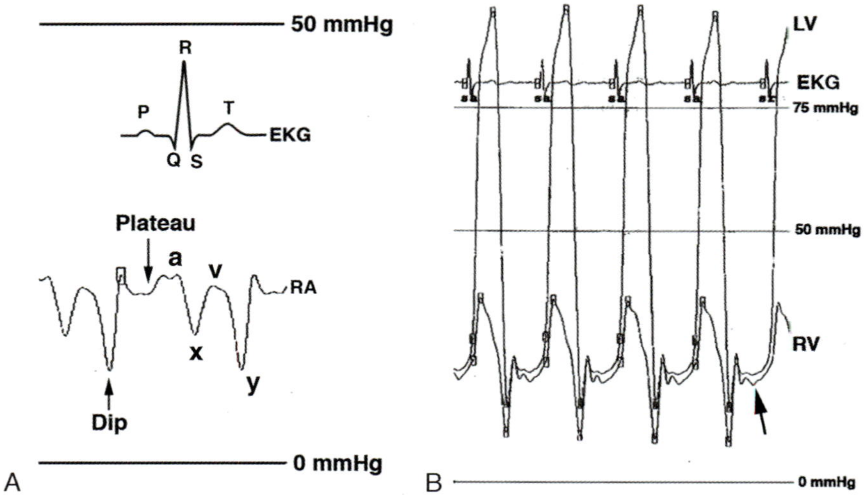

Fig 9.14 **(A)** Right atrial pressure tracing. Early diastolic dip and later diastolic plateau form square-root sign (√), typical in constrictive pericarditis. **(B)** There is equalization of RV and LV diastolic pressure *(arrow)*, also typical in constrictive pericarditis.

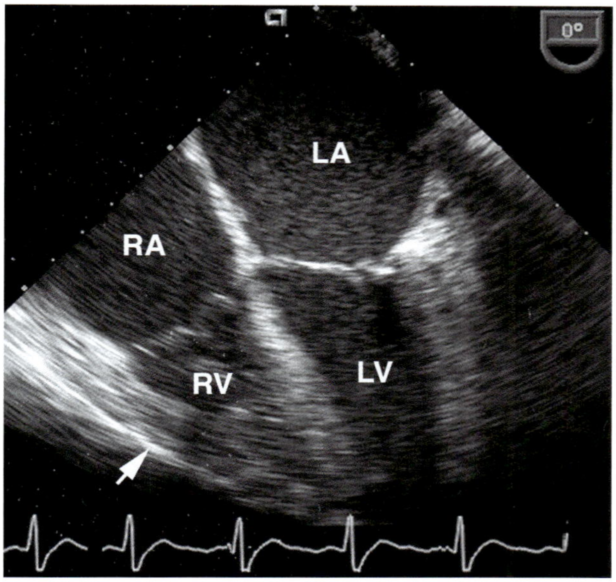

Fig 9.15 In this four-chamber view, atria are enlarged and ventricular chambers are small, as expected with pericardial constriction. Area of pericardial thickening along right ventricular free wall is seen *(arrow)*.

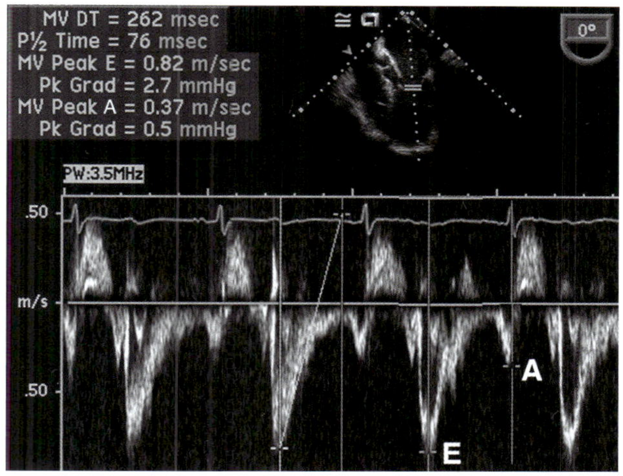

Fig 9.16 Left ventricular diastolic filling pattern shows high E/A ratio and steep deceleration slope. This pattern of diastolic filling is consistent with rapid early diastolic filling, with impaired late diastolic filling due, in this case, to pericardial constriction. This pattern of diastolic filling is also seen with severe left ventricular diastolic dysfunction due to decreased compliance

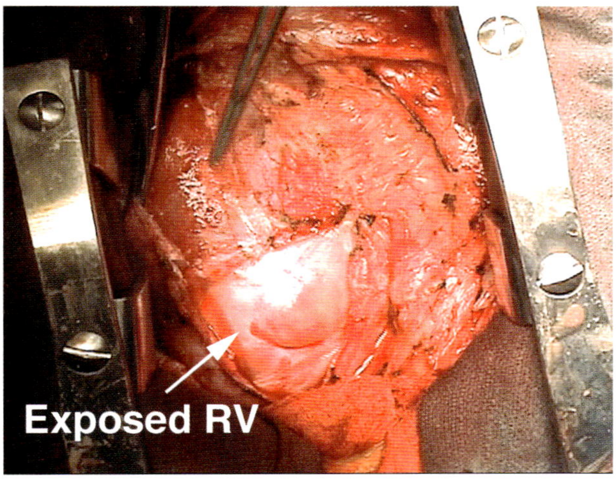

Fig 9.17 At surgery, pericardium was severely thickened and calcified. Pericardium was stripped from phrenic nerve to phrenic nerve laterally.

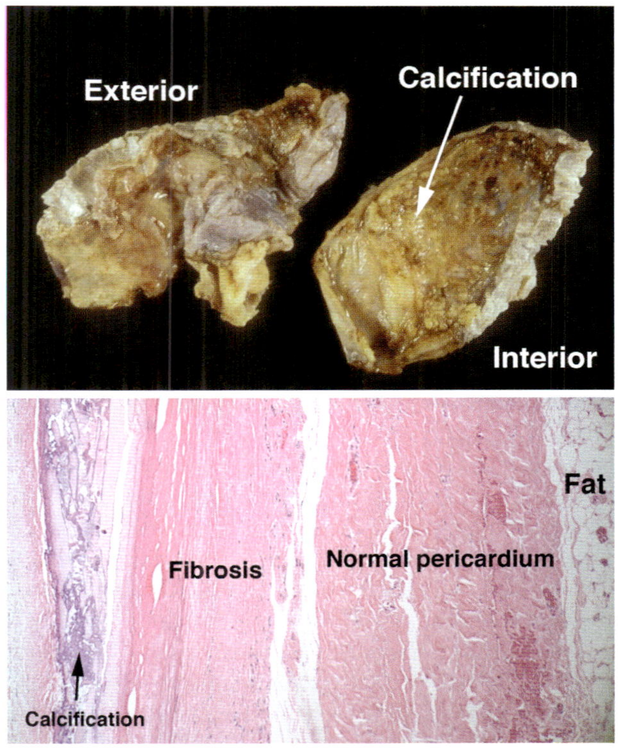

Fig 9.18 Gross findings on pathology were segments of fibrotic pericardium, with thickness ranging from 0.3 to 1.4 cm. Microscopic examination showed fibrosis, calcification, and patchy chronic inflammation consistent with constrictive pericarditis.

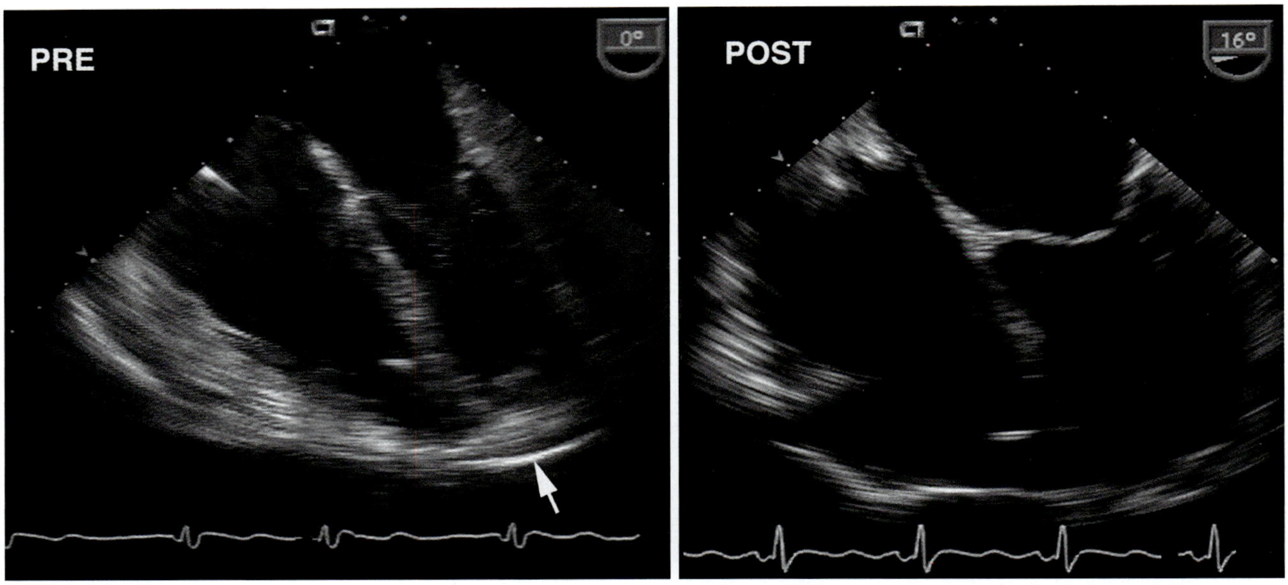

Fig 9.19 Comparison of preoperative *(left)* and postpericardiectomy *(right)* four-chamber views using small depth scale shows increased size of ventricular chambers after relief of constrictive physiology. Arrow indicates thickened pericardium.

Comments

Constrictive pericarditis may be due to prior infectious pericarditis (tuberculous or viral), trauma or cardiac surgery, rheumatologic disorders, neoplasia, or mediastinal radiation, but in many cases a cause is not found. The basic pathophysiology of constriction is that the adherence, thickening, and fibrosis of the pericardium result in the ventricles being unable to fill adequately in diastole. The primary problem in clinical diagnosis is distinguishing pericardial constriction from a restrictive cardiomyopathy. Both are characterized by small ventricles with normal systolic function, abnormal diastolic filling patterns, biatrial enlargement, and an elevated central venous pressure. However, with restrictive cardiomyopathy, pulmonary pressures are often elevated, the pericardium is normal in thickness, and the diastolic pressures in the right and left ventricles are not equal.

The hallmark of pericardial constriction is a thickened pericardium, as in this case. Although echocardiography often first suggests the diagnosis of constriction, evaluation of the presence and severity of pericardial thickening by echocardiography is limited. Both CT and MRI provide better definition of pericardial anatomy and should be considered when echocardiography suggests this diagnosis.

With both pericardial constriction and restrictive cardiomyopathy, the pattern of ventricle filling on a single cardiac cycle is characterized by a rapid early diastolic filling phase, and a reduced atrial contribution to filling. However, when multiple beats are examined, there are no significant respiratory changes in patients with restrictive cardiomyopathy. In contrast, in patients with pericardial constriction, there are marked reciprocal respiratory changes in left and right ventricular diastolic filling. The rigid adherent pericardium limits the total cardiac volume so that as right-sided filling increases with inspiration, the left ventricle is compressed and left-sided filling decreases. The opposite changes occur with expiration. (These changes are not reliable in patients receiving positive pressure ventilation.) Tissue Doppler evaluation is also helpful for diagnosis of constrictive pericarditis.

At cardiac catheterization, there is equalization of the diastolic pressures in the cardiac chambers with pericardial constriction. The demonstration that right and left ventricle diastolic pressures are equal (within 5 mm Hg of each other) after volume loading is diagnostic for constriction. The diastolic pressure curve also classically shows an early diastolic dip, due to the initial high-pressure gradient from atrium to ventricle, followed by rapid equalization of pressures as the constricted ventricle quickly fills to capacity. The late diastolic plateau phase is flat, as there is no further ventricular filling and no change in ventricular pressure. This results in the pressure curve looking like the mathematical symbol for a square root.

Suggested Reading

1. Amaki M, Savino J, Ain DL, et al: Diagnostic concordance of echocardiography and cardiac magnetic resonance-based tissue tracking for differentiating constrictive pericarditis from restrictive cardiomyopathy, Circ Cardiovasc Imaging 7(5): 819–827, 2014.
2. Alraies MC, Kusunose K, Negishi K, et al: Relation between echocardiographically estimated and invasively measured filling pressures in constrictive pericarditis, Am J Cardiol 113(11): 1911–1916, 2014.
3. Welch TD, Ling LH, Espinosa RE, et al: Echocardiographic diagnosis of constrictive pericarditis: Mayo Clinic criteria, Circ Cardiovasc Imaging 7(3):526–534, 2014.

CASE 9-3
Pericardial Tamponade During Percutaneous Coronary Intervention

This 78-year-old man had a history of CABG 8 years before his admission to our hospital. In the last several months he had been bothered by increasing chest pain and shortness of breath. A myocardial perfusion scan revealed evidence of ischemia in the inferior wall. His symptoms persisted despite optimal medical management, and therefore he was taken for coronary angiography. The vein graft to the right coronary artery was found to have a 90% focal stenosis in the body of the graft. A drug-eluting stent was deployed to the midsaphenous vein graft; however, he became diaphoretic, hypoxic, hypotensive, and developed ST elevations in the inferior leads. The vein graft defect was stented, without clinical improvement. He was endotracheally intubated, and a TEE was performed.

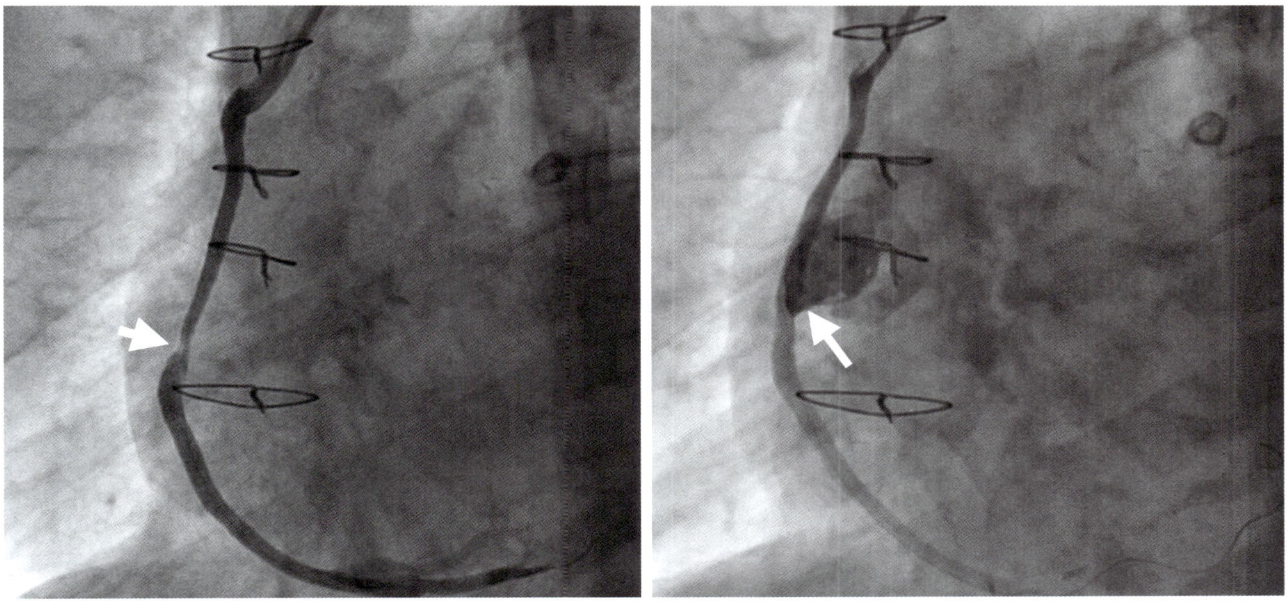

Fig 9.20 On left, arrow indicates focal stenosis in vein graft to right coronary artery. On right, free extravasation of contrast is seen.

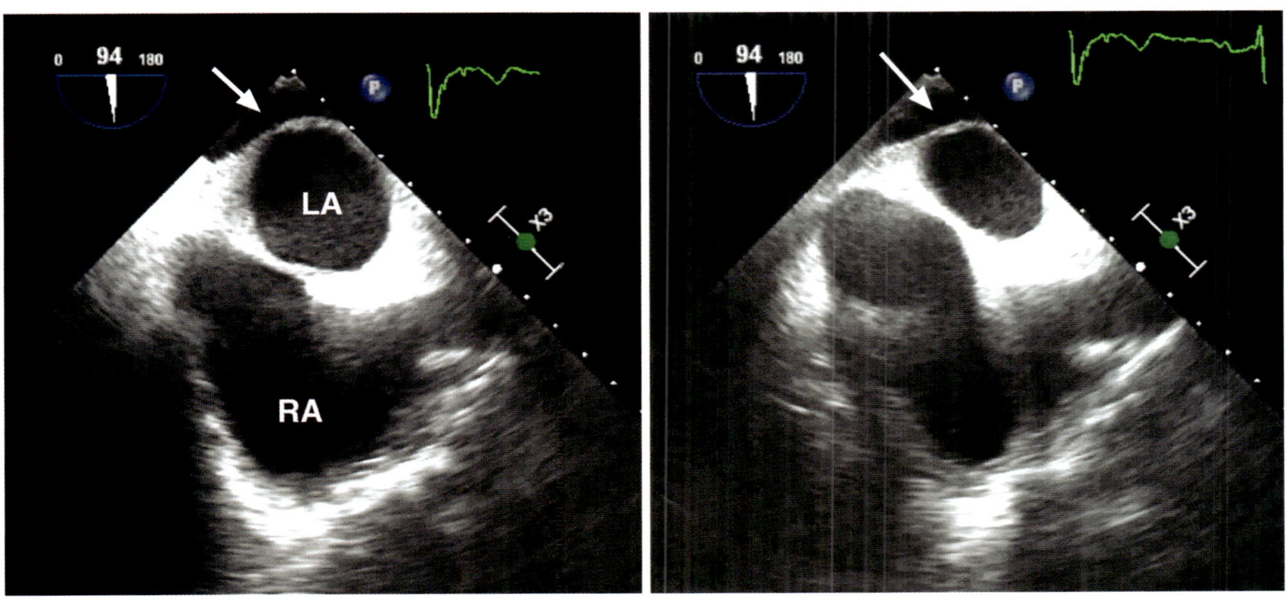

Fig 9.21 A midesophageal bicaval view was obtained. There is pericardial effusion behind left atrium *(arrow)*; left atrial collapse is present.

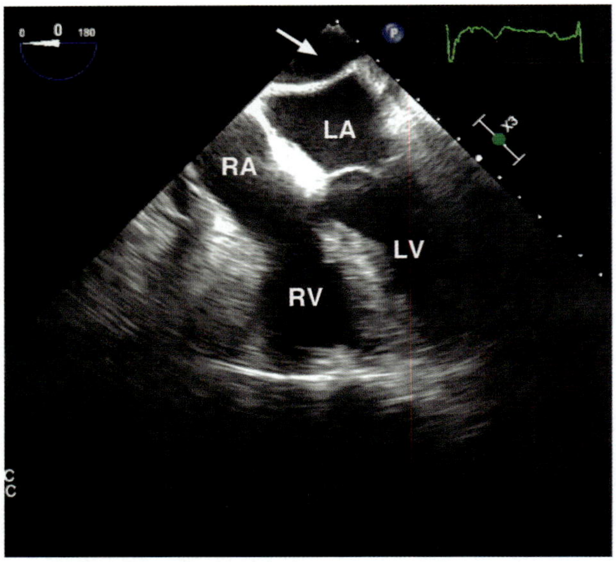

Fig 9.22 In midesophageal four-chamber view, there is compression of left atrium posteriorly by pericardial effusion.

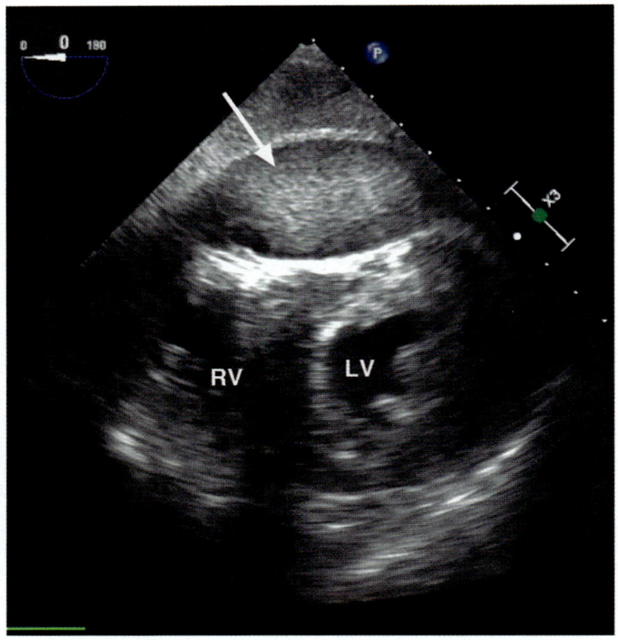

Fig 9.23 In this transgastric short-axis view, collection is seen *(arrow)*. There is compression of LV and RV. Patient was taken to surgery. After sternotomy and drainage of pericardial blood, there was immediate hemodynamic improvement. New saphenous vein graft was placed to right coronary artery.

Comments

As this case illustrates, a localized acute pericardial effusion can result in tamponade-like physiology even in the absence of circumferential pericardial fluid. Localized effusions may be difficult to recognize for several reasons. First, because the effusion is due to acute bleeding into the pericardial space, spontaneous contrast due to low velocity flow and thrombus formation in the acute effusion may be mistaken for a mass, instead of pericardial fluid. Second, multiple views are needed to identify the fluid because the effusion is localized. Third, in some cases the effusion may invert the atrial wall so severely that the fluid itself appears to be the atrium, with the atrial wall lying next to the atrial septum and atrioventricular valve. In this situation, color Doppler may show the slit-like atrial chamber. If the diagnosis is still uncertain, saline or left-sided echo contrast can be used to opacify the cardiac chambers. The possibility of a localized effusion compressing one or more cardiac chambers should be considered in all surgical and interventional procedures with a sudden unexplained deterioration in hemodynamics.

Suggested Reading

1. Aggarwal C, Varghese J, Uretsky BF: Left atrial inflow and outflow obstruction as a complication of retrograde approach for chronic total occlusion: report of a case and literature review of left atrial hematoma after percutaneous coronary intervention, Catheter Cardiovasc Interv 82(5):770–775, 2013.
2. Bagur R, Bernier M, Kandzari DE, et al: A novel application of contrast echocardiography to exclude active coronary perforation bleeding in patients with pericardial effusion, Catheter Cardiovasc Interv 82(2):221–229, 2013.

10 Diseases of the Great Vessels

Pseudoaneurysms

CASE 10-1
Aortic Pseudoaneurysm after AVR with Anterior Extension

This 41-year-old man with Reiter's syndrome underwent mechanical aortic valve replacement 9 years ago for aortic regurgitation. Four months ago he developed prosthetic valve endocarditis. He was treated with antibiotics and repeat aortic valve replacement with that procedure complicated by a paravalvular abscess requiring placement of a pericardial patch in the periannular region. Postoperatively, he had persistent paravalvular regurgitation and repeat echocardiography showed "rocking" of the prosthesis and a possible pseudoaneurysm. A preoperative transesophageal echocardiogram demonstrated valve dehiscence with blood flow from the aorta into an anterior echo-free space that also communicated with the left ventricle. He was referred for surgery.

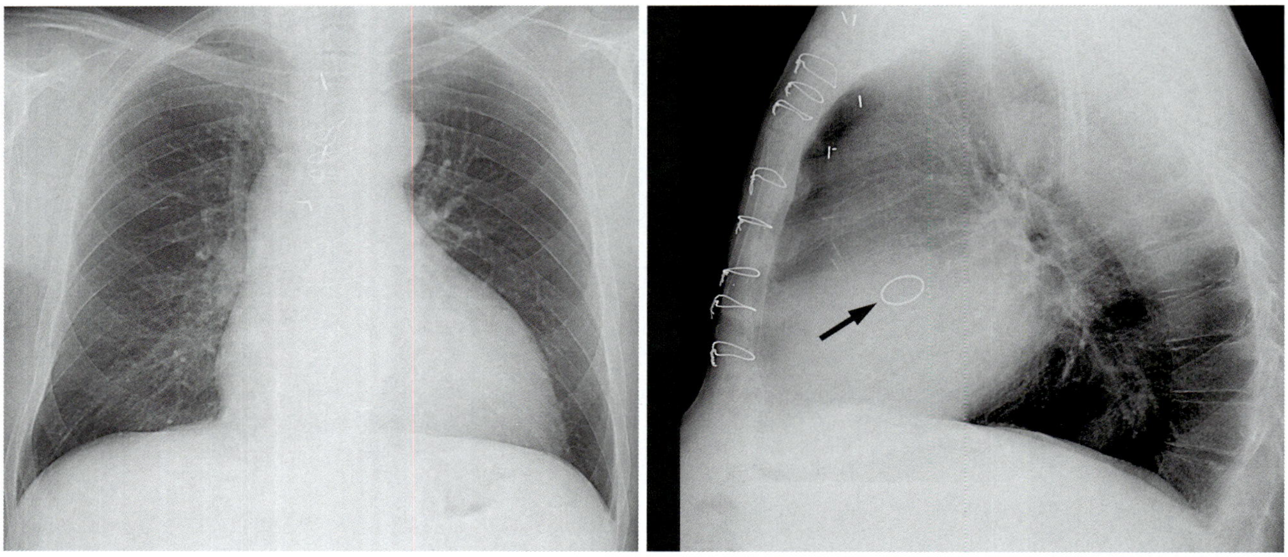

Fig 10.1 Chest radiography shows prominence of ascending aorta. Lateral view demonstrates enlarged ascending aorta with opacification of retrosternal space, and presence of radio-opaque ring of prosthetic valve *(arrow)*.

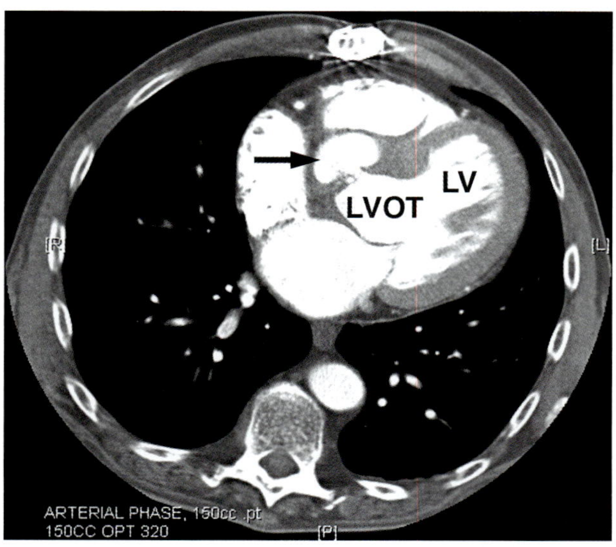

Fig 10.2 Chest CT with contrast at level of left ventricle shows abnormal area *(arrow)* filled with contrast, that communicates anteriorly with LVOT.

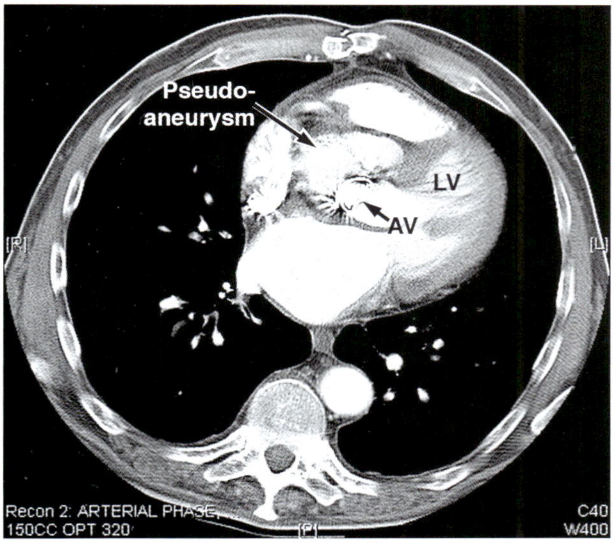

Fig 10.3 Chest CT with contrast at level of prosthetic aortic valve (AV). Anterior to prosthetic aortic valve is collection of contrast with irregular borders, which is extraluminal and measuring 2.3 × 4.2 cm. These findings are consistent with aortic pseudoaneurysm.

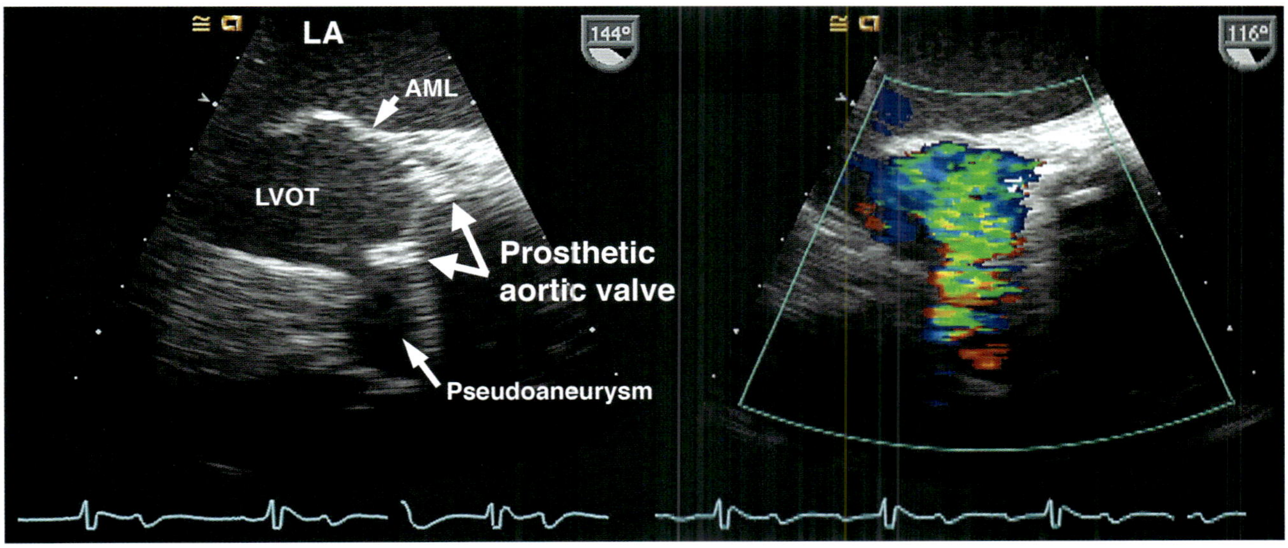

Fig 10.4 In TEE long-axis plane (at 144 degrees rotation), pseudoaneurysm is seen anterior to prosthetic aortic valve. Color Doppler *(right)* demonstrates flow in and out of pseudoaneurysm from LV outflow tract.

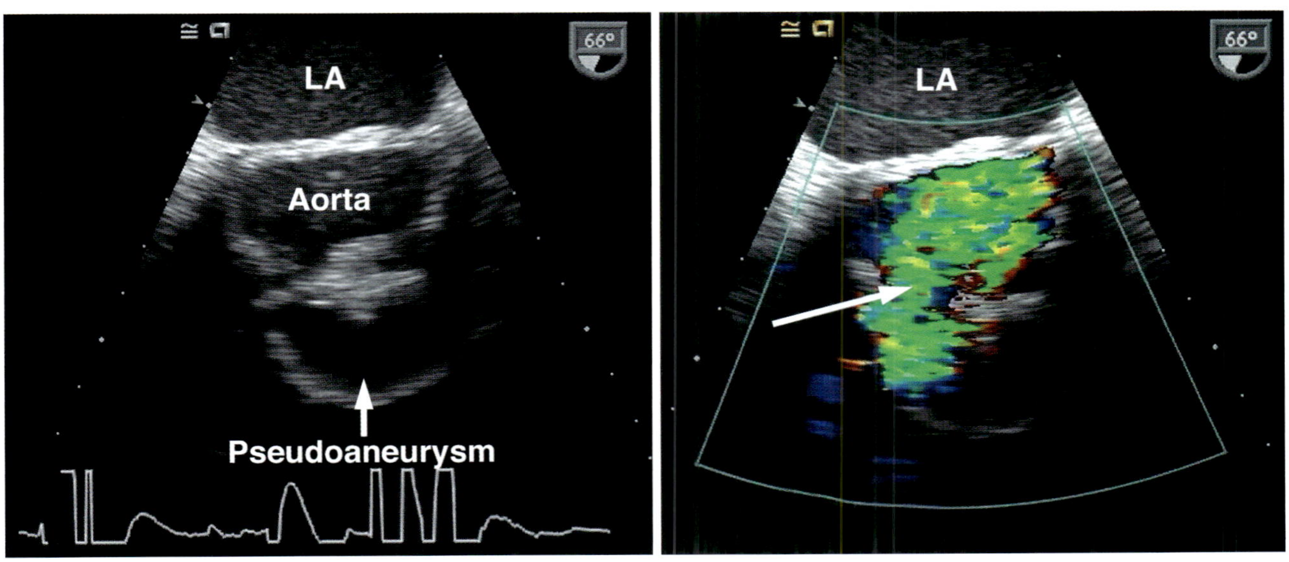

Fig 10.5 In short-axis TEE view at level of ascending aorta, large echo-free space with irregular borders, consistent with pseudoaneurysm is seen.

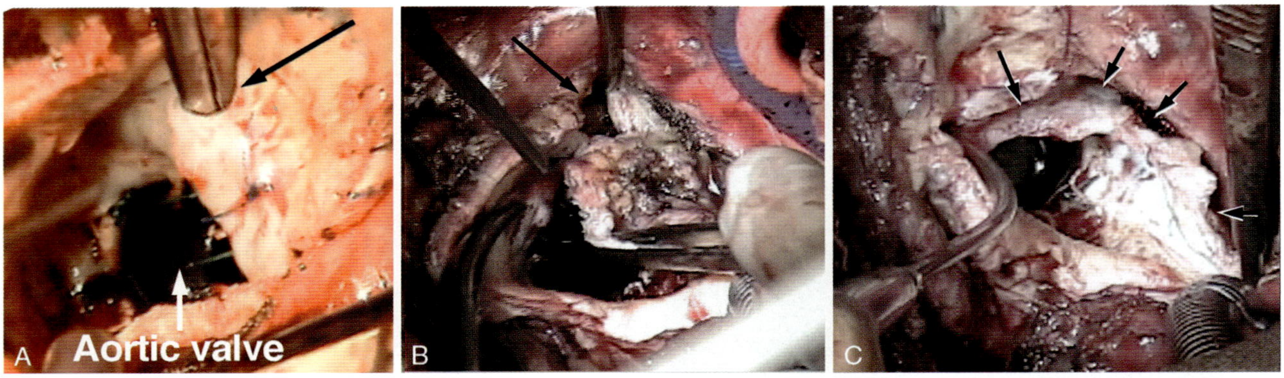

Fig 10.6 At surgery, opening aorta revealed orifice of right coronary artery *(arrow)* just above prosthetic aortic valve **(A)**. In **(B)**, anterior aortic wall has been retracted to reveal entrance into pseudoaneurysm *(arrow)*. After removal of anterior aortic wall **(C)**, very large pseudoaneurysm was appreciated *(arrows)*, originating from underneath right main coronary artery and extending down to middle of noncoronary sinus.

CASE 10-2
Aortic Pseudoaneurysm after AVR with Posterior Extension

12 years prior to admission, this 44-year-old male underwent bioprosthetic AVR for endocarditis. Seven years later he underwent redo sternotomy and second replacement for aortic valve bioprosthesis failure. Four days prior to this admission he developed increasing shortness of breath, and presented to the Emergency Department where examination showed pulmonary edema and lab data including an elevated B-type natriuretic peptide level of 386 pg/mL (Normal <101). TTE and TEE revealed a dilated LV with severe aortic regurgitation and an unstable bioprosthesis with posterior dehiscence and a posterior aortic pseudoaneurysm. His EF was 50-55%. He denied chest pain, syncope, PND, orthopnea, swelling, significant DOE, fevers, chills, nausea, vomiting, diarrhea, and rash. At surgery, the prosthetic valve was explanted, the opening to the pseudoaneurysm patched, and a new bioprosthetic valve placed.

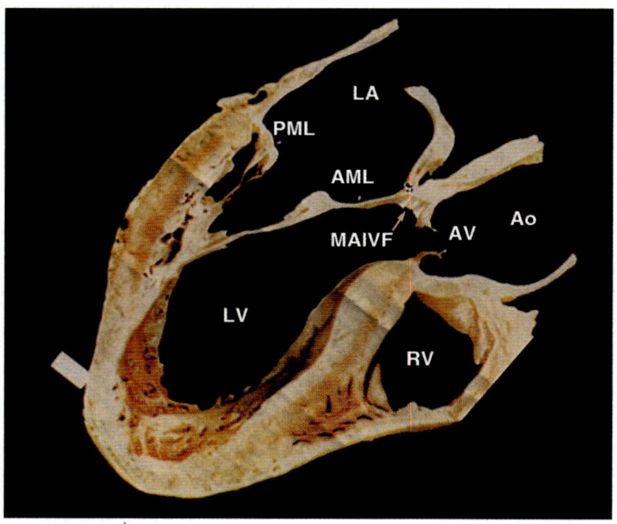

Fig 10.7 This normal anatomic specimen is oriented in the long-axis plane. Note that the fibrous skeleton of the heart is characterized by continuity between the posterior wall of the aortic root and the base of the anterior mitral leaflet. With infection of this region, an aneurysm can form that extends posterior to the aortic root. (Reproduced with permission from Karalis DG et al: Transesophageal echocardiographic recognition of subaortic complications in aortic valve endocarditis. Circulation 1992; 86:353–623, 1992 American Heart Association.)

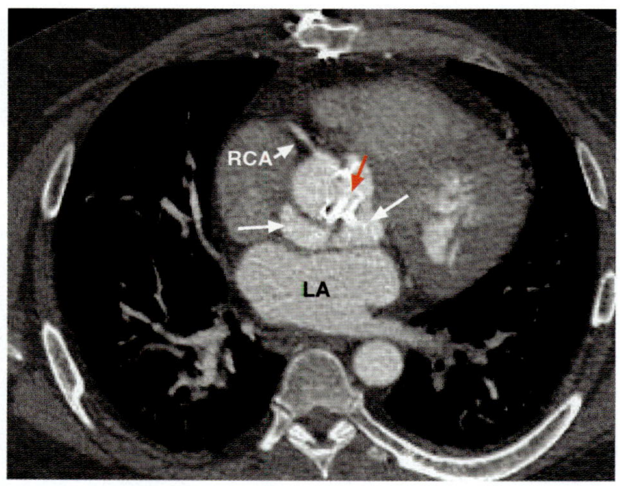

Fig 10.8 Preoperative CT scan. Red arrow indicates valve prosthesis. White arrows indicate posterior pseudoaneurysm, which appears to have two separate areas of fluid collection and impinges on left atrium.

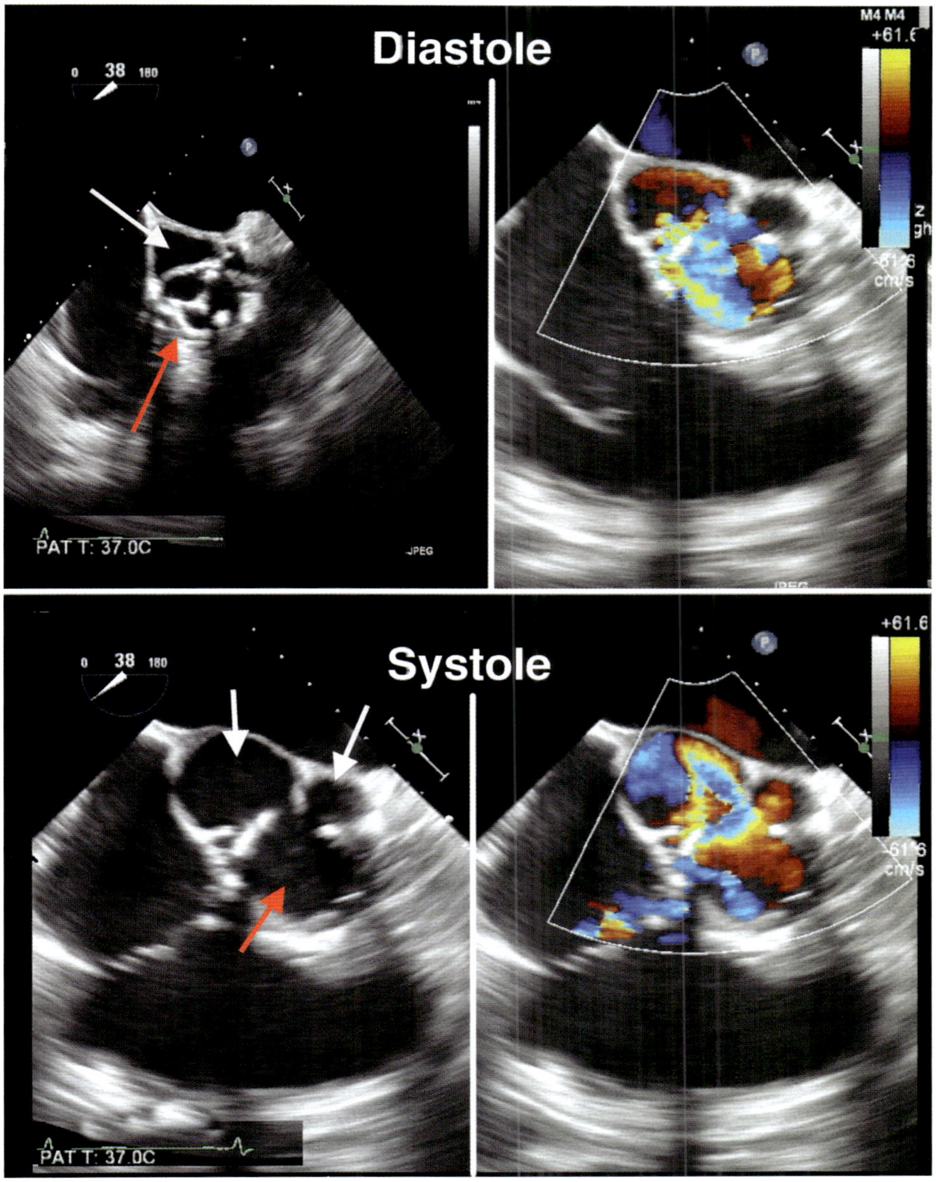

Fig 10.9 Midesophageal short-axis view. In the upper left panel, the red arrow indicates the prosthetic aortic valve, and the white arrow the pseudoaneurysm. The upper right panel shows diastolic flow originating from both the regurgitant valve and the emptying of the pseudoaneurysm into the LV outflow tract. In systole, color Doppler shows the pseudoaneurysm *(white arrows)* filling from the LVOT, which is indicated by the red arrow.

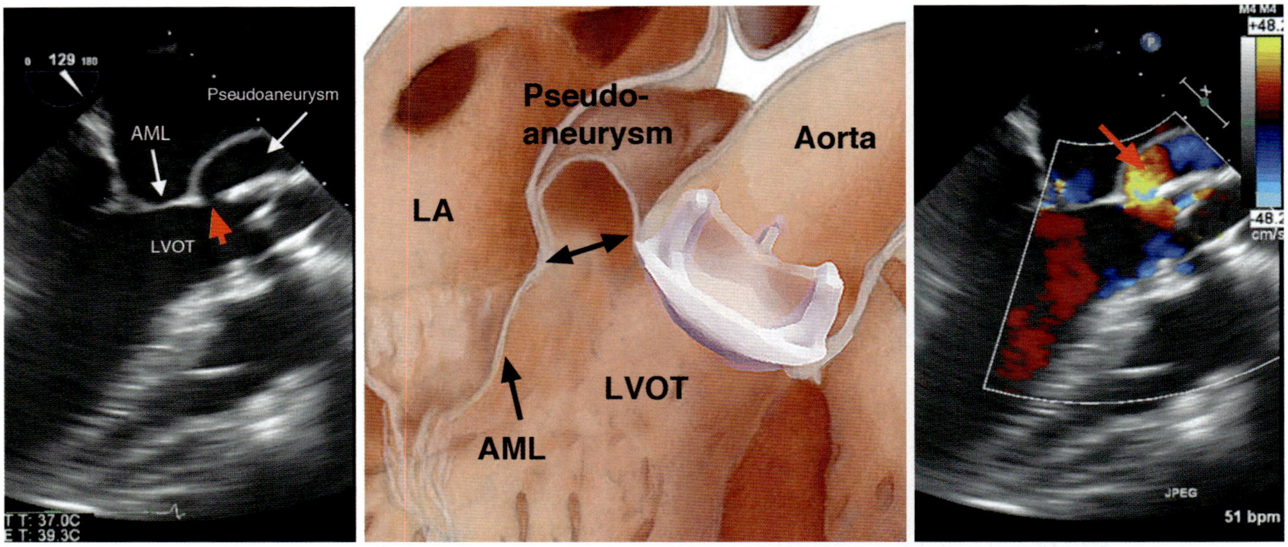

Fig 10.10 In left panel, midesophageal long-axis view demonstrates area of dehiscence between prosthetic aortic valve and native annulus *(red arrow)*. This suggests that in addition to aortic pseudoaneurysm, patient has aneurysm of aortic-mitral intravalvular fibrosa with additional cavity adjacent to aortic pseudoaneurysm, with communication between these cavities. This is graphically demonstrated in the middle panel. In right panel, color Doppler demonstrates flow between LVOT and pseudoaneurysm *(red arrow)*. (Figure from Zoghbi W: Echocardiographic recognition of unusual complications after surgery on great vessels and cardiac valves. In Otto CM, editor: The practice of clinical echocardiography, ed 3, 2007, Elsevier, p 618.)

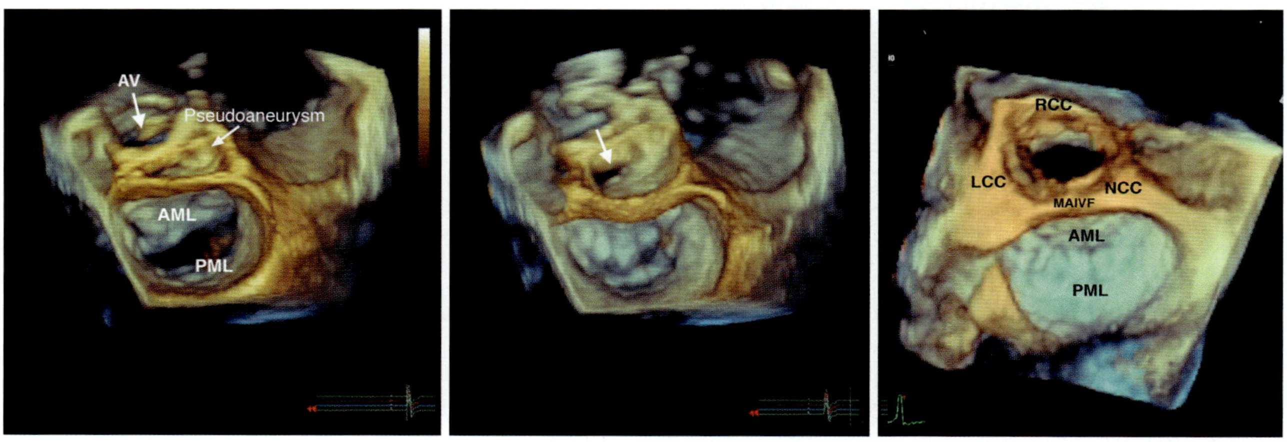

Fig 10.11 In these 3D TEE images, dome of left atrium and pseudoaneurysm have been cropped away. At left in diastole, pseudoaneurysm is compressed between aortic valve prosthesis and left atrium. In middle during systole, pseudoaneurysm expands and communication between pseudoaneurysm and LV outflow tract is seen *(white arrow)*. This is seen more clearly in corresponding video clip. On right is normal image for comparison. Note close approximation of aortic and mitral valves in normal heart compared with separation of aortic valve from mitral valve by pseudoaneurysm in this case.

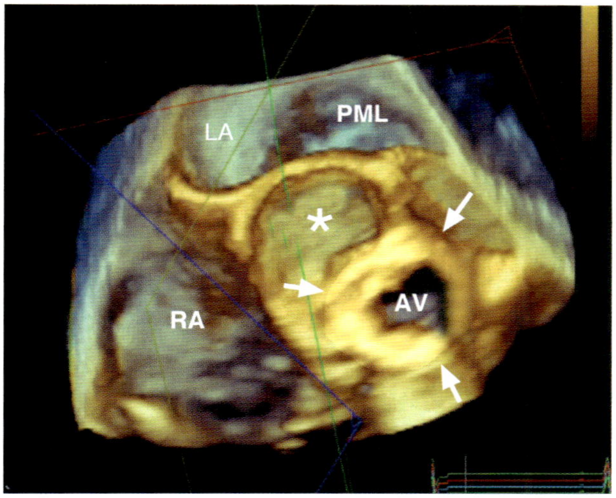

Fig 10.12 From anterior perspective, during systole, aortic valve prosthesis is indicated by three white arrows and pseudoaneurysm by asterisk.

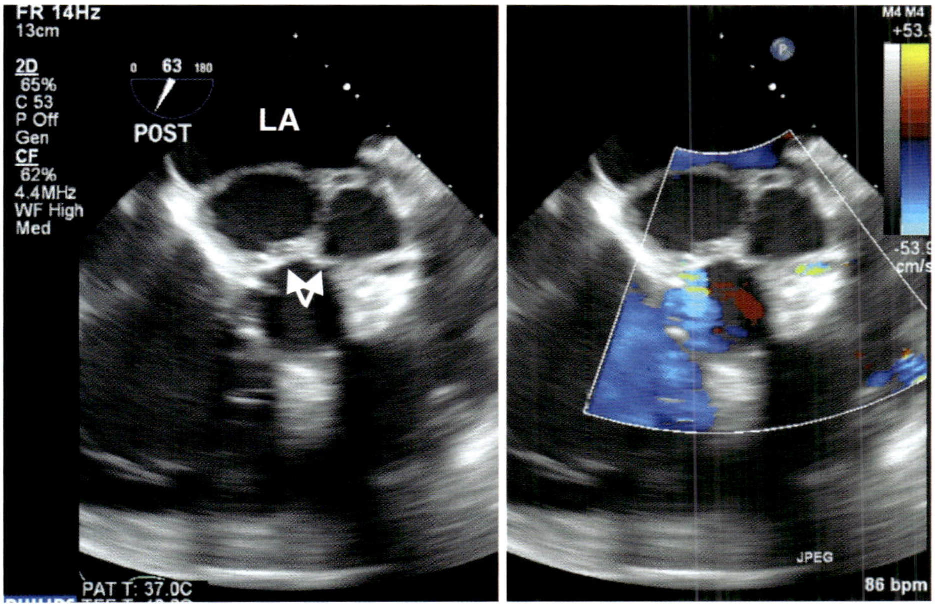

Fig 10.13 Patient was taken to OR. Ascending aortotomy was performed and aortic valve prosthesis explanted. Entry to pseudoaneurysms were patched, and new tissue prosthesis was placed. In midesophageal short-axis view, patches are indicated by arrows. On color Doppler, there is minimal communication seen.

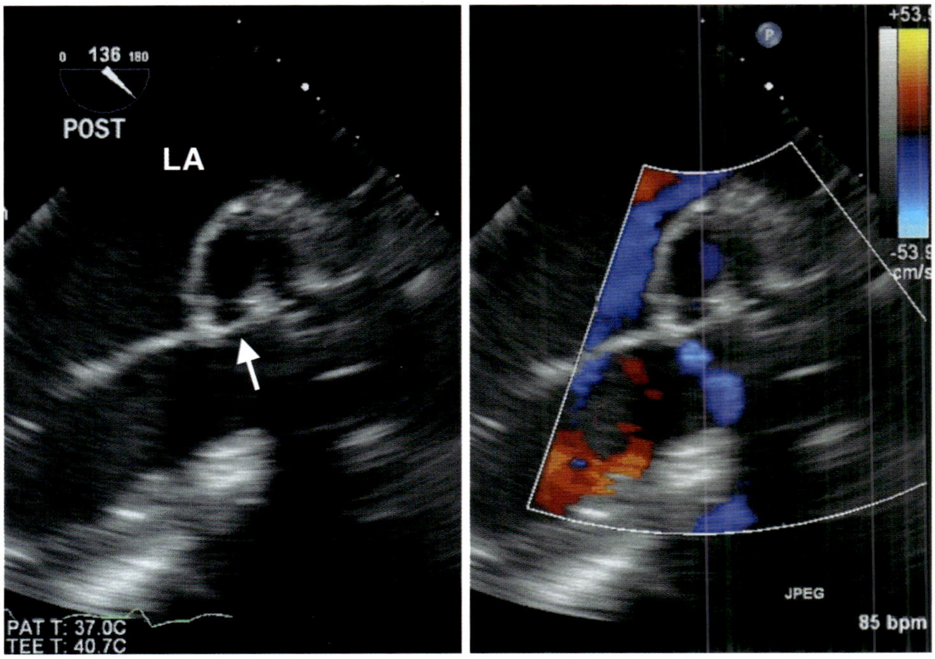

Fig 10.14 In corresponding midesophageal long-axis view, patch again is seen *(white arrow)*. On color Doppler, there was no residual flow between aorta or LV and pseudoaneurysm cavity.

CASE 10-3
Aortic Pseudoaneurysm after Ascending Aortic Graft Dehiscence

This 43-year-old male originally presented 2 years before the current admission with an acute Type A aortic dissection that originated above the aortic valve and extended to the iliac bifurcation. At that time his ascending aorta was replaced with a tube graft and the native aortic valve preserved. He was readmitted to our institution with chest pain and Staph aureus bacteremia. CT scan revealed a large mediastinal hematoma; anterior and posterior pseudoaneurysms were seen at the proximal end of the aortic graft.

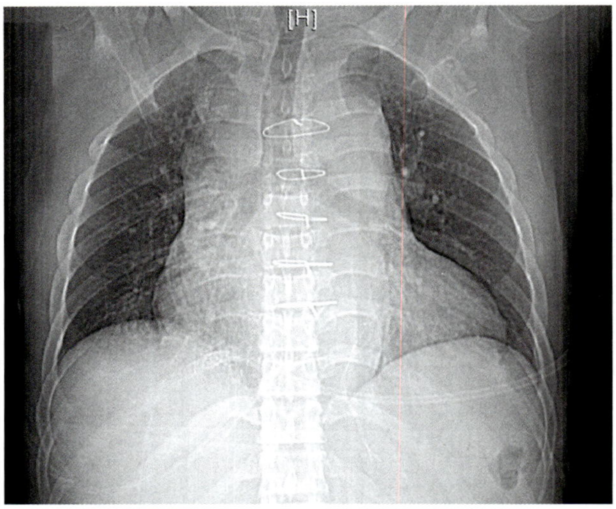

Fig 10.15 PA chest x-ray shows enlarged mediastinum.

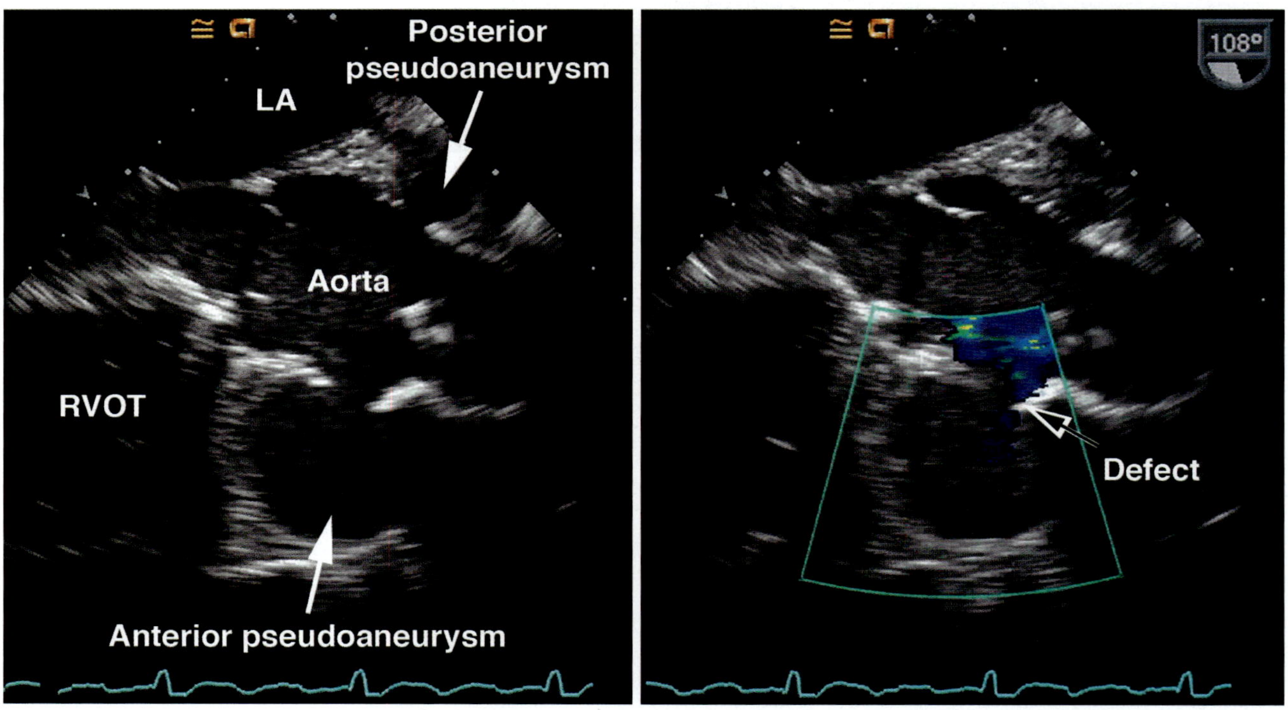

Fig 10.16 Long-axis view of aortic valve and ascending aorta shows dehiscence of proximal end of aortic graft, and both anterior and posterior pseudoaneurysms. Color Doppler *(right)* reveals flow from aorta, through defect and into anterior pseudoaneurysm.

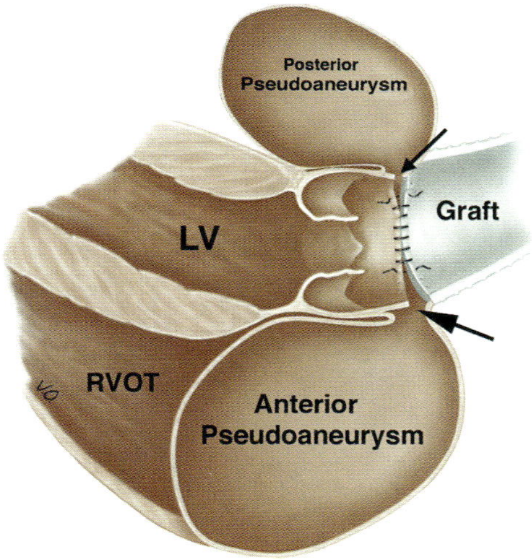

Fig 10.17 This drawing, corresponding to long-axis TEE in Fig 10.16, demonstrates origin *(arrows)* of anterior and posterior pseudoaneurysms.

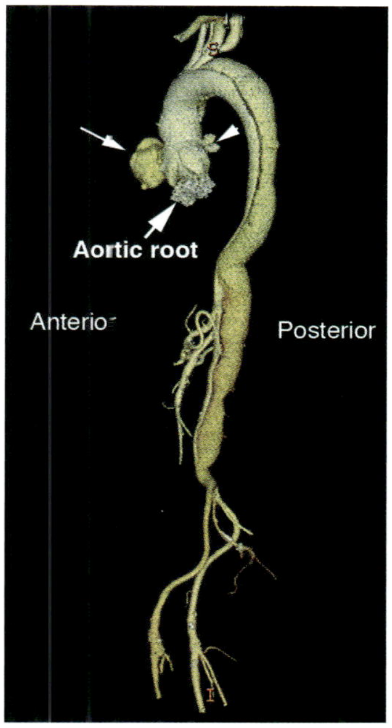

Fig 10.18 3D CT reconstruction shows pseudoaneurysms *(arrows)* in relation to aortic root.

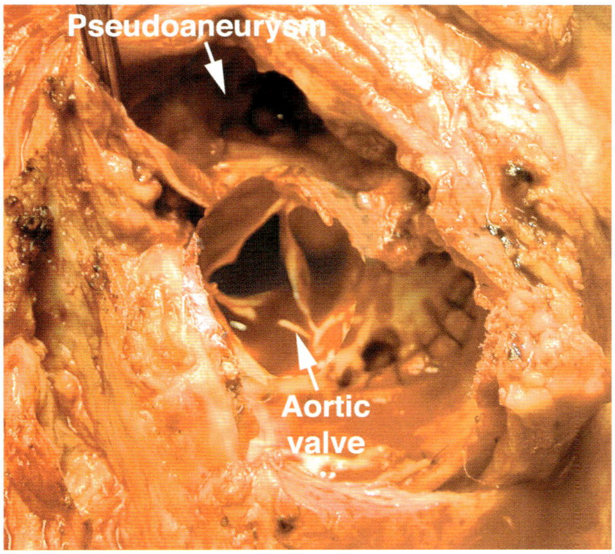

Fig 10.19 At surgery, large pseudoaneurysm was seen anterior to aortic root.

Comments

A pseudoaneurysm is a contained aortic rupture that may be due to infection of an aortic valve prosthesis with abscess formation and tissue destruction or to dehiscence of a suture line at the anastomosis of an aortic tube graft. At the site of rupture, adhesions and scarring limit the extravasation of blood resulting in a contained space. In most cases, the only communication is from the aorta into the pseudoaneurysm space. However, when valve dehiscence extends both above and below the valve plane, blood enters the pseudoaneurysm from the aorta, and exits into the LV outflow tract, simulating aortic regurgitation. In contrast to a true aneurysm, the walls of a pseudoaneurysm are not composed of aortic tissue. Because a pseudoaneurysm is due to rupture of the aorta, albeit "contained," treatment is surgical.

Suggested Reading

1. Evangelista A: Imaging aortic aneurysmal disease, Heart 100:909–915, 2014.
2. Ekici F, Kocabaş A, Aktaş D, Çetin I, Eminoğlu S: Native aortic valve endocarditis complicated by pseudoaneurysm of mitral-aortic intervalvular fibrosa, Echocardiography 31:E60–E63, 2014.

Aortic Dissection

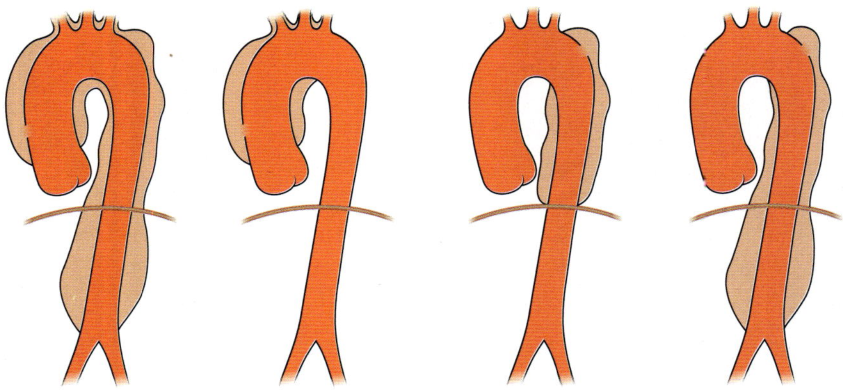

Stanford	A	A	B	B
DeBakey	I	II	IIIa	IIIb
Penn Extent	a	a	a	a
	b	b	b	b
	c	c	c	c
	b&c	b&c	b&c	b&c

Fig 10.20 Stanford, DeBakey, and Penn classification schemes for aortic dissection. In Penn classification, Stanford Type A aortic dissection is integrated with DeBakey I (with descending aortic involvement) and DeBakey II (without descending aortic involvement). Similarly, for Stanford Type B aortic dissection, extension in descending aortic may be in thorax alone (DeBakey III extent A) or in both thorax and abdomen (DeBakey III extent B). Further categorization is based on extension of clinical presentation with postischemic profile: a, absence of ischemia; b, branch vessel malperfusion; c, circulatory collapse; and b and c, both branch vessel malperfusion and circulatory collapse. Within Stanford Type B or DeBakey III, Penn class category may be subdivided into high risk (Type I) or low risk (Type II) of complications depending on echo-anatomic features. (From Tan CN, Fraser AG: Perioperative transesophageal echocardiography for aortic dissection. *Can J Anesth* 61:362–378, 2014. With permission.)

CASE 10-4
Ascending and Aortic Arch Dissection

This 57-year-old male patient presented to an outside hospital with the sudden onset of substernal chest pain, described as constant, nonradiating, and worse with movement. He had not had similar pain in the past. He denied trauma, shortness of breath, nausea, vomiting, numbness, tingling, weakness, back pain, abdominal pain, or syncope. His only risk factor for coronary disease was hypertension. He was taken urgently to the cardiac catheterization laboratory for what was suspected acute myocardial infarction and was found to have a normal left coronary system. The right coronary system could not be engaged; however, a dissection flap was seen in the ascending aorta. The patient urgently underwent computed tomographic angiography (CTA) of the aorta demonstrating an acute Type A aortic dissection extending from the aortic sinuses into the ascending aorta, around the arch and down into the descending thoracic aorta. The diameter of the aortic sinuses was severely enlarged at 5.3 cm. At the time of the CTA scan, there was no significant pericardial effusion or involvement of the head vessels. The patient was transferred to our institution for definitive management. At surgery, the aortic sinuses and ascending aorta were resected, and replaced with a composite valve, root, and aortic graft. The coronary arteries were implanted into the graft.

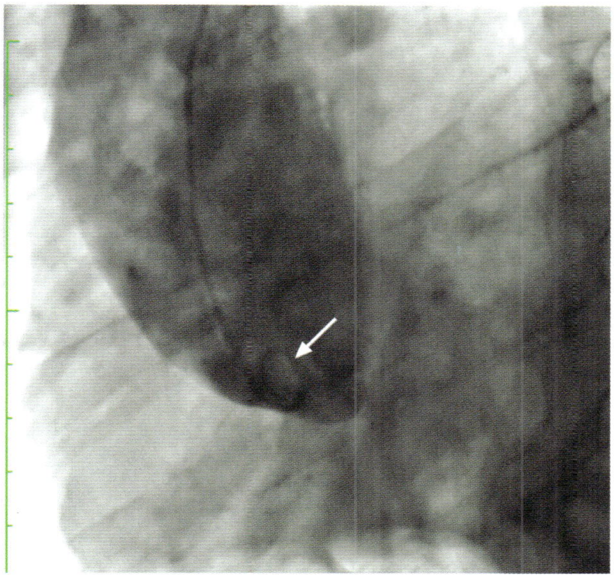

Fig 10.21 Aortic root injection with pigtail catheter *(arrow)* fails to opacify sinuses, suggesting that catheter is in false lumen of aortic dissection, with aortic sinuses connected to true lumen.

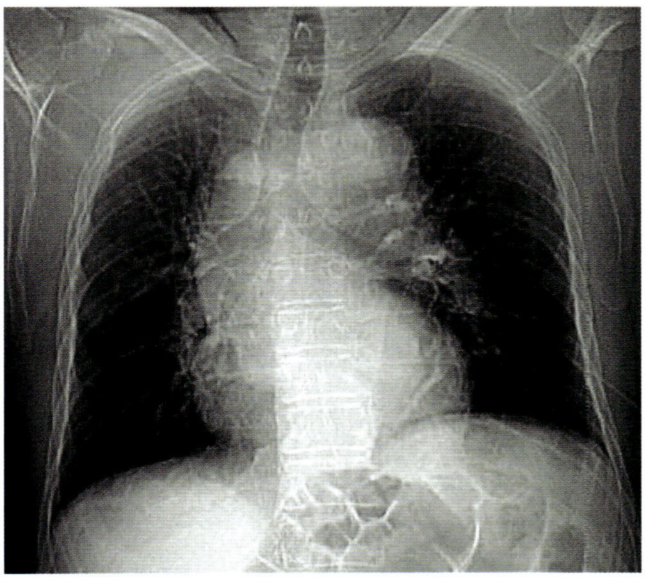

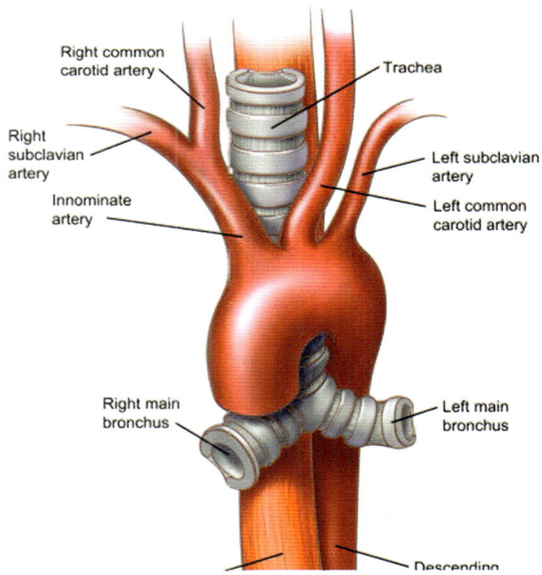

Fig 10.22 Chest x-ray shows widened mediastinum, and obtuse angulation of mainstem bronchi, as result of pressure by enlarged ascending aorta. (Right image from Minnich DJ. Mathisen, DJ: Anatomy of the trachea, carina, and bronchi, Thorac Surg Clin 17:571–585, 2007. With permission.)

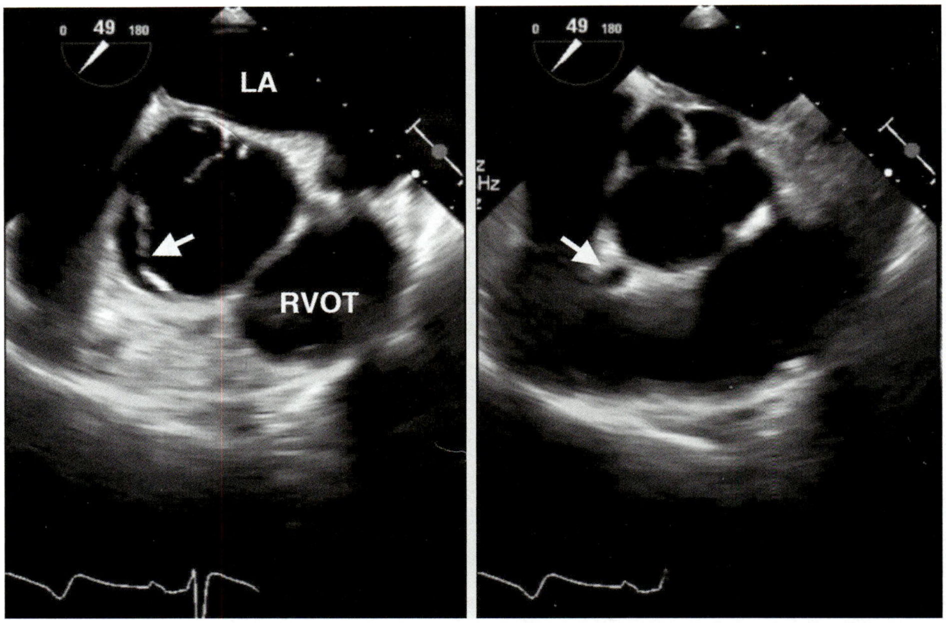

Fig 10.23 In this midesophageal short-axis view, fenestrated dissection flap is seen during systole *(arrow, left)*. In diastole *(right)*, right coronary artery is seen *(arrow)*.

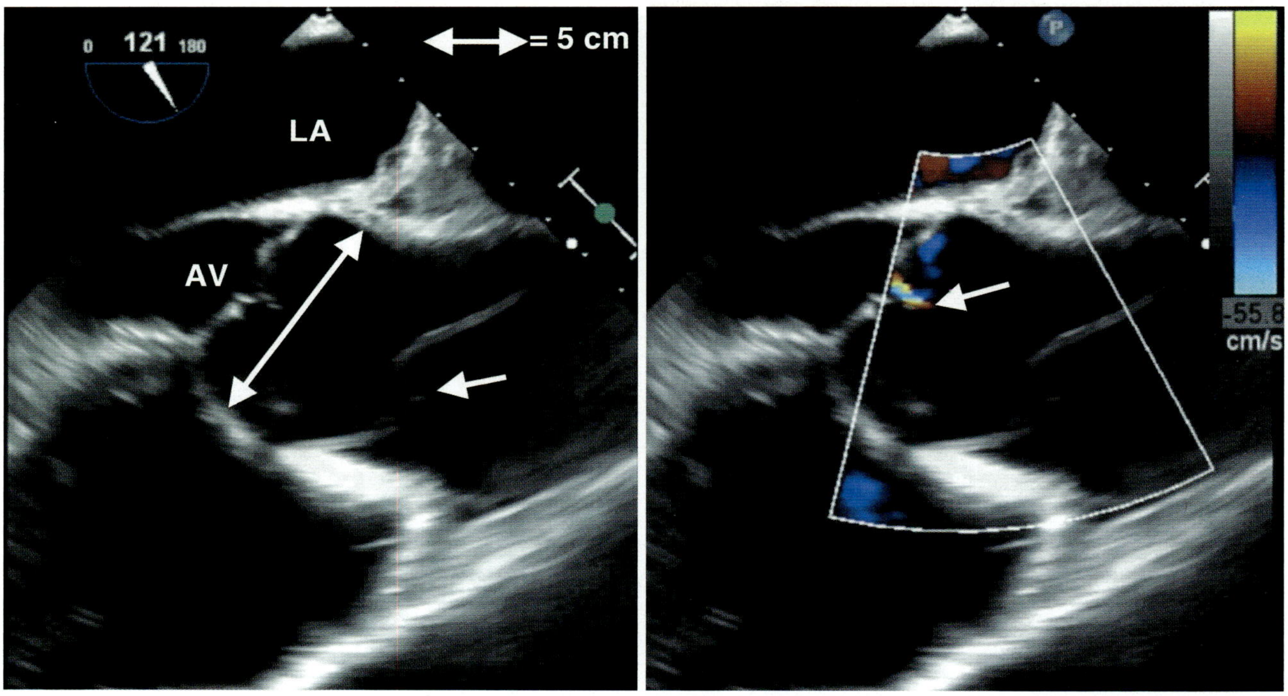

Fig 10.24 In this midesophageal long-axis view, left image clearly shows dissection flap *(arrow)*. In addition, aortic diameter at level of sinuses of Valsalva is enlarged at 5 cm. On right, arrow indicates trace aortic regurgitation.

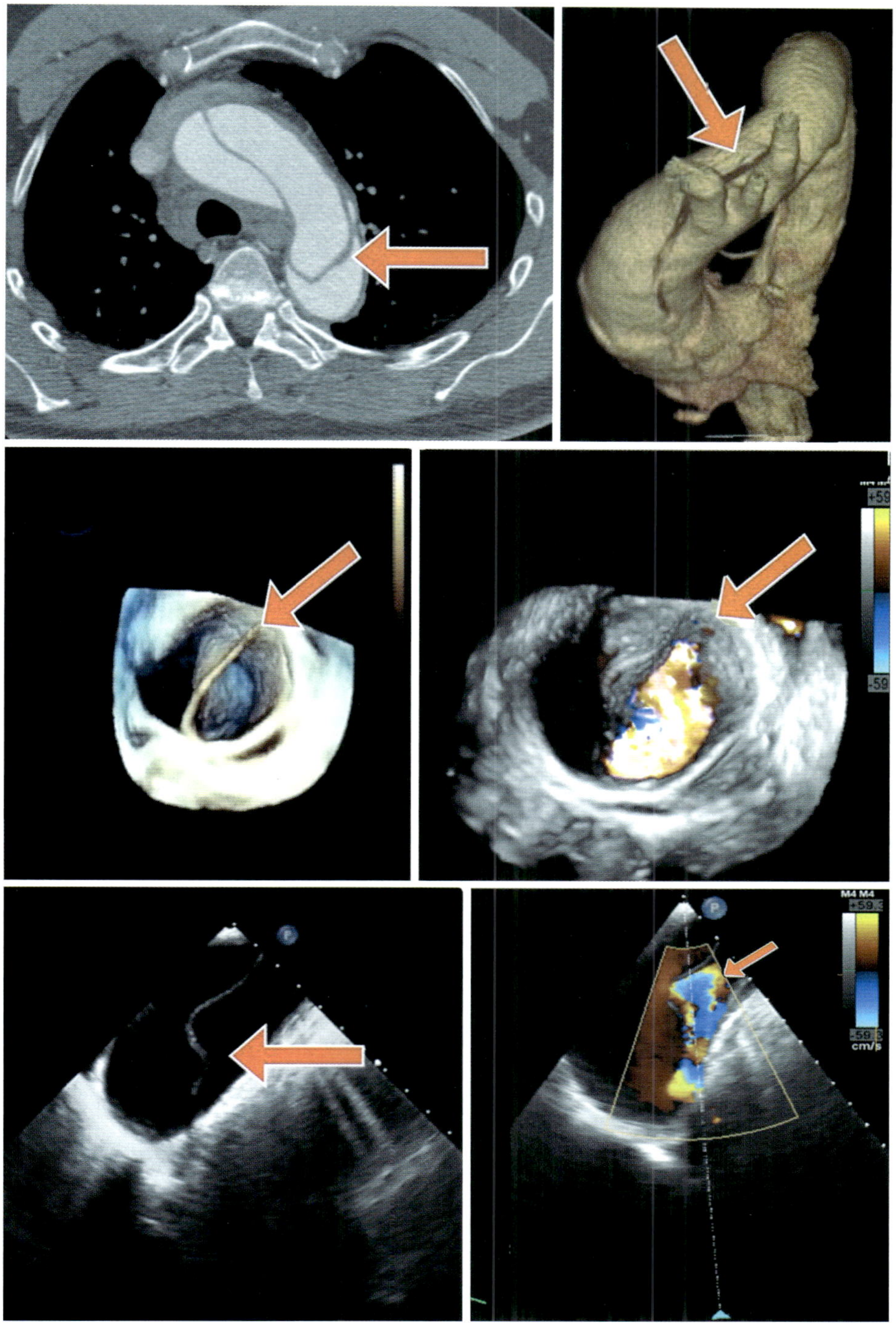

Fig 10.25 Multimodal imaging of aortic arch. In each instance red arrow indicates dissection flap. Top two images are CT scan as well as 3D reconstructed CT. Middle two images are 3D TEE representations of arch, with color Doppler filling what is presumably false lumen; in real time, undulating motion of flap is appreciated. Lower two images are 2D TEE images of arch; on right, turbulent color Doppler is again filling what is presumably false lumen, which is better appreciated in real time.

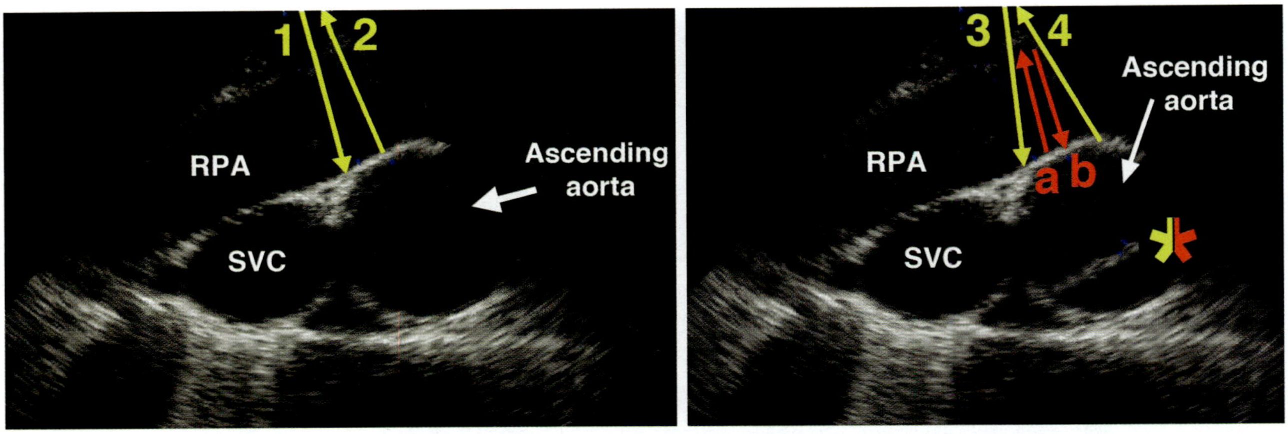

Fig 10.26 Reverberation artifact. Left frame: In this high esophageal short-axis image from a different patient, ultrasound is emitted *(yellow arrow 1)* and reflected off the interface of the anterior wall of the right pulmonary artery (RPA) and posterior wall of the ascending aorta. Most echoes return to the transducer *(yellow arrow 2)*. Right frame: After ultrasound is emitted *(yellow arrow 3)*, some returning echoes *(red arrow a)* are reflected off the posterior wall of the RPA before reaching the transducer. These reflecting echoes *(red arrow b)* then return to the interface between the anterior RPA and the posterior wall of the ascending aorta before finally returning to the transducer *(yellow arrow 4)*. The transducer interprets these echoes as coming from a depth equal to the sum of the red and yellow arrows. This artifact *(yellow and red asterisk)* may be interpreted as aortic dissection flap. With epiaortic scanning, artifact was no longer seen.

Comments

The initial diagnosis of acute aortic dissection often is made with CTA imaging because this modality is rapidly available 24/7 at most medical centers with an ED. Both CTA and MRI are equivalent to TEE in terms of sensitivity and specificity and both have the advantage of allowing evaluation of distal vessels and a wide field of view in the mediastinum. The choice of diagnostic modality in an individual patient often depends on the speed with which the study can be obtained and the expertise of each particular institution. Once the diagnosis is made, the patient is rapidly transferred or moved to the OR with minimal additional interim evaluation.

The echocardiographic diagnosis of aortic dissection is based on visualization of a linear mobile echogenic structure within the aortic lumen, such as the initial flap. It is particularly important to evaluate the ascending aorta because treatment of a dissection that involves the ascending aorta (Type A) is surgery whereas treatment of a dissection limited to the descending aorta (Type B) often is medical.

On echocardiography, imaging artifacts may share some features of an aortic dissection so the echocardiographer should ensure that the mobile intraluminal echo is not due to reverberations. Dissection flaps may be missed if image quality is poor or if there is limited visualization of any aortic segment. The interface between the innominate vein and the aortic arch may be mistaken for a dissection flap. However, with a careful examination by an experienced echocardiography, TEE has a sensitivity of about 98% with a specificity of 98% for diagnosis of aortic dissection.

The TEE performed in the OR thus is critical in defining the exact location and extent of dissection, involvement of the coronary artery ostia, and the presence of a pericardial effusion (implying impending aortic rupture). The TEE also can evaluate aortic valve anatomy to identify those with a bicuspid valve and to evaluate the degree of aortic regurgitation. Even if evaluated before arriving in the OR, the clinical situation changes rapidly with aortic dissection so that reevaluation is critical. The baseline TEE is also helpful in surgical planning: when severe sinus dilation is present as in this case, the possibility of a connective tissue disorder (such as Marfan syndrome) must be considered. These patients require a Bentall procedure with stabilization of the aortic annulus, replacement of the sinuses as well as ascending aorta, valve replacement, and coronary reimplantation. In patients with an ascending aortic dissection but normal sinuses, the native aortic valve may be resuspended at the proximal anastomosis of the ascending aorta graft repair.

Suggested Reading

1. Tan CN, Fraser AG: Perioperative transesophageal echocardiography for aortic dissection, Can J Anesth 61:362–378, 2014.
2. Pape LA, Awais M, Woznicki EM, et al: Presentation, diagnosis, and outcomes of acute aortic dissection: 17-year trends from the International Registry of Acute Aortic Dissection, J Am Coll Cardiol 66:350–358, 2015.

CASE 10-5
Bicuspid Valve and Aortic Dissection

This 50-year-old man presented with the acute onset of bilateral leg weakness and numbness when lifting weights. His initial examination was unremarkable and he was discharged from the ED. Several days later he once again presented to hospital with persistent symptoms, but also with nausea and vomiting and bloody stools. Laboratory work revealed acute renal injury and elevated liver function tests. CTA revealed an aortic dissection flap that extended from the ascending aorta to the iliac bifurcation.

The patient underwent an aortic root and valve replacement using a composite graft with an aortic valve bioprosthesis and coronary reimplantation.

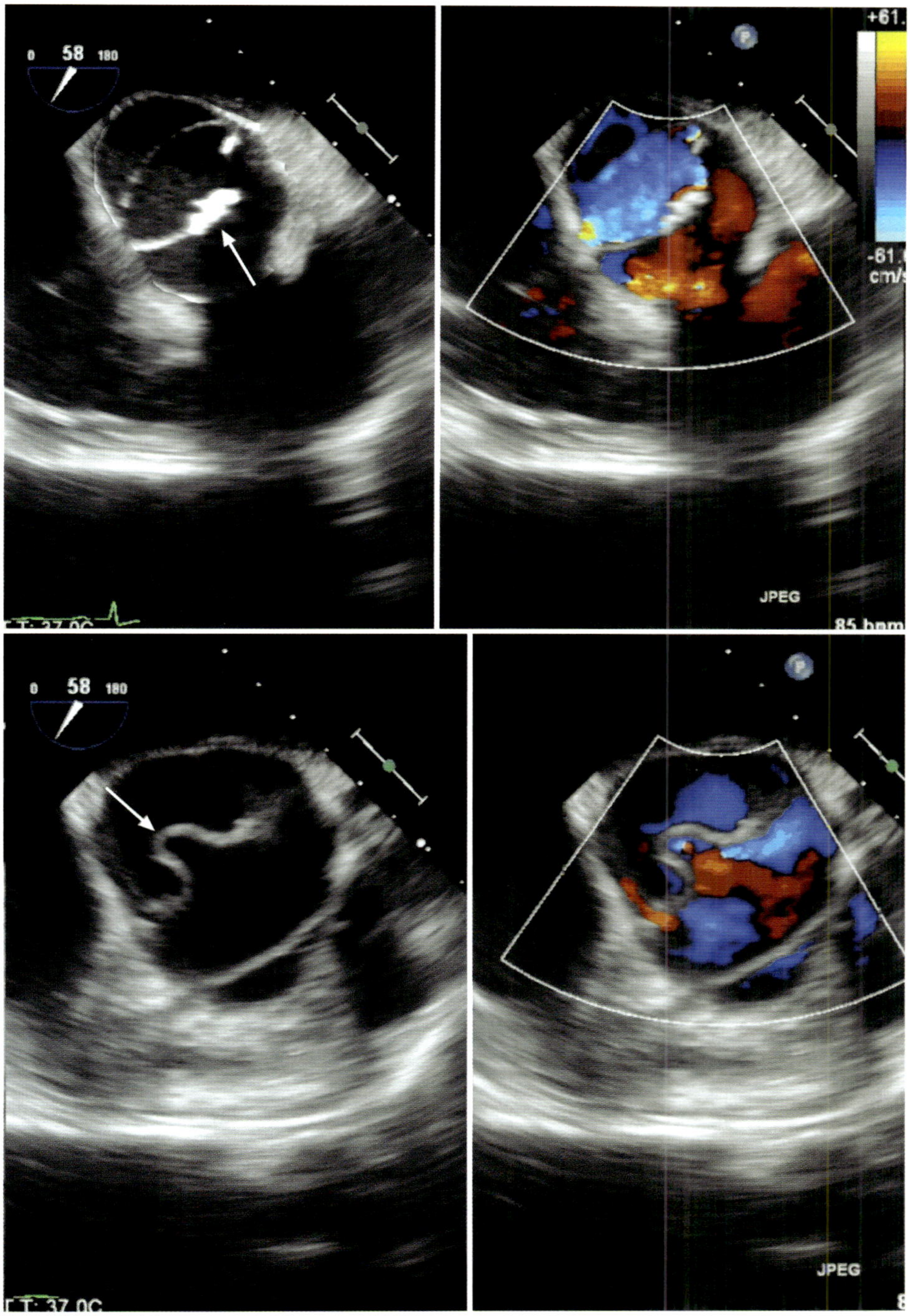

Fig 10.27 In this midesophageal short-axis view, top two frames are in systole. Valve is bicuspid with fusion of right and left coronary cusps. There is raphe *(arrow)*, partially shadowed. In the bottom two frames during diastole, dissection flap *(arrow)* prolapses toward, and thus obscures visualization of valve.

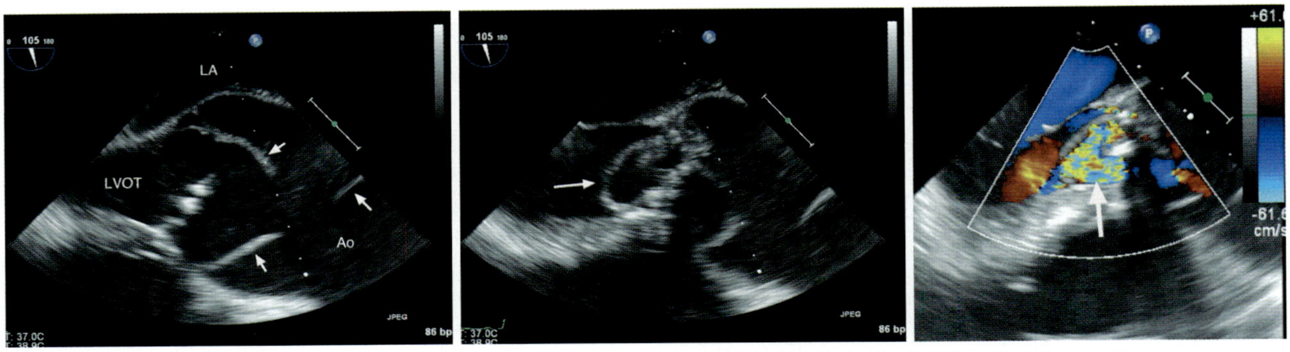

Fig 10.28 In this midesophageal long-axis view, left frame shows valve in systole. Valve leaflet is bright calcified structure adjacent to LV outflow tract (LVOT), not complex dissection flap which is indicated by arrows. Dissection flap close to aortic valve can sometimes be mistaken for valve leaflets on CT or TEE imaging. Correct diagnosis can be made by ascertaining insertion site of leaflets into aortic annulus, examining pattern of motion and using color Doppler to identify diagnostic flow patterns. In middle frame, flap *(arrow)* prolapse through valve during diastole. In right frame, color Doppler indicates flow regurgitating through valve and being somewhat contained by dissection flap *(arrow)*.

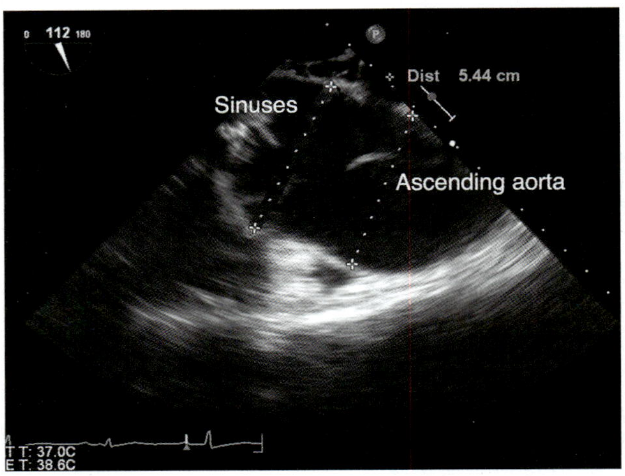

Fig 10.29 Sinuses and ascending aorta are both severely dilated with diameter of 5.4 cm.

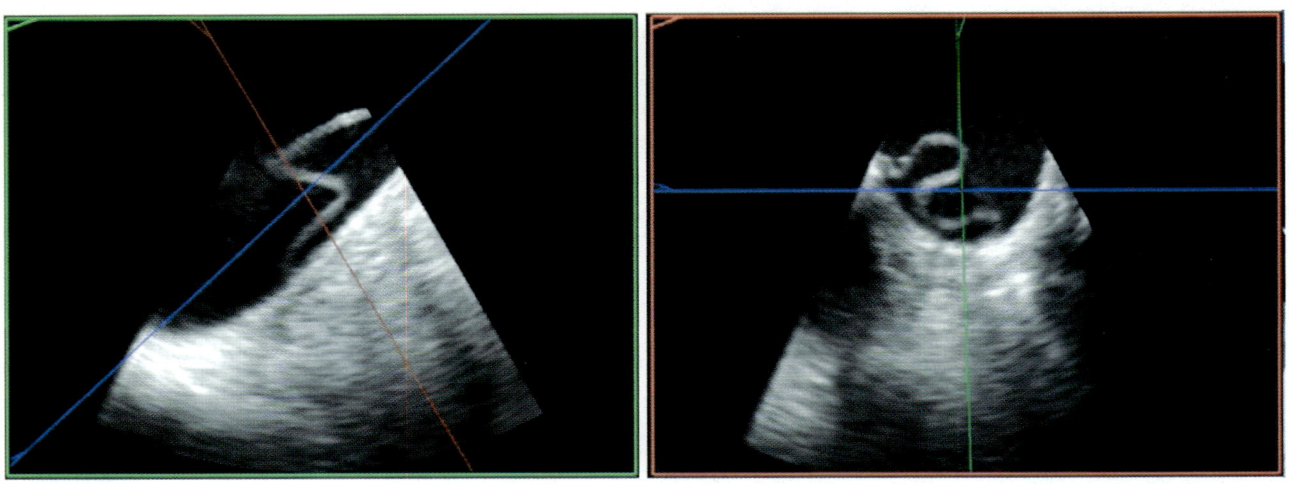

Fig 10.30 Orthogonal views in aortic arch show serpiginous flap.

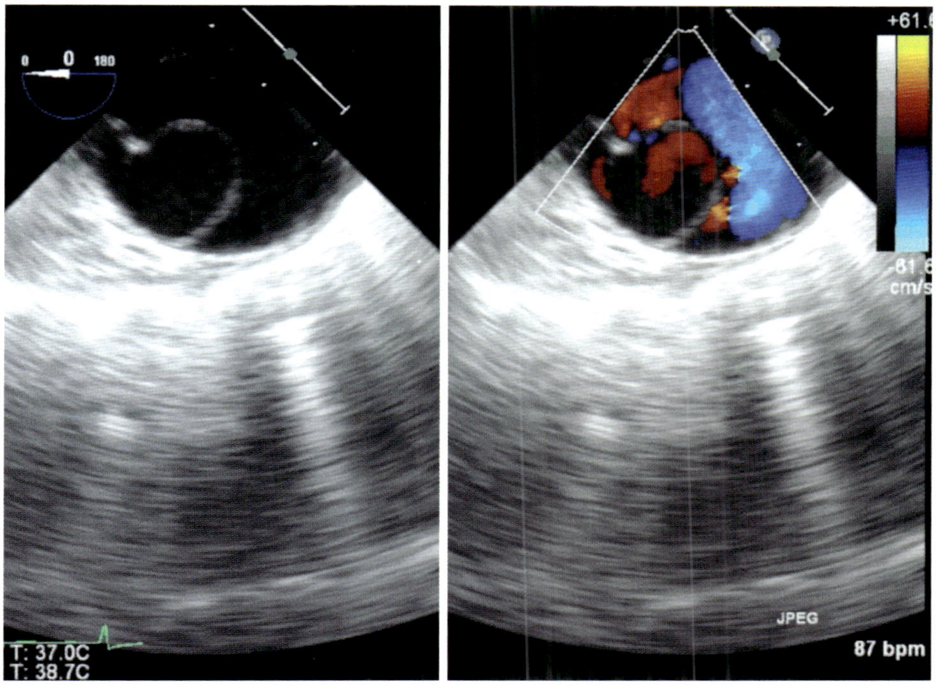

Fig 10.31 Flap is seen in descending aorta. Color Doppler pattern makes it difficult to discern which is true lumen and which is false. However, true lumen is usually smaller than the false lumen.

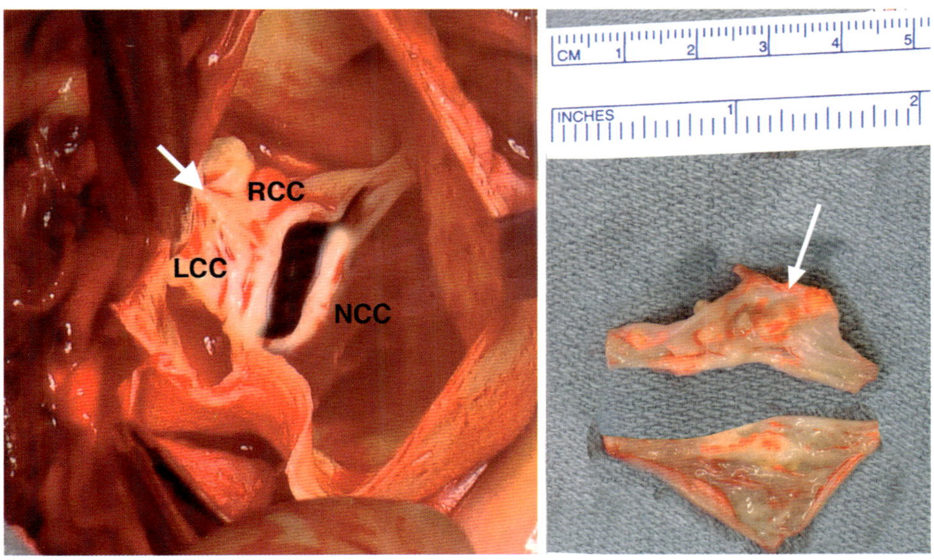

Fig 10.32 Aortic valve in vivo *(left)* showing fusion of the RCC and the LCC. On the right, the leaflets are seen following explantation. Arrows indicate raphe.

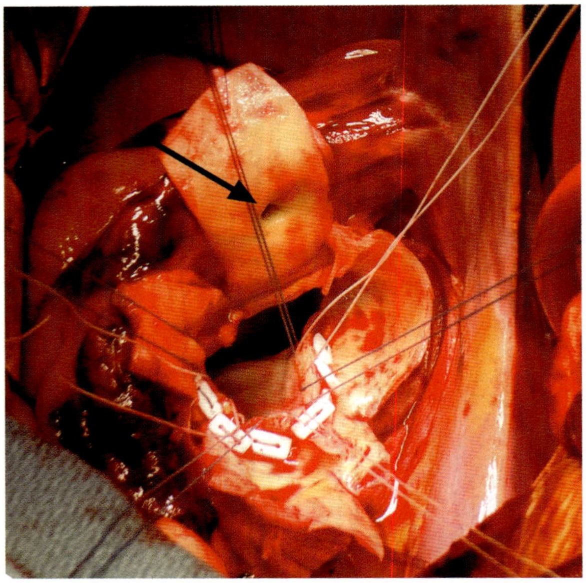

Fig 10.33 Aortic valve and root have been resected. Arrow indicates one of coronary buttons before trimming. (See Fig 10.34, frame (A).)

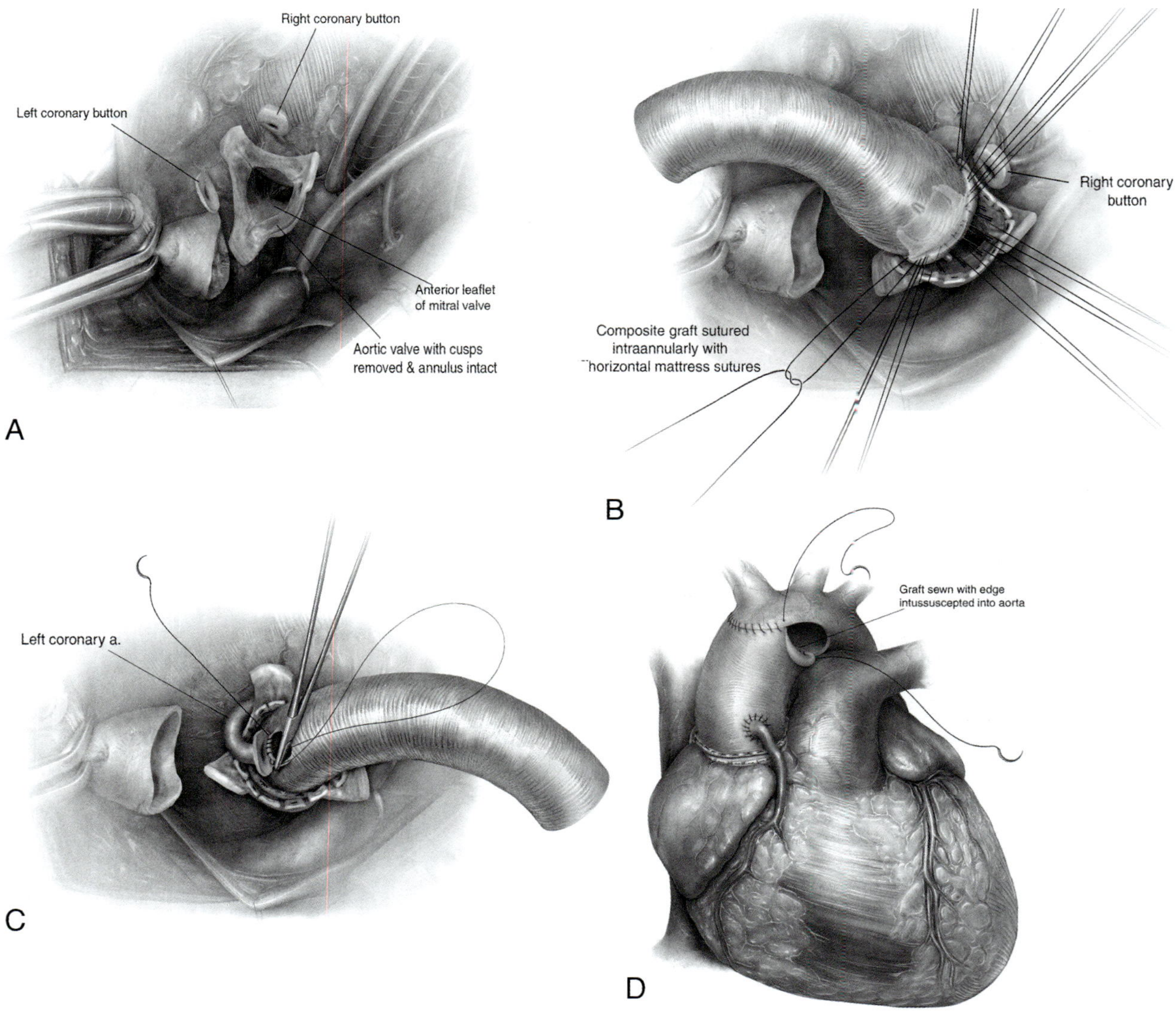

Fig 10.34 In (A), cross-clamp has been applied, and diseased ascending aorta including sinuses of Valsalva and aortic valve have been resected; all that remains are coronary buttons and annulus. In (B), valved conduit with tissue bioprosthesis at that distal end, is sutured to aortic annulus. In (C) two holes are made in graft to accommodate coronary buttons, and in (D), heart with tube graft and one coronary button visible. a = artery. (From Gleason TG: Aortic root replacement with composite valved conduit, Operat Techn Thorac Cardiovasc Surg 13:161–171, 2008. With permission.)

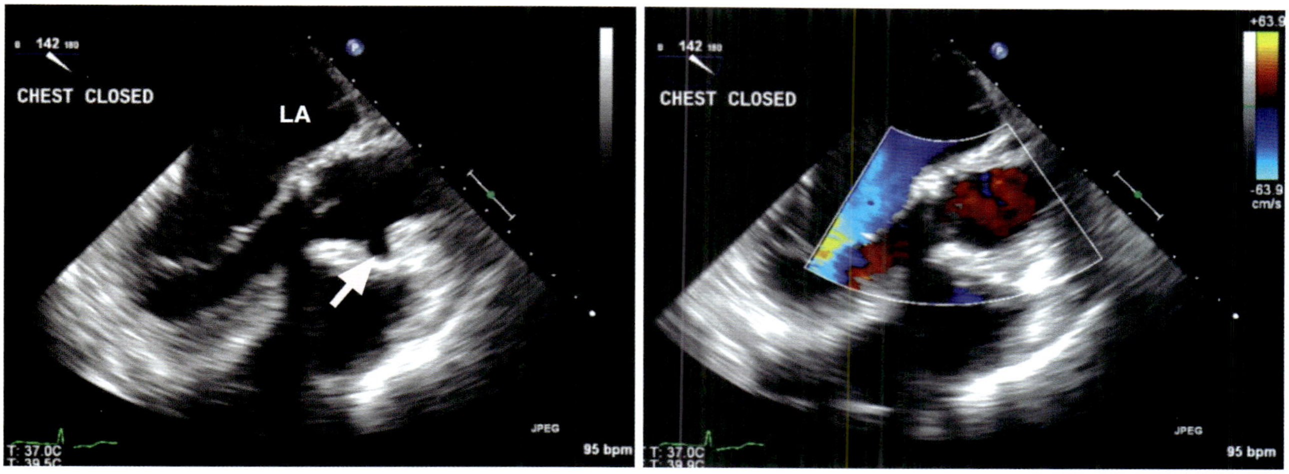

Fig 10.35 After procedure, there is no aortic regurgitation seen in midesophageal long-axis view. Arrow indicates right coronary button.

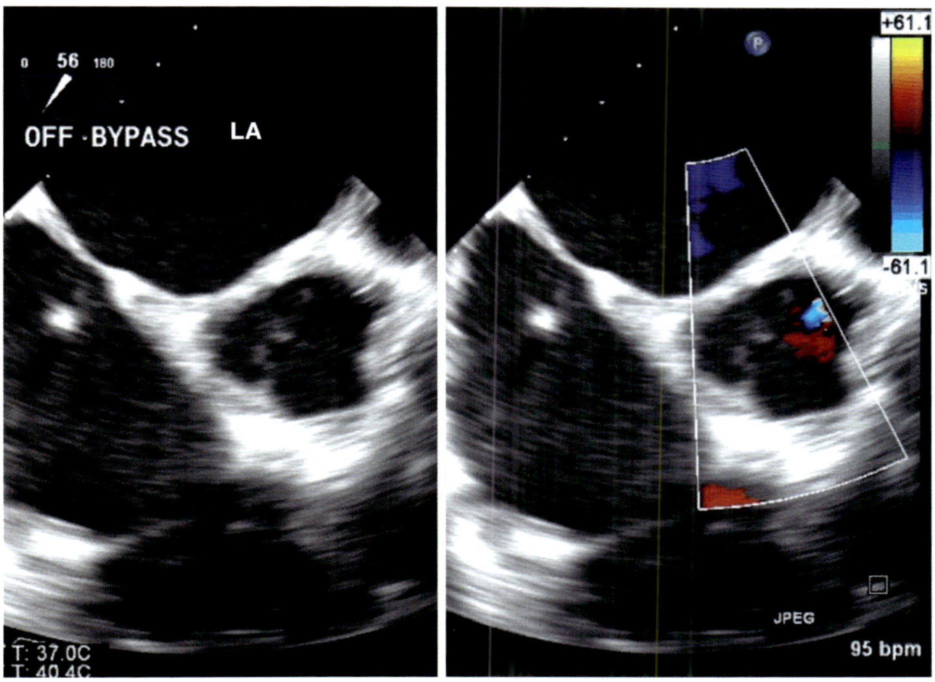

Fig 10.36 Similarly, in midesophageal short-axis view, valve is competent.

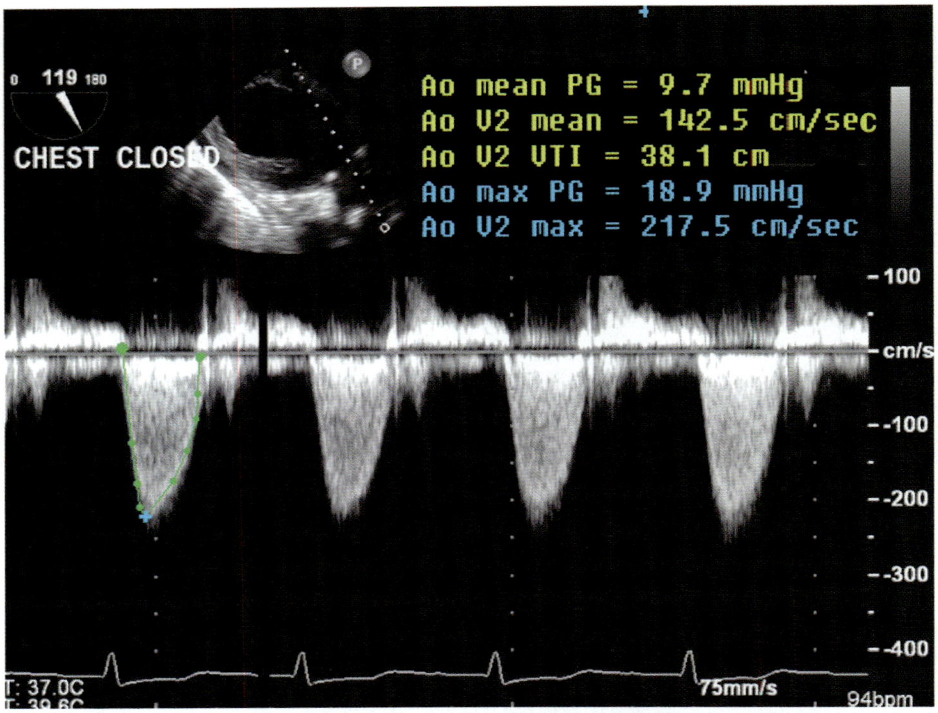

Fig 10.37 Continuous wave Doppler from transgastric long-axis view shows minimal gradients, consistent with nonobstructive prosthetic valve.

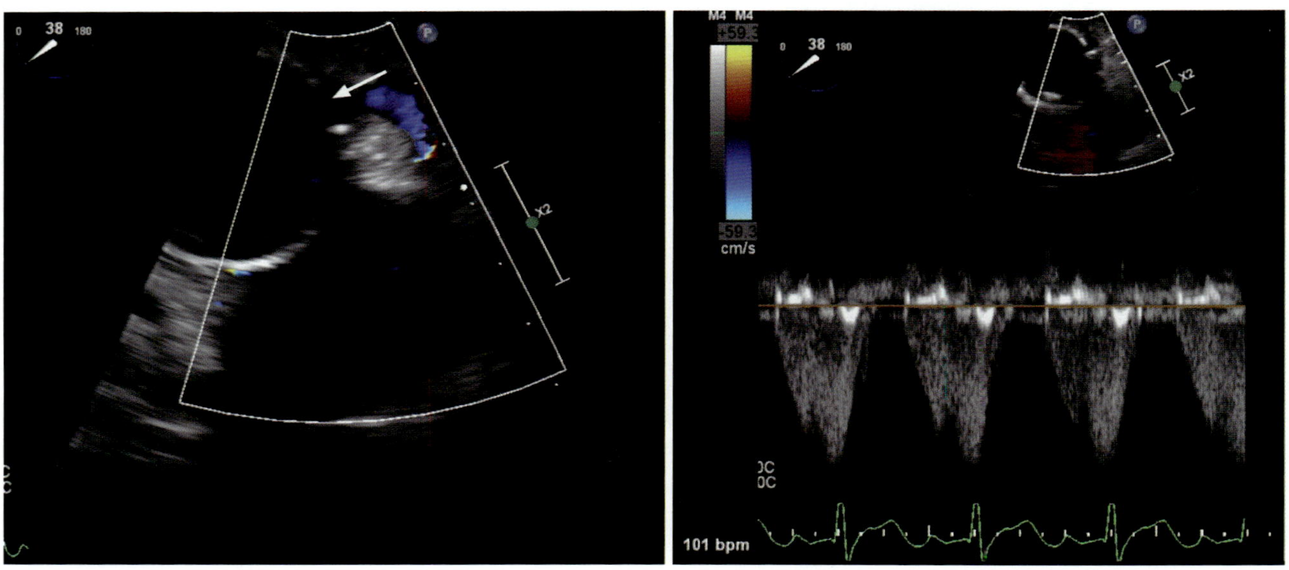

Fig 10.38 Left coronary button is imaged *(arrow)* and pulsed wave Doppler shows flow during diastole.

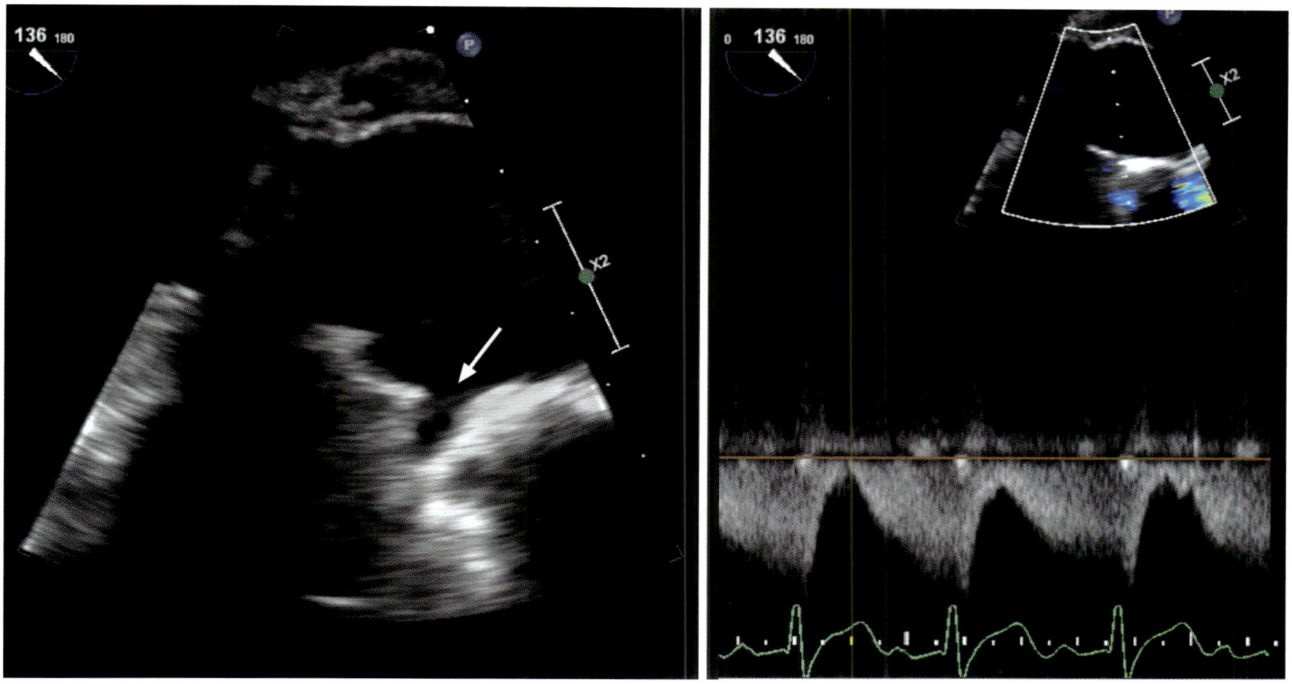

Fig 10.39 Right coronary button is imaged *(arrow)* and pulsed wave Doppler shows flow primarily during diastole.

Comments

A congenitally bicuspid aortic valve is present in 1% to 2% of the entire population. Bicuspid aortic valve disease is not confined to the valve leaflets; the aorta also is abnormal. Histopathologic studies now support an underlying connective tissue disease process with elastin fragmentation, irregularities in smooth muscle integrity, and increased collagen deposition. Compared with normal adults with a trileaflet aortic valve, bicuspid aortic valve patients have larger dimensions of the aortic sinuses and ascending aorta, abnormal aortic elasticity, are at risk for progressive aortic dilation, and have an estimated age-adjusted relative risk of dissection of 8.4 compared with patients with a trileaflet valve, corresponding to an absolute risk of 3.1 cases per 10,000 patient-years. The risk factors for aortic dissection in bicuspid valve patients remain unclear but may include the specific morphology of the valve, in addition to a family history of dissection. In patients with a known bicuspid valve, periodic imaging is recommended for assessment of aortic size either with echocardiography (if the aorta is well seen) or with CT or MRI imaging. Prophylactic aortic root replacement is recommended when aortic diameter exceeds 5.5 cm if there are no other risk factors, and 5.0 cm if there is rapid progression or a family history of dissection.

Suggested Reading

1. Wojnarski CM, Svensson LG, Roselli EE, et al: Aortic dissection in patients with bicuspid aortic valve-associated aneurysms, Ann Thorac Surg 100:1666–1674, 2015.
2. Adamo L, Braverman AC: Surgical threshold for bicuspid aortic valve aneurysm: a case for individual decision-making, Heart 101:1361–1367, 2015.
3. Detaint D, Michelena HI, Nkomo VT, et al: Aortic dilatation patterns and rates in adults with bicuspid aortic valves: a comparative study with Marfan syndrome and degenerative aortopathy, Heart 100:126–134, 2014.
4. Michelena HI, Khanna AD, Mahoney D, et al: Incidence of aortic complications in patients with bicuspid aortic valves, JAMA 306:1104–1112, 2011.
5. Schaefer BM, Lewin MF, Stout KK, et al: The bicuspid aortic valve: an integrated phenotypic classification of leaflet morphology and aortic root shape, Heart 94:1634–1638, 2008.

Complications of Aortic Dissection

CASE 10-6
Aortic Dissection with Severe Aortic Regurgitation

This 44-year-old woman with a history of obesity, hypertension, and diabetes, presented to the ED with chest pain. A diastolic murmur was appreciated on physical examination.

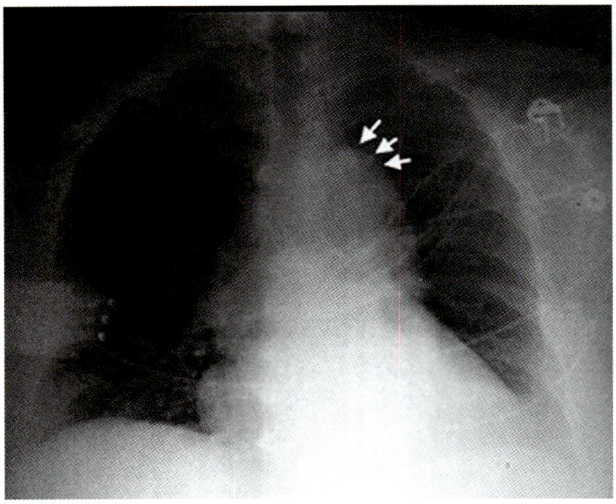

Fig 10.40 PA chest radiography shows wide mediastinum with prominence of aortic arch *(arrows)*.

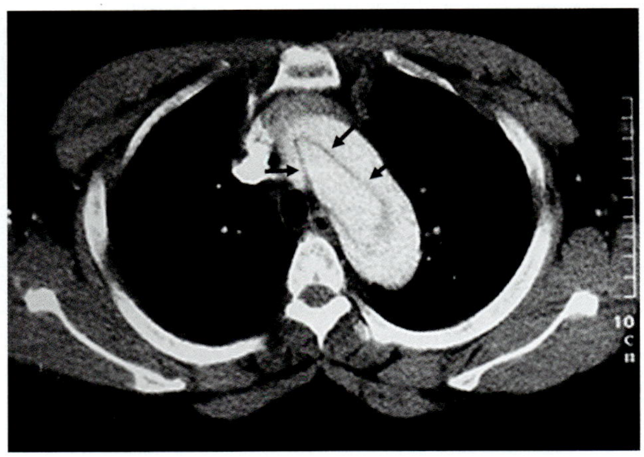

Fig 10.41 Chest CT with contrast demonstrates enlarged aortic arch with linear density inside lumen consistent with dissection flap *(arrows)*.

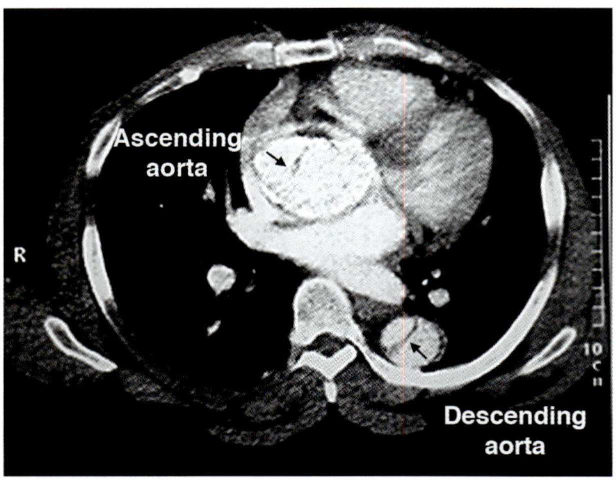

Fig 10.42 Chest CT at level of left atrium, shows dilated ascending aorta with distorted contour and intraluminal density consistent with dissection flap *(arrow)*. Although descending thoracic aorta is normal in size, linear dissection flap is present in lumen *(arrow)*.

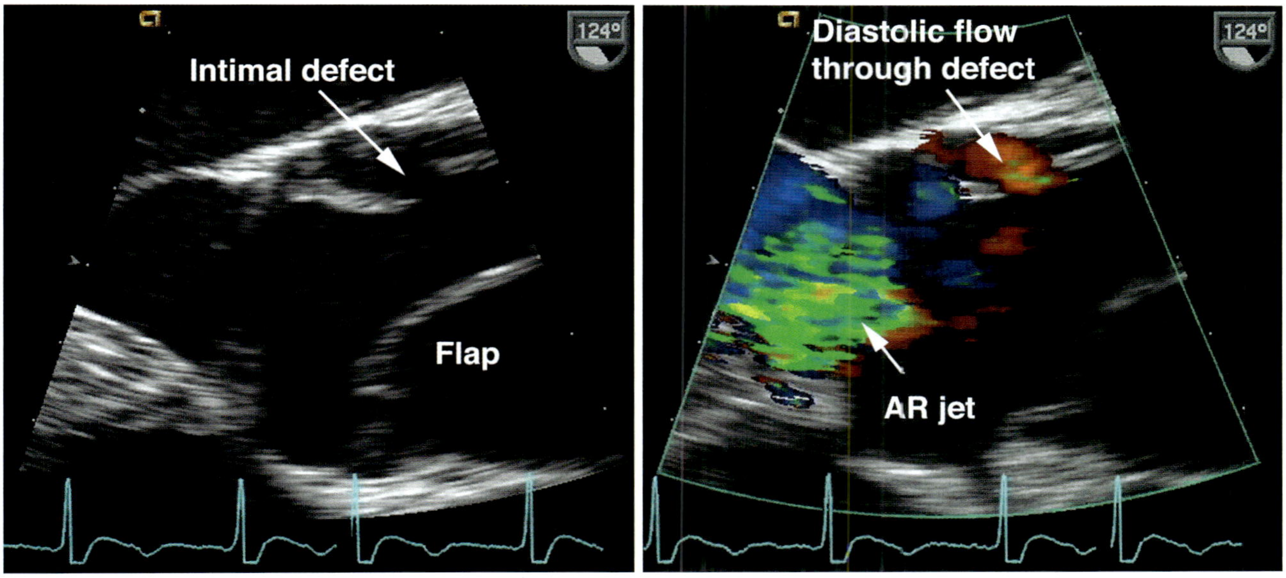

Fig 10.43 Intraoperative TEE images in magnified long-axis view of ascending aorta shows dissection flap about 1 cm distal to aortic valve leaflets. Along posterior aspect of aorta, area of discontinuity in flap is seen. Color flow imaging *(right)* shows flow into false lumen via this defect and shows severe aortic regurgitation.

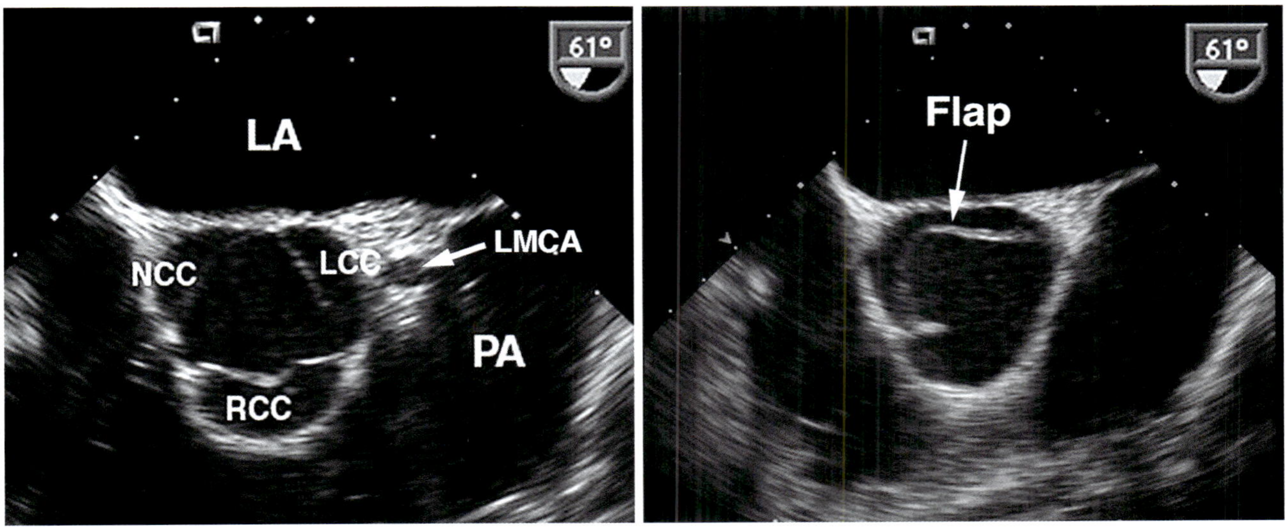

Fig 10.44 Short-axis TEE view of aortic valve shows normal trileaflet valve open in systole *(left)*. Left main coronary artery (LMCA) is seen adjacent to left coronary cusp (LCC). In diastole *(right)*, dissection flap prolapses proximally into image plane.

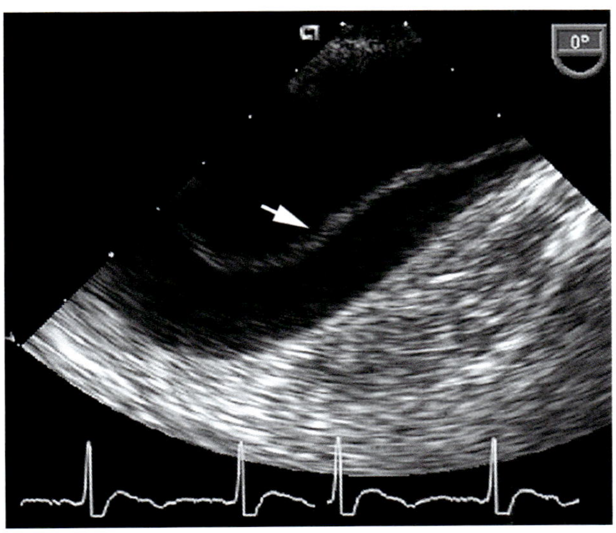

Fig 10.45 High TEE view of aortic arch shows intraluminal flap *(arrow)*. In real time, motion of intimal flap, independent from motion of aortic wall, can be appreciated.

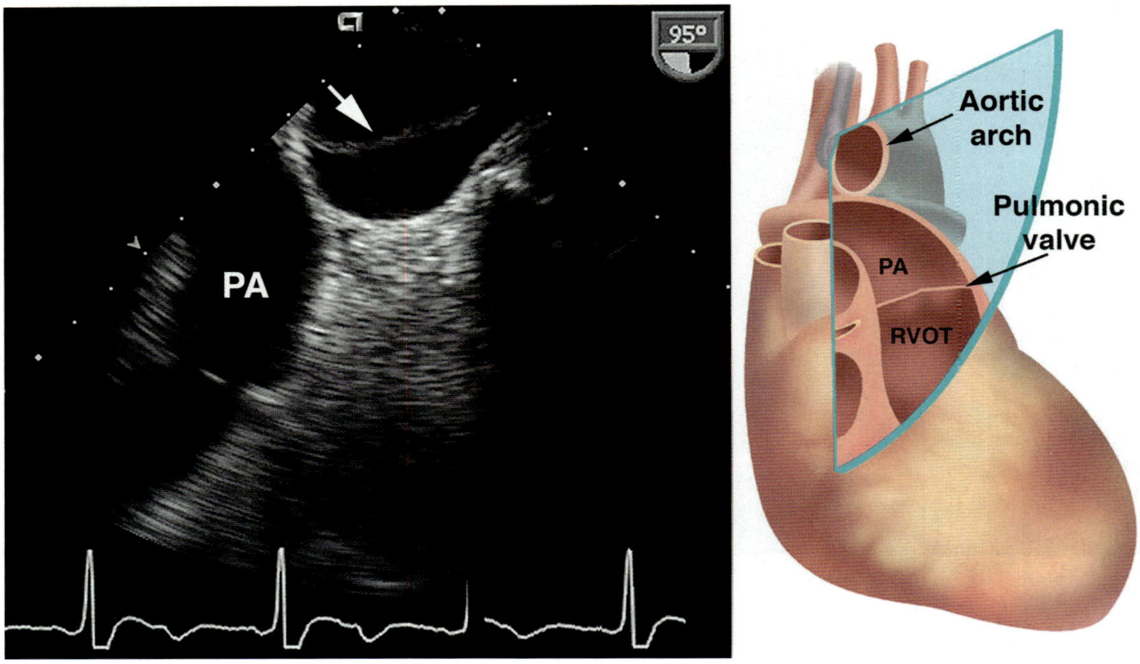

Fig 10.46 From same transducer position as Fig 10.45, image plane is rotated to 95 degrees to obtain this short-axis view of aortic arch, with intimal flap *(arrow)* seen. On right is graphic representation of how view is obtained.

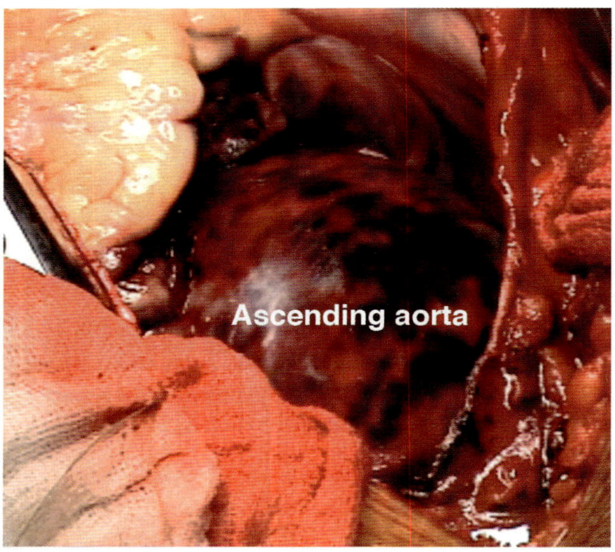

Fig 10.47 At surgery, enlarged ascending aorta shows discoloration typical for dissection.

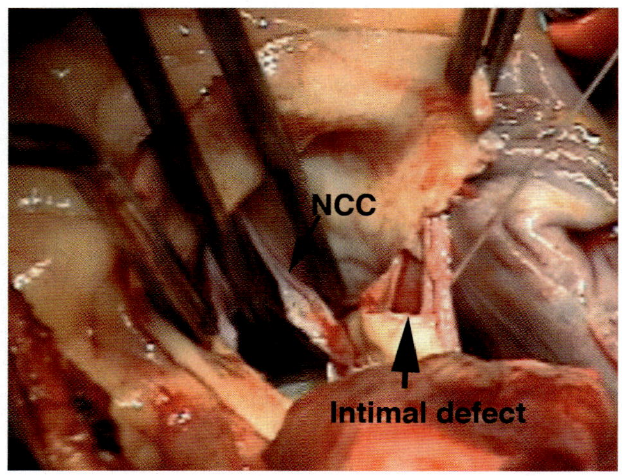

Fig 10.48 After opening aorta, intimal defect *(arrow)* in close proximity to aortic valve noncoronary cusp (NCC) is appreciated. Aortic valve was resuspended in 28-mm Dacron tube graft replacement of ascending aorta.

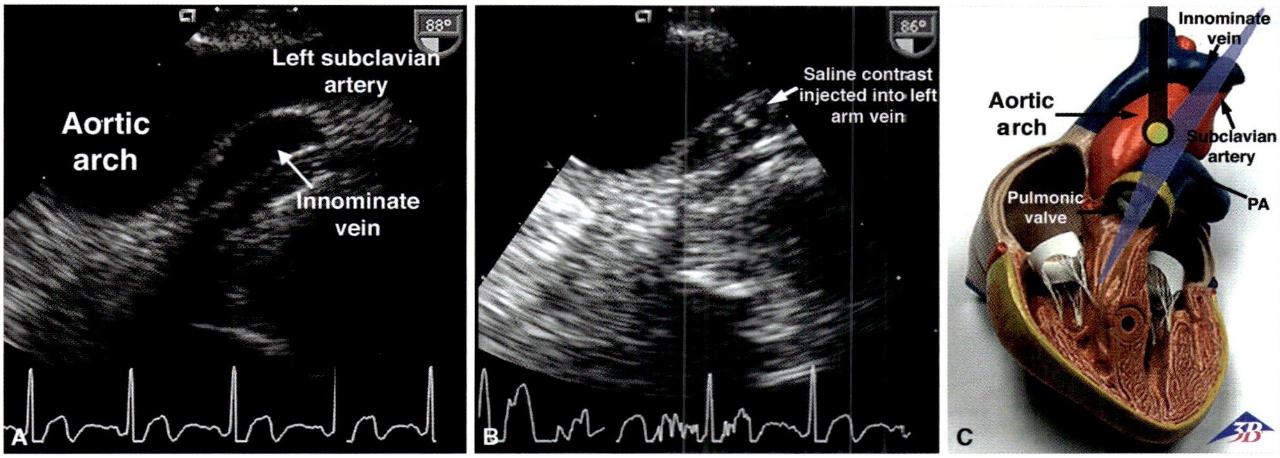

Fig 10.49 Panel (**A**) shows high esophageal view of distal arch at 88 degrees, with left subclavian artery clearly delineated. Innominate vein is anterior to arch. Interface between innominate vein and arch may be mistaken for dissection flap. Agitated saline contrast injected through left arm vein (panel (**B**)) opacifies innominate vein. In panel (**C**), anatomy is illustrated in model. (Based on Economy Heart Model 3B Scientific®.)

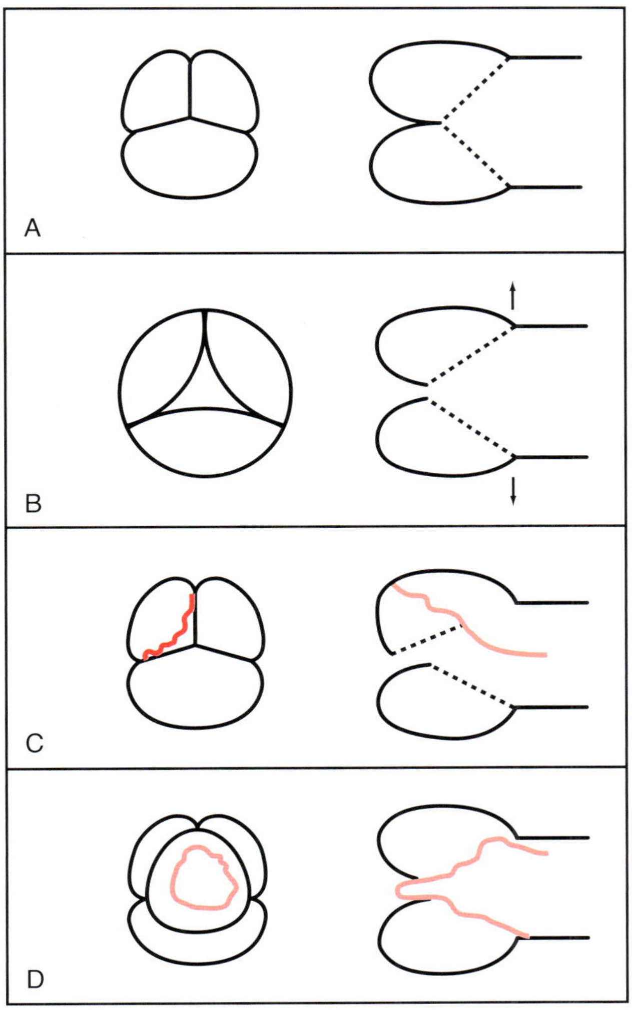

Fig 10.50 Different mechanisms of aortic regurgitation in Type A aortic dissection are illustrated. Further description is found in comments. (Reproduced with permission from Movsowitz HD et al, Transesophageal echocardiographic description of mechanisms of aortic regurgitation in acute Type A aortic dissection: Implications for aortic valve repair, J Am Coll Cardiol 36:884, 2000. ©Elsevier Inc.)

Comments

Aortic regurgitation in patients with an aortic dissection may be due to one of several mechanisms as illustrated in Fig 10.50, with frame (A) being normal. Compared with patients with normal aortic anatomy, aortic regurgitation may be due to (B) dilation of the sinuses of Valsalva with incomplete central coaptation of the leaflets, (C) extension of the dissection into the layers of the valve leaflet resulting in a flail leaflet with severe regurgitation, or (D) distortion of the valve commissures by the dissection flap leading to asymmetric leaflet closure and an eccentric regurgitant jet. Mechanisms (B) and (D) are usually managed with valve resuspension inside a prosthetic graft; mechanism (C) usually necessitates valve replacement, either in addition to a prosthetic graft, or as part of a valved aortic conduit.

Suggested Reading

1. Thorsgard ME, Morrissette GJ, Sun B, et al: Impact of intraoperative transesophageal echocardiography on acute type-A aortic dissection, J Cardiothorac Vasc Anesth 28:1203–1207, 2014.
2. Wang CJ, Rodriguez Diaz CA, Trinh MA: Use of real-time three-dimensional transesophageal echocardiography in Type A aortic dissections: advantages of 3D TEE illustrated in three cases, Ann Card Anaesth 18:83–86, 2015.

CASE 10-7
Pericardial Effusion and Tamponade

This 60-year-old man presented with chest pain to an outside hospital 48 hours before transfer to our medical center. Coronary angiography was attempted but the right coronary artery could not be identified and he became hypotensive. A chest CT showed an ascending aortic dissection and he was transferred for emergency surgery.

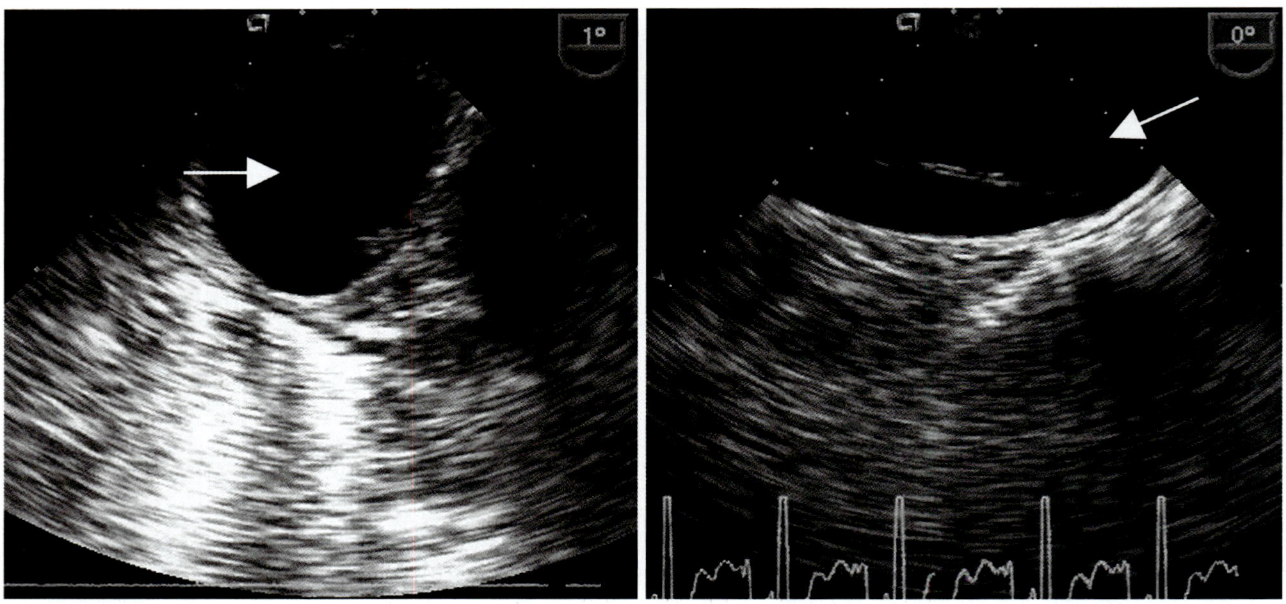

Fig 10.51 TEE short- and long-axis views of descending thoracic aorta show prominent dissection flap *(arrow)*.

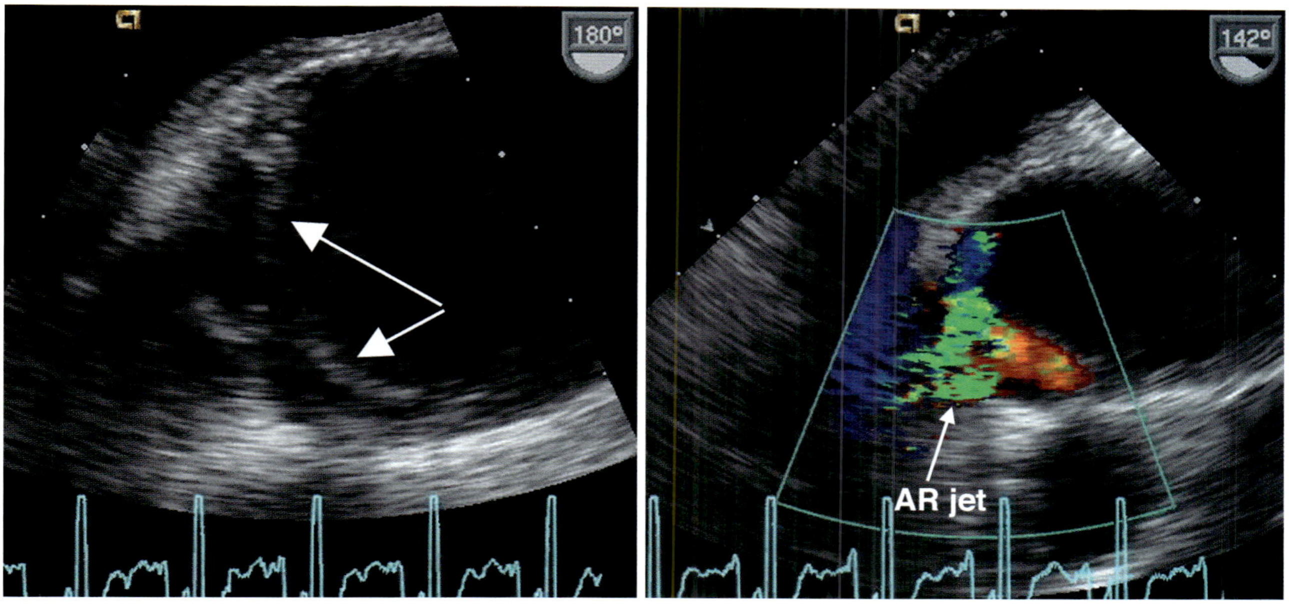

Fig 10.52 Long-axis view at 180 degrees of ascending aorta showing complex dissection flap *(arrows)*. Color Doppler *(right)* shows aortic regurgitation.

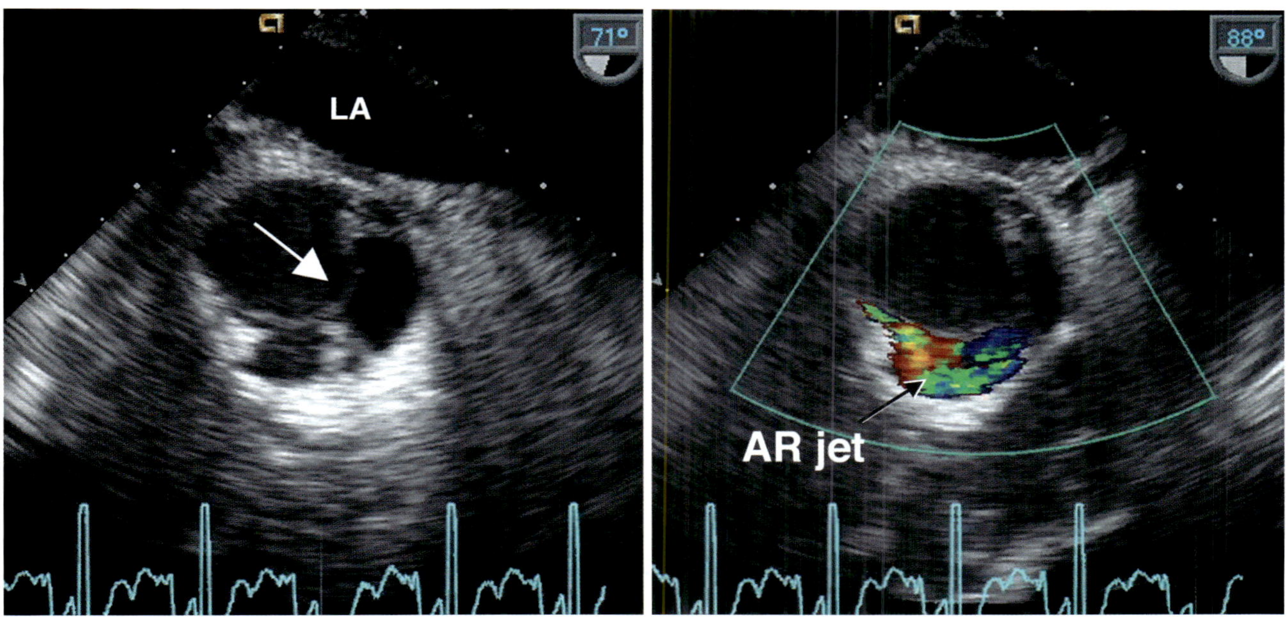

Fig 10.53 Rotation of image plane to 71 degrees provides short-axis view of ascending aorta with complex intimal flap *(arrow)* that on still-frame images might be mistaken for aortic valve leaflets. Real-time images show erratic motion characteristic of dissection flap. Color flow *(right)* demonstrates AR.

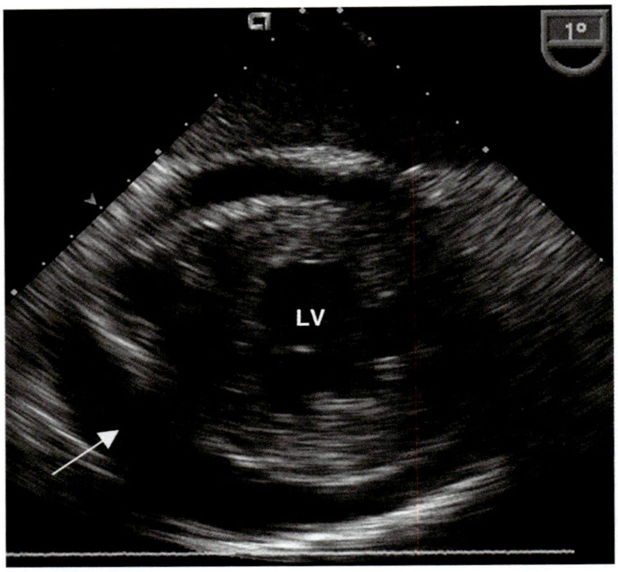

Fig 10.54 Transgastric short-axis view showing circumferential pericardial effusion *(arrow)*. In real time, there is right ventricular collapse.

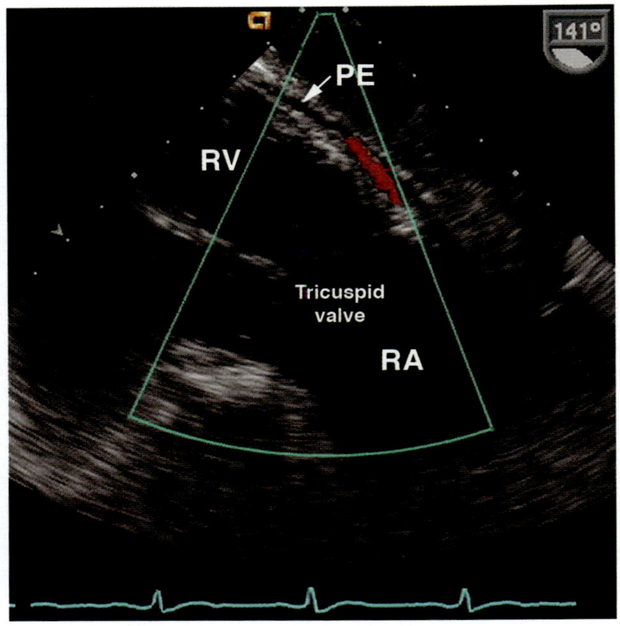

Fig 10.55 Transgastric long-axis imaging of right-sided cardiac structures reveals color Doppler flow in pericardial space.

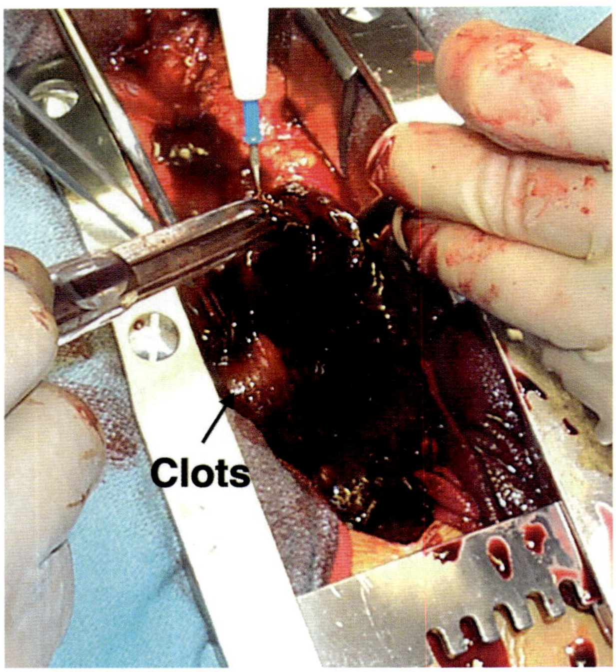

Fig 10.56 At surgery, pericardium was tense and about 500 to 700 cc of old blood and clot were removed from pericardial space.

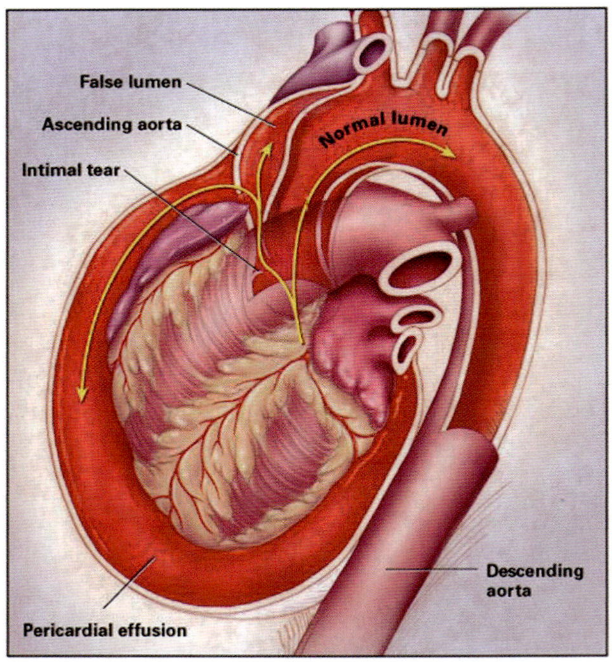

Fig 10.57 This drawing illustrates how blood entering false lumen can enter pericardial space via defect in aortic wall at its base. (Reproduced from Nallamothu B, et al, Of nicks and time, N Engl J Med 345:359–363, 2001. ©Massachusetts Medical Society.)

Comments

An aortic dissection may cause a pericardial effusion by leakage from the aorta into the pericardium. The normal pericardium extends a small distance up the great vessels with a potential pericardial space posterior to the aorta and pulmonary artery; this space is known as the transverse sinus of the pericardium. If the dissection extends into the base of the aorta, a small tear in the wall allows blood to enter the pericardial space via the transverse sinus (Fig 10.57). Thus, the finding of a pericardial effusion in a patient with suspected aortic dissection, especially in the presence of color Doppler flow in the pericardial space, is an ominous sign. If the leakage increases, pericardial tamponade may occur due to rapid accumulation of blood in the pericardial space.

Although women account for only about one third of aortic dissection, they tend to be older and most often have signs suggestive of rupture, including pericardial effusion, periaortic hematoma, and pleural effusions. Women are more likely than men to be hypotensive and to have pericardial tamponade and the surgical mortality in women is 32% compared with 22% in men.

Suggested Reading

1. Hoff E, Eagle T, Pyeritz RE, et al: Pulse pressure and type A acute aortic dissection in-hospital outcomes (from the International Registry of Acute Aortic Dissection), Am J Cardiol 113:1255–1259, 2014.
2. Nienaber CA, Fattori R, Mehta RH, et al: Gender-related differences in acute aortic dissection, Circulation 109:3014–3021, 2004.

CASE 10-8
Right Coronary Artery Compromise

This 50-year-old man with a history of hypertension, presented with 4 days of intermittent chest pain. He was treated with a beta-blocker and heparin and an ECG was obtained.

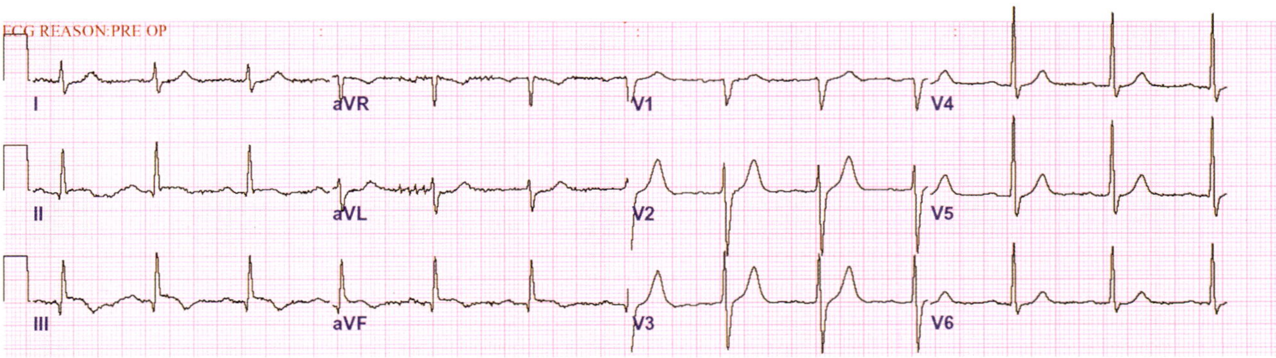

Fig 10.58 12 lead ECG with 1-mm ST-elevation, T-wave inversion, and small Q-waves in leads II, III, and aVF, suggesting inferior myocardial infarction. Because of these ECG changes, he was taken promptly to catheterization laboratory.

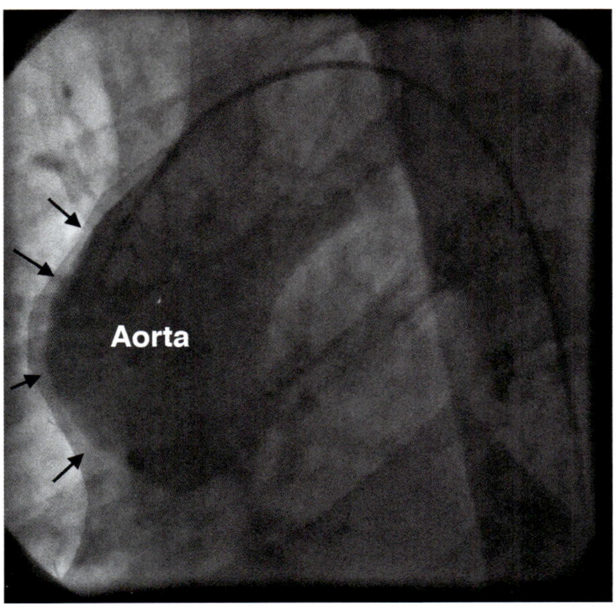

Fig 10.59 At catheterization, aortography shows irregularity in anterior contour of ascending aorta *(arrow)* with contrast seen outside aortic silhouette. Because of concern for ascending aortic dissection, chest CT study was performed.

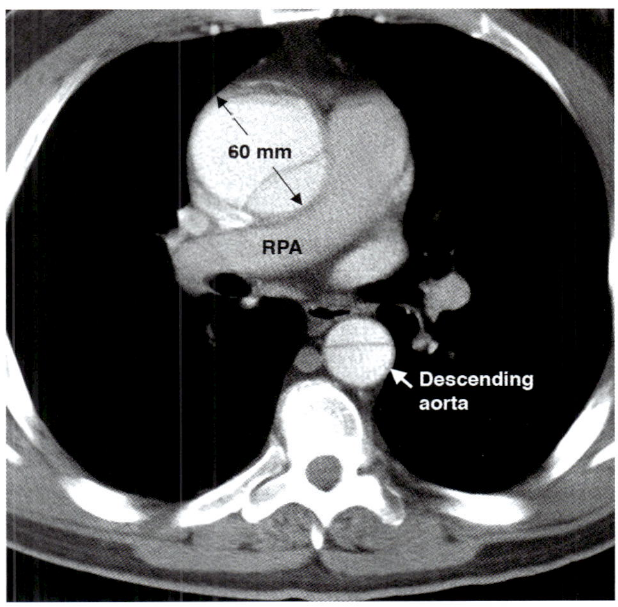

Fig 10.60 Chest CT with contrast at level of right pulmonary artery (RPA) shows dilated ascending aorta (60 mm) with prominent dissection flap. Flap is also seen in descending aorta.

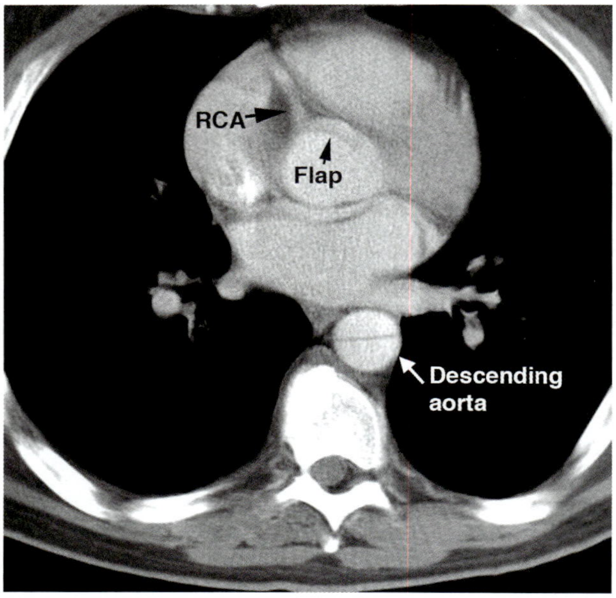

Fig 10.61 In this chest CT at level of right coronary artery (RCA), dissection flap is seen in descending thoracic aorta. Ascending aorta shows dissection flap crossing origin of right coronary artery, resulting in compromise of coronary blood flow.

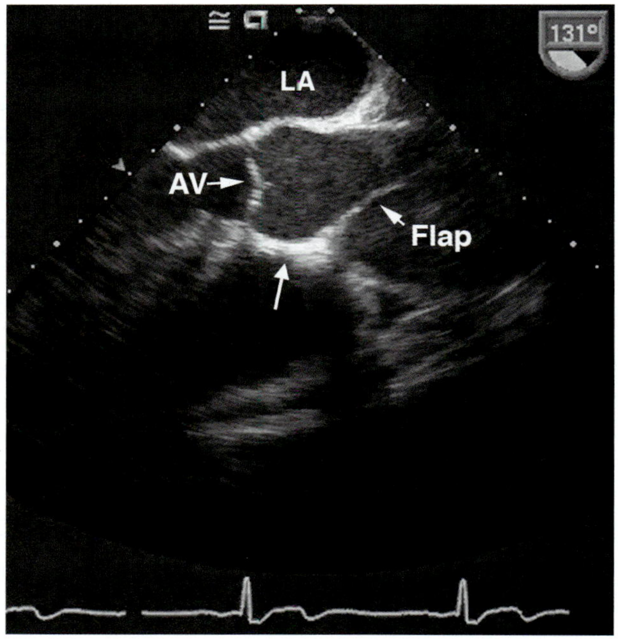

Fig 10.62 Intraoperative long-axis TEE images of ascending aorta demonstrate enlarged aorta with intimal flap that begins at sinotubular junction, about 2 cm superior to aortic valve (AV). Note proximity of flap to site of origin of right coronary artery *(arrow)*.

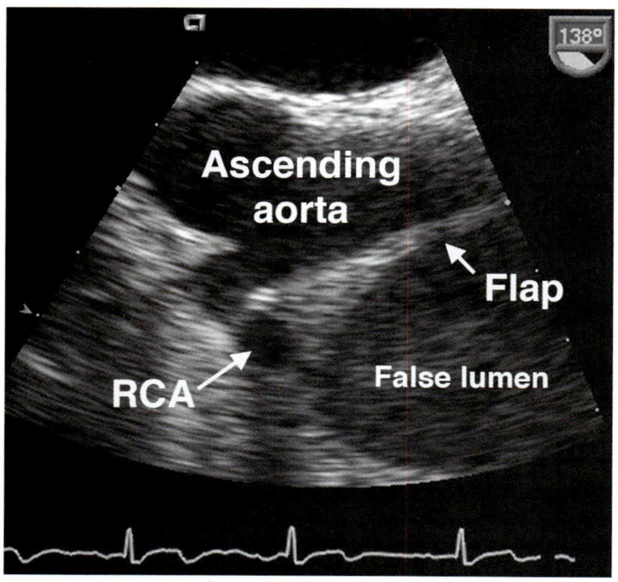

Fig 10.63 Close-up of long-axis TEE image better shows relationship of dissection flap and right coronary ostium.

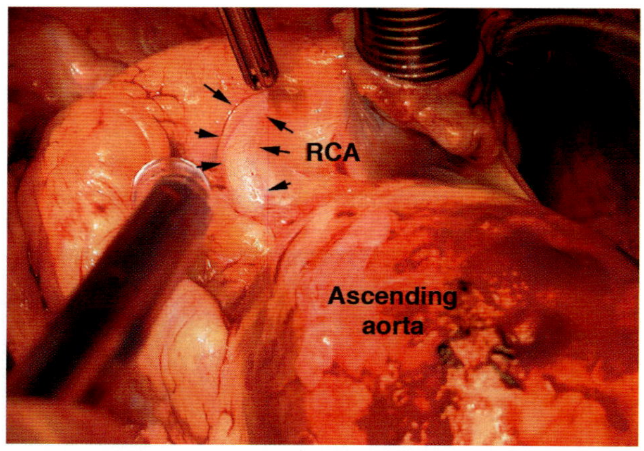

Fig 10.64 At surgery, enlarged ascending aorta is at bottom right of photograph. Right coronary artery (RCA) is of normal caliber.

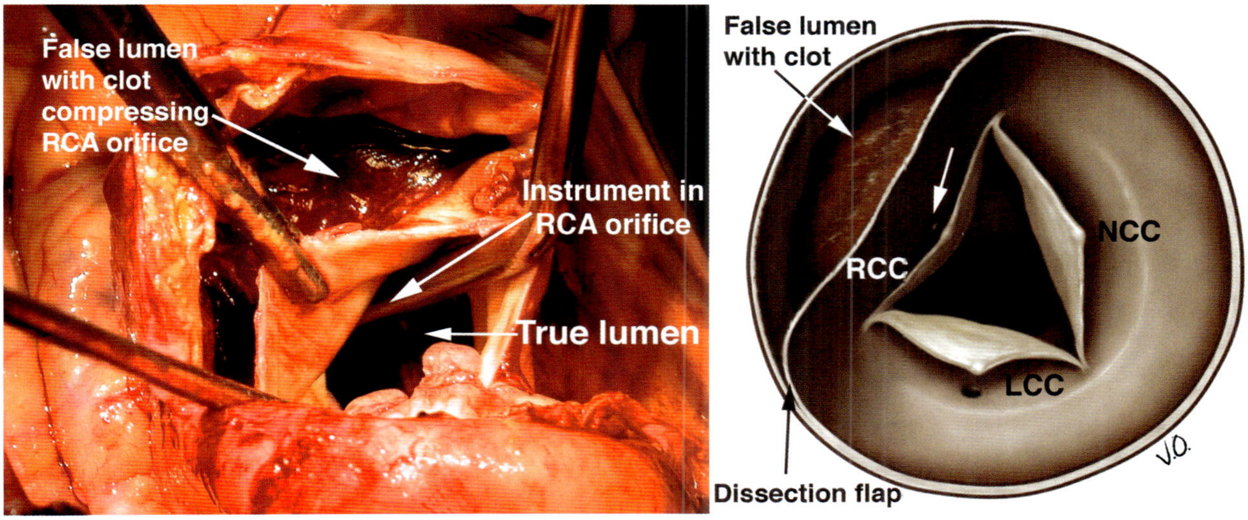

Fig 10.65 With aorta opened, false lumen with clot is seen compressing aorta in vicinity of right coronary cusp *(left)*. With slight retraction of dissection flap, distorted right coronary ostium is visualized *(right, arrow)*. Ascending aorta was replaced with 28-mm Dacron graft, aortic valve was resuspended, and saphenous vein graft was placed to distal right coronary artery.

Comments

An aortic dissection may induce myocardial ischemia or infarction by compromising the blood flow in the coronary artery. The mechanism of impaired coronary blood flow may be extension of the dissection into the coronary artery itself or occlusion of the orifice by the dissection flap or a hematoma, as in this case. This case emphasizes the importance of considering aortic dissection in the differential diagnosis of chest pain, even when coronary ischemia is present.

Suggested Reading

1. Boettcher BT, Irish SM, Algahim M, et al: Acute, severe chest pain in the presence of known coronary artery disease: new myocardial ischemia, aortic dissection, or some other evolving cardiovascular catastrophe? J Cardiothorac Vasc Anesth 30: 861–864, 2015.
2. Kawahito K, Adachi H, Murata S, Yamaguchi A, Ino T: Coronary malperfusion due to type A aortic dissection: mechanism and surgical management, Ann Thorac Surg 76:1471–1476, 2003.

CASE 10-9
Right Coronary and Aortic Valve Involvement

This 55-year-old man suddenly collapsed when at work. He was resuscitated by the emergency medical technicians but remained hypotensive and did not regain consciousness. Chest CT showed a Type A aortic dissection and he was transferred to our medical center.

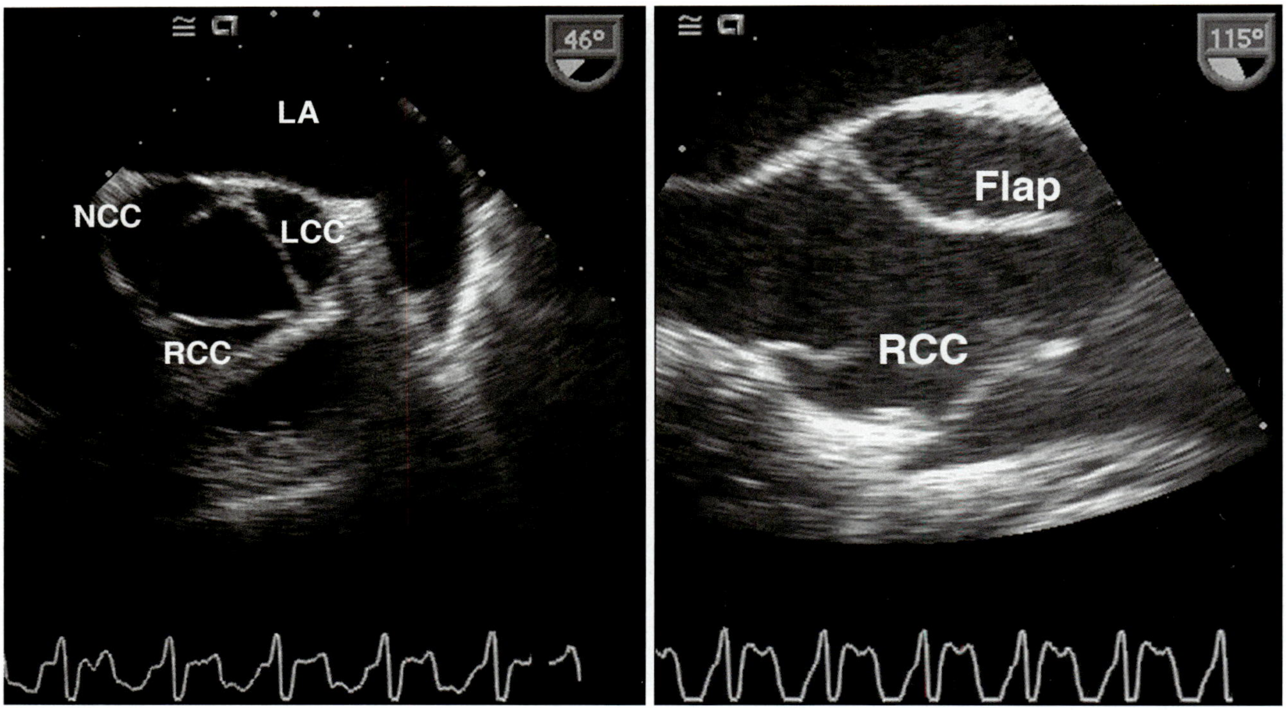

Fig 10.66 TEE images of aortic valve show trileaflet valve but in real time, distortion of shape of noncoronary sinus of Valsalva is seen. In long-axis view *(right)*, complex dissection flap is seen in close proximity to valve leaflets.

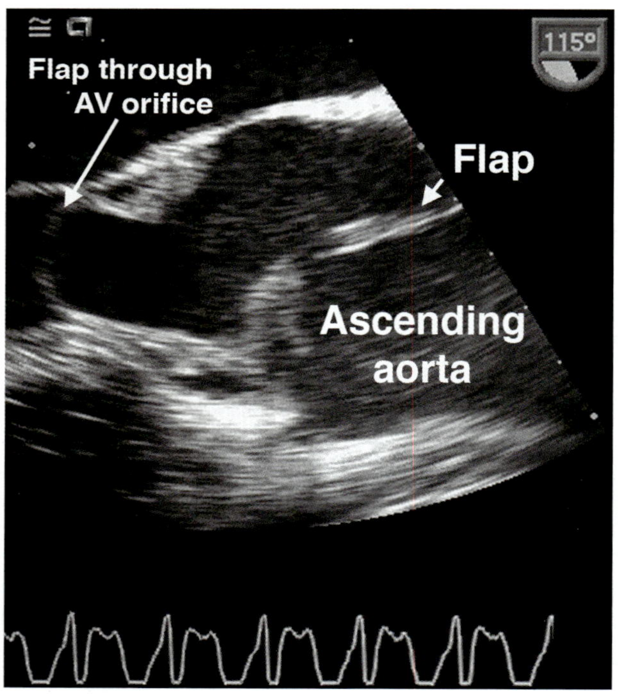

Fig 10.67 In magnified long-axis view of ascending aorta at 115 degrees, angulated medially, dissection flap is seen to prolapse across aortic valve in diastole.

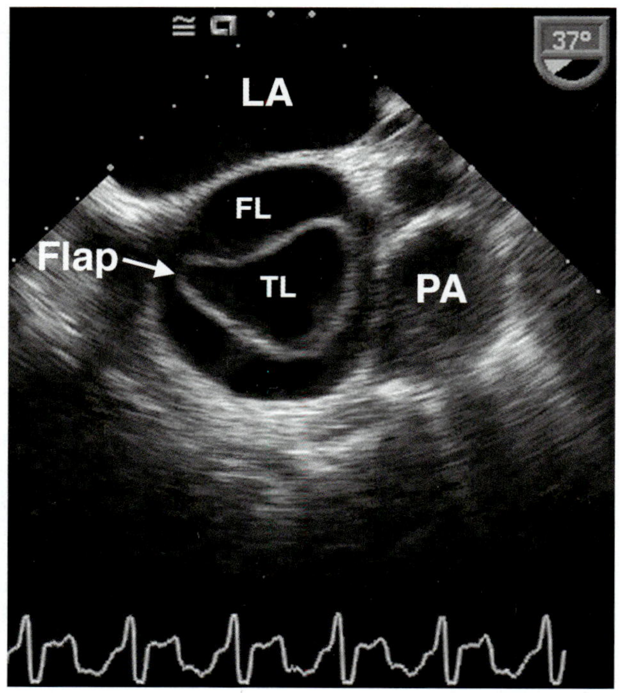

Fig 10.68 High TEE view of ascending aorta shows circumferential dissection flap. True lumen (TL) is in center. FL = false lumen.

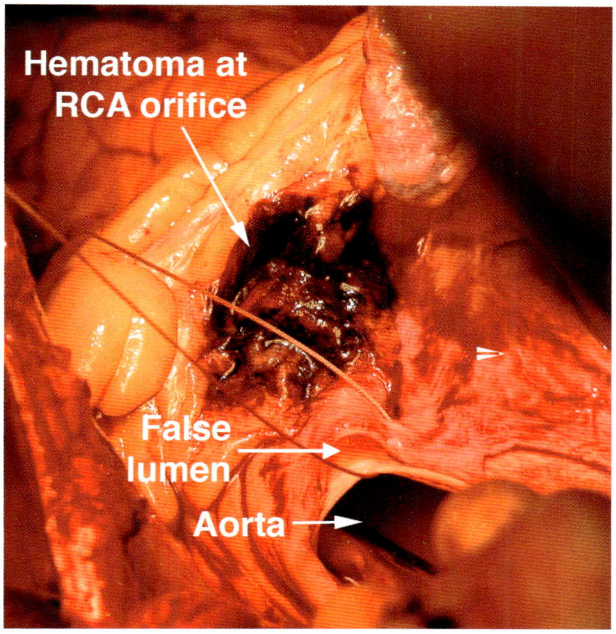

Fig 10.69 Surgical view of opened aorta showing extensive hematoma at site of right coronary orifice.

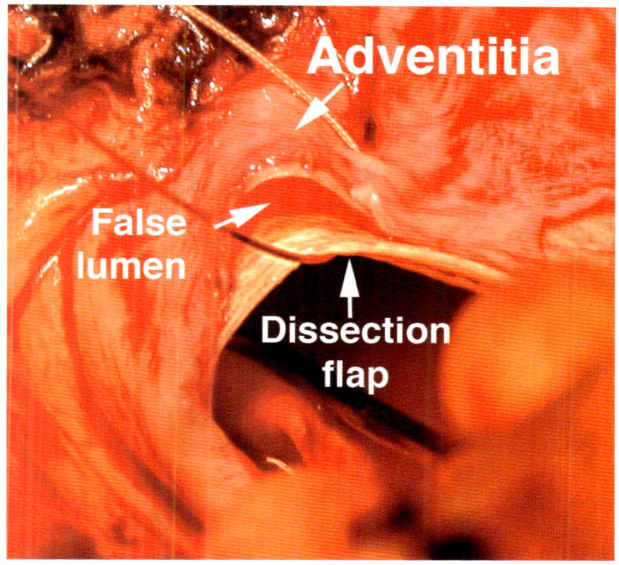

Fig 10.70 Close-up photograph of aortic wall illustrating dissection flap, false lumen, and adventitia.

Comments

This patient had compromise of right coronary blood flow due to compression of the coronary artery by the aortic hematoma. Sudden collapse was due to ventricular fibrillation, most likely secondary to myocardial ischemia induced by the right coronary artery compression. The mild central aortic regurgitation was due to dilation of the sinuses of Valsalva with relatively normal aortic leaflet motion despite the proximity of the dissection flap to the valve. Delineation of the origin and extent of the dissection flap may help the surgeon in planning the operative procedure, even with images obtained in the OR by the anesthesiologist as the surgery is starting.

Suggested Reading

1. Lentini S, Perrotta S: Aortic dissection with concomitant acute myocardial infarction: from diagnosis to management, J Emerg Trauma Shock 4:273–278, 2011.

Sinus of Valsalva Aneurysms

CASE 10-10
Right Coronary Sinus of Valsalva Aneurysm with RVOT Obstruction

This 65-year-old male presented to his primary care provider after a brief flu-like illness. He was otherwise completely asymptomatic. Physical examination revealed a murmur and he was referred for echocardiography, which revealed a sinus of Valsalva aneurysm. Surgical repair was planned.

The aneurysm was resected and patched via the right ventricle, and the aortic root and aortic valve excised and replaced with a valved conduit.

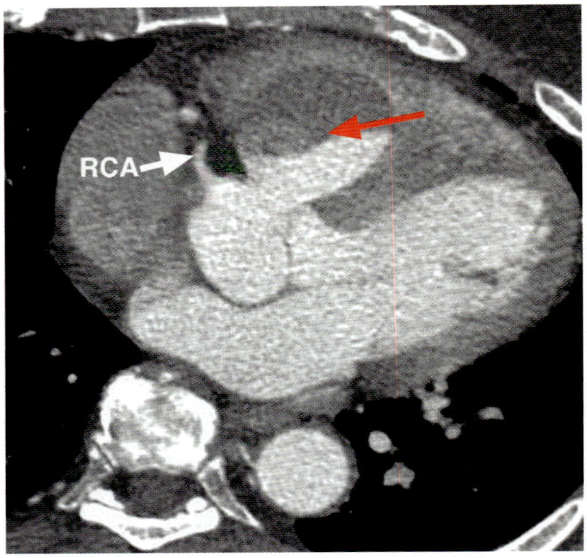

Fig 10.71 In this CT scan, right coronary artery (RCA) and sinus of Valsalva aneurysm *(red arrow)* both emanate from right coronary sinus. Aneurysm appears partly thrombosed with contrast filling only part of aneurysm.

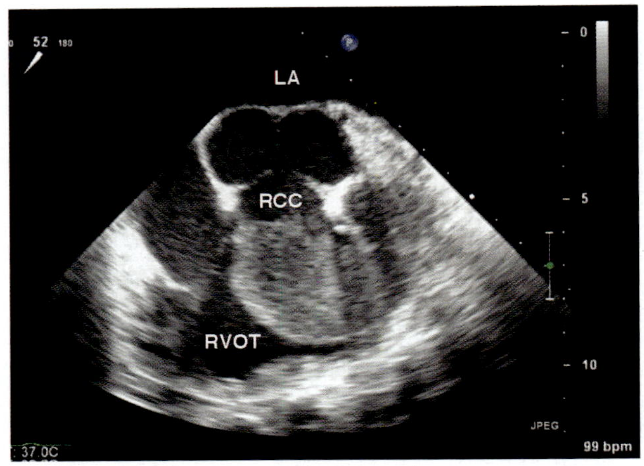

Fig 10.72 In this midesophageal short-axis view, aneurysm is seen protruding into RVOT. Echodensity of space suggests low flow state inside large aneurysm.

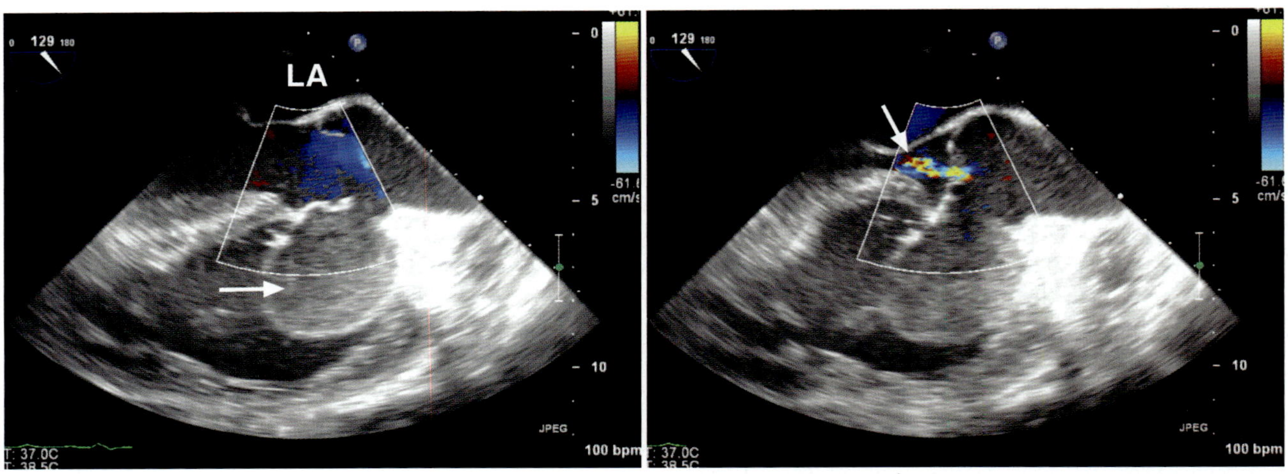

Fig 10.73 In this midesophageal long-axis view, aneurysm *(white arrow)* is again seen protruding into RVOT. On left, systole is seen; on right during diastole, jet of mild AR is seen *(arrow)*.

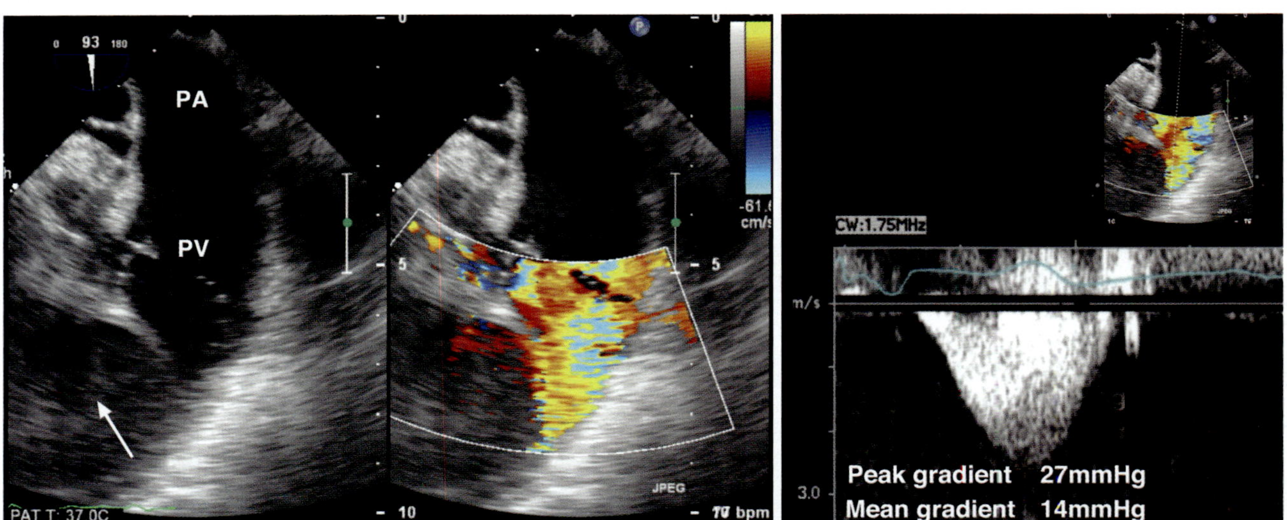

Fig 10.74 In this high esophageal long-axis view, aneurysm *(arrow)* is appears to obstruct RVOT. Turbulent color flow Doppler is seen. Continuous wave Doppler shows peak and mean pressure gradients of 27 and 14 mm Hg, consistent with significant obstruction.

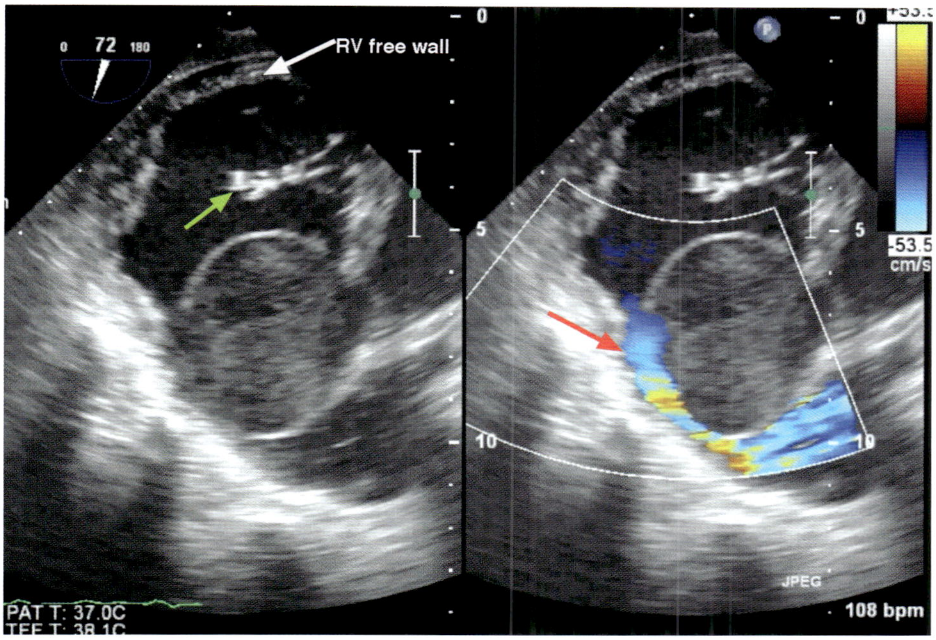

Fig 10.75 In this transgastric "inflow-outflow" view, similar color Doppler pattern is seen *(red arrow)*. Green arrow indicates tricuspid valve. Right ventricular hypertrophy of 7 mm is noted.

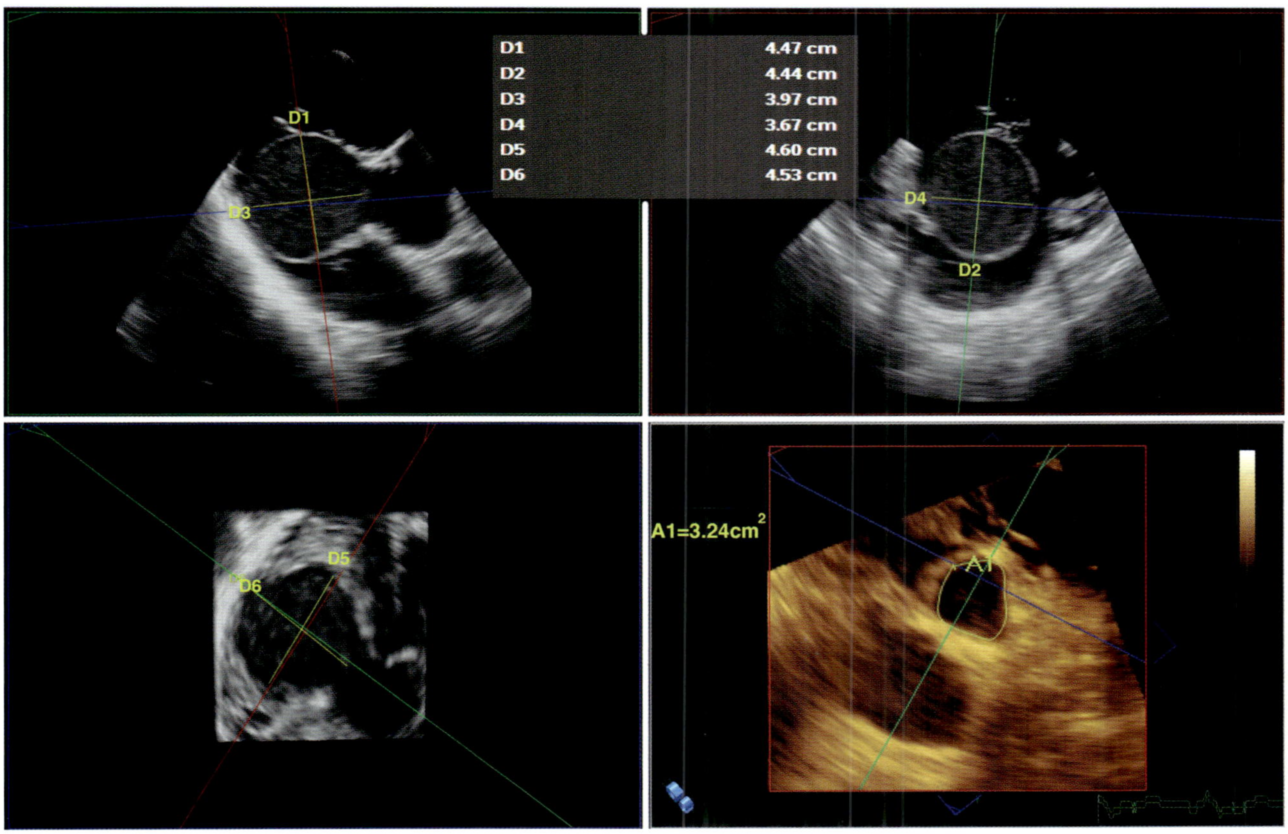

Fig 10.76 Multiplanar reconstruction was performed. Multiple diameters were obtained and show aneurysm to be largely spherical. Neck of aneurysm was measured at 3.24 cm.

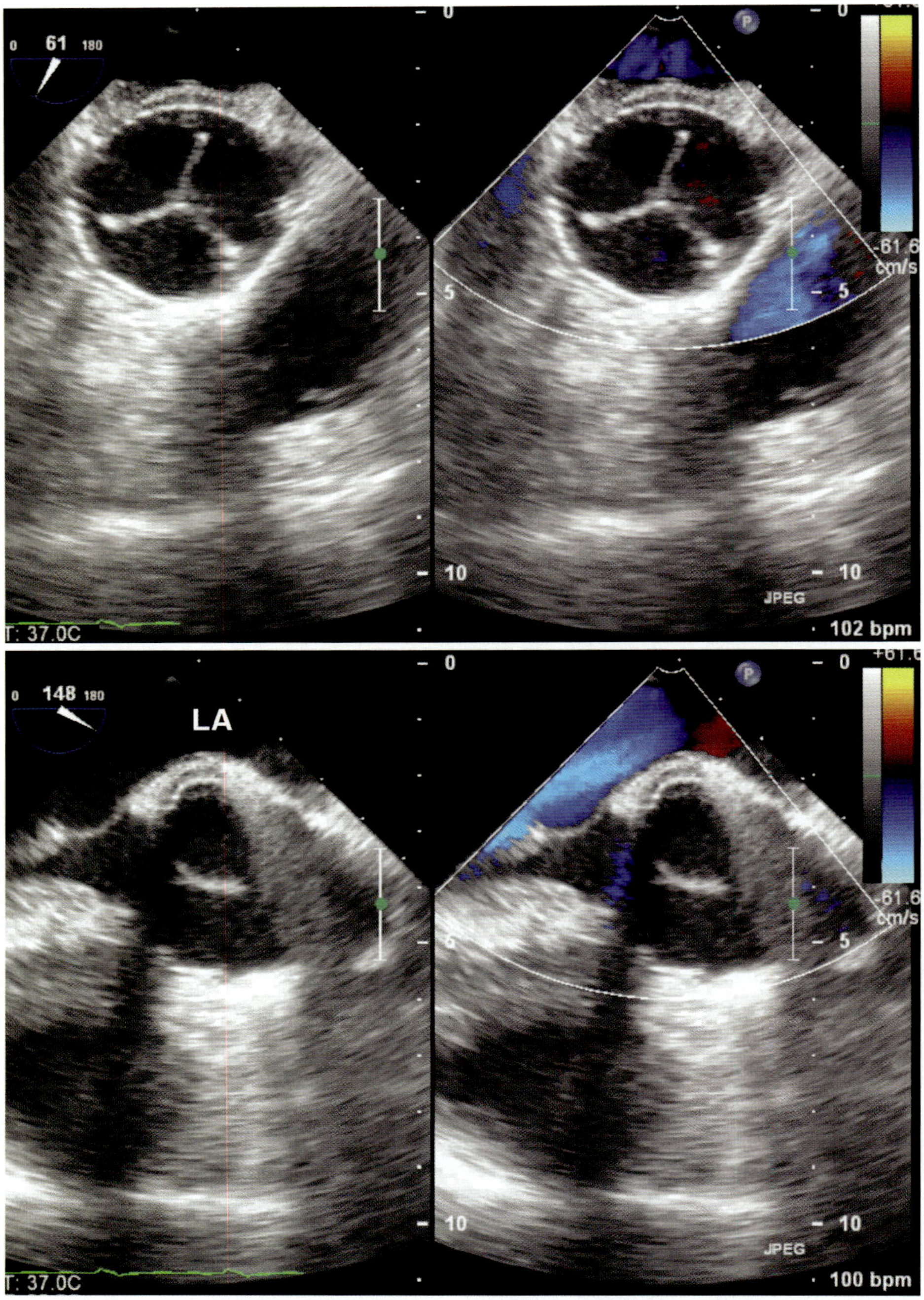

Fig 10.77 Aneurysm was resected, and defect in right coronary sinus patched. Aortic valve was replaced with composite graft and bioprosthetic valve because aortic root could not be adequately reconstructed. These changes are seen in midesophageal short-axis *(top two frames)* and long-axis *(bottom two frames)* views.

CASE 10-11
Right Coronary Sinus of Valsalva Aneurysm with Rupture into the RVOT

Seven years before admission, this 35-year-old patient was noted to have a murmur and outside imaging suggested the diagnosis of an outlet ventricular septal defect. She underwent a more dedicated workup with echo, MRI, TEE, and cardiac catheterization at her home hospital and was sent to our center. After evaluation, it was clear that the murmur and abnormal flow seen on imaging was not due to a ventricular septal defect and instead was consistent with a sinus of Valsalva rupture with left-to-right shunting into the right ventricular outflow tract. At surgery, the ruptured sinus of Valsalva aneurysm was resected, the anterior cusp of the pulmonic valve was repaired, and the RV outflow tract defect was closed with an autologous pericardial patch.

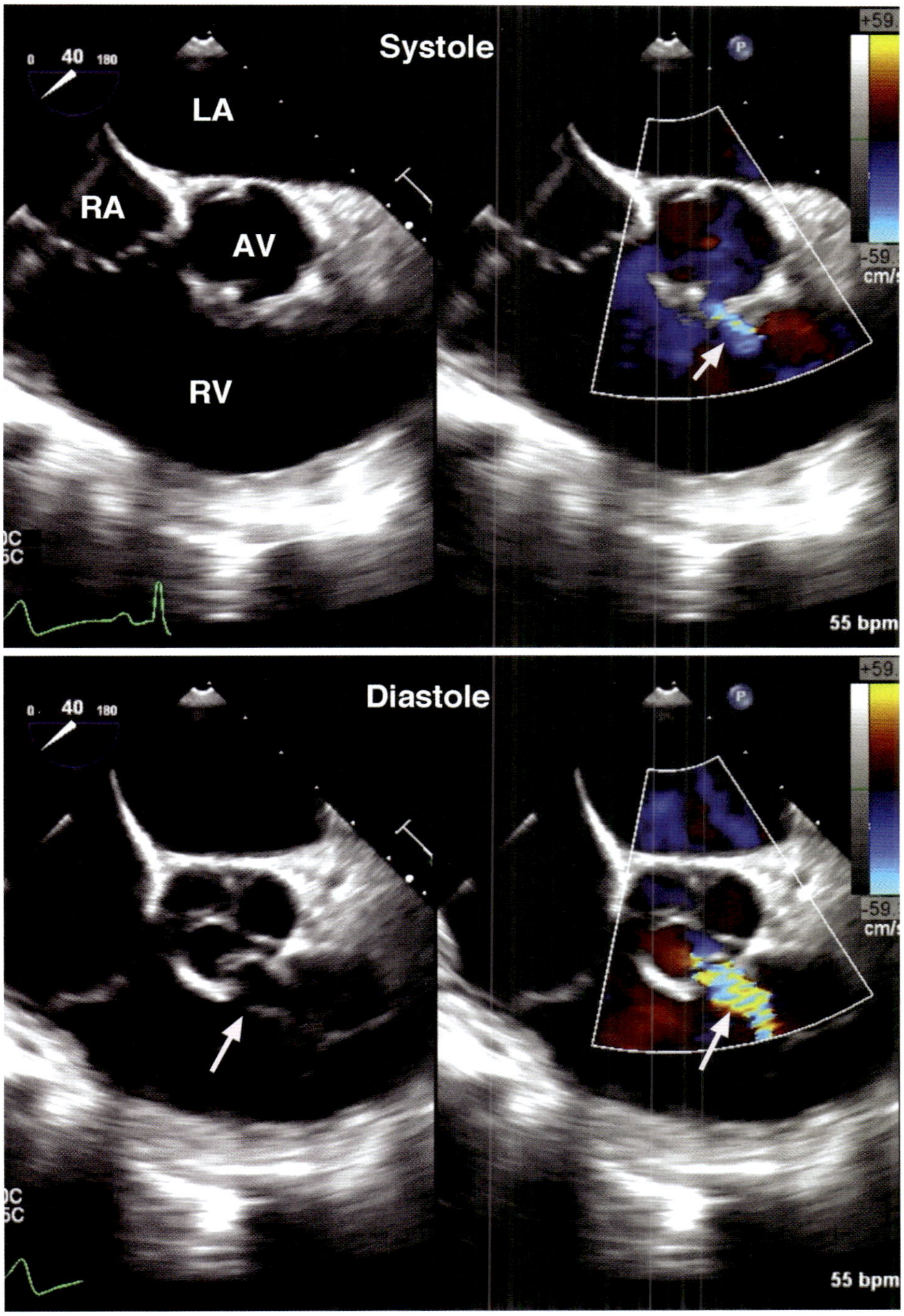

Fig 10.78 In this midesophageal short-axis, top two frames are in systole. Small jet is seen entering RVOT from right coronary cusp. In lower two frames, in diastole, jet is again seen.

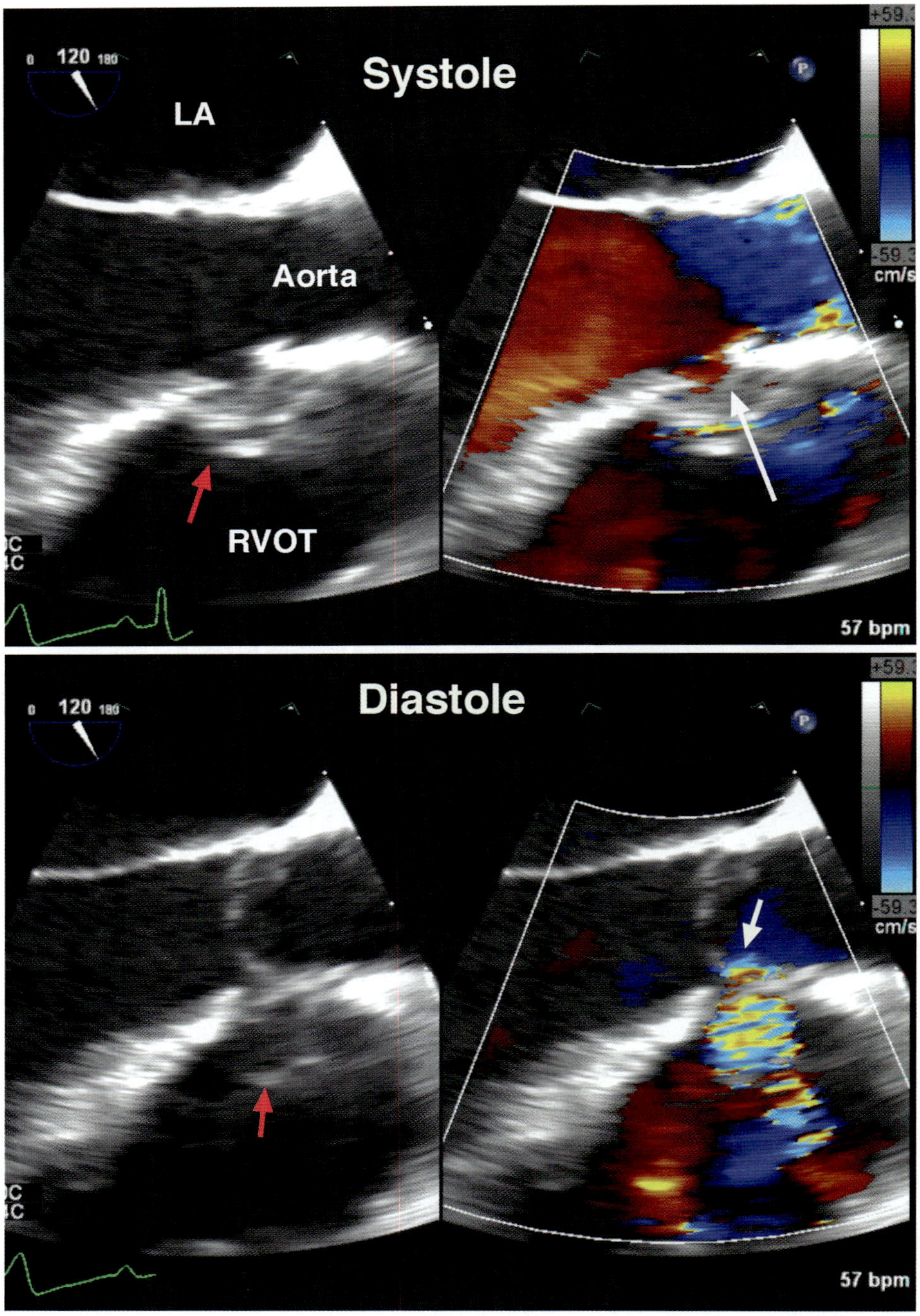

Fig 10.79 Similar findings are seen in midesophageal long-axis view. Red arrows indicate windsock. Again, jet is more pronounced in diastole *(white arrow)*.

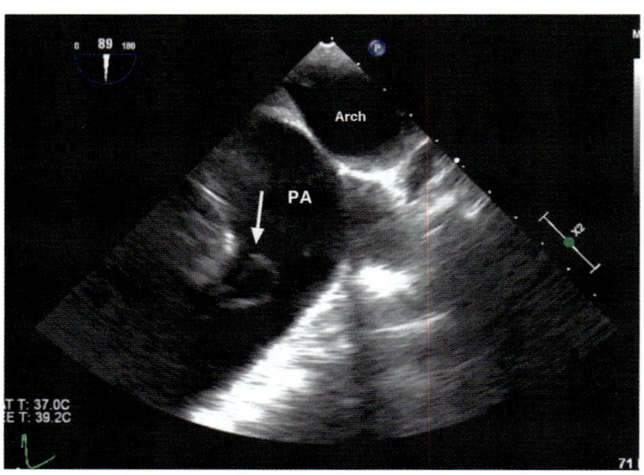

Fig 10.80 In upper esophageal long axis, windsock is seen adjacent to where pulmonic valve lies. There was neither pulmonic regurgitation nor stenosis.

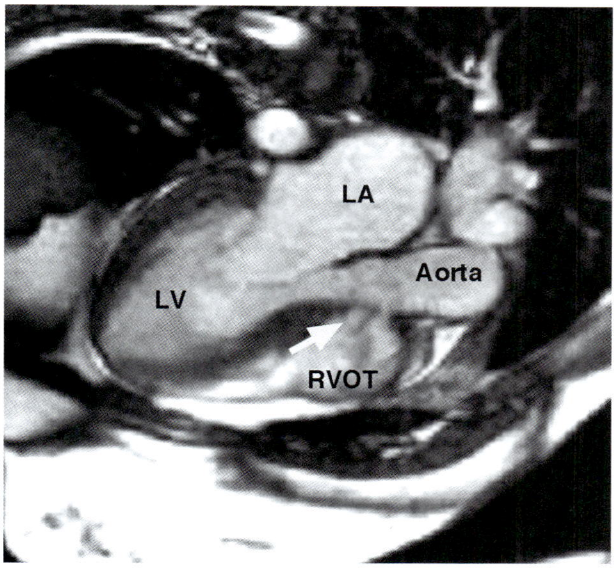

Fig 10.81 In this MRI, view analogous to midesophageal long axis is presented. Small jet is seen in RVOT during diastole *(arrow)* which is better appreciated in real time.

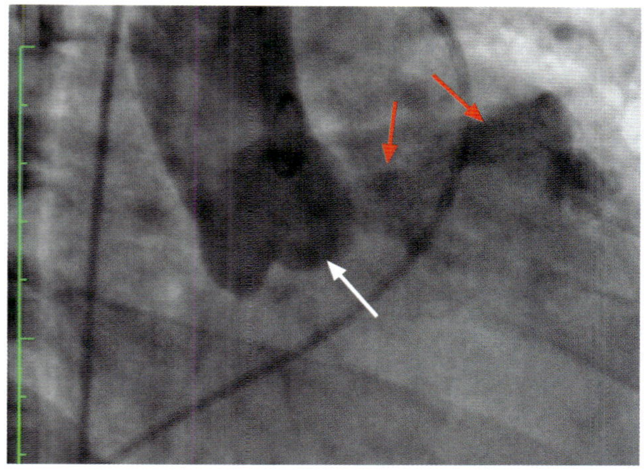

Fig 10.82 Patient was referred for coronary arteriography. With aortic root injection, right coronary cusp is seen *(white arrow)*, as is angiographic dye entering RVOT *(red arrows)*.

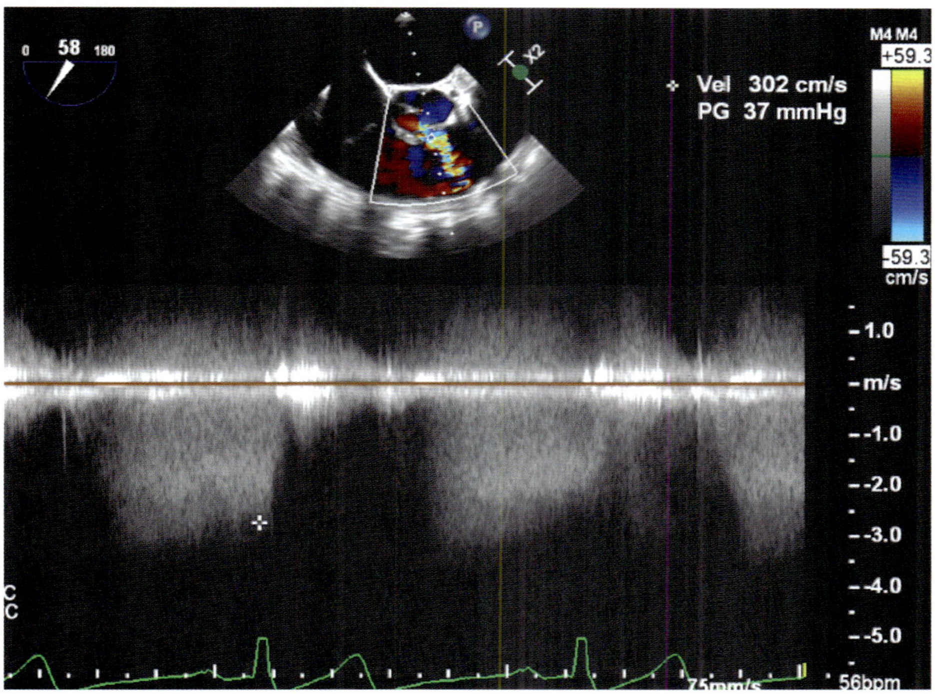

Fig 10.83 Continuous wave Doppler of jet shows end diastolic gradient of 37 mm Hg. Flow is primarily in diastole, but also seen in systole. Velocity at end diastole of about 3.5 m/s is consistent with 50 mm Hg difference between aortic diastolic and RV diastolic pressure.

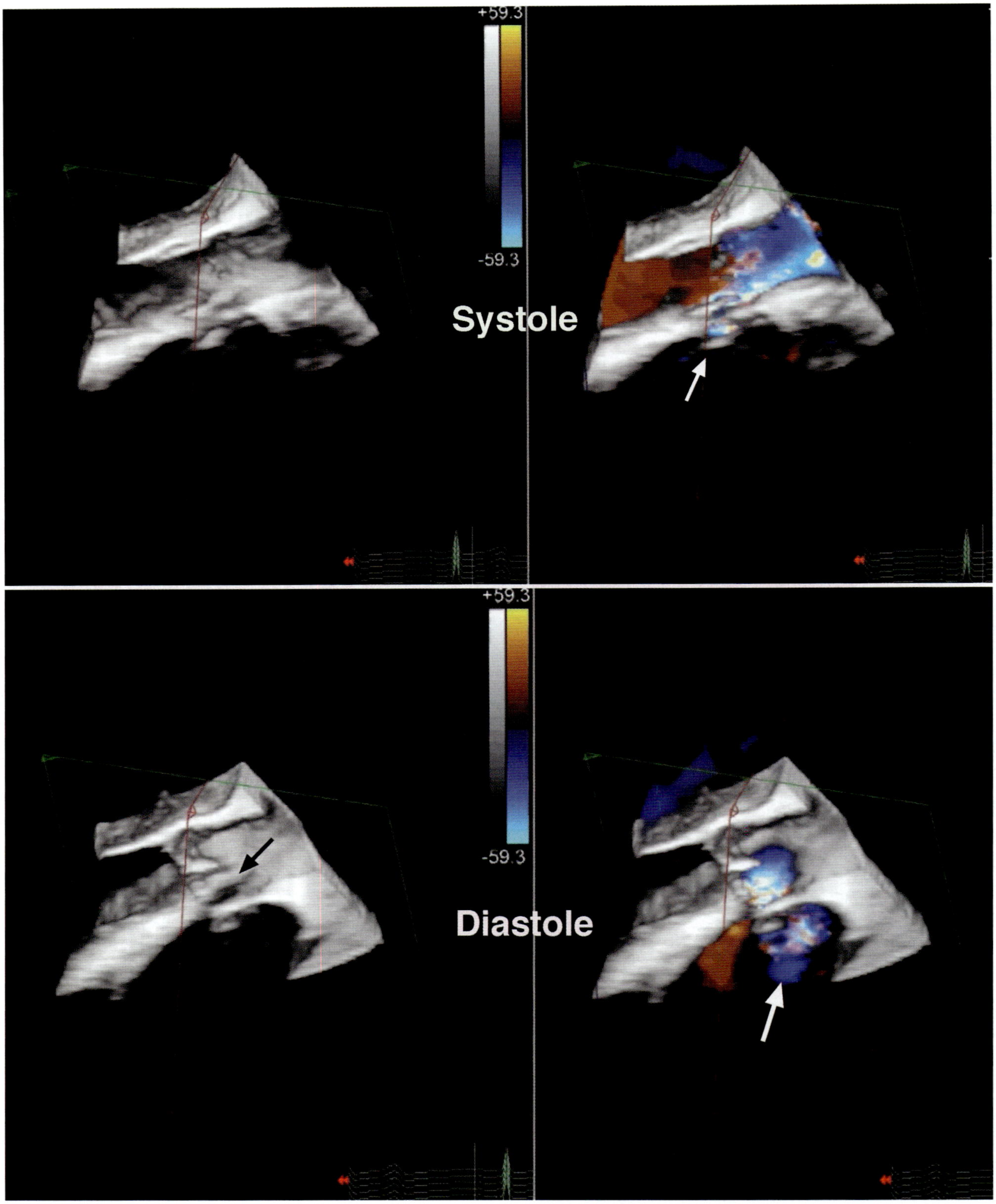

Fig 10.84 In this 3D midesophageal view, jet *(white arrows)* as well as sinus defect *(black arrow)* are seen.

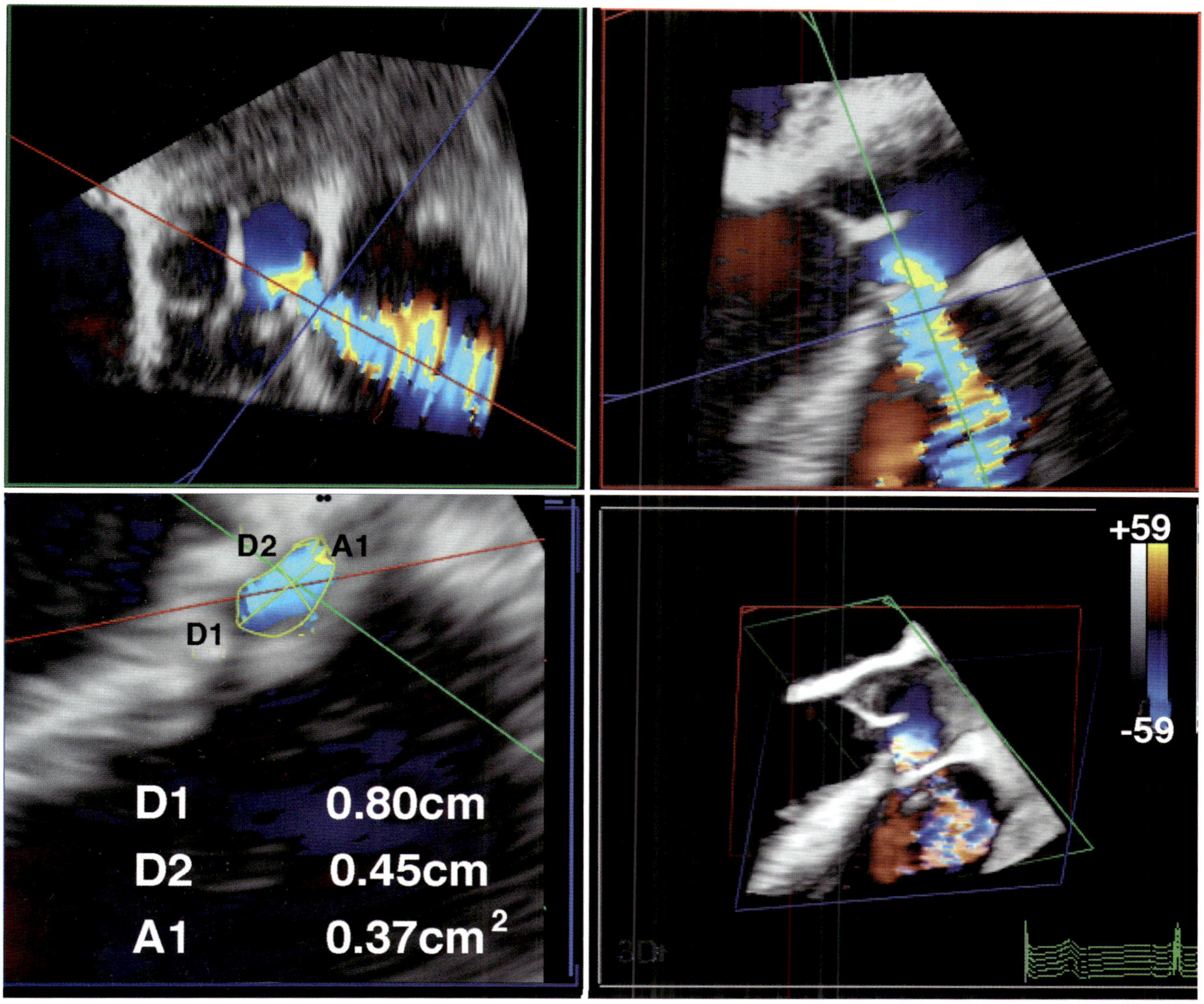

Fig 10.85 Using multiplanar reconstruction, cross sectional dimensions of windsock are presented.

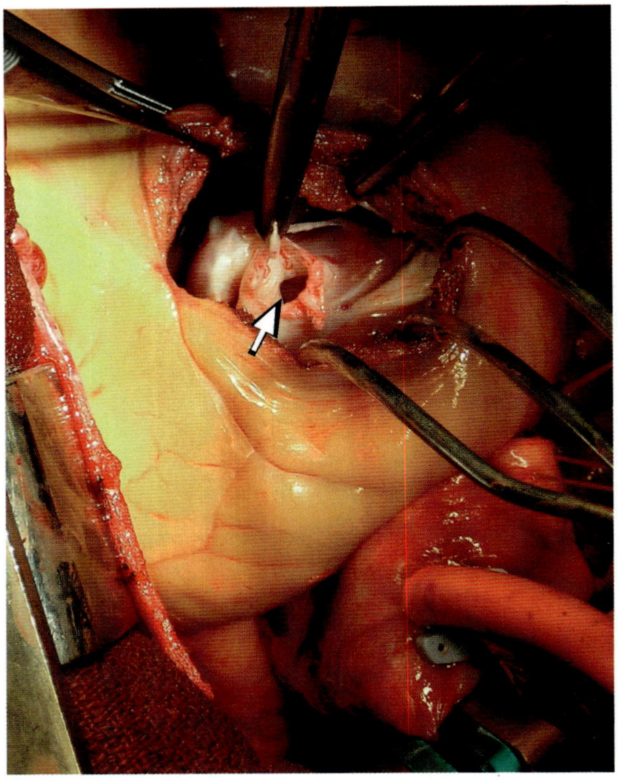

Fig 10.86 After initiating cardiopulmonary bypass, RVOT was opened, and windsock of sinus of Valsalva aneurysm was seen with defect *(arrow)* that allowed communication between RVOT and right coronary sinus of Valsalva.

Comments

A sinus of Valsalva aneurysm (SVA) may be congenital, as in this case, or may be acquired as a complication of endocarditis with paravalvular extension of the infection resulting in aortic sinus dilation and rupture. A congenital sinus of Valsalva aneurysm typically appears as a thin, irregular, undulating, tubular structure (similar in shape and motion to a windsock used at airfields to show wind direction and speed) that communicates with one of the aortic sinuses. A congenital SVA is asymptomatic with diagnosis on echocardiography requested for unrelated reasons. However, spontaneous rupture of the SVA can occur resulting in a communication from the aorta into the RV outflow tract (for the right coronary sinus), the left atrium (for the left coronary sinus), or the right atrium (for the noncoronary sinus). Flow from the high-pressure aorta into the low-pressure right heart or left atrium results in a high-velocity flow signal in both systole and diastole, in most patients, although some have predominant diastolic flow as in this case. Closure of a ruptured SVA typically is undertaken to relieve left-to-right shunting and to reduce the risk of endocarditis long term.

Suggested Reading

1. Moustafa S, Mookadam F, Cooper L, et al: Sinus of Valsalva aneurysms—47 years of a single center experience and systematic overview of published reports, Am J Cardiol 99:1159–1164, 2007.
2. Vadivelu R, Rohit MK, Yadav M: Ruptured sinus of Valsalva aneurysm from left coronary sinus into right atrium: a rare anomaly with an odd presentation, BMJ Case Rep 25:2013, 2013.
3. Afshar AH, Kolesnikov S, Pourafkari L, et al: Right Valsalva sinus aneurysm protruding into the right ventricle: a case report, J Cardiovasc Thorac Res 7:126–128, 2015.

Other Aortic Pathology and Procedures

CASE 10-12
Aortic Atheroma

This 78-year-old woman was referred for aortic valve replacement for severe aortic stenosis with congestive heart failure.

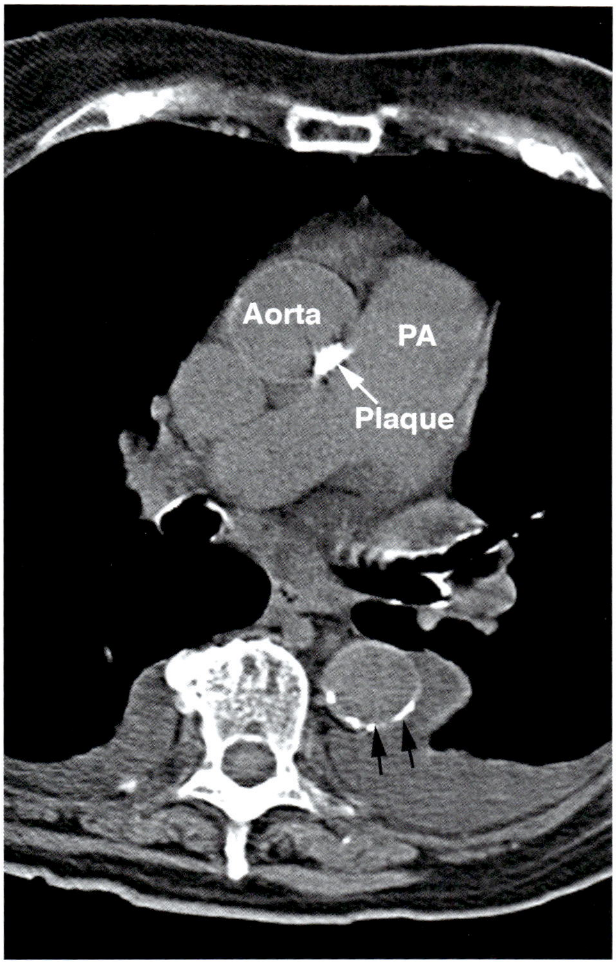

Fig 10.87 Chest CT shows area of calcification, consistent with atherosclerotic plaque along posterior aspect of ascending aorta *(arrow)*.

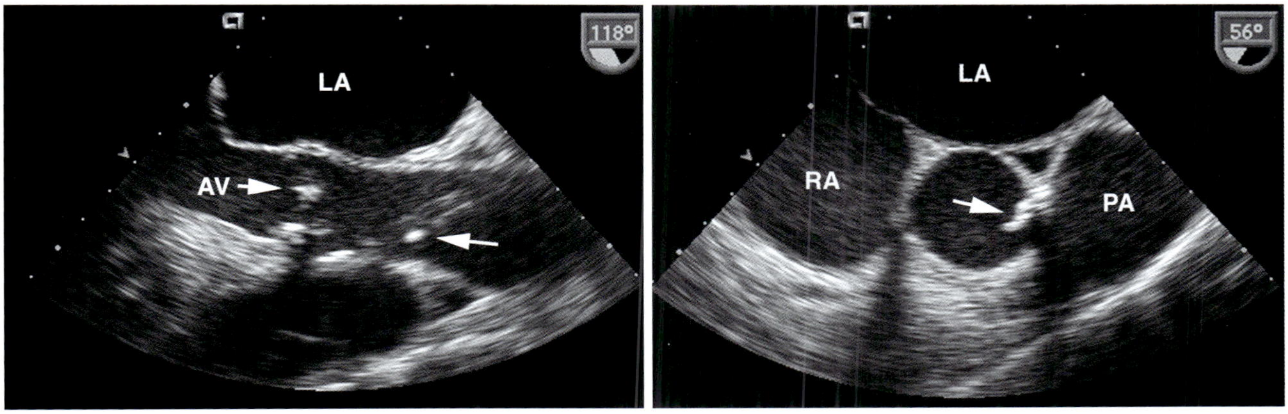

Fig 10.88 On left, long-axis view of aortic valve and ascending aorta shows calcification of aortic valve (AV) leaflets and area of calcification in ascending aorta *(arrow)*. On right, short-axis view of ascending aorta shows protruding atheroma *(arrow)*.

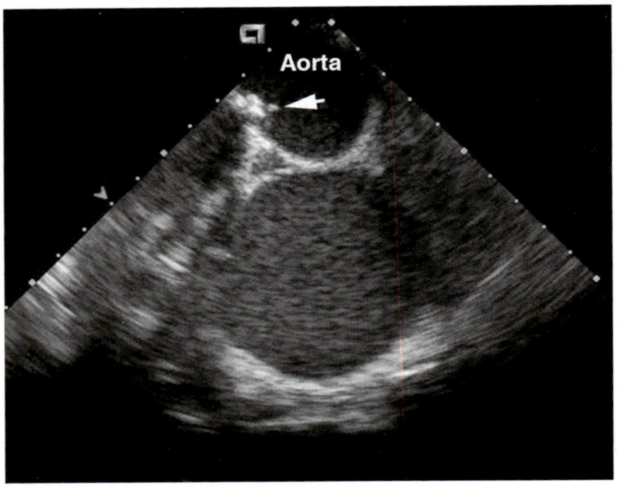

Fig 10.89 Surgeon used sterile epiaortic scanning to carefully locate area of atherosclerosis in ascending aorta. This allowed surgeon to avoid this area during cannulation for cardiopulmonary bypass and to avoid placing proximal vein graft anastomosis at this site.

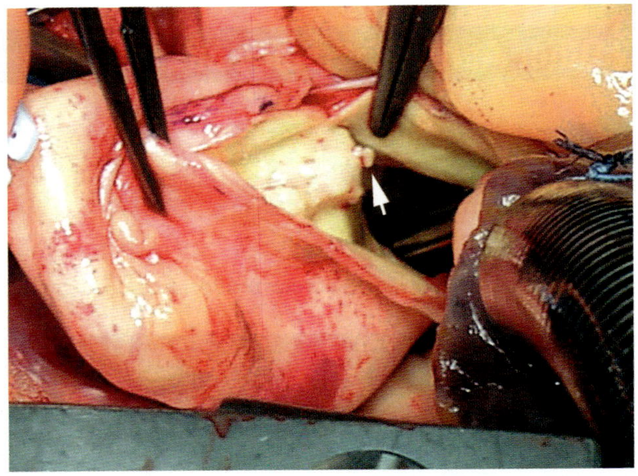

Fig 10.90 With aorta opened, protruding atheroma is visualized *(arrow)*. Aortic valve was replaced with biologic tissue prosthesis and aortic atheroma was resected.

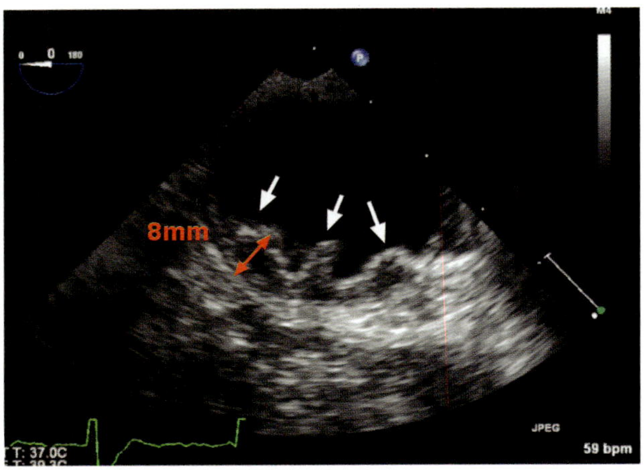

Fig 10.91 In another patient with aortic stenosis who presented for TAVR, middescending aorta showed extensive atheroma formation *(white arrows)*.

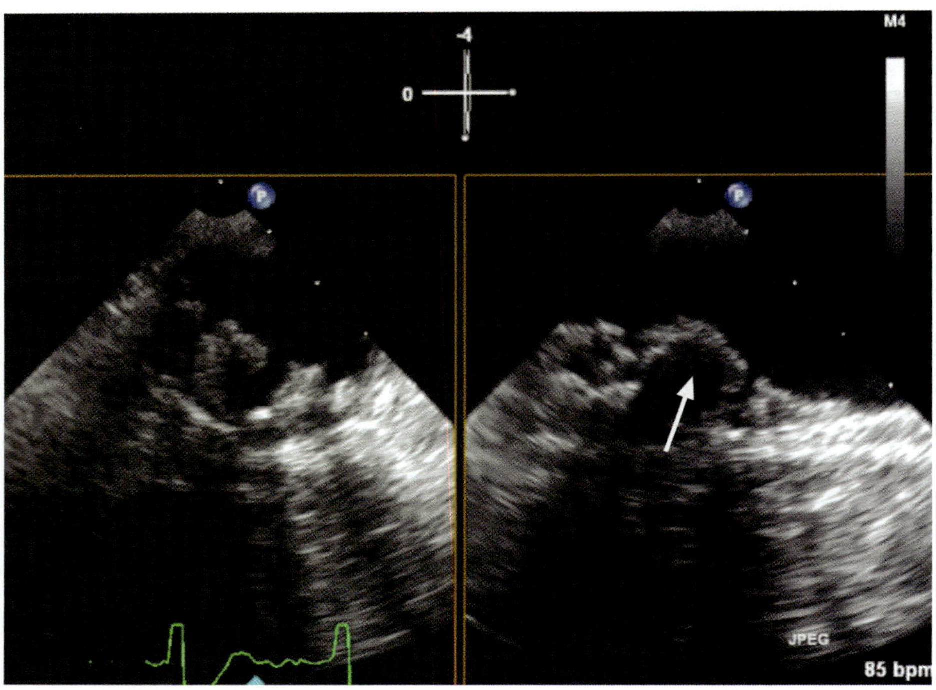

Fig 10.92 At 10 cm proximally, biplane imaging of descending thoracic aorta again showed extensive atheromatous change with mobility of some portions. White arrow indicates shadowing secondary to calcium deposits.

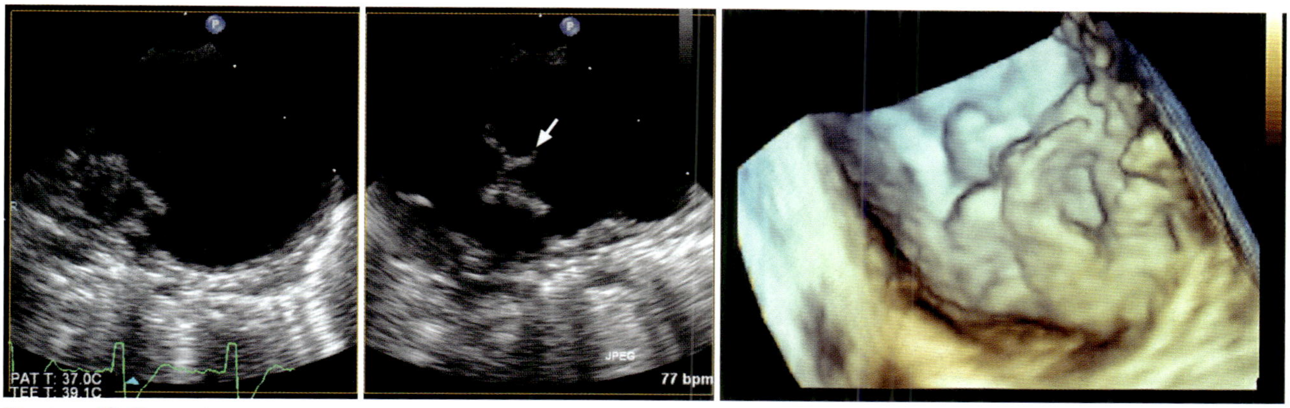

Fig 10.93 Further proximally, there is again mobile plaque *(white arrow)*. 3D TEE imaging shows atheromatous change to be fairly broad based.

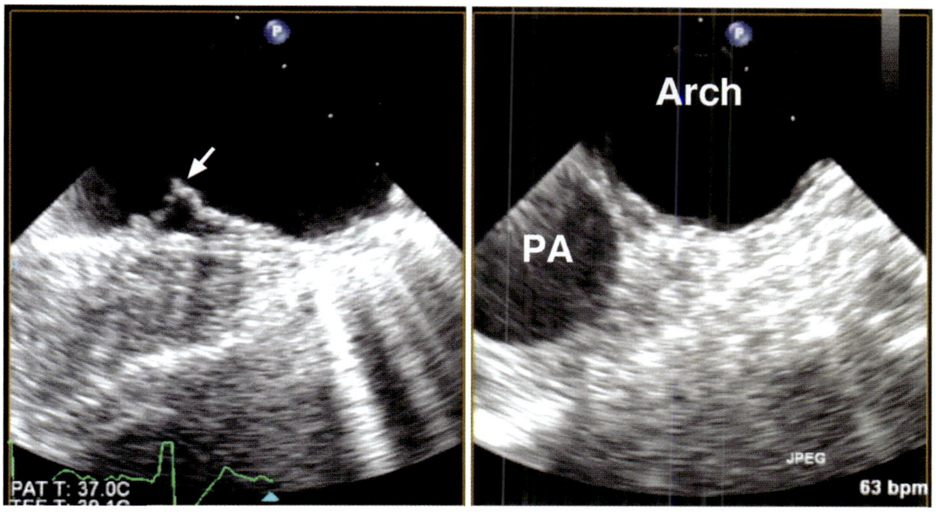

Fig 10.94 In distal arch, biplane imaging shows atheromatous change with mobile components *(arrow)*, better appreciated in real time.

Comments

Aortic atheromas are identified on TEE imaging as irregular areas of variable echodensity that may follow the contour of the aortic wall or may protrude into the aortic lumen. Calcified areas in the plaques are identified by echodensity and shadowing. Atheromas that protrude into the lumen may rupture and be associated with localized thrombus formation.

The finding of aortic atheroma in the descending thoracic aorta is associated with the presence of coronary artery disease. In addition, plaque complexity predicts clinical outcome with a 15% annual risk of death or a cerebral embolic event in patients with a complex plaque (thickness greater than or equal to 4 mm or any mobile components) compared to those with a noncomplex plaque.

At the time of cardiac surgery, epiaortic scanning may be used, as in this case, to avoid cross-clamping, cannulation, or placement of bypass grafts in atherosclerotic regions of the vessel.

Suggested Reading

1. Weissler-Snir A, Greenberg G, Shapira Y, et al: Transoesophageal echocardiography of aortic atherosclerosis: the additive value of three-dimensional over two-dimensional imaging, Eur Heart J Cardiovasc Imaging 16:389–394, 2015.
2. Denny JT, Pantin E, Chiricolo A, et al: Increasing severity of aortic atherosclerosis in coronary artery bypass grafting patients evaluated by transesophageal echocardiography, J Clin Med Res 7:13–17, 2015.

CASE 10-13
Penetrating Ulcer of the Ascending Aorta

A 24-year-old male with a known history of a bicuspid aortic valve, presented with chest pain and underwent CT scanning. CT revealed an intramural hematoma of his ascending aorta with a small pericardial effusion. He had no evidence of aortic insufficiency, coronary insufficiency, or tamponade. He was brought semiurgently to the OR for repair of his intramural hematoma.

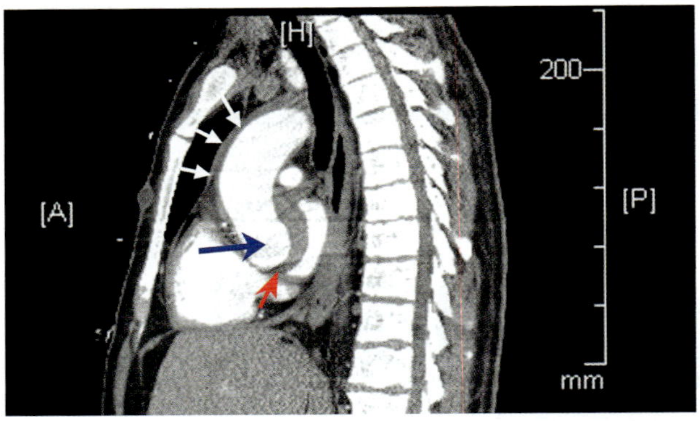

Fig 10.95 Preoperative CT scan showed both posterior *(red arrow)* and anterior *(white arrows)* periaortic hematoma. Blue arrow indicates ascending aorta.

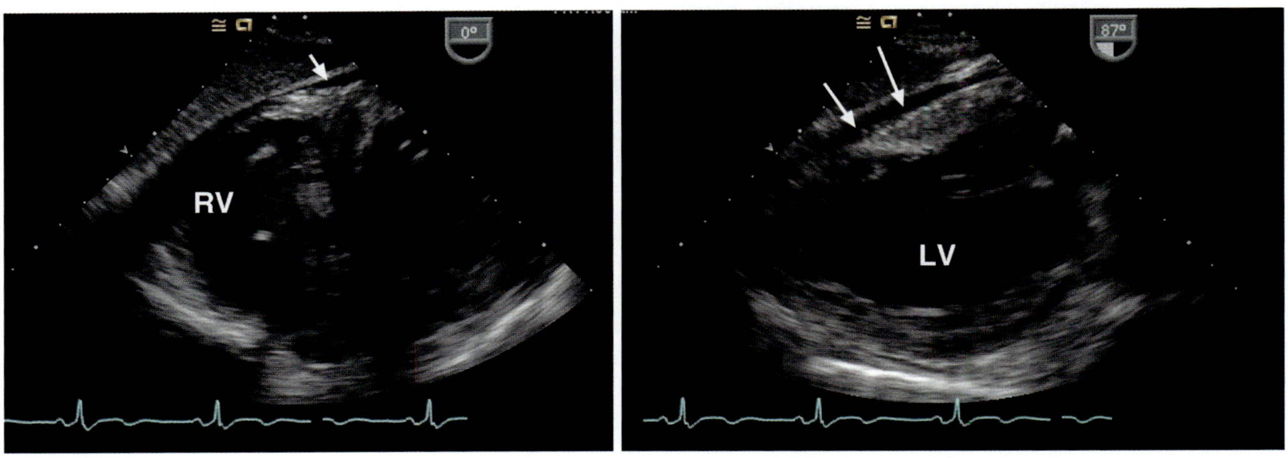

Fig 10.96 Transgastric biplane imaging of ventricles revealed small posterior pericardial effusion *(white arrows)*.

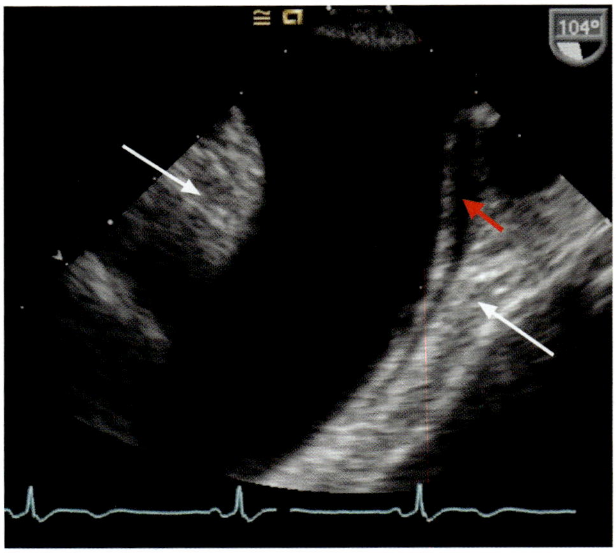

Fig 10.97 From high esophageal position with rightward turning of probe, ascending aorta is seen. Periaortic hematoma is indicated by white arrows, and pericardial fluid by the red arrow.

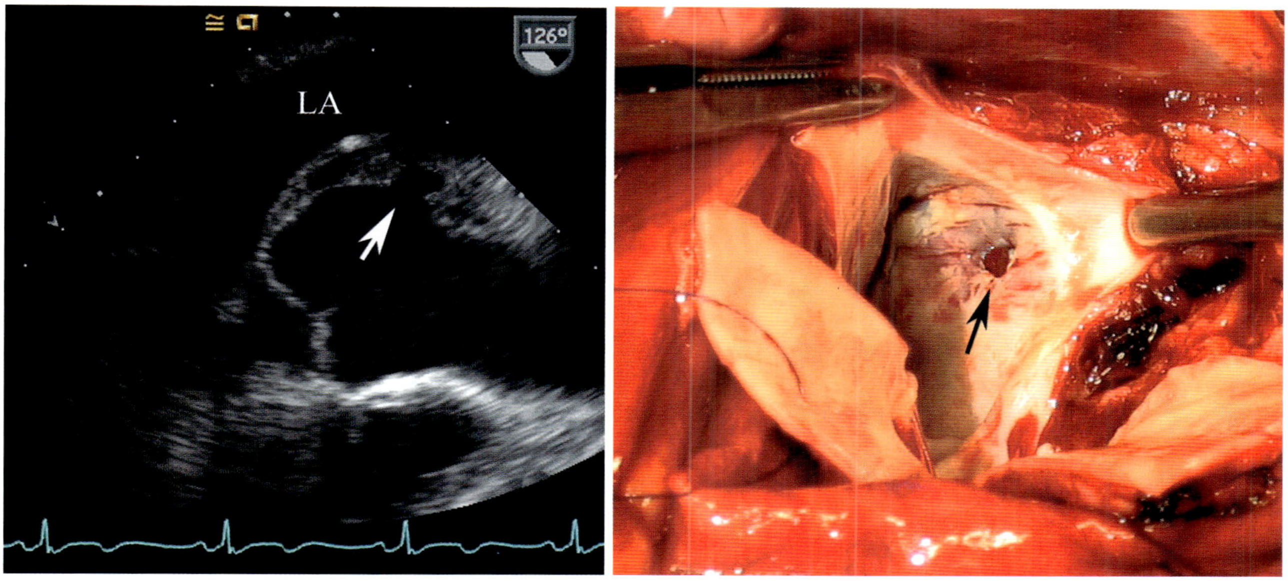

Fig 10.98 On left, midesophageal long-axis view of ascending aorta is seen. White arrow indicates penetrating ulcer, which is surrounded by hematoma. On right, after aorta is cross-clamped and ascending aorta opened; penetrating ulcer is clearly visible *(arrow)*. This defect in aortic wall is superior to coronary ostia, which were identified separately in other images.

Comments

Instead of the classic presentation of an aortic dissection, a limited tear in the aortic wall may allow hematoma formation in the wall of the aorta, which is called an aortic intramural hemorrhage. On echocardiography, an aortic intramural hemorrhage appears as a crescent shaped area of increased echodensity around the aorta. The prognosis and treatment of aortic intramural hematoma is similar to aortic dissection.

Another clinical variant, known as penetrating aortic "ulcer," is weakening of the aortic wall at the site of an atherosclerotic plaque with a contained rupture of the aorta into the surrounding tissue. The contained rupture, or pseudoaneurysm, is identified as an irregular blood-filled space adjacent to the aorta, with or without a demonstrable connection between the aorta and the pseudoaneurysm. Treatment is surgical to replace the ruptured segment of the aorta.

Suggested Reading

1. Chou AS, Ziganshin BA, Charilaou P, et al: Long-term behavior of aortic intramural hematomas and penetrating ulcers, J Thorac Cardiovasc Surg 151:361–372, 2016.
2. Matsushita A, Fukui T, Tabata M, et al: Preoperative characteristics and surgical outcomes of acute intramural hematoma involving the ascending aorta: a propensity score-matched analysis, J Thorac Cardiovasc Surg 151:351–358, 2016.

CASE 10-14
Aortic Valve Replacement With Coronary Artery Reimplantation (David Procedure)

This 29-year-old female had been clinically diagnosed with Marfan's syndrome 20 years previously, and recently underwent genetic testing in which a likely pathogenic variant in one allele of FBN1, the gene that encodes fibrillin-1, was identified.

Although the patient was asymptomatic, there was concern that her aortic size had increased and was quite large when indexed for body size with a ratio of the observed to expected root diameter of 1.36 (normal is 1.0 or less). There was only mild aortic regurgitation.

In light of the fact that she was contemplating pregnancy, a surgical opinion was sought and she was scheduled for aortic root replacement with aortic valve repair or replacement.

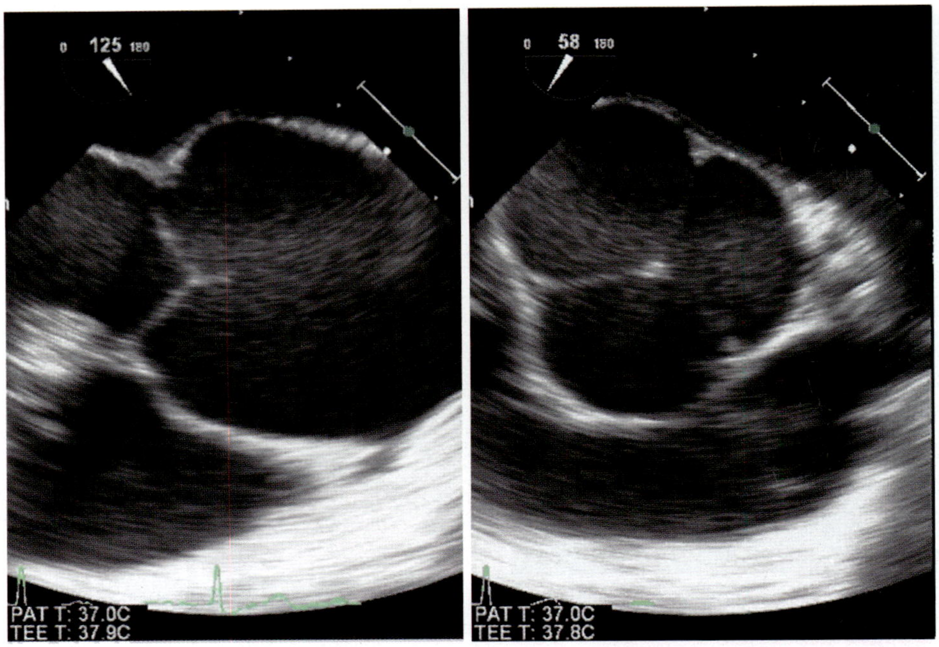

Fig 10.99 TEE long-axis *(left)* and short-axis *(right)* view of ascending aorta shows marked dilation of sinuses of Valsalva, and thin aortic leaflets. There is no aortic regurgitation.

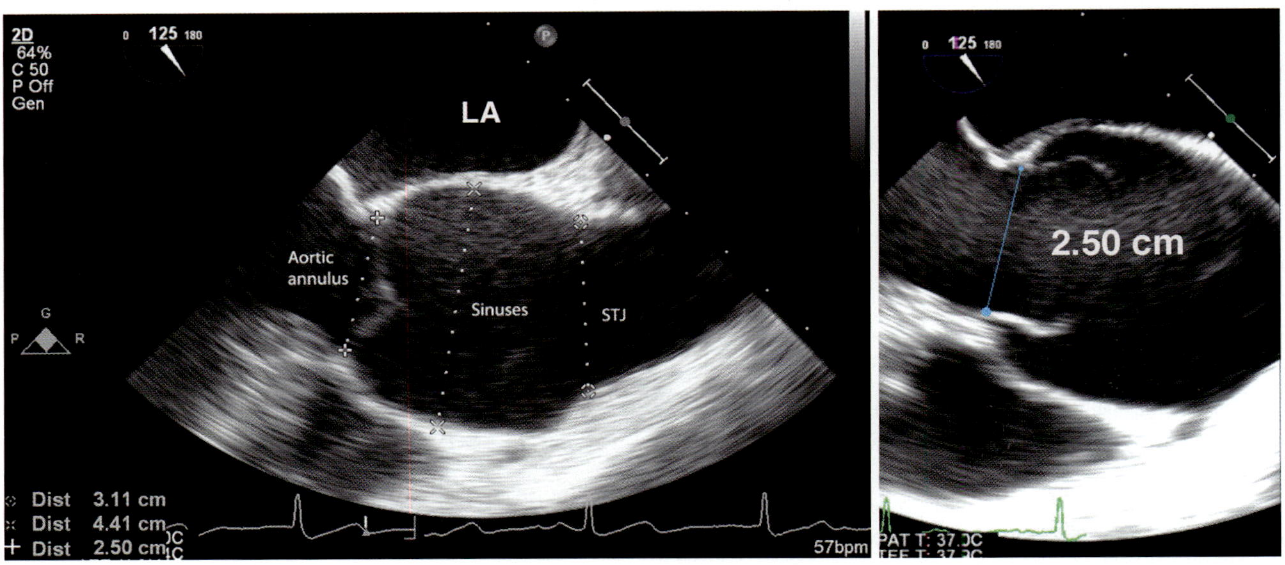

Fig 10.100 Measurements show dilation of sinuses and sinotubular junction, but normal-sized aortic annulus in diastole and systole *(right)*.

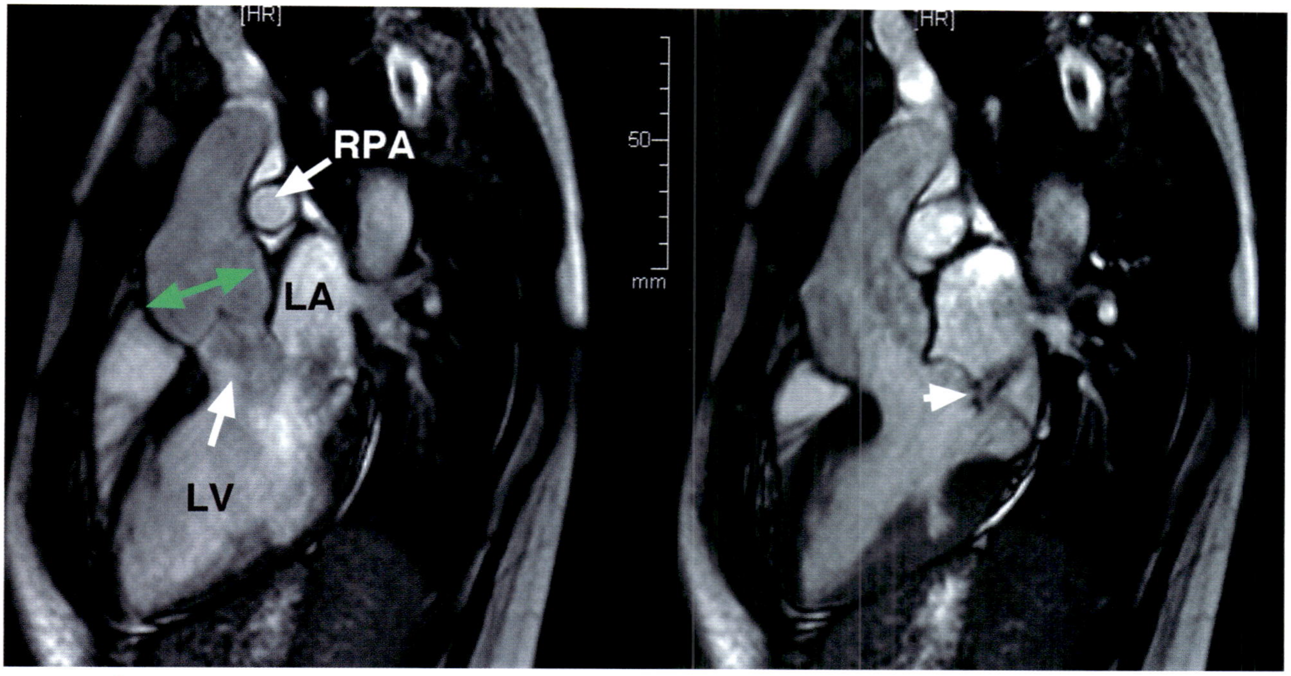

Fig 10.101 Cardiac MRI in diastole *(left)* shows small amount of aortic regurgitation *(white arrow)*. Sinuses are measured at 50 mm *(green arrow)*. In systole *(right)*, white arrow indicates small amount of MR. In real time, jets are better appreciated.

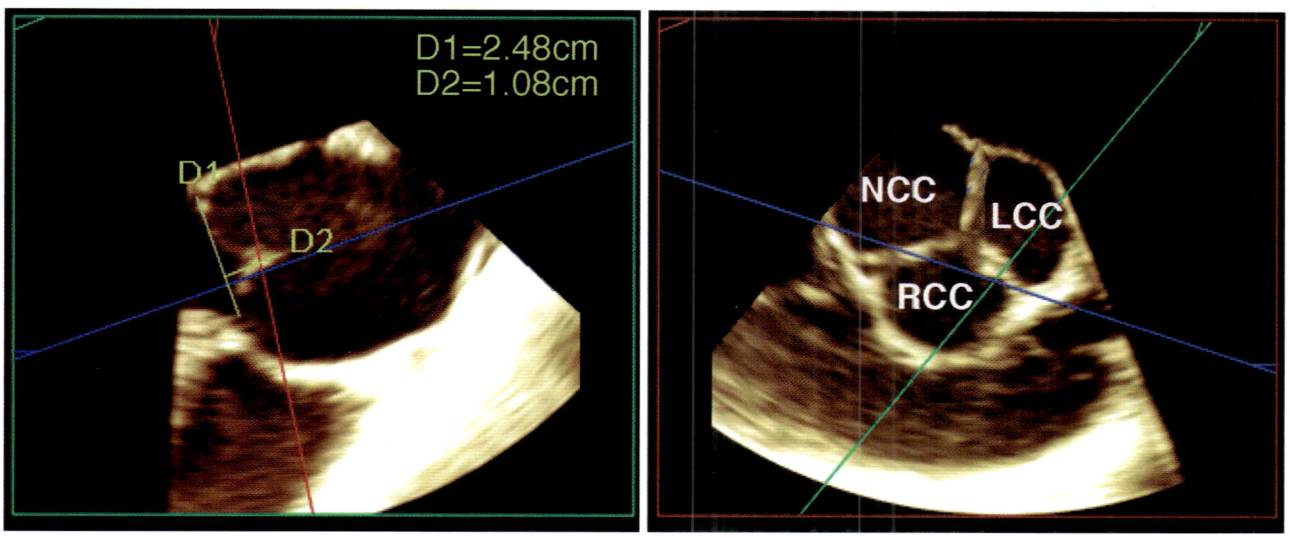

Fig 10.102 Using multiplanar reconstruction, height of lateral aspect of coaptation between left and right coronary cusps is found to be 1.08 cm above annular plane. Similar results were found for two other coaptation combinations. This information may aid surgeon in planning repair.

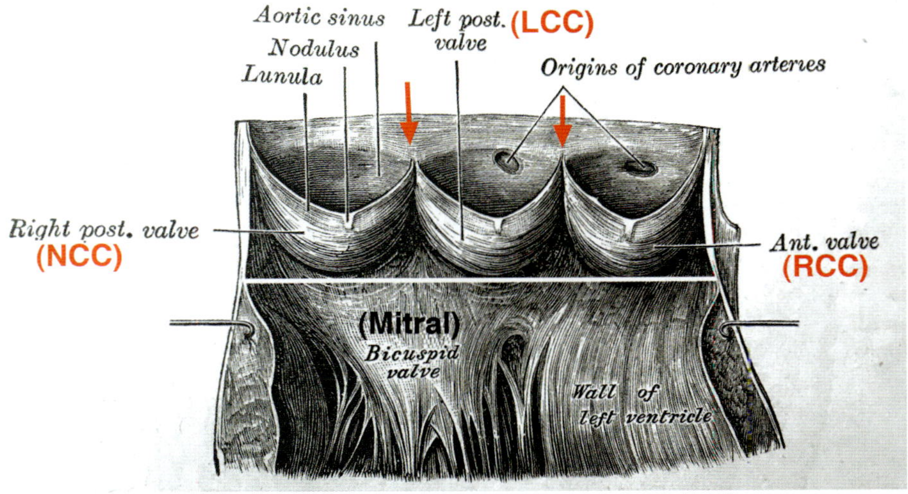

Fig 10.103 With aortic valve "opened up" between right and non (posterior) cusp, points of coaptation *(red arrows)* are seen as they attach to sinotubular junction. White line indicates basal attachments of cusps, which form surgical aortic annulus. (From Gray H: Anatomy of the human body, Philadelphia, 1918, Lea & Febiger.)

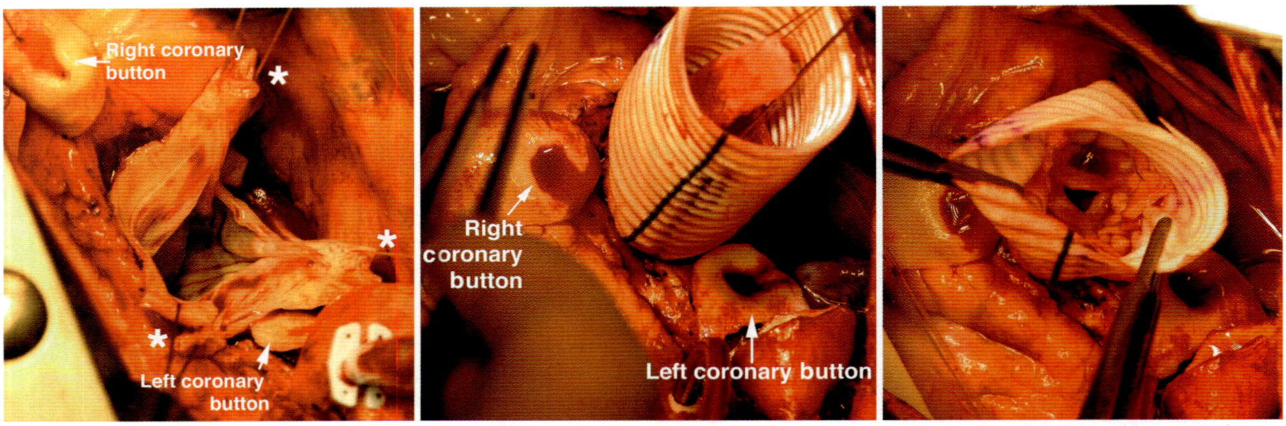

Fig 10.104 These images are taken from patient who had similar expression of Marfan's syndrome and operation. Left panel: Ascending aorta was resected, with preservation of aortic valve, including small "posts" of ascending aorta *(asterisks)* corresponding to coaptation points of three commissures of aortic valve. Right and left coronary ostia were isolated with small circle of aortic tissue, called "buttons." Middle panel: Dacron tube graft replacement for ascending aorta has been positioned around valve. Aortic annulus end of graft is scalloped to provide "neo-sinuses." Base of graft at annular level is stabilized to prevent later dilation in patient with Marfan syndrome. Right panel: View of valve inside graft with commissural posts positioned for resuspension of valve. After valve procedure is complete, coronary buttons are then reimplanted onto graft.

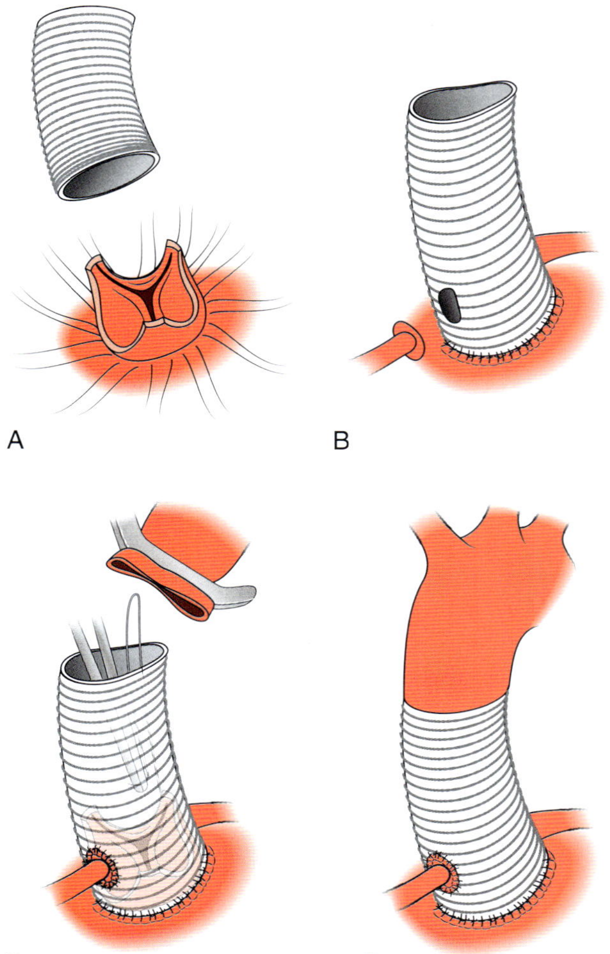

Fig 10.105 In this graphic representation of important components of this technique, entire aortic valve along with its annulus and 3 to 5-mm rim of aortic wall is secured inside appropriately sized synthetic tube graft. Graft is first secured to aortic annulus just below level of valve leaflets. Preserved aortic valve is then "implanted" inside graft by sewing 3 to 5-mm rim of remaining aortic wall to graft. Finally, coronary buttons are sewn to tube graft, which in turn is sewn to distal ascending aorta. (From Feindel C, David T: Aortic valve sparing operations: basic concepts, Int J Cardiol 97:61–66, 2004. With permission.)

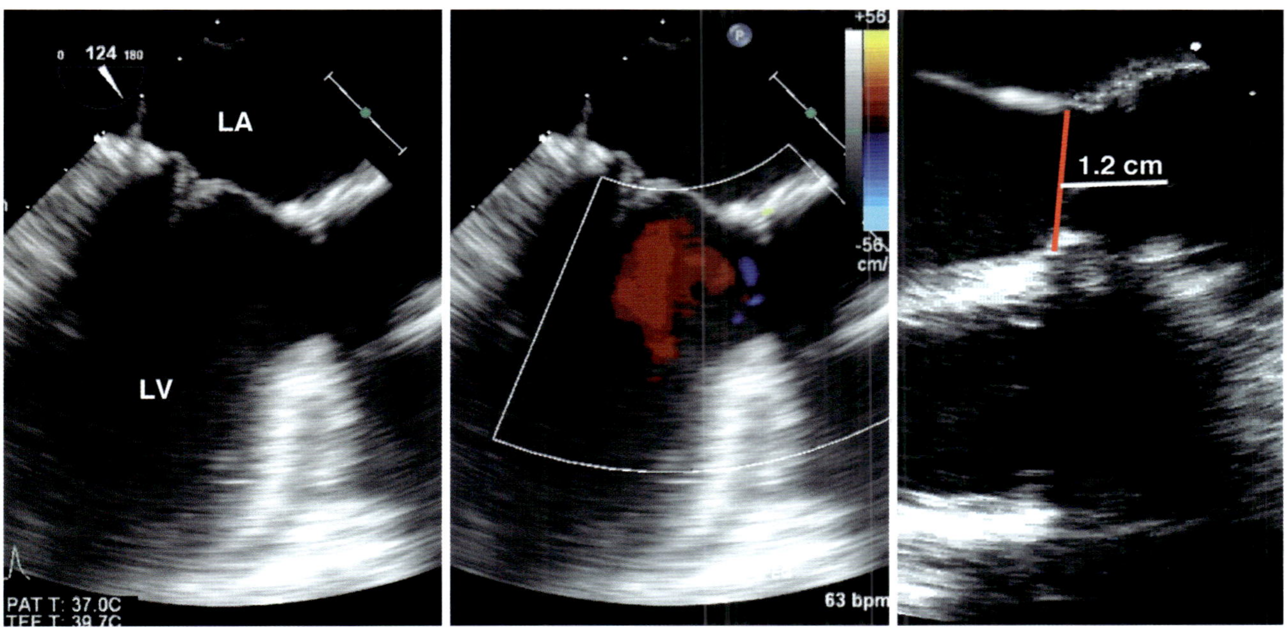

Fig 10.106 Postbypass TEE long-axis images of aortic valve show normal closure in diastole with no aortic regurgitation on color Doppler imaging. Right panel shows coaptation height of 1.2 cm.

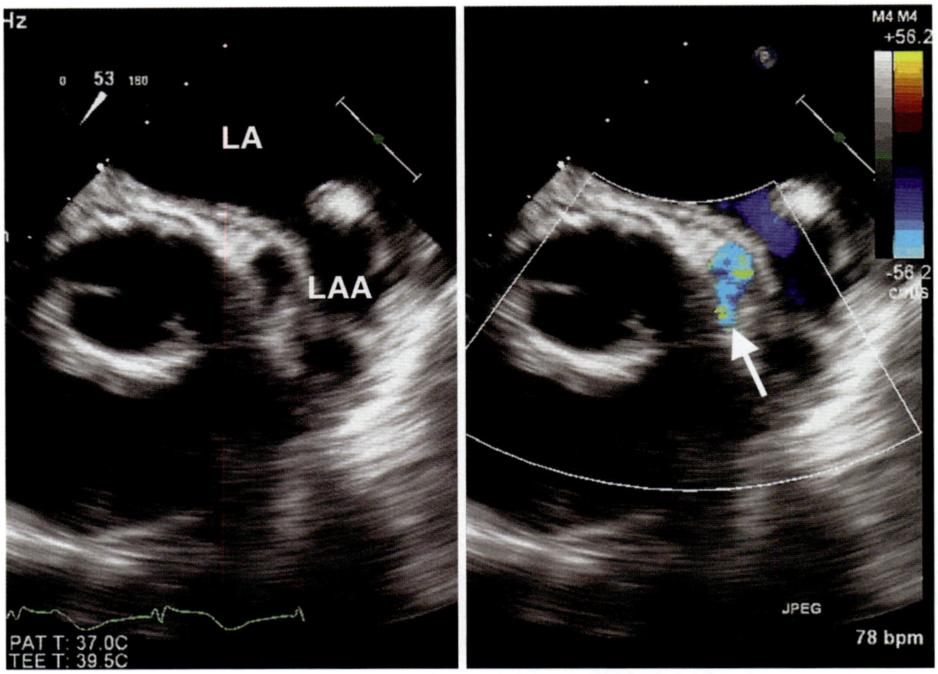

Fig 10.107 Short-axis view of aortic valve at 53 degrees shows trileaflet native valve *(left)* in diastole with no aortic regurgitation. White arrow indicates flow in left coronary artery.

Comments

The pattern of aortic dilation in patients with Marfan syndrome is characterized by loss of the normal contour of the sino-tubular junction with dilation extending form the aortic annulus without interruption into the ascending aorta. Because the genetic defect affects the entire aorta, the surgical procedure includes resection and replacement of the sinuses of Valsalva all the way down to the annulus level. This necessitates reimplantation of the coronary arteries.

When the aortic valve leaflets are abnormal, a valved conduit is used. However, if the aortic valve appears anatomically normal, many surgeons prefer to retain the native aortic valve. The normal relationships of the commissures and leaflets are restored by resuspension of the valve within the aortic conduit. The combination of a smaller diameter at the level of the commissures along with stabilization of the aortic annulus, results in a competent valve and the leaflets are no longer stretched across an enlarged annulus. Because of the redundancy of leaflet tissue, the reimplanted valve often does not look classically trileaflet.

Suggested Reading

1. Van Dyck MJ, Watremez C, Boodhwani M, et al: Transesophageal echocardiographic evaluation during aortic valve repair surgery, Anesth Analg 111:59–70, 2010.
2. Kim TY, Alfirevic A, Wallace LK: Transesophageal echocardiography for tricuspid aortic valve repair, Anesth Analg 110:370–372, 2010.

Pulmonary Artery Pathology

CASE 10-15
Pulmonary Thrombo-Endarterectomy

This 51-year-old man had a 7-year history of dyspnea and was found to have recurrent pulmonary emboli. He had progressive symptoms and a decline in functional status, despite appropriate anticoagulation and placement of an inferior vena cava filter. He now was referred for pulmonary thrombo-embolectomy surgery.

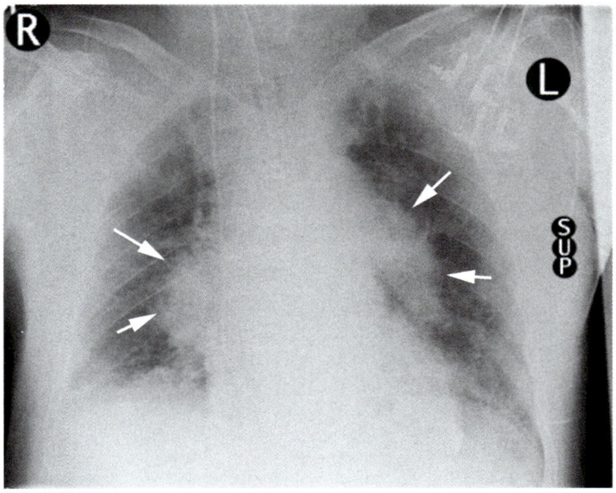

Fig 10.108 Chest radiography shows enlargement of right and left pulmonary arteries consistent with chronic pulmonary hypertension *(arrows)*.

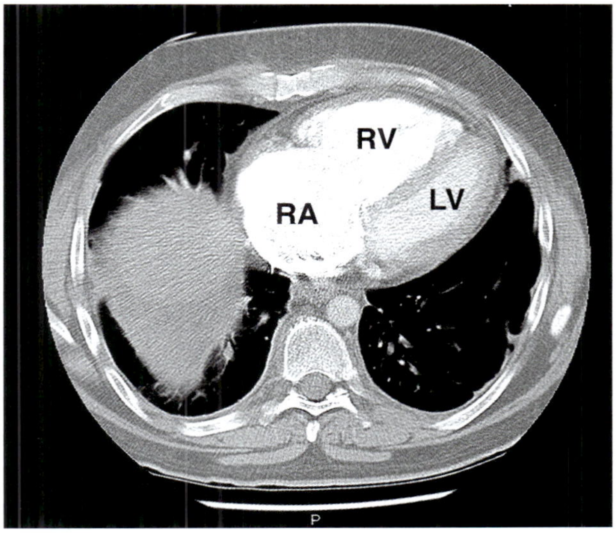

Fig 10.109 Chest CT with contrast at level of ventricles shows severe right ventricular and right atrial enlargement.

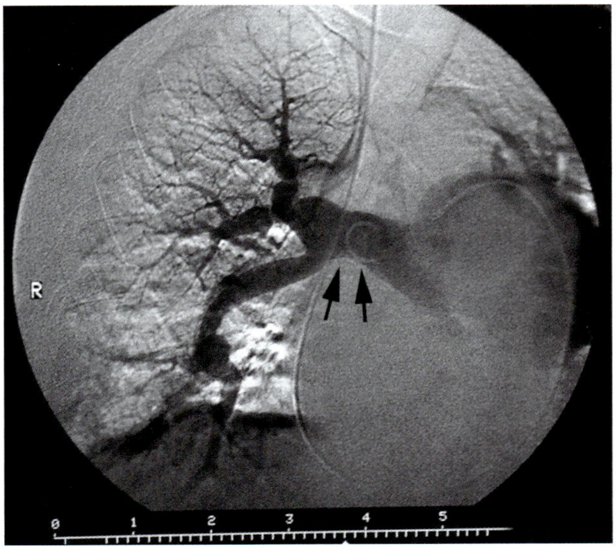

Fig 10.110 Selective right pulmonary angiogram shows irregular contour along inferior aspects of dilated artery *(arrows)* consistent with intraluminal thrombus. Other areas of irregularity and stenosis are seen distally in pulmonary vascular bed.

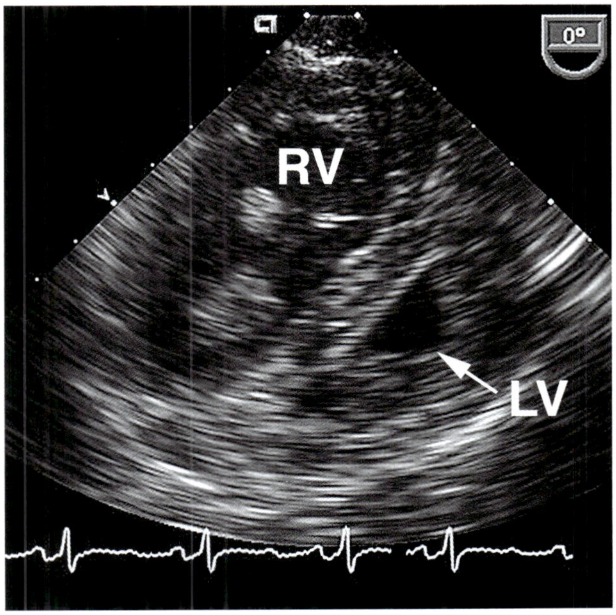

Fig 10.111 Transgastric short-axis view shows severely enlarged and hypokinetic right ventricle with septal flattening consistent with right ventricular pressure and volume overload.

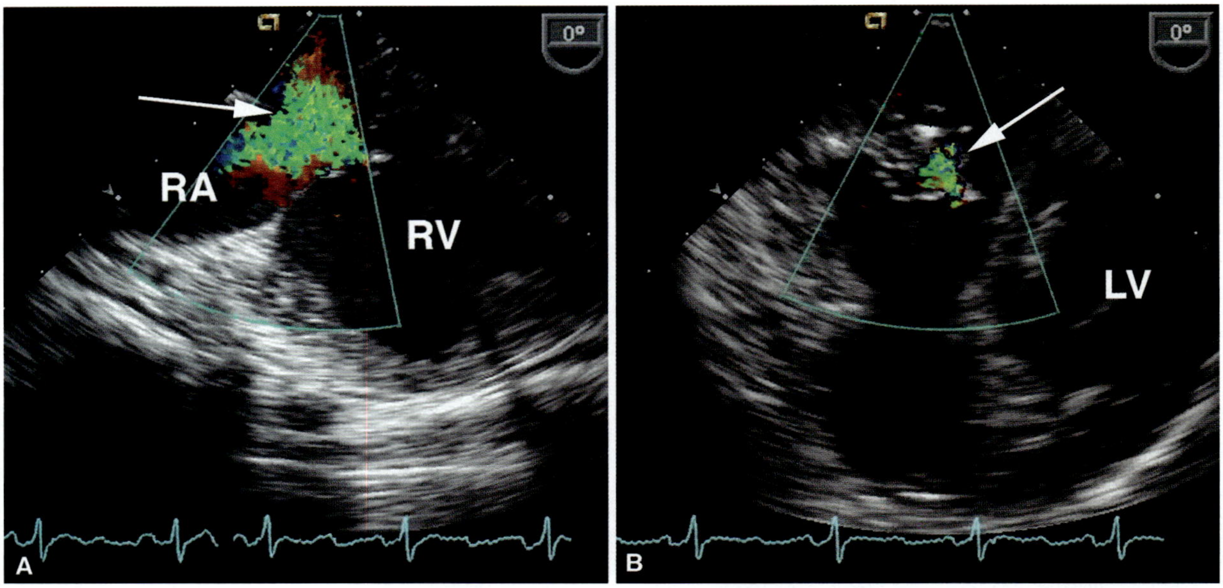

Fig 10.112 View of right ventricle (RV) and right atrium (RA) at zero degrees (**A**) shows moderate tricuspid regurgitation *(arrow)*, in addition to severe right ventricular dilation. Right ventricular free wall is thickened, consistent with long-standing pulmonary hypertension. Transgastric imaging of tricuspid valve in short axis, shows tricuspid regurgitation jet *(arrow)* to be central (**B**).

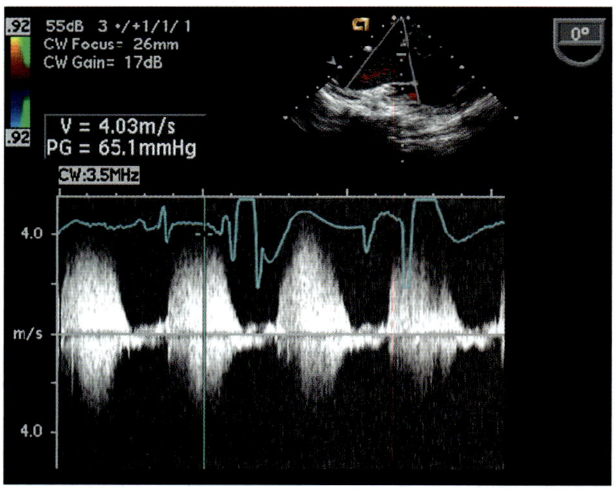

Fig 10.113 Continuous wave Doppler interrogation of tricuspid regurgitation jet shows velocity of 4 m/s. Although this may be underestimated due to nonparallel intercept angle, this velocity indicates right ventricular to right atrial pressure difference of 64 mm Hg in systole. If right atrial pressure is 10 mm Hg, estimated pulmonary artery systolic pressure is 74 mm Hg.

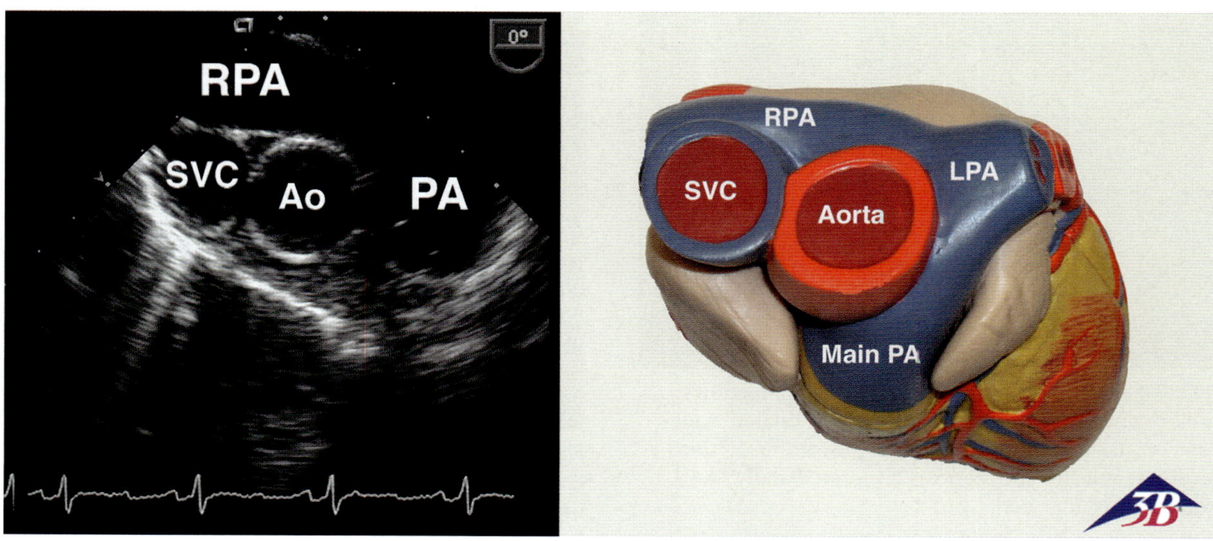

Fig 10.114 High esophageal TEE view at zero degrees in normal subject shows pulmonary artery (PA), right pulmonary artery (RPA), superior vena cava (SVC), and aorta *(left)*. Model shows more detail *(right)*. (Based on Economy Heart Model 3B Scientific®.)

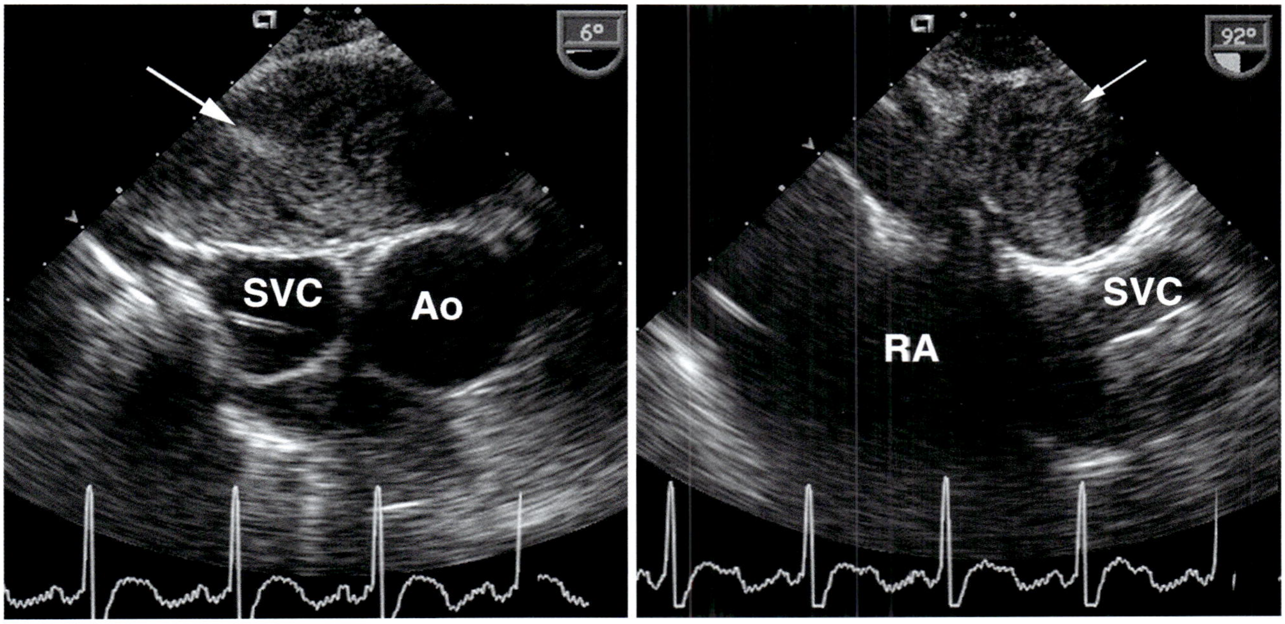

Fig 10.115 In our patient, same TEE view (*left*) as Fig 10.114 shows severely dilated right pulmonary artery with spontaneous contrast *(arrow)* consistent with stasis of blood flow. Catheter is present in superior vena cava (SVC). Rotating image plan to 92 degrees *(right);* similar findings are seen in enlarged right pulmonary artery *(arrow).*

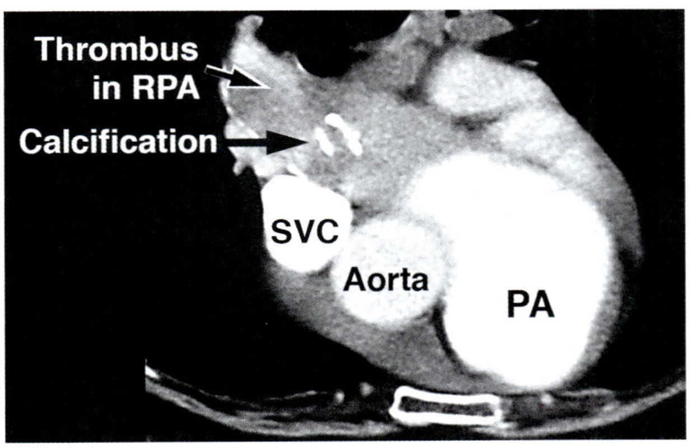

Fig 10.116 CT scan contrast with image oriented to correspond to TEE view in Fig 10.115 shows severe dilated pulmonary artery with chronic thrombus (and calcification) in right pulmonary artery *(arrow).*

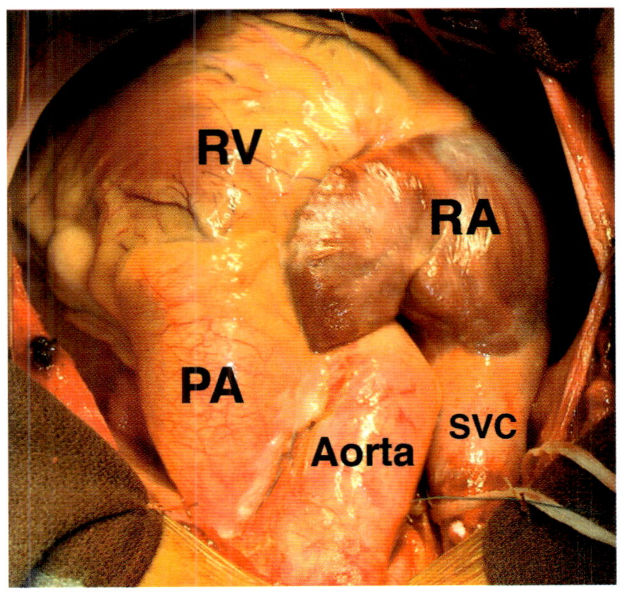

Fig 10.117 Intraoperative view of heart showing relationships between great vessels. All right-sided structures are dilated.

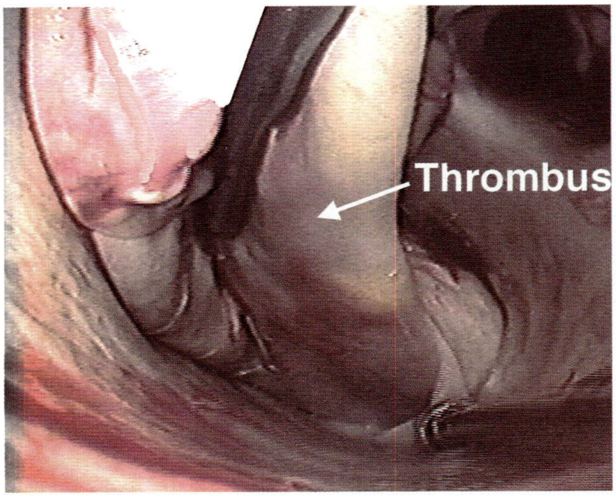

Fig 10.118 With pulmonary artery opened, chronic thrombus was identified and endarterectomy of right pulmonary vascular bed was performed. Left pulmonary artery was also opened and endarterectomy performed.

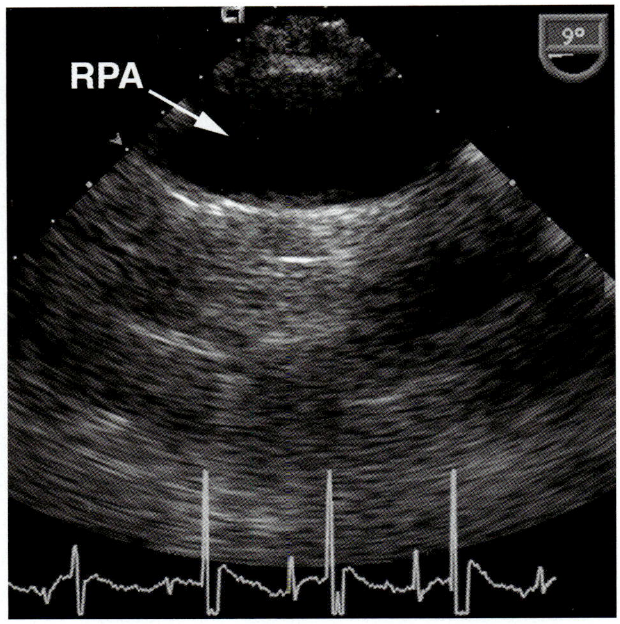

Fig 10.119 TEE view of right pulmonary artery (RPA) after completion of procedure.

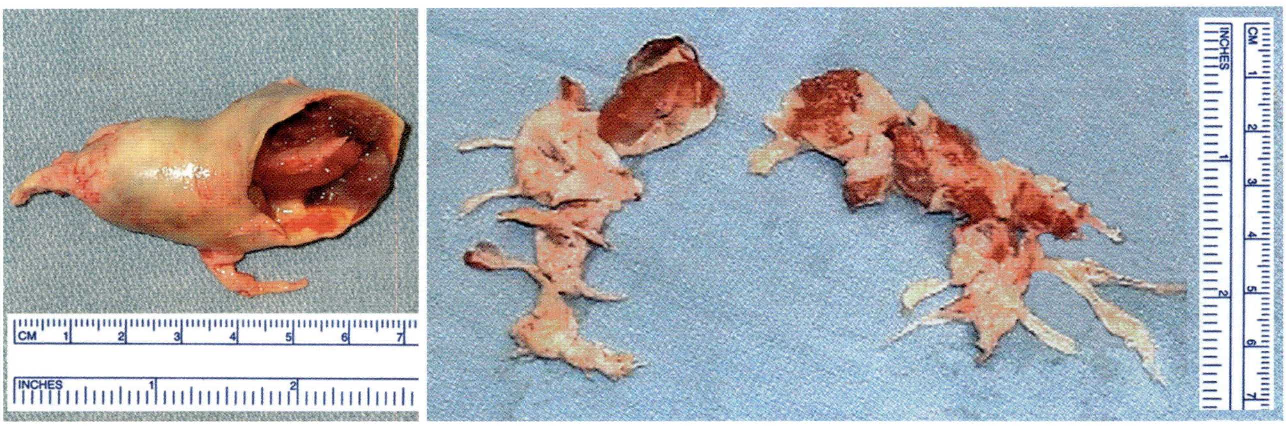

Fig 10.120 Portion of resected thrombus *(left)* corresponding to area seen on TEE imaging. Histologic examination revealed laminated thrombotic material with focal areas of atherosclerosis. At right, "cast" of pulmonary circulation is formed after surgeon lays whole specimen out.

Comments

TEE is not used as a primary diagnostic approach to evaluation of pulmonary embolism. It is unusual to directly visualize thrombi in the pulmonary arteries, even with TEE imaging, although these findings have a high specificity when present, as in this case.

However, echocardiography provides indirect evidence of pulmonary vascular disease and often is the first test to suggest that pulmonary emboli be considered in the differential diagnosis. In patients with pulmonary hypertension, typical findings include right ventricular dilation, hypertrophy, and systolic dysfunction with a characteristic pattern of septal motion toward the right ventricle (instead of toward the center of the left ventricle) in systole. With right sided pressure overload, the reversed contour of the ventricular septum persists in both systole and diastole. In contrast, with right sided volume overload, the reverse curvature of the septum is most prominent in diastole.

Echocardiography provides reliable estimated of pulmonary systolic pressure based on the velocity in the tricuspid regurgitation jet (right ventricular to right atrial systolic pressure difference equals 4 times the tricuspid regurgitant velocity squared) plus the estimated right atrial pressure (based on the size and respiratory variation of the inferior vena cava in spontaneously breathing patients, or by direct measurement of RA pressure in mechanically ventilated patients).

In patients undergoing pulmonary thrombo-endarterectomy, TEE is useful for detection of extrapulmonary thrombi; for example, in the superior or inferior vena cava, the right atrium or right ventricle. Detection of extrapulmonary thrombi altered surgical management in 10% of cases in a surgical series of 50 patients.

Suggested Reading

1. Mediratta A, Addetia K, Medvedofsky D, et al: Echocardiographic diagnosis of acute pulmonary embolism in patients with McConnell's sign, Echocardiography 33:696–702, 2016.
2. Jasudavisius A, Arellano R, Martin J, et al: A systematic review of transthoracic and transesophageal echocardiography in noncardiac surgery: implications for point-of-care ultrasound education in the operating room, Can J Anaesth 63:480–487, 2016.

CASE 10-16
Two Cases of Pulmonary Artery Donor–Recipient Mismatch after Orthotopic Heart Transplantation

1. Anastomotic stenosis. This 51-year-old women with Class III/IV heart failure due to restrictive cardiomyopathy underwent heart transplantation. However, when attempting to wean from cardiopulmonary bypass, she was noted to have a right ventricular pressure of 70/40 mm Hg and the right heart catheter could not be advanced into the pulmonary artery.

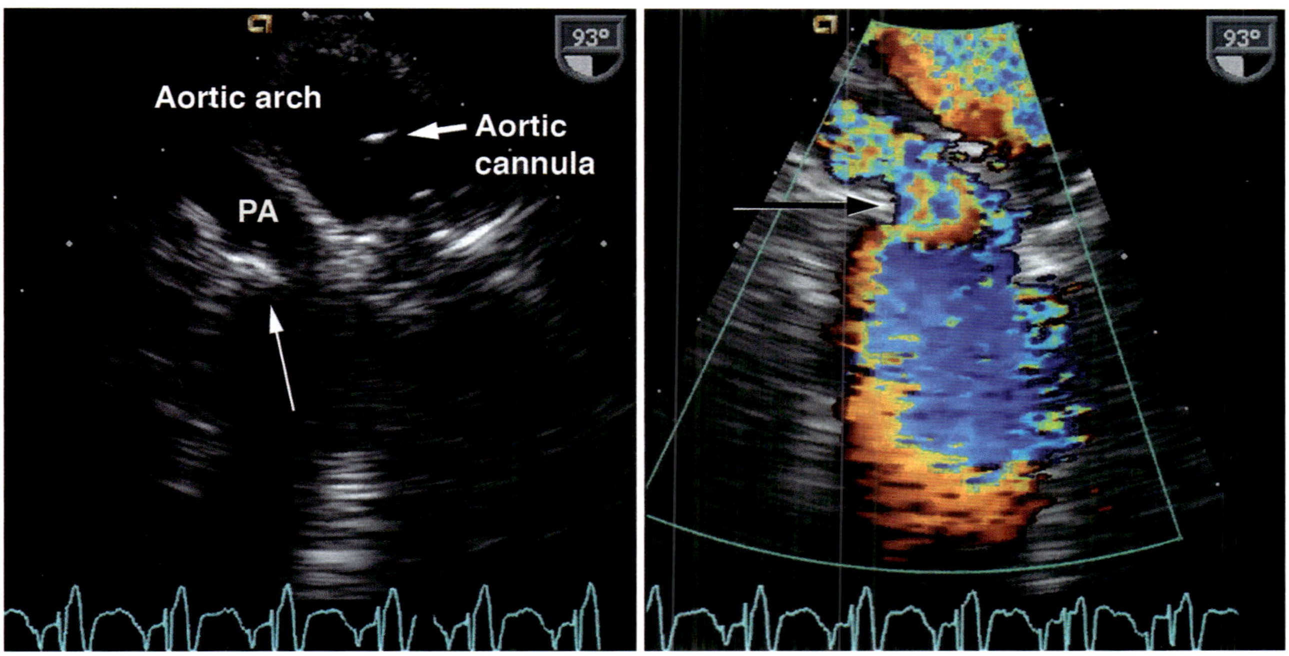

Fig 10.121 In this high esophageal view, posterior ridge at pulmonary artery (PA) anastomosis is seen *(left, arrow)*, causing narrowing of main pulmonary artery. Color Doppler shows increase in velocity at ridge level *(right, arrow)*.

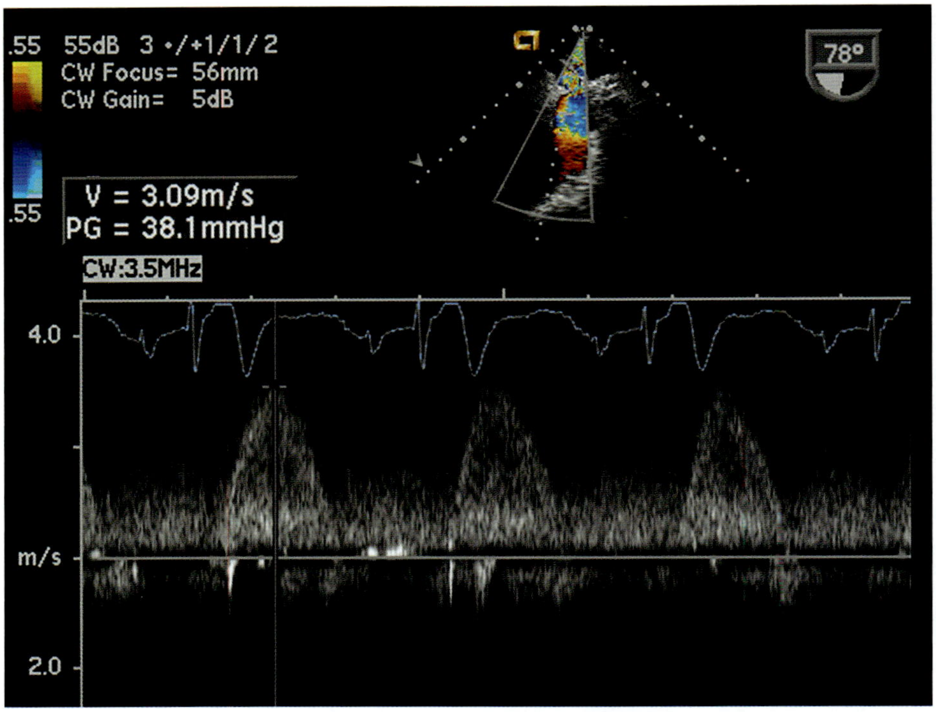

Fig 10.122 Continuous wave Doppler shows velocity of 3.1 m/s across pulmonary artery anastomosis, consistent with maximum systolic gradient of 38 mm Hg.

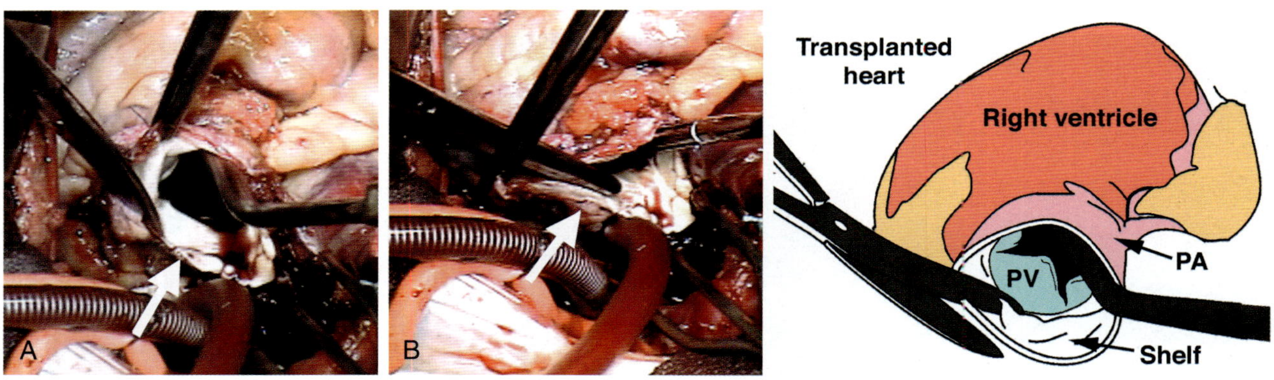

Fig 10.123 At surgery, after reopening PA anastomosis, pulmonic valve was normal but posterior shelf of tissue was distorting shape of pulmonary artery (*arrow*, **A**). After this tissue was removed (*arrow*, **B**), right ventricular pressures were normal as cardiopulmonary bypass was weaned. Illustration demonstrates resection of shelf.

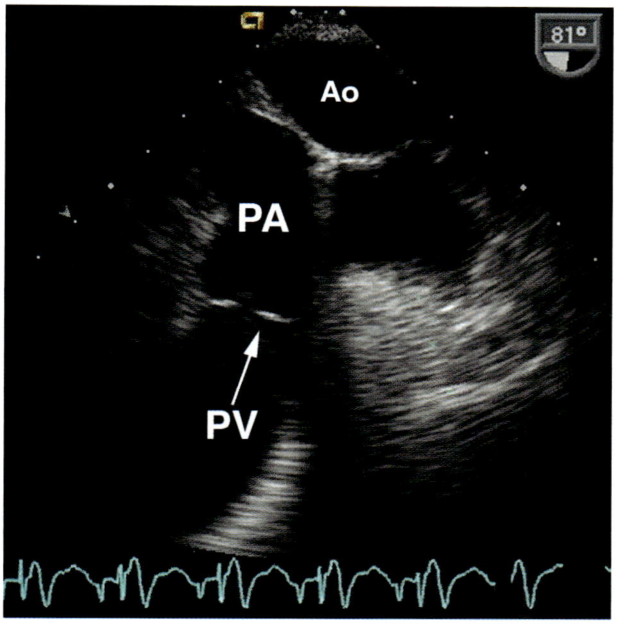

Fig 10.124 After surgical repair, same view as Fig 10.121 shows normal diameter of pulmonary artery.

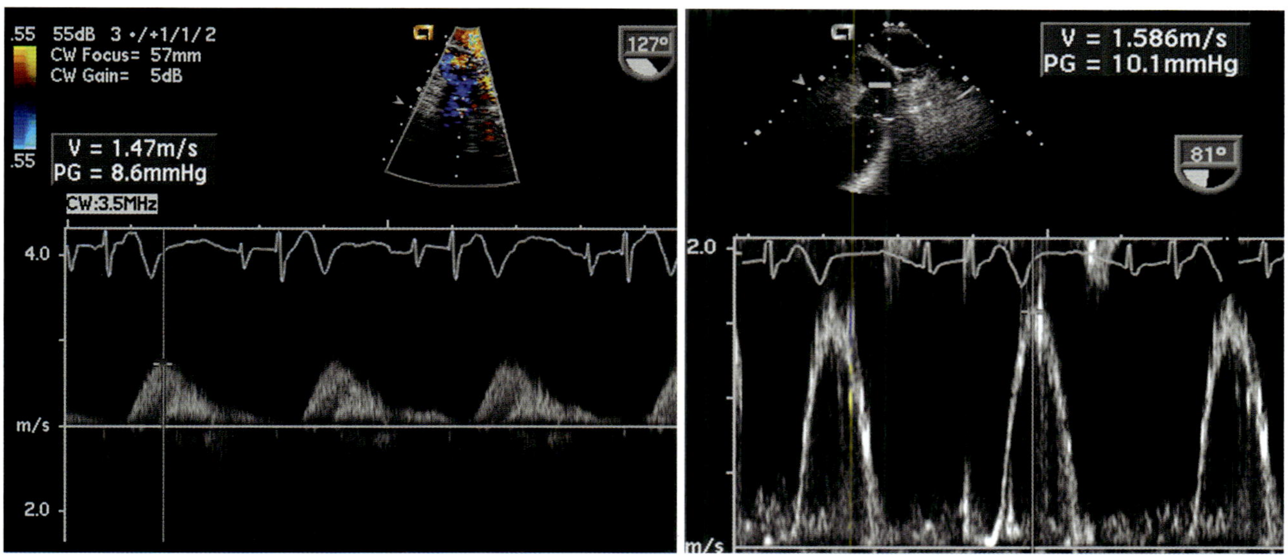

Fig 10.125 Continuous wave Doppler recordings confirm velocity of 1.5 m/s. Pulsed Doppler interrogation of pulmonary artery flow at anastomotic site shows laminar flow signal with maximum velocity of only 1.6 m/s.

2. Pulmonic regurgitation. This is a 47-year-old male who had undergone an orthotopic heart transplant 1 week previously. He had a clinically uneventful perioperative course; however, on serial echo imaging, he was noted to have severe pulmonic regurgitation. Because of the poor long-term prognosis of this finding, he was brought to the OR for exploration, and possible repair or replacement of his pulmonic valve. The valve was carefully examined and there was no evidence of perforation and the leaflets all appeared healthy. Because the length of the anastomosis was slightly long, 5 mm was circumferentially trimmed from both the donor and recipient ends. The donor pulmonary artery was reoriented about 20 degrees counterclockwise from its previous location. The patient was weaned from cardiopulmonary bypass without difficulty.

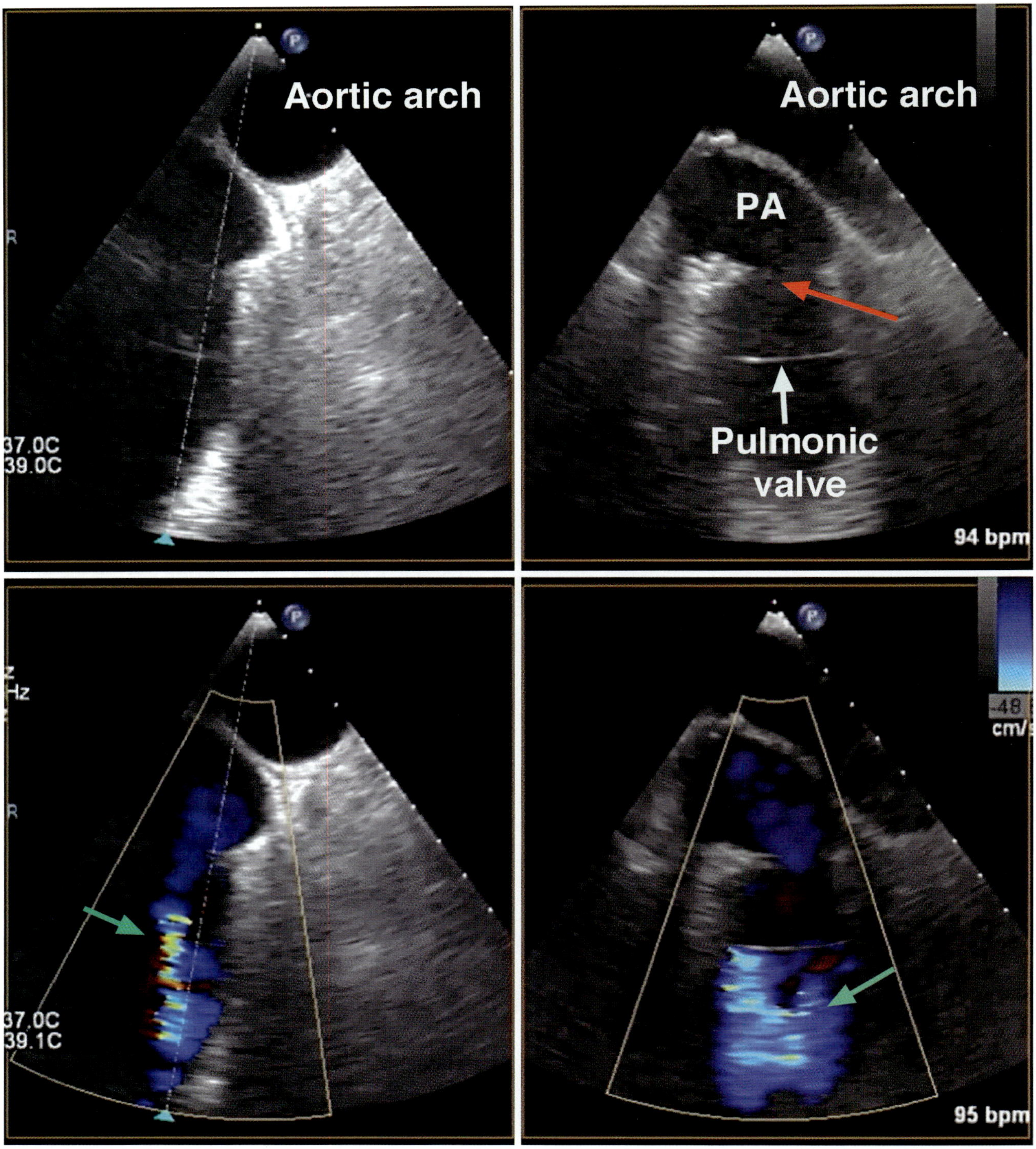

Fig 10.126 In this four-quadrant image, biplane imaging from high esophageal view shows what appears to be narrowing of anastomotic site *(red arrow)*. Pulmonic valve appears structurally normal; however, there is significant pulmonic regurgitation by color Doppler *(green arrow)*.

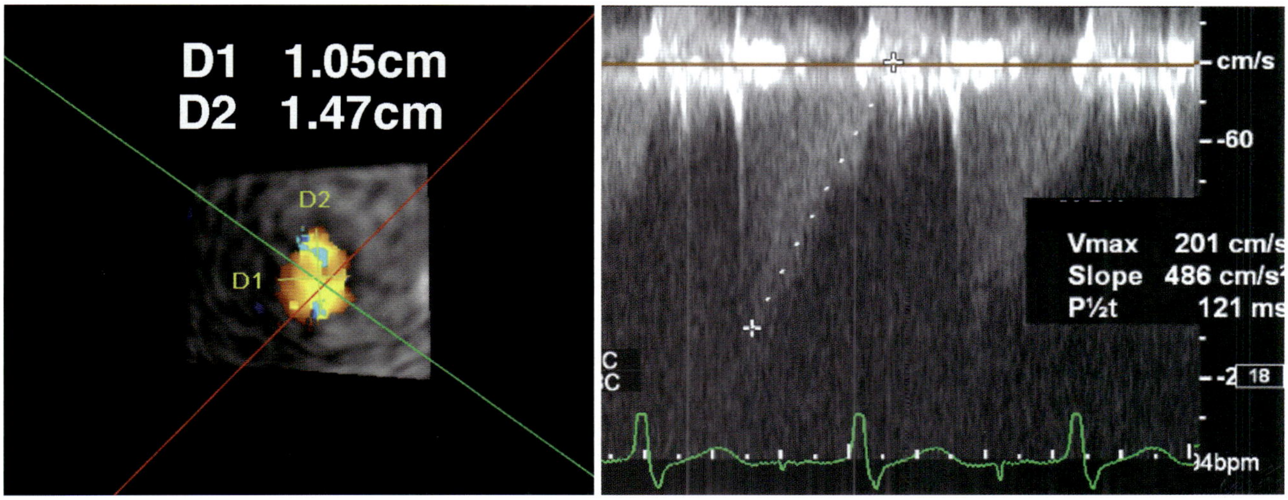

Fig 10.127 Using multiplanar reconstruction, vena contracta measured 1.05 cm by 1.47 cm. Pressure half-time of pulmonic regurgitation jet is 121 msec.

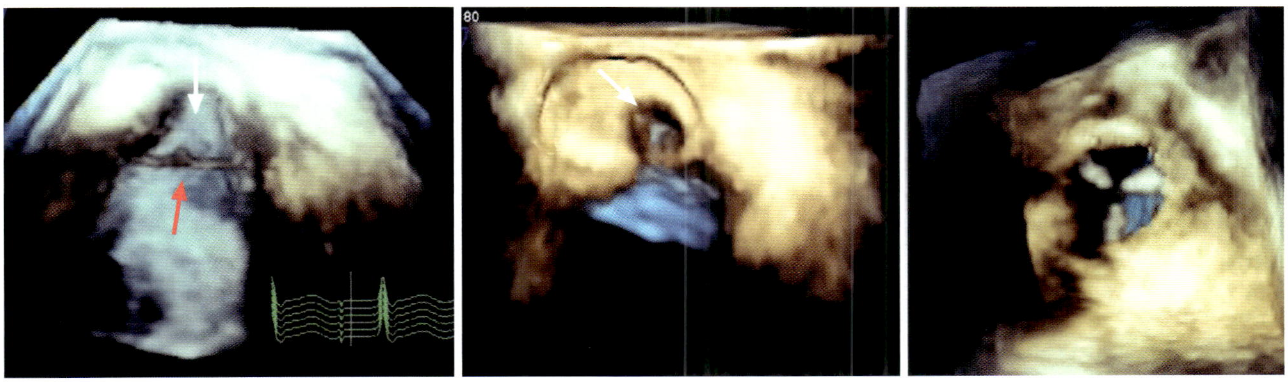

Fig 10.128 High esophageal 3D imaging with anterior aspect of pulmonary artery cropped away shows normal appearing pulmonic valve *(red arrow)* and anastomotic site *(white arrow)* that appears narrowed *(left)*. In center image, anastomotic site is examined from superior vantage point. Cropping farther down shows trileaflet pulmonic valve that appears symmetrically closed in diastole.

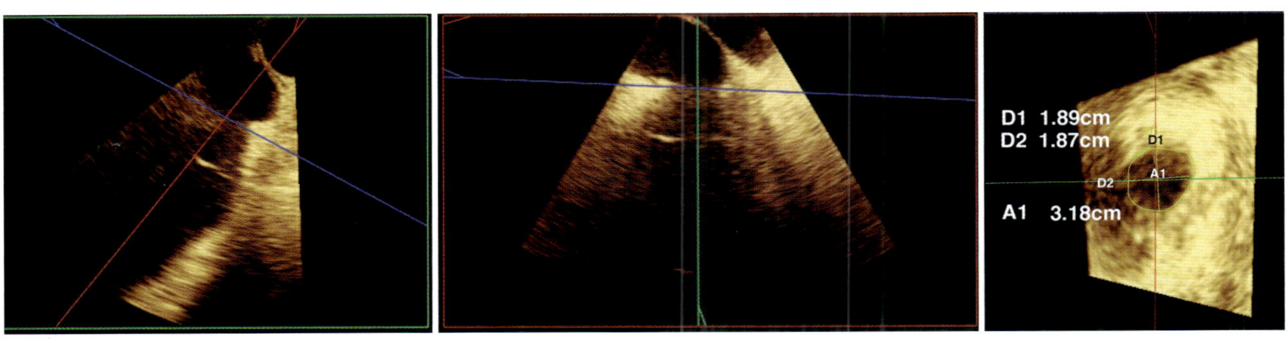

Fig 10.129 Multiplanar reconstruction of anatomic site shows diameters of 1.89 cm and 1.87 cm, with area of 3.18 cm^2. Diameter of pulmonic annulus was 3.22 cm.

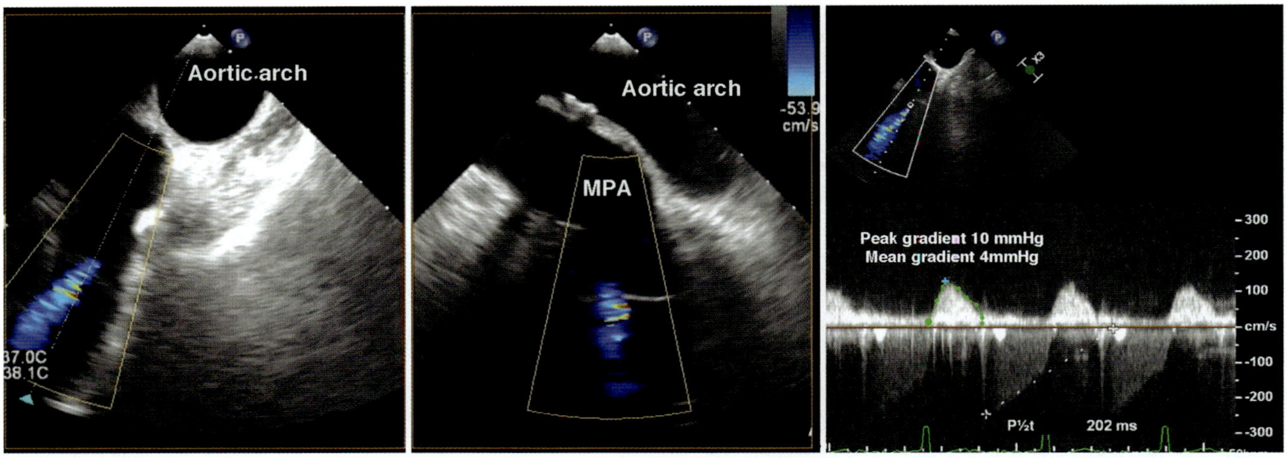

Fig 10.130 The narrowed anastomosis was revised. Postbypass biplane imaging shows reduced amount of pulmonic regurgitation, now with vena contracta of 0.3 cm, and pressure half-time of 202 msec. Peak and mean systolic gradients are not different than preoperative measurements.

Comments

In both these patients, the pliable pulmonary artery had normal flow immediately after the transplant procedure. However, in the first case, when the chest wall was closed, the pulmonary artery was pushed posteriorly against a ridge of tissue resulting in apparent pulmonary artery obstruction with a high antegrade flow velocity, and pressure gradient. In the second case, closing the chest wall resulted in distortion of the normal pulmonic valve anatomy resulting in inadequate leaflet coaptation and severe pulmonic regurgitation. On reoperation, in the first case, removal of the tissue ridge relieved pulmonary artery obstruction. In the second case, resection of the excess length of the pulmonary artery allowed normal pulmonic leaflet motion with resolution of regurgitation. The possibility of extrinsic compression causing distortion of normal valve anatomy or pseudostenosis should be considered when there is an acute change in hemodynamics, either stenosis or regurgitation, particularly in the immediate perioperative period.

Suggested Reading

1. Wu AH, Kolias TJ: Cardiac transplantation: pre- and posttransplant evaluation. In Otto CM, editor: The practice of clinical echocardiography, ed 5, Philadelphia 2016, Elsevier.

11 Masses

Normal variants

Case 11-1 Left atrial appendage
Case 11-2 Eustachian valve
Case 11-3 Lipomatous hypertrophy of the interatrial septum
Case 11-4 Spinal cord
Case 11-5 Lambl's excrescence

Thrombi

Case 11-6 Left atrial appendage thrombus
Case 11-7 Left ventricular thrombus

Primary cardiac tumors

Case 11-8 Pulmonic valve mass
Case 11-9 Aortic valve fibroelastoma
Case 11-10 Atrial myxoma
Case 11-11 Obstruction of LV filling by myxoma
Case 11-12 Pulmonary artery leiomyosarcoma
Case 11-13 Angiosarcoma

Secondary tumors

Case 11-14 Renal cell carcinoma with extension to right atrium
Case 11-15 Renal cell carcinoma with tumor embolization to pulmonary artery
Case 11-16 Right ventricular melanoma

Pleural Effusion

Case 11-17 Left and right pleural effusions

Normal Variants

CASE 11-1
Left Atrial Appendage

TEE is often requested before electrical cardioversion or catheter ablation for atrial fibrillation to evaluate the left atrial appendage for the presence of thrombus. Adequate visualization of the atrial appendage requires at least two orthogonal views, using a high-frequency (5 MHz or higher) transducer and with the image zoomed to show the appendage anatomy. This case shows normal views of the left atrial appendage in a patient undergoing coronary artery bypass grafting surgery.

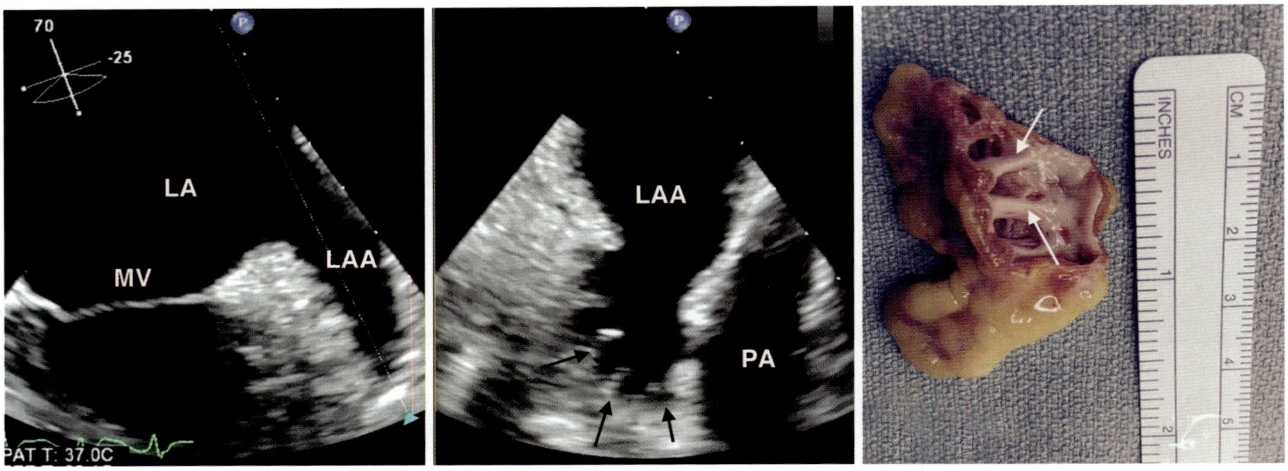

Fig 11.1 In this midesophageal biplane view, atrial appendage is visualized in two-chamber plane *(left)* with mitral valve obliquely cut. Note normal curved triangular shape of atrial appendage. Using biplane mode, line for second image plane is aligned in center of atrial appendage to show orthogonal view *(middle panel)*. In far right image, normal left atrial appendage has been opened. White arrows (as well as *black arrows in middle TEE image*) indicate normal pectinate muscles or trabeculations; it is important to recognize normal variation in size and appearance of these so as not to mistake them for atrial thrombi.

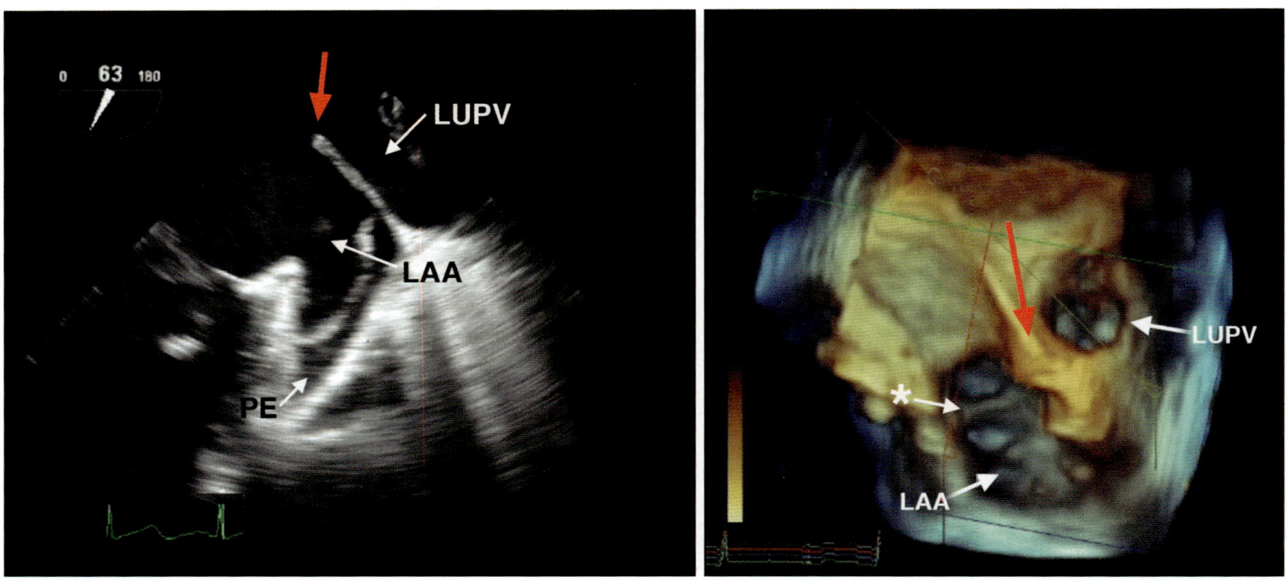

Fig 11.2 With probe rotated to patient's left side, left upper pulmonary vein as well as prominent ridge of tissue between appendage and left upper pulmonary vein *(red arrows)* are seen. This ridge can be very prominent in some patients and may cause reverberation artifacts that might be mistaken for thrombus in appendage. Small pericardial effusion (PE) around lateral wall of appendage is noted. In right frame, corresponding 3D image is seen; in video, appendage is noted to be fibrillating. Asterisk indicates pectinate muscle.

CASE 11-2
Eustachian Valve

In a patient undergoing cardiopulmonary bypass, baseline echocardiographic images were obtained before cannulation of the inferior vena cava via the right atrium.

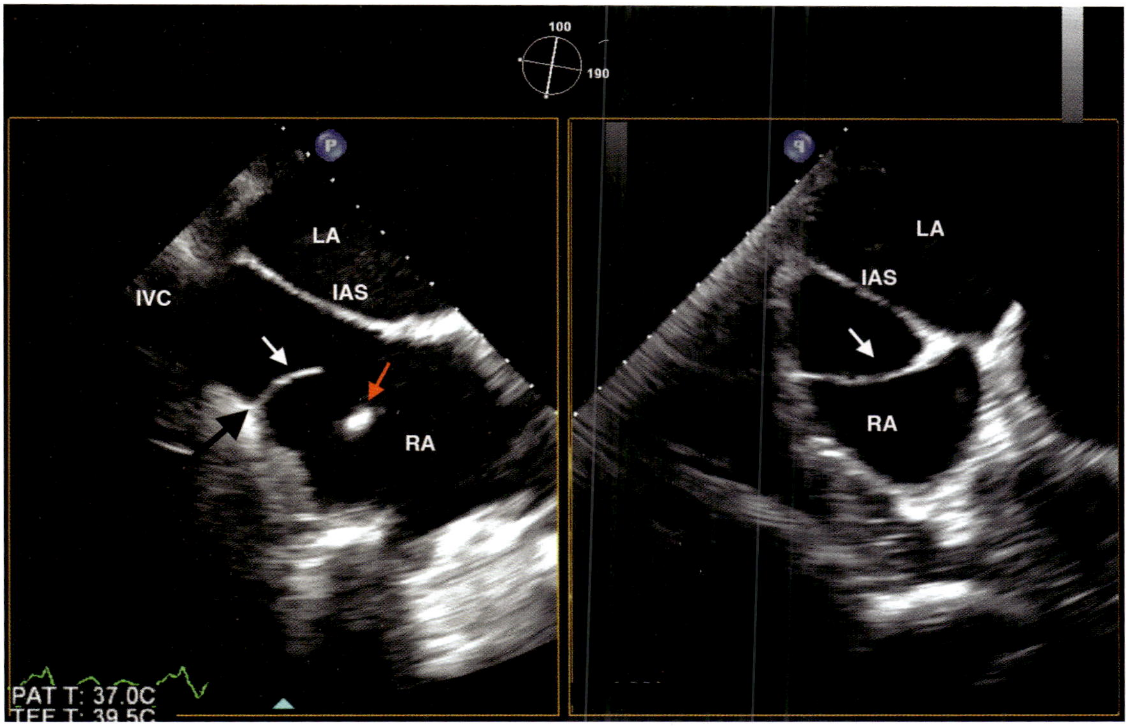

Fig 11.3 In TEE bicaval view *(left)* with transducer advanced toward gastroesophageal junction, a view of the IVC is obtained with better visualization of the Eustachian valve *(black arrow)* originating at the IVC-RA junction and extending into the right atrium; the linear strand *(white arrow)* extending from the valve is part of the Chiari network. With biplane imaging *(right)*, the Chiari network *(white arrow)* is seen to traverse right atrium, joining Eustachian valve on the left to Thebesian valve (valve of coronary sinus) on the right. Red arrow indicates pacing wire in right atrium.

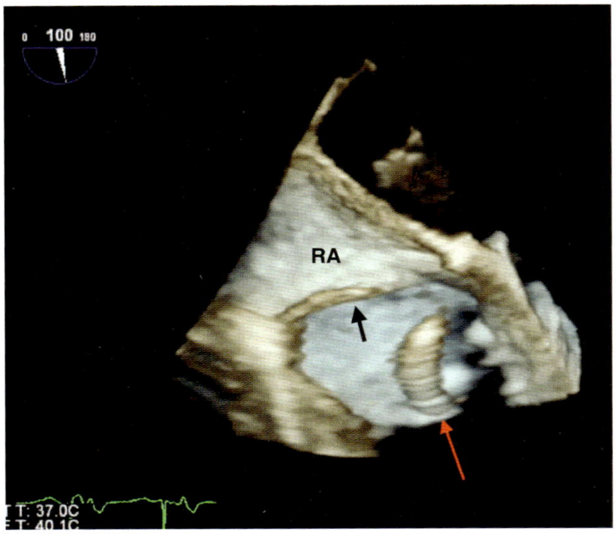

Fig 11.4 3D TEE imaging shows Chiari network and Eustachian valve in greater detail *(black arrow)*. Pacing wire *(red arrow)* is seen coming into RA from inferior vena cava.

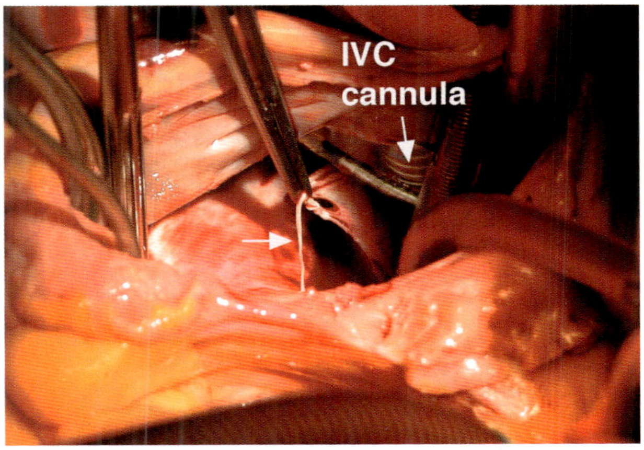

Fig 11.5 In intraoperative photograph from different patient, right atrium has been opened for placement of IVC cannula. Forceps are grasping edge of Eustachian valve and portion of Chiari network *(arrow)* is also seen. IVC = inferior vena cava.

CASE 11-3
Lipomatous Hypertrophy of the Interatrial Septum

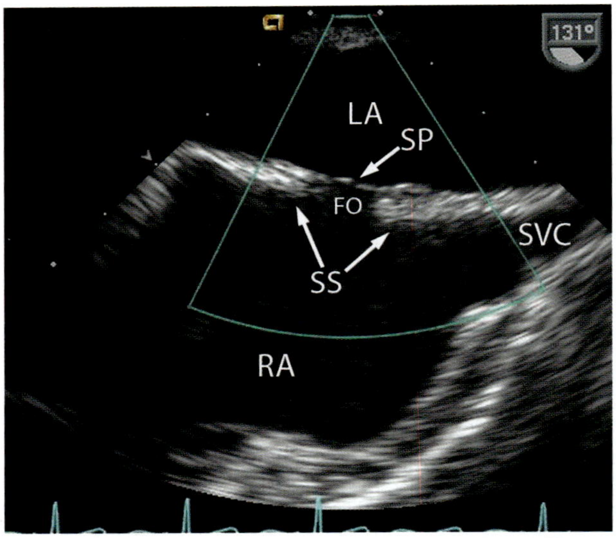

Fig 11.6 This bicaval view shows normal relationships of interatrial septum. In center are septum primum (SP), fossa ovalis (FO), and septum secundam (SS). SVC = superior vena cava.

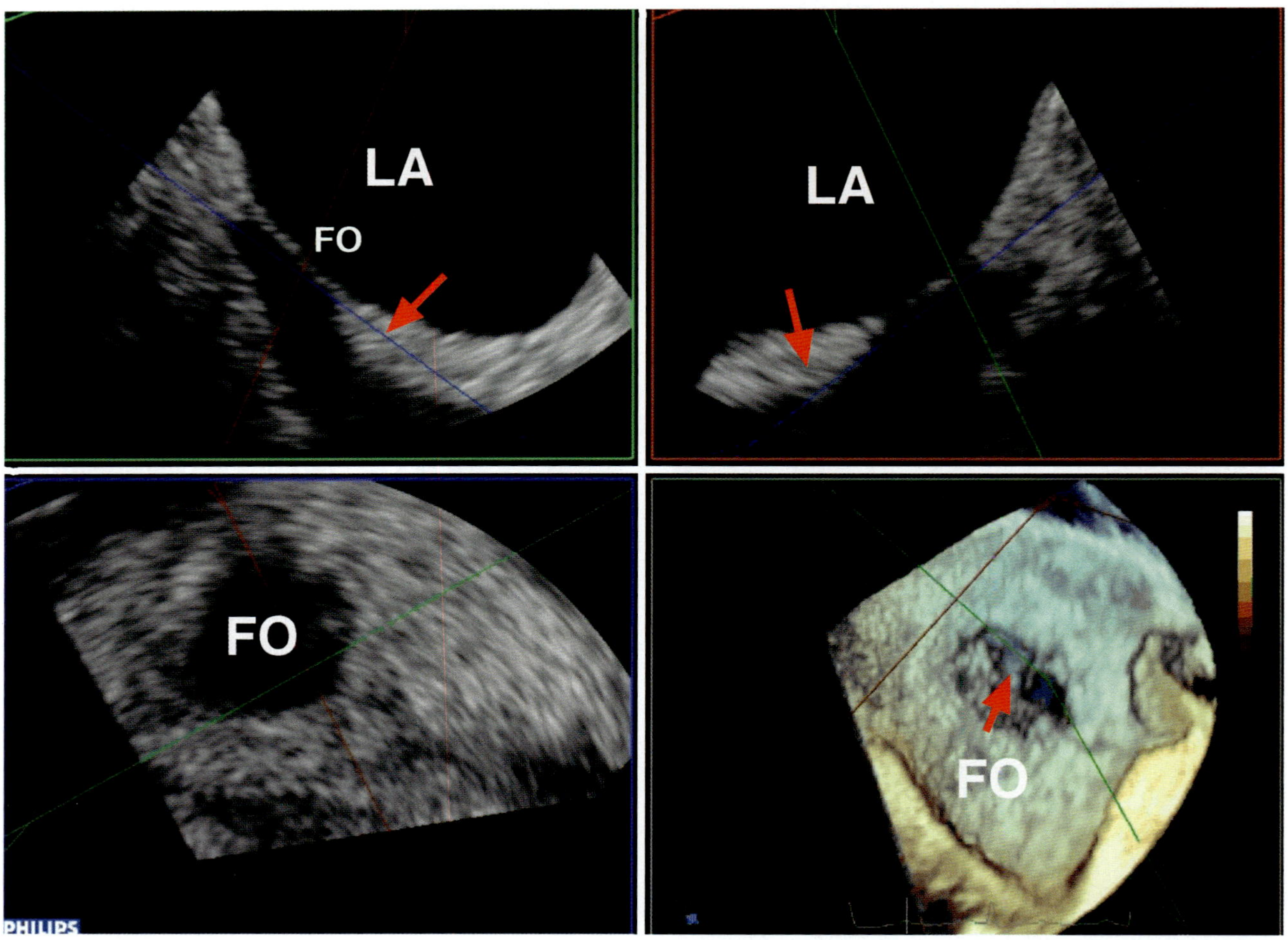

Fig 11.7 This multiplanar reconstruction shows increase width of septum secundum, most likely from fatty deposition. Fat is not actually infiltrating septum, but occupies space where during embryogenesis superior part of common atrium invaginates, forming septum secundum. (From Anderson RH, Brown NA, Webb S: Development and structure of atrial septum. Heart 88:104–110, 2002.) In top two orthogonal images, red arrows indicate fatty deposition, whereas in 3D image seen from left atrial perspective *(bottom right)*, red arrow indicates fossa ovalis, which is somewhat circular as seen in bottom left image.

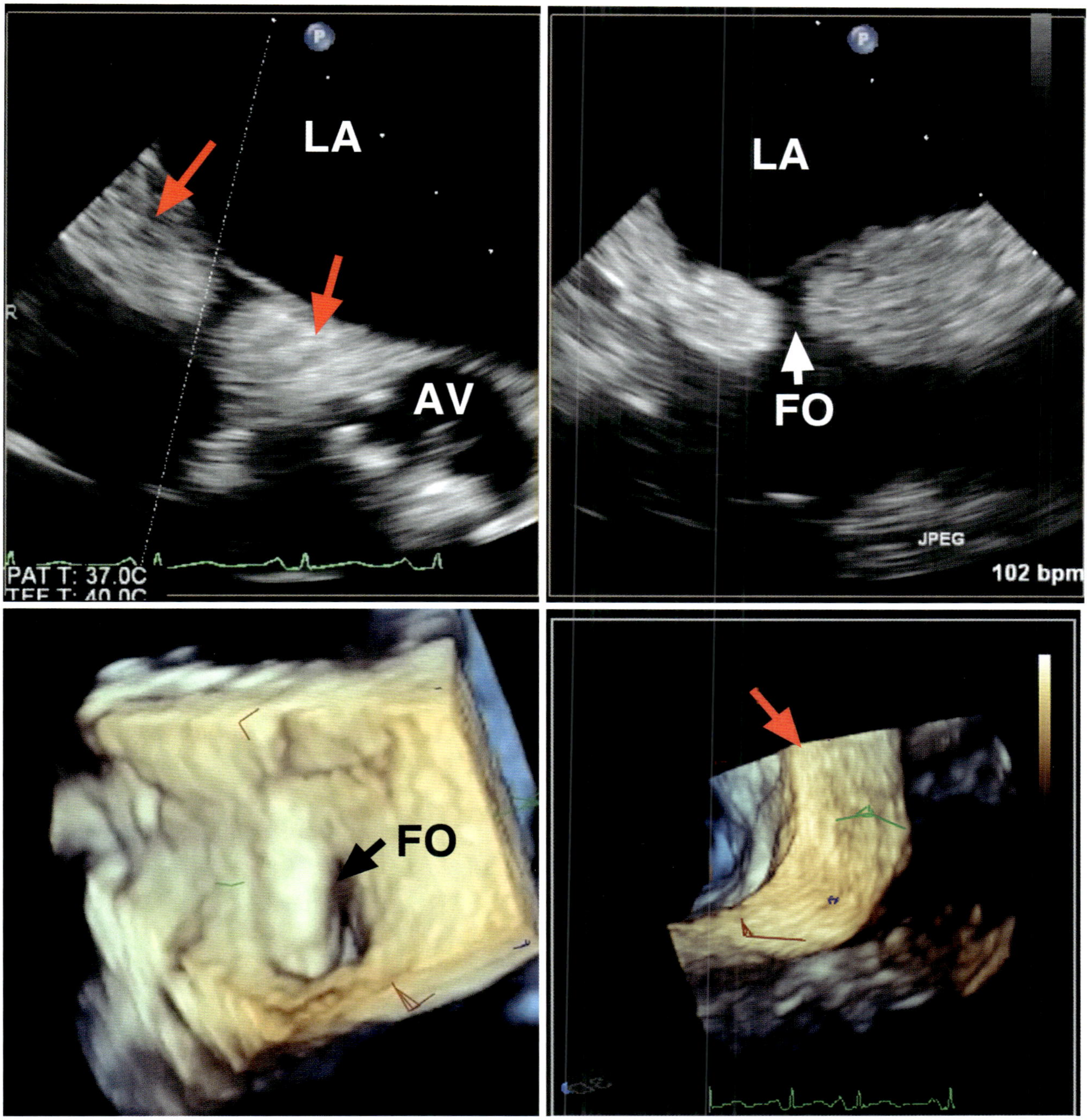

Fig 11.8 In this patient who presented for TAVR, fatty deposition was more pronounced *(red arrows),* and fossa ovalis is more slit-like in appearance. Bottom right image was obtained by rotating bottom left image counterclockwise along its horizontal axis.

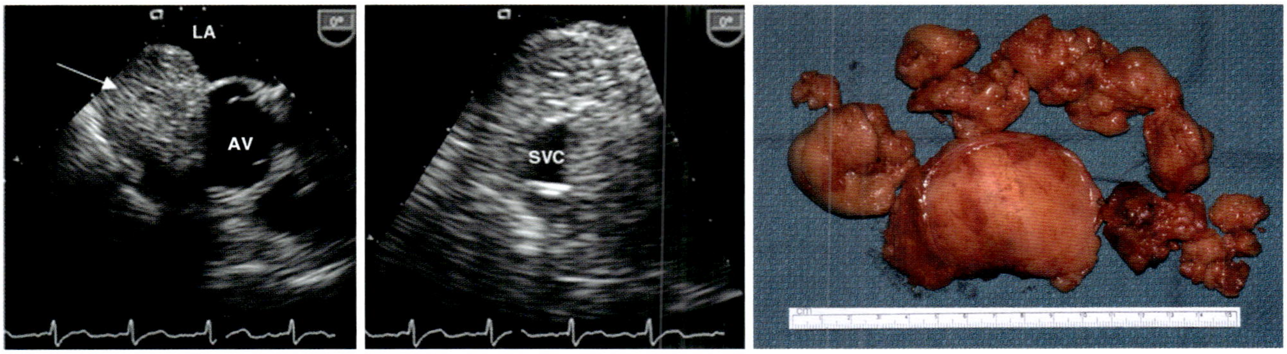

Fig 11.9 This patient had massive deposition of fat that extended cephalad to envelop SVC, and produce venous congestion of head and neck. At surgery, large amounts of fat were excised and atrial septum reconstructed.

CASE 11-4
Spinal Cord

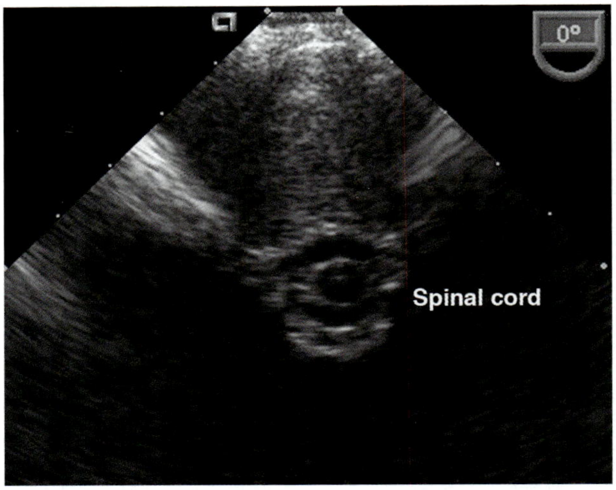

Fig 11.10 With TEE probe rotated posteriorly to image descending thoracic aorta, spinal cord may be seen and should not be mistaken for abnormal finding.

CASE 11-5
Lambl's Excrescence

This 71-year-old woman presented for aortic valve replacement because of severe aortic insufficiency.

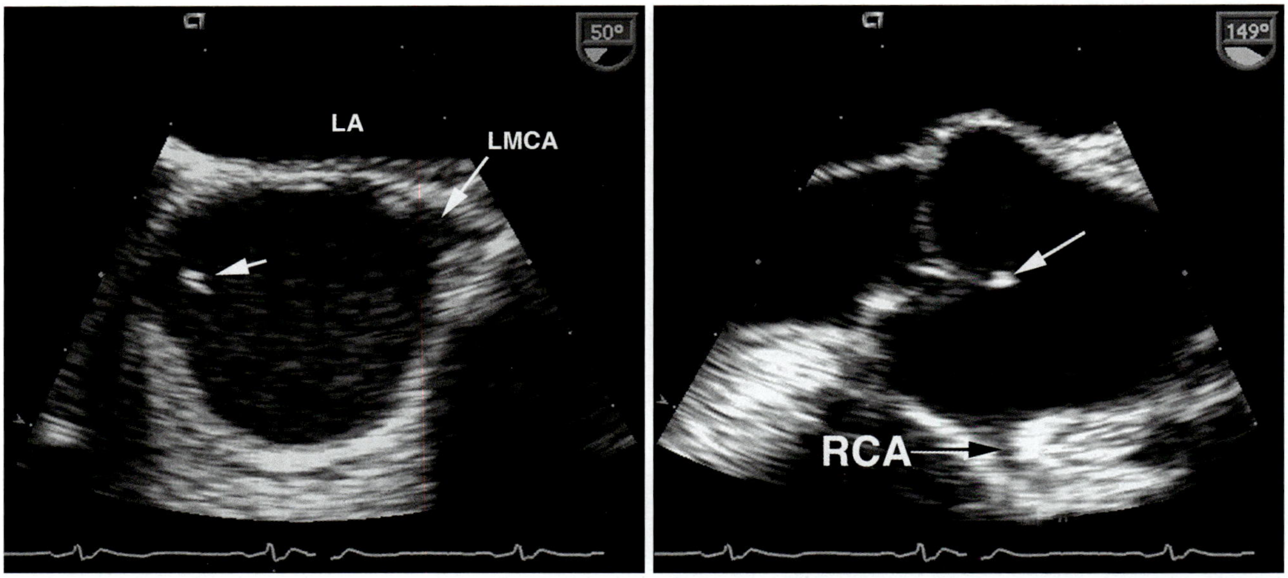

Fig 11.11 Preoperative TEE in long- and short-axis views revealed small mobile density *(arrows)* approximately 3 mm in diameter, which appeared to be attached to edge of a valve leaflet.

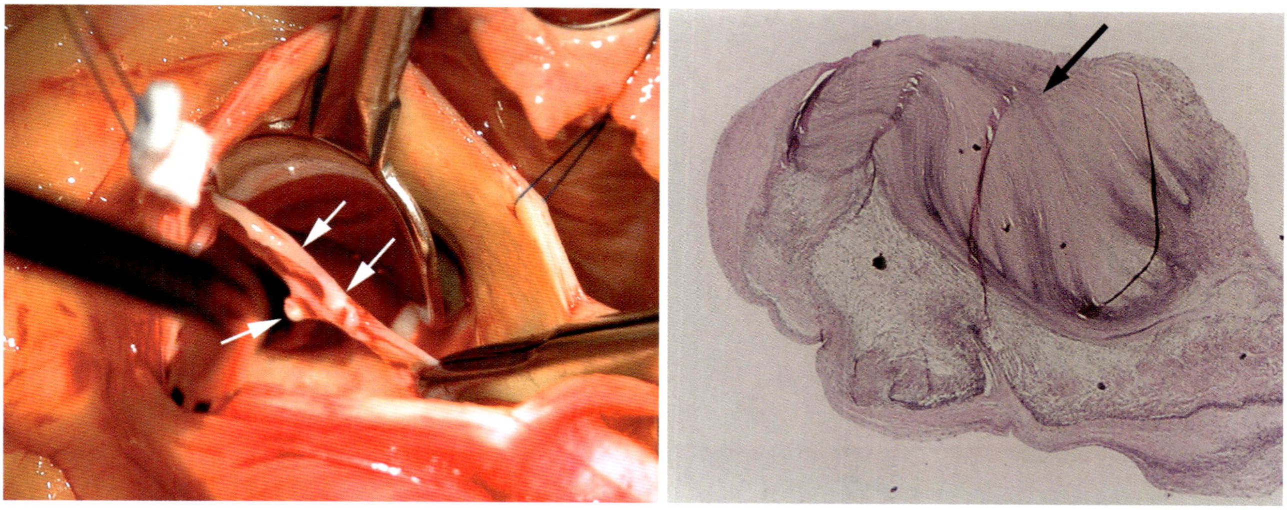

Fig 11.12 In left panel, double arrow indicates noncoronary cusp of aortic valve. Single arrow indicates mass seen on TEE. Microscopic examination *(right panel)* of one of aortic leaflets shows fibroelastic thickening of free edge, with sheets of fibroelastic tissue *(arrow)*, consistent with long-standing aortic regurgitation.

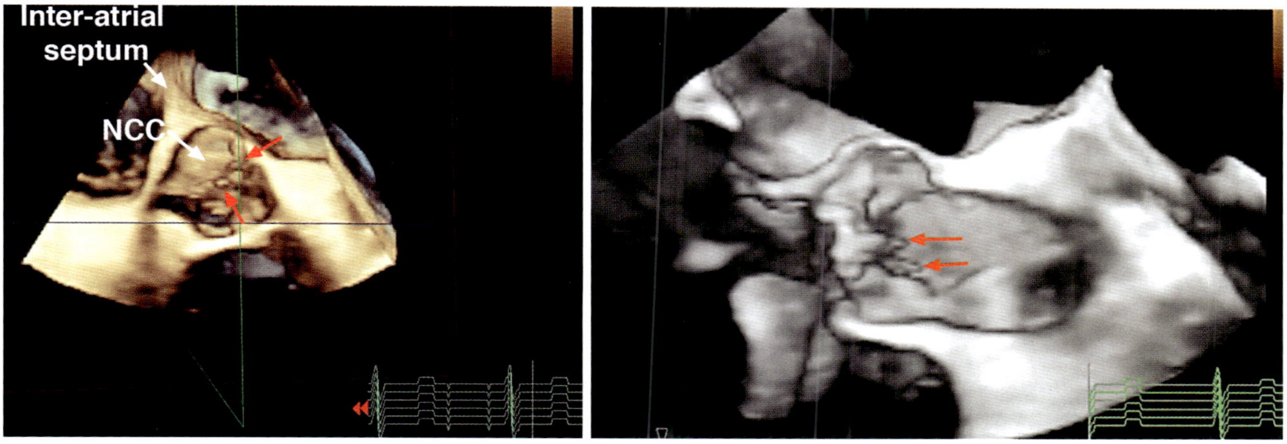

Fig 11.13 In this 3D TEE, short axis of aortic valve from aortic perspective *(left)* and long axis *(right)*, shows calcified valve, with red arrows indicating excrescences. In real time, their mobility is appreciated.

Comments

Small valve strands that microscopically are fibroelastic tissue are normal components of the aortic and mitral valve that increase in frequency with age. These small strands, often called Lambl's excrescence, appear as small, linear mobile echoes that are most often attached to the upstream side of the valve (ventricular side of the aortic and atrial side of the mitral valve). However, they are also seen attached to the nodules of Arantius at the tip of the valve cusps, on the aortic side of the valve, as in this case. The clinical importance of valve strands is unclear, with some studies suggesting an association with stroke but other data suggesting that these are an incidental finding associated with age but without clinical consequences.

Suggested Reading

1. Leitman M, Tyomkin V, Peleg E, et al: Clinical significance and prevalence of valvular strands during routine echo examinations, Eur Heart J Cardiovasc Imaging 15(11):1226–1230, 2014.
2. Jaffe W, Figueredo VM: An example of Lambl's excrescences by transesophageal echocardiogram: a commonly misinterpreted lesion, Echocardiography 24(10):1086–1089, 2007.

Thrombi

CASE 11-6
Left Atrial Appendage Thrombus

This 42-year-old woman was diagnosed with rheumatic heart disease as a child and at the age of 16 had an open mitral valvotomy via thoracotomy. She had been relatively well, but recently became more symptomatic, and was found to have severe mitral stenosis She was referred for mitral valve replacement with a concurrent maze procedure to treat atrial fibrillation.

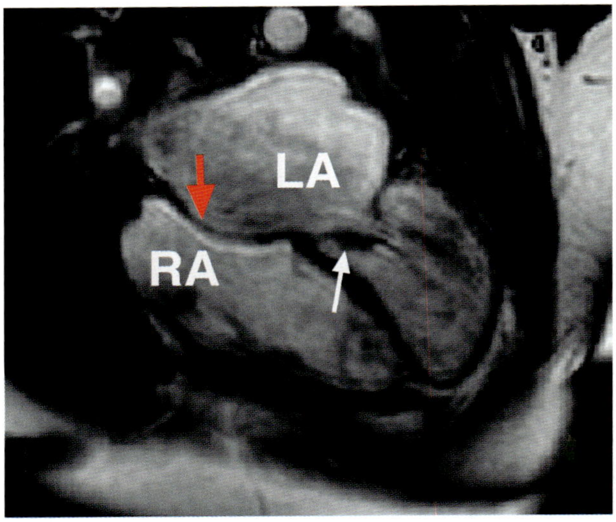

Fig 11.14 In this cardiac MRI, there is severe LA enlargement, and thickened mitral valve with restricted opening during diastole *(white arrow)*. Interatrial septum *(red arrow)* is bowed to right, indicative of elevated LA pressure

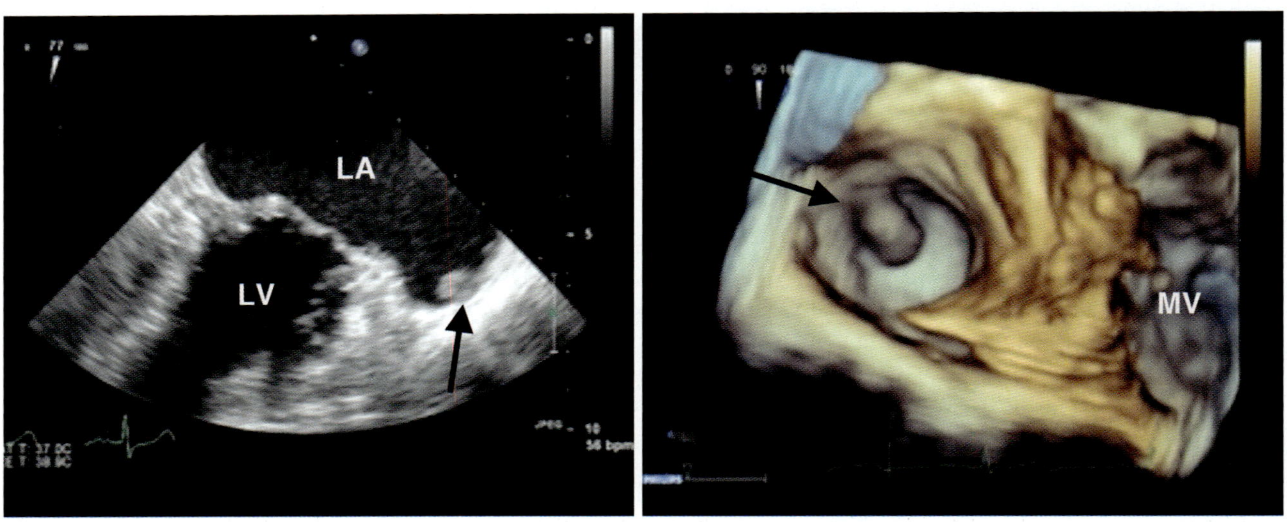

Fig 11.15 Intraoperative echocardiography from midesophageal two-chamber view, with careful angulation and rotation to optimize image of left atrium, shows echodensity consistent with thrombus *(left, arrow)*. Spontaneous contrast is also present in appendage. Sensitivity of TEE for detection of left atrial thrombus is highest when high-frequency transducer (typically 7 MHz) and instrument's magnification (or resolution) mode is utilized. On the right, 3D TEE from the left atrial perspective shows the appendage and thrombus *(arrow)*.

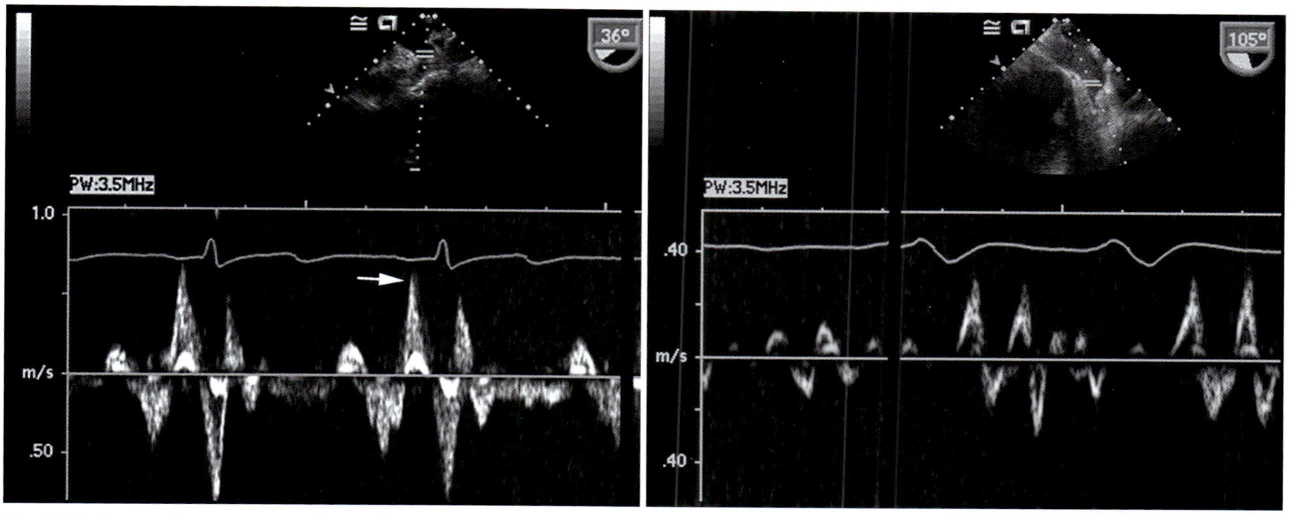

Fig 11.16 In another patient with similar presentation, flow in atrial appendage is examined by placing pulsed Doppler sample volume about 1 cm from mouth of appendage. In normal sinus rhythm *(left)*, flow velocity after atrial contraction of at least 0.4 cm/sec toward transducer is normal *(arrow)*. In atrial fibrillation, as in this case, lower-velocity, more frequent flow signals are seen *(right)*.

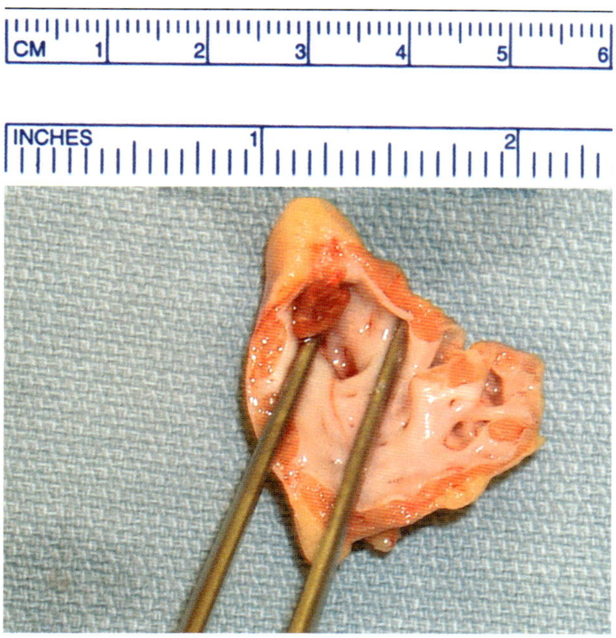

Fig 11.17 Because of presence of atrial appendage thrombus in patient undergoing maze procedure, left atrial appendage was resected. Surgical specimen (from another patient with similar presentation) shows red thrombus and paler normal trabeculation of atrial appendage. Trabeculations must be distinguished from thrombus on TEE imaging.

Comments

Patients with atrial fibrillation are at risk of systemic embolic events due to thrombus formation in the fibrillating left atrium. Most left atrial thrombi occur in the atrial appendage, which is not well visualized on transthoracic imaging. The sensitivity of transthoracic echocardiography for detection of left atrial thrombus is only about 50%. TEE provides high-resolution images of the left atrium and, with an experienced operator, has a sensitivity and specificity of nearly 100% for detection of atrial thrombi.

Imaging of the left atrial appendage should be performed in at least two orthogonal views, typically at 0 and 90 degrees, using a high-frequency transducer and a zoom high-resolution imaging mode. The use of biplane imaging, supplemented by 3D imaging or 2D imaging with minor changes in angulation and rotation from this image plane, are useful approaches to distinguish normal appendage trabeculations, which move with and connect with the atrial wall, from thrombi, which often protrude and have independent motion. Less often, thrombi occur in the body of the atrium, so that careful examination in multiple image planes of the entire atrium, including the atrial septal region, is needed.

Suggested Reading

1. Prutkin J, Akoum N: The role of echocardiography in patients with atrial fibrillation and flutter. In Otto CM, editor: The practice of clinical echocardiography, ed 5, Philadelphia, 2016, Elsevier.
2. Yamamoto M, Seo Y, Kawamatsu N, et al: Complex left atrial appendage morphology and left atrial appendage thrombus formation in patients with atrial fibrillation, Circ Cardiovasc Imaging 7(2):337–343, 2014.

CASE 11-7
Left Ventricular Thrombus

This 19-year-old male presented to his local ED with a 9-day history of progressive fatigue, and shortness of breath on exertion. Echocardiography at that time revealed a profound impairment of right and left ventricular systolic function. He was transferred to our hospital and taken to the cath laboratory, where after normal coronary angiography an intraaortic balloon pump was placed for cardiogenic shock. He then was taken to the operating room for placement of cannulae for veno-arterial extracorporeal membrane oxygenation (ECMO).

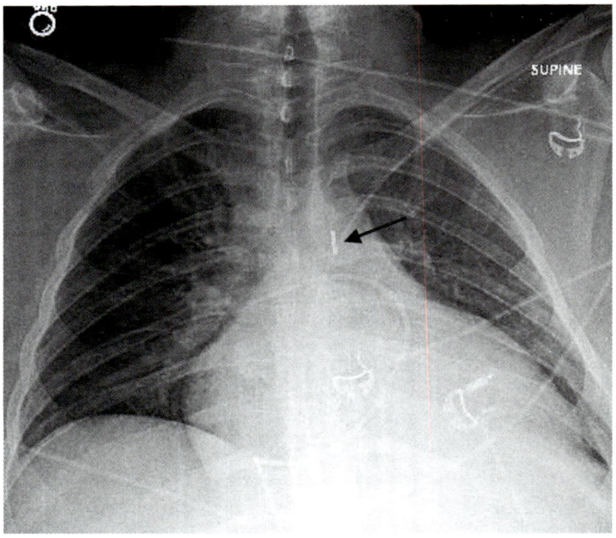

Fig 11.18 Chest x-ray revealed generalized cardiomegaly. Intraaortic balloon pump is in good position; arrow indicates tip.

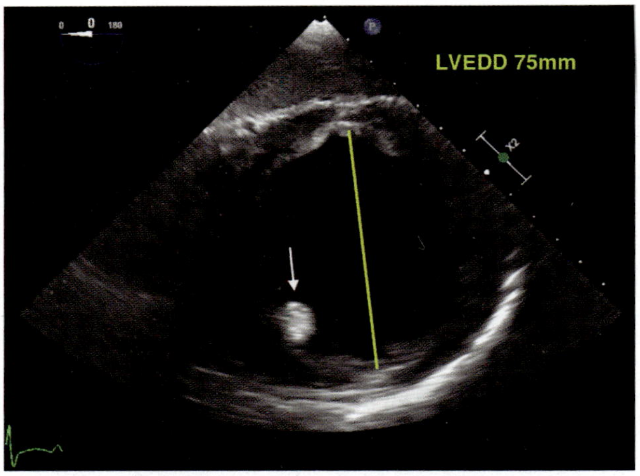

Fig 11.19 Transgastric short axis demonstrates dilated LV with end diastolic dimension of 75 mm. Arrow indicates spherical, echo-dense, LV mass along anterior wall. Video images show global LV hypokinesis with severely reduced overall systolic function, as well as larger, less echo-dense, mobile mass adjacent to brighter mass. These findings are consistent with LV thrombus. Other possibilities are unlikely given concurrent LV dilation and dysfunction. Normal structures, such as papillary muscle or trabeculations, would have same echodensity and motion as myocardium.

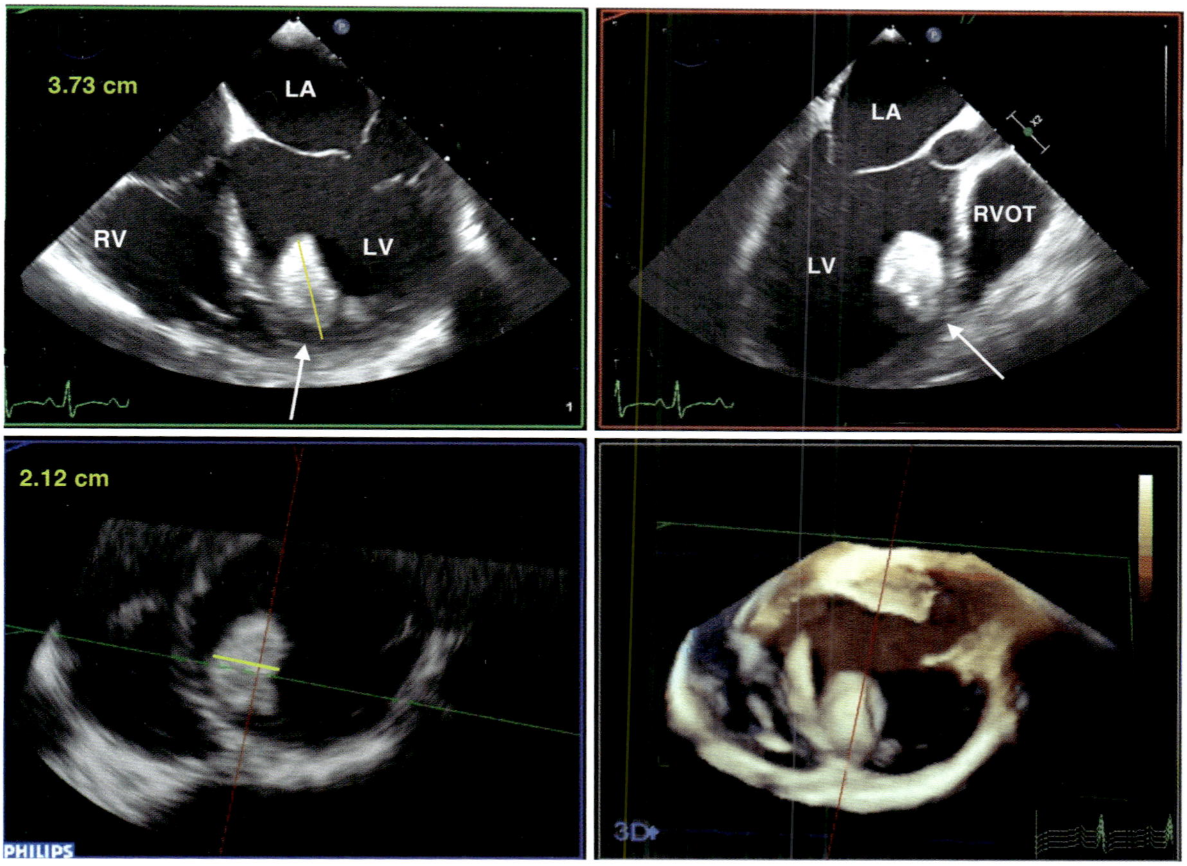

Fig 11.20 Multiplanar reconstruction from 3D volumetric image acquisition is used to further visualize and measure dimensions of mass. In bottom right frame, full 3D volume demonstrates mass in same view as blue plane (shown in 2D image for measurement in lower left image). Green line shows orientation of image plane shown in upper left, and red shows location of image plane shown in upper right panel. Given clinical history, arrows most likely indicate thrombus, which appears to be attached to junction of anterior wall and anterior portion of interventricular septum.

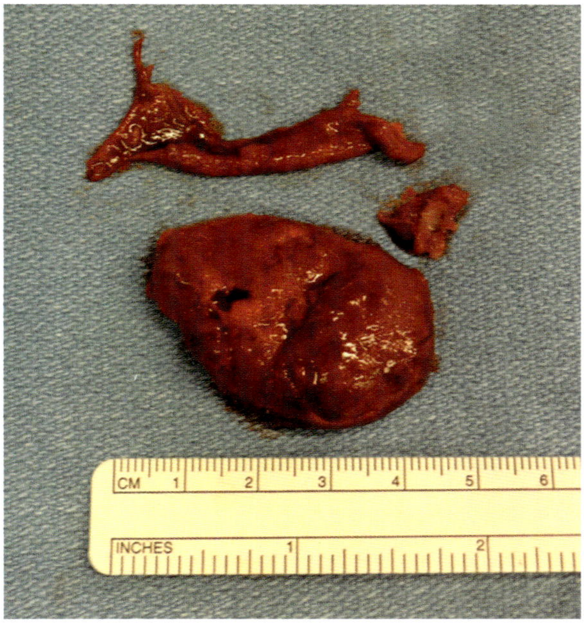

Fig 11.21 At time of ventriculotomy and LV assist device placement, thrombotic material was removed.

Comments

Left ventricular thrombus is most often seen in the setting of myocardial infarction and cardiomyopathy, and is sometimes associated with hypercoaguable diatheses. Although many diagnostic modalities are used, TTE is the most commonly employed, with or without echo contrast.

Knowledge of the presence of a thrombus is especially important in the workup of an embolic event, and in the patient whose heart is to be manipulated by a cardiac surgeon or interventionalist. TEE is not as sensitive as TEE, as the apex of the LV, where many thrombi reside, may not be well visualized. In this case, the size of the mass allowed easy detection. The clinical context suggested that it was thrombotic material; confirmation came at the time of LVAD placement.

Suggested reading

1. Carpenter K, Adams D: Apical mural thrombus: Technical pitfalls. Heart 80:S6–S8, 1998.
2. Delewi R, Zijlstra F, Jan Piek J: Left ventricular thrombus formation after acute myocardial infarction. Heart 98:1743–1749, 2012.

Primary Cardiac Tumors

CASE 11-8
Pulmonic Valve Mass

This 73-year-old woman was referred for closure of a sinus venosus septal defect and a tricuspid valve annuloplasty for symptoms of congestive heart failure with progressive RV dilation and tricuspid regurgitation.

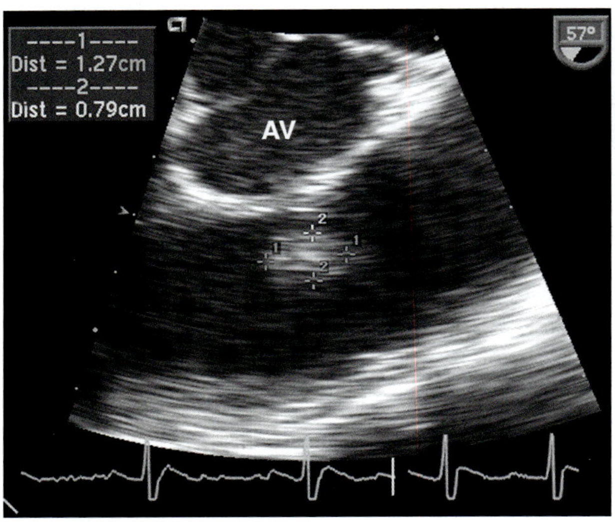

Fig 11.22 Incidental finding on intraoperative TEE was mobile mass in region of pulmonic valve measuring 1.3 by 0.8 cm in diameter.

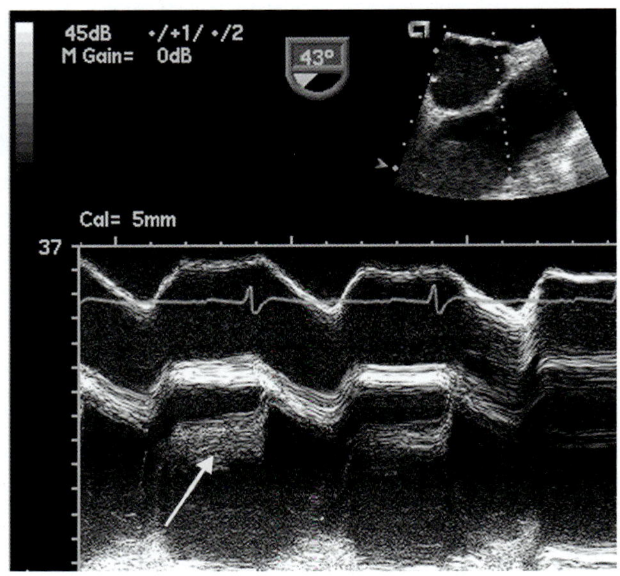

Fig 11.23 M-mode recording of this mass *(arrow)* shows motion that parallels motion of pulmonic valve.

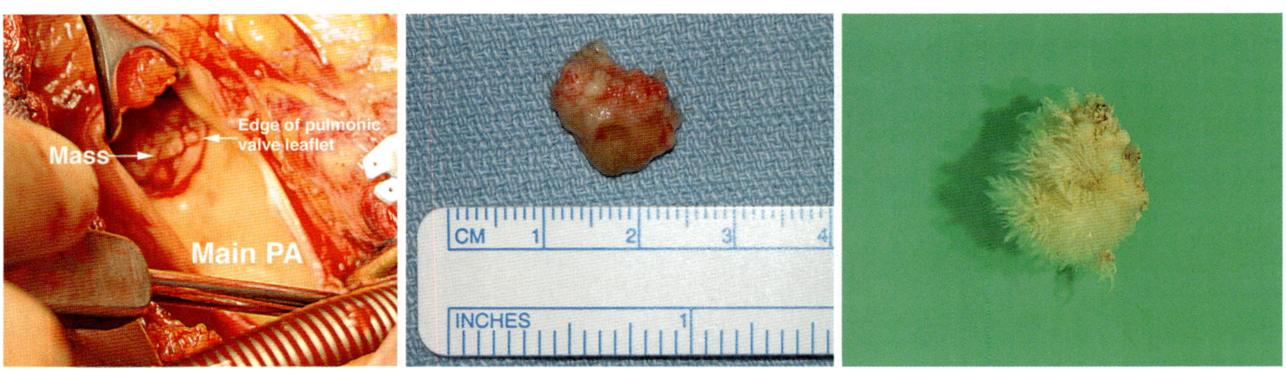

Fig 11.24 Surgical inspection of pulmonic valve showed discrete mass on leaflet that was carefully excised without damage to valve leaflet. Excised mass on histologic examination was consistent with papillary fibroelastoma *(center panel)*. The frond-like in-vivo appearance of these tumors can only be demonstrated on excised tissue by suspending mass in water *(right panel)*.

CASE 11-9
Aortic Valve Fibroelastoma

This 60-year-old woman was referred for placement of a mitral annuloplasty ring for treatment of severe mitral regurgitation due to a dilated cardiomyopathy with congestive heart failure symptoms.

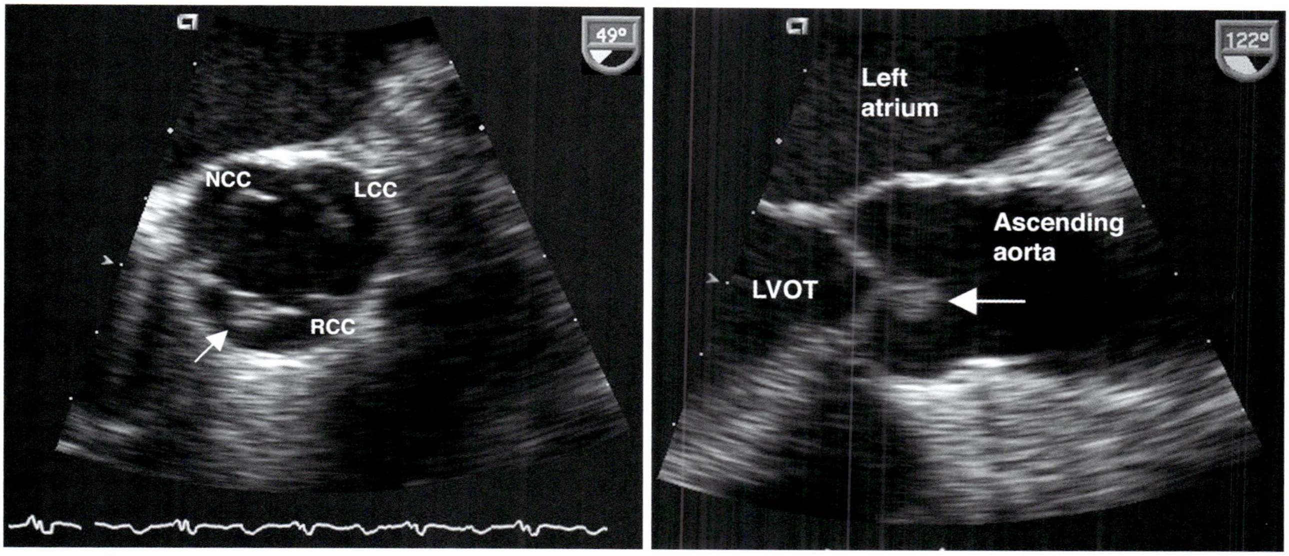

Fig 11.25 Incidental finding on intraoperative TEE, shown in short-axis *(left)* and long-axis *(right)* views of aortic valve, was small, globular mass on tip of right coronary cusp *(arrows)*.

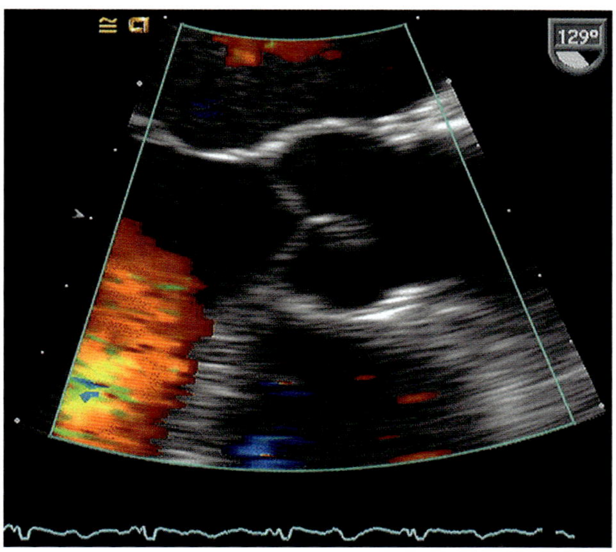

Fig 11.26 Color flow imaging in long-axis view shows no aortic regurgitation.

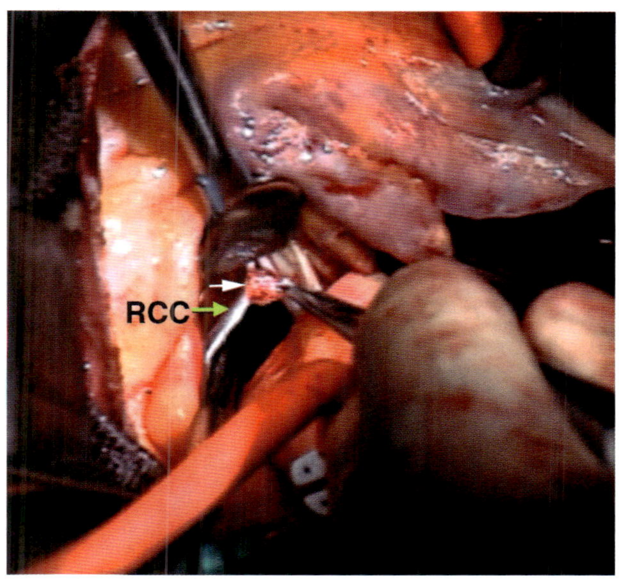

Fig 11.27 At surgery, small verrucous mass *(white arrow)* was excised from right coronary cusp of aortic valve. There was no injury to valve leaflets and no aortic regurgitation on postpump TEE. Pathology was consistent with papillary fibroelastoma.

Comments for Cases 11-8 and 11-9

A papillary fibroelastoma is a benign cardiac tumor that typically occurs on the aortic or mitral valve. Unlike valvular vegetations, these tumors tend to be located on the downstream (instead of upstream) side of the valve and are not associated with destruction of the underlying valve disease. The macroscopic appearance of these tumors is a frond-like mass, sometimes with superimposed thrombus. Microscopically, there is abundant elastic and fibrous tissue—similar to the normal component of the valve leaflet. The prevalence of papillary fibroelastomas increases with age, although the gender distribution is about equal. The most common valve sites (in order of prevalence) are aortic (44%), mitral (35%), tricuspid (13%), and pulmonic (8%) valves, with size at the time of detection ranging from 2 to 70 mm.

The optimal management of these tumors is controversial; many are found incidentally on echocardiography requested for other reasons, as in this case. In others, the tumor appears to be related to cerebrovascular events, myocardial infarction, sudden death, or peripheral embolic events. Clearly, in patients with embolic events or other symptoms, excision is appropriate and recent data suggest that recurrent stroke is more common in patients who do not undergo excision of these small valve tumors. With smaller asymptomatic masses, there is disagreement about optimal management, although risk factors for events include size and mobility of the mass. As echocardiographic image quality improves, it is likely that more, smaller fibroelastomas will be detected as incidental findings.

Suggested Reading

1. Gowda RM, Khan IA, Nair CK, et al: Cardiac papillary fibroelastoma: a comprehensive analysis of 725 cases, Am Heart J 146:404–410, 2003.
2. Tamin SS, Maleszewski JJ, Scott CG, et al: Prognostic and bioepidemiologic implications of papillary fibroelastomas, J Am Coll Cardiol 65:2420–2429, 2015.

CASE 11-10
Atrial Myxoma

This 52-year-old woman with endometrial stromal sarcoma, who had been treated with radiation therapy, underwent a chest CT scan and MRI as part of the evaluation before surgical resection of the endometrial tumor. A 4-cm left atrial mass was noted and confirmed on TEE. She had no other evidence of metastatic disease and was referred for cardiac surgery.

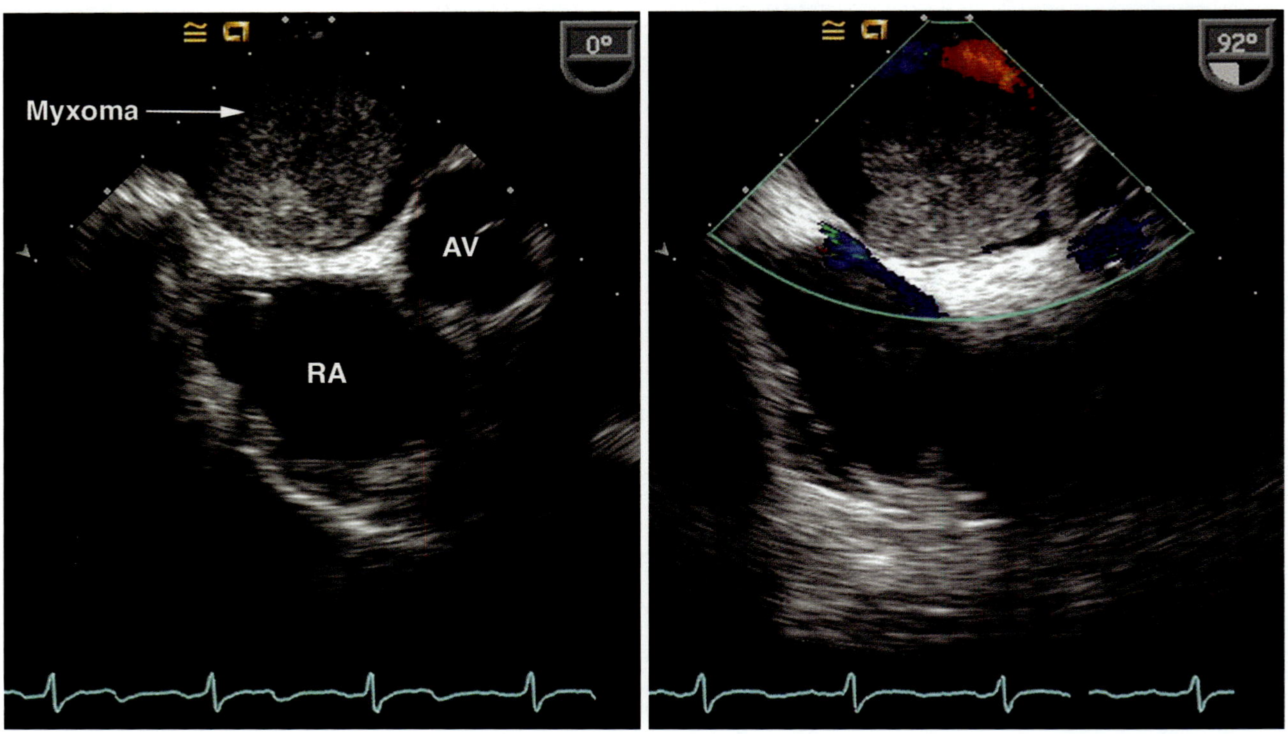

Fig 11.28 High transesophageal view at 0 degrees shows large, slightly heterogeneous mass that appears to arise from fossa ovalis region of atrial septum *(left)*. Color Doppler shows flow around mass but without significant obstruction to blood flow *(right)*.

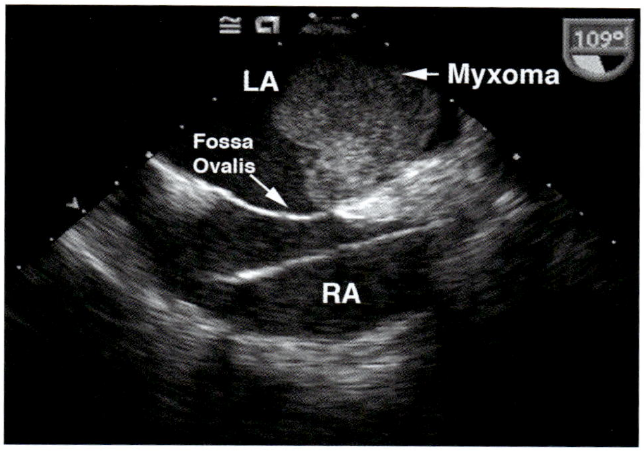

Fig 11.29 Rotation of image plane to 109 degrees provides better visualization of attachment of mass via narrow base to superior aspect of fossa ovalis.

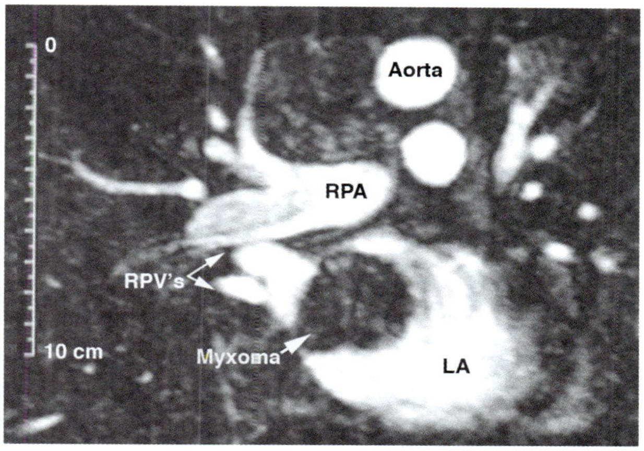

Fig 11.30 MRI scan shows mass in left atrium. RPVs = right pulmonary veins.

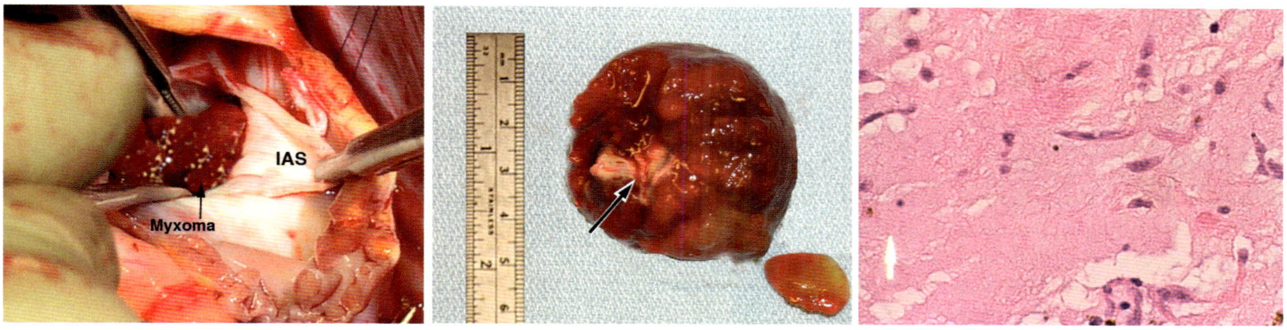

Fig 11.31 Surgical approach was via right atrium, with incision from right atrium through fossa ovalis after careful palpation to identify base of tumor. Entire base in atrial septum was excised, along with mass, and atrial septum was repaired. Postoperative TEE showed no residual tumor or atrial septal defect. IAS = interatrial septum. Excised mass is typical for atrial myxoma, which has relatively smooth surface with gelatinous appearance *(center panel)*. Arrow indicates attachment site of tumor to fossa ovalis. Microscopic examination with hematoxylin and eosin (H&E) stain is typical for myxoma, which has scattered cells with abundant intercellular material *(right panel)*.

Comments

Most primary cardiac tumors are benign, with myxomas accounting for about 30% of them. Cardiac myxomas originate in the left atrium in 75% of cases, with less common sites including the right atrium (about 10%), and left ventricle and right ventricle (each about 5%). Atrial myxomas are usually attached to the fossa ovalis region of the interatrial septum. An atrial myxoma may present with systemic symptoms such as fever, malaise, and embolic events. However, even a pathologically benign tumor may be hemodynamically malignant if there is obstruction to intracardiac blood flow. Large left atrial tumors may obstruct left ventricular filling, with a clinical presentation that mimics mitral stenosis. With the increasing use of noninvasive imaging techniques, cardiac tumors are more often diagnosed earlier in the disease course, on studies ordered for other indications, as in this case.

Suggested Reading

1. Bruce CJ: Cardiac tumors. In Otto CM, editor: The practice of clinical echocardiography, ed 5, Philadelphia, 2016, Elsevier.
2. Shah IK, Dearani JA, Daly RC, et al: Cardiac myxomas: a 50-year experience with resection and analysis of risk factors for recurrence, Ann Thorac Surg 100 495–500, 2015.

CASE 11-11
Obstruction of LV Filling by Myxoma

This 56-year-old woman presented with palpitations, orthopnea, fatigue, and dizziness. Transthoracic imaging revealed a large left atrial pedunculated tumor with intermittent obstruction of the mitral valve. Given symptoms and imaging findings suggesting a myxoma, she was referred for surgical intervention.

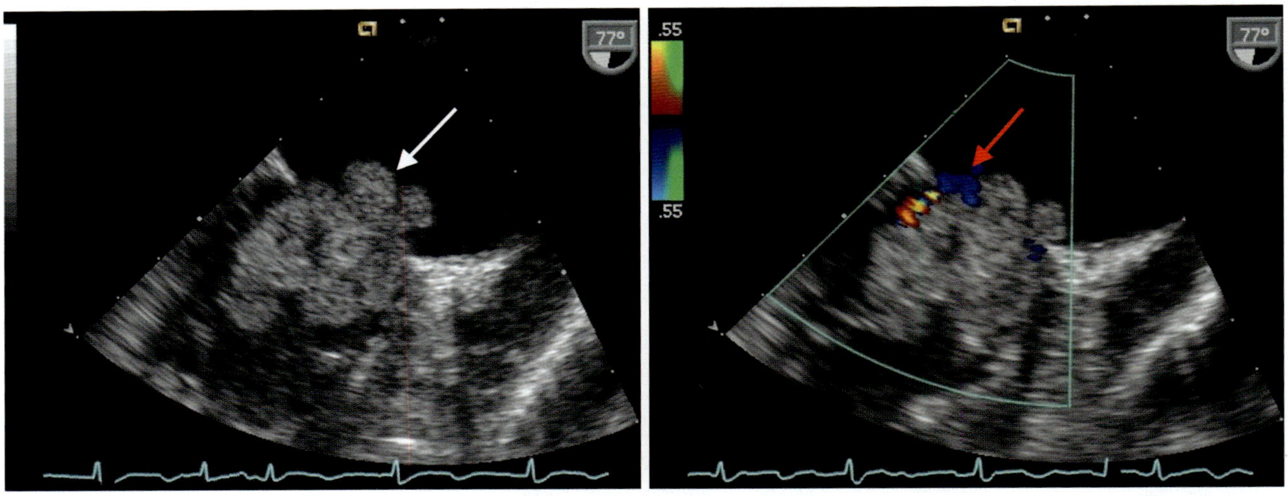

Fig 11.32 2D imaging in midesophageal two-chamber view *(left)* during diastole shows tumor *(white arrow)* engaging mitral orifice. Color Doppler *(right),* shows small amount diastolic inflow *(red arrow)* Doppler. LA = left atrium, LV = left ventricle. In video clip, "plopping" of tumor into mitral orifice during diastole is seen.

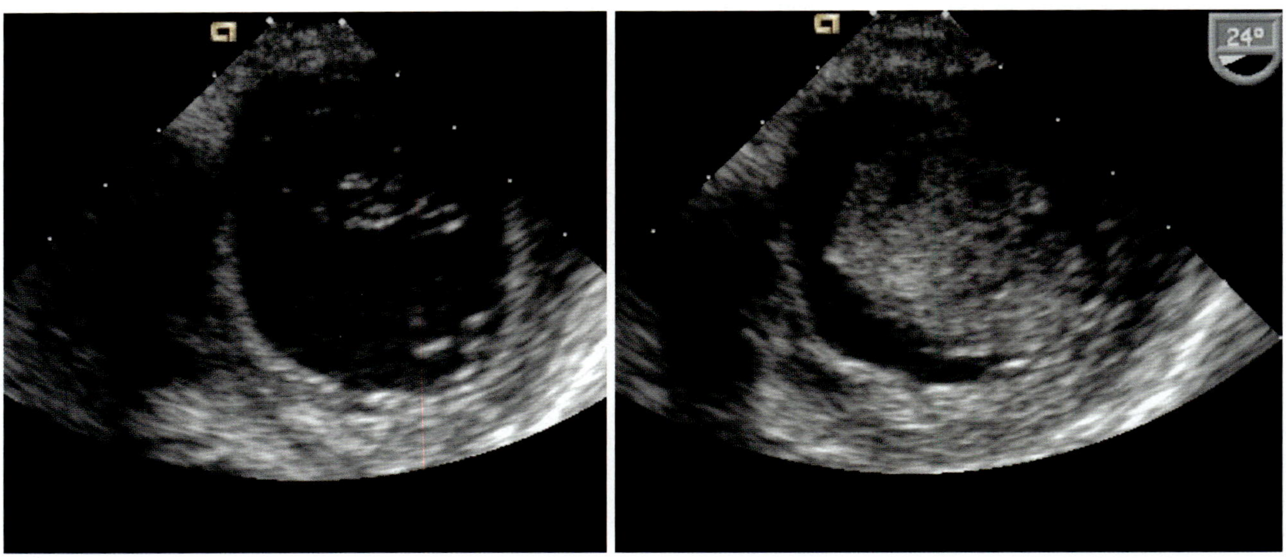

Fig 11.33 In this transgastric short-axis view, mitral valve appears normal during systole *(left),* and is obstructed by tumor prolapsing into orifice during diastole *(right).*

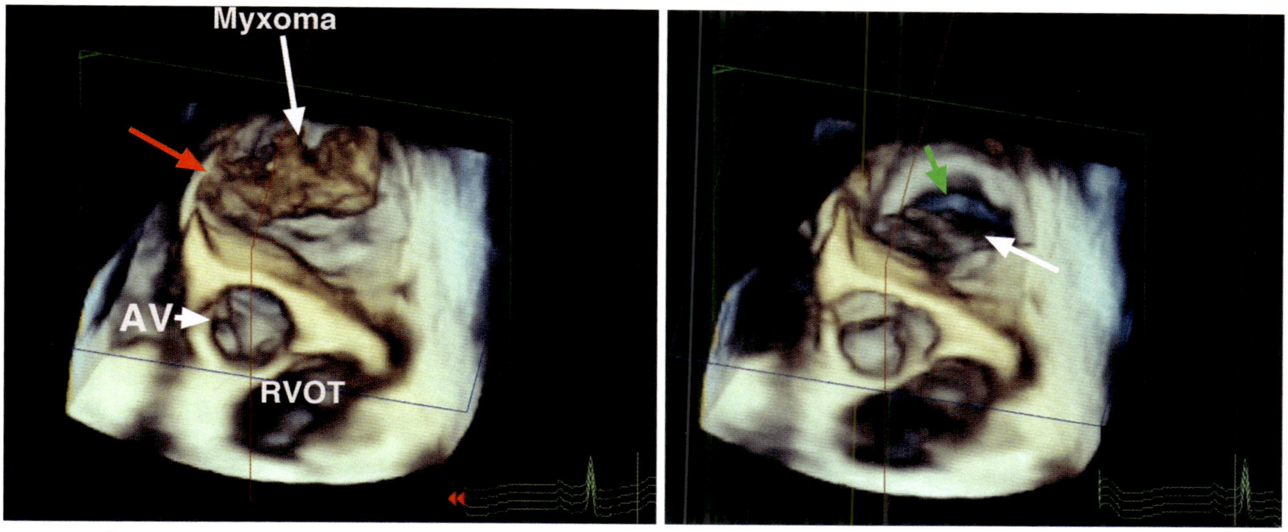

Fig 11.34 In patient with similar presentation, TEE was obtained at time of surgery. On left, in systole and with roof of left atrium cropped away, mass is seen with its attachment to interatrial septum *(red arrow)*. Aortic valve is open. On right during diastole, mass has prolapsed though mitral inlet, although space is observed between mass and posterior wall of LA *(green arrow)*.

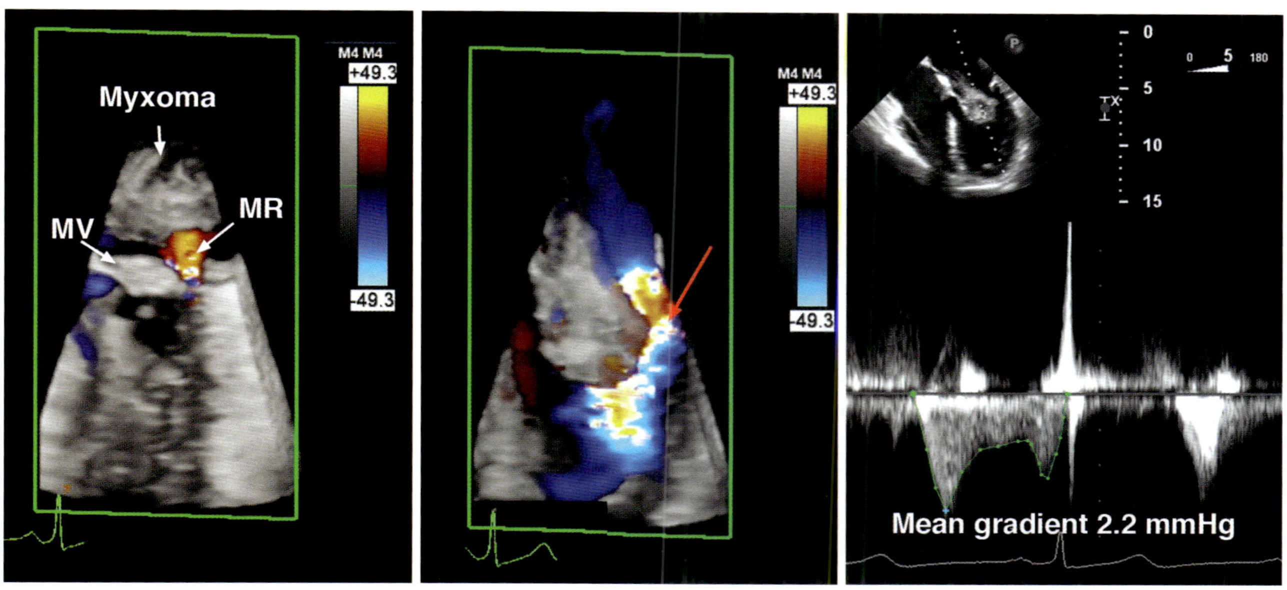

Fig 11.35 In same patient as in previous Fig 11.34, on left in systole, 3D color Doppler shows small jet of MR; in center, 3D color Doppler demonstrates mitral inflow going around prolapsing myxoma *(red arrow)*. On right, mean inflow gradient is 2.2 mm Hg.

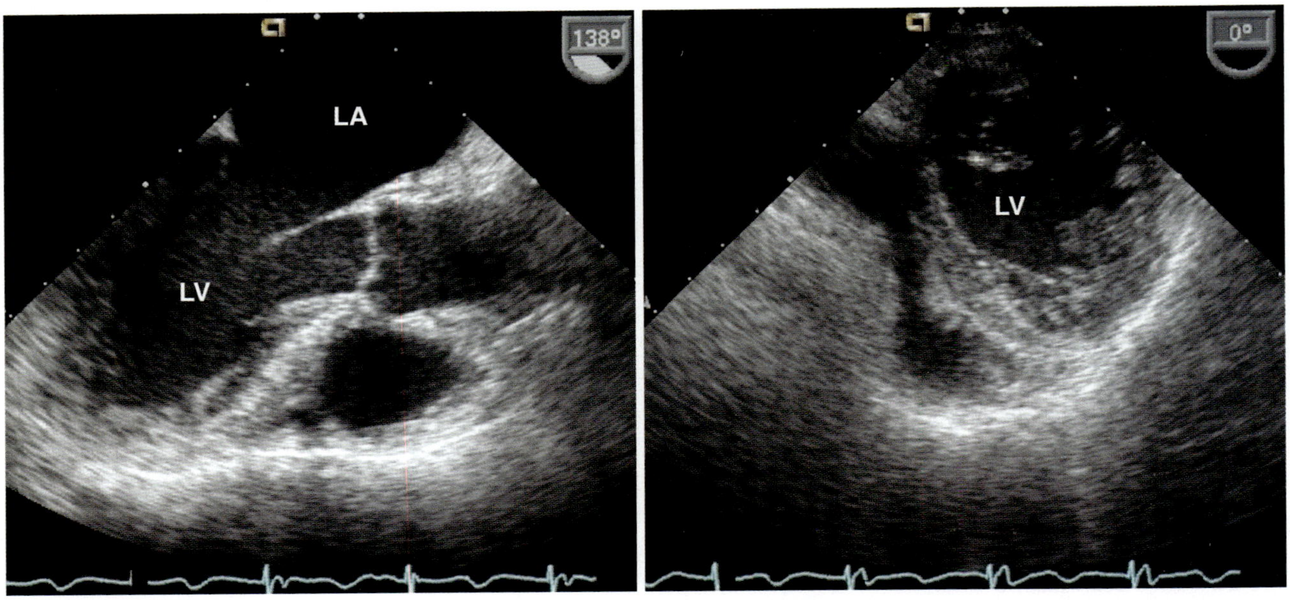

Fig 11.36 Postoperatively, there is no evidence of residual tumor in midesophageal long axis *(left panel)* and transgastric short axis *(right panel)*.

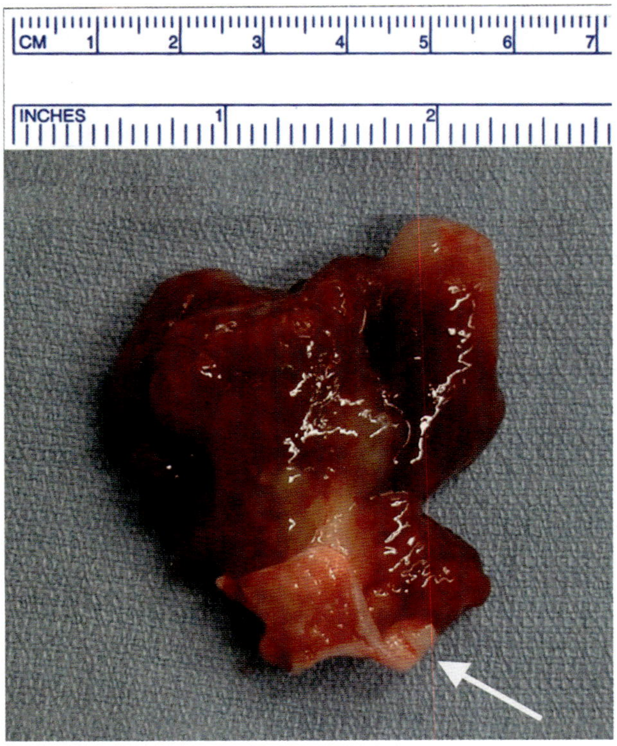

Fig 11.37 Excised specimen. Arrow indicates tumor attachment to interatrial septum.

Comments

Even though this tumor is a pathologically benign atrial myxoma, from a physiologic point of view the mass is malignant because it obstructs left ventricular inflow. Any further increase in size of the tumor will result in hemodynamics similar to mitral valve stenosis with an elevated left atrial pressure and pulmonary pressures resulting in symptoms of shortness of breath, decreased exercise tolerance, and pulmonary edema. Thus it is important for the echocardiographer to evaluate the physiologic consequences of an intracardiac mass, in addition to defining the anatomy.

Tumors can cause cardiovascular compromise via several mechanisms:

- Obstruction to flow (as in this case)
- Compression of cardiac chambers
- Production of pericardial fluid with tamponade physiology
- Invasion of myocardium
- Tumor embolization

CASE 11-12
Pulmonary Artery Leiomyosarcoma

A 44-year-old, otherwise healthy woman, with history of progressive shortness of breath was diagnosed with acute pulmonary embolus at an outside hospital and treated with systemic anticoagulation. Two months later, she was transferred to our institution for consideration of pulmonary embolectomy and endarterectomy due to worsening shortness of breath despite therapeutic anticoagulation.

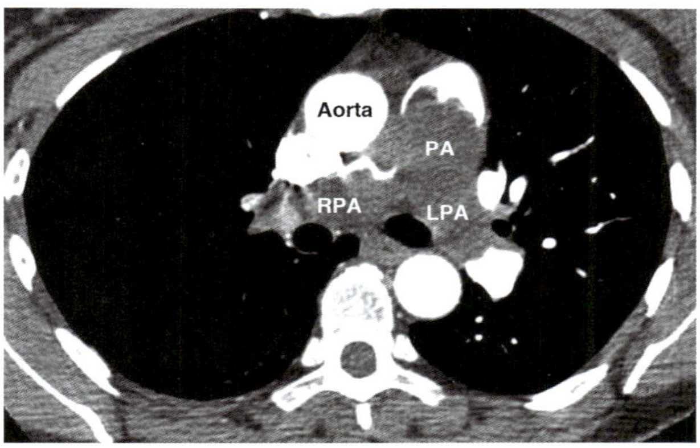

Fig 11.38 This CT scan shows main pulmonary artery and bifurcation filled with mass.

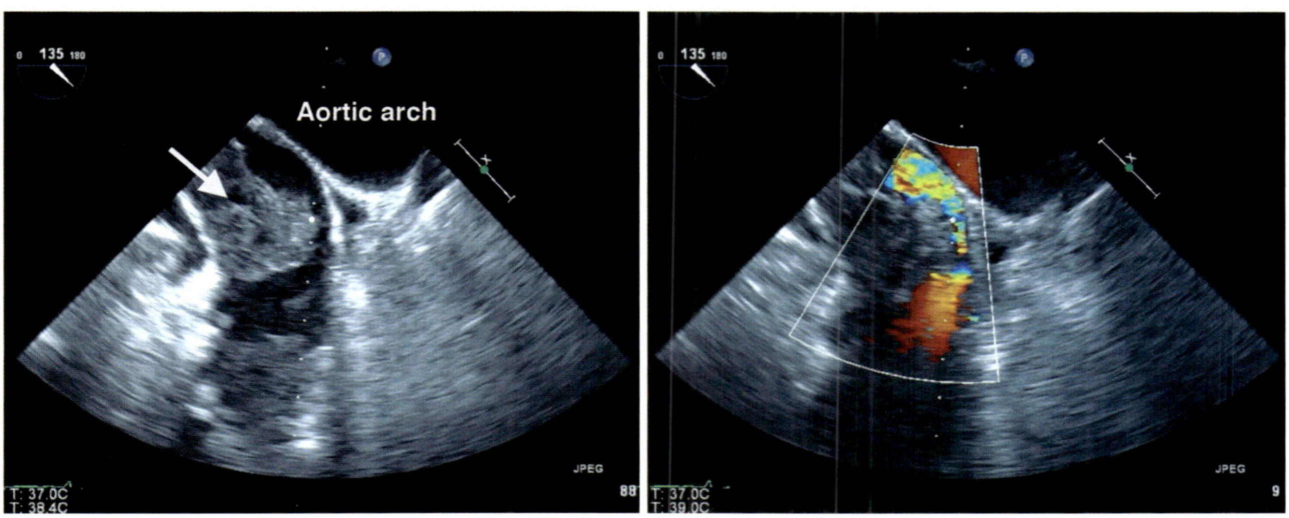

Fig 11.39 From upper esophageal window aortic-arch short-axis view, mass is visualized in main pulmonary artery *(left panel).* In right panel, aliasing of narrow jet of color flow is seen during systole. In real time, "tumor plop" during diastole mitigates any pulmonic regurgitation.

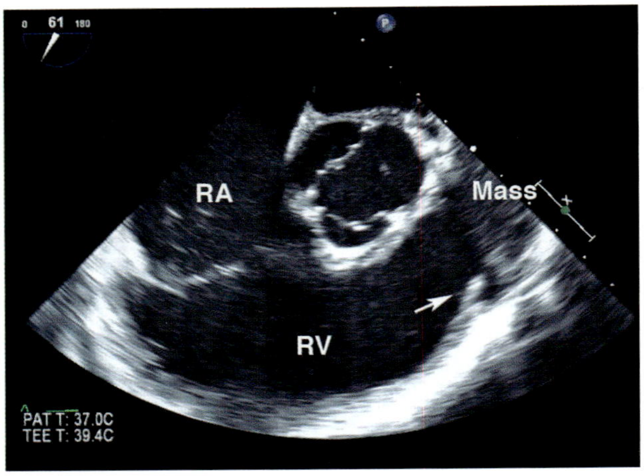

Fig 11.40 From midesophageal right ventricle inflow–outflow view, grossly abnormal and nonfunctioning pulmonary valve leaflet *(arrow)* is seen. As this image is in systole, mass is barely seen from this window. Previous destruction of valvular architecture speaks to process that is more likely malignant than embolic.

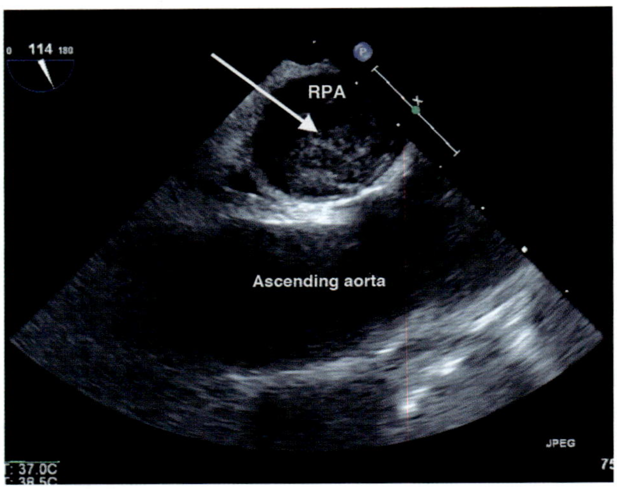

Fig 11.41 From midesophageal long-axis window, probe is slowly withdrawn until right pulmonary artery is seen. Mass fills lumen *(arrow)*. RPA = right pulmonary artery.

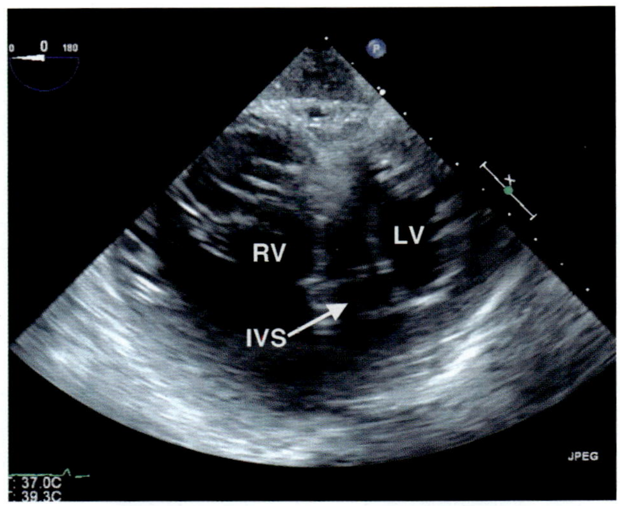

Fig 11.42 This transgastric short-axis image shows right ventricular enlargement, and "D"-shaped septum, consistent with right ventricular pressure overload. RV = right ventricle, LV = left ventricle, IVS = interventricular septum.

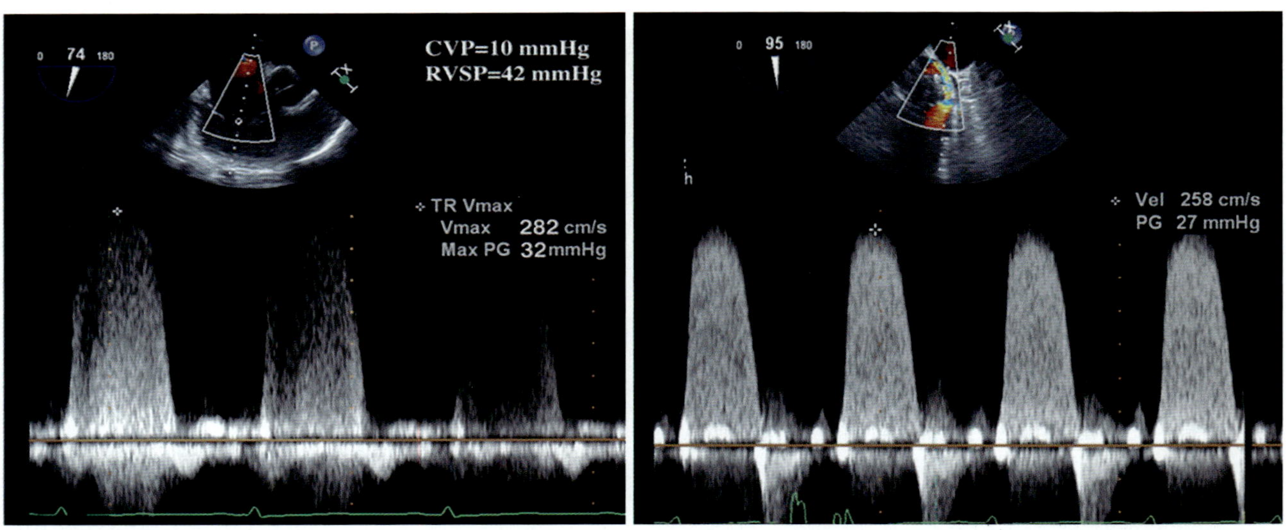

Fig 11.43 Continuous wave Doppler of tricuspid regurgitation jet *(left)* is consistent with pressure gradient between right atrium and right ventricle of 32 mm Hg. Adding central venous pressure of 10 mm Hg yields estimated RV systolic pressure of 42 mm Hg. Pulmonic valve antegrade velocity in systole *(right)* is 2.6 m/sec, which according to modified Bernoulli equation equals pressure gradient of 27 mm Hg between right ventricle and pulmonary artery; therefore pulmonary artery systolic pressure is approximately 15 mm Hg. CVP = central venous pressure, RVSP = right ventricular systolic pressure.

Comments

Malignant primary cardiac tumors are rare, accounting for about 15% of primary cardiac tumors. Most primary malignant cardiac tumors are sarcomas with rare cases of primary cardiac lymphoma or pericardial mesothelioma. Sarcomas can arise in any part of the heart, with left heart involvement most common, and typically present in patients between the 3rd and 5th decades of life. The various histologic subtypes of sarcoma do not have distinct echocardiographic features but diagnosis often is first suspected by echocardiography as the clinical features are also nonspecific.

Suggested Reading

Simpson L, Kumar SK, Okuno SH, et al: Malignant primary cardiac tumors: review of a single institution experience, Cancer 112(11): 2440–2446, 2008.

CASE 11-13
Angiosarcoma

This 33-year-old man presented with hemoptysis and dyspnea and was found to have a pericardial effusion and diffuse pulmonary nodules on chest CT imaging. Echocardiography shows an RA mass with apparent involvement of the RA free wall. He was referred for surgical intervention for a tissue diagnosis and resection of the mass.

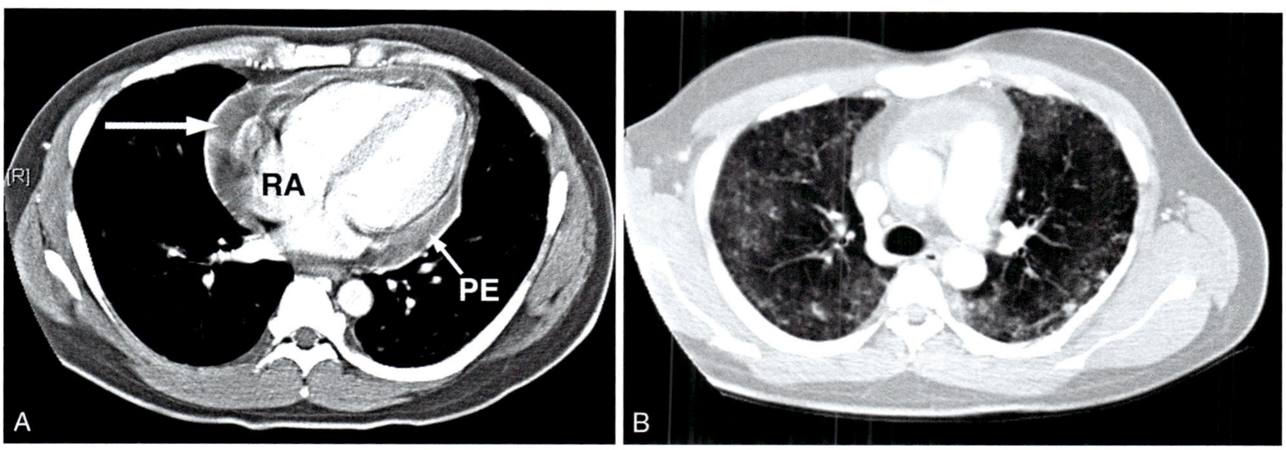

Fig 11.44 **(A)** CT scan shows mass abutting right atrium *(arrow)* and pericardial effusion (PE). **(B)** Lungs show diffuse, widespread pulmonary ground-glass opacities in miliary nodular pattern, most consistent with hematogenous spread of metastases.

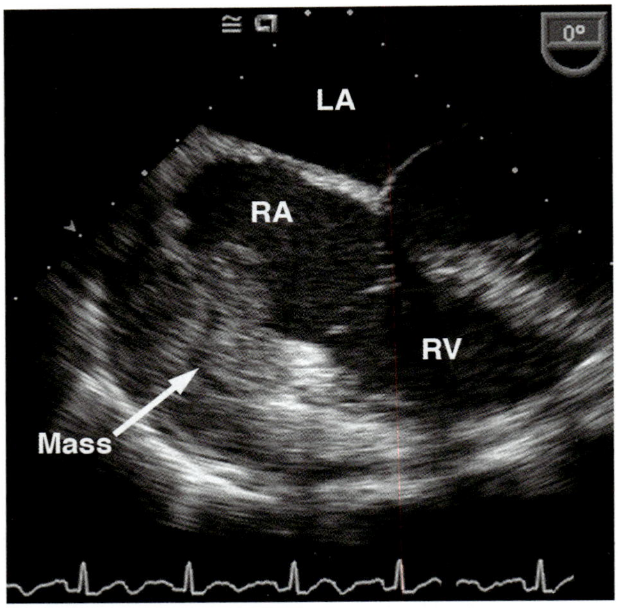

Fig 11.45 Midesophageal four-chamber TEE shows mass infiltrating right atrial wall, with intracavitary extension. Tricuspid valve appears uninvolved.

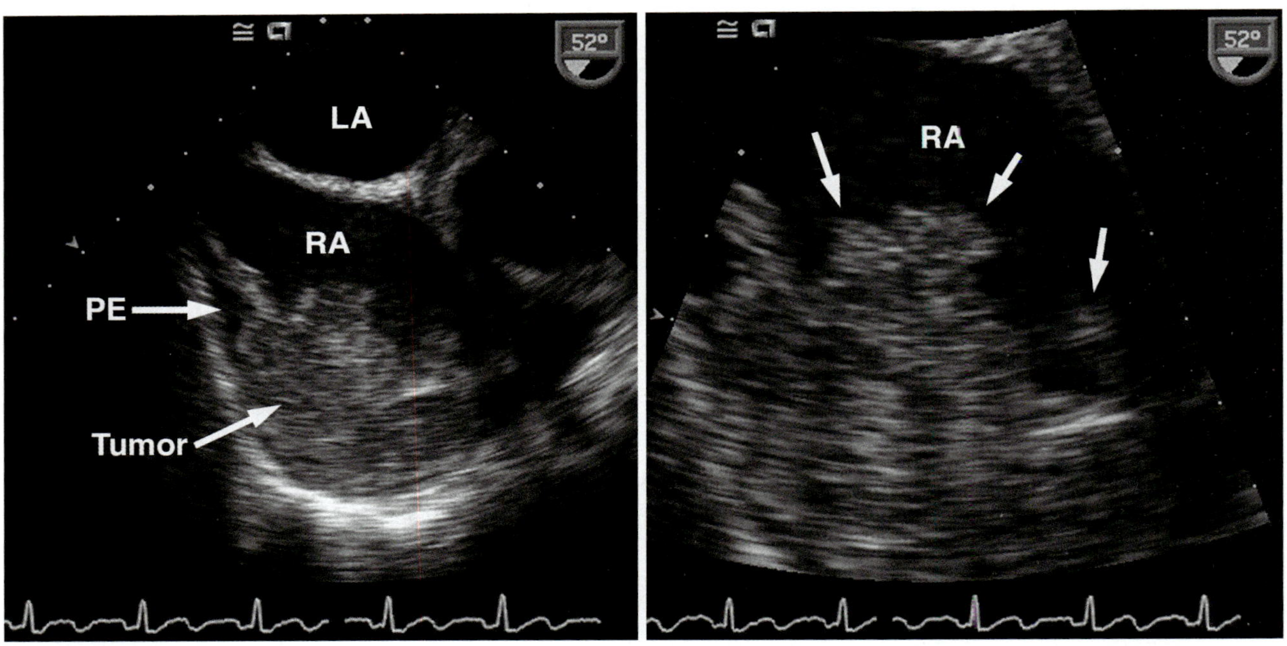

Fig 11.46 Rotating probe to 52 degrees shows mass again. In real time, intracavitary components are quite mobile *(arrows)*. Mass is densely adherent to right atrial wall, and is surrounded by pericardial effusion.

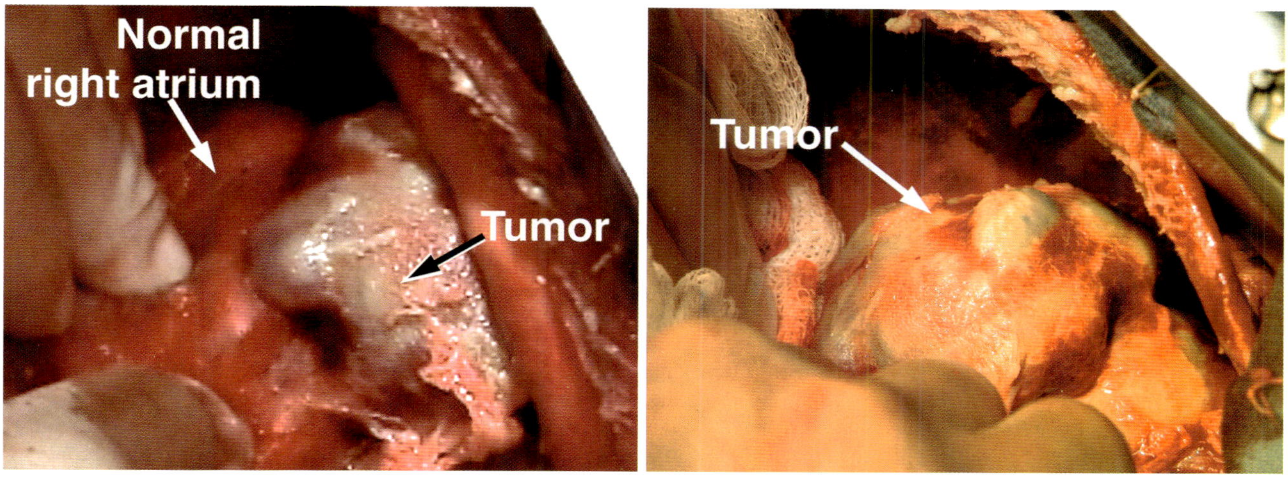

Fig 11.47 After sternotomy, medial retraction of heart reveals densely adherent tumor. Further retraction of heart reveals full extent of tumor.

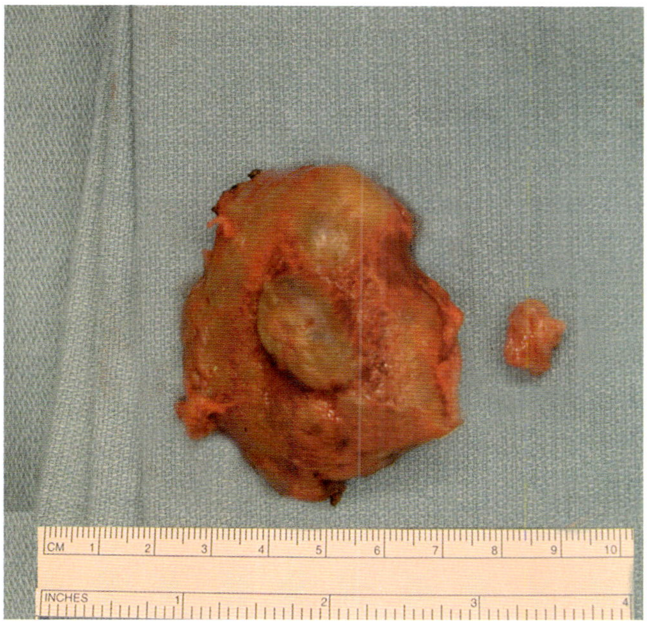

Fig 11.48 Two components of tumor are shown—the tumor itself on left and smaller mass on right, which was one of mobile components within RA on TEE.

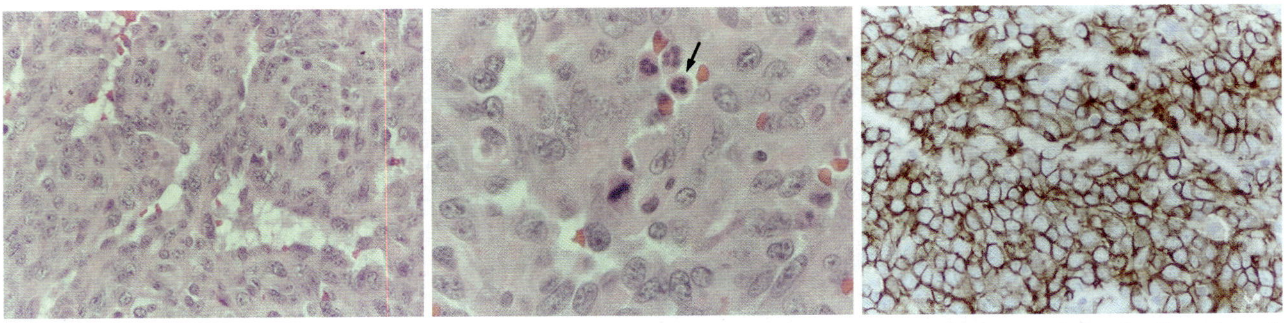

Fig 11.49 Microscopic examination of tumor using hematoxylin and eosin (H&E) shows spindled to epithelioid cells with oval to elongated, enlarged, hyperchromatic nuclei with prominent nucleoli. Cells are arranged in sheets that form anastomosing, slit-like vascular spaces *(left panel)*. In center panel, high-power view of histology shows mitotic figure *(arrow)*. There were up to 41 mitotic figures per 10 high-power fields. Approximately 50% of neoplasm was necrotic. Using specific immunohistochemical stain marker for vascular endothelial cells (CD31) shows prominent vascular tissue consistent with angiosarcoma *(right panel)*.

Comments

The differential diagnosis of a right atrial mass includes thrombus, either of local origin or in transit from a peripheral vein, an atypical infected vegetation or a tumor. Tumors may represent direct extension from a noncardiac primary tumor (most often lung, breast, or lymphoma) or may be cardiac in origin. Most primary cardiac tumors are benign, with 18% of cardiac myxomas presenting in the right atrium. Malignant cardiac tumors account for only about one-quarter of all primary cardiac tumors, with the proportions of all cardiac tumors about 9% for angiosarcomas, 5% for rhabdosarcomas, 4% for mesotheliomas, and 3% for fibrosarcomas.

In patients with a cardiac tumor, the echocardiographic examination focuses on the location and extent of the tumor, the physiologic consequences (e.g., valve obstruction or regurgitation), and any associated findings, such as pericardial effusion. The appearance of this mass was suggestive of a primary malignant cardiac tumor. The mass appeared to invade the right atrial free wall, had an irregular appearance within the right atrium and was associated with a pericardial effusion. However, this tumor did not result in hemodynamic compromise; instead, clinical manifestations were related to pulmonary embolic events.

Suggested Reading

1. Habertheuer A, Laufer G, Wiedemann D, et al: Primary cardiac tumors on the verge of oblivion: a European experience over 15 years, J Cardiothorac Surg 10:56, 2015.
2. Hoffmeier A, Sindermann JR, Scheld HH, et al: Cardiac tumors—diagnosis and surgical treatment, Dtsch Arztebl Int 111(12): 205–211, 2014.

Secondary Tumors

CASE 11-14
Renal Cell Carcinoma with Extension to Right Atrium

This 55-year-old man with renal cell carcinoma extending into the right atrium underwent surgery for en bloc removal of the right kidney and mass with cooperation of urologic, liver, and cardiac surgeons.

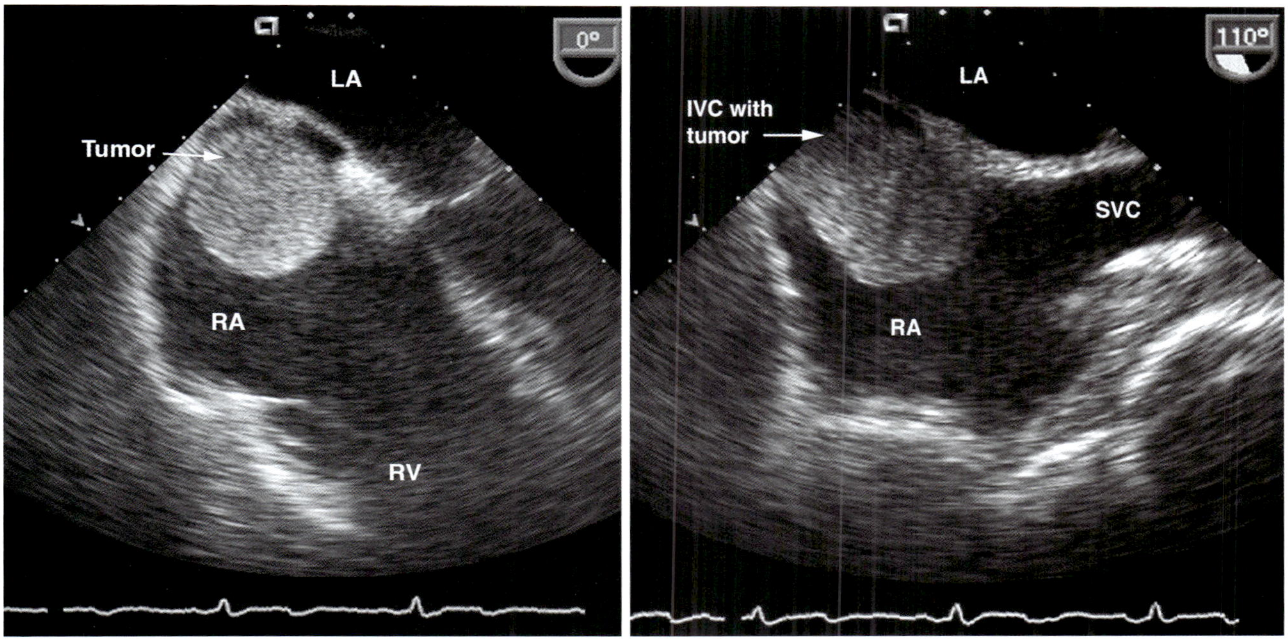

Fig 11.50 TEE images in four-chamber view show large spherical mass in right atrium that appears adjacent, but not attached, to atrial septum *(left panel)*. As image plane is rotated to bicaval view of right atrium (RA) and superior vena cava (SVC), mass is seen extending from inferior vena cava (IVC) into RA *(right panel)*

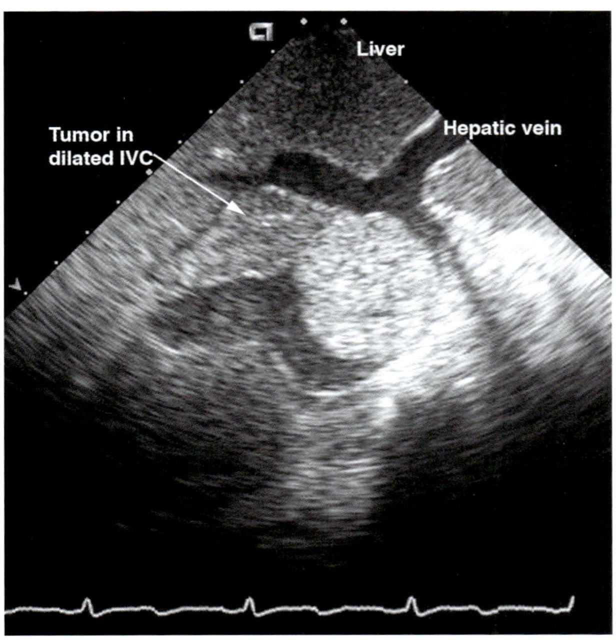

Fig 11.51 Placing sterile sheathed surfaced probe directly on liver provides image of tumor mass filling inferior vena cava. Hepatic veins are also dilated.

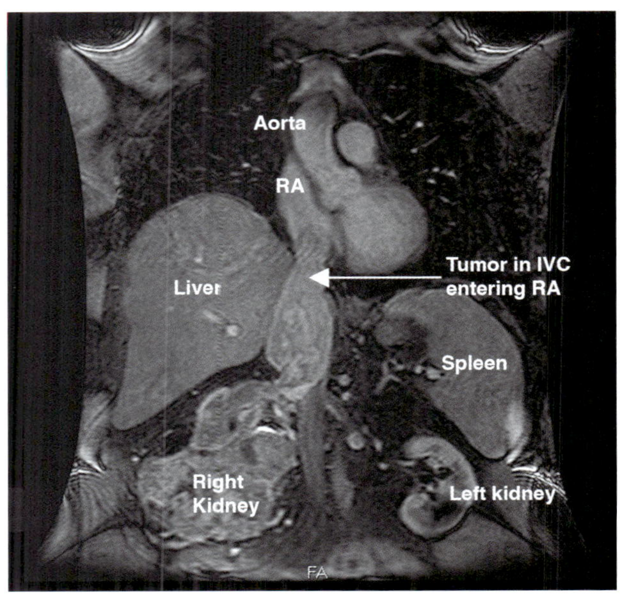

Fig 11.52 Sagittal plane MR image demonstrated extent of tumor from right kidney into inferior vena cava and right atrium.

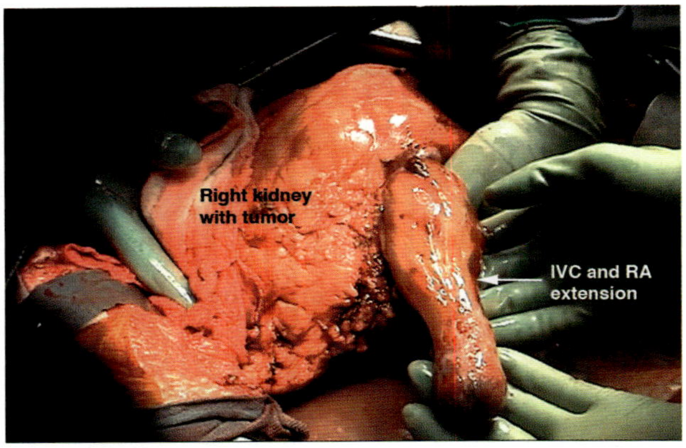

Fig 11.53 Excised kidney with tumor extension into IVC and RA was removed en bloc.

CASE 11-15
Renal Cell Carcinoma with Tumor Embolization to Pulmonary Artery

This 54-year-old man with a right renal tumor with extensive vena caval thrombosis presented with pulmonary embolism. At baseline in the operating room for en bloc resection of renal tumor, a mobile tumor was seen in the right atrium extending from the inferior vena cava into the right atrium, with diastolic prolapse into the right ventricle. During the procedure, the extension of tumor into the heart disappeared.

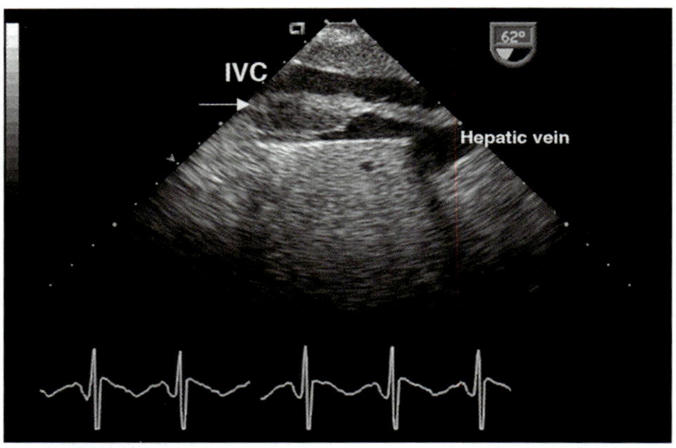

Fig 11.54 Transgastric images of inferior vena cava (IVC) show mass *(arrow)* extending along length of vessel.

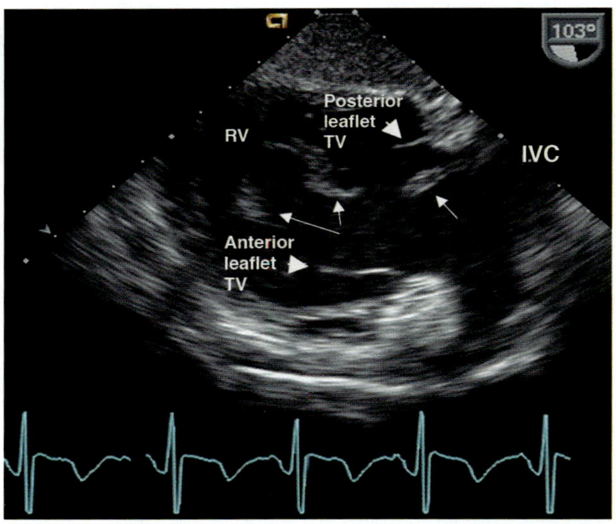

Fig 11.55 Transgastric right ventricular inflow view shows that mass *(arrows)* extends from inferior vena cava (IVC) across right atrium, and crosses tricuspid valve (TV) into right ventricle.

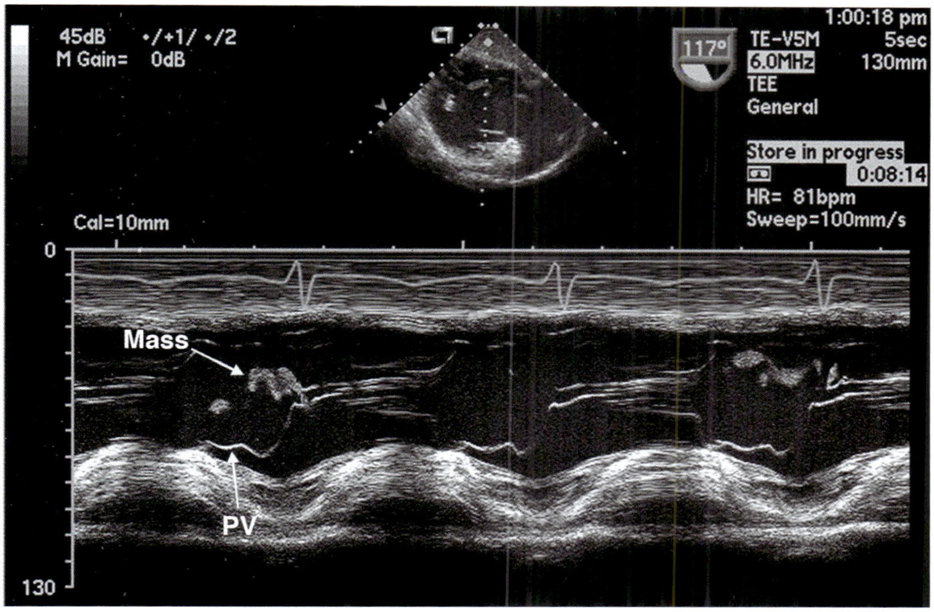

Fig 11.56 M-mode from this position confirms that mass moves independently (i.e., with different pattern of motion) from tricuspid valve, with motion that varies from beat to beat.

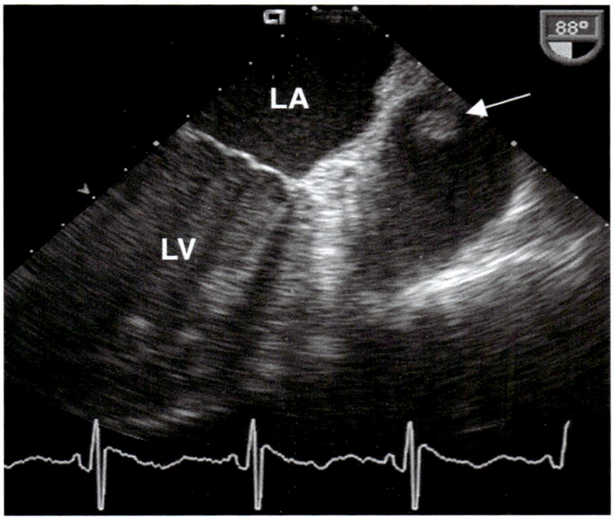

Fig 11.57 TEE two-chamber view shows that mass *(arrow)* is also present in pulmonary artery.

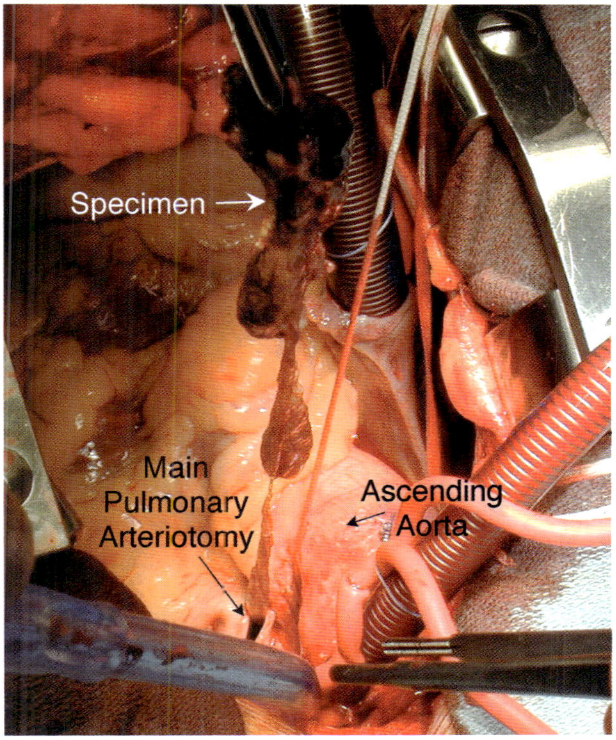

Fig 11.58 At surgery, single irregular string-like mass was removed en bloc—it extended from inferior vena cava through right heart and into pulmonary artery.

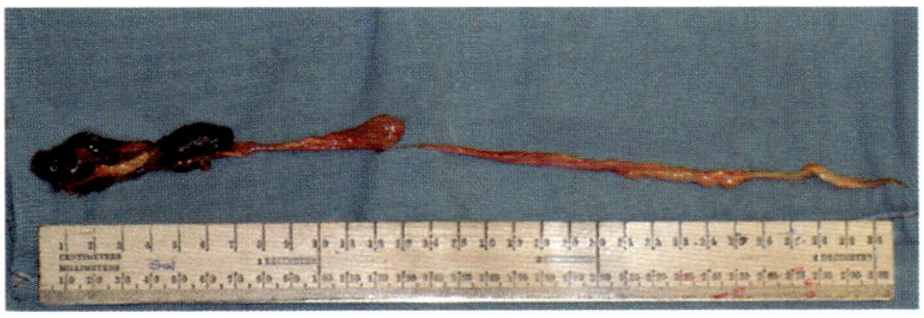

Fig 11.59 Excised mass was over 24 cm in length, with histology consistent with renal cell carcinoma.

Comments for Cases 11-14 and 11-15

Renal cell carcinoma may spread by direct extension up the inferior vena cava into the right atrium. Tumor extension into the right atrium demonstrates a typical appearance, as illustrated by these two cases. TEE allows precise delineation of the size and location of tumor extension into the right atrium and allows confirmation that the tumor does not attach to the atrial wall or involve the tricuspid valve. With a complete anatomic definition of the tumor, the surgical resection is often performed "en bloc," with collaboration between the renal and cardiac surgeons. Intraoperative TEE is essential for guiding the surgical approach and documenting the absence of tumor and normal right heart function after resection.

Suggested Reading

1. Colwell EM, Gandhi SD, Iqbal Z, et al: Use of multimodal imaging in the management of tumor embolism from the inferior vena cava through the right heart in a patient with renal cell carcinoma, J Cardiothorac Vasc Anesth 28(5): 1421–1424, 2014.
2. George J, Grebenik K, Patel N: The importance of intraoperative transoesophageal monitoring when operating on renal cancers that involve the right atrium. Ann R Coll Surg Engl 96(6): e18–e19, 2014.

CASE 11-16
Right Ventricular Melanoma

The patient, a 49-year-old woman, had 6 years previously undergone surgery for an eyelid melanoma. This most recent presentation was because of increasing shortness of breath and fatigue. A CT scan demonstrated a mass in the RV. At surgery, the mass was excised from its attachment to the interventricular septum and anterior free wall.

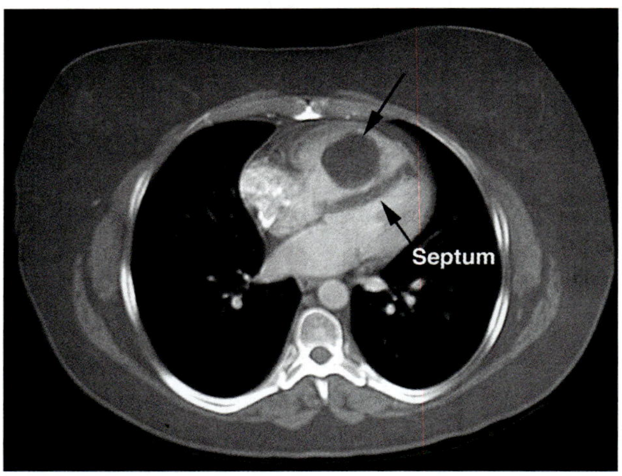

Fig 11.60 CT scan demonstrated mass in enlarged right ventricle *(arrow)*. Shape of interventricular septum is noted to be flat or curved toward LV, instead of normal curvature toward RV.

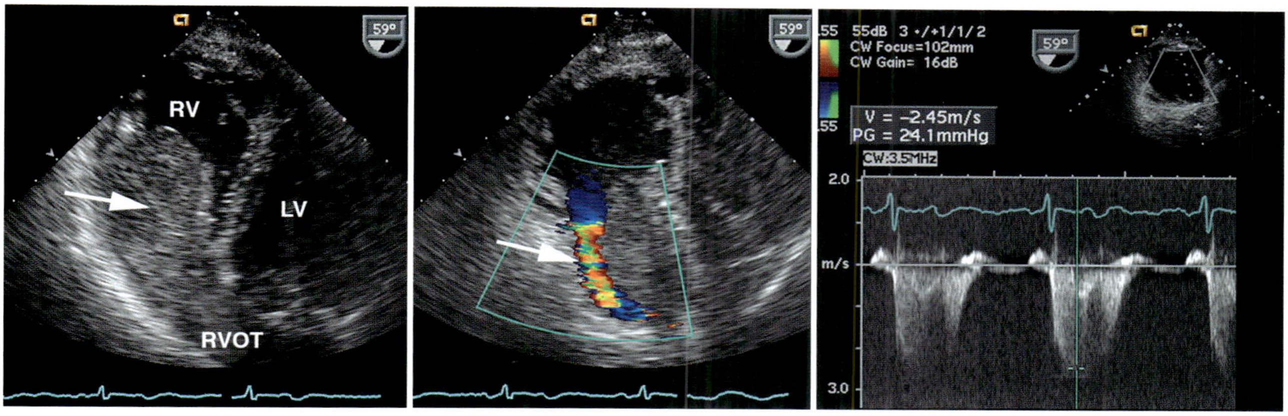

Fig 11.61 On transgastric 2D view *(left)*, probe has been rotated to patient's right, and scanning angle rotated to image RV outflow tract. Color Doppler *(center)* shows very narrowed flow stream from RV into outflow tract, secondary to obstruction by tumor. Continuous wave Doppler *(right)* demonstrates RV outflow tract gradient of 24 mm Hg.

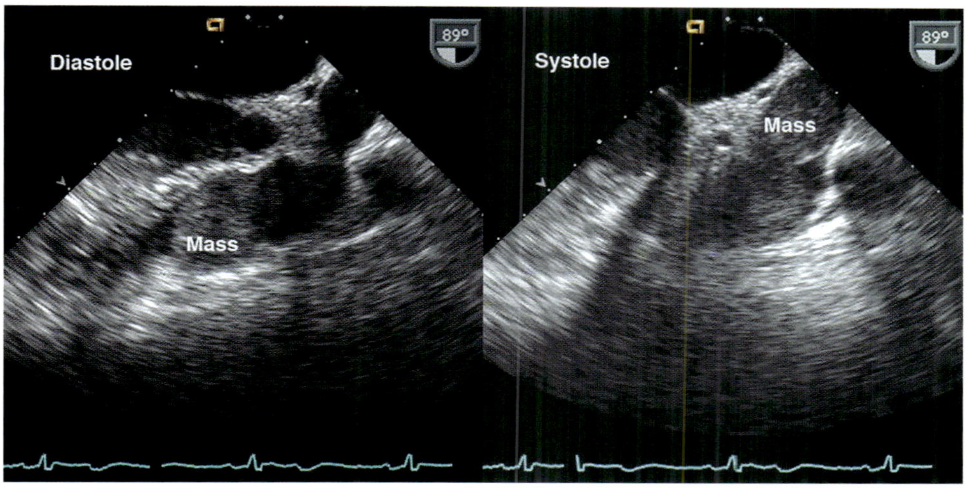

Fig 11.62 This midesophageal view shows RV outflow tract and main pulmonary artery. In diastole *(left)* tumor has prolapsed into outflow tract, and during systole *(right)* tumor is propelled into main pulmonary artery.

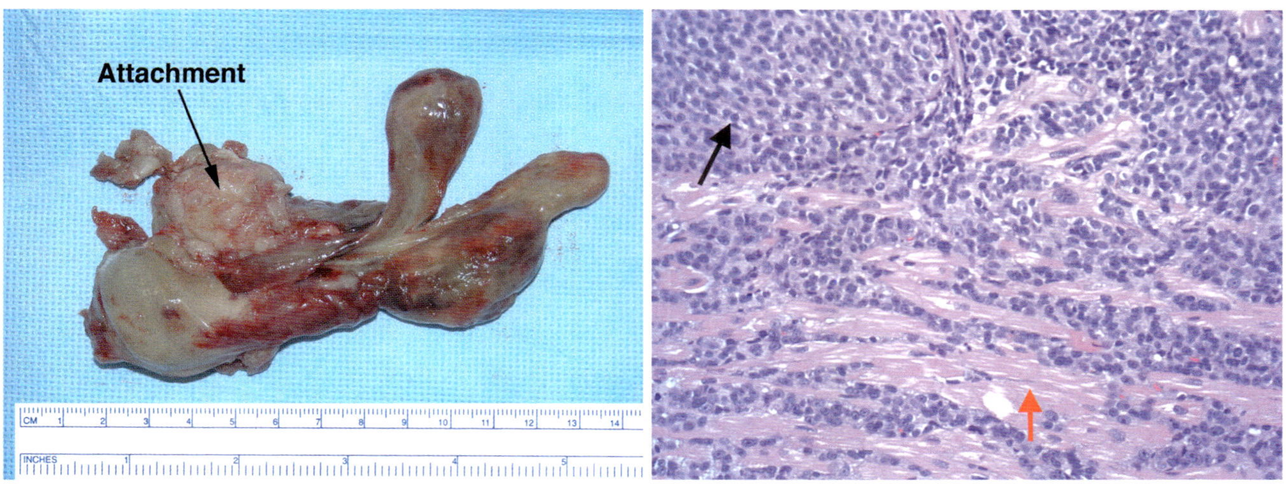

Fig 11.63 Excised tumor *(left)* with arrow indicating where it was attached to anterior RV free wall and interventricular septum. Multilobulated appearance is consistent TEE imaging findings. Microscopic examination *(right)* reveals tumor cells *(black arrow)* interspersed with muscle *(red arrow)*.

Comments

Noncardiac tumors that invade the heart (called secondary tumors) are 30 times more common than primary cardiac tumors. In autopsy series of patients dying of malignant disease, up to 20% have cardiac involvement. Noncardiac tumors can affect the heart by direct extension from adjacent tumor masses (e.g., with lung or breast cancer), by intravascular extension (e.g., renal cell), or by hematogenous (e.g., melanoma) or lymphatic spread (e.g., lymphoma). Although melanoma is less common than lung or breast cancer, cardiac metastases are found in about 50% of autopsy cases. Metastatic melanoma can involve any cardiac chamber or the pericardium.

Suggested Reading

1. Allen BC, Mohammed TL, Tan CD, et al: Metastatic melanoma to the heart, Curr Probl Diagn Radiol 41(5):159–164, 2012.
2. Fontana A, Corsi D, Viganò E, et al: Added value of real time three-dimensional echocardiography in the diagnosis of an apical right ventricular metastasis from malignant melanoma, Echocardiography 30(1):E16–E20, 2013.

Pleural Effusions

CASE 11-17
Left and Right Pleural Effusions

Pleural effusions are commonly encountered in the perioperative period. If clinically significant, TEE can guide the surgeon in draining the collection; its relationship to the descending aorta is key; if the effusion is posterior to the aorta it is pleural, whereas if it insinuates itself between the aorta and the left atrium, it is pericardial.

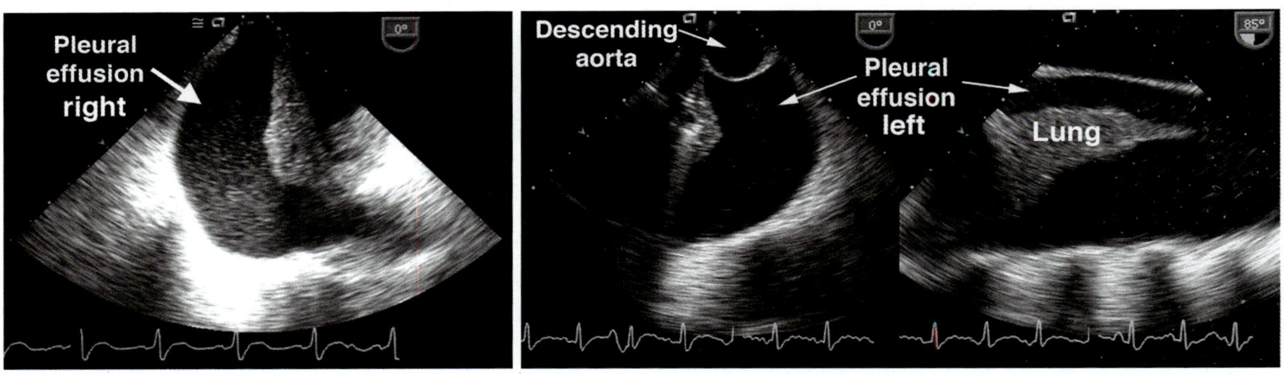

Fig 11.64 Right-sided pleural effusion is best seen by rotating probe to patient's right, while advancing it from midesophageal position. Left-sided effusion is best seen by rotating posteriorly until descending aorta is seen, and then withdrawing and advancing it to appreciate its size.

12 Mechanical Circulatory Support

In addition to standard cardiopulmonary bypass during cardiac surgery, there now are several options for longer-term mechanical circulatory support ranging from a simple intraaortic balloon pump to a total artificial heart. Some of these devices are used in the hospital setting because of the external components of the device and need for continuous monitoring, including the intraaortic balloon pump (IABP), percutaneous assist devices, and use of an external corporal membrane oxygenator (ECMO). Others are designed for long-term use in the outpatient setting, including implanted ventricular assist devices and a total artificial heart (TAH).

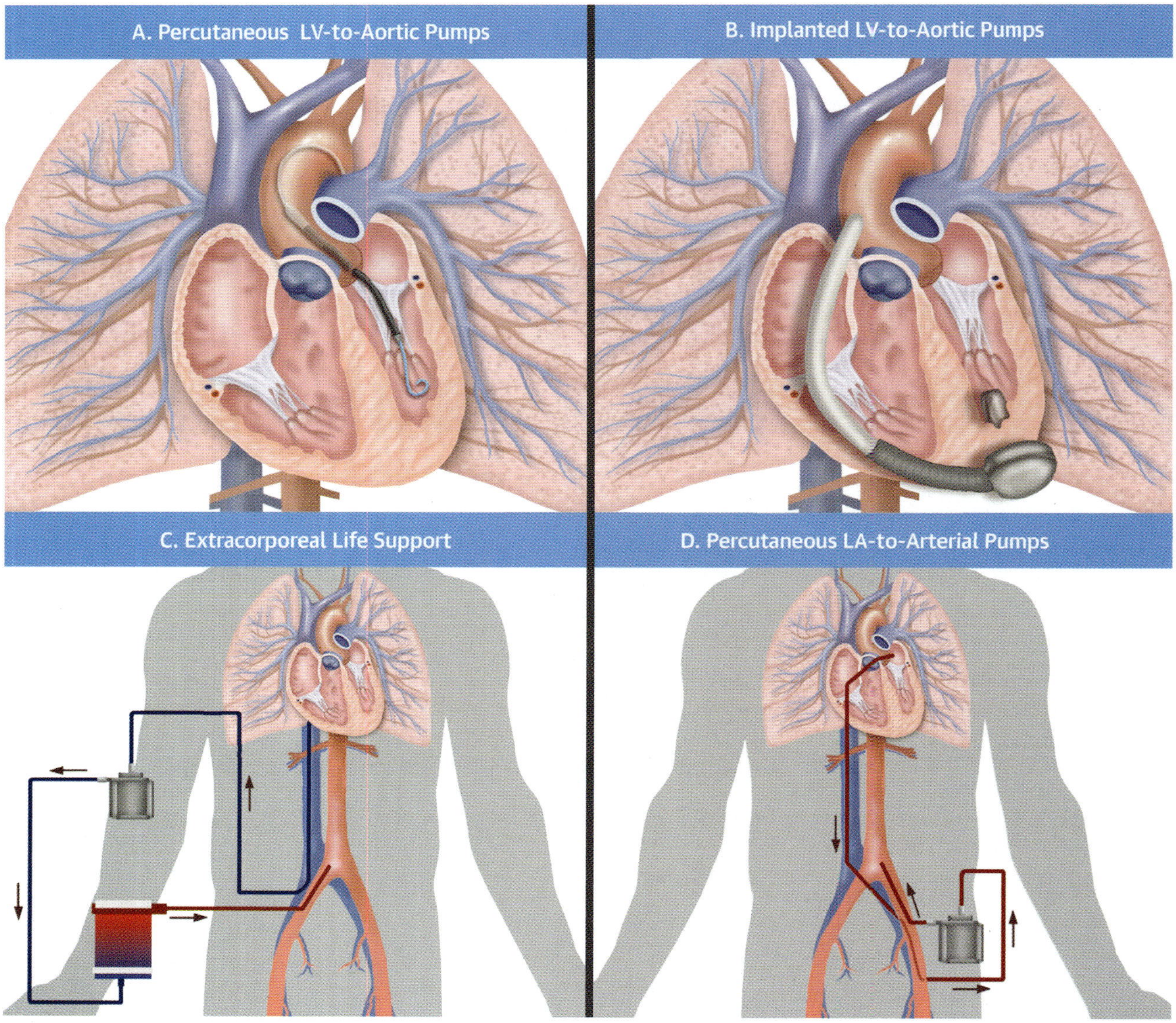

Fig 12.1 Although all forms of mechanical circulatory support return blood to arterial system, they differ with respect to site from which they draw blood. These differences underlie differences in their hemodynamic effects. Percutaneous axial flow devices **(A)** (Impella®) and durable ventricular devices **(B)** (surgically implanted LVAD) that take blood from the LV have similar physiology. Extracorporeal membrane oxygenation (ECMO) withdraws blood from right atrium or venous system and utilizes a blood gas exchange unit **(C)**. Percutaneous devices can also achieve LA sourcing of blood (without need for gas exchange unit) **(D)** (TandemHeart®). LA = left atrium/atrial; LV = left ventricle/ventricular. (From Burkhoff D, Sayer G, Doshi D, Uriel N: Hemodynamics of mechanical circulatory support, J Am Coll Cardiol 66:2663–2674, 2015.)

CASE 12-1
Intraaortic Balloon Pump

An intraaortic balloon pump (IABP) may be positioned before surgery in patients with hemodynamic compromise or with critical coronary artery disease or may be placed at the end of the procedure to facilitate weaning from cardiopulmonary bypass in patients with severely impaired left ventricular systolic function. The catheter is inserted via a femoral artery, and positioned in the descending thoracic aorta, with the catheter tip just distal to the left subclavian artery.

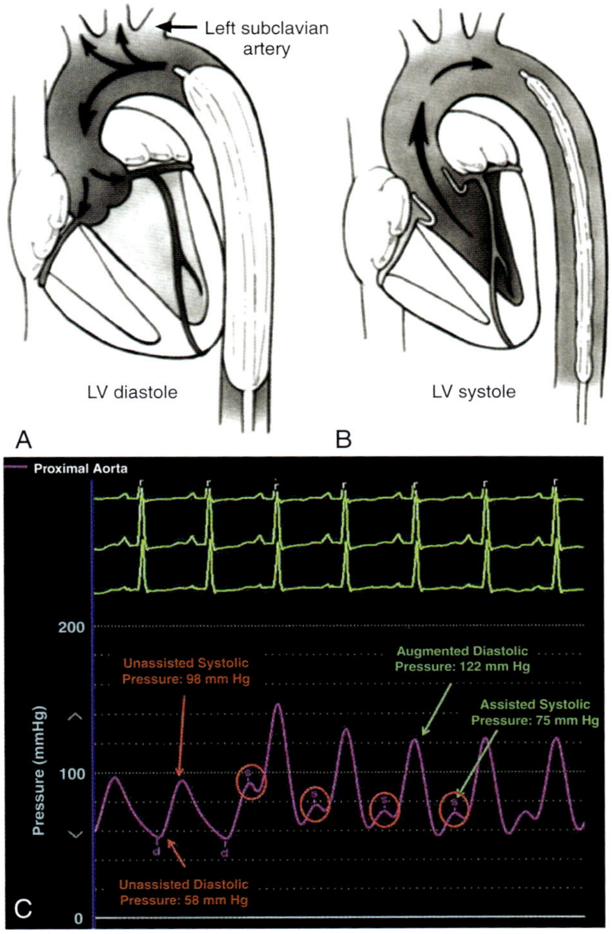

Fig 12.2 IABP is positioned distal to left subclavian origin and inflates in diastole **(A)**, increasing aortic root and coronary perfusion, then deflates in systole **(B)**, reducing LV afterload. **(C)** Hemodynamic tracing of proximal aortic pressure at time of IABP activation shows reduction in systolic pressure and augmented diastolic pressure. Reduced aortic systolic pressure is an indicator of mechanical unloading of left ventricular pressure. (A and B reproduced with permission from Jones HA, et al: J Invasive Cardiol 24(10):544–550, 2012. C reproduced with permission from Kapur NK, Esposite M: Hemodynamic support with percutaneous devices in patients with heart failure, Heart Fail Clin 11:215–230, 2015.)

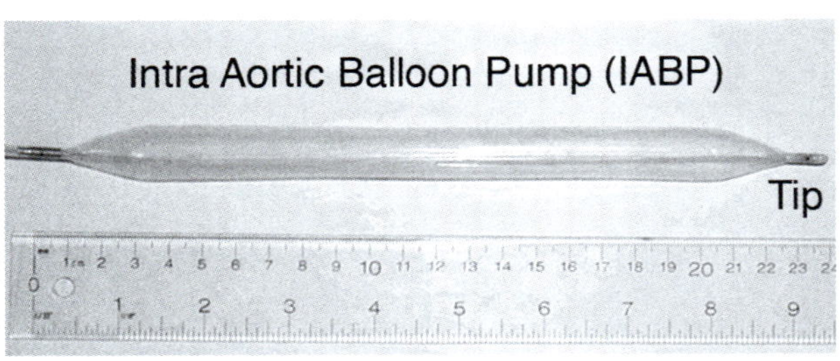

Fig 12.3 Photograph of an intraaortic balloon pump (IABP), demonstrating tip and length of balloon that is placed in the descending aorta. IABP tip has a radiopaque marker to aid in positioning. Proximal end of catheter is off the image at left.

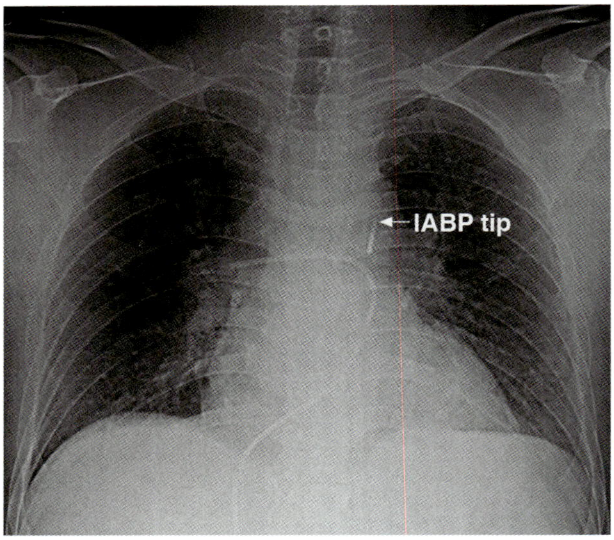

Fig 12.4 Chest radiograph demonstrating the tip of the IABP just distal to the aortic arch. Right heart catheter is also present.

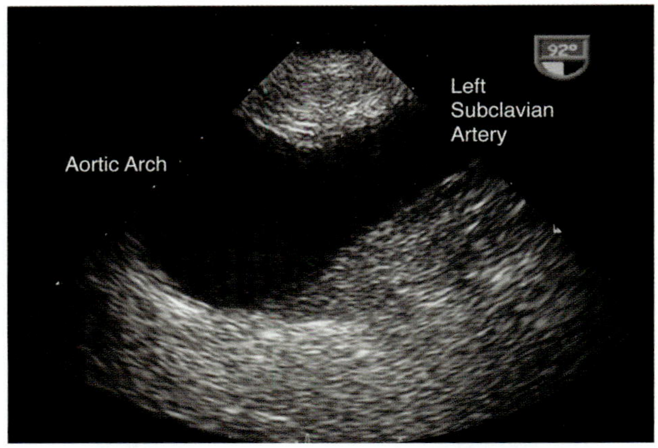

Fig 12.5 This view of the aortic arch and left subclavian artery is obtained from a very high TEE position, with probe turned to patient's left side and image plane rotated to about 90 degrees. This view is helpful for confirming correct positioning of the IABP, which will be seen if the tip is advanced too far into the aorta.

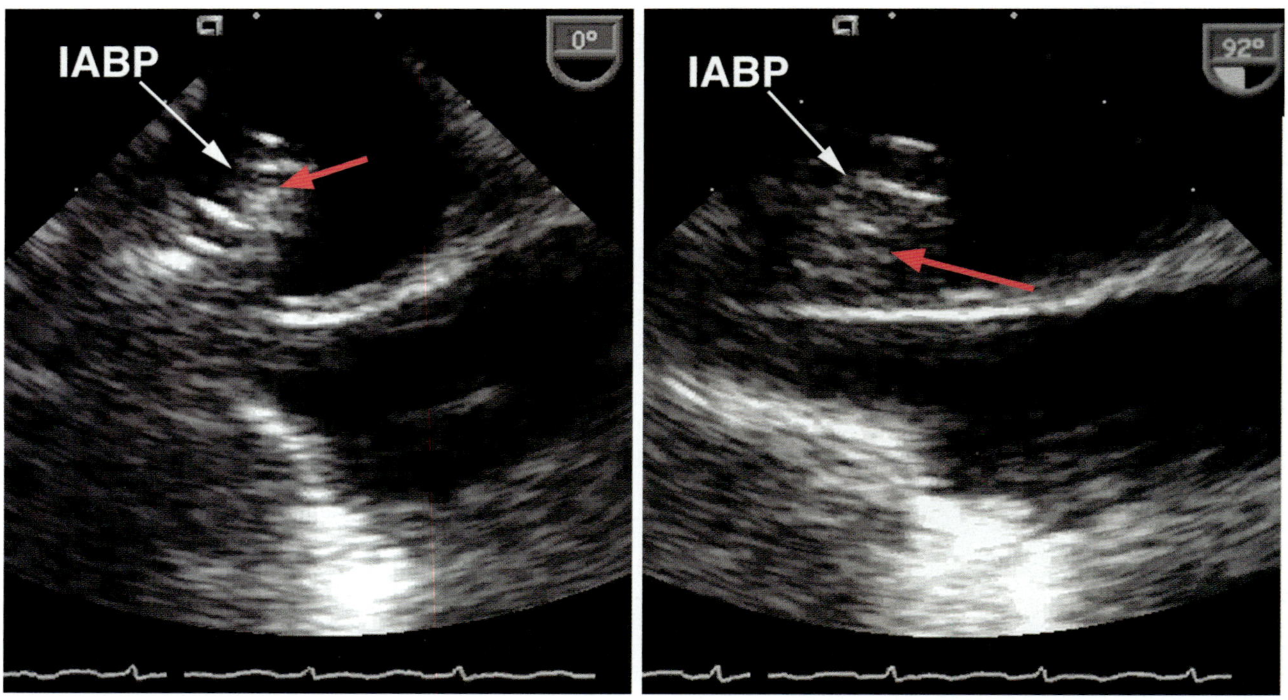

Fig 12.6 This view of the descending thoracic aorta reveals typical appearance in short-axis view *(left)* and long-axis view *(right)* of intraaortic balloon pump. In real time, the device is seen to pulsate in synchrony with the heartbeat. There are multiple reverberations from inflated balloon *(red arrow)*.

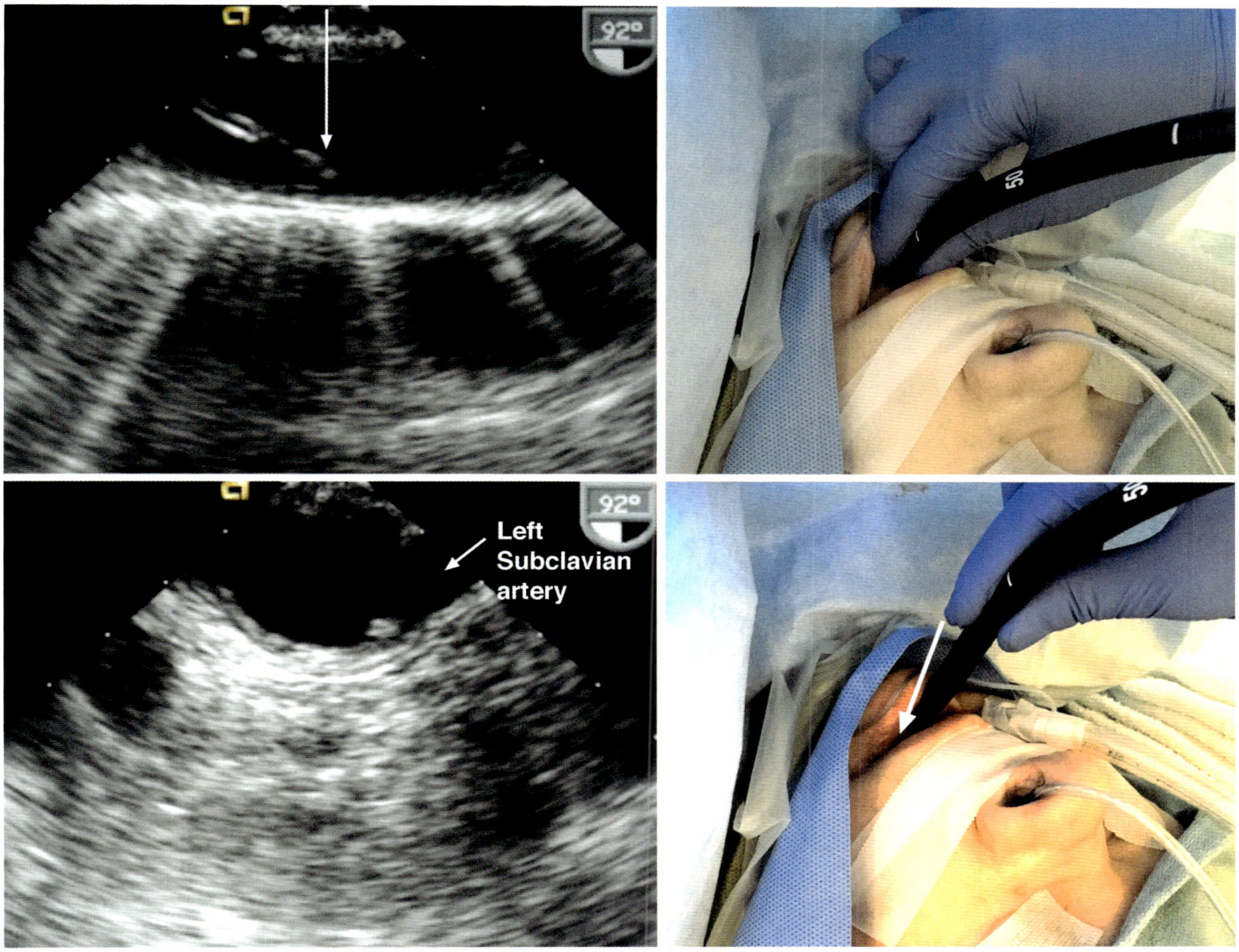

Fig 12.7 Technique for determining position of the IABP. With balloon preferably suspended and descending thoracic aorta visualized in the long axis, operator withdraws probe until tip is in middle of sector, and places a finger where probe meets patient's teeth (upper two images). Probe is slowly withdrawn with finger held in place until left subclavian artery is seen, at which point the operator stops and measures distance from finger to teeth (*lower two images*). (With the assistance of Heather Reed MD).

Comments

The purpose of an IABP is to improve both forward cardiac output in systole and coronary flow in diastole. The balloon inflates during diastole and deflates during systole, with timing based on an arterial pressure waveform and/or the electrocardiogram. Balloon inflation in diastole improves coronary artery blood flow, which occurs mainly in diastole, by increasing the coronary perfusion pressure. Balloon deflation in systole effectively decreases left ventricular afterload resulting in an increase in forward cardiac output.

An IABP is contraindicated in patients with significant aortic regurgitation, as diastolic balloon inflation increases the volume of backflow across the aortic valve.

Suggested Reading

1. De Silva K, Lumley M, Kailey B, et al: Coronary and microvascular physiology during intraaortic balloon counterpulsation, JACC Cardiovasc Interv 7:631–640, 2014.

CASE 12-2
External Centrifugal Pump Devices

This patient was taken to the cardiac catheterization laboratory for placement of a TandemHeart® percutaneous assist device (Cardiac-Assist®, Pittsburgh, PA) for circulatory support after an acute myocardial infraction and percutaneous coronary intervention with acute heart failure.

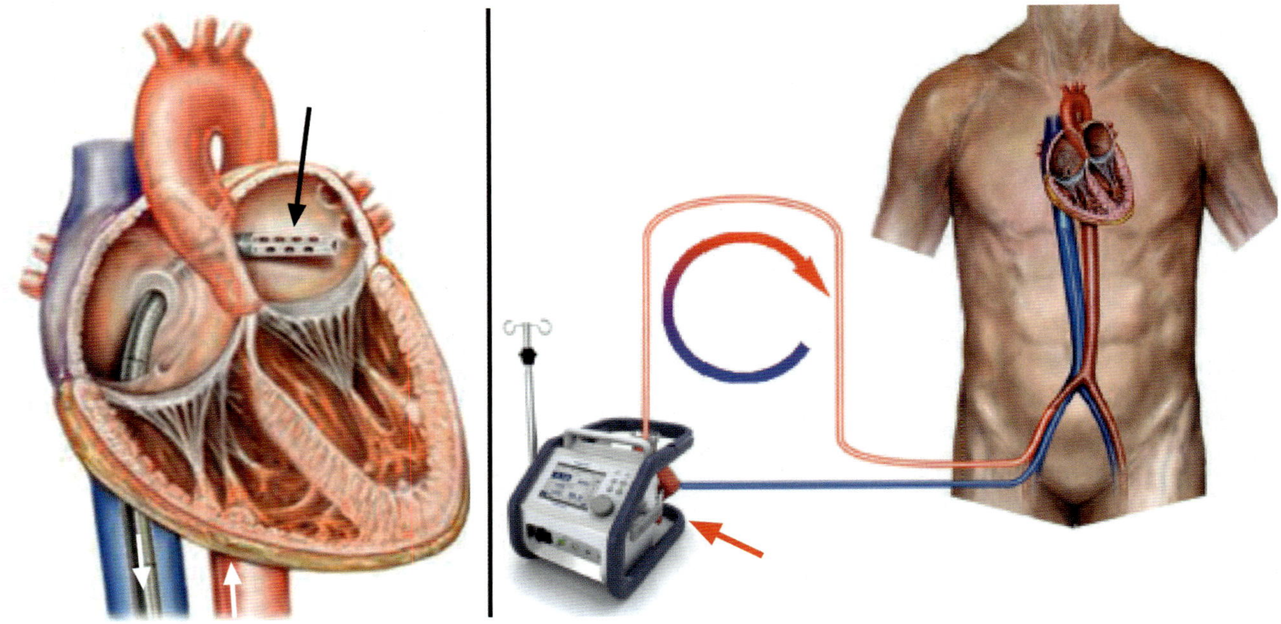

Fig 12.8 Schematic of device. Oxygenated blood is removed from left atrium via multiorifice transseptal cannula *(black arrow)*, and with use of centrifugal pump *(red arrow)* is delivered to a cannula in the femoral artery. (From Myat A, Patel N, Tehrani S, et al: Percutaneous circulatory assist device for high-risk coronary intervention, J Am Coll Cardiol Interv 8:229–244, 2015. With permission.)

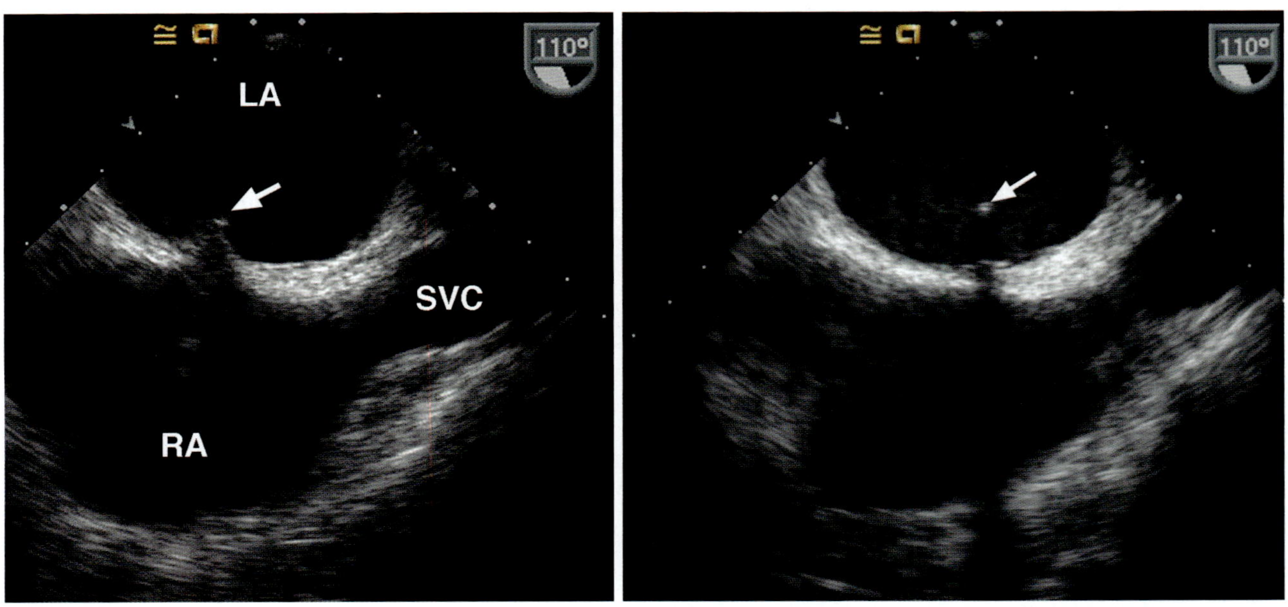

Fig 12.9 Transseptal puncture. Interatrial septum is first tented with needle *(left)*, and then punctured *(right)*. White arrows indicate puncture needle.

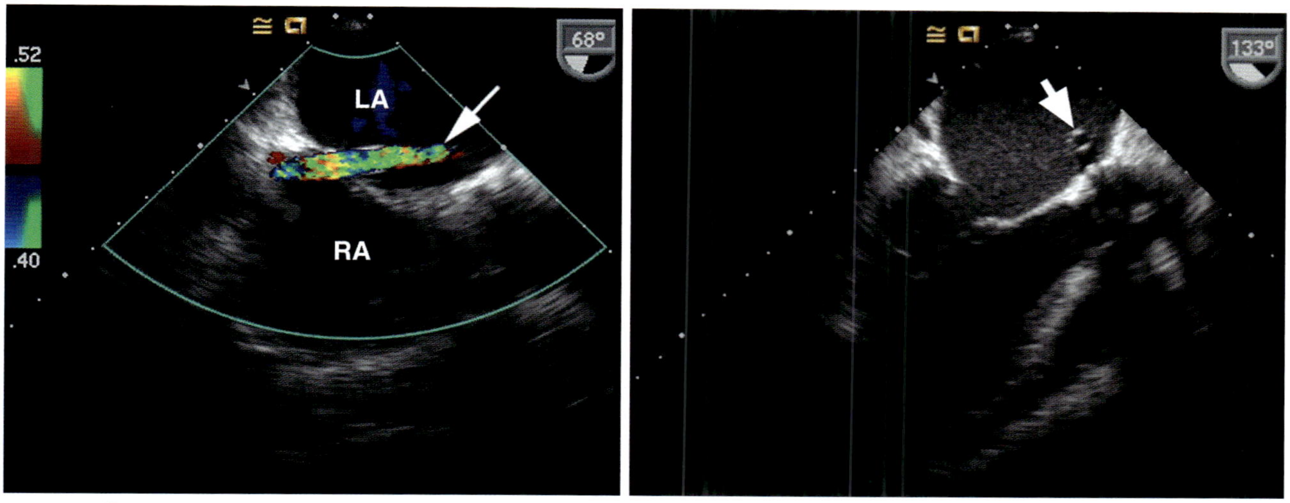

Fig 12.10 In left frame, cannula with color flow is seen to cross interatrial septum into LA. On right, cannula is seen in cross section.

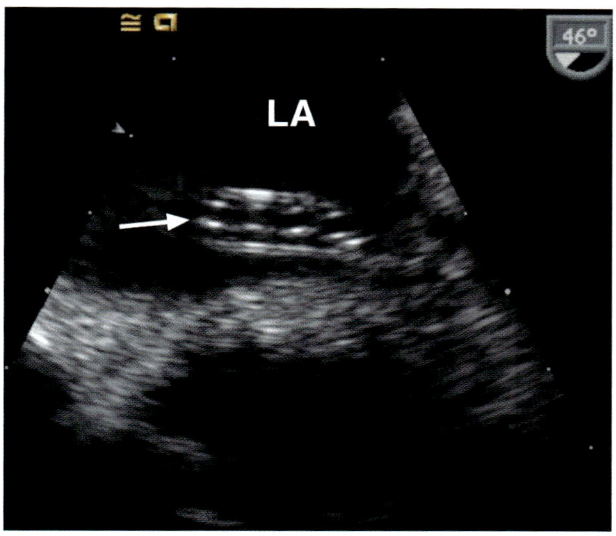

Fig 12.11 Close-up of end of inflow cannula in left atrium. Multiple orifices are seen. Position of distal end of inflow cannula is important; if too close to interatrial septum, it may retract into right atrium causing flow of right atrial blood to device and significant shunt.

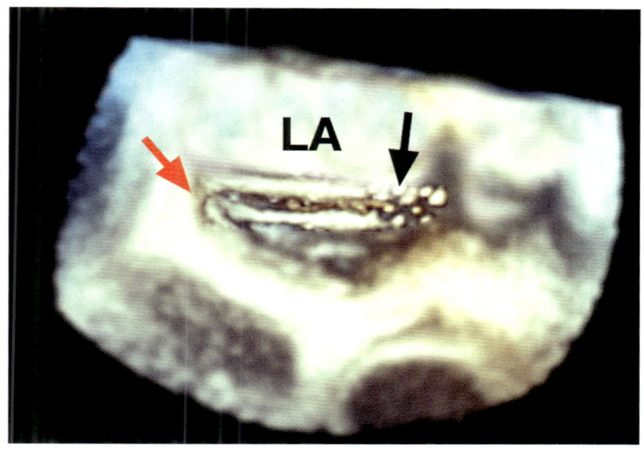

Fig 12.12 3D TEE of left atrium shows cannula crossing interatrial septum *(red arrow)*. Multiorificed tip is indicated by black arrow.

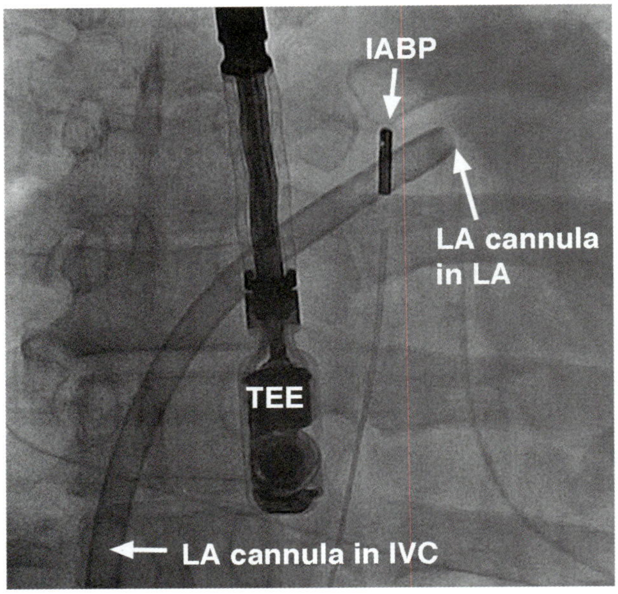

Fig 12.13 On x-ray, position of LA cannula crossing interatrial septum to provide inflow into TandemHeart® is visible. This patient also has IABP with radiopaque tip in descending aorta, behind LA. In real time normal inflation–deflation of IABP can be appreciated.

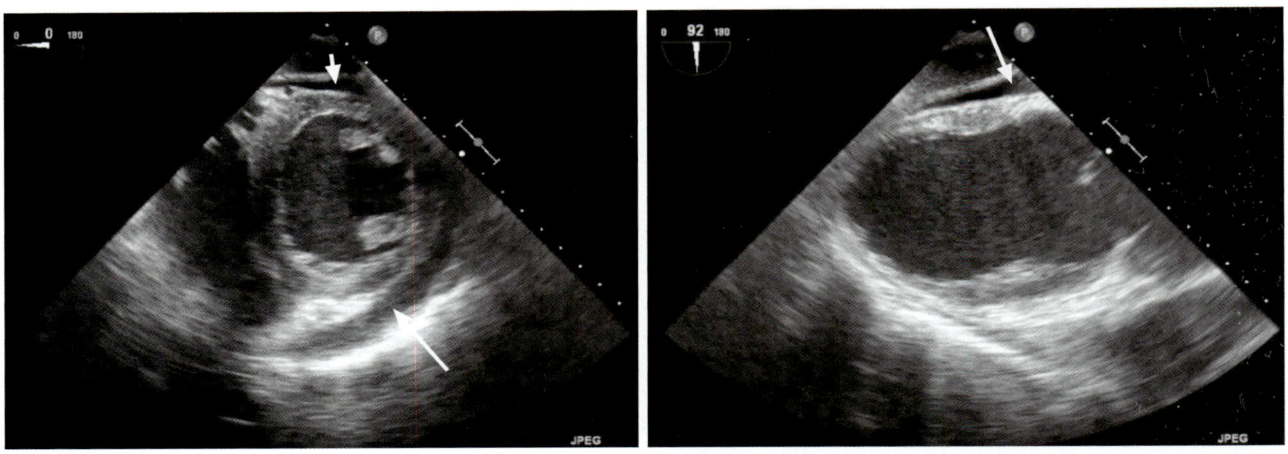

Fig 12.14 In different case, this 50-year-old man with preexisting heart failure was brought to cath lab following major myocardial infarction. In real time, profound hypokinesis is seen in all major ventricular segments. Left ventricle is seen in transgastric short axis and long axis. Arrow indicates collection of pericardial effusion. In real time, ventricles are severely hypokinetic.

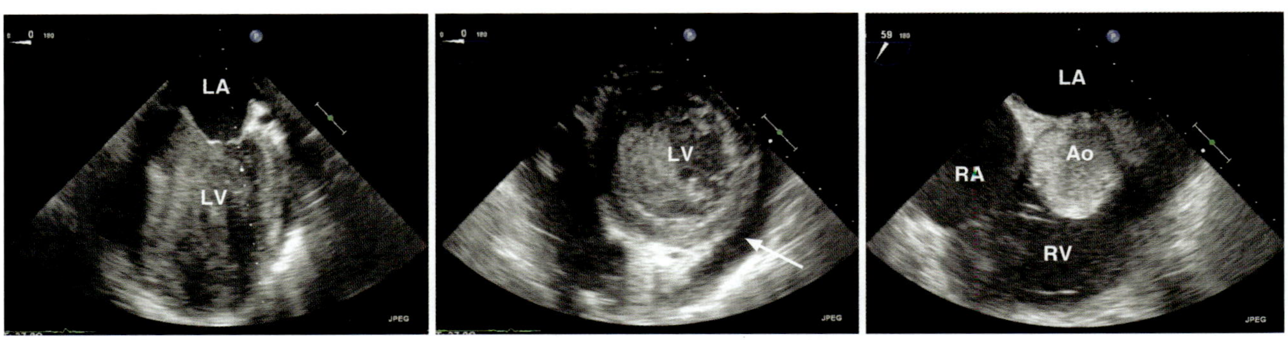

Fig 12.15 In same patient as seen in Fig 12.14, TandemHeart® cannulae were placed and flow from LA to aorta was initiated. After initiating flow, significant echo contrast in left ventricle and aortic root was seen, which did not clear. This phenomenon was secondary to extremely low native left ventricular stroke volume. The arrow indicates pericardial fluid.

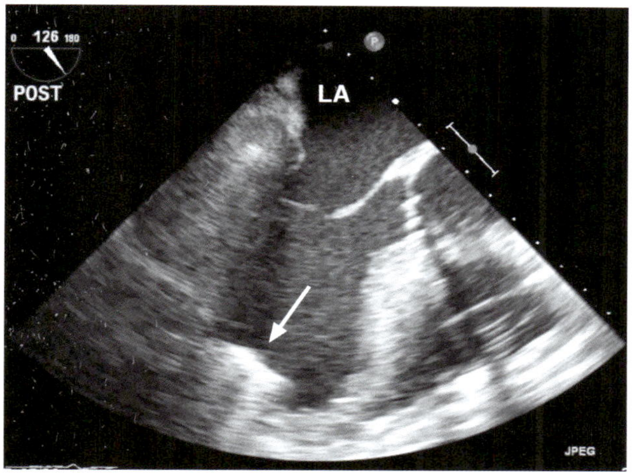

Fig 12.16 In same patient as Fig 12.14, because of concern for risk of left-sided thrombosis, even with anticoagulation, patient was taken to OR where implanted left ventricular assist device was placed and percutaneous device removed. Arrow indicates inflow cannula to device.

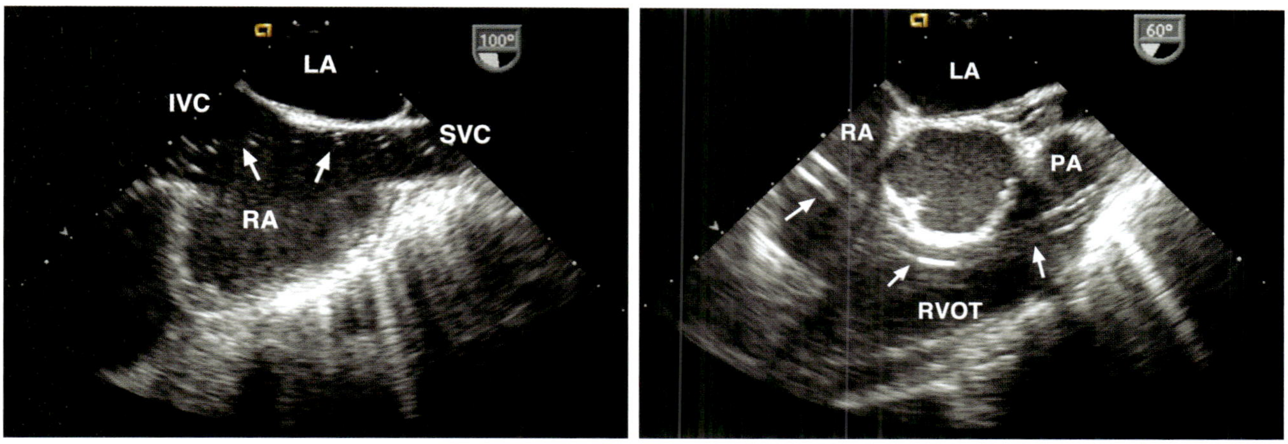

Fig 12.17 Another example of support with TandemHeart® is this 57-year-old man who suffered right ventricular infarction resulting in cardiogenic shock. He was taken urgently to the cath lab where a right-sided TandemHeart® device was placed. Inflow cannula to the device, a multiorifice catheter similar to femoral venous cannula used for bypass, was placed via right internal jugular vein *(left)*. Outflow cannula to patient was placed via femoral vein, and through right atrium, tricuspid valve, and pulmonic valve into main PA *(middle, arrows)* thereby passing failing right ventricle.

Comments

Cardiac mechanical support with an external centrifugal pump devices or percutaneous axial flow assist device is primarily used for acute heart failure in the hospital setting where rapid recovery of ventricular function is likely, such as with a high-risk percutaneous coronary intervention. This approach also may be utilized for acute support, followed by placement of a device intended for longer term support or as a bridge to heart transplantation.

Suggested Reading

1. Kowalczyk AK, Mizuguchi KA, Couper GS, et al: Use of intraoperative transesophageal echocardiography to evaluate positioning of TandemHeart® percutaneous right ventricular assist, Anesth Analg 118:72–75, 2014.
2. Kirkpatrick J: Cardiac assist devices: normal findings, device failure and weaning parameters. In Otto CM, editor: The Practice of Clinical Echocardiography, ed 5, Philadelphia, 2016, Elsevier.

CASE 12-3
Percutaneous Axial Flow Assist Devices

Newer percutaneous or centrally placed axial flow assist devices are available for temporary ventricular support (Impella®, Abiomed, Danvers, MA). Placement is retrograde through the aortic valve. These devices offer temporary support for a failing heart as a bridge to recovery, transplant decision, or a more durable device. They are also placed during some procedures such as high-risk percutaneous coronary intervention (PCI) or ventricular tachycardia ablation procedures.

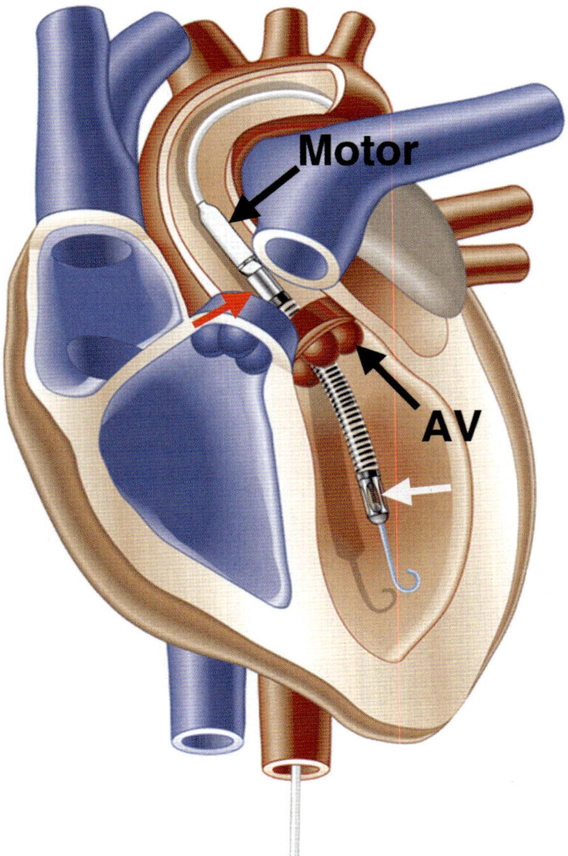

Fig 12.18 Schematic shows device being passed retrograde through aortic valve. Inlet port to device is seen in left ventricle *(white arrow)*, and outflow port in ascending aorta *(red arrow)*.

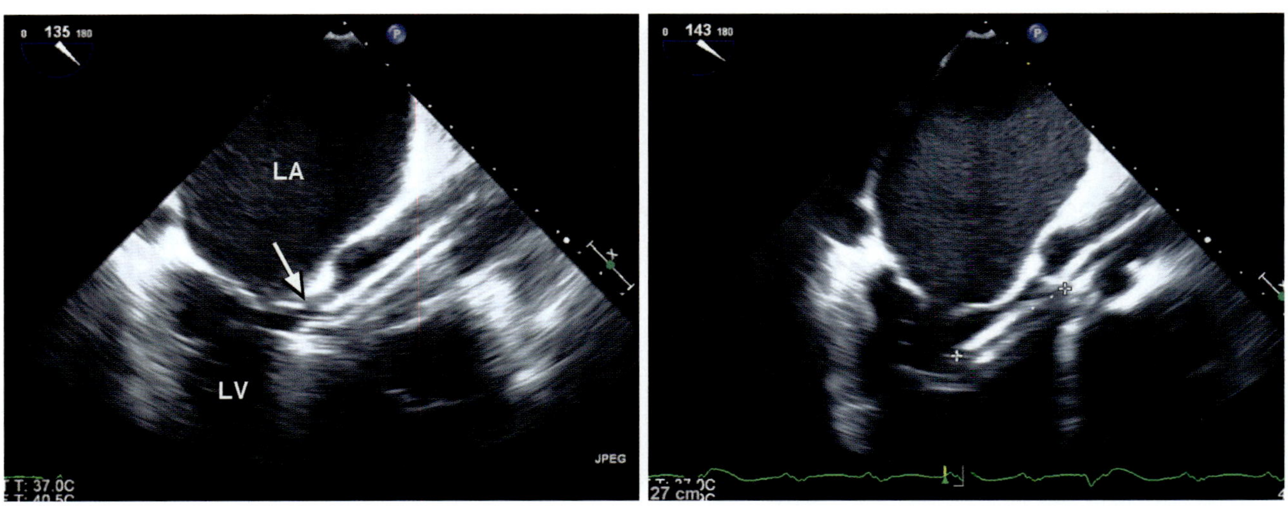

Fig 12.19 On left, ventricular side of device *(arrow)* is seen passing through aortic valve, and on right, device is advanced to its final position. In order to ensure that outlet is positioned optimally just above aortic valve, inlet should be 3–4 cm on LV side of aortic annulus. Inlet is identified on echocardiography as discontinuity in parallel lines of cannula with echoes from cannula tip and pigtail visible more apically in LV chamber.

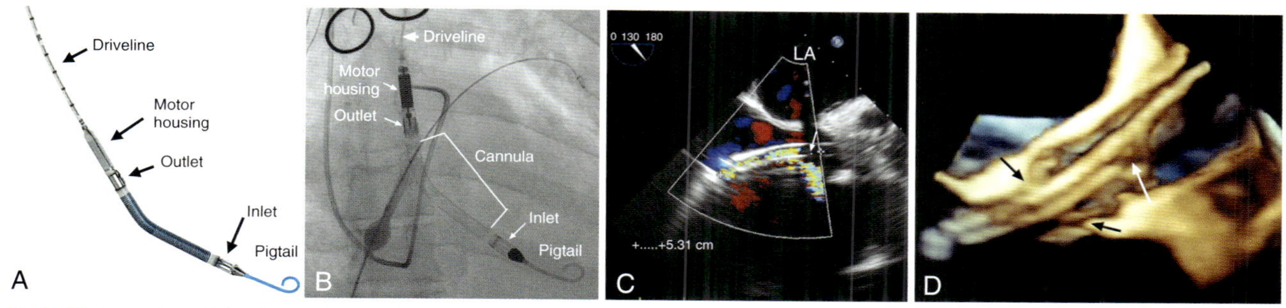

Fig 12.20 A model of the device **(A)** and an image from cardiac catheterization **(B)** illustrates the components of the device: The driveline that is attached to the motor housing, the inlet and outlet ports, and the cannula itself. The 2D TEE **(C)** shows flow in the device; the positions of the ports relative to the aortic valve can be ascertained as can the depth into the left ventricle. It is imperative that the outlet port (white arrow) be above the aortic valve. The 3D TEE **(D)** is a closer look at the outlet port *(white arrow)* and its relationship to the aortic annulus *(black arrows)*.

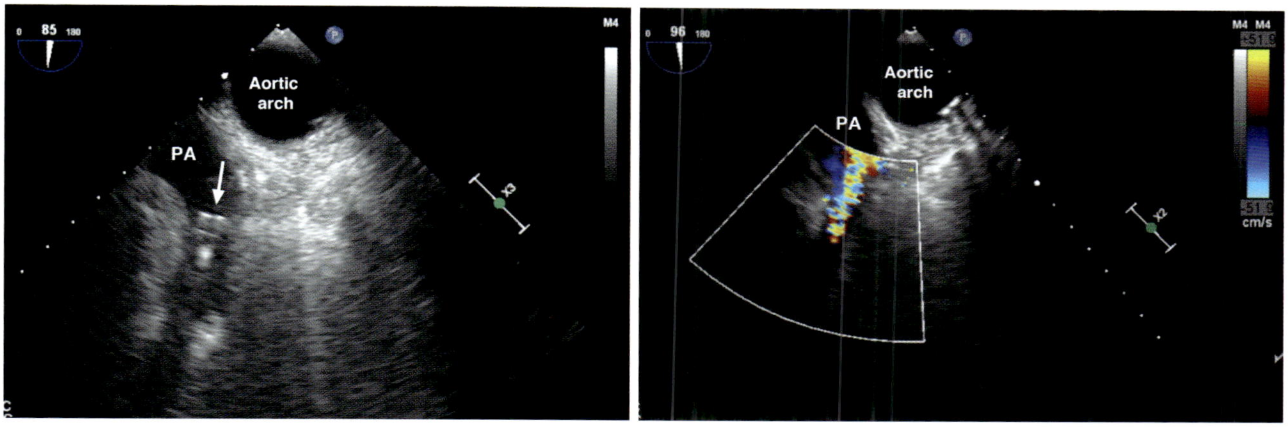

Fig 12.21 Modification of original Impella® allows use on right side of heart for up to 14 days, delivering 4 L/min of flow. Inflow comes from the right atrium, and outflow is delivered to the main pulmonary artery. These findings are illustrated in different patient with acute right heart failure. At left, high esophageal TEE shows cannula to be in pulmonary artery *(arrow)*, and on right, color flow Doppler shows outflow to pulmonary artery.

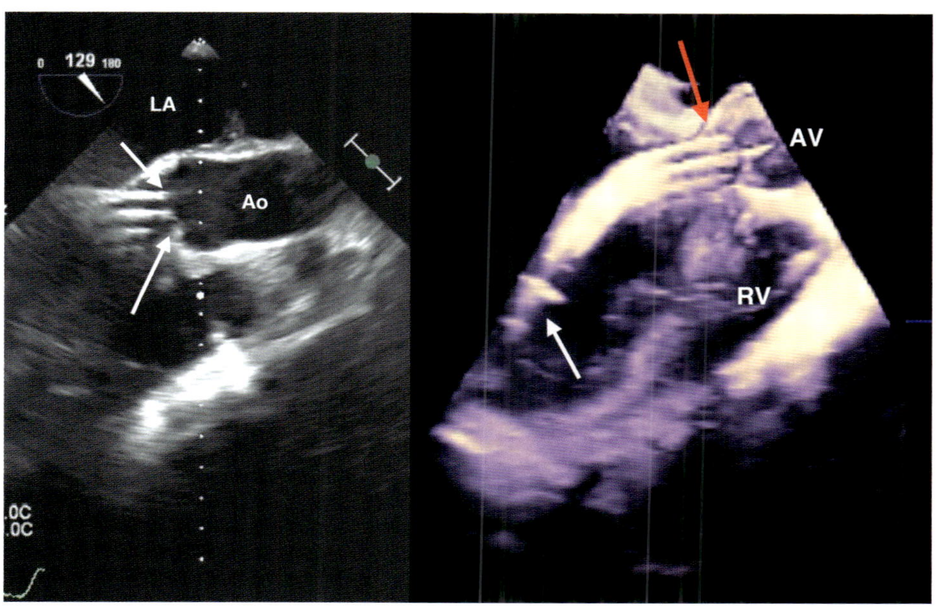

Fig 12.22 In this patient, a 42-year-old male, Impella support was needed after an acute myocardial infarction. On the third day, the device stopped functioning properly so he was taken to the cath lab for assessment. The left image is a midesophageal long-axis view showing the aortic valve *(white arrows)* and the Impella completely within the ventricle. The right image is a 3D TEE at the same depth, showing the aortic valve and the end of Impella beneath it *(red arrow)*, and the inlet portion of the device deep in the LV cavity. Compare this to the normal appearance of the device in Figs 12.18, 12.19, and 12.20.

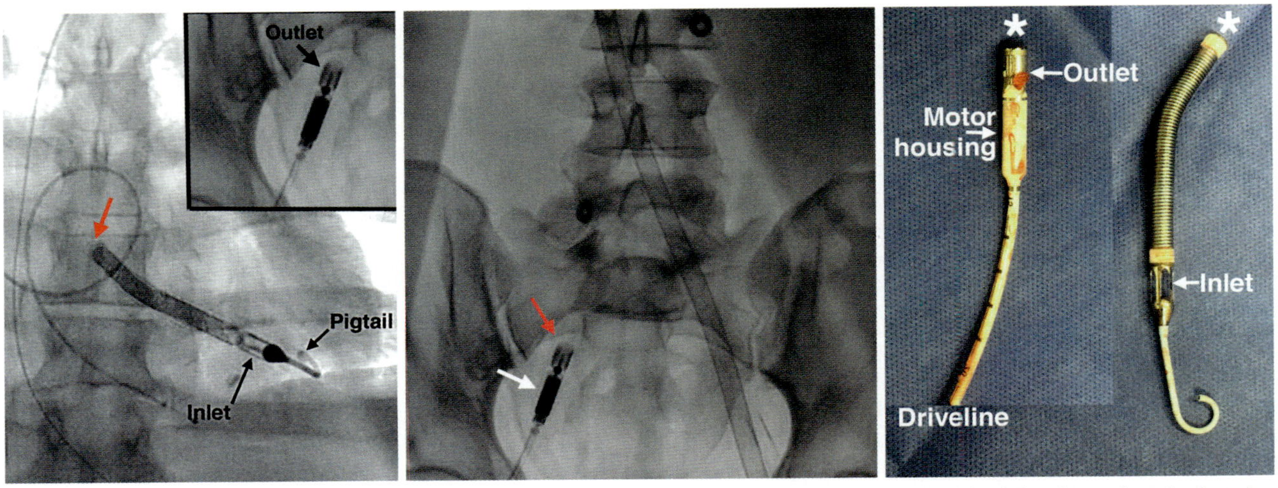

Fig 12.23 In the left image, the device is seen to have fractured. The inset shows the piece which has been detached, and as can be seen in the center image, sits in the right femoral artery. The ends indicated by the two red arrows would normally be connected, and the white arrow indicates the motor housing. The pelvic portion was easily removed, and the interventionalist extracted the intracardiac portion, best appreciated in the corresponding video. On the right, the portions of the device are seen. Compare these images to the normal appearance in Fig 12.20.

Comments

The transcatheter axial flow device is available in several sizes; the smaller devices can be placed percutaneously, via a 14 Fr sheath and provide flow rates about 2.5 L/min. A larger device requires surgical implantation but provides up to 5.0 L/min of flow. Echo assessment prior to implantation should focus on ventricular function, as well as the presence of aortic valve disease; stenotic valves might make passage more difficult as well as making the stenosis worse, whereas regurgitation may increase in severity with the device in place. Echo guidance for placement can aid in appropriate placement into the left ventricle as well as evaluation of impingement on the mitral valve apparatus leading to mitral valve dysfunction. The midesophageal long-axis view is typically the best when measuring depth, and evaluation of the mitral valve at multiple angles is necessary to rule out mitral valve dysfunction caused by the device.

Suggested Reading

1. Patel KM. Sherwani SS, Baudo AM, et al: The use of transesophageal echocardiography for confirmation of appropriate Impella 5.0 device placement, Anesth Analg 14:82–85, 2012.

CASE 12-4
Extracorporeal Membrane Oxygenation

This 24-year-old woman with cystic fibrosis was awaiting lung transplantation, but despite tracheostomy and mechanical ventilation, she had profound hypercarbia. It was decided to proceed to veno-venous (V-V) extracorporeal membrane oxygenation (ECMO) in an attempt to optimize gas exchange prior to transplant. She was taken to the OR where her right internal vein was cannulated with a double-lumen V-V ECMO cannula (Avalon©, Maquet, Rastatt, Germany). Three weeks later she underwent successful double-lung transplantation.

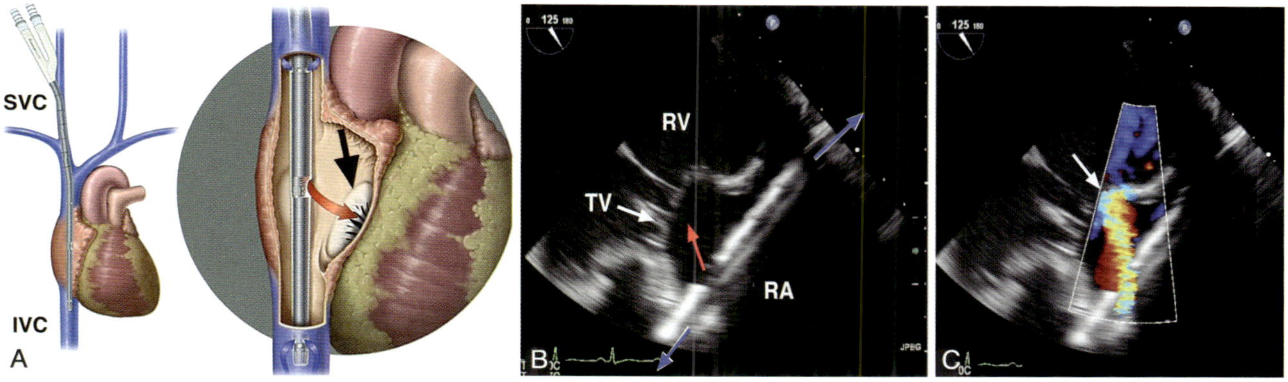

Fig 12.24 Veno-venous ECMO cannula positioning. Panel A illustrates Avalon© (Maquet, Rastatt, Germany) bicaval dual-lumen cannula for veno-venous extracorporeal membrane oxygenation. Catheter is seen entering internal jugular vein, and advanced to facilitate drainage of venous blood from IVC and SCV, with outflow lumen placed opposite tricuspid valve *(black arrow)*. Transgastric long-axis view of right atrium and right ventricle; in panel B, venous blood leaving patient is represented by blue arrows, and oxygenated blood exiting cannula is directed to tricuspid valve *(red arrow)*. In panel C, color Doppler illustrates flow from cannula through tricuspid valve. Examination of the distal portion of the cannula is recommended to ensure that a hepatic vein has not been entered. (Panel A reprinted from Souilamas R, Souilamas J, Alkhamees K, et al: Extracorporal membrane oxygenation in general thoracic surgery: A new single veno-venous cannulation, J Cardiothorac Surg 6:52–54, 2011. With permission.)

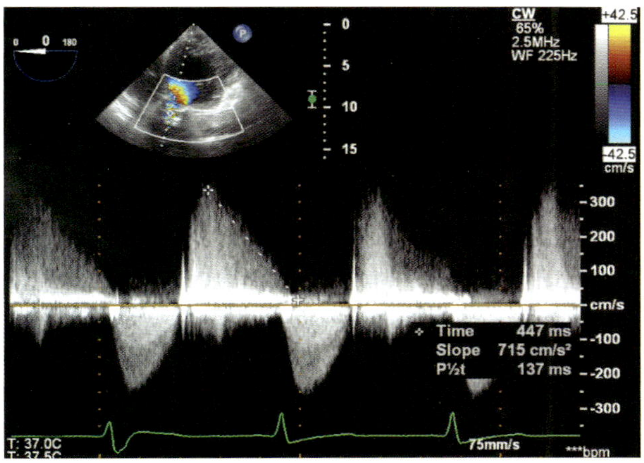

Fig 12.25 This 39-year-old man underwent Bentall procedure for severe aortic regurgitation and aortic dilation. Baseline intraoperative TEE before Bentall showed severe aortic regurgitation. Color Doppler and continuous wave Doppler tracings were obtained from deep transgastric position. Pressure half time of aortic regurgitation jet is extremely short at 137 msec, indicative of severe aortic regurgitation.

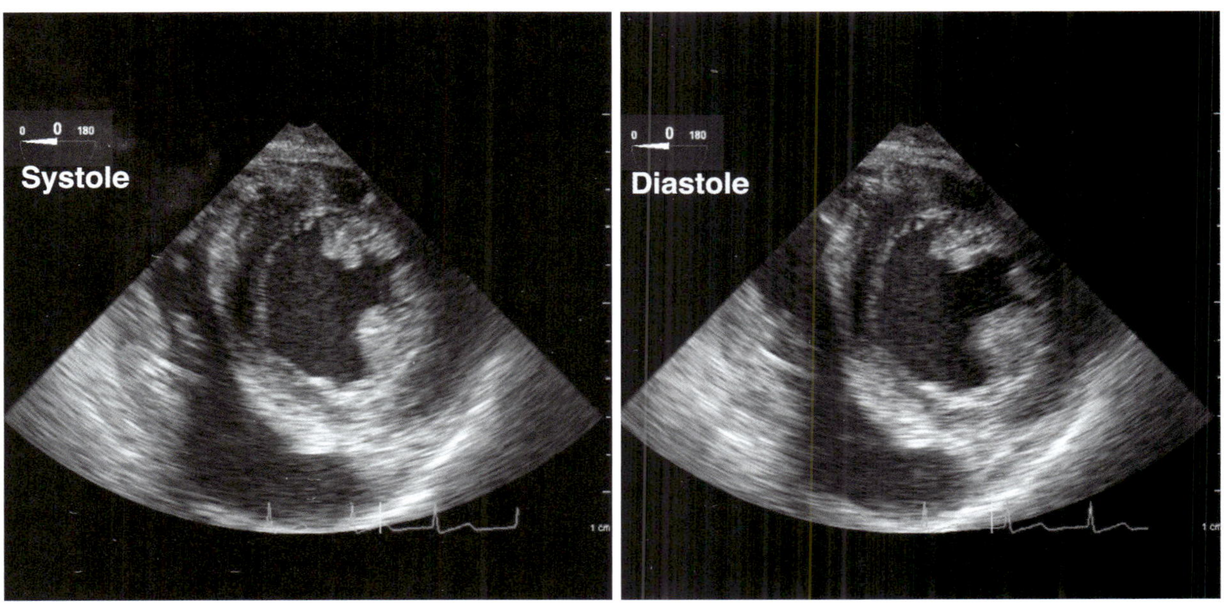

Fig 12.26 Surgery was complex, and cardiopulmonary bypass pump time was long. Although left ventricular function was only mildly reduced preoperatively, it deteriorated significantly after procedure. Despite large doses of inotropes and intraaortic balloon pump support, patient could not be weaned from bypass, and was placed on V-A ECMO support. Systolic and diastolic frames after attempt at separation from bypass are indicative of very low fractional area of change, better appreciated when real-time clip is observed.

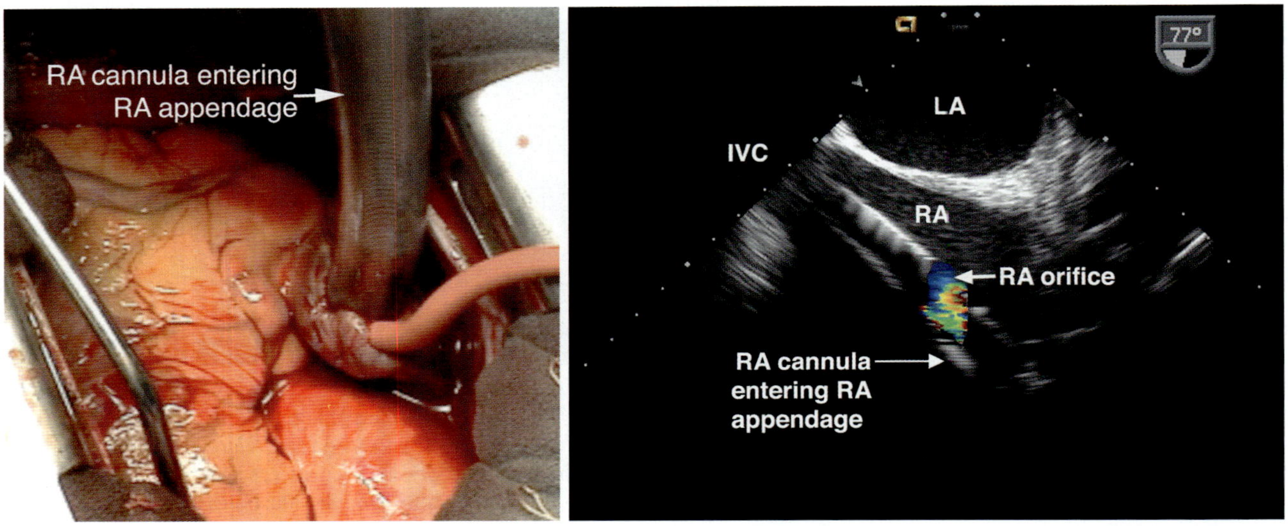

Fig 12.27 Venous cannula for ECMO circuit was preexisting right atrial line used during bypass. Cannula had been inserted into right atrial appendage and advanced into inferior vena cava. "Two-stage cannula" drains blood from IVC with its distal orifice, and from right atrium and superior vena cava from right atrial orifice.

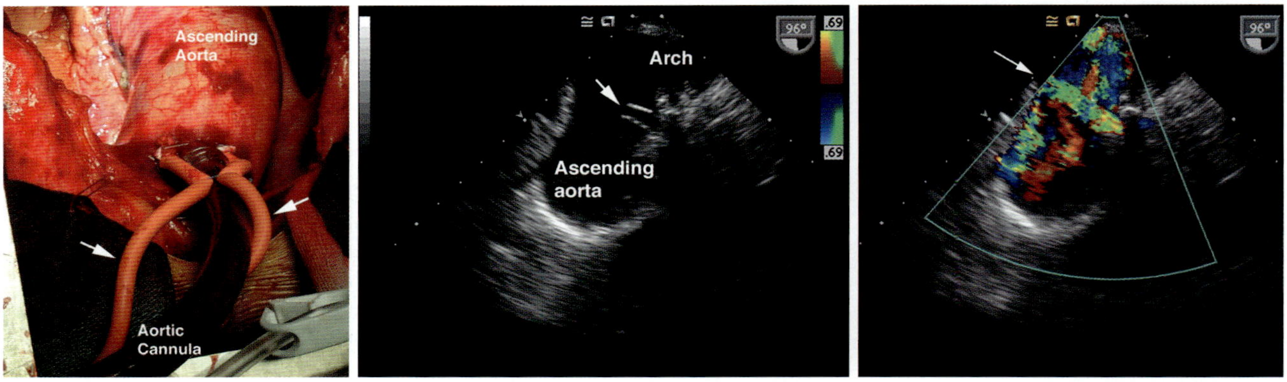

Fig 12.28 Aorta had been cannulated via femoral artery during surgery; however, since chest was going to be left open, aorta was cannulated centrally. In real-time TEE, high-velocity jet emanating from aortic cannula is seen to hit back wall of aorta.

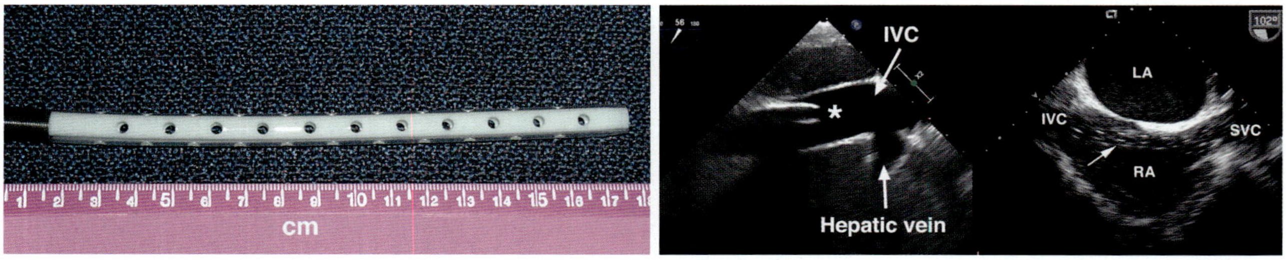

Fig 12.29 In circumstances where chest has not been opened and V-A ECMO support is required, femoral artery is cannulated for arterial access, and multiorifice femoral venous cannula *(left frame)* is advanced to right atrium so that tip is just into superior vena cava. In center frame, transgastric view with probe turned to patient's right shows cannula tip *(*)* as it ascends inferior vena cava. On right, cannula is shown in its final position.

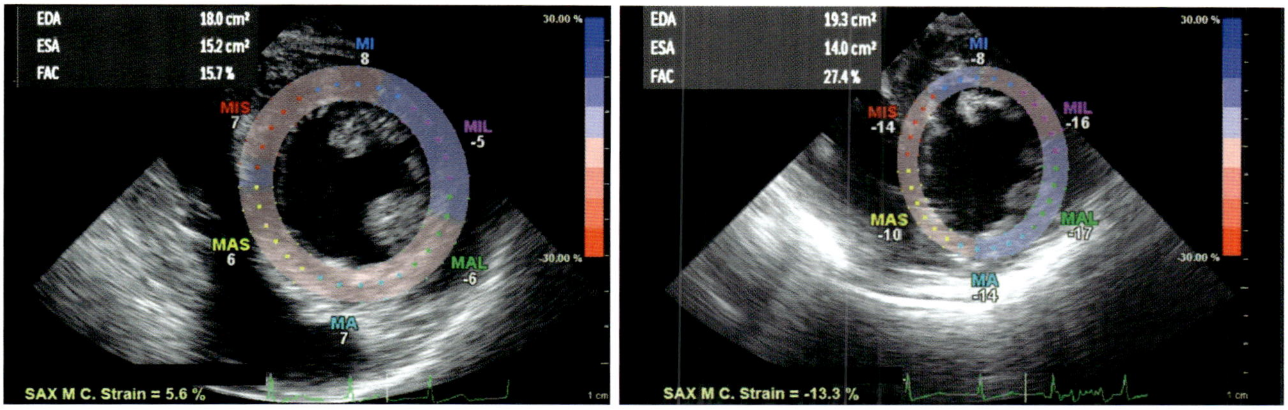

Fig 12.30 Over next 4 days LV systolic function improved and patient was decannulated from ECMO with inotropic and intraaortic balloon pump support. Speckle tracking strain imaging shows a grossly abnormal strain and fractional area of change after initial attempts to separate from bypass, and much improved values at time of ECMO decannulation 4 days later.

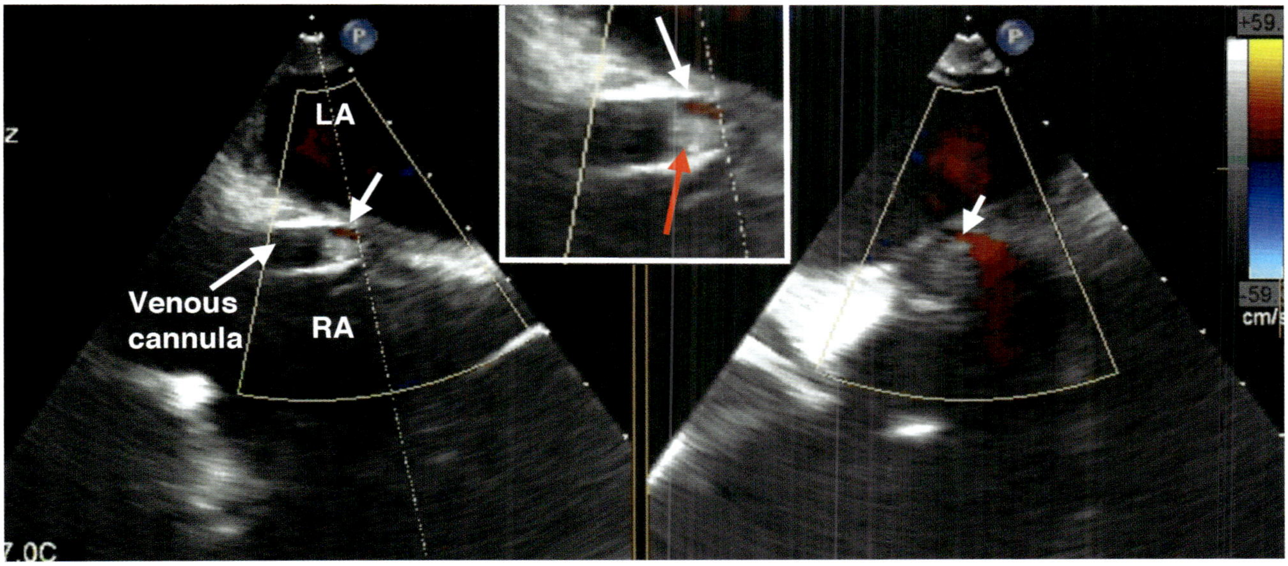

Fig 12.31 In another patient on V-A ECMO, low flows prompted a TEE. On the left, the venous cannula can be seen abutting the interatrial septum; the image is magnified in the inset, with the red arrow indicating a thrombus, and the white arrow indicating a small amount of inflow. On the right, orthogonal imaging shows another perspective of the compromised inflow.

Comments

In patients with respiratory failure refractory to ventilator management in whom cardiac function is adequate, veno-venous (V-V) ECMO can be used to support lung function. A double-lumen cannula is placed via the internal jugular vein into the right atrium. Venous blood is drawn to the device, oxygenation and carbon dioxide occurs, and the blood is pumped back into the right atrium. TEE is used to position this later orifice opposite the tricuspid valve to ensure that the oxygenated blood enters the right ventricle and does not recirculate through the device.

Veno-arterial (V-A) ECMO provides both a continuous flow pump that provides biventricular support and a membrane oxygenator to improve oxygenation and carbon dioxide exchange. The advantage of V-A ECMO compared to other short-term assist device options include the ability to place cannulas and initiate treatment at the bedside at centers experienced with this approach.

Suggested Reading

1. Saffarzadeh A, Bonde P: Options for temporary mechanical circulatory support, J Thorac Dis 7:2102–2011, 2015.

CASE 12-5
Left Ventricular Assist Device

This 30-year-old man had a long history of familial, nonischemic cardiomyopathy, has had difficulty with volume overload, shortness of breath, and paroxysmal nocturnal dyspnea, all of which had been worsening over the previous several months. Several days prior to admission he described an exercise tolerance of about a half-block before stopping due to shortness of breath. His weight was 10 kg over his dry weight. He was admitted for left ventricular assist device (LVAD) placement.

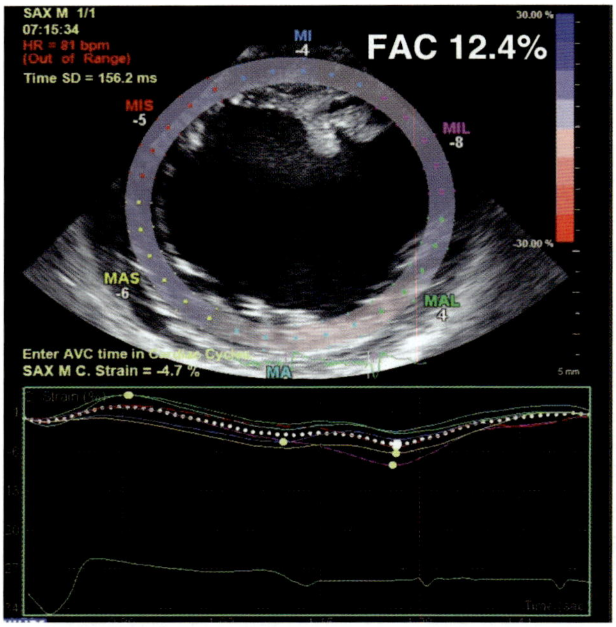

Fig 12.32 Circumferential strain measured from transgastric midpapillary view is severely diminished, consistent with patient's cardiomyopathy.

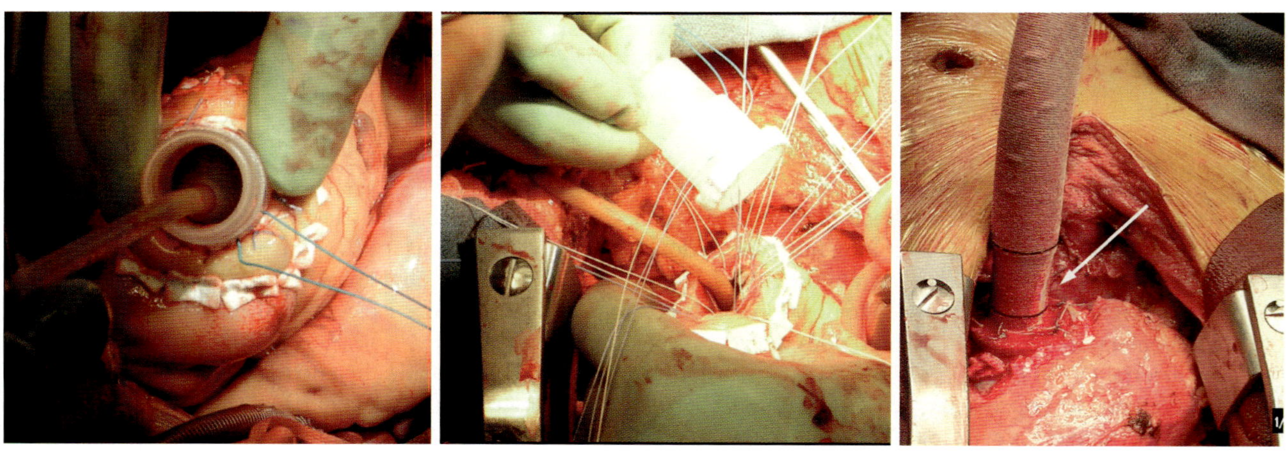

Fig 12.33 At the time of surgery, an inflow cannula is placed at the left ventricular apex. On the left, a circular piece of the apex is resected, an adaptor sewn on, and a Foley catheter placed through the orifice into the LV cavity. This serves to prevent entrainment of air as well as decreasing blood from the LV entering the field. In the middle frame, the apex is prepared for the attachment of the inflow cannula, and the final result is seen in the right frame.

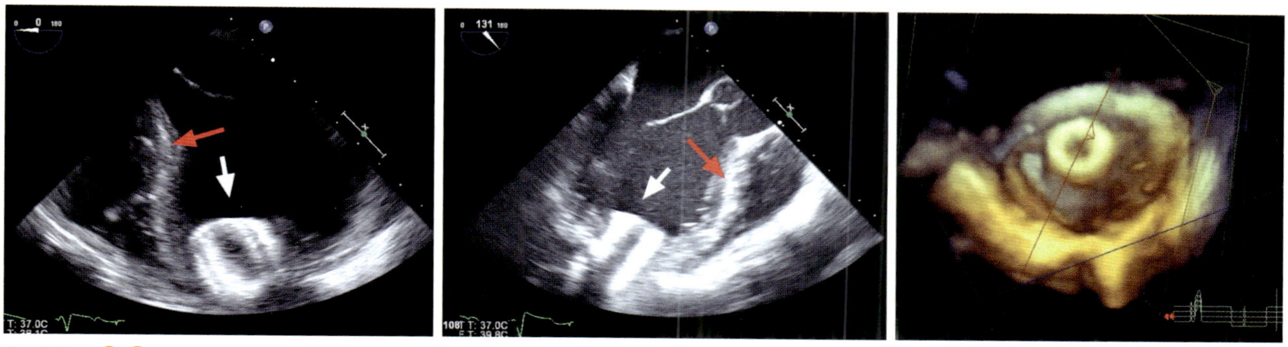

Fig 12.34 Orthogonal 2D images show the end of the inflow cannula *(white arrow)* is clear of the interventricular septum *(red arrow)*. In the 3D TEE on the right, the orifice of the inflow is seen to be free of any contact with the LV walls.

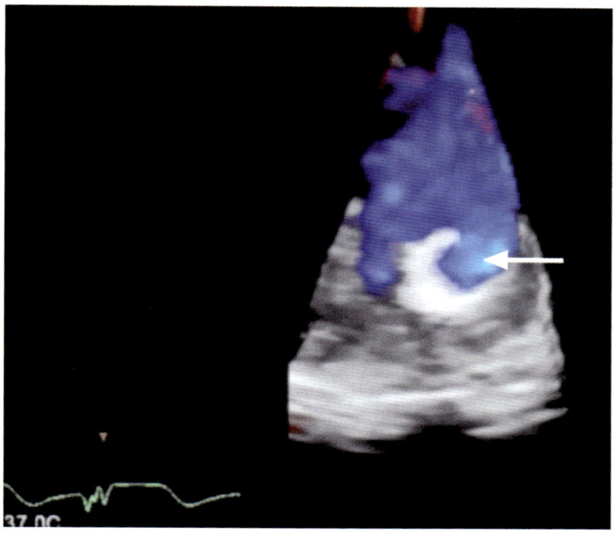

Fig 12.35 3D color TEE shows flow going into the orifice of the inflow cannula.

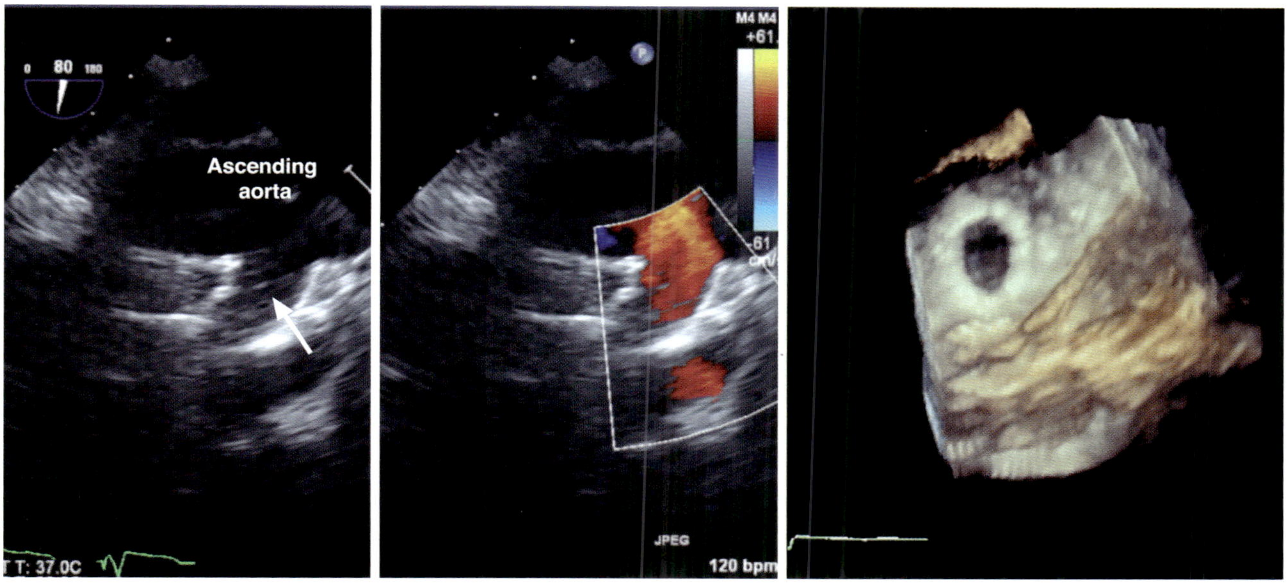

Fig 12.36 The outflow cannula and its anastomosis to the ascending aorta are seen in this midesophageal long-axis image. On the far right, a 3D image acquired from the same view shows the outflow cannula orifice opening into the ascending aorta.

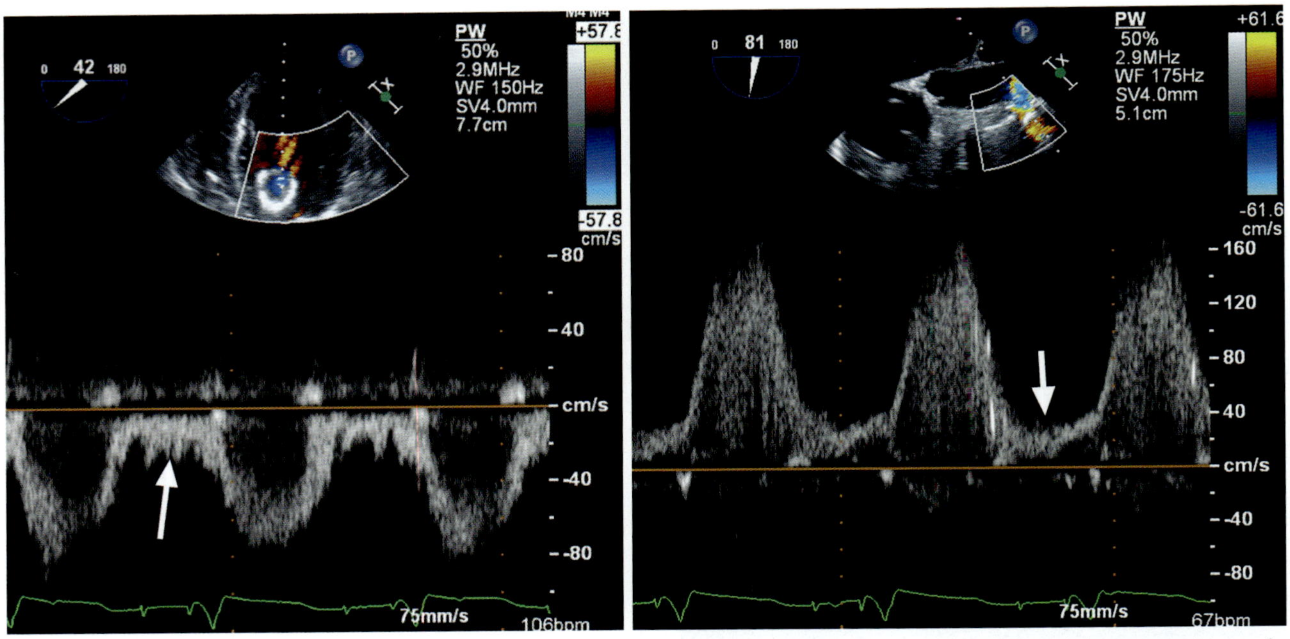

Fig 12.37 Spectral Doppler of the inflow cannula *(left)* and outflow cannula *(right)*. There is a basal flow *(white arrows)* in each. Pulsatile flow is concurrent with LV contraction, which drives blood the LVAD and augments the flow.

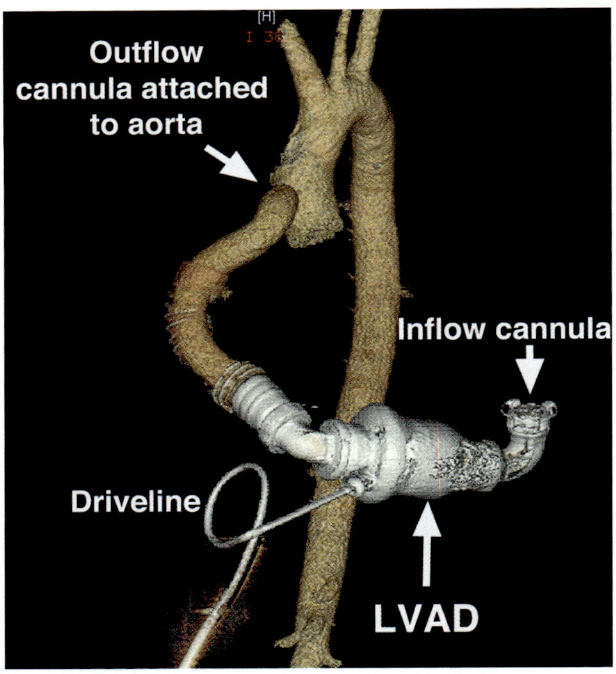

Fig 12.38 A postoperative CT scan show the outflow cannula connected to the aorta just above the sinuses of Valsalva and in inflow cannula at the LV apex, with the LV assist device (LVAD) implanted under the skin of the upper abdomen. The driveline exits the skin to attach to the external power source.

The next 4 images show specific issues seen in the pre and post bypass assessment of the LVAD patient.

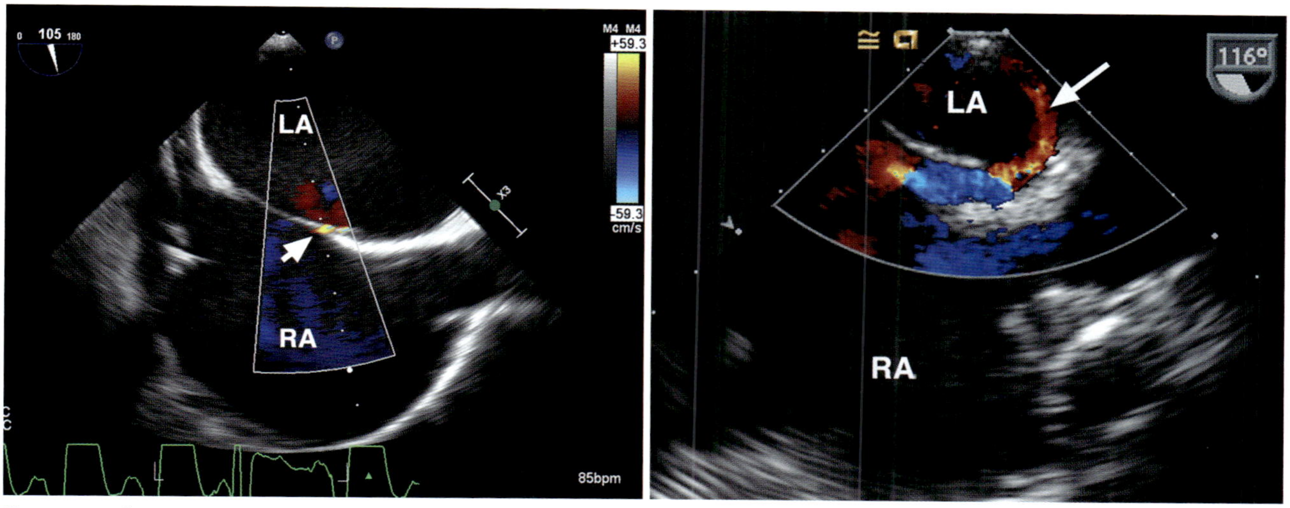

Fig 12.39 Left: Preoperative imaging demonstrates a small patent foramen ovale (PFO). This was closed on bypass. Right: In a different patient in whom an LVAD was placed, and a small PFO with left-to-right shunt left alone, postbypass hypoxemia developed. Color Doppler imaging of the PFO in the midesophageal bicaval view revealed it to be larger, with right-to-left shunting *(arrow)*.

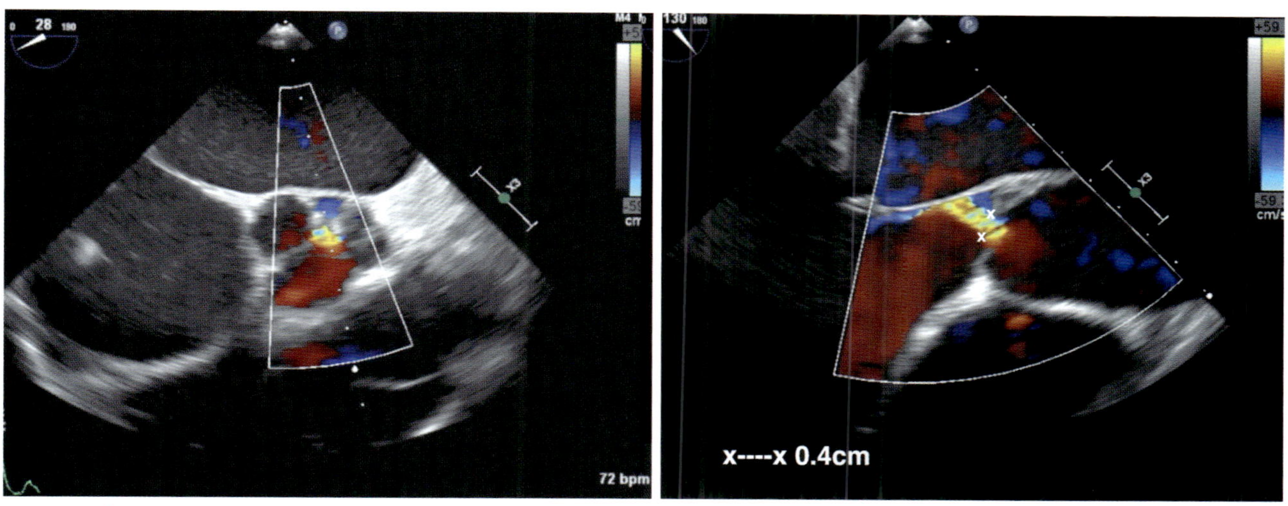

Fig 12.40 Preoperative imaging also demonstrates a moderate amount of aortic regurgitation. Concurrent with the placement of an LVAD, a bioprosthetic AV was placed.

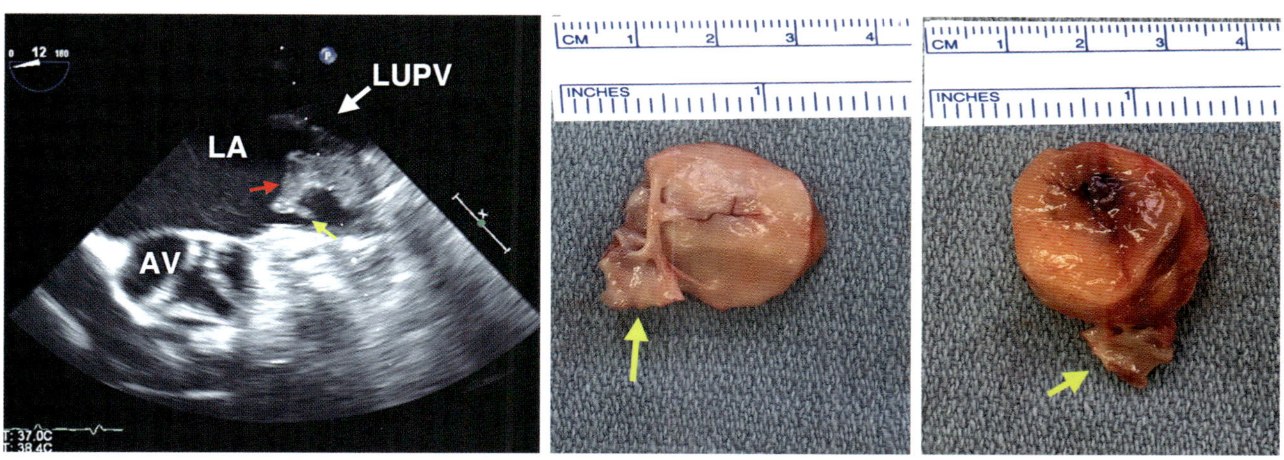

Fig 12.41 This 62-year-old male with severe reduction in systolic function and chronic atrial fibrillation presented for LVAD placement. Prebypass TEE revealed the presence of a large thrombus *(red arrow)* with mobile elements *(yellow arrow)* better appreciated in real time. There was also spontaneous echo contrast in the LA. In the center panel, the excised thrombus is seen from the left atrial side, and on the right, from the perspective of the LAA apex. The yellow arrows indicate the corresponding mobile portions seen on TEE.

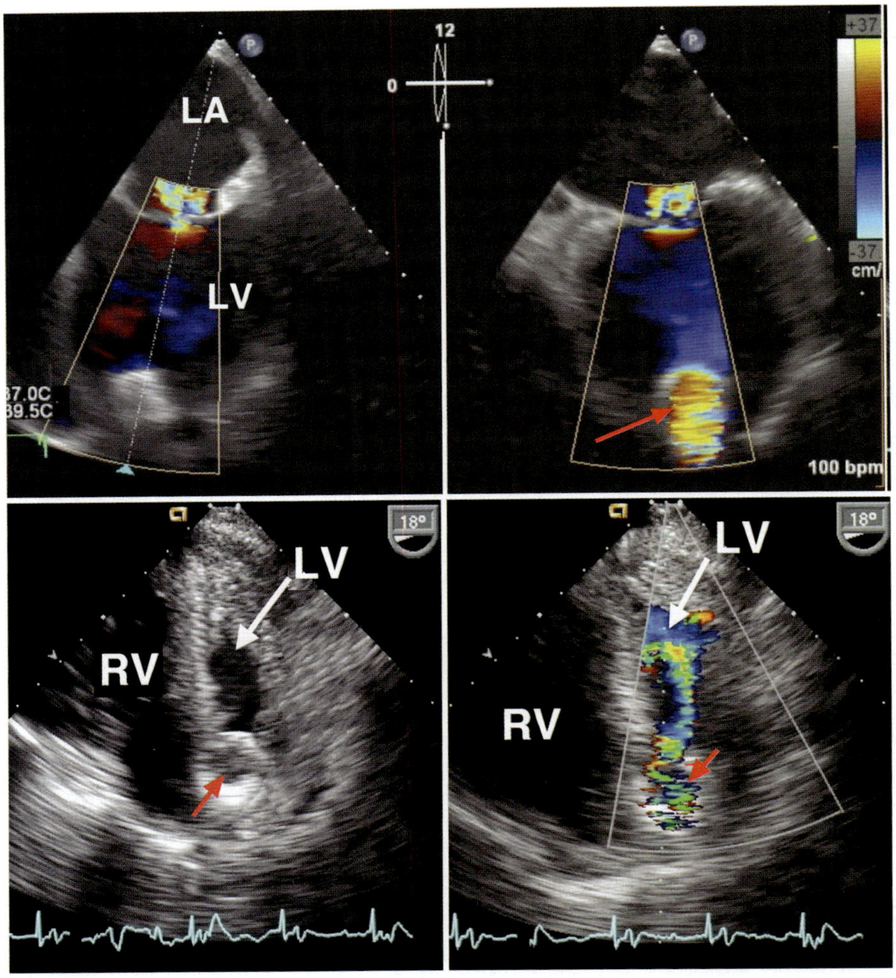

Fig 12.42 In the top 2 panels, color flow Doppler demonstrates unobstructed flow from LA and LV through inflow cannula *(red arrow)*. The lower two panels demonstrate a "suction event"; inadequate volume in the LV causes obstruction of the inflow cannula orifice *(red arrow)* by the collapsing left ventricular walls.

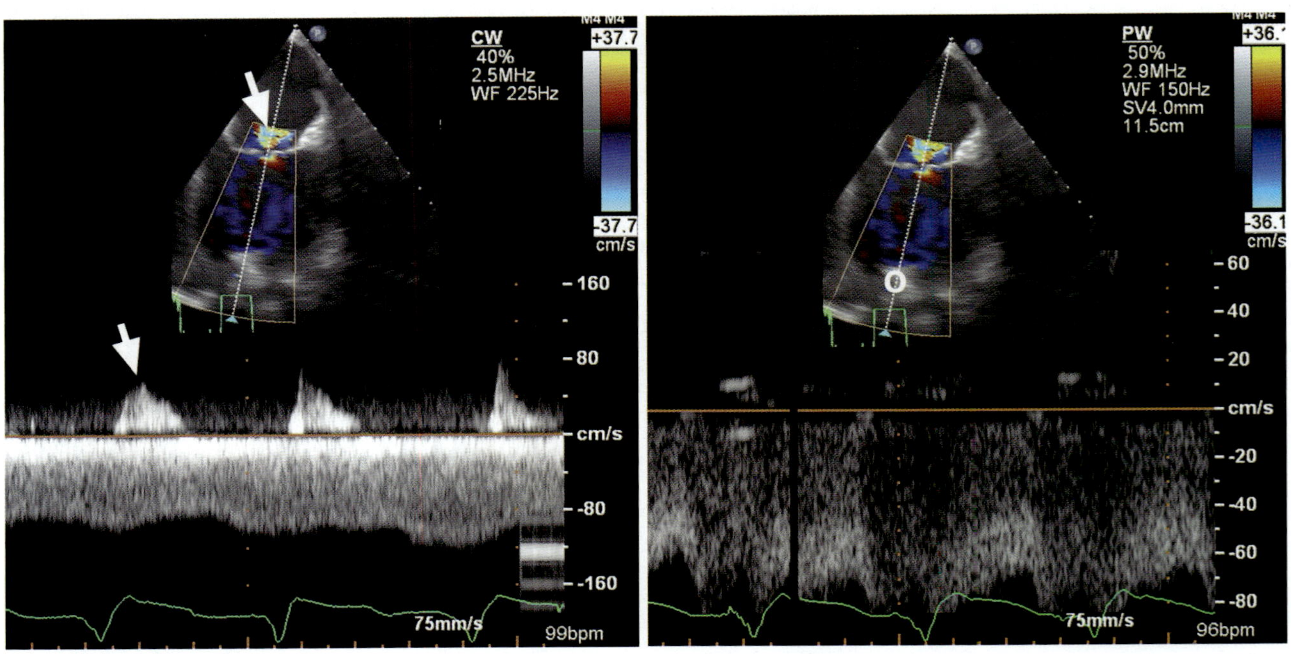

Fig 12.43 At left continuous wave Doppler shows steady nonpulsatile flow into LVAD *(below baseline)*; however, portion of MR jet is also picked up *(arrow)*. At right, use of pulsed wave Doppler with gate placed right at orifice of inflow cannula only shows flow into LVAD.

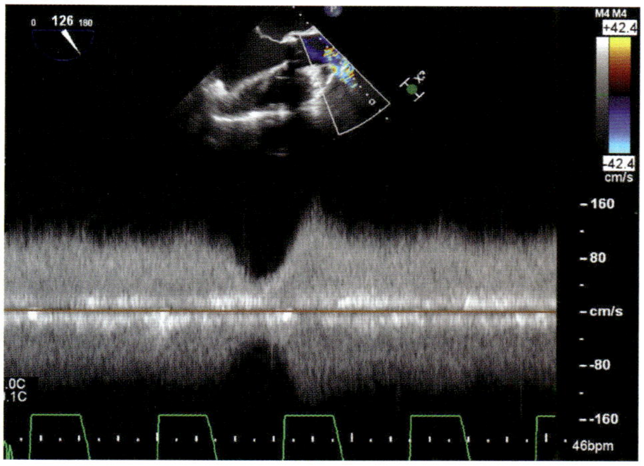

Fig 12.44 Continuous wave Doppler of outflow cannula shows nonpulsatile flow above baseline, with some mirror imaging below baseline.

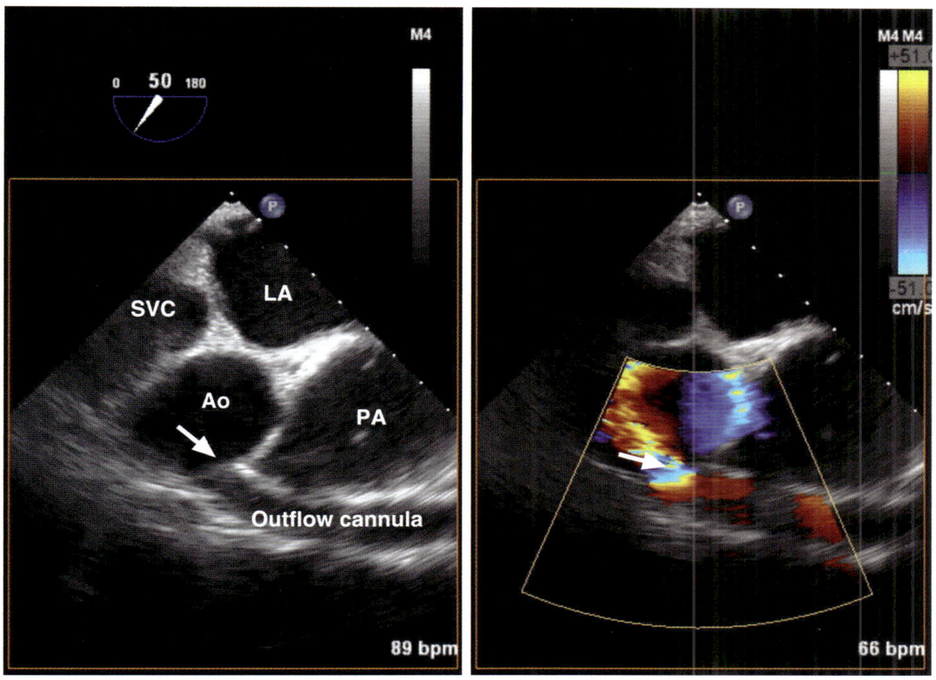

Fig 12.45 Outflow cannula is seen entering aorta in midesophageal short-axis view.

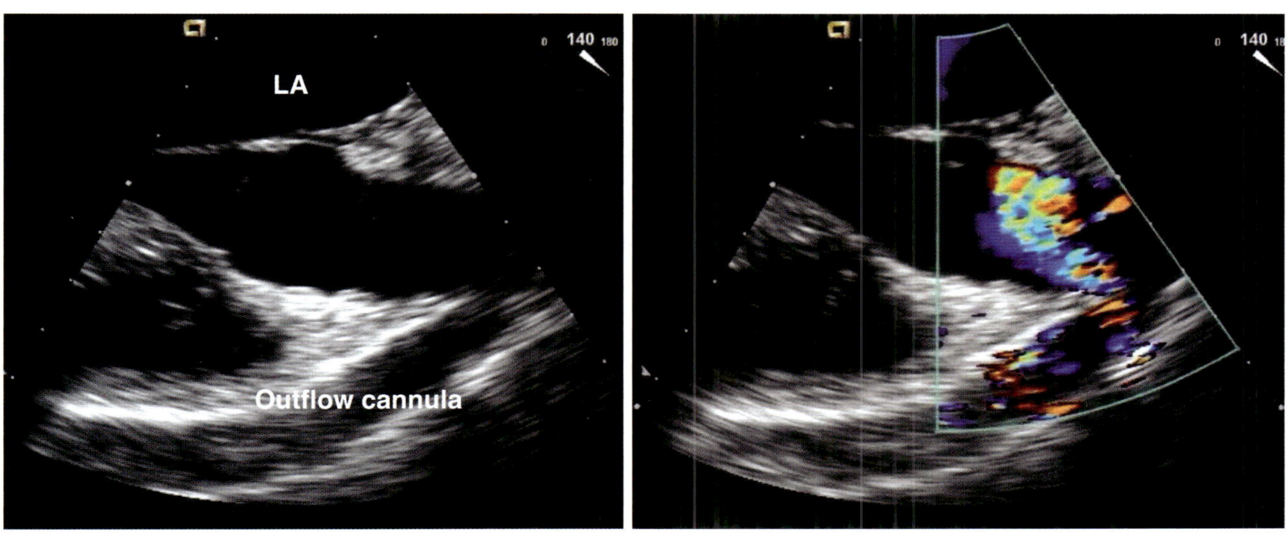

Fig 12.46 Outflow cannula is seen entering aorta in midesophageal long-axis view.

Comments

As the LVAD withdraws blood from the left ventricle, left atrial (LA) pressure falls below right atrial (RA) pressure. It is important to determine prebypass whether a patent foramen ovale is present, because right-to-left shunting will invariably occur if it is not closed. Any thrombi detected on the left side of the heart must be dealt with before instituting flow through the device to avoid systemic embolization. A mechanical aortic valve, even if functional, should be replaced with a bioprosthetic valve to minimize the increased risk of valvular thrombosis and possible embolization. Mitral stenosis, if significant, may limit the ability of blood to be removed to the device by the inflow cannula.

Right ventricular function as well as the degree of tricuspid regurgitation must be ascertained and closely followed to ensure adequate delivery of volume to the left side of the heart. The orifice of the ventricular apical cannula (inflow cannula) should be imaged in the four- and two-chamber views, and if available, a 3D image should show the cannula tip sitting within the ventricular cavity. Lack of obstruction by adjacent walls should be ascertained. Because the outflow cannula terminates in the ascending aorta, it is important to rule out significant aortic regurgitation; this would lead to LV distension during aortic flow as well as diminished blood flow to the body due to recirculation through the pump. If the intravascular volume is too low, or the RV function diminishes to a critical level, a suction event may occur in which the walls of the LV are drawn inwards blocking the inflow cannula. The treatment involves turning down the speed of the pump drawing blood out of the LV, giving volume, and supporting RV function. Patients may return to the OR because of LVAD malfunction. The TEE exam should focus on possible causes: intracardiac thrombi, or problems with the cannulae themselves.

Suggested Reading

1. Stainback RF, Estep JD, Agler DA, et al: Echocardiography in the management of patients with left ventricular assist devices: Recommendations from the American Society of Echocardiography, J Am Soc Echocardiogr 28:853–909, 2015.
2. Kirkpatrick JN, Wieselthaler G, Strueber M, et al: Ventricular assist devices for treatment of acute heart failure and chronic heart failure, Heart 101:1091–1096, 2015.
3. Dandel M, Hetzer R: Myocardial recovery during mechanical circulatory support: Weaning and explantation criteria, Heart Lung Vessel 7:280–288, 2015.

CASE 12-6
Right Ventricular Assist Device

This 75-year-old woman, who had previously undergone aortic valve replacement for endocarditis, presented following follow-up CT with an ascending aortic diameter of 62 mm, as well as dilation of the sinuses of Valsalva. She was taken to surgery where a Bentall procedure (replacement of ascending aorta and aortic valve, and reimplantation of the coronary arteries) was performed with technical difficulties because of her previous surgery. She suffered a postoperative right ventricular infarction, and returned to the OR where cannulas were placed in her pulmonary artery and right atrium to facilitate a right ventricular assist device. In the ensuing 3 days she showed little clinical improvement and returned to the OR for chest exploration. TEE showed that outflow cannula had migrated in to the right pulmonary artery. It was removed, and an end-to-side graft to the main pulmonary was placed, resulting in immediate clinical improvement.

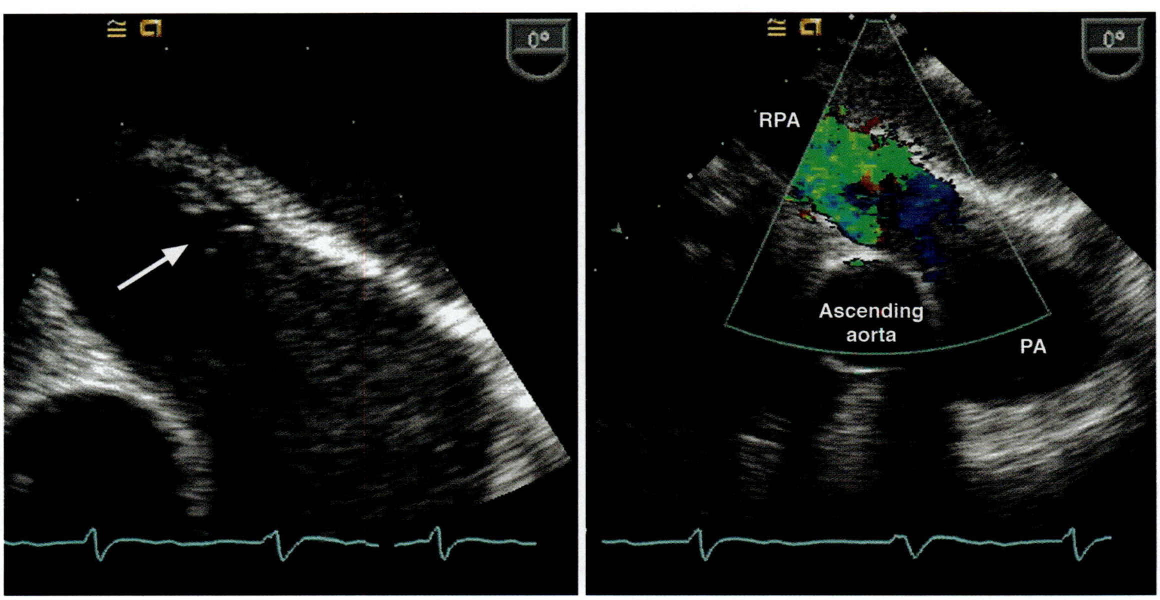

Fig 12.47 At left is zoomed image of outflow cannula terminating in right pulmonary artery. At right, color flow Doppler shows that flow is directed solely to right pulmonary artery.

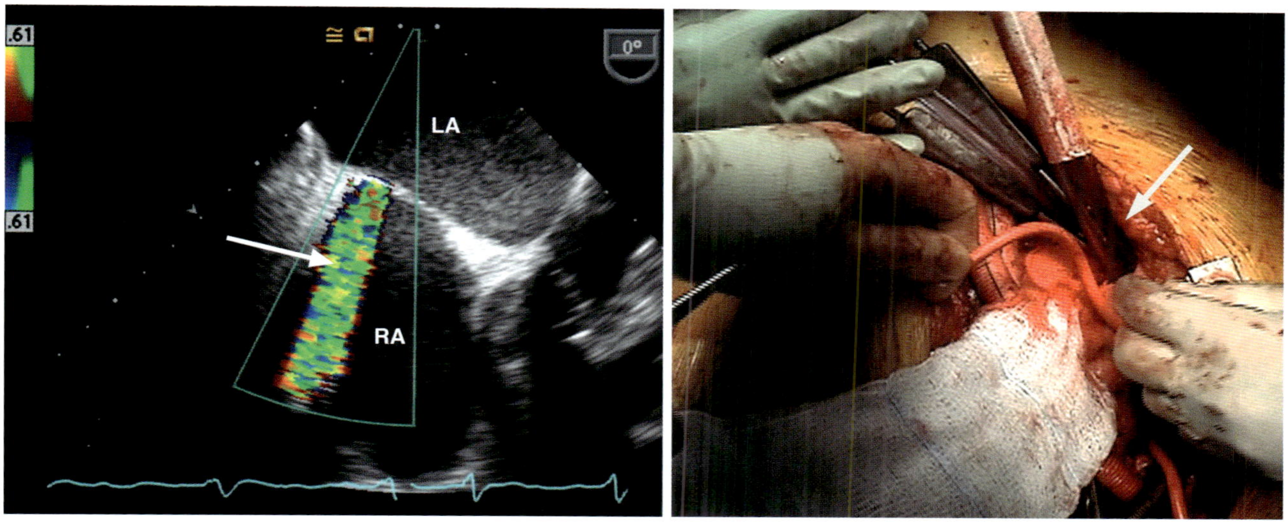

Fig 12.48 In midesophageal four-chamber imaging, flow is seen in inflow cannula *(arrow)* present in right atrium. On right, cannula is seen in surgical field *(arrow)*.

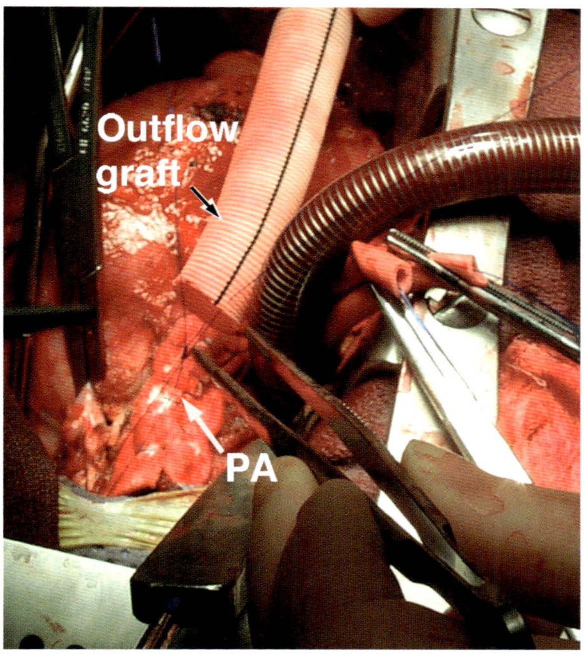

Fig 12.49 Outflow graft is seen being anastomosed to main pulmonary artery.

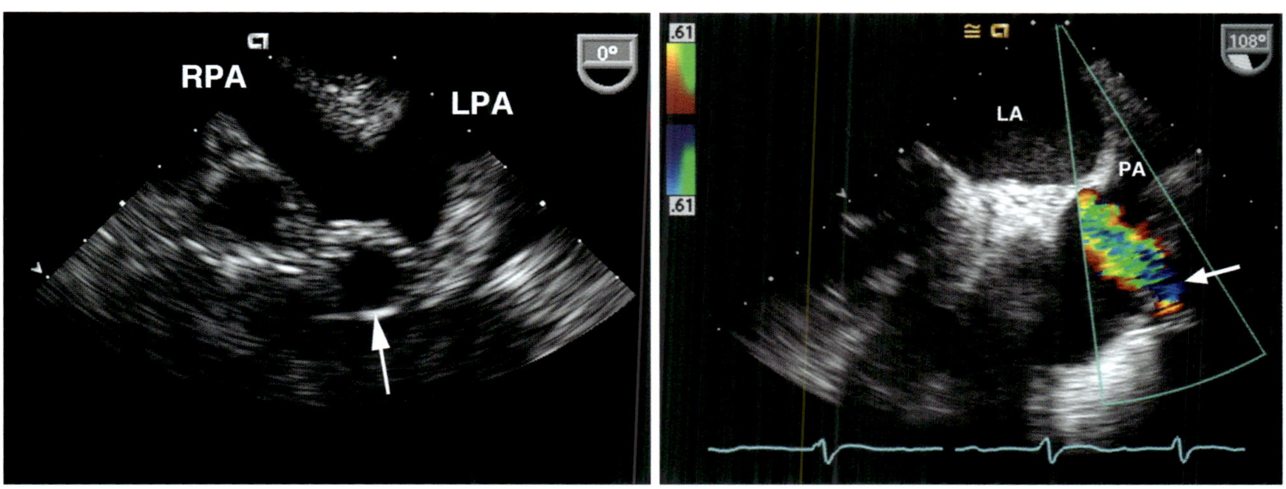

Fig 12.50 At left, outflow cannula *(arrow)* is seen in high esophageal short axis of pulmonary artery bifurcation. At right, midesophageal view at 108 degrees with color Doppler shows flow entering main pulmonary artery *(arrow)*.

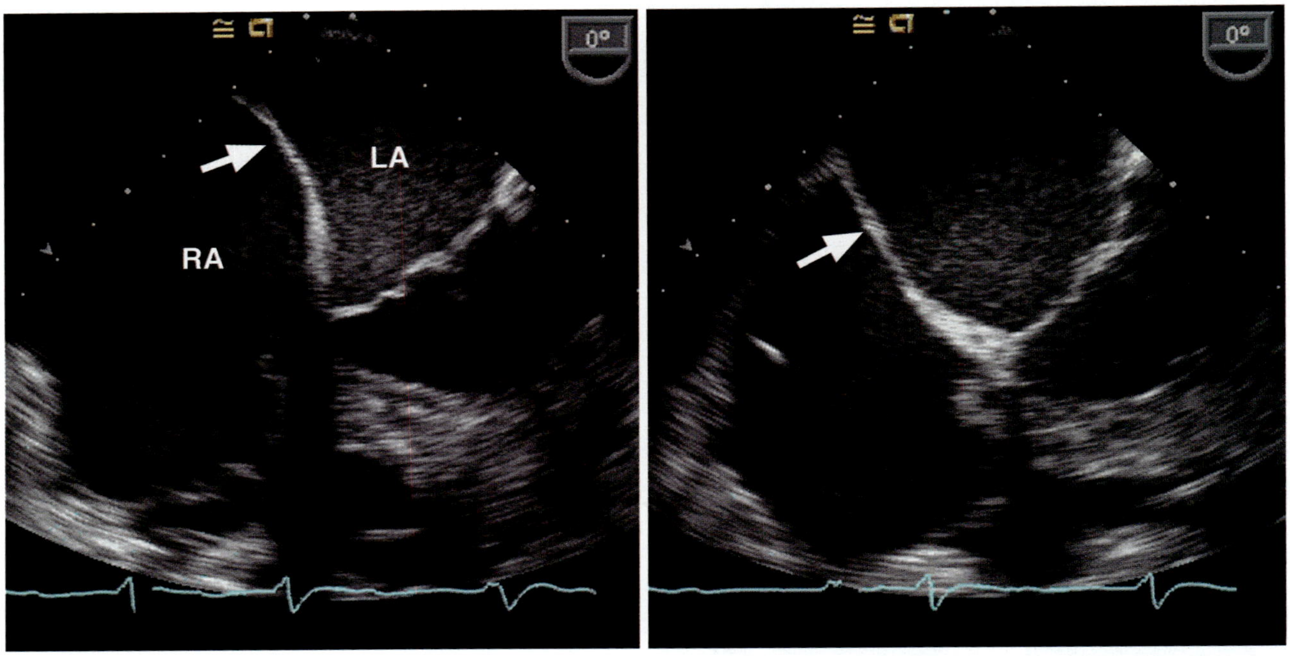

Fig 12.51 Two midesophageal four-chamber images. Image at left is taken prior to outflow cannula revision. Interatrial septum *(arrow)* is bulging toward left, indicating elevated right atrial pressure. Following outflow cannula revision, the interatrial septum has moved back toward right, indicating reduction in right atrial pressure.

Comments

A right ventricular assist device bypasses the right heart with systemic venous return from the right atrium directed through the assist device and back into the pulmonary artery. It is important to rule out significant PR as this will lead to right ventricular distention when the device is active.

Suggested Reading

1. Dandel M, Krabatsch T, Falk V: Left ventricular vs. biventricular mechanical support: Decision making and strategies for avoidance of right heart failure after left ventricular assist device implantation, Int J Cardiol 198:241–250, 2015.

CASE 12-7
Total Artificial Heart

This 40-year-old woman with a history of coarctation repair (as a child), and bicuspid aortic stenosis treated with mechanical aortic valve replacement 8 years ago, was admitted to our hospital with an acute coronary syndrome likely related to complex abscess/dehiscence of her prosthetic aortic valve. Because of a low ejection fraction (35%) and advanced endocarditis, she was scheduled for a total artificial heart (TAH).

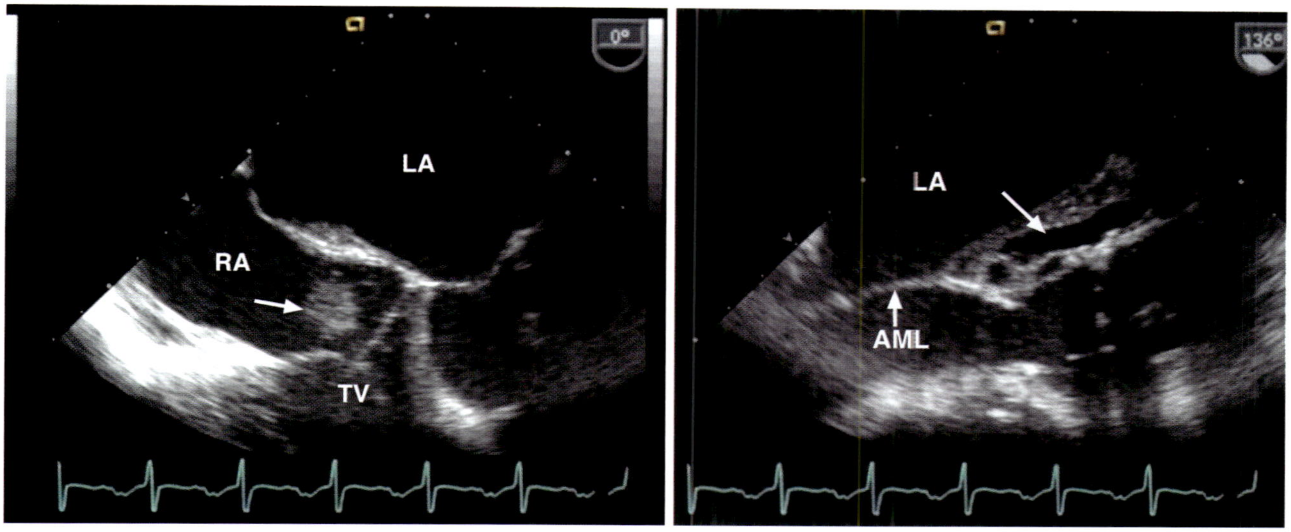

Fig 12.52 Baseline intraoperative TEE shows large tricuspid valve vegetation *(left, arrow)* in four-chamber view and complex aortic abscess *(right, arrow)* in long-axis view.

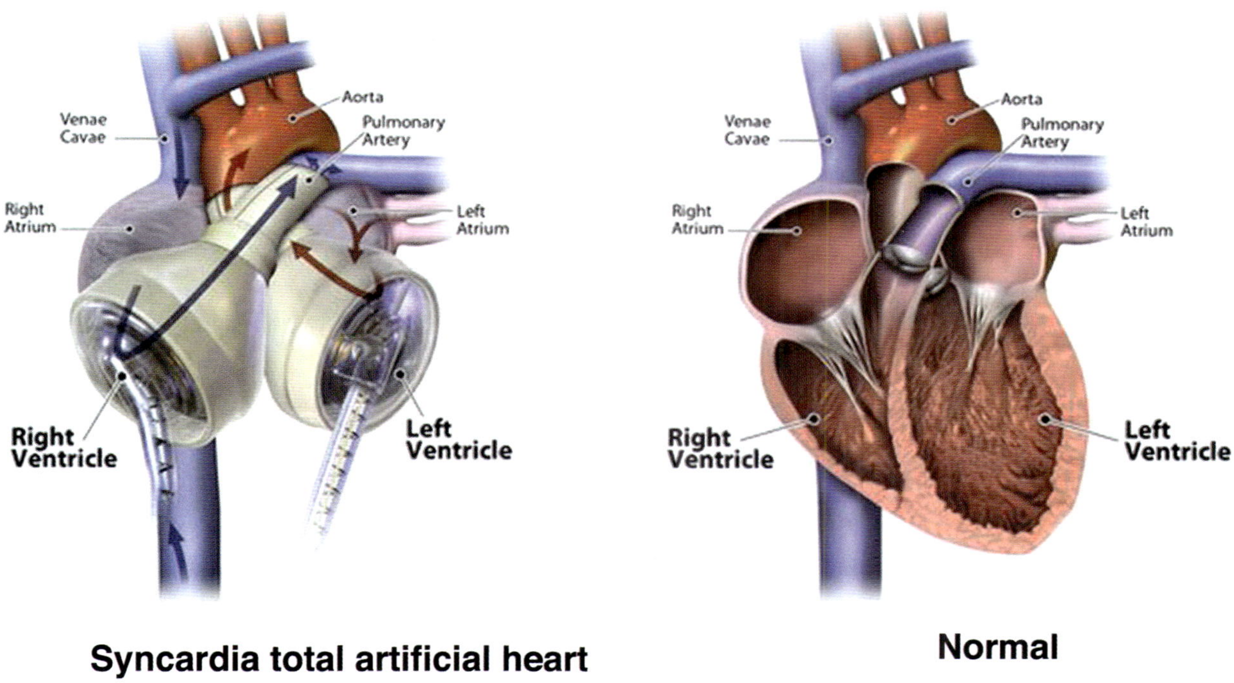

Fig 12.53 Schematics of SynCardia total artificial heart are demonstrated. Right and left atrial cuffs are anastomosed to "ventricles," whose filling is controlled by tilting disc valves. Ventricles then eject blood into aorta and pulmonary artery, again controlled by tilting disc valves.

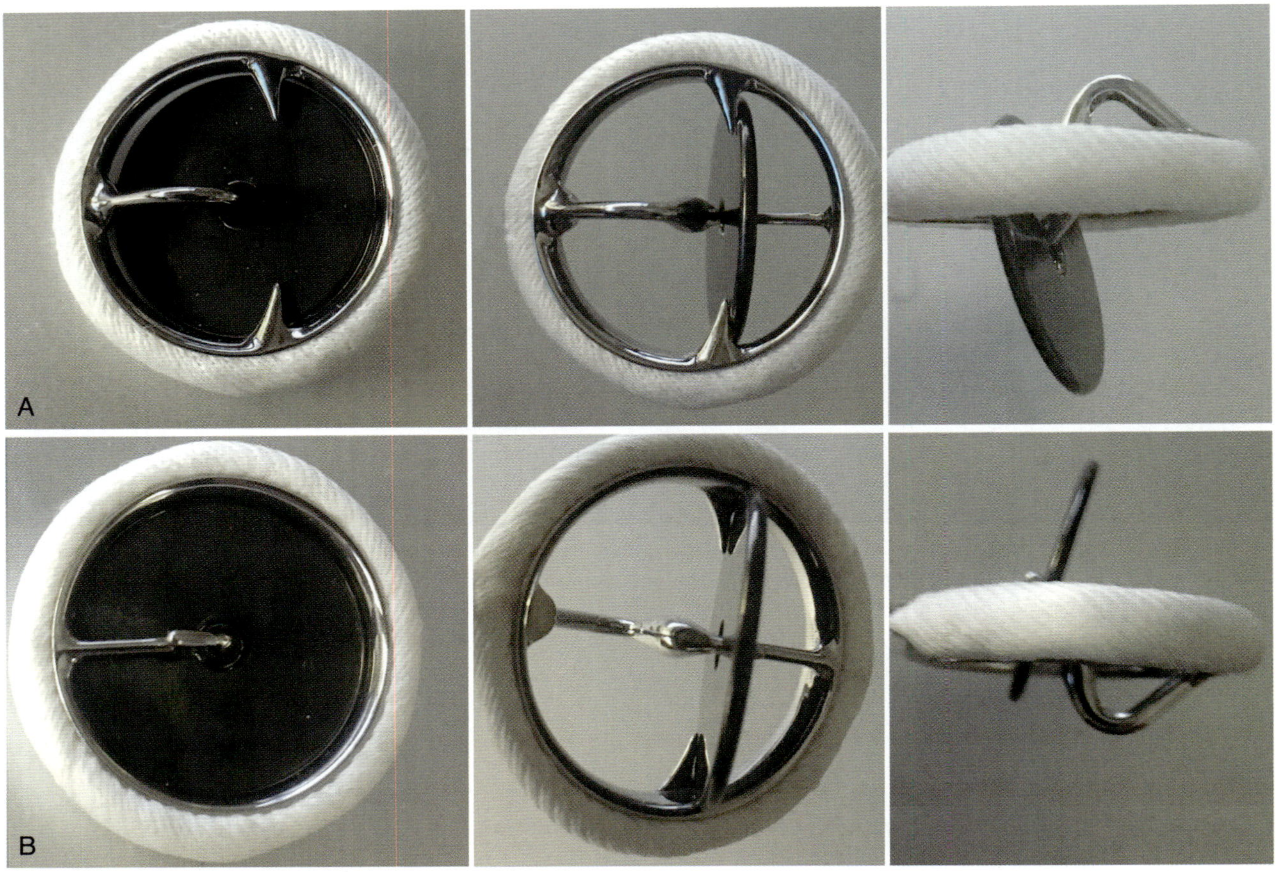

Fig 12.54 In top three panels (**A**), atrio-ventricular tilting disc valve is seen from left atrial perspective in *(from left to right)* closed and open position, as well as from side. In lower three panels, valve subtending great vessel is seen from aortic (or pulmonary arterial) side again in *(from left to right)* closed and open position, as well as from side.

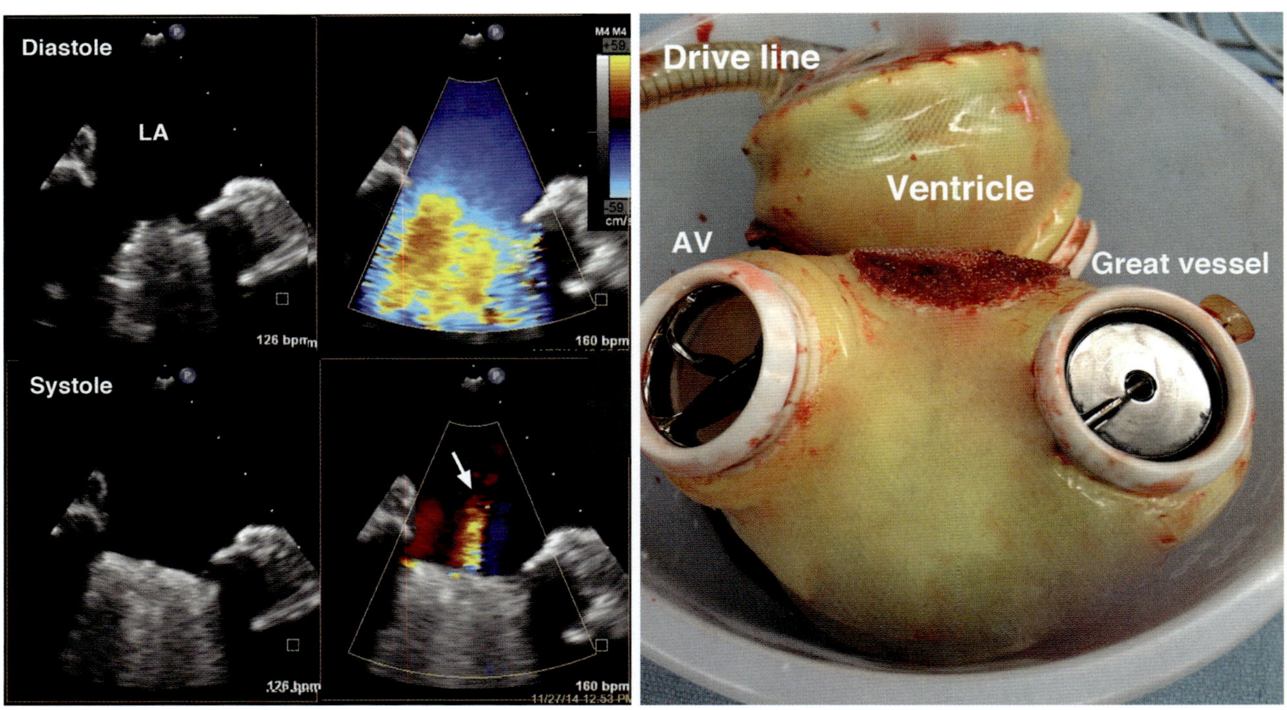

Fig 12.55 With total artificial heart, ventricles and atrioventricular valves are excised and atria connected to artificial heart. At left, TEE shows adequate function of tilting disc prosthetic mitral valve, with cleaning jet seen during systole *(arrow)*. In right panel, left side of artificial heart explanted prior to heart transplantation; mitral valve is at left and aortic prosthetic valve at right.

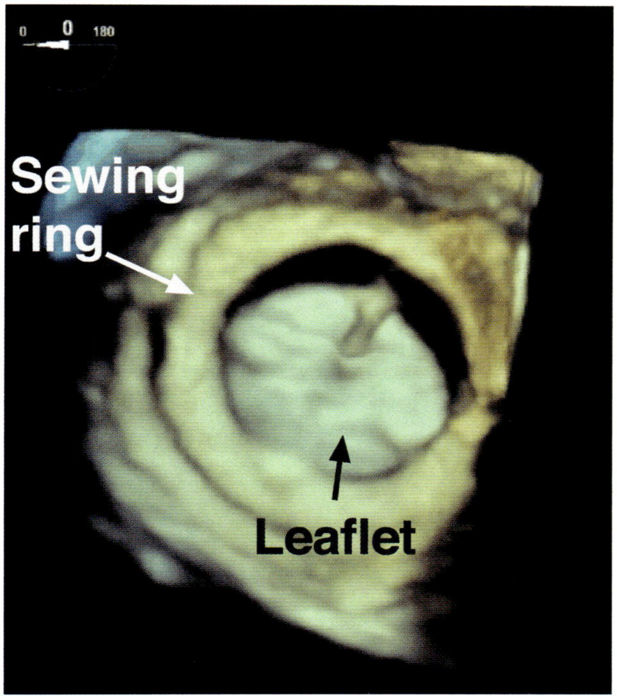

Fig 12.56 Prosthetic mitral valve is shown in 3D TEE.

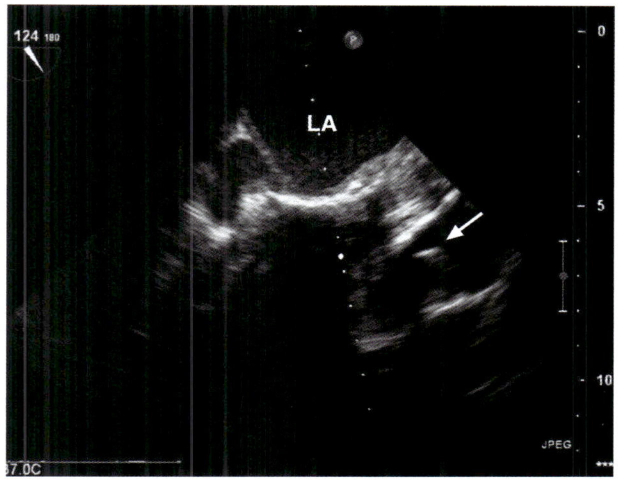

Fig 12.57 Prosthetic cutflow valves (aortic, pulmonic) are difficult to image secondary to interference by components of device. Here aortic valve *(arrow)* is incompletely seen within graft that connects ventricle to ascending aorta.

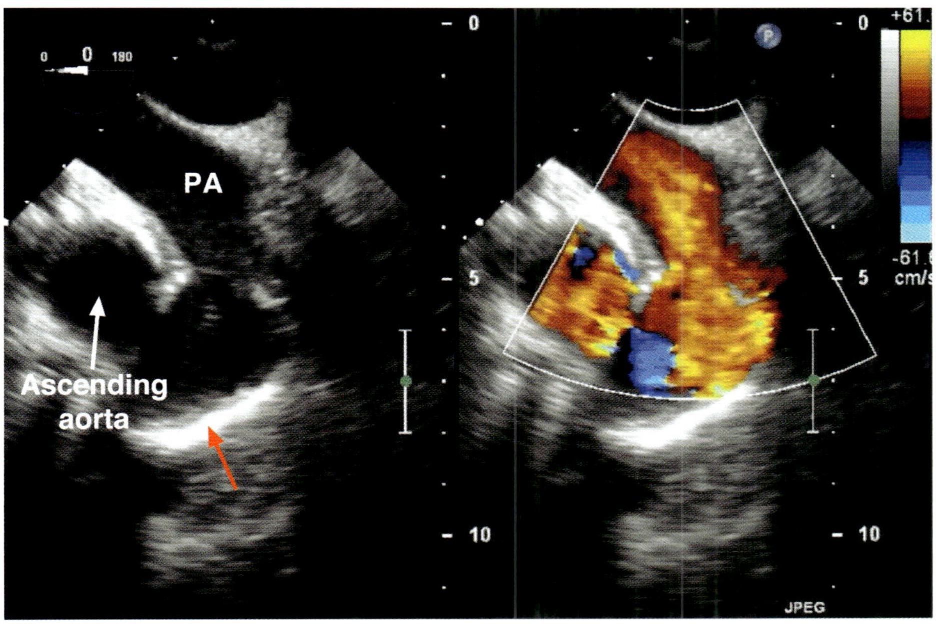

Fig 12.58 Red arrow indicates graft material from device to pulmonary artery. Color Doppler imaging *(right)* shows flow into the pulmonary artery. Pulmonic valve is not visualized.

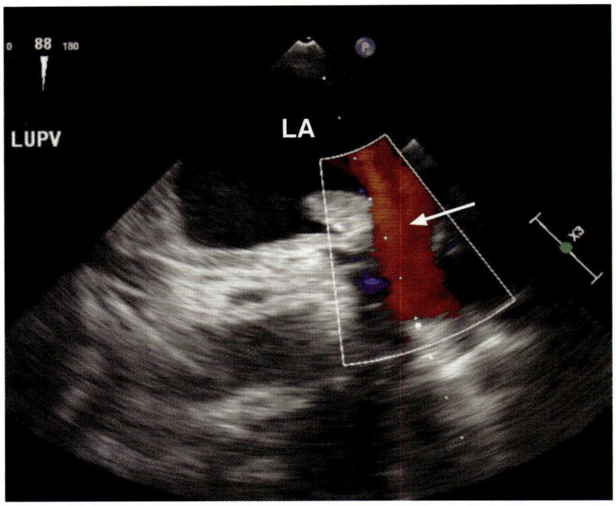

Fig 12.59 It is important to determine adequacy of connections to native atria. Here widely patent left upper pulmonary vein is seen.

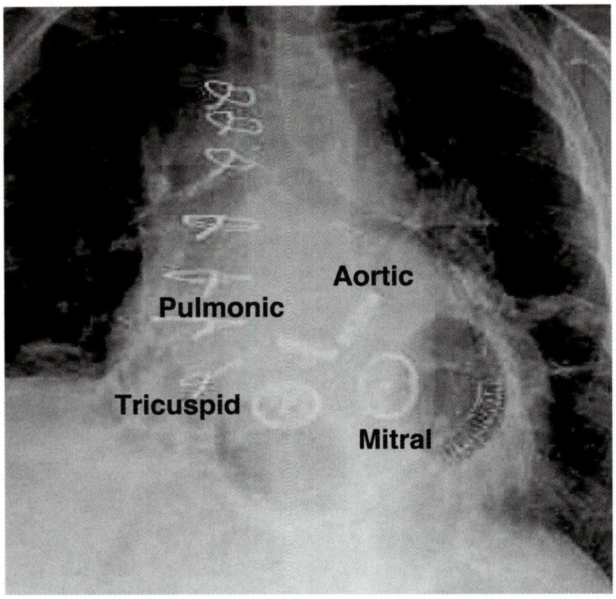

Fig 12.60 On postoperative chest x-ray, four tilting disc valves are seen.

Options for end-stage biventricular heart failure include mechanical support of only the LV with an LVAD plus medical optimization of the right heart function, placement of both left and right ventricular assist devices (Bi-VADs), or a total artificial heart. Echocardiographic imaging of a total artificial heart from transthoracic windows is of limited value due to inability to image the mechanical heart with ultrasound. Even from a TEE approach, imaging is limited due to shadowing and reverberations from the four mechanical valves. However, the native atria remain intact and tamponade can occur. Dysfunction of the mechanical valves also can occur. Thus, TEE is useful for (1) evaluation of the mechanical tricuspid and mitral valves from the atrial perspective, and (2) evaluation of the right and left atrium to exclude compression due to a localized posterior pericardial effusion.

Suggested Reading

1. Mizuguchi KA, Padera RF, Kowalczyk A, et al: Transesophageal echocardiography imaging of the total artificial heart, Anesth Analg 117:780–784, 2013.

13 Transcatheter Valve Therapies

Transcatheter Aortic Valve Replacement

Since the first transcatheter bioprosthetic aortic valve was implanted, changes have included smaller and more flexible delivery systems for use in smaller vessels; lower frame height in order to minimize interference with coronary blood flow, mitral valve function, and atrioventricular heart block; a basal skirt to minimize paravalvular regurgitation; and greater variety of valve sizes to accommodate different annular dimensions. Figs 13.8, 13.20, and 13.21 show the designs in common use today.

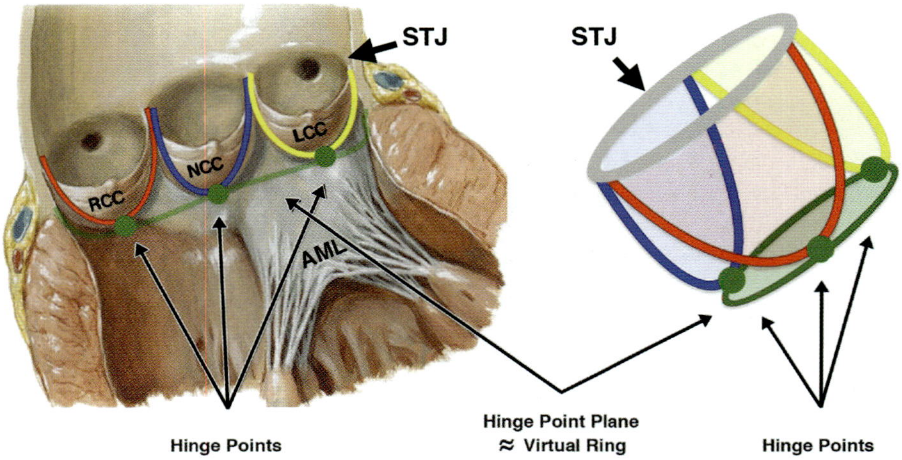

Fig 13.1 Normal anatomy of aortic annulus. The aortic leaflets insert into aorta in crown-like fashion *(red, blue, and yellow)*, with high point being sinotubular junction. For purposes of annular sizing, the aortic annulus is defined as a virtual ring *(green line)* with three anatomical anchor points at nadir *(green points)* of each of the attachments of the three aortic leaflets. (From Kasel AM, Cassese S, Bleiziffer S, et al: Standardized imaging for aortic annular sizing: Implications for transcatheter valve selection, JACC Cardiovasc Imaging 6:249–262, 2013. With permission.)

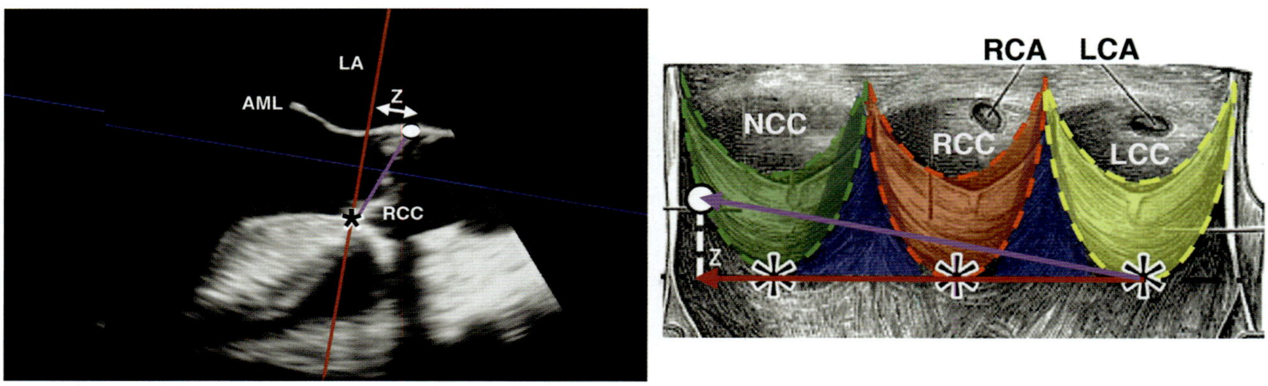

Fig 13.2 A common error that occurs with 2D estimation of aortic annulus is illustrated. Leaflet hinge points seen on 2D mid-esophageal long-axis image *(left)* represent the interface of the leaflet and left ventricular wall at either nadir of leaflet or basal plane *(red line)* or at a point *(white circle, purple line)* that is a highly variable distance *(z)* above the basal plane. Use of 3D TEE reconstructive techniques obviates the issue. (From Jilaihawi H, Kashif M, Fontana G, et al: Cross-sectional computed tomographic assessment improves accuracy of aortic annular sizing for transcatheter aortic valve replacement and reduces incidence of paravalvular aortic regurgitation, JACC 59:1275–1286, 2012.)

CASE 13-1
Balloon Expandable Bioprosthetic Aortic Valve

This 82-year-old man with a history of remote CABG for coronary artery disease, type 2 diabetes, and severe COPD, had a 6-month history of progressive dyspnea on exertion, lightheadedness, and substernal chest pain. On TTE he was found to have severe aortic stenosis. Because of his high surgical risk and comorbidities, he was scheduled for transcatheter aortic valve replacement (TAVR).

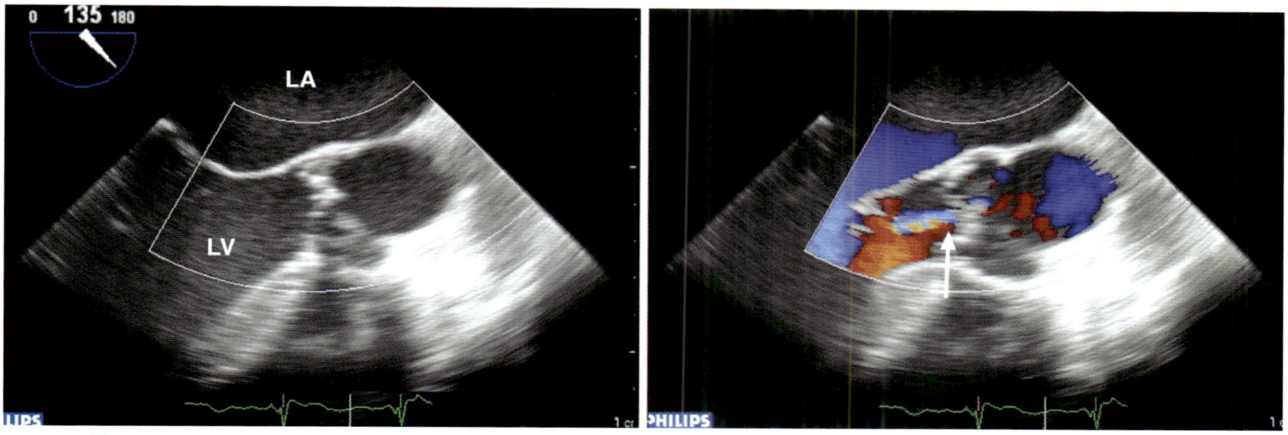

Fig 13.3 Midesophageal long-axis view shows a heavily calcified aortic valve with mild aortic regurgitation *(arrow)*. Video images show limited leaflet motion without color Doppler flow acceleration proximal to the valve. LV systolic function was normal, and there was only mild, central mitral regurgitation.

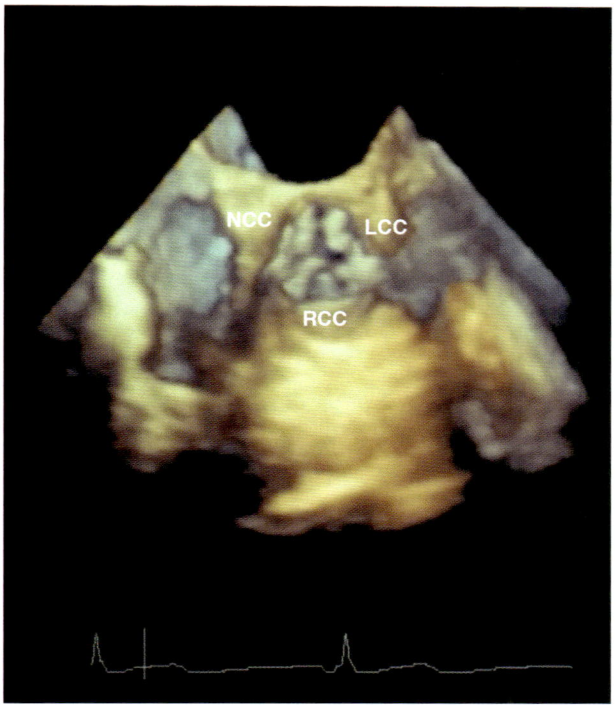

Fig 13.4 3D TEE from aortic side of the valve shows heavily calcified leaflets with a small systolic orifice area.

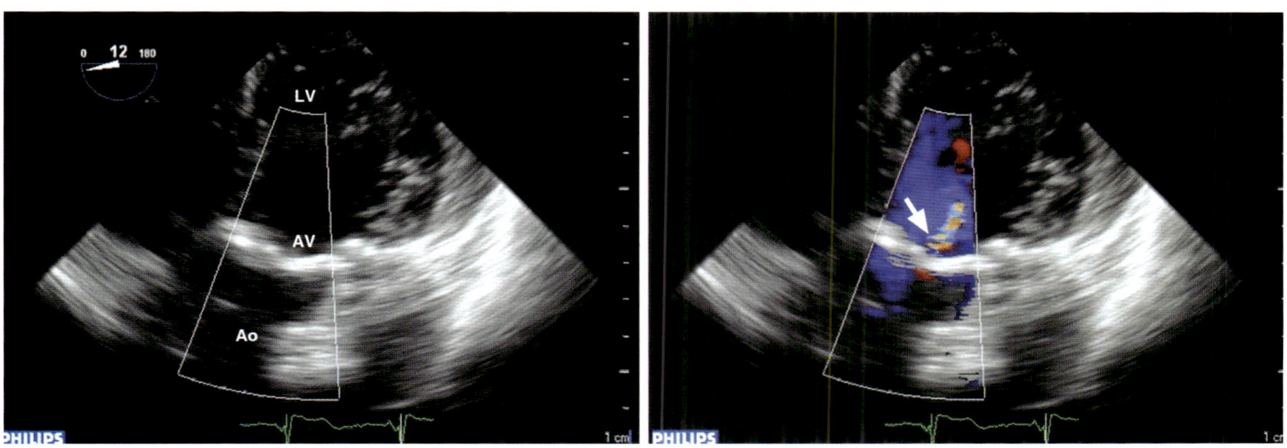

Fig 13.5 Deep transgastric image demonstrates the small jet of central aortic regurgitation. In cases of echo dropout from the esophageal window, gastric views offer an alternative.

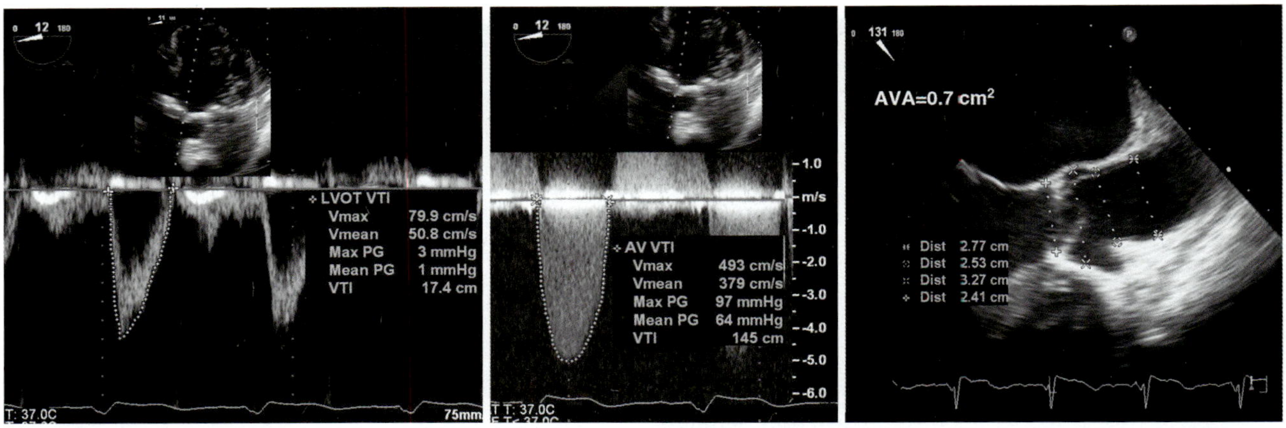

Fig 13.6 Using the continuity equation, the aortic valve area is calculated at 0.7 cm^2.

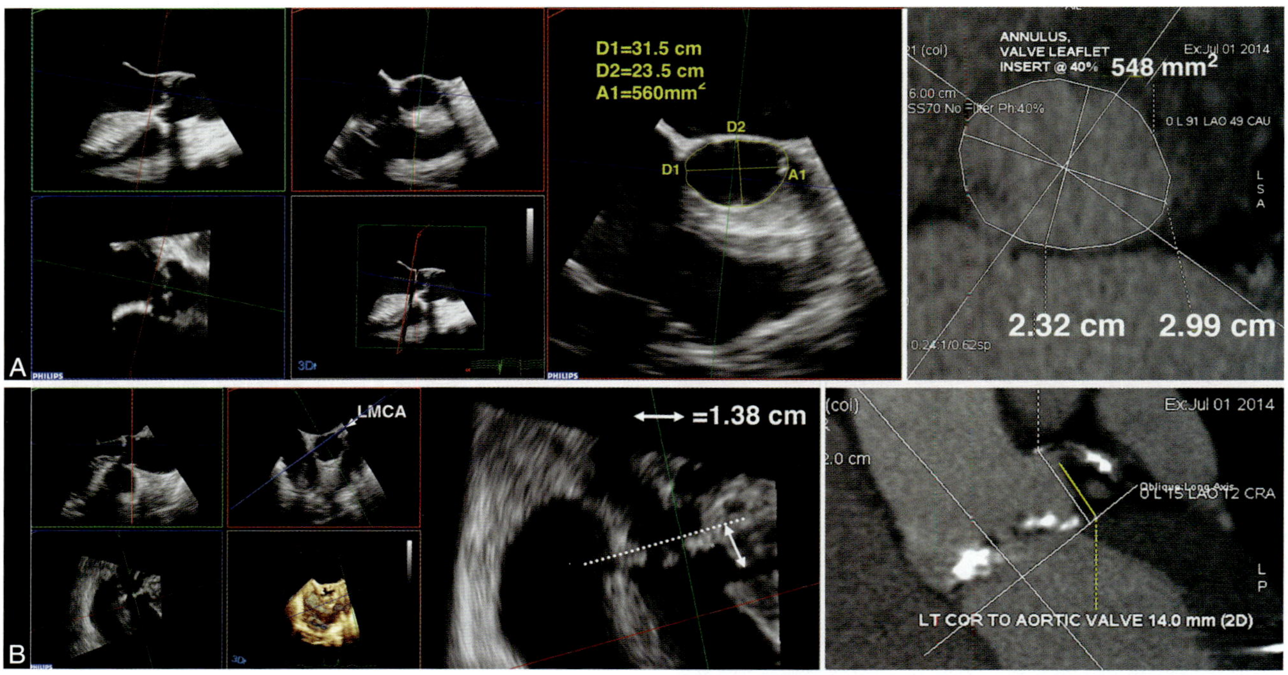

Fig 13.7 The top images show the use of multiplanar reconstruction *(left)* in deriving the cross-sectional diameters and area of the left ventricular outflow tract, which are consistent with those obtained by CT scan *(right)*. The bottom images show the use of multiplanar reconstruction *(left)* to derive the distance of the left main coronary ostium from the aortic annulus. This distance is consistent with those obtained by CT scan *(right)*. The risk of coronary artery occlusion by the native leaflets following valvuloplasty is higher with smaller coronary ostia-aortic annular distances. These measurements are made predeployment in an attempt to prevent either the frame of the implanted valve or the native coronary leaflet from extending to the upper margin of the coronary ostium.

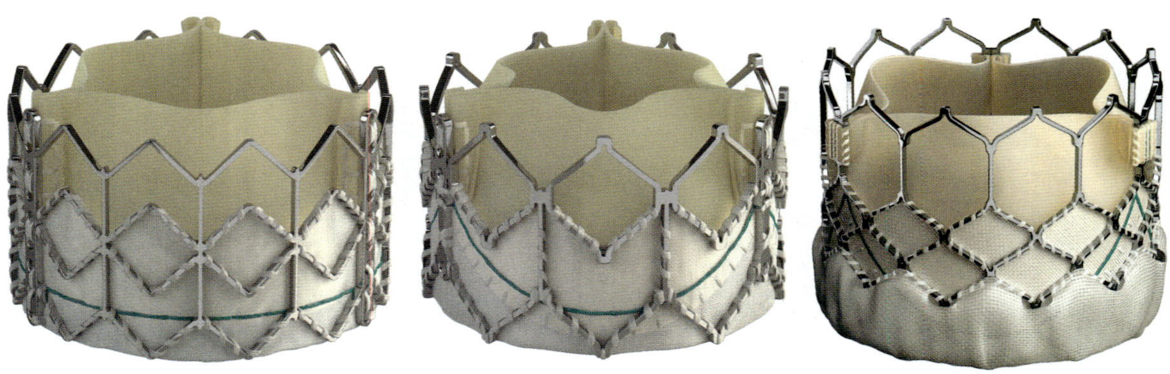

Fig 13.8 *(Left)* The Edwards SAPIEN transcatheter heart valve. *(Middle)* The Edwards SAPIEN XT transcatheter heart valve. *(Right)* The Edwards SAPIEN 3 transcatheter heart valve; this newest iteration has a basal skirt designed to minimize paravalvular regurgitation. Courtesy of Edwards Lifesciences LLC, Irvine, CA.

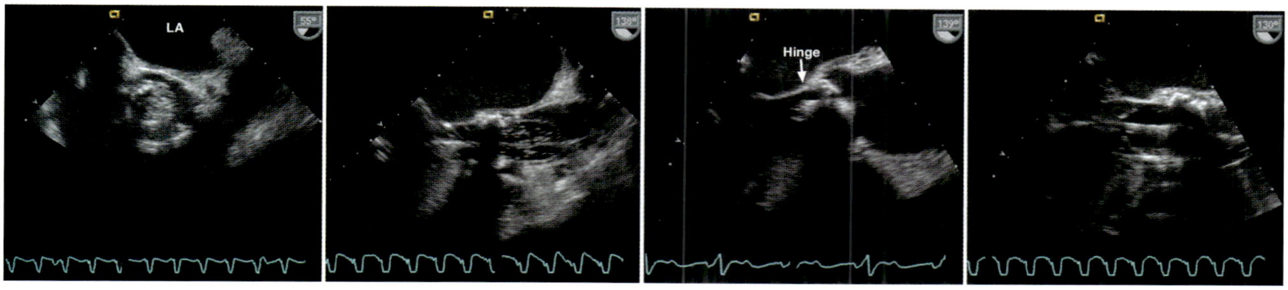

Fig 13.9 In another patient also having a TAVR, three components of deployment are seen. In the left two frames, balloon commissurotomy is performed; in the right two frames, the crimped valve is positioned 2–3 mm past the hinge point of the aortic and mitral valves and then deployed. Rapid ventricular pacing is used during balloon inflation.

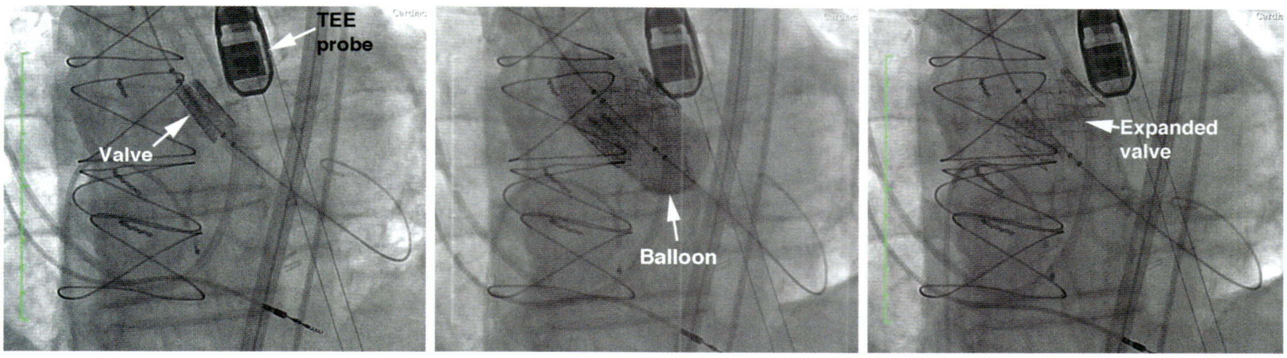

Fig 13.10 Subsequent images are from the original patient. With fluoroscopy, the crimped valve is seen in position *(left)*. In center, the balloon and valve have been expanded, and on right, the balloon has been deflated, leaving the valve in situ.

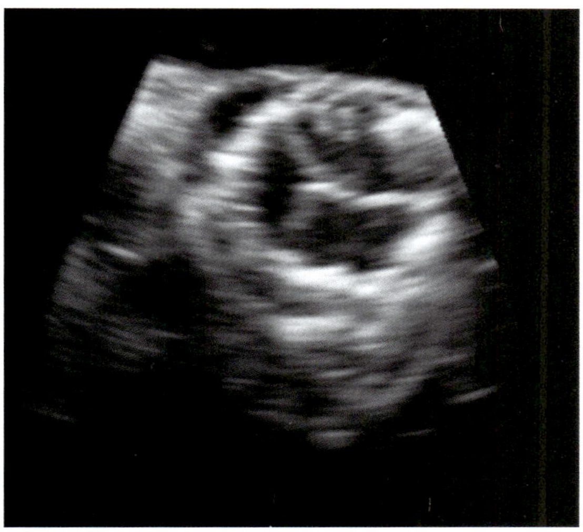

Fig 13.11 Midesophageal short-axis imaging shows the valve to be in good position, with no evidence of aortic regurgitation seen on color Doppler.

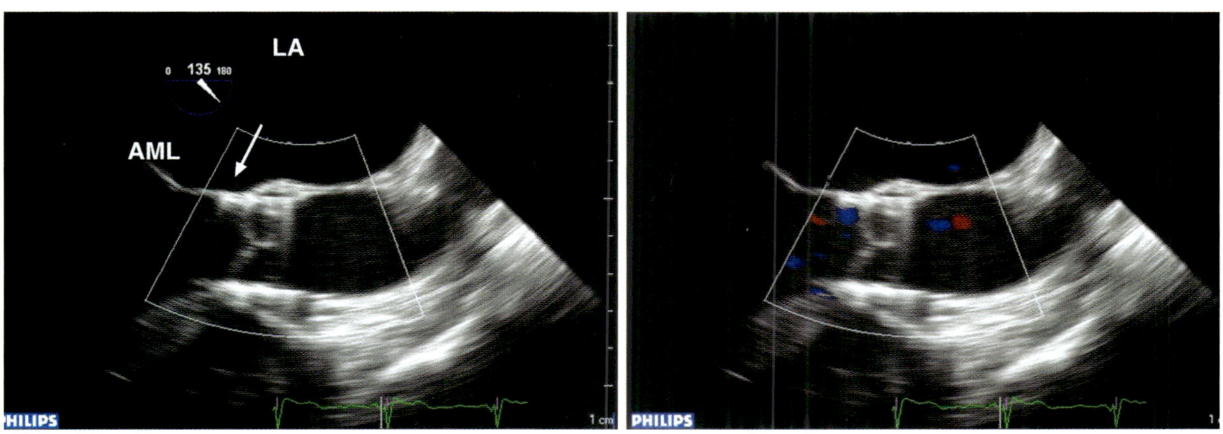

Fig 13.12 Midesophageal long-axis imaging also shows valve to be in good position, with no evidence of aortic regurgitation. There was no impingement of the valve on the anterior mitral leaflet nor was there worsening of preprocedural mitral regurgitation.

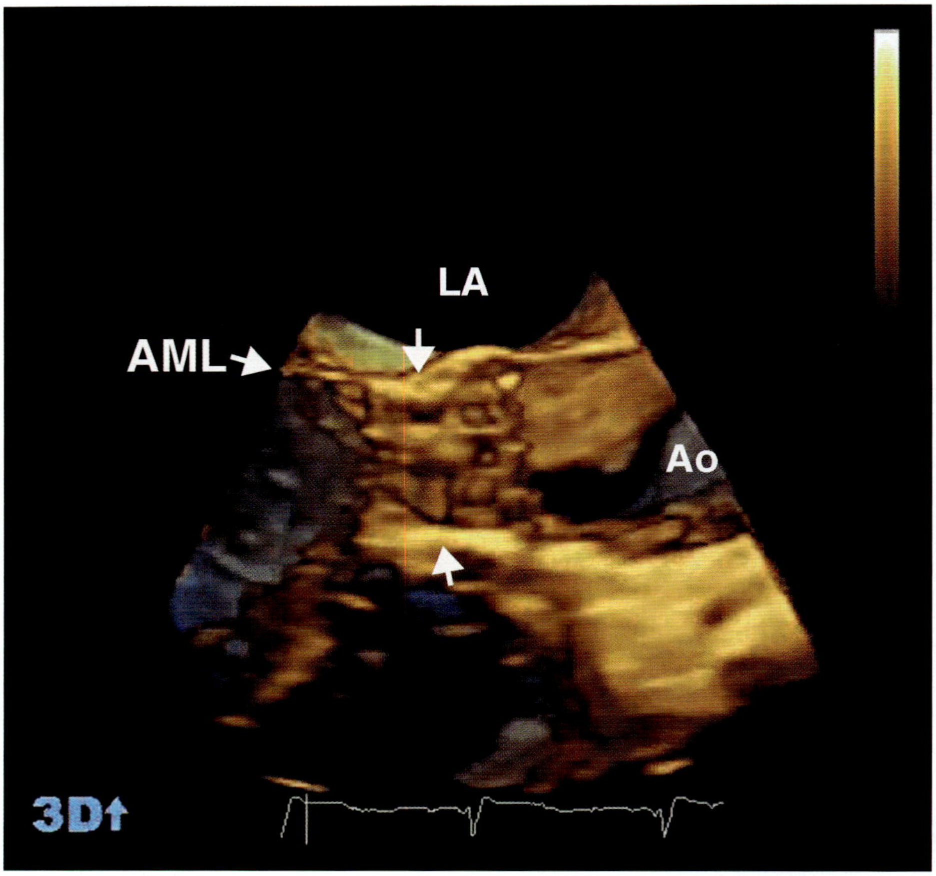

Fig 13.13 3D long axis shows the valve in the appropriate position.

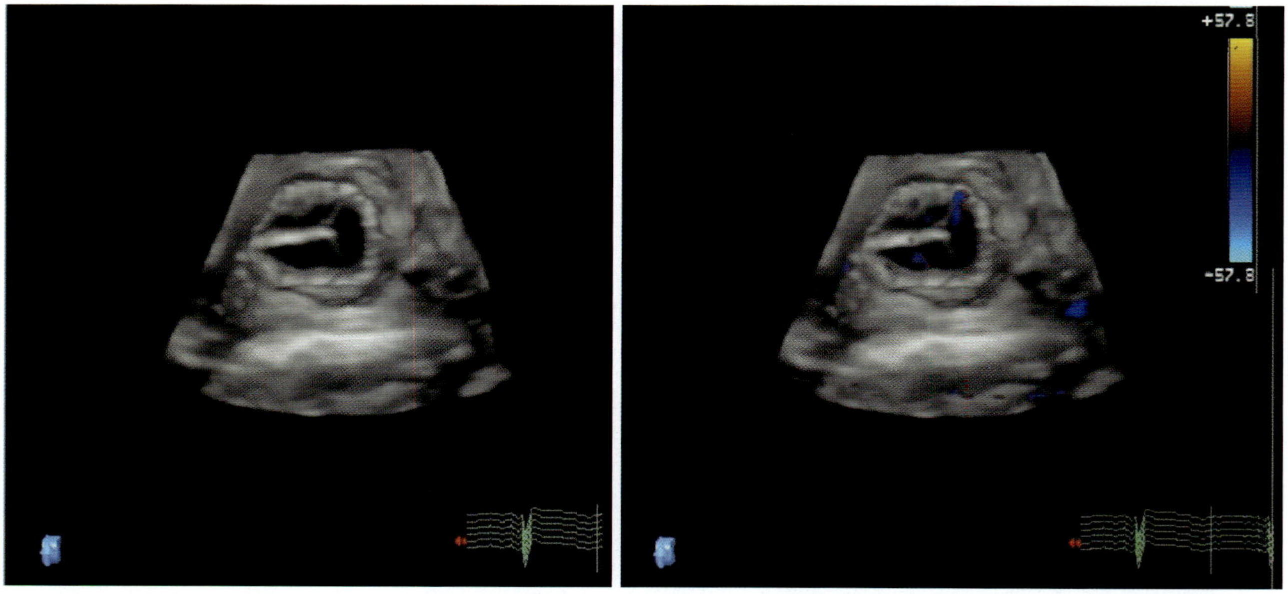

Fig 13.14 Valve is seen in 3D from the left ventricular outflow tract perspective. There is no evidence of aortic regurgitation. Postdeployment gradients across the new valve were dramatically reduced. There was no change in the mild amount of mitral regurgitation after deployment of valve.

CASE 13-2
Transapical Balloon Expandable Bioprosthetic Aortic Valve Replacement

This 76-year-old man presented with increasing dyspnea and fatigue over a 6-month period. Severe aortic stenosis with an aortic valve area of 0.6 cm^2 was diagnosed by TTE. The patient had comorbidities that included severe PVD with iliac stents, as well as a previous CABG with patent LIMA graft.

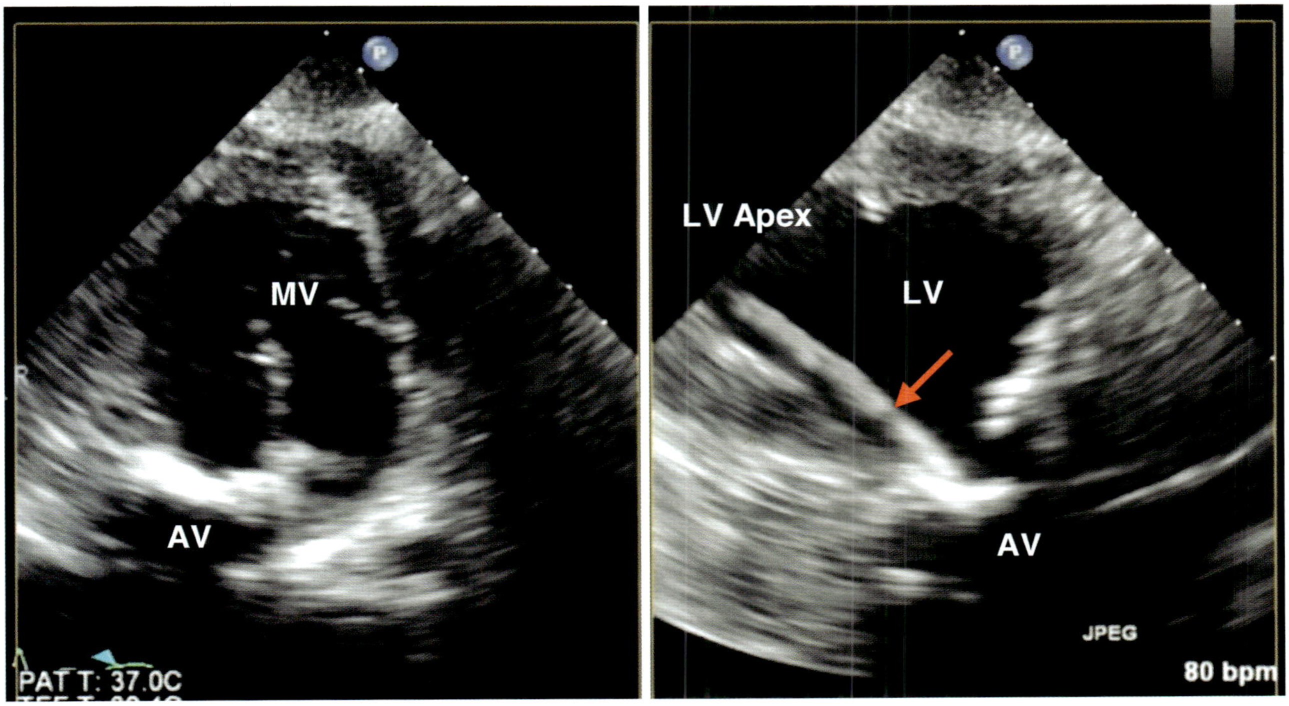

Fig 13.15 In patients in whom lower extremity arteries are unable to accommodate the delivery system, a small thoracotomy may be performed to facilitate delivery through left ventricular apex. In this biplane image, a deep transgastric image is seen on left and orthogonal view on right. A guide wire *(red arrow)* has been introduced into left ventricle via apex, and has been advanced through LVOT and aortic valve.

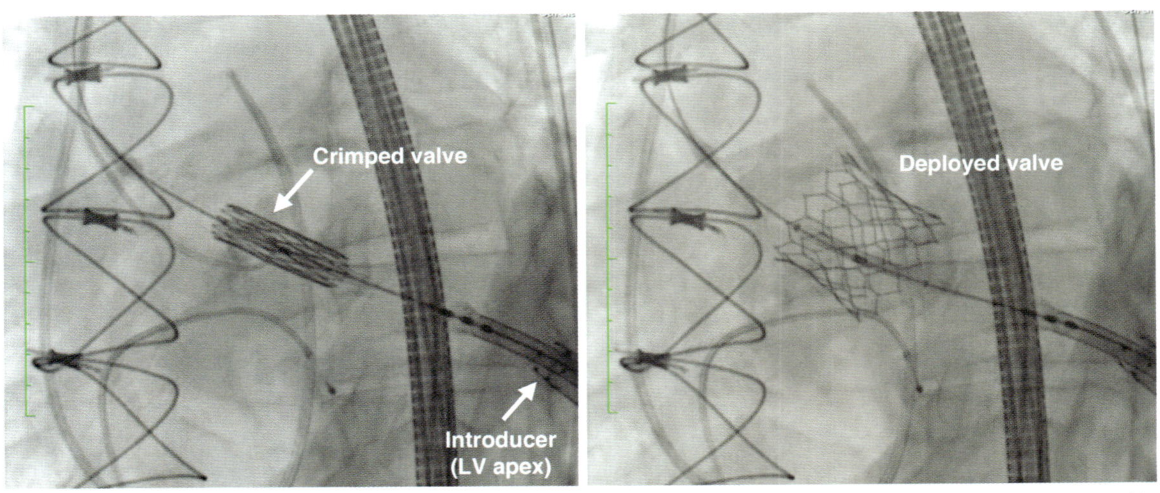

Fig 13.16 As visualized with fluoroscopy, the delivery apparatus has been introduced into left ventricle via apex *(left)* and valve deployed *(right)*.

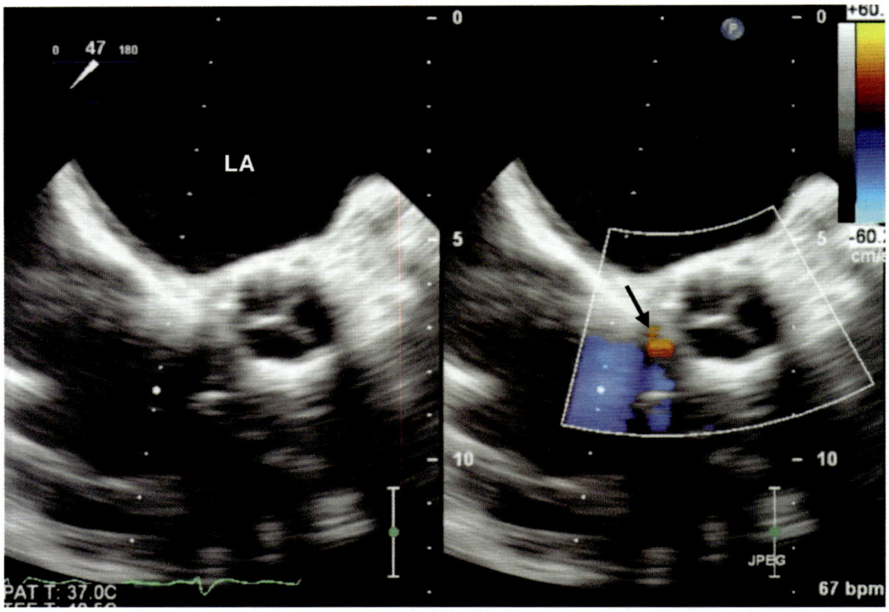

Fig 13.17 In midesophageal short axis, deployed valve shows only mild paravalvular regurgitation *(arrow)*.

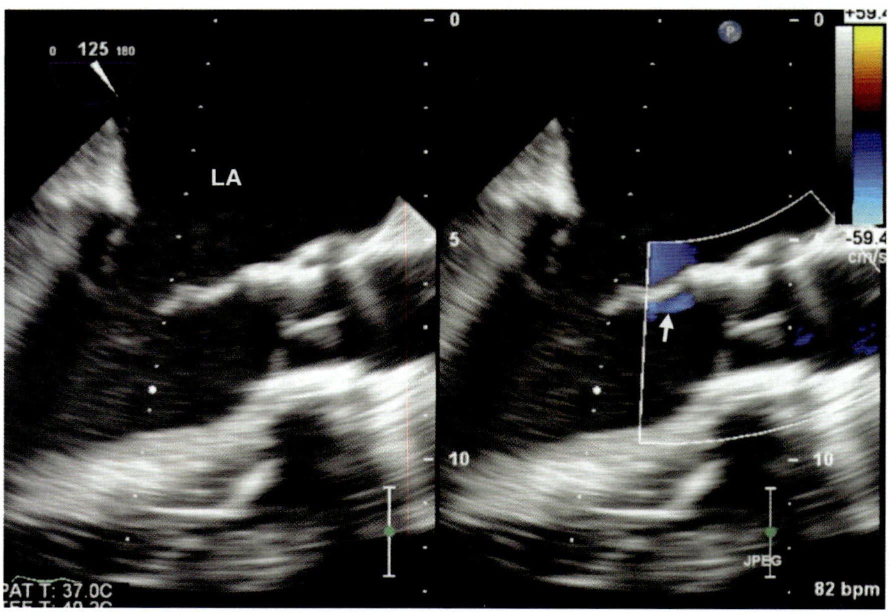

Fig 13.18 In midesophageal long axis, deployed valve shows only mild paravalvular regurgitation *(arrow)*. Valve is slightly more ventricular than desired, without any significant effect on mitral valve function.

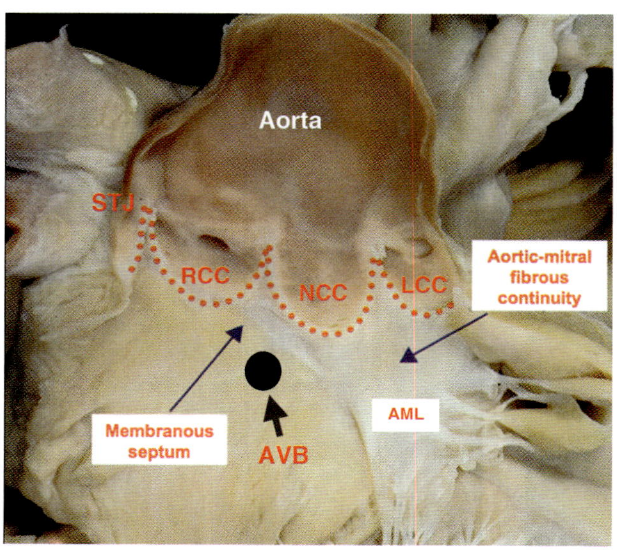

Fig 13.19 Aortic valvar complex, including aortic valve, annulus, sinuses, aorta, coronary arteries, membranous septum, and mitral valve. Dotted red line indicates insertion of aortic leaflets, from basal ring to sinotubular junction. The proximity of the atrioventricular bundle (AVB) explains why heart block is more common with prostheses that extend further into left ventricle. (From Leon MB, Piazza N, Nikolsky E, et al: Standardized endpoint definitions for transcatheter aortic valve implantation clinical trials: A consensus report from the Valve Academic Research Consortium, Eur Heart J 32:205–217, 2011. With permission.)

CASE 13-3
Self-Expanding Bioprosthetic Aortic Valve

The patient is an 85-year-old man with severe symptomatic aortic stenosis and multiple comorbidities. TAVR was recommended as treatment.

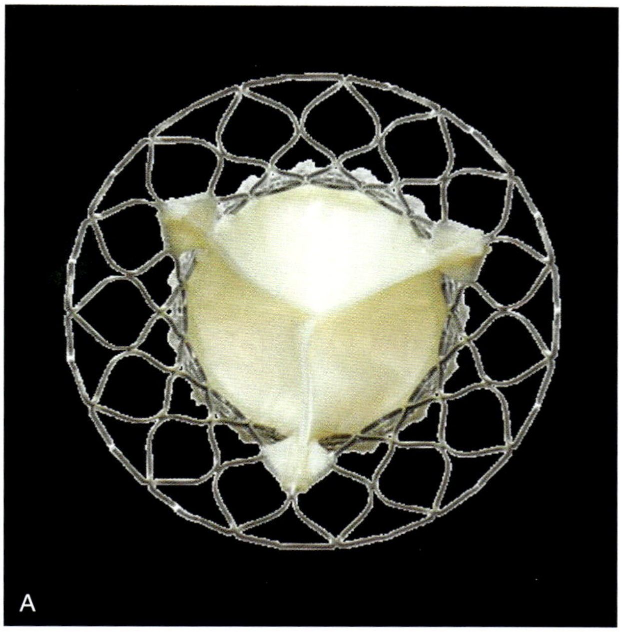

Fig 13.20A Medtronic CoreValve (Medtronic, Minneapolis, Minnesota), top view. Trileaflet porcine valve is sewn into nitinol wire frame.

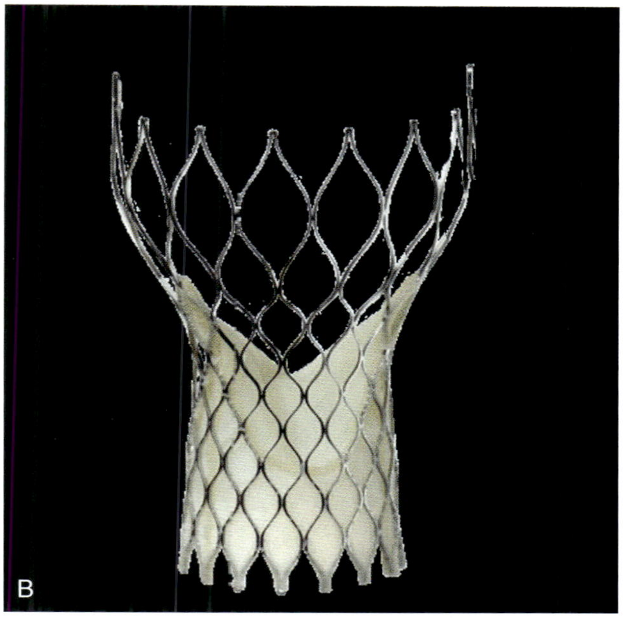

Fig 13.20B Medtronic CoreValve (Medtronic, Minneapolis, Minnesota), side view

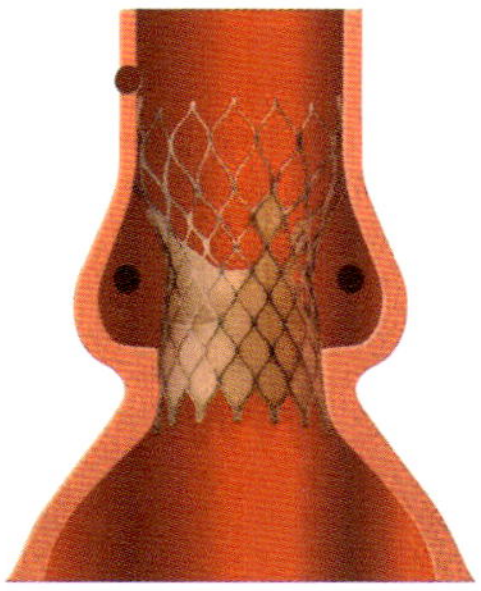

Fig 13.21 Medtronic CoreValve positioned in aortic root.

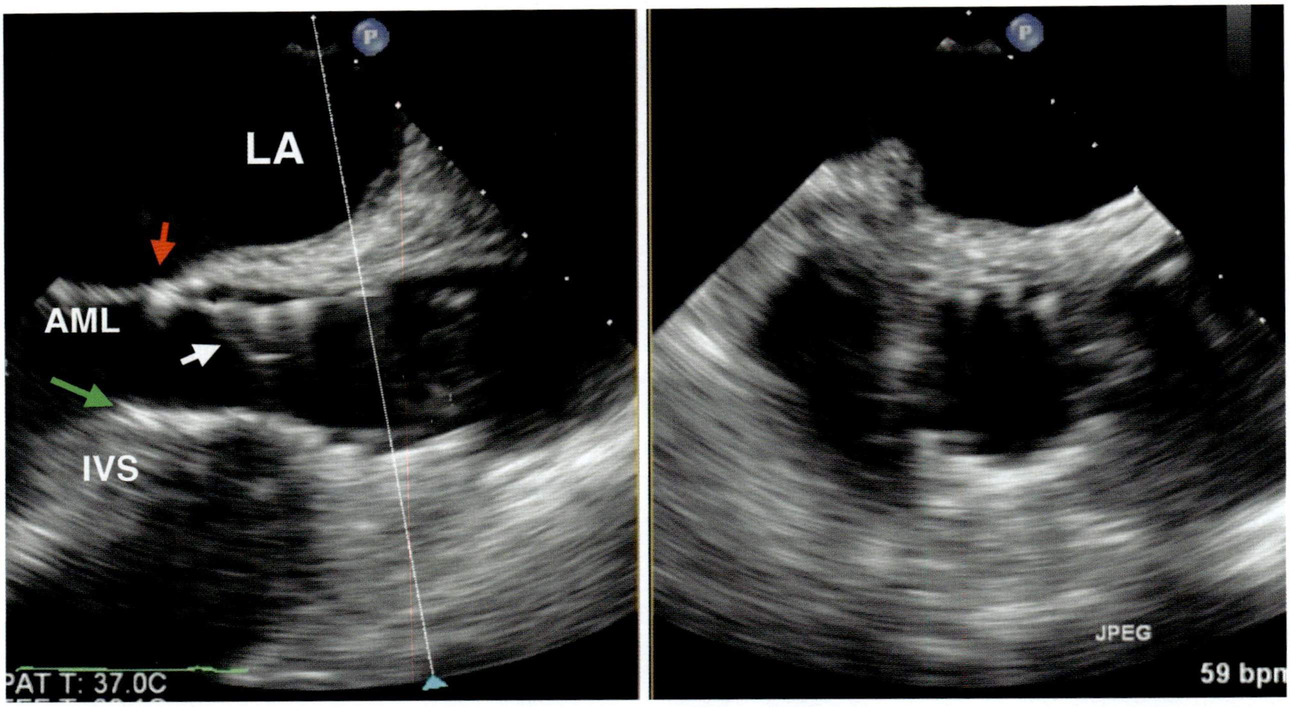

Fig 13.22 Biplane imaging of deployed valve is seen in this midesophageal long-axis view. White arrow indicates the valve itself, which is above the annulus, which is indicated by the red arrow. Green arrow shows the ventricular portion of the frame abutting the interventricular septum.

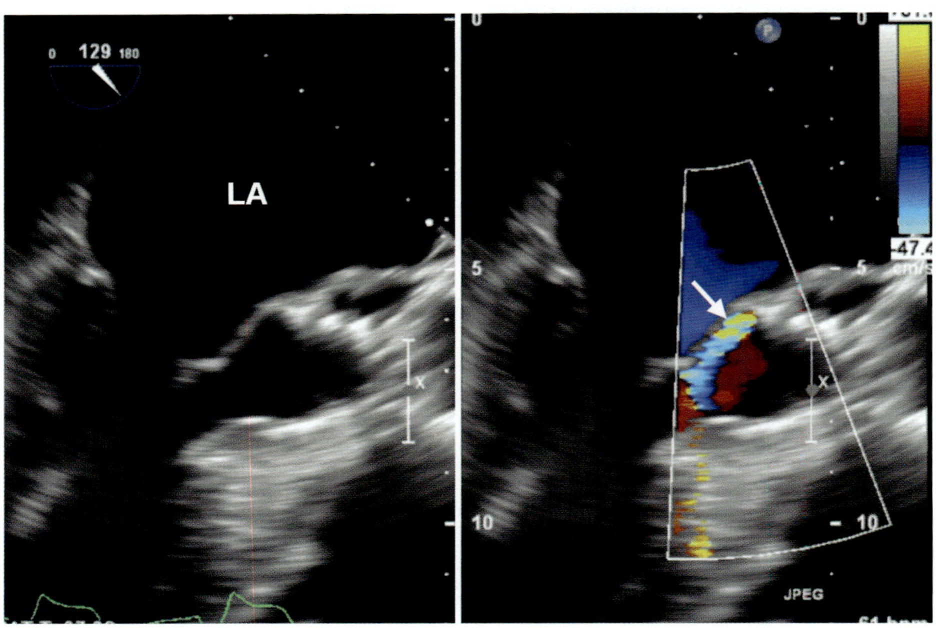

Fig 13.23 Color Doppler imaging shows a jet of paravalvular regurgitation *(white arrow).*

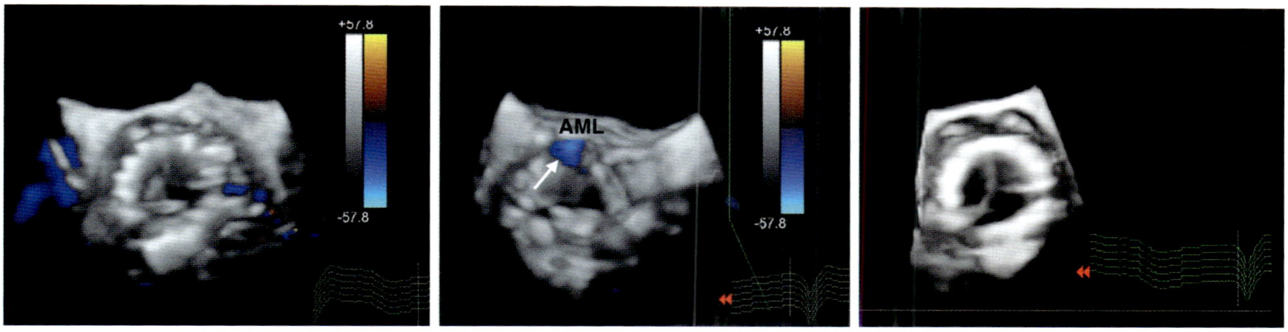

Fig 13.24 3D TEE with color Doppler. Left frame is from left atrial perspective, and center frame is from left ventricular perspective. White arrow indicates anterior paravalvular jet, which is between the anterior mitral leaflet and the prosthetic valve. In right frame, three leaflets of the CoreValve are seen.

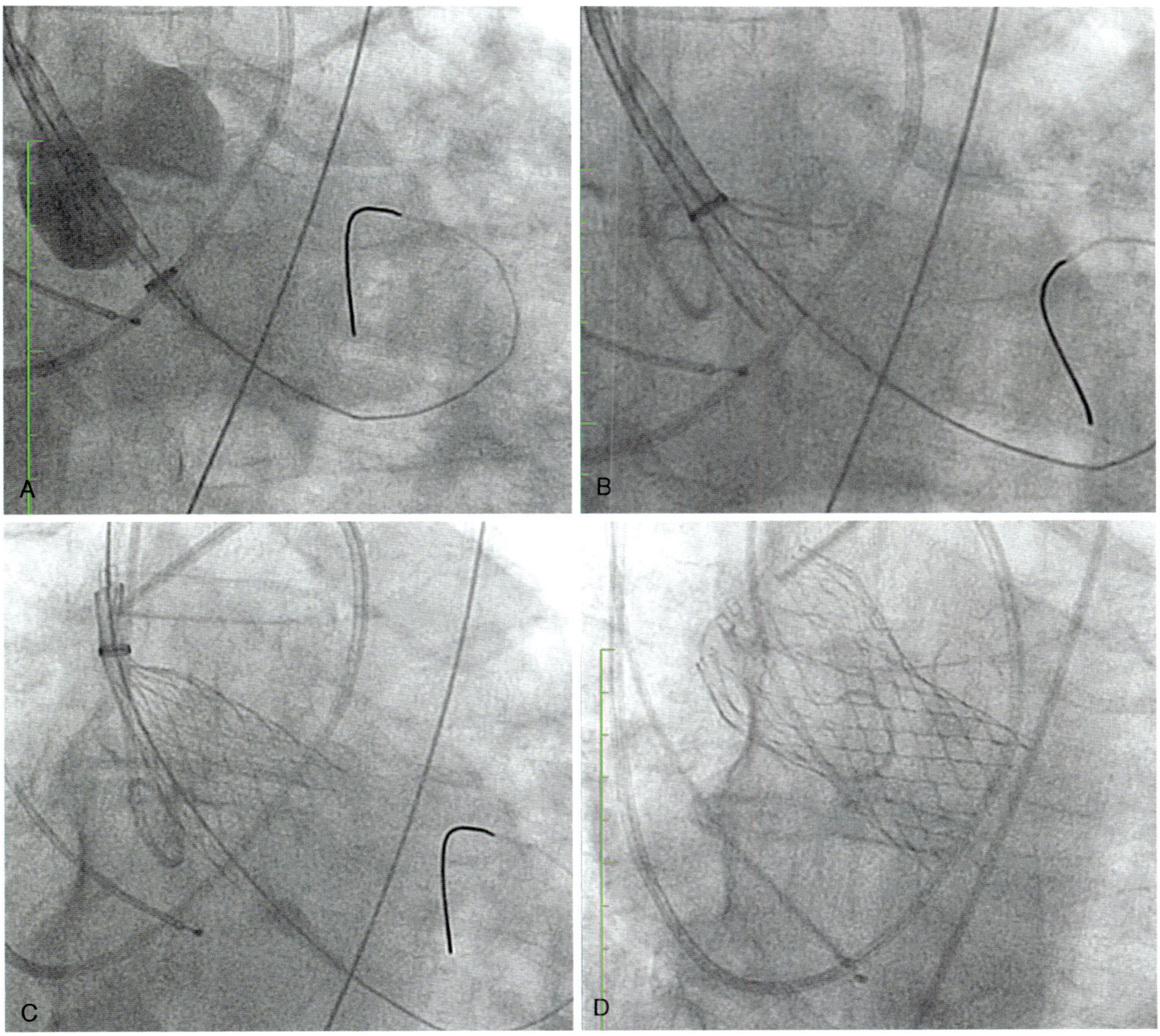

Fig 13.25 This series of fluoroscopic images shows the stages of valve deployment. In **(A)**, the undeployed valve has been positioned across the native aortic valve. In **(B)** valve is allowed to expand from the ventricular side, and this process is carried on in **(C)**. In **(D)**, valve is completely deployed. Subsequent angiography showed coronary circulation to be normal.

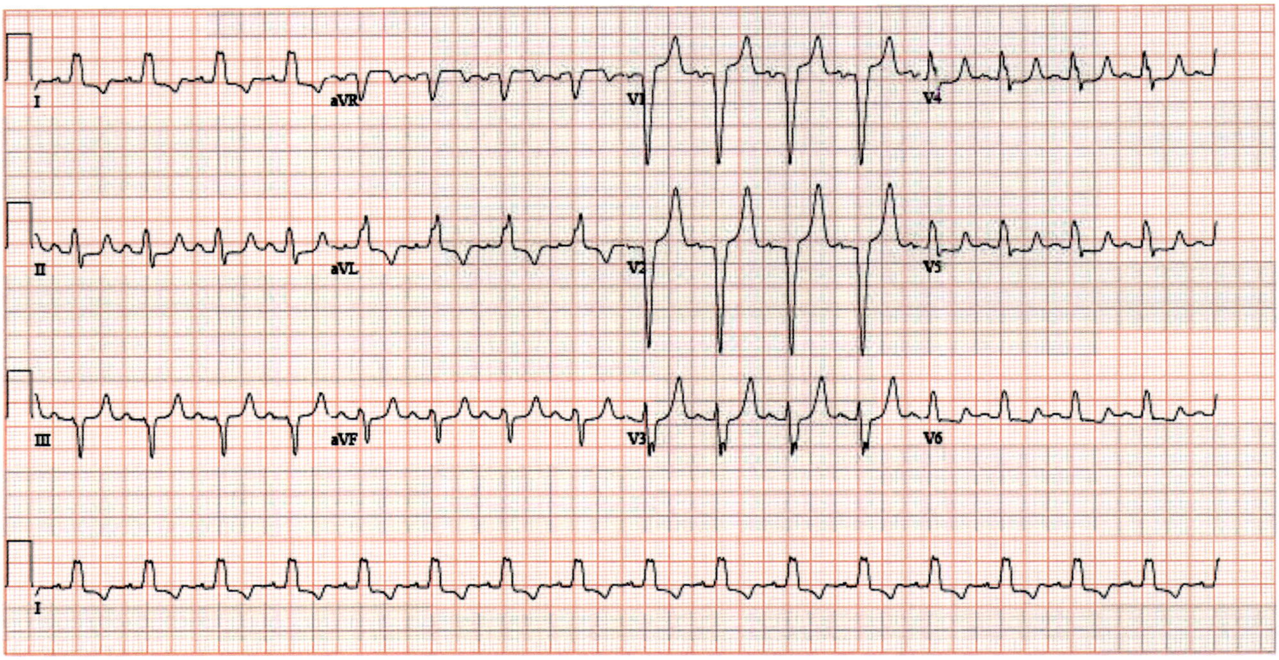

Fig 13.26 Following deployment, the patient developed a new left bundle branch block, which resolved in 24 h.

Comments

Transcatheter aortic valve replacement (TAVR) is now a standard approach to treatment of adults with severe symptomatic aortic stenosis (AS) who have a high or prohibitive risk for surgical valve replacement. Echocardiography is essential for determining that AS is severe and for evaluation of ventricular size and function and other concurrent cardiac conditions before the procedure. Currently, transesophageal echocardiography (TEE) often is used during the procedure to assist in valve positioning and for rapid detection of complications after the procedure, as in these examples. In some cases, 3D TEE imaging of the LV outflow tract and aortic annulus may be helpful for valve sizing; however, CT imaging before the procedure is recommended for optimal valve sizing. TEE is feasible when general anesthesia is used for the TAVR procedure. As experienced centers transition to moderate sedation for TAVR procedures, transthoracic imaging may replace intraprocedural TEE with fluoroscopy used to guide placement of the prosthetic valve.

Suggested Reading

1. Hahn RT, Little SH, Monaghan MJ, et al: Recommendations for comprehensive intraprocedural echocardiographic imaging during TAVR, JACC Cardiovasc Imaging 8(3):261–287, 2015.
2. Patel PA, Gutsche JT, Vernick WJ, et al: The functional aortic annulus in the 3D era: Focus on transcatheter aortic valve replacement for the perioperative echocardiographer, J Cardiothorac Vasc Anesth 29(1):240–255, 2015.
3. Wang H, Hanna JM, Ganapathi A, et al: Comparison of aortic annulus size by transesophageal echocardiography and computed tomography angiography with direct surgical measurement, Am J Cardiol 115(11):1568–1573, 2015.

CASE 13-4
Paravalvular Regurgitation after TAVR Deployment

The patient is a 64-year-old man who over the previous 2 years had become increasingly short of breath, with frequent syncope. He was diagnosed with severe aortic stenosis. Because of hepatic cirrhosis, he was offered TAVR.

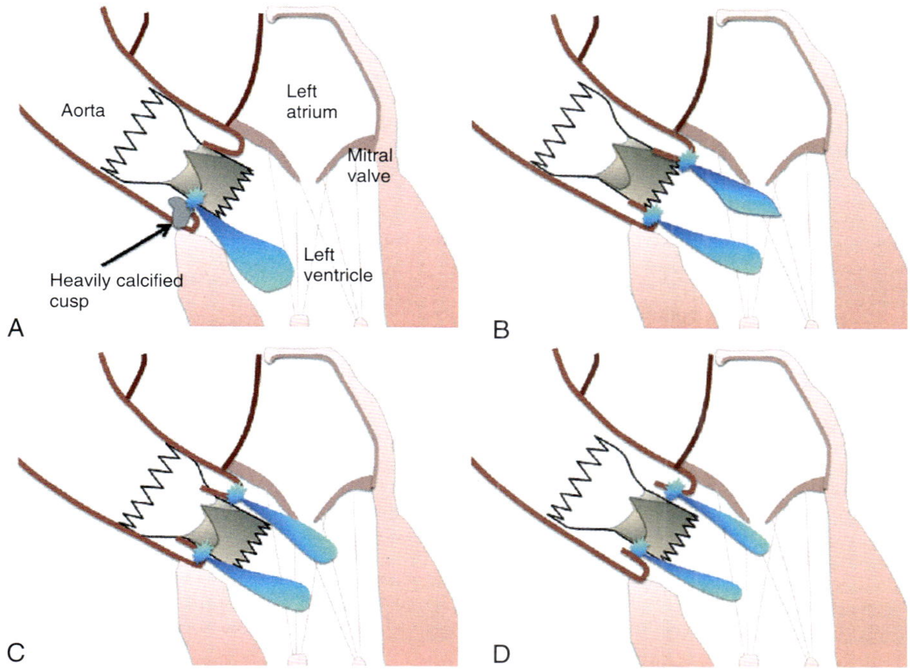

Fig 3.27 Mechanisms of para-prosthetic aortic regurgitation. After transcatheter aortic valve implantation, paravalvular leaks can result from underexpansion of prosthesis stent frame, which might be caused by calcifications of the annulus or cusps of the native valve **(A),** valve malposition with too shallow **(B)** or too deep **(C)** implantation depth of the prosthesis, and/or annulus-prosthesis size mismatch **(D)**. (From Sinning JM, Hammerstingl C, Vasa-Nicotera M, et al: Aortic regurgitation index defines severity of peri-prosthetic regurgitation and predicts outcome in patients after transcatheter aortic valve implantation, JACC 59:1134–1141, 2012. With permission.)

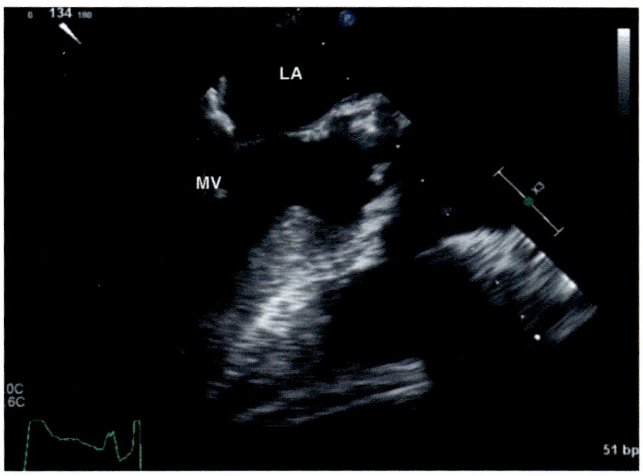

Fig 13.28 Preoperative midesophageal long-axis imaging showed a heavily calcified aortic valve.

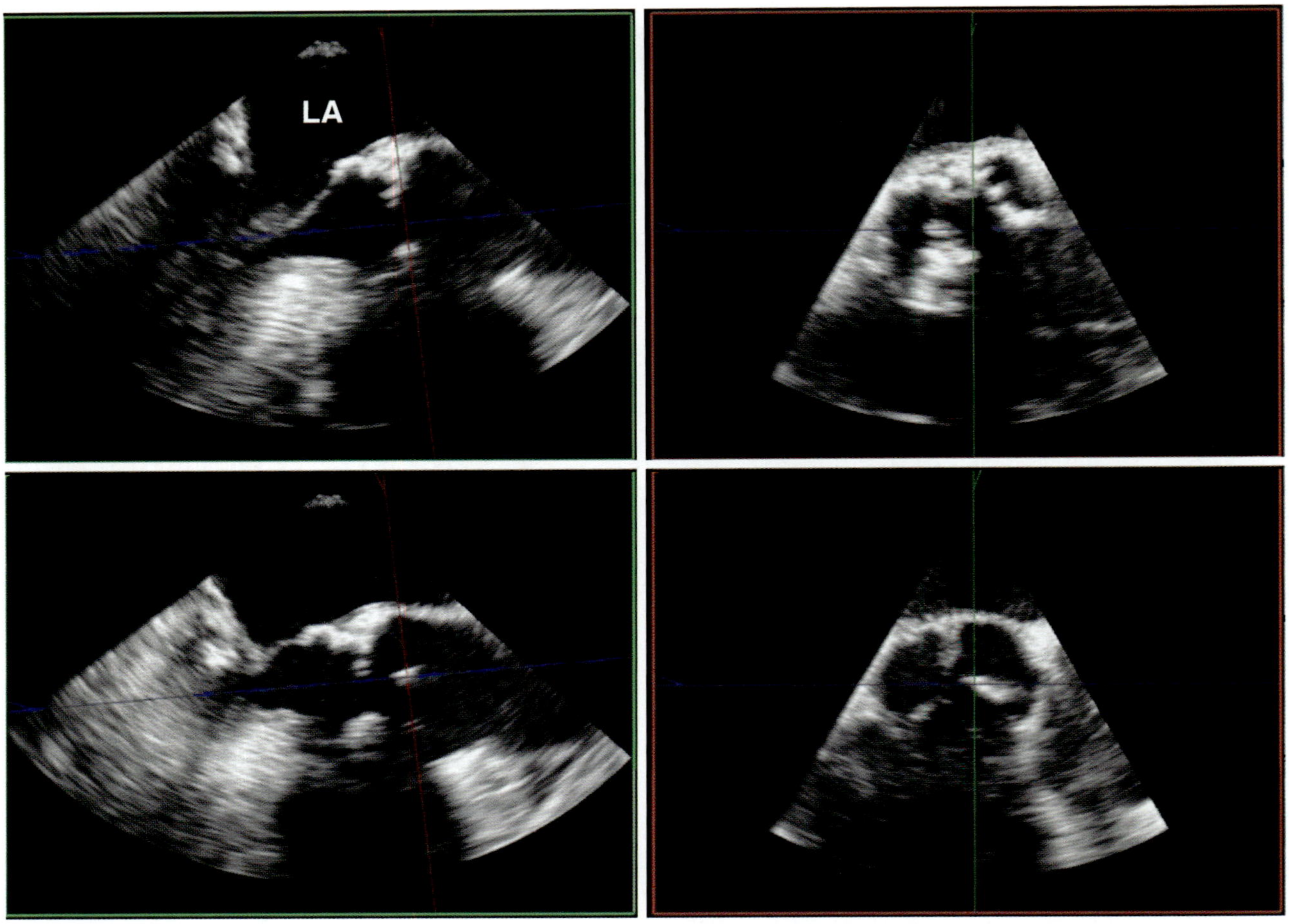

Fig 13.29 Using multiplanar reconstruction, the top two images showed a heavily calcified valve at the level of the leaflet bodies, whereas the bottom two images show less calcification at the leaflet edges.

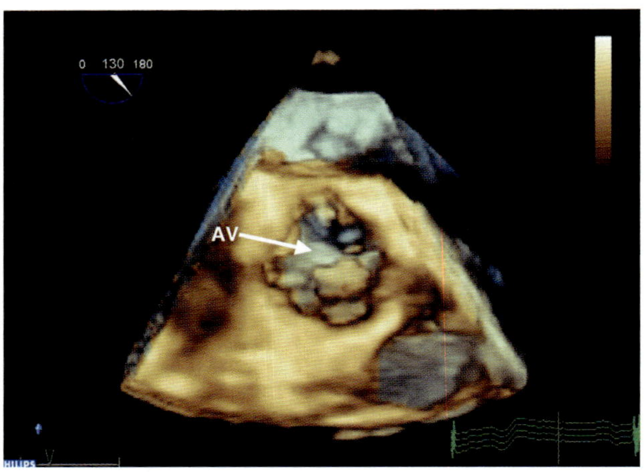

Fig 13.30 3D TEE from the aortic perspective shows heavy calcification, with most of remaining leaflet tissue shadowed.

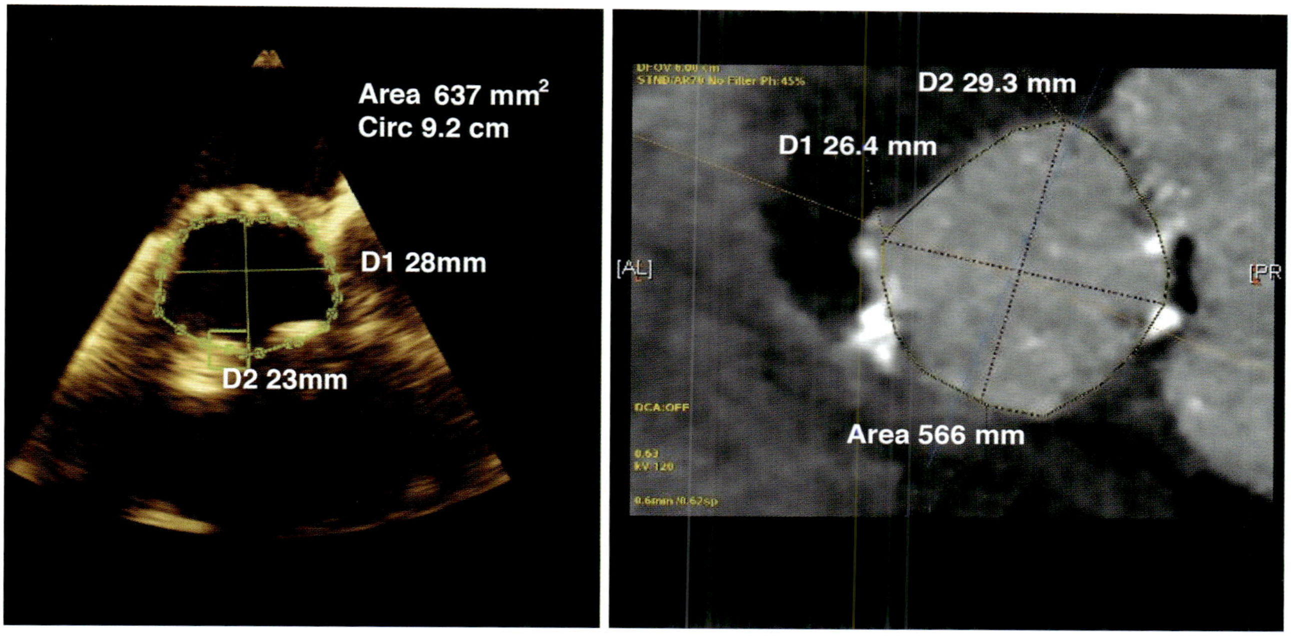

Fig 13.31 Using multiplanar reconstruction, diameter and area measurements were made. Corresponding CT measurements at right. Currently, CT measurements are recommended for clinical decision making about the type and size of TAVR valve.

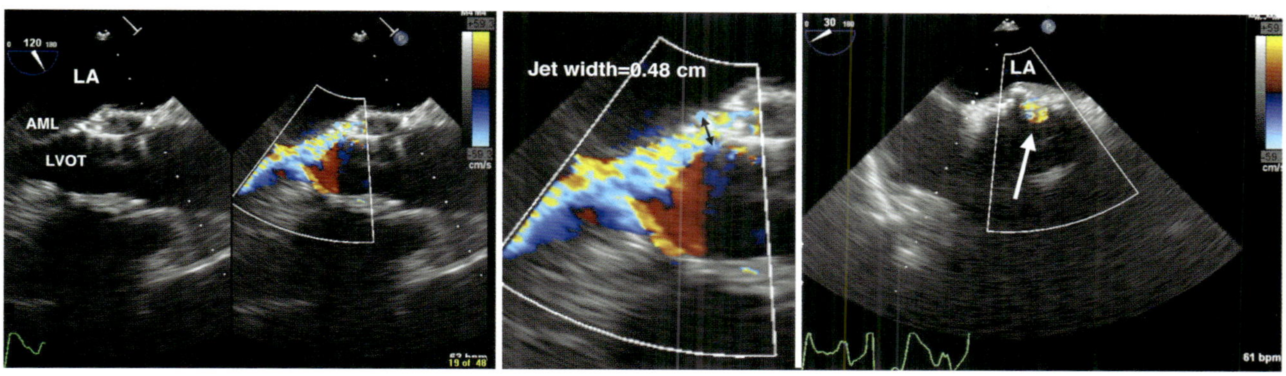

Fig 13.32 In left panel is a midesophageal long-axis view with CD, showing paravalvular regurgitant jet. Middle panel is a zoomed image with the jet width measured at 0.48 cm. On right, the jet in short axis is seen. Location is posterior, and hugs anterior mitral leaflet. Quantification is difficult because the true vena contract is not evident. The jet width suggests a moderate degree of paravalvular regurgitation.

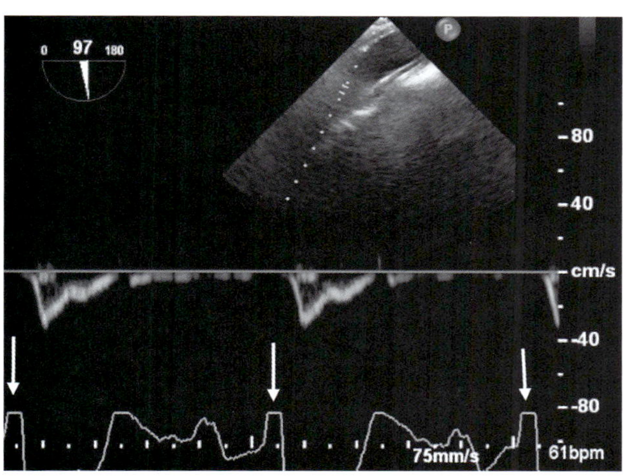

Fig 13.33 Pulsed Doppler of descending aorta does not show diastolic flow reversal. Arrows indicate QRS with systolic flow signal seen below zero baseline.

Suggested Reading

1. Abdelghani M, Soliman OI, Schultz C, et al: Adjudicating paravalvular leaks of transcatheter aortic valves: A critical appraisal, Eur Heart J 2016 Apr 13.
2. Oh JK, Little SH, Abdelmoneim SS, et al: CoreValve U.S. Pivotal Trial Clinical Investigators: Regression of paravalvular aortic regurgitation and remodeling of self-expanding transcatheter aortic valve: An observation from the CoreValve U.S. Pivotal Trial, JACC Cardiovasc Imaging 8(12):1364–1875, 2015.
3. Pibarot P, Hahn RT, Weissman NJ, et al: Assessment of Paravalvular Regurgitation Following TAVRA Proposal of Unifying Grading Scheme. JACC Cardiovasc Imaging 8(3): 340–360, 2015.

CASE 13-5
Transcatheter Bioprosthetic Valve Prolapse

This 78-year-old man with symptomatic aortic stenosis presented with multiple comorbidities, including three previous sternotomies for coronary artery disease. He was offered TAVR as an alternative to sternotomy and surgical aortic valve replacement.

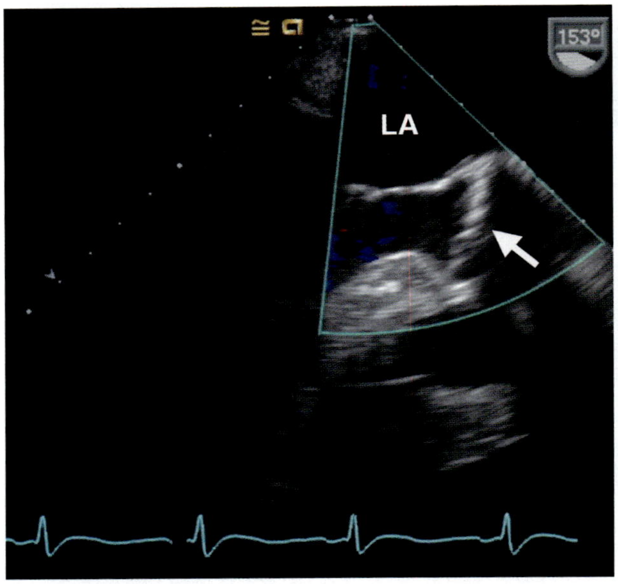

Fig 13.34 In this midesophageal long-axis view, there is obvious calcification of aortic leaflets.

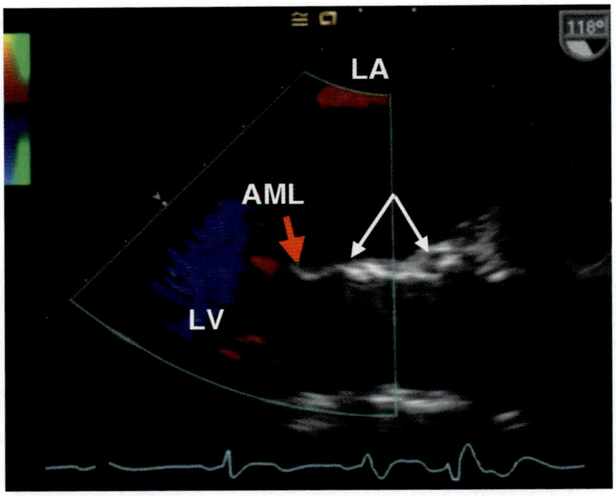

Fig 13.35 Balloon commissurotomy was performed and the balloon expandable valve was deployed. It appeared to be in good position. White arrows indicate the valve frame.

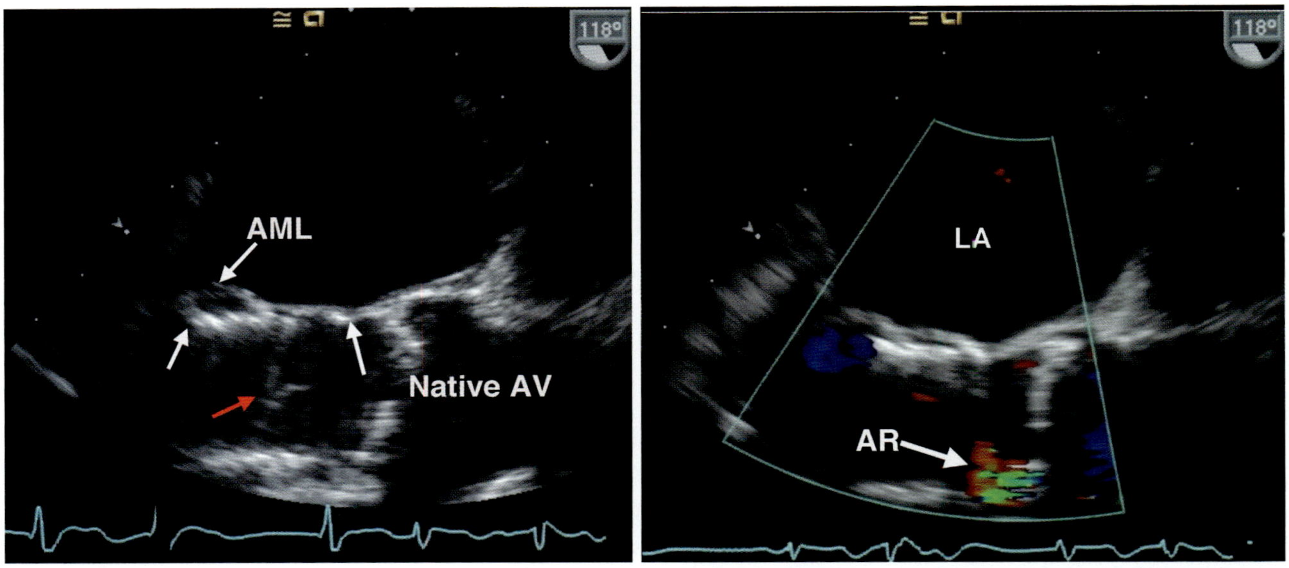

Fig 13.36 Within seconds, the prosthetic valve had prolapsed back into the LVOT, and was now completely covering the anterior mitral leaflet. Red arrow indicates the new leaflets. Although there was no interference with mitral valve function, the native, stenotic valve is now evident. With color Doppler, aortic regurgitation is now seen, probably worsened by balloon commissurotomy.

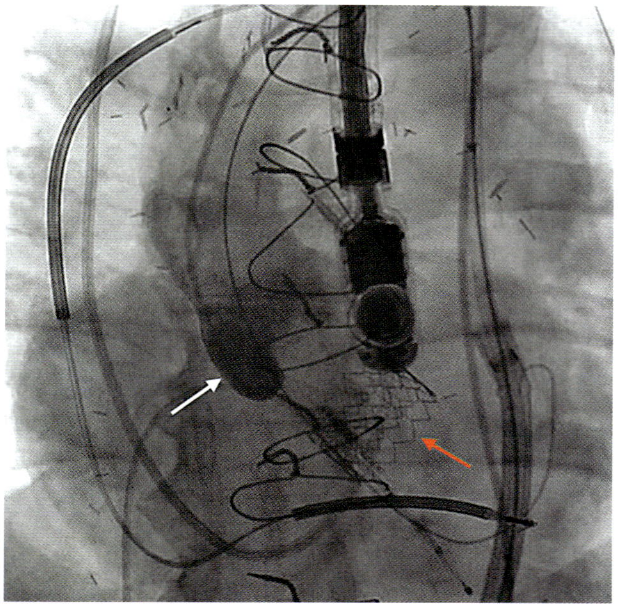

Fig 13.37 Angiography shows the new valve *(red arrow)* to be well below the aortic sinuses *(white arrow)*.

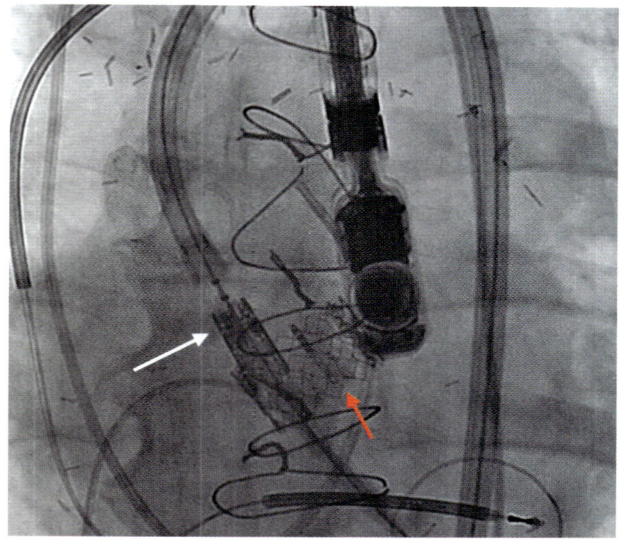

Fig 13.38 Following an attempt at pulling the first balloon expandable valve back with inflated balloon, a second balloon expandable valve is introduced through the first.

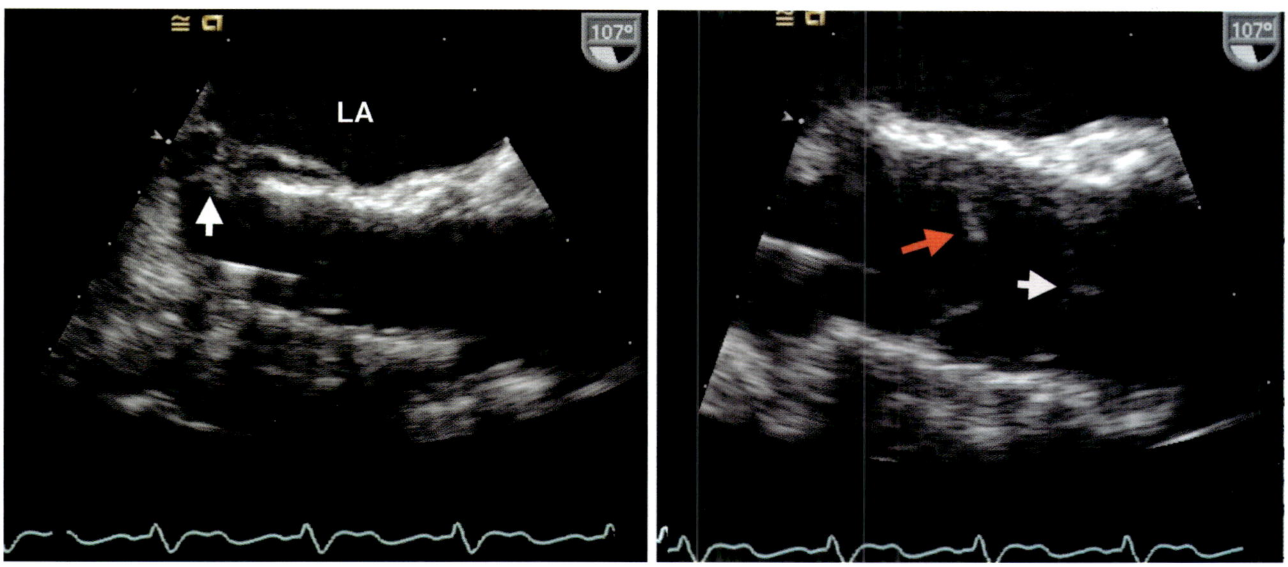

Fig 13.39 Following deployment of second valve, there was less contact with anterior mitral leaflet *(left)*. White arrow indicates the coaptation point of mitral leaflets. On right, the red arrow indicates the first valve whose leaflets are no longer functional, and white arrow indicates the new transcatheter balloon expandable valve that was deployed overlapping the top end of the first valve.

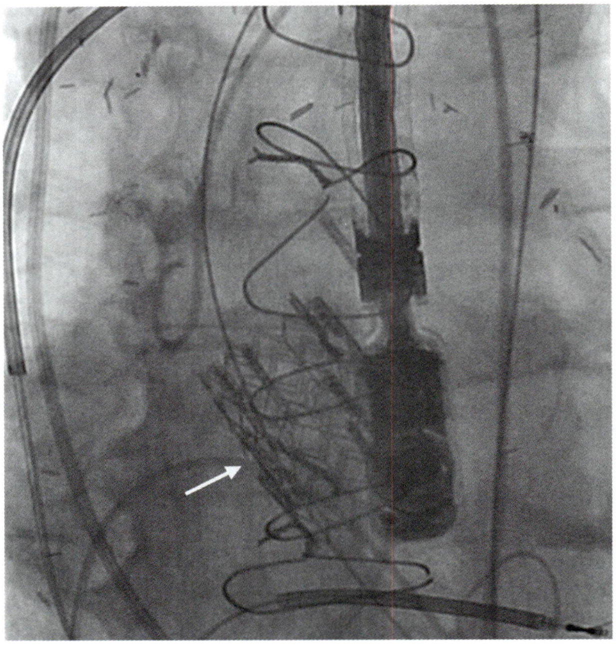

Fig 13.40 On fluoroscopic imaging, the combination of valves is indicated by white arrow. In real time, no aortic regurgitation is seen.

CASE 13-6
Annular Rupture After Valve Deployment

This 77-year-old man with symptomatic severe aortic stenosis was referred for TAVR because of his comorbidities, the most important of which was hepatic insufficiency.

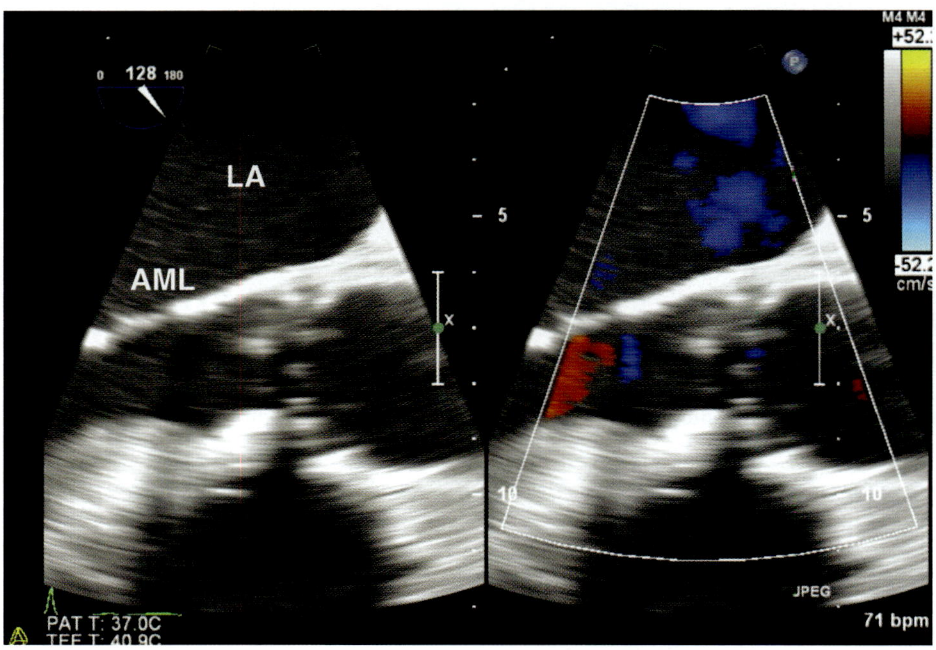

Fig 13.41 Preoperative midesophageal long axis shows a heavily calcified aortic valve without regurgitation.

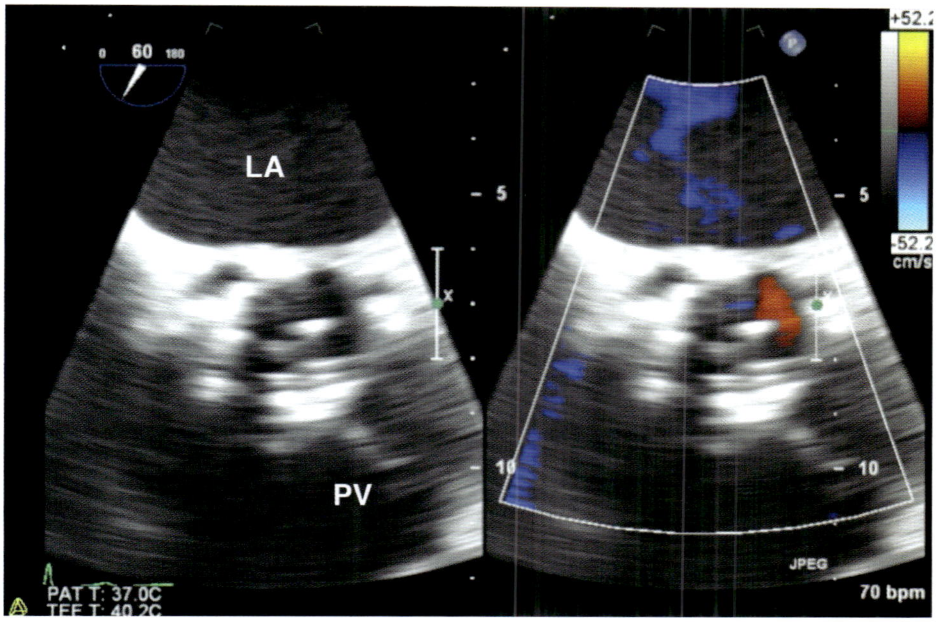

Fig 13.42 Preoperative midesophageal short axis shows a heavily calcified aortic valve without regurgitation.

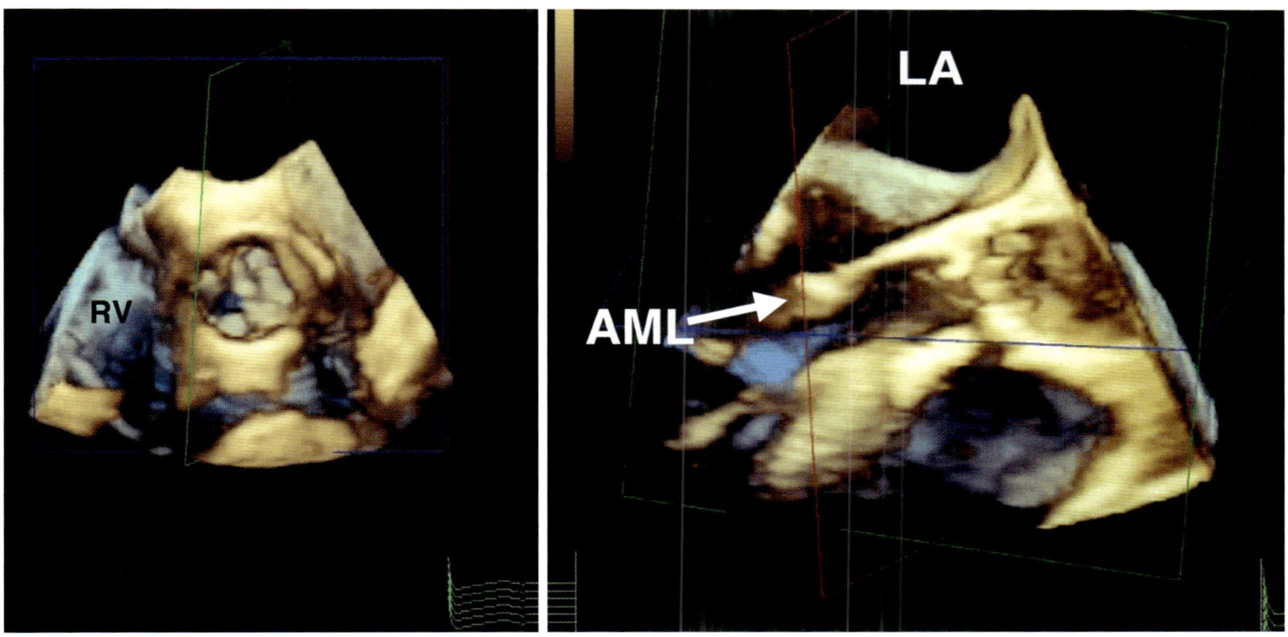

Fig 13.43 3D TEE shows similar findings. In real time, valve leaflet excursion is minimal.

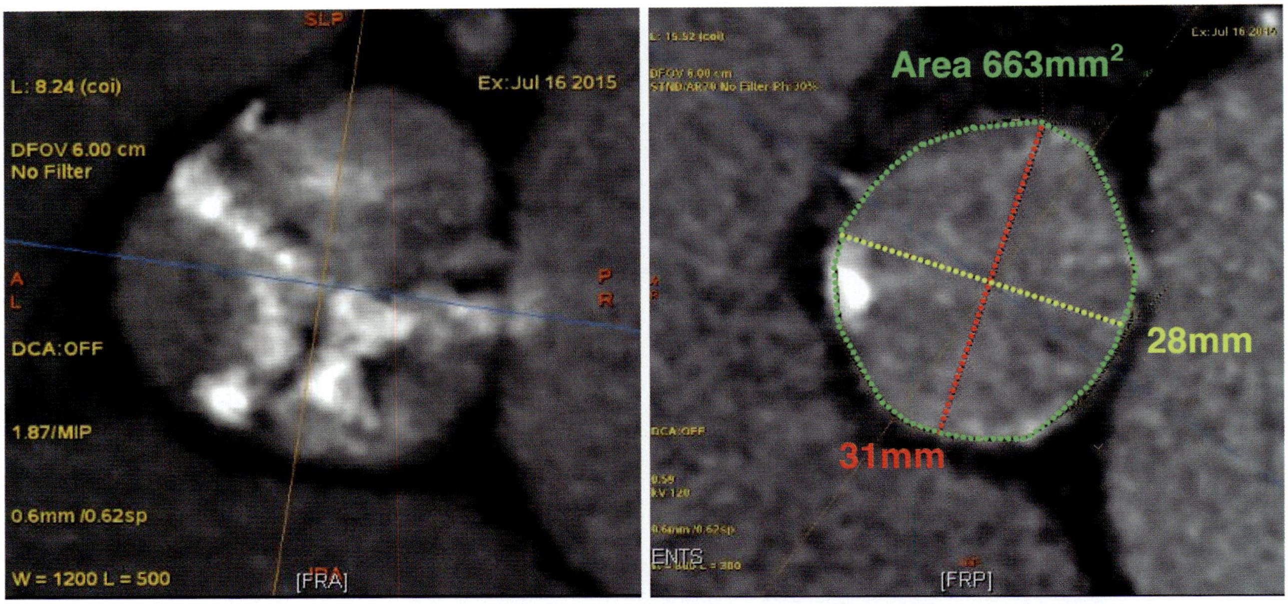

Fig 13.44 Preoperative CT scanning was undertaken to facilitate valve sizing. On left, heavily calcified valve is seen. On right, diameters at the leaflet insertion points are 28 mm by 31 cm, and the area is measured at 663 mm². Based on manufacturer's recommendations (Table 13.1), 29-mm SAPIEN valve was chosen.

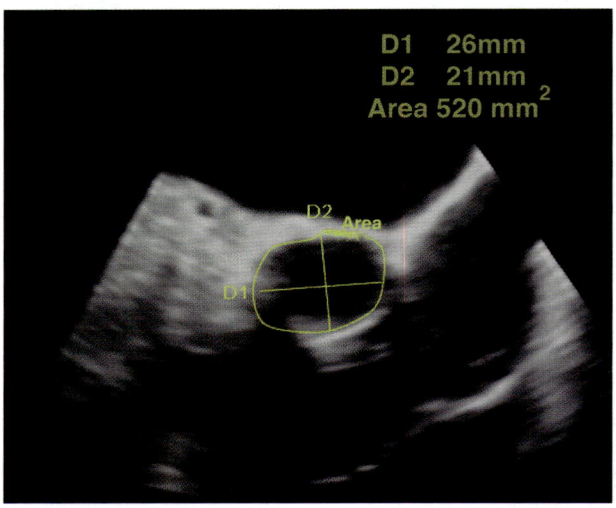

Fig 13.45 3D imaging with multiplanar reconstruction (MPR) of aortic annulus showed diameters at the leaflet insertion points are 26 mm by 31 mm, and the area is measured at 520 mm².

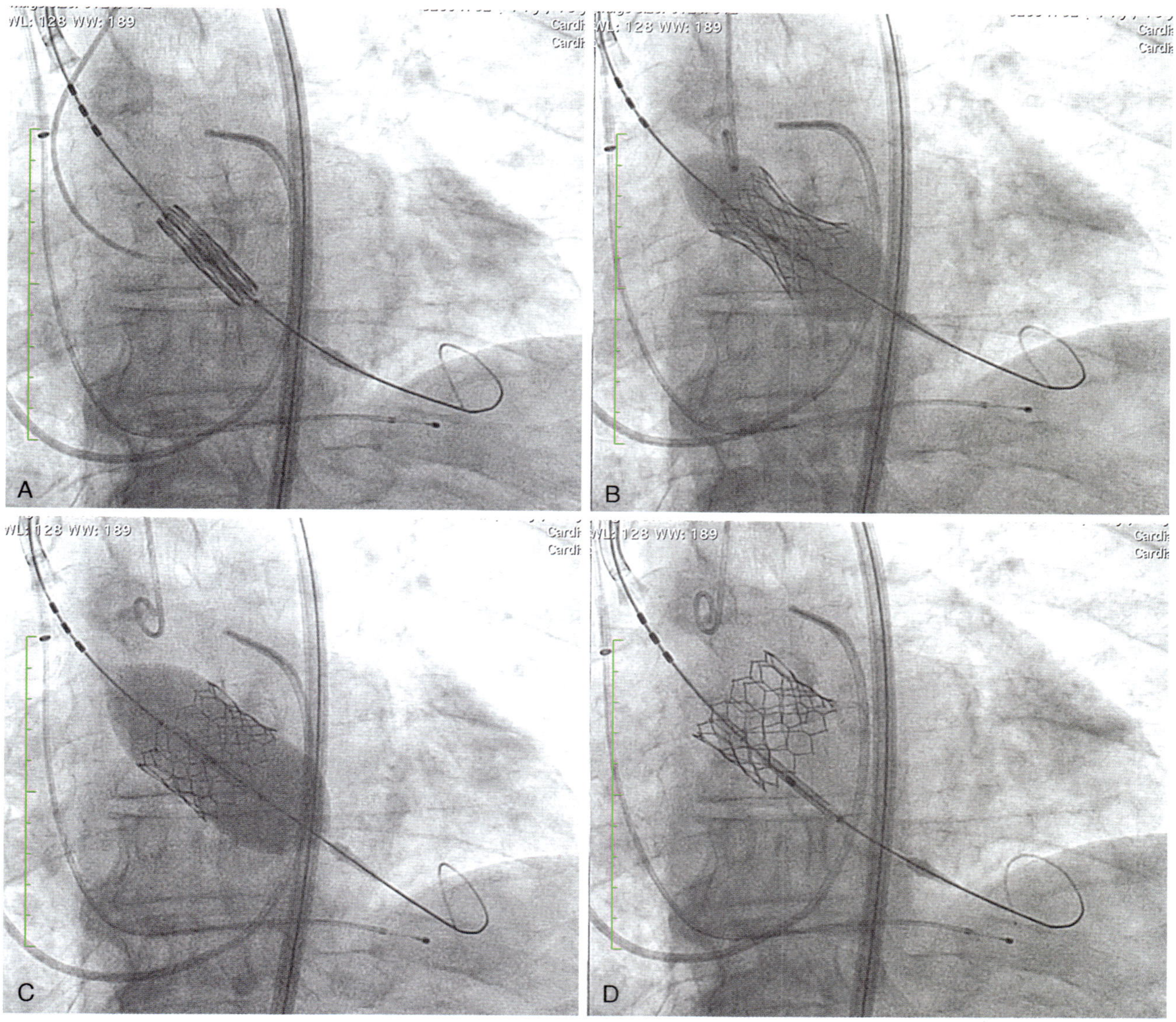

Fig 13.46 These fluoroscopy images show (**A**) the valve positioned, (**B**) start of balloon inflation, (**C**) balloon fully inflated and valve deployed, and (**D**) balloon deflated.

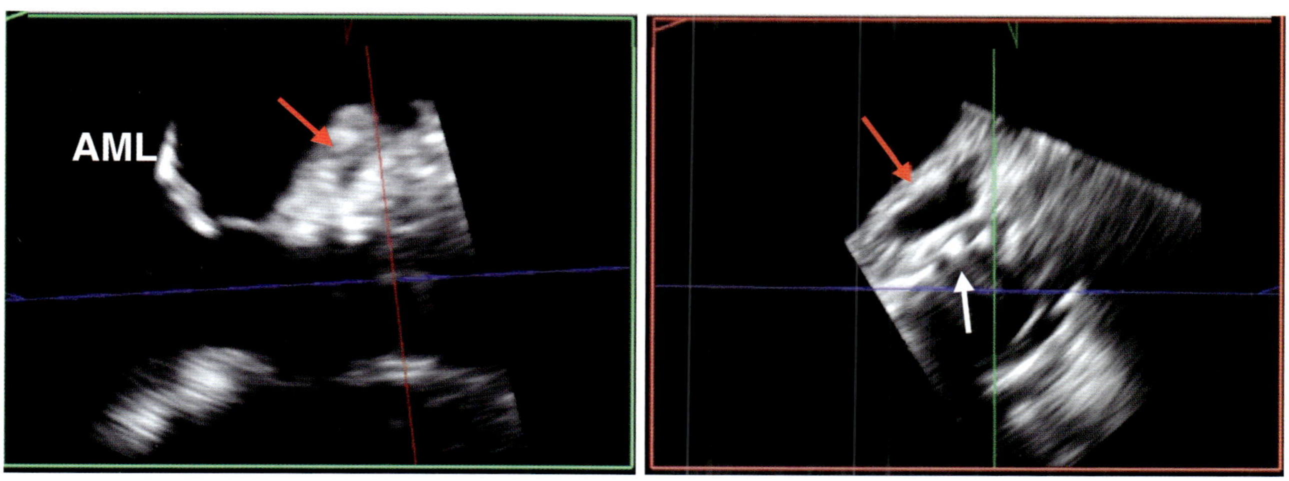

Fig 13.47 3D imaging with MPR is shown with midesophageal long axis on left and short axis on right. White arrow indicates the valve frame; however, in both views, there is what appears to be a periaortic hematoma *(red arrows)*.

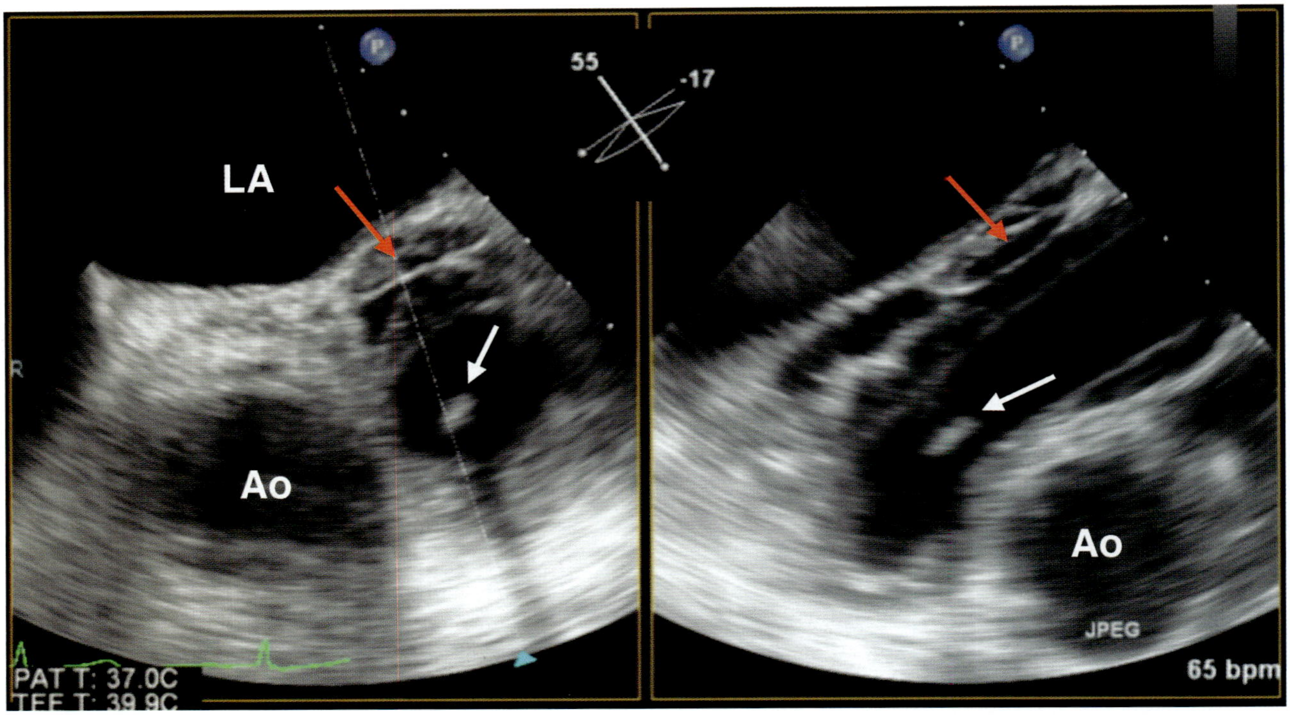

Fig 13.48 Biplane of aortic root again shows para-aortic hematoma *(red arrows)*. White arrows indicate PA catheter. In real time the PA is compressed.

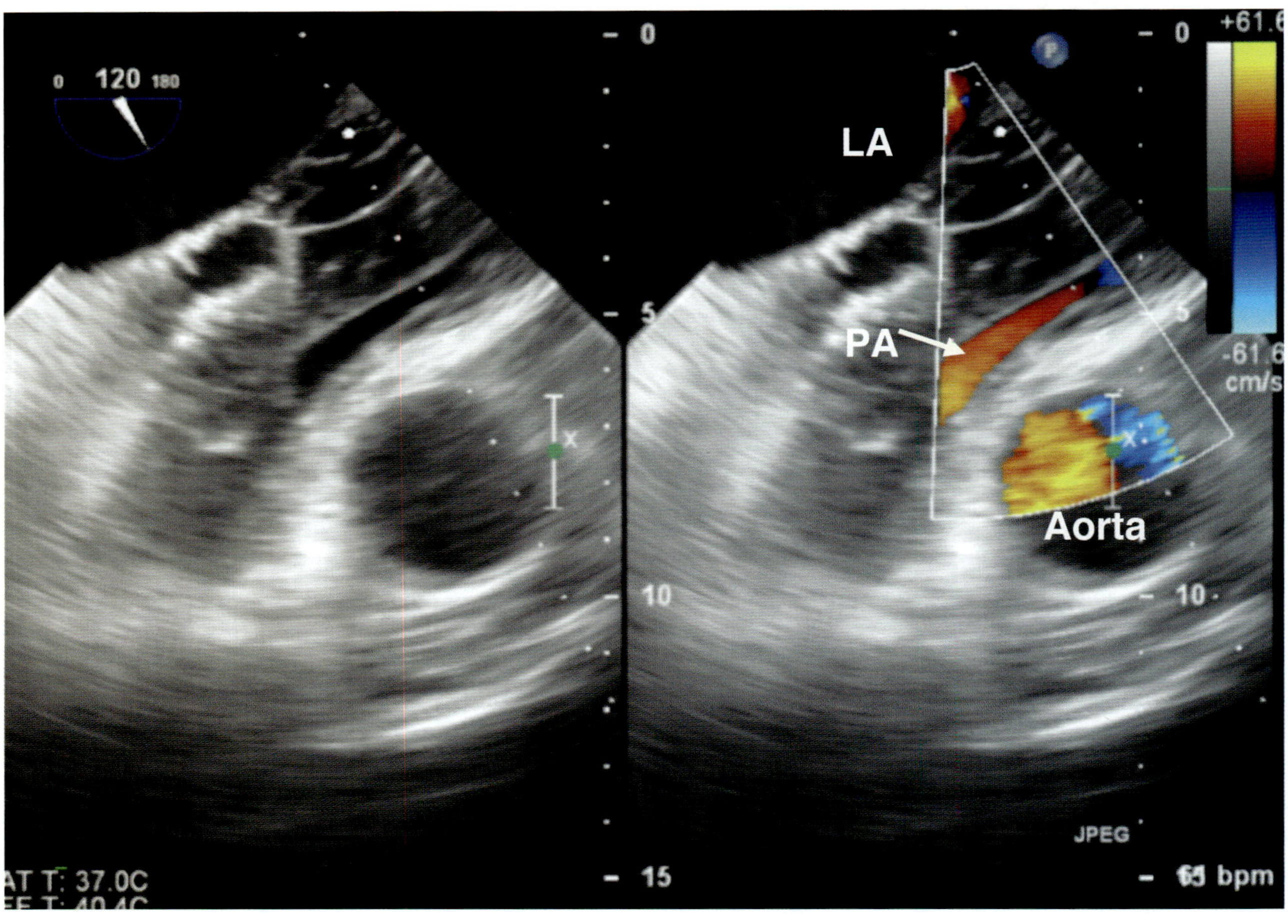

Fig 13.49 Color-flow Doppler demonstrates pulmonary artery compression.

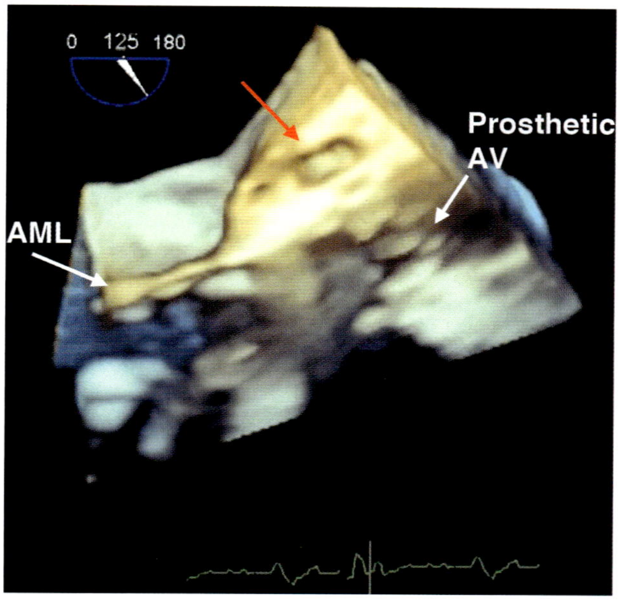

Fig 13.50 3D long-axis view also indicates the para-aortic hematoma *(red arrow)*.

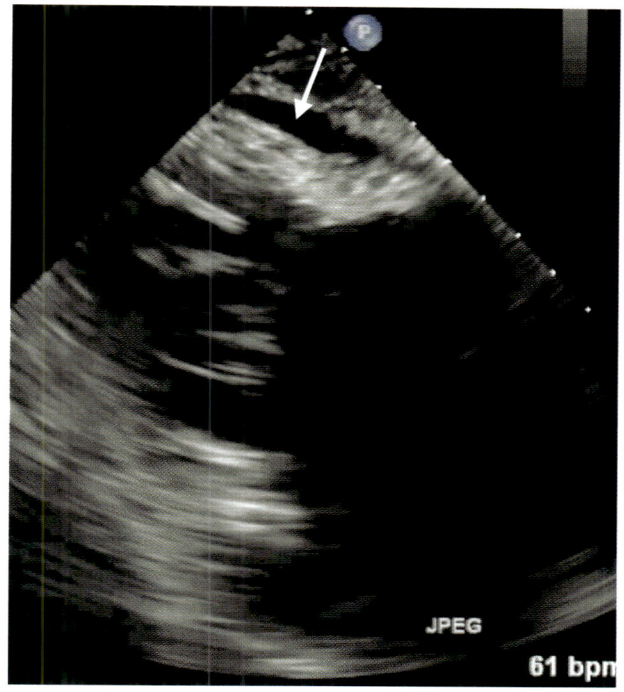

Fig 13.51 Transgastric long-axis imaging of the left ventricle shows a new pericardial effusion.

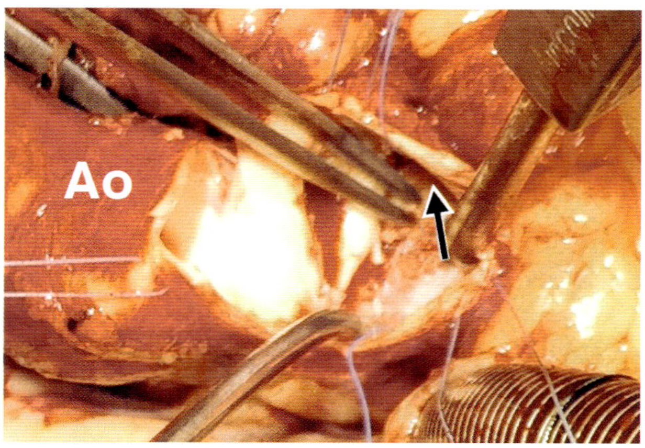

Fig 13.52 The decision was made to do a sternotomy, go on to CPB, and assess the aorta for injury. Following aortotomy, the valve was explanted, revealing an aortic annular rupture *(arrow)* under the noncoronary cusp. This was repaired, and a tissue aortic valve was placed.

TABLE 13-1
Manufacturer's Recommendations for S3 Valve Sizing

Valve size	20 mm	23 mm	26 mm	29 mm
Inflation volume	11 mL	17 mL	23 mL	33 mL
Diameter TEE	16–19 mm	18–22 mm	21–25 mm	24–28 mm
Area CT	273–345 mm^2	338–430 mm^2	430–546 mm^2	540–683 mm^2

Comments

Valve prolapse (or embolization) can occur with an undersized device or incorrect placement. In this case the valve was deployed in the correct position but then prolapsed into the LV outflow tract because of an undersized valve or inadequate anchoring by the calcified native aortic valve. In this situation, some valve types can be recaptured and redeployed; alternatively, a second TAVR device can be placed within and adjacent to the original TAVR device as shown here. Annular rupture is a rare, but life-threatening, complication of TAVR most often the result of oversizing the device. TEEs allow rapid recognition of this complication based on the presence of a rapidly expanding pericardial effusion with tamponade physiology. Treatment is immediate pericardial drainage followed by prompt surgical repair.

Suggested Reading

1. Hahn RT, Gillam LD, Little SH: Echocardiographic imaging of procedural complications during self-expandable transcatheter aortic valve replacement, JACC Cardiovasc Imaging 8(3):319–336, 2015.
2. Hahn RT, Kodali S, Tuzcu EM, et al: Echocardiographic imaging of procedural complications during balloon-expandable transcatheter aortic valve replacement, JACC Cardiovasc Imaging 8(3):288–318, 2015.
3. Bloomfield GS, Gillam LD, Hahn RT, et al: A practical guide to multimodality imaging of transcatheter aortic valve replacement, JACC Cardiovasc Imaging 5:441–455, 2015.
4. Kasel AM, Cassese S, Bleiziffer S, et al: Standardized imaging for aortic annular sizing: Implications for transcatheter valve selection, JACC Cardiovasc Imaging 6:249–262, 2013.

CASE 13-7
Valve-in-Valve Therapy for Bioprosthetic Mitral Regurgitation

Five months before this admission, the patient had undergone CABG and bioprosthetic mitral valve replacement for triple vessel disease and severe mitral regurgitation. The patient had previously undergone thoracic irradiation for Hodgkin's lymphoma, which made the operative dissection extremely difficult. Placement of the valve was challenging because of extensive mitral annular calcification, and postbypass there was still moderate mitral regurgitation. The surgeon attributed this later finding to stent distortion during seating of the valve. Because symptoms had not abated, and the reoperative risk prohibitive, he was offered a percutaneous valve-in-valve procedure.

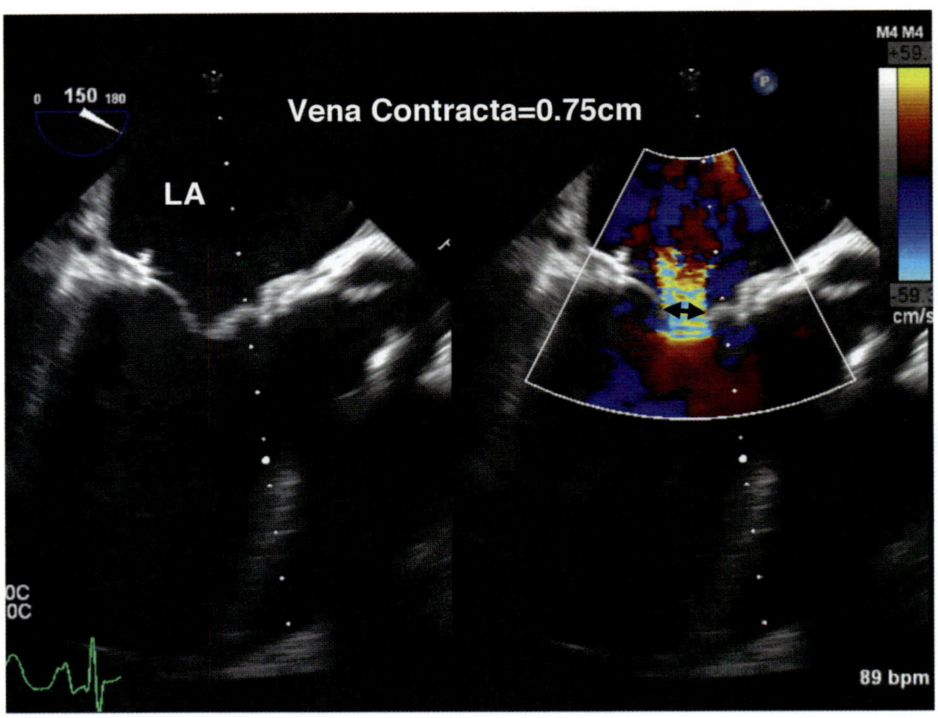

Fig 13.53 Midesophageal long-axis imaging showed prosthetic mitral regurgitation with a vena contracta of 0.75 cm.

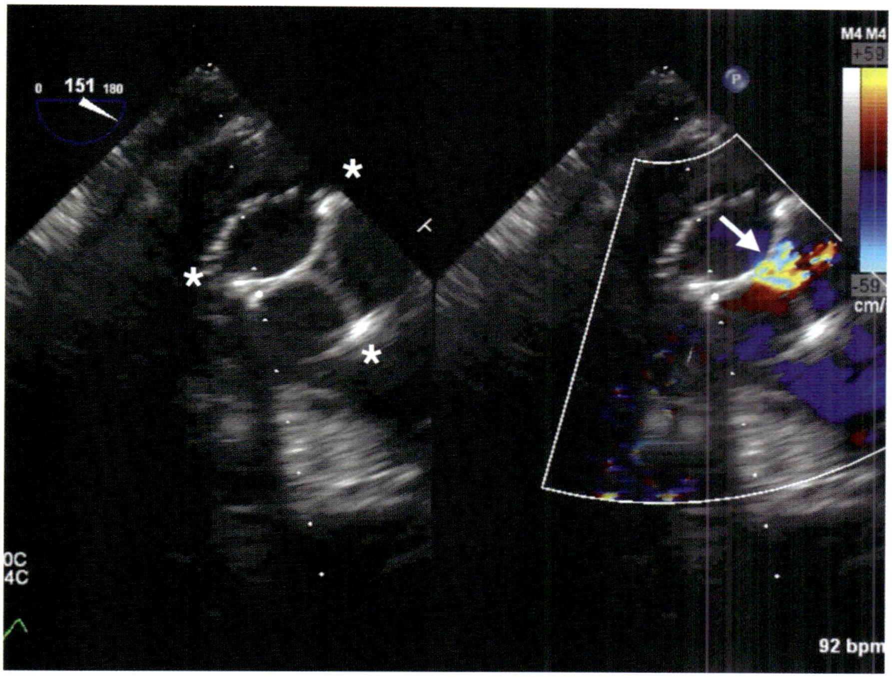

Fig 13.54 Transgastric long-axis imaging with probe turned to patient's left shows the mitral prosthesis, with three posts *(asterisks)* and central jet of mitral regurgitation.

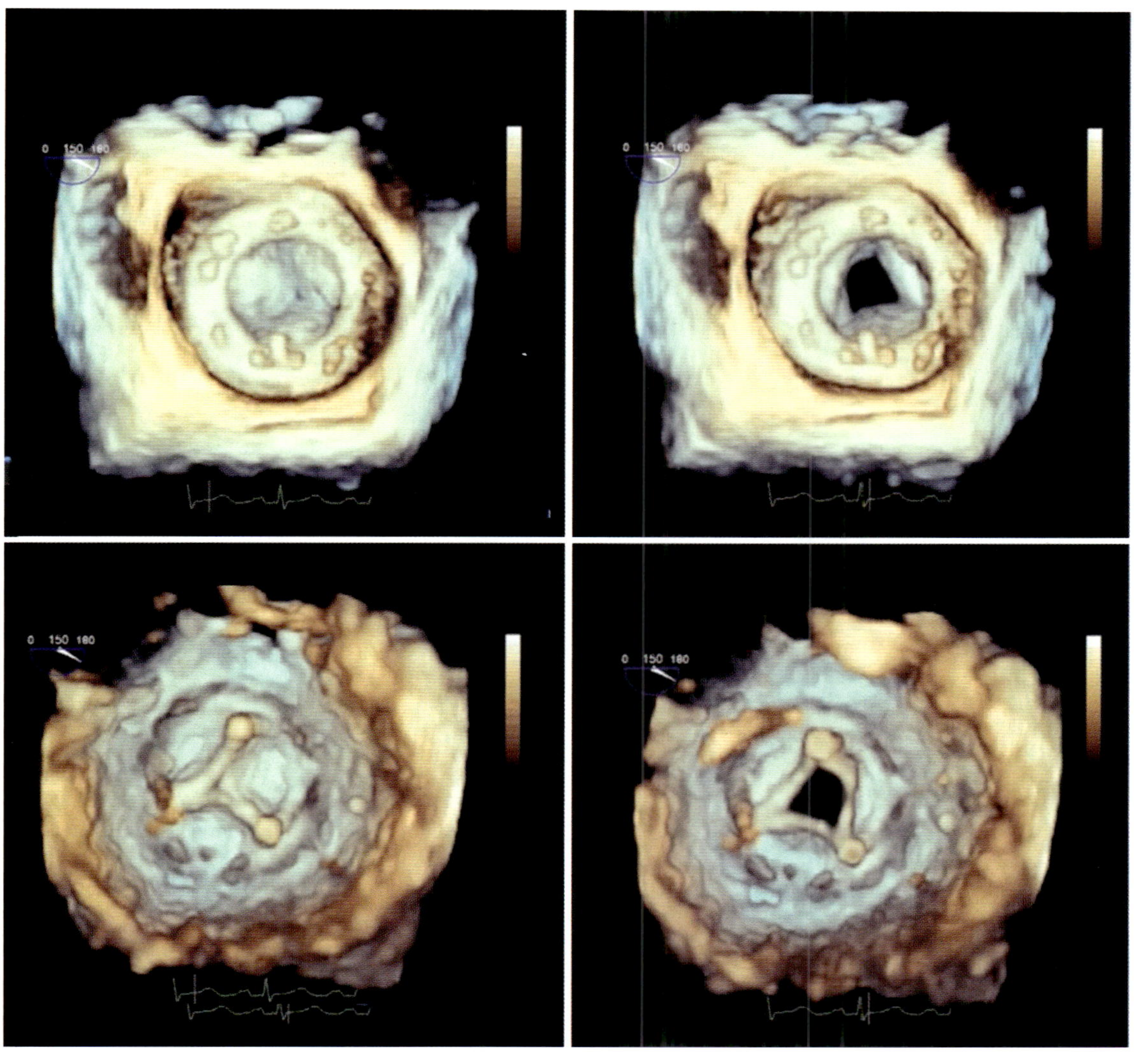

Fig 13.55 In top two frames, prosthetic valve is seen from the left atrial perspective; systole on left and diastole on right. In the lower two frames, prosthetic valve is seen from left ventricular perspective, systole on left and diastole on right. In real time, all leaflets show restricted motion.

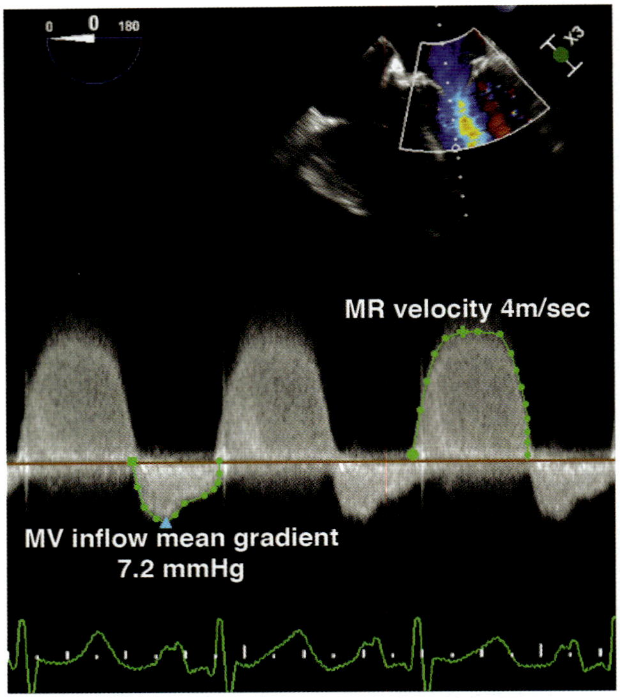

Fig 13.56 Continuous wave Doppler showed a dense velocity profile of mitral regurgitation, while mean inflow gradient was 7.2 mmHg.

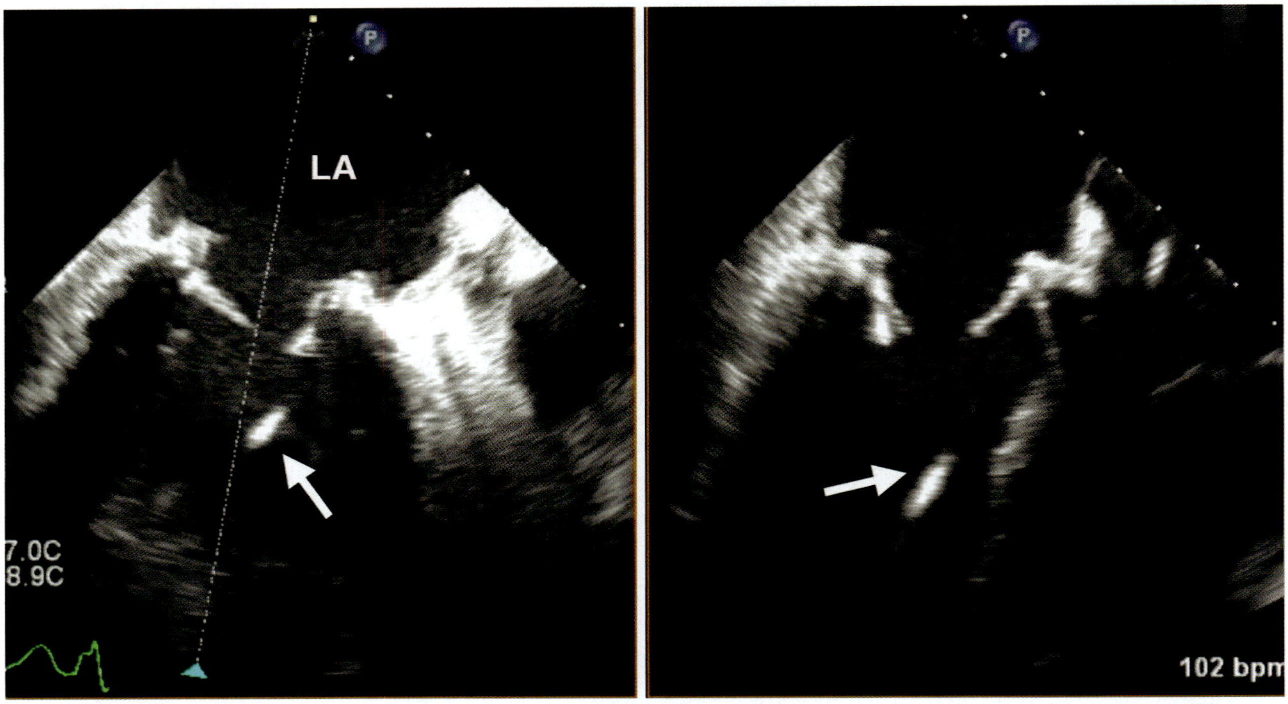

Fig 13.57 Midesophageal biplane imaging shows a guide wire *(arrows)* approaching the prosthetic valve, having been percutaneously introduced via left ventricular apex.

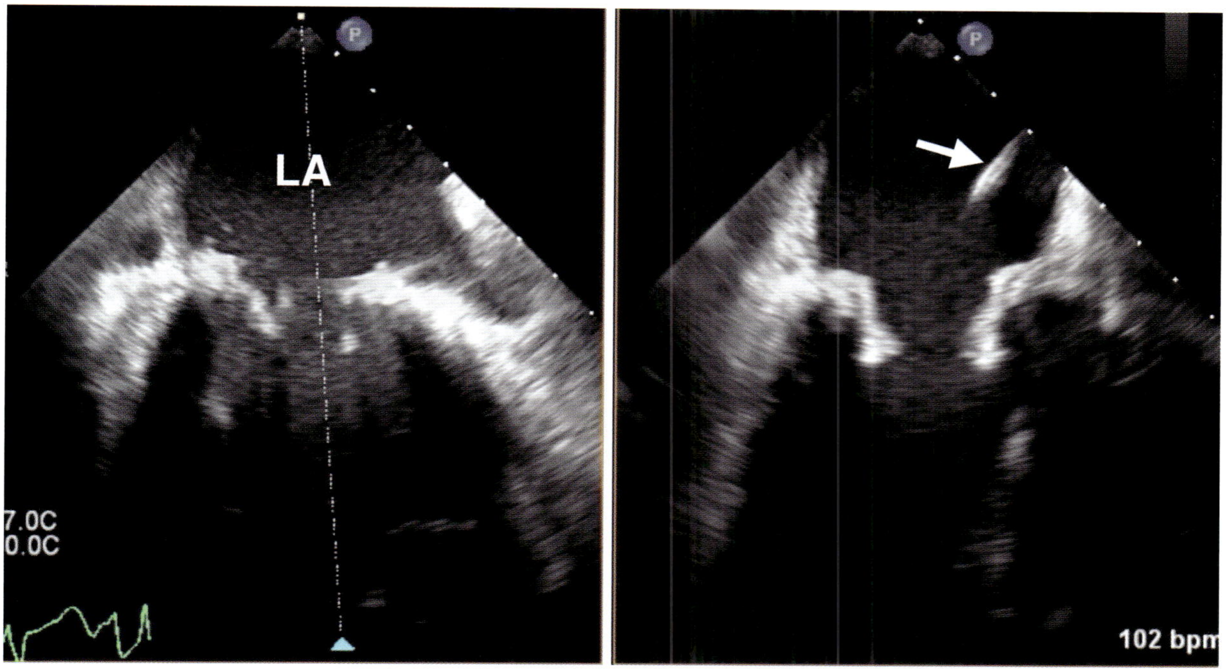

Fig 13.58 ▶ Midesophageal biplane imaging shows the guide wire *(arrow)* now in the left atrium.

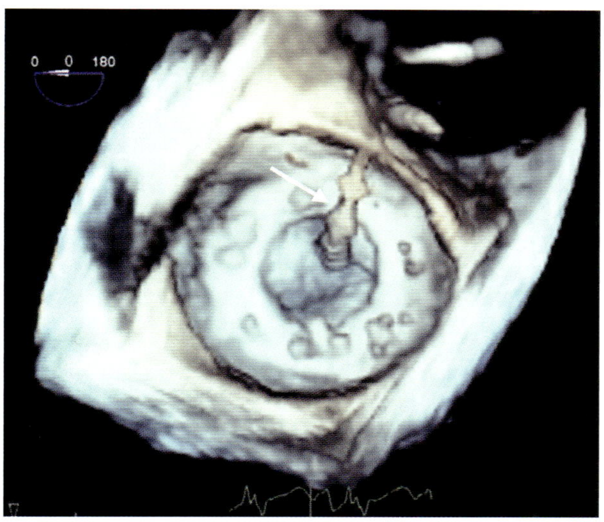

Fig 13.59 ▶ 3D TEE from the left atrial perspective shows the delivery device guide coming through the mitral prosthesis and into the left atrium.

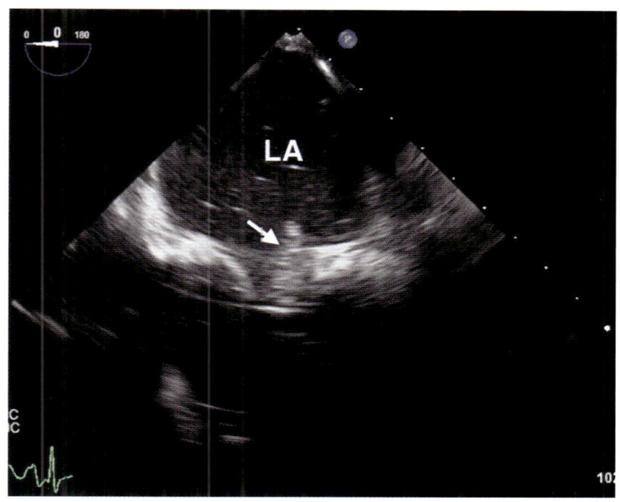

Fig 13.60 ▶ From midesophageal position, the valve housing has been advanced across the bioprosthetic mitral valve.

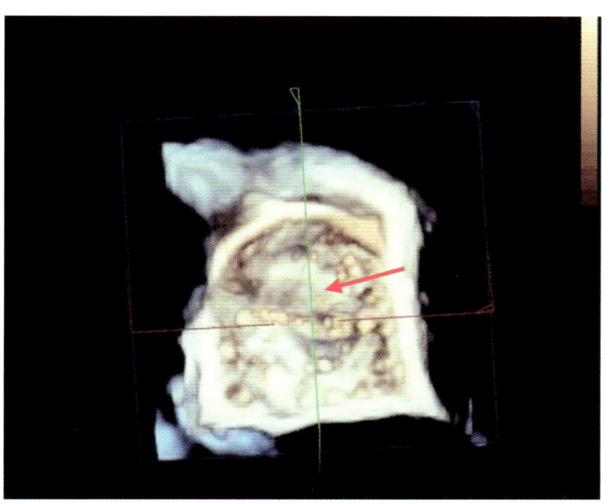

Fig 13.61 ▶ 3D TEE from the left atrial perspective shows the deployment balloon fully inflated *(red arrow)*.

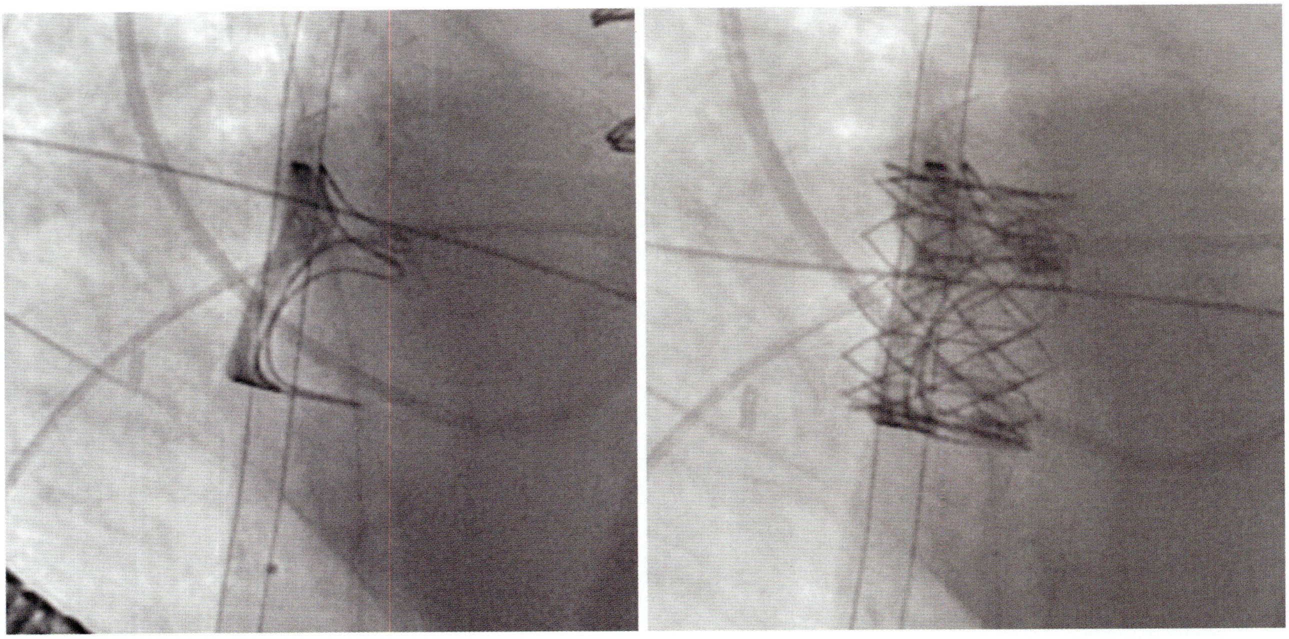

Fig 13.62 At left, fluoroscopy shows the 29 bioprosthetic mitral valve. At right, 29 SAPIEN 3 valve (Edwards SAPIEN prosthesis, Edwards Lifesciences, Irvine, California) has been deployed inside of it.

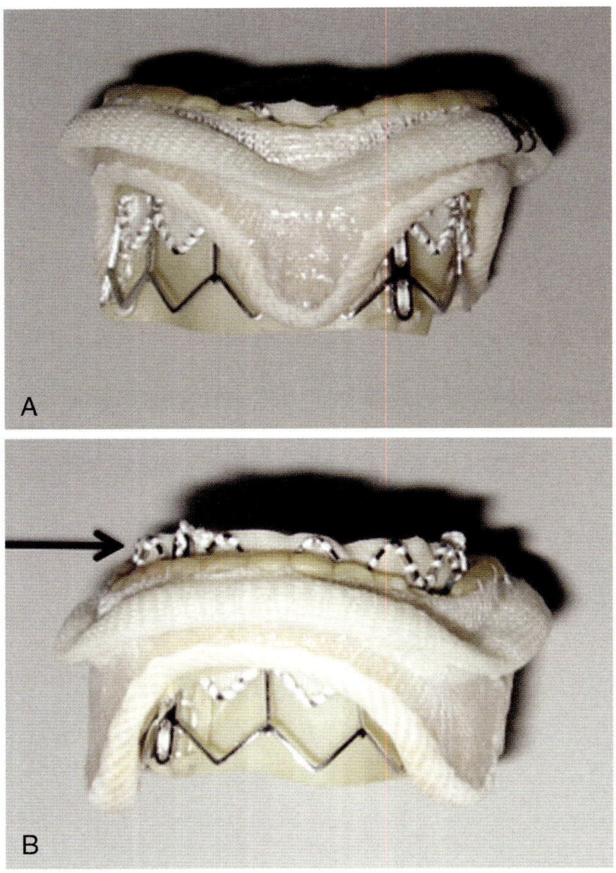

Fig 13.63 In vitro demonstration of transcatheter valve (Edwards SAPIEN) implanted within Carpentier Edwards valve. **(A)** Incorrect positioning: transcatheter valve is implanted too high within outflow tract of surgical valve. This may result in splaying of surgical valve posts and transcatheter valve embolization. **(B)** Correct valve positioning: transcatheter valve *(arrow)* is implanted such that it overlaps surgical sewing ring, allowing better anchoring and more secure position. (Webb J.G., Wood D.A., Ye J.; Transcatheter valve-in-valve implantation for failed bioprosthetic heart valves. Circulation. 121 2010:1848–1857.)

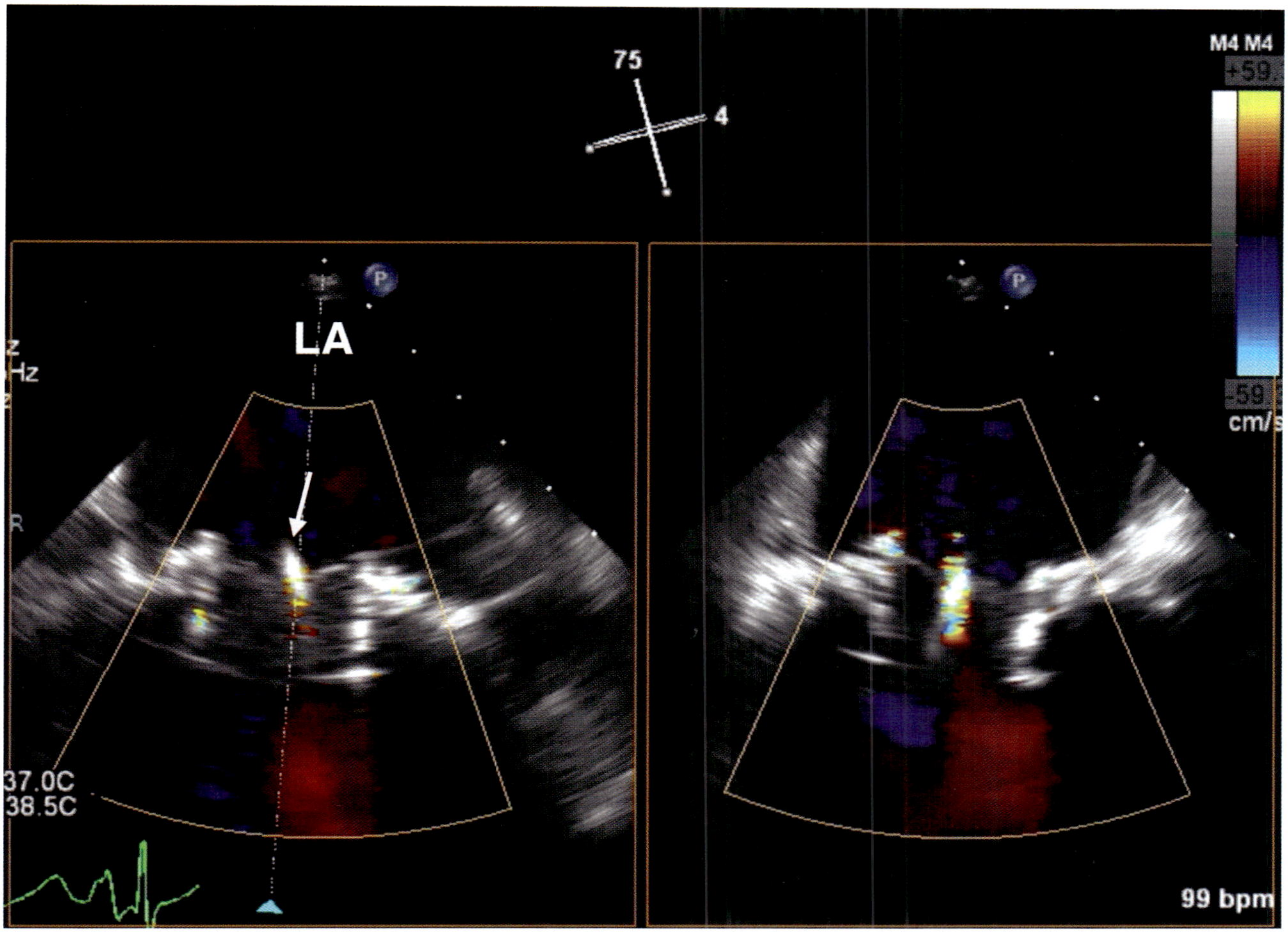

Fig 13.64 Midesophageal biplane imaging with color Doppler shows the valve deployed without regurgitation.

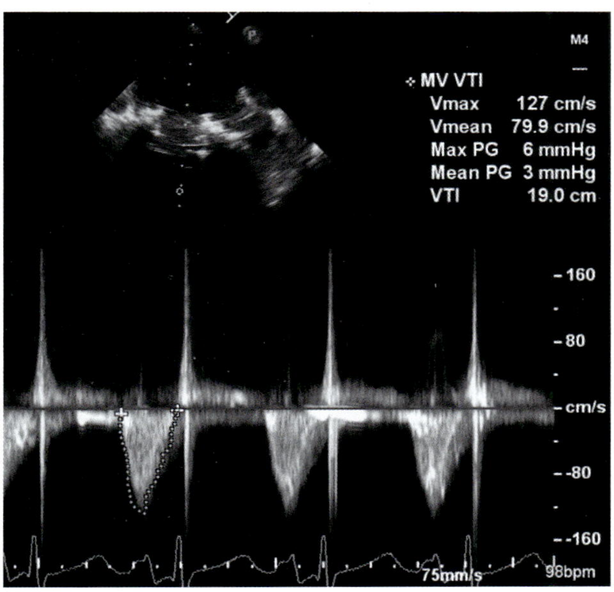

Fig 13.65 Continuous wave Doppler showed reduction in mean inflow gradient to 3 mmHg.

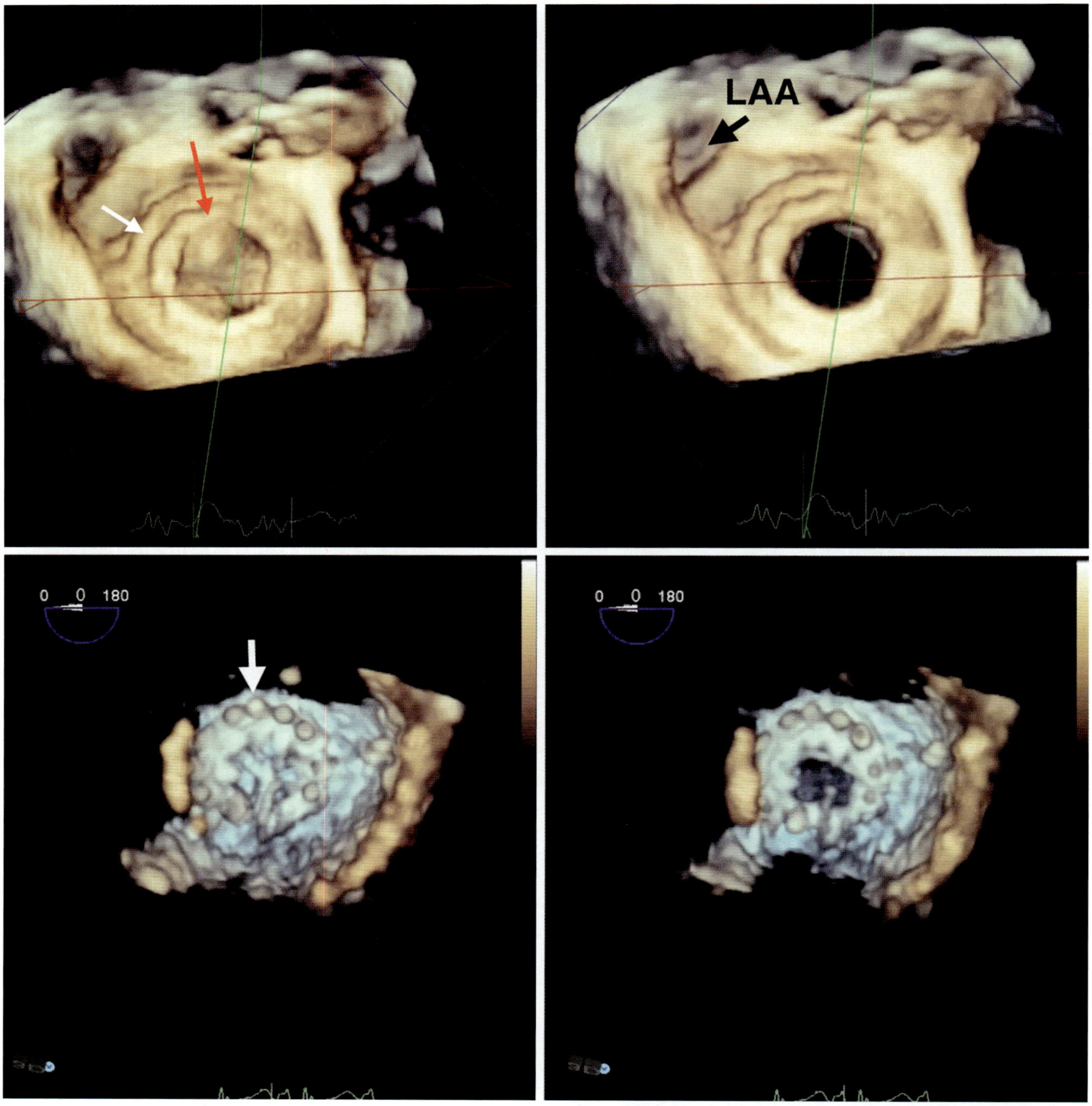

Fig 13.66 In top two frames, the newly deployed valve in prosthetic valve is seen from left atrial perspective, with systole on left and diastole on right. White arrow indicates old bioprosthetic valve, and red arrow indicates newly deployed valve. In lower two frames, prosthetic valve is seen from left ventricular perspective; systole on left and diastole on right. Arrow indicates characteristic frame of SAPIEN valve.

Comments

Bioprosthetic valve regurgitation may occur gradually because of leaflet calcification or may be acute because of valve rupture adjacent to an area of calcification (as in Case 13-6) or endocarditis with leaflet destruction or paravalvular infection. Paravalvular regurgitation also may result from suture dehiscence with a calcified or fibrotic annulus, even in the absence of infection. Indications for intervention for prosthetic valve regurgitation included symptoms because of severe valve leakage, intractable anemia derived from hemolysis, or progressive LV dilation and systolic dysfunction as per guidelines for native valve regurgitation. The first step in patient evaluation is to determine whether active infection is present; blood cultures should be obtained in all patients with new prosthetic valve regurgitation. The next step is to determine whether regurgitation is valvular or paravalvular, which often requires both transthoracic and transesophageal imaging because the prosthetic valve shadow obscures circumferential imaging from either approach alone. 3D color Doppler is particularly helpful for localizing the site of regurgitation. Paravalvular regurgitation requires either surgical intervention or closure with a transcatheter device, whereas valvular regurgitation might be amenable to placement of a transcatheter valve within the surgical prosthetic valve, such as a valve-in-valve procedure. Next, the severity of valvular regurgitation should be determined using standard Doppler approaches. During the procedure, TEE guidance is helpful in optimal positioning of the device. In the mitral position, it is important to ensure that the transcatheter device does not protrude into the LV outflow tract causing subaortic obstruction. In the aortic position, it is important to ensure the coronary ostia are not blocked by the transcatheter valve (see case 13-9).

Suggested Reading

1. Hamid NB, Khalique OK, Monaghan MJ, et al: Transcatheter valve implantation in failed surgically inserted bioprosthesis: Review and practical guide to echocardiographic imaging in valve-in-valve procedures, JACC Cardiovasc Imaging 8(8): 960–979, 2015.
2. Paradis JM, Del Trigo M, Puri R, et al: Transcatheter valve-in-valve and valve-in-ring for treating aortic and mitral surgical prosthetic dysfunction, J Am Coll Cardiol 66(18): 2019–2037, 2015.

CASE 13-8
Valve-in-Valve Therapy for Bioprosthetic Mitral Stenosis

The patient is an 80-year-old woman with history of significant progressive and highly symptomatic bioprosthetic mitral valve stenosis 10 years after mitral valve replacement with a 25-mm Carpentier Edwards (CE) bioprosthetic valve (Edwards Lifesciences, Irvine, California). Her history also includes aortic valve replacement with a bioprosthetic valve (currently without significant regurgitation or stenosis) and coronary artery bypass graft surgery for multivessel coronary atherosclerosis. Noncardiac conditions include chronic obstructive pulmonary disease with severe pulmonary hypertension, immunosuppression with long-term methotrexate treatment for severe psoriasis, type 2 diabetes mellitus, and advanced chronic kidney disease. Because her surgical risk was high with an STS PROM score of 28%, she was offered transcatheter mitral valve-in-valve replacement using the Melody transcatheter pulmonary valve (Medtronic, Minneapolis, Minnesota) as compassionate use.

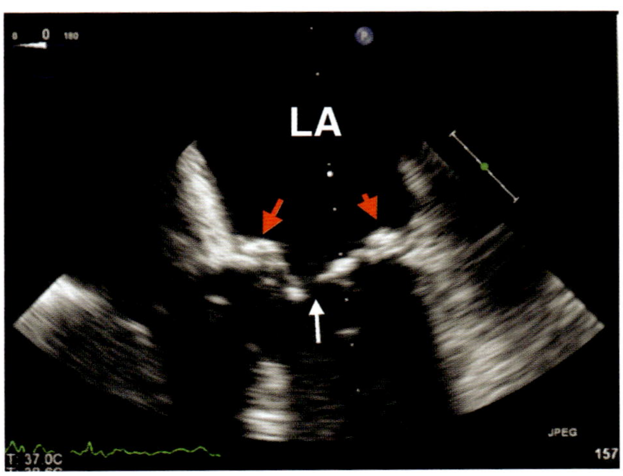

Fig 13.67 In this midesophageal four-chamber view, red arrows indicate the sewing ring of the bioprosthetic mitral valve. Leaflets are thickened and calcified, with a small maximal excursion during diastole *(white arrow)*.

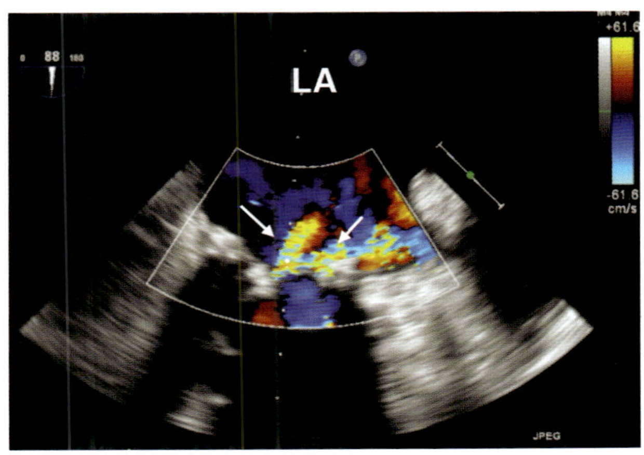

Fig 13.68 In this midesophageal two-chamber image, color Doppler shows a complex jet of mitral regurgitation *(white arrows)*.

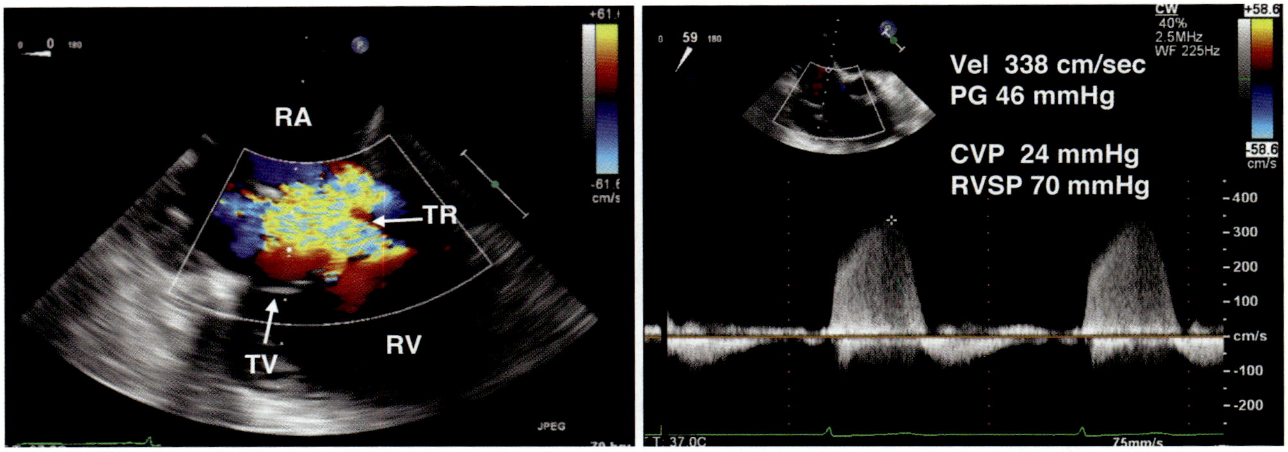

Fig 13.69 Severe tricuspid regurgitation, thought to be secondary to elevated pulmonary artery pressures and annular dilation, is seen in this midesophageal view. Continuous wave Doppler yields an estimated right ventricular systolic pressure of 70 mmHg.

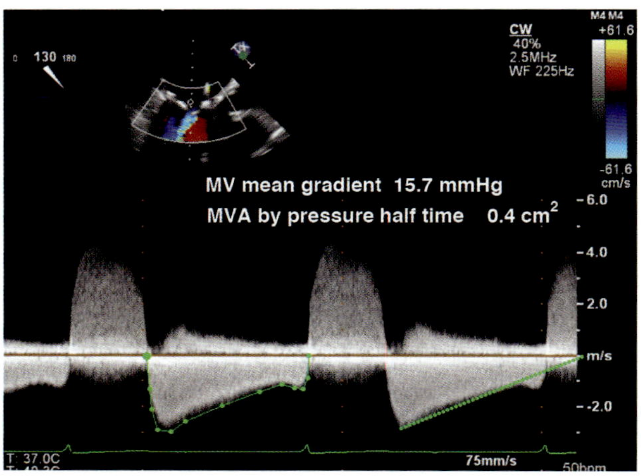

Fig 13.70 Continuous wave Doppler of mitral inflow shows a mean gradient of 15.7 mmHg. By the pressure half time method, the mitral valve area is 0.4 cm^2.

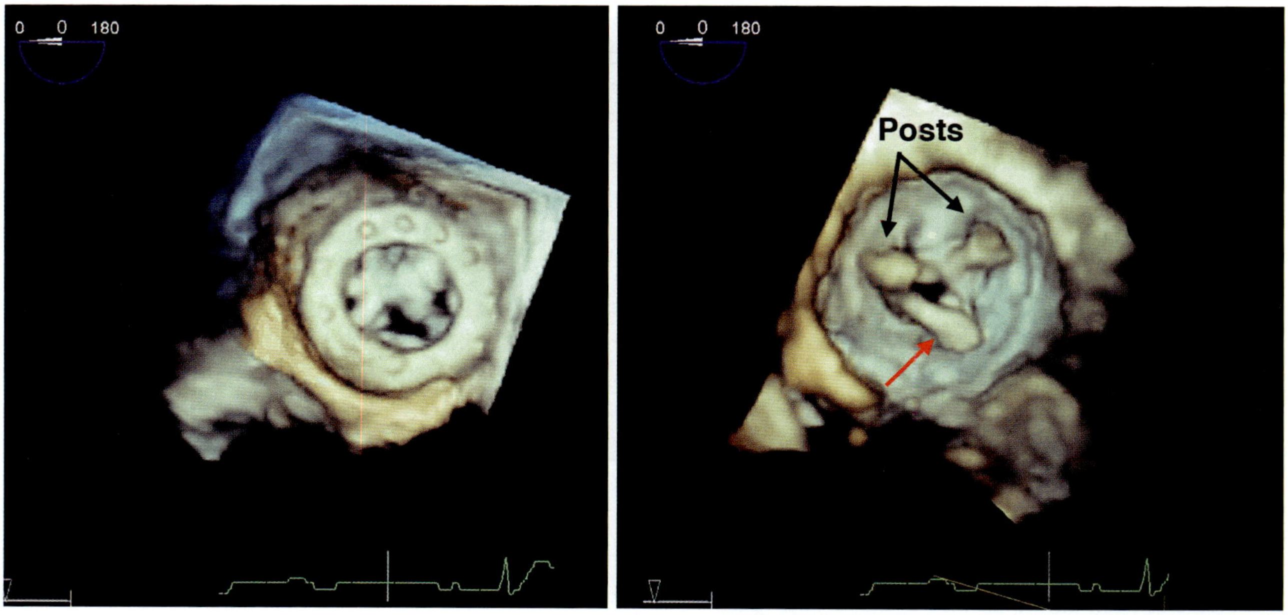

Fig 13.71 Tissue prosthesis is seen in 3D from left atrial perspective *(left)* and left ventricular perspective *(right)*. Leaflet thickening is evident. Red arrow indicates leaflet tissue that is mobile when visualized in real time.

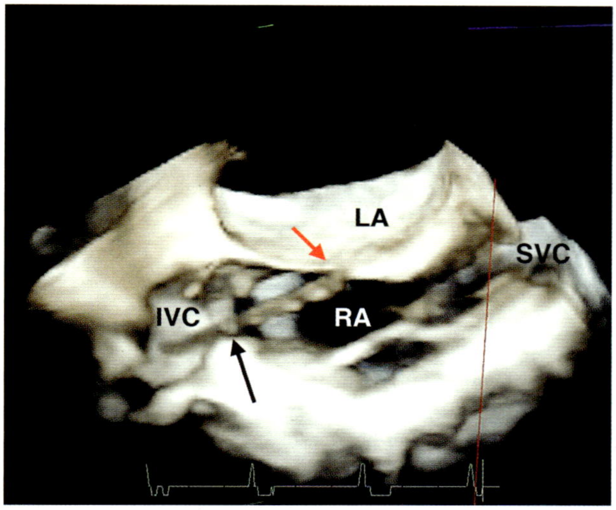

Fig 13.72 3D TEE showing transseptal puncture *(red arrow)* following advancement into right atrium via IVC *(black arrow)*.

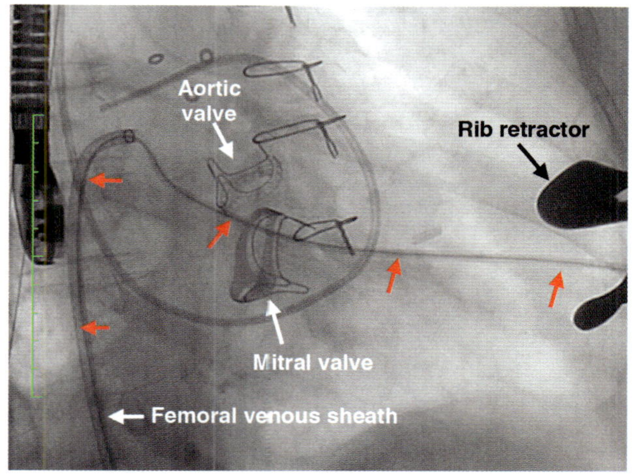

Fig 13.73 A "transapical rail" was created. Briefly, through exchange of catheters and wires, a wire in LV that had been introduced via LV apex was advanced through the mitral bioprosthesis into the left atrium. A 25-mm gooseneck snare was advanced transseptally secured the apical ventricular wire in the left atrium. LV wire was then exteriorized via the femoral vein *(red arrows)*. This transapical rail was then used to introduce the Melody valve across prosthetic mitral valve.

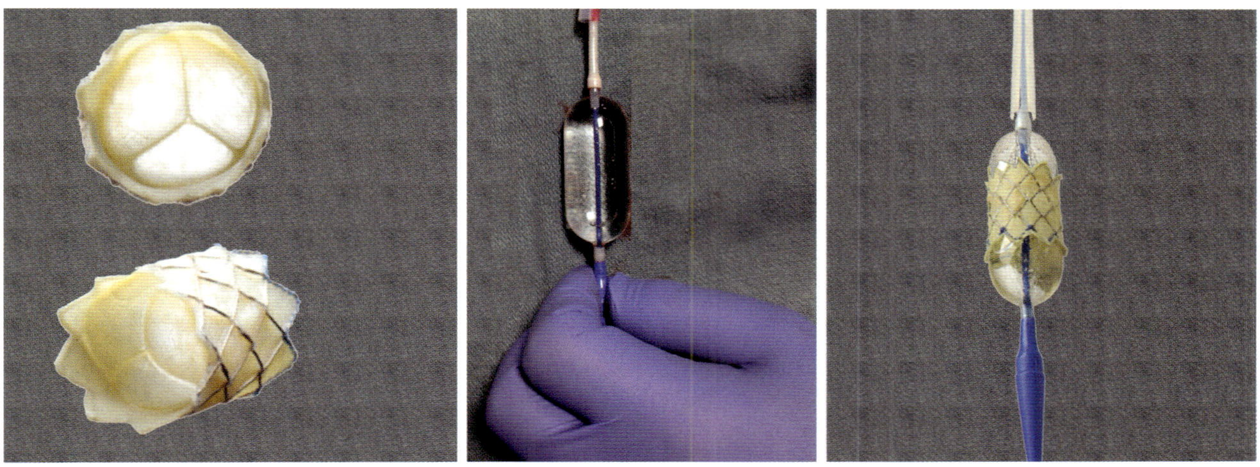

Fig 13.74 Melody valve. On left, valve is seen from top and from side. Delivery balloon inflated appears in center frame, and at right is delivery system and valve as it would appear when fully deployed.

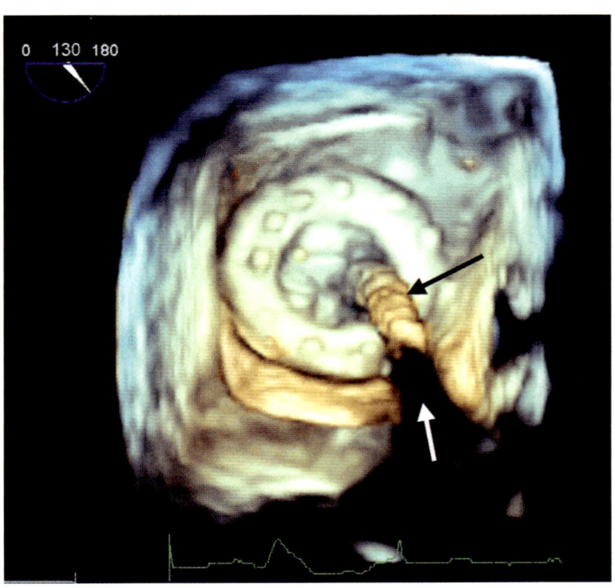

Fig 13.75 In this 3D TEE from left atrial perspective, the delivery apparatus *(black arrow)* has just engaged the prosthetic mitral valve. Dark space indicated by the white arrow is dropout or shadowing by the apparatus.

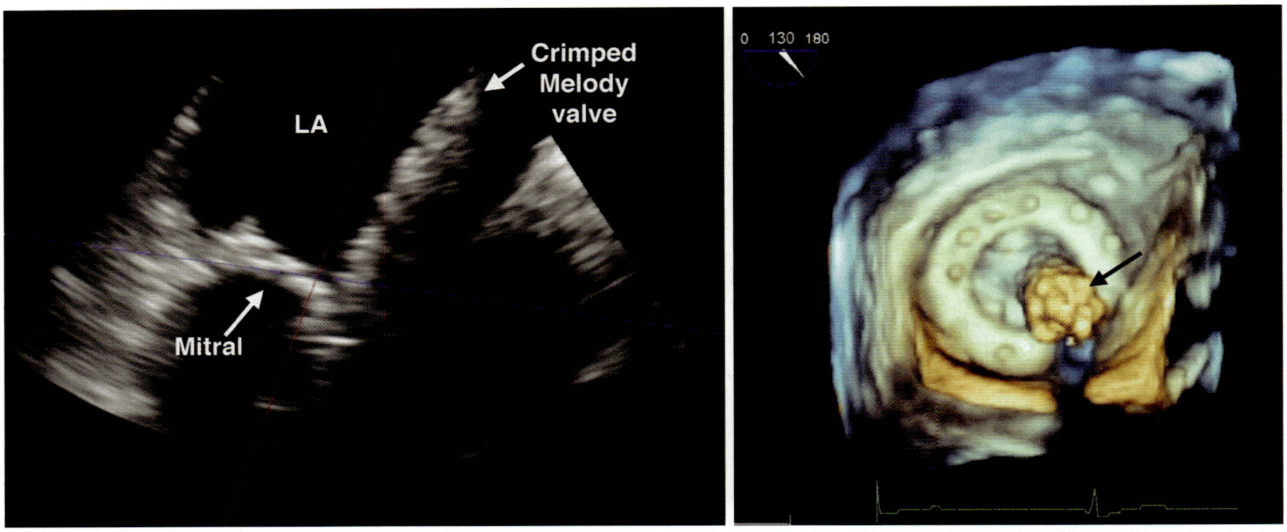

Fig 13.76 On left is two-chamber midesophageal view, showing crimped Melody valve engaging bioprosthetic mitral valve. On right is a 3D TEE from left atrial perspective showing the portion of the crimped valve *(black arrow)* in left atrium.

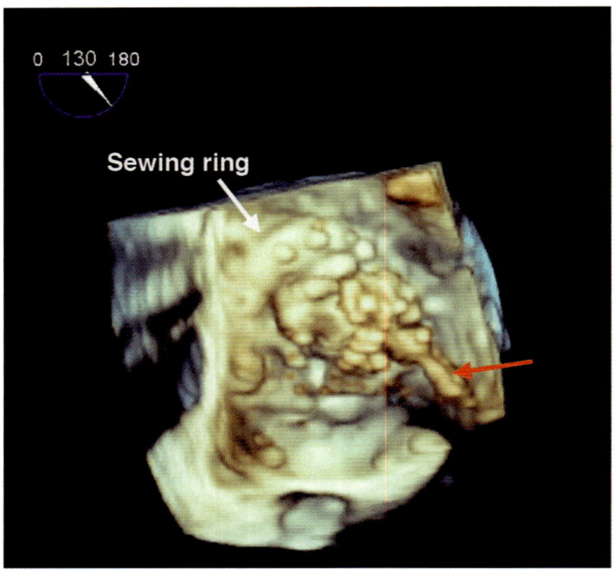

Fig 13.77 3D TEE from left atrial perspective shows the balloon being inflated inside the bioprosthetic mitral sewing ring.

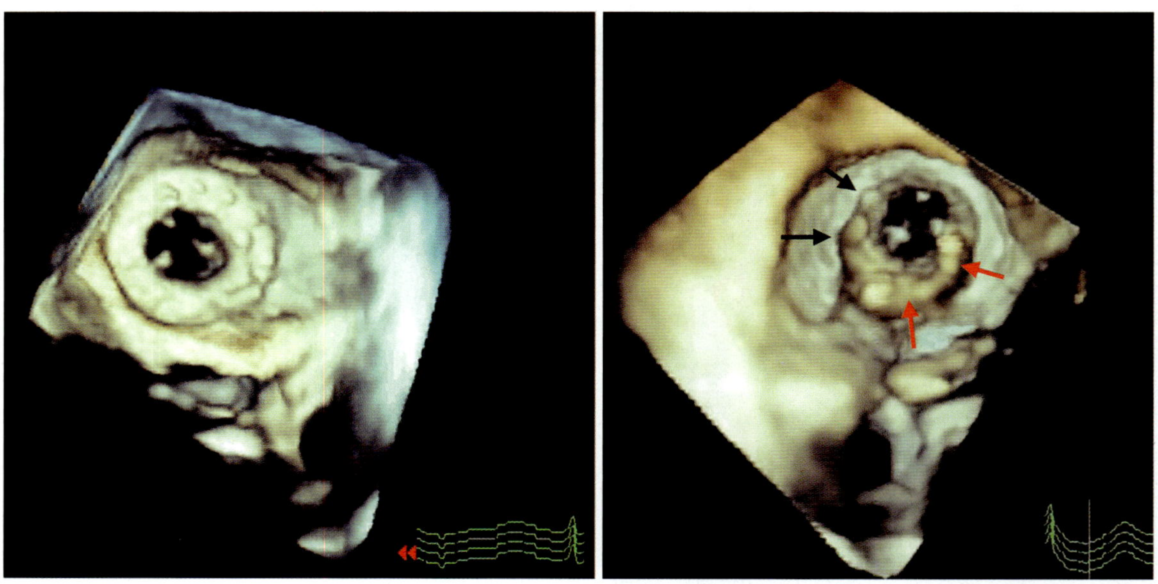

Fig 13.78 On left is a 3D TEE from left atrial perspective showing the native sewing ring, with the Melody valve deployed within. From left ventricular perspective, familiar appearance of cage *(black arrows)* is seen. Red arrows indicate probable artifact.

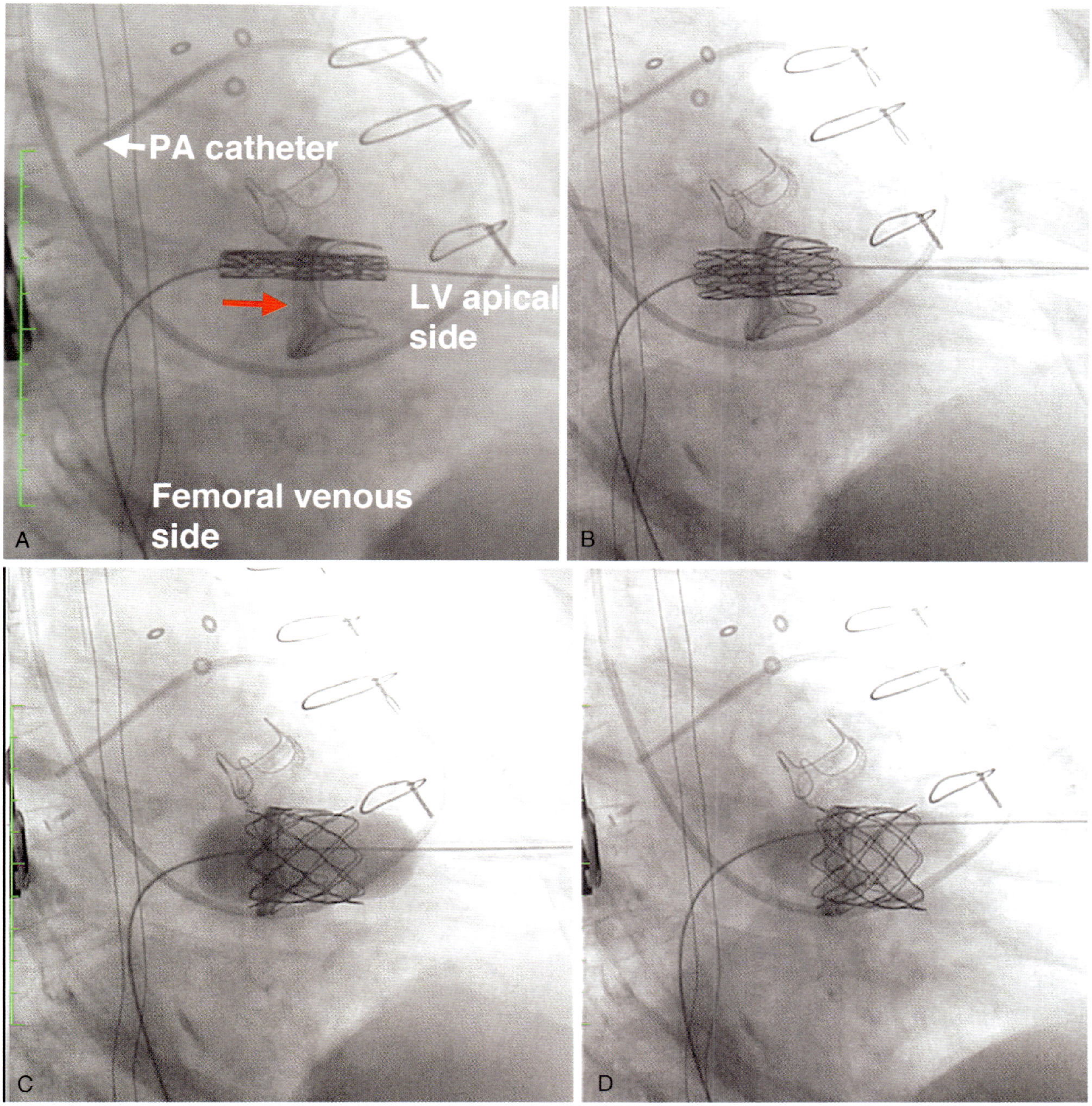

Fig 13.79 Fluoroscopy of Melody valve deployment. **(A)** Crimped valve has engaged the bioprosthetic mitral valve *(red arrow)*. **(B)** Inflation of balloon has begun. **(C)** Inflation of balloon is complete and the valve has been fully deployed. **(D)** Balloon has been deflated leaving the Melody valve in place.

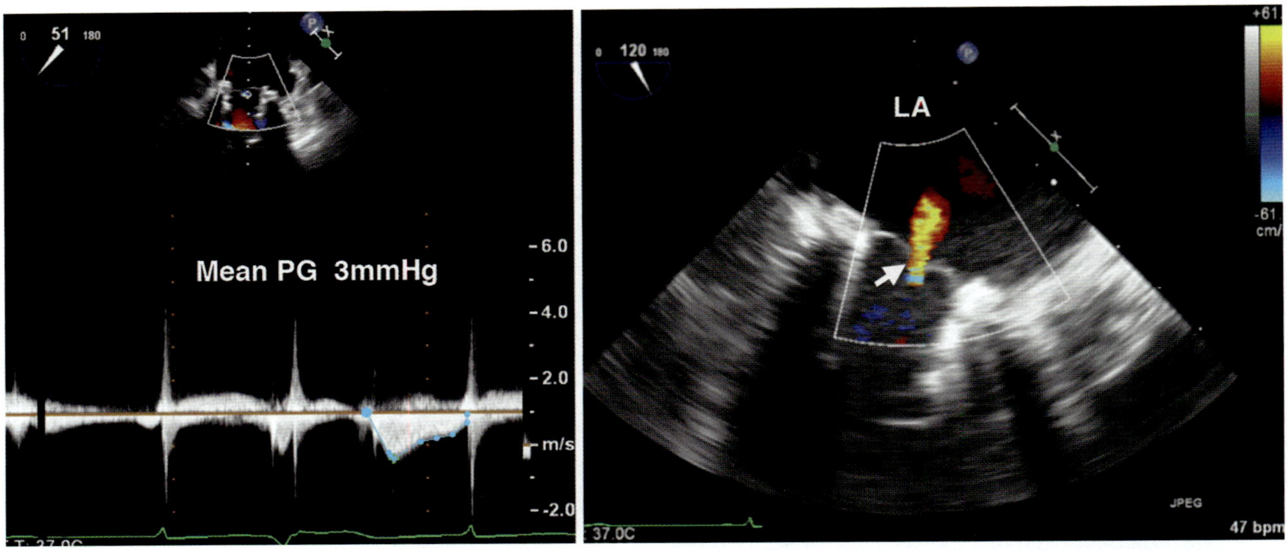

Fig 13.80 Mean gradient across the Melody valve was 3 mmHg. Color Doppler showed a small amount of central regurgitation.

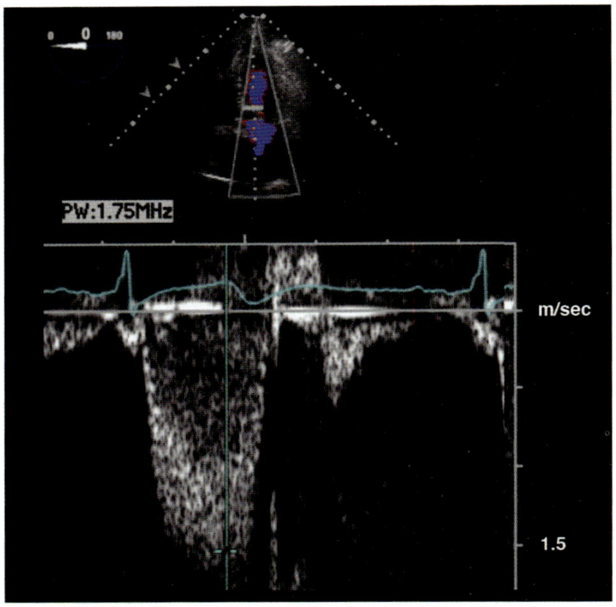

Fig 13.81 Because the Melody valve protrudes to some extent into the left ventricular outflow tract, pulsed wave Doppler from a deep transgastric view was used to measure the peak gradient, which was 9 mmHg.

CASE 13-9
Valve-in-Valve Therapy for Bioprosthetic Aortic Stenosis

The patient is a 77-year-old man who 12 years previously had an AVR with a Hancock II bioprosthesis for aortic stenosis. Five days previously he had developed dyspnea on exertion, lower extremity edema, and chest "achiness." One day before presentation, a new diastolic heart murmur was appreciated and urgent TTE revealed a torn aortic cusp and focal area of increased echodensity along the anterior portion of the aortic valve. He had a negative workup for endocarditis, and because of multiple comorbidities was offered TAVR valve-in-valve therapy.

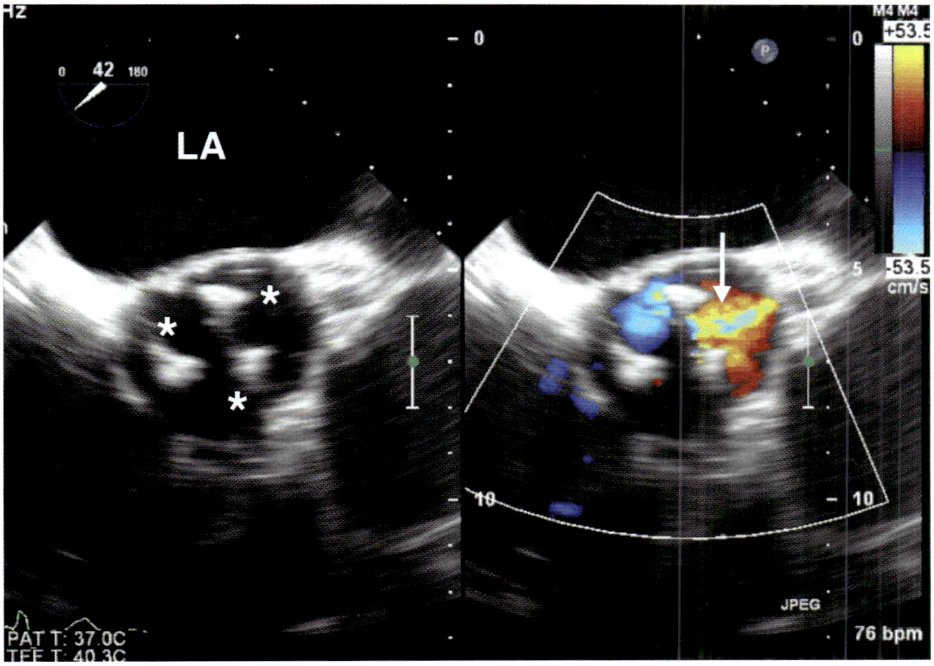

Fig 13.82 In this midesophageal short-axis view, the asterisks identify three posts of prosthetic valve. White arrow indicates a jet of aortic regurgitation.

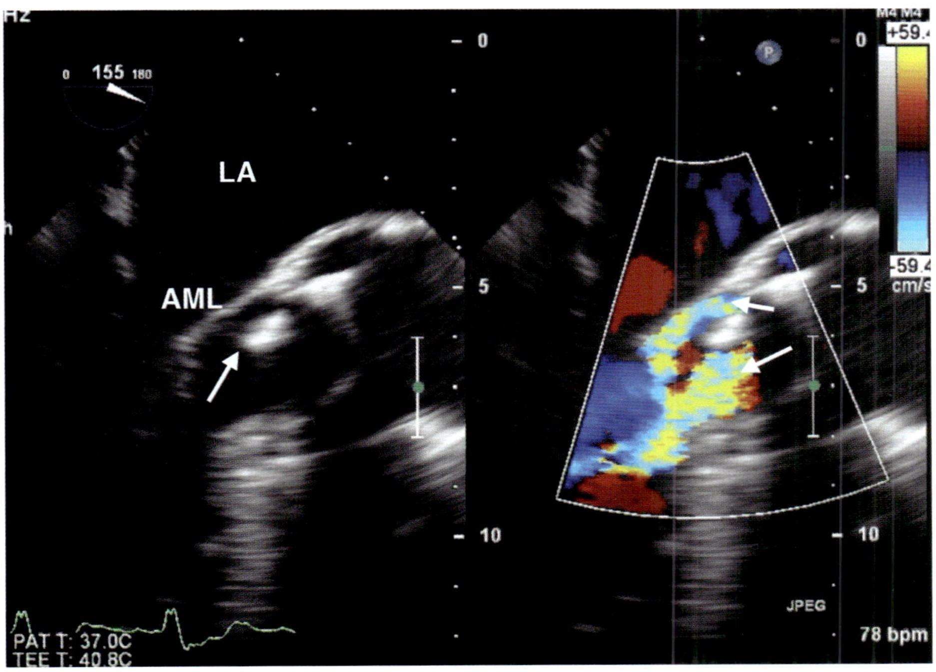

Fig 13.83 In this midesophageal long-axis view, white arrow in the left frame indicates a mass, which, given the clinical findings, is in keeping with prolapse of a portion of the prosthetic aortic valve. In the right frame, the arrows indicate componenets of the jet of AR.

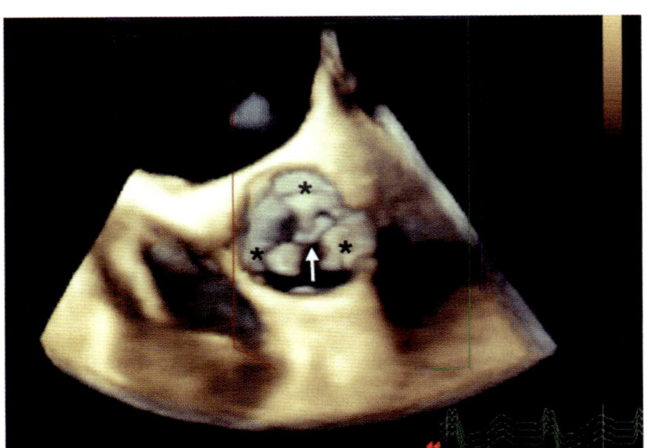

Fig 13.84 In this 3D TEE from left atrial perspective, the asterisks again indicate the valve posts. White arrow indicates the prolapsing mass, which can be better appreciated by the real time video.

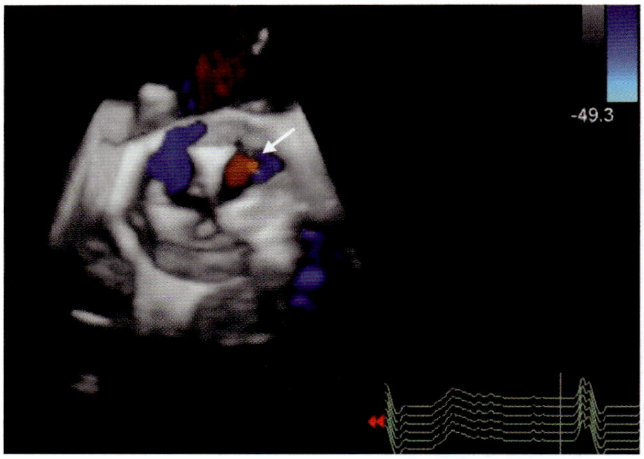

Fig 13.85 A corresponding 3D color Doppler image shows the jet of aortic regurgitation.

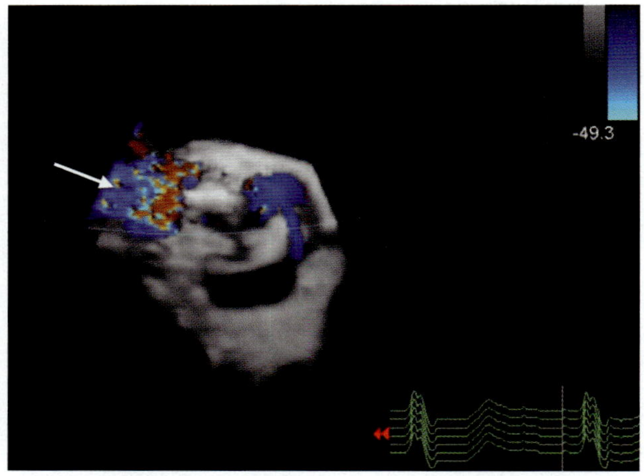

Fig 13.86 With the 3D color image flipped 180 degrees on its horizontal axis, the white arrow indicates the jet of aortic regurgitation.

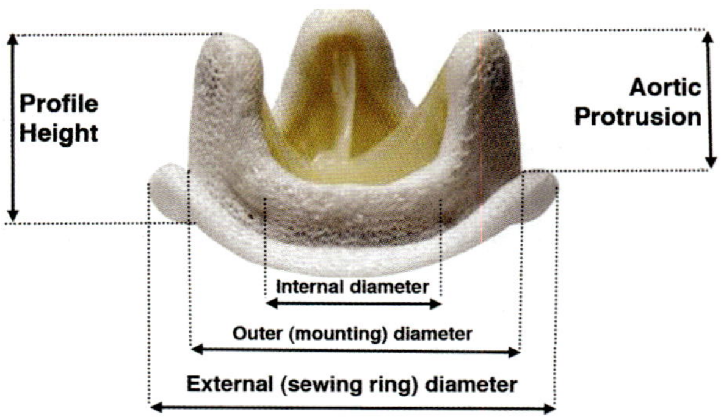

Fig 13.87 Dimensions of stented bioprosthetic valves, in this case the Hancock II porcine valve. The labeled value size generally corresponds to the outer diameter. For valve-in-valve procedures, the internal diameter is more relevant. Stented prosthesis was 25 mm, so 23-mm SAPIEN XT valve in valve was placed.

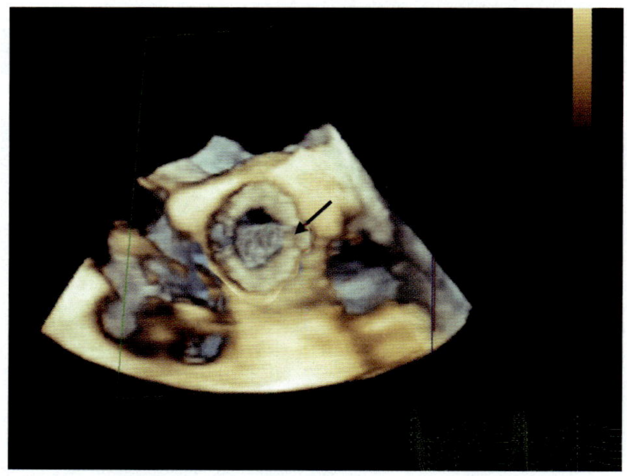

Fig 13.88 SAPIEN 23-mm valve has been deployed *(arrow)*, as seen from left atrial perspective.

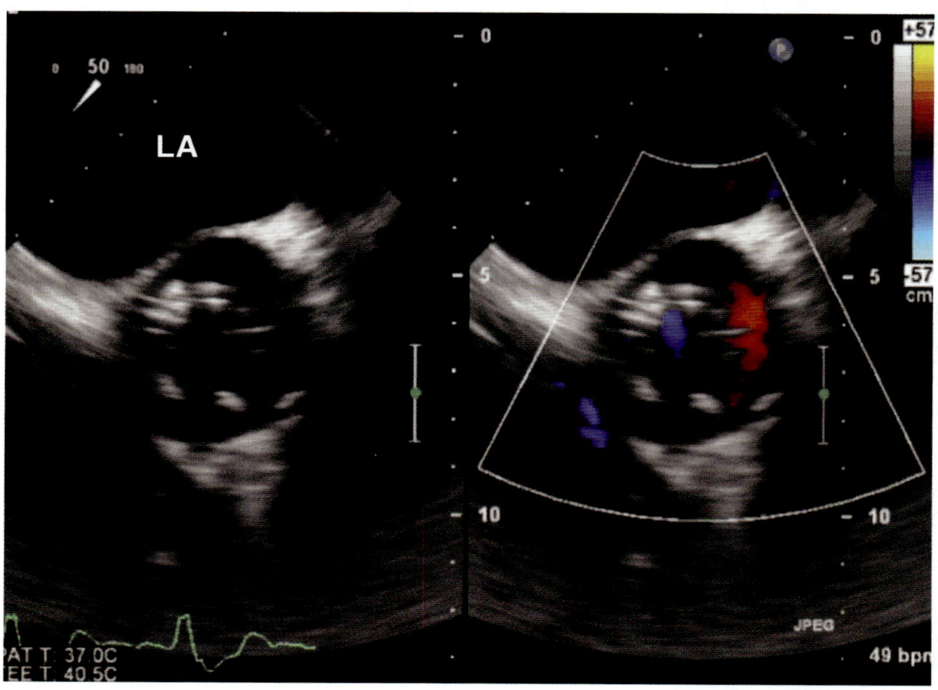

Fig 13.89 In this midesophageal short-axis view, SAPIEN valve masks posts. There is no residual regurgitation.

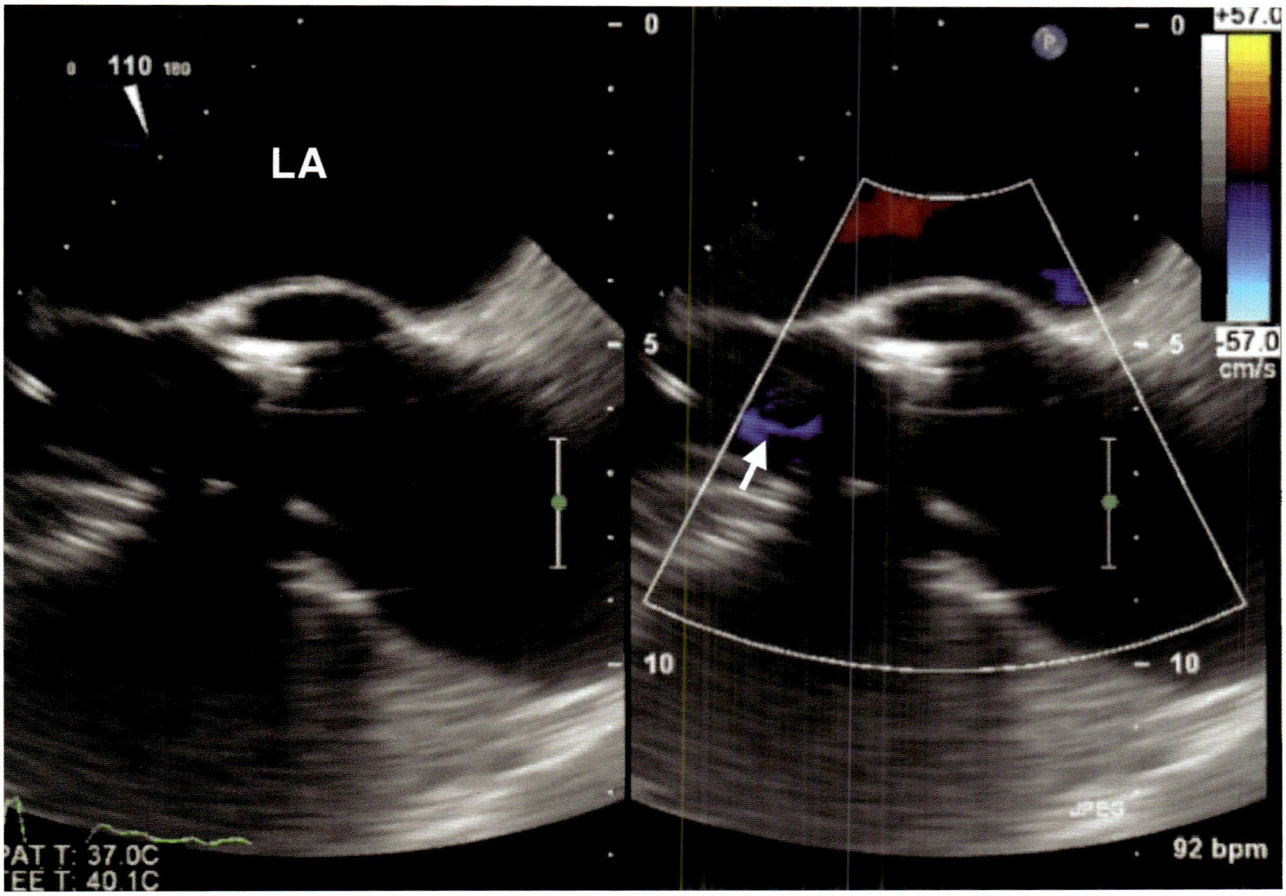

Fig 13.90 In this midesophageal long-axis view, there is trace residual regurgitation *(white arrow)*.

Comments

Bioprosthetic valves leaflets may become calcified and fibrotic over time resulting in gradually progressive stenosis. Indications for intervention for prosthetic valve stenosis are similar to the indications for treatment of native valve disease. With severe symptomatic prosthetic valve stenosis, repeat surgical valve replacement may be appropriate in many patients, depending on surgical risk, patient age and life expectancy, and patient values and preferences. Another treatment option is placement of a transcatheter valve inside the surgical bioprosthetic valve as in the examples of prosthetic mitral and aortic stenosis shown here. TEE is helpful for documenting the severity of stenosis, placement of the valve-in-valve prosthesis, and hemodynamic evaluation after device implantation.

Suggested Reading

1. Attizzani GF, Ohno Y, Latib A, et al: Transcatheter aortic valve implantation under angiographic guidance with and without adjunctive transesophageal echocardiography, Am J Cardiol 116(4):604–611, 2015.
2. Phan K, Zhao DF, Wang N, et al: Transcatheter valve-in-valve implantation versus reoperative conventional aortic valve replacement: A systematic review, J Thorac Dis 8(1):E83–E93, 2016.

Transcatheter Mitral Valve Therapies

CASE 13-10
Mitral Balloon Commissurotomy

The patient, a 43-year-old woman at 22 6/7 weeks gestation was admitted with hypotension, tachycardia, and a new diagnosis of severe mitral stenosis.

The patient felt well until approximately 2 weeks before admission, when she developed a cough with yellow sputum and shortness of breath. Over the previous 2 to 3 days she had subjective fevers and chills, with possible rigors. On the day before admission, she presented to outside ER, where she was found to be hypotensive and tachycardic; a TTE demonstrated a new diagnosis of severe mitral valve stenosis and pulmonary hypertension. She was transferred to this hospital where she received antibiotics, diuretics, and small doses of a beta blocker for heart rate control. She was deemed suitable for mitral balloon commissurotomy, which was scheduled urgently for the next day.

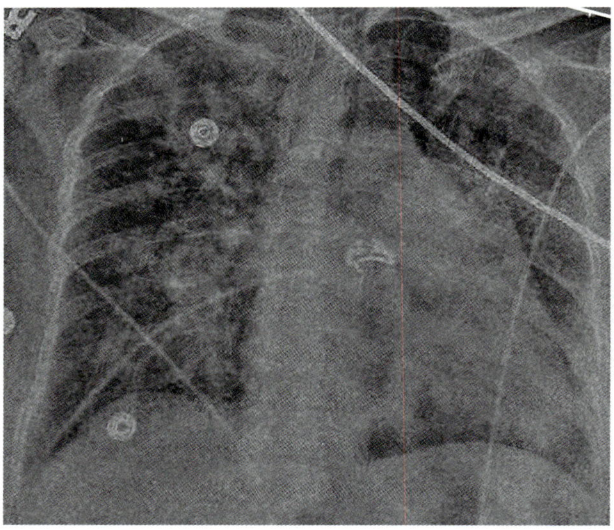

Fig 13.91 CXR on admission showed large left atrium and diffuse bilateral pulmonary infiltrates.

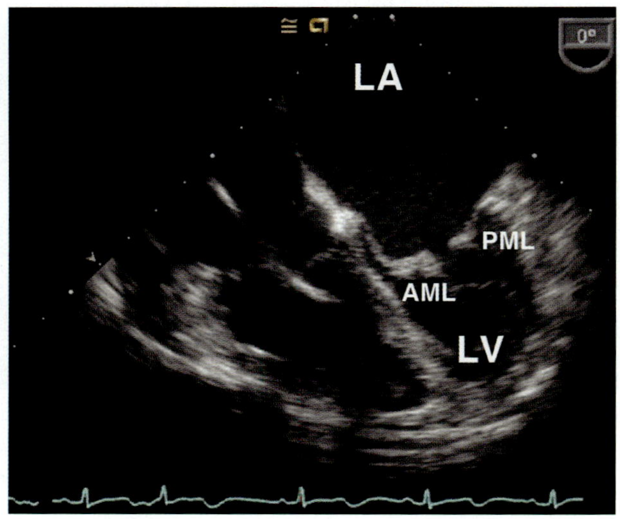

Fig 13.92 In this midesophageal four-chamber view, the mitral valve shows the typical findings of rheumatic mitral stenosis with a "hockey-stick" appearance of the anterior mitral leaflet. In real time, the posterior leaflet is fixed.

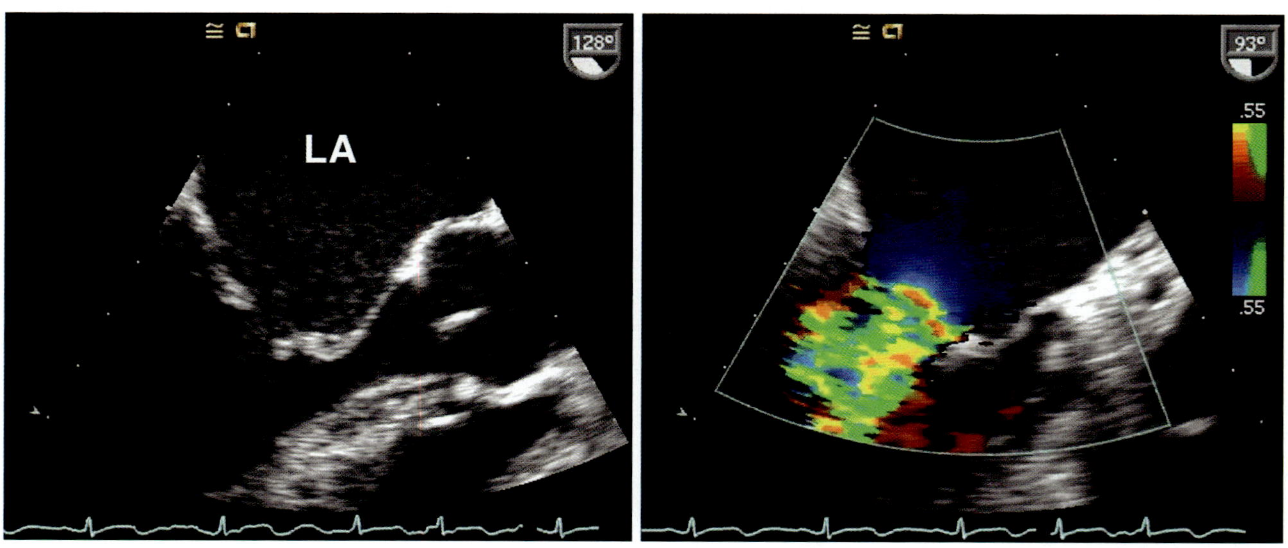

Fig 13.93 Similar findings are seen in midesophageal long-axis view. There is aliasing of inflow signal and no significant mitral regurgitation. There is severe left atrial enlargement. Imaging of left atrial appendage revealed no thrombus. There is no significant calcification of the mitral leaflets, which are reasonably mobile and not thickened. Aortic valve is normal, and no significant aortic regurgitation was seen.

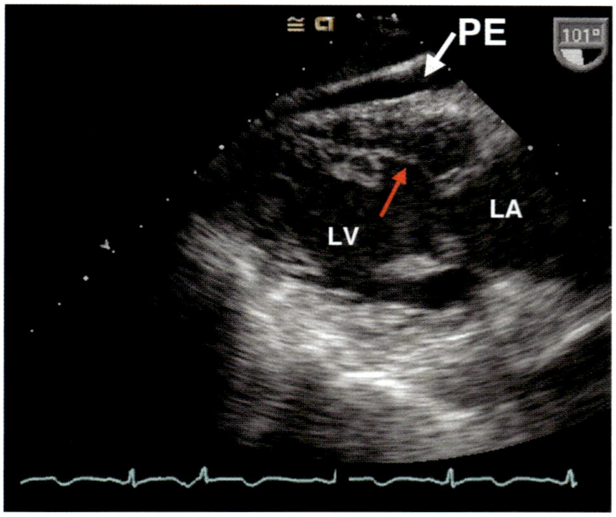

Fig 13.94 From the transgastric long-axis view of the left ventricle, subvalvular apparatus appears normal. Red arrow indicates thin, nonshortened chord. There is a small posterior pericardial effusion.

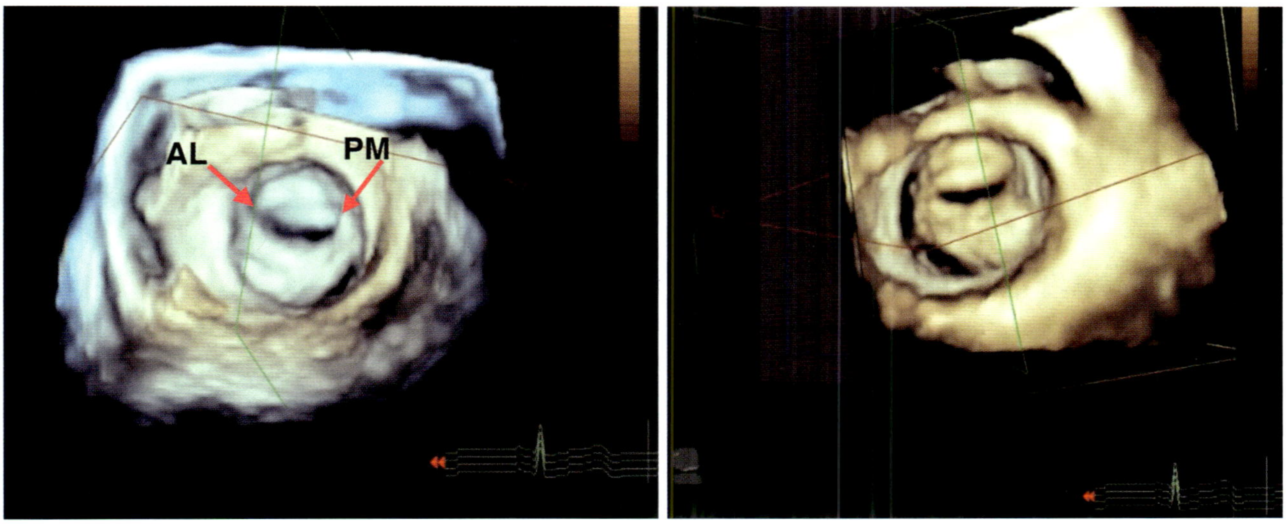

Fig 13.95 In another patient presenting for commissurotomy with similar clinical picture, 3D TEE showed a typical rheumatic mitral valve with antero-lateral and postero-medial commissural fusion. Left atrial perspective is on left and ventricular perspective on right.

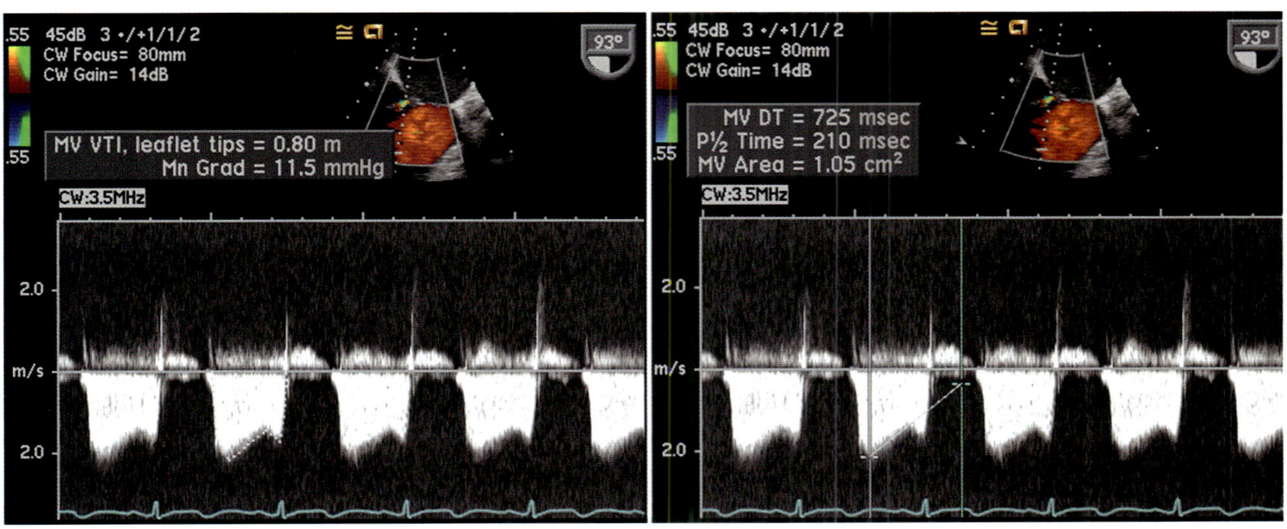

Fig 13.96 Preprocedural mitral inflow Doppler measurements show a mean transmitral pressure of 11.5 mmHg, and MVA of 1.05 cm^2 by pressure half-time method.

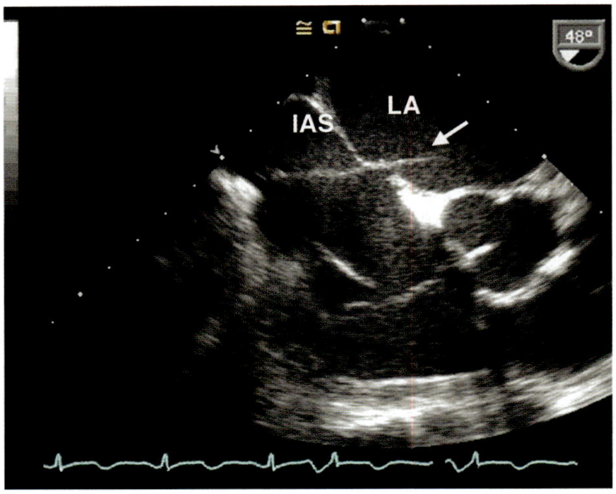

Fig 13.97 In this right ventricular inflow–outflow view, wire has been passed across interatrial septum.

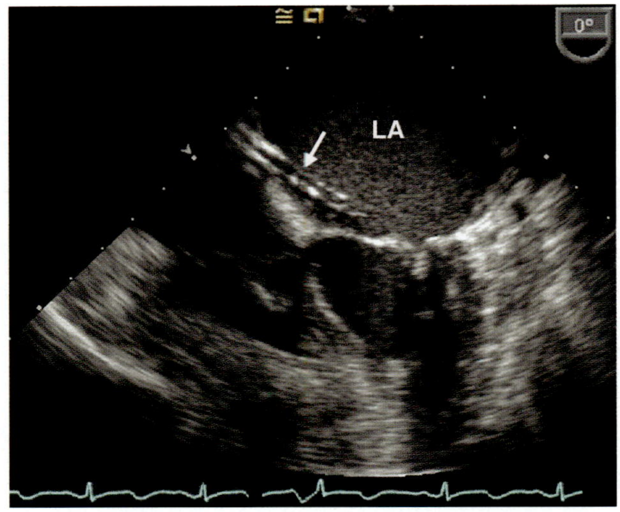

Fig 13.98 In this midesophageal four-chamber view, catheter has been advanced into left atrium; this will accommodate the commissurotomy balloon.

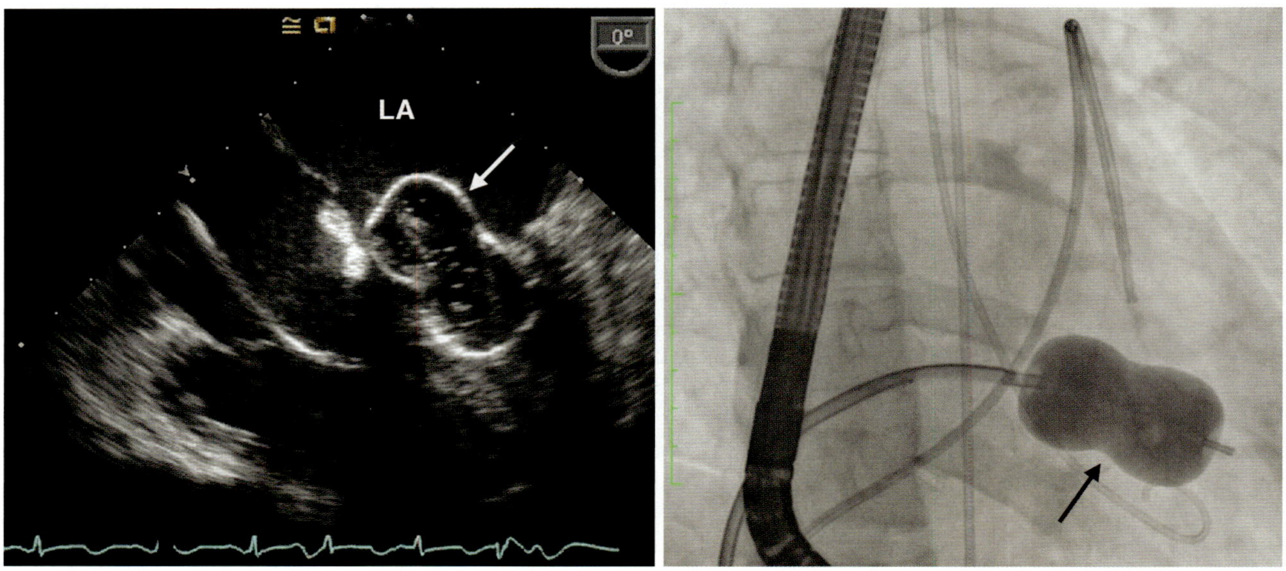

Fig 13.99 Midesophageal four-chamber *(left)* and fluoroscopy *(right)* show balloon *(arrows)* at maximal inflation.

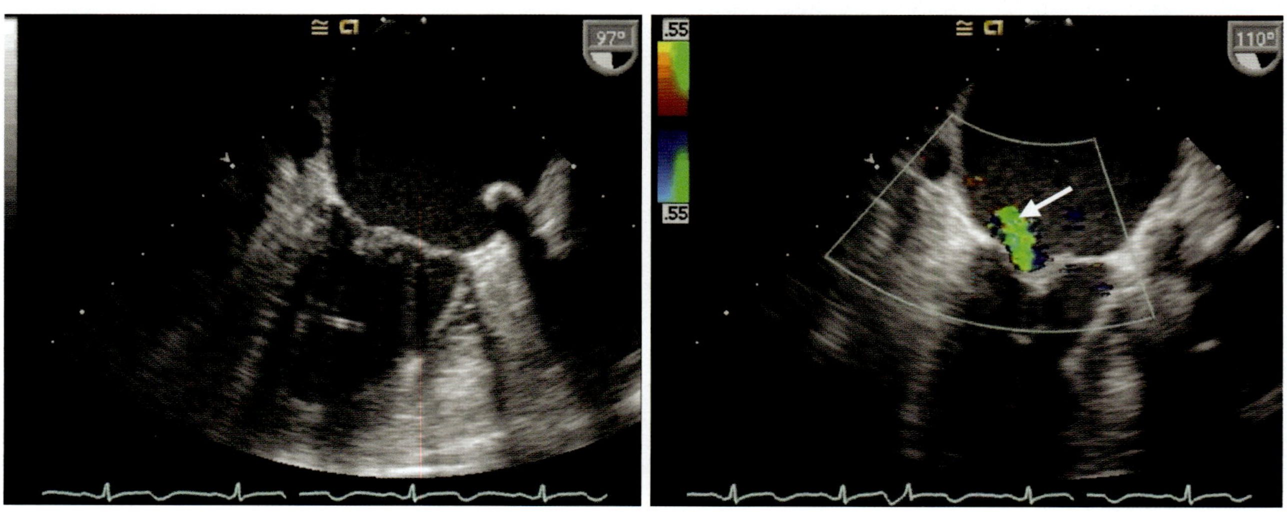

Fig 13.100 After several dilations, a new, small jet of mitral regurgitation was seen in this midesophageal two-chamber view.

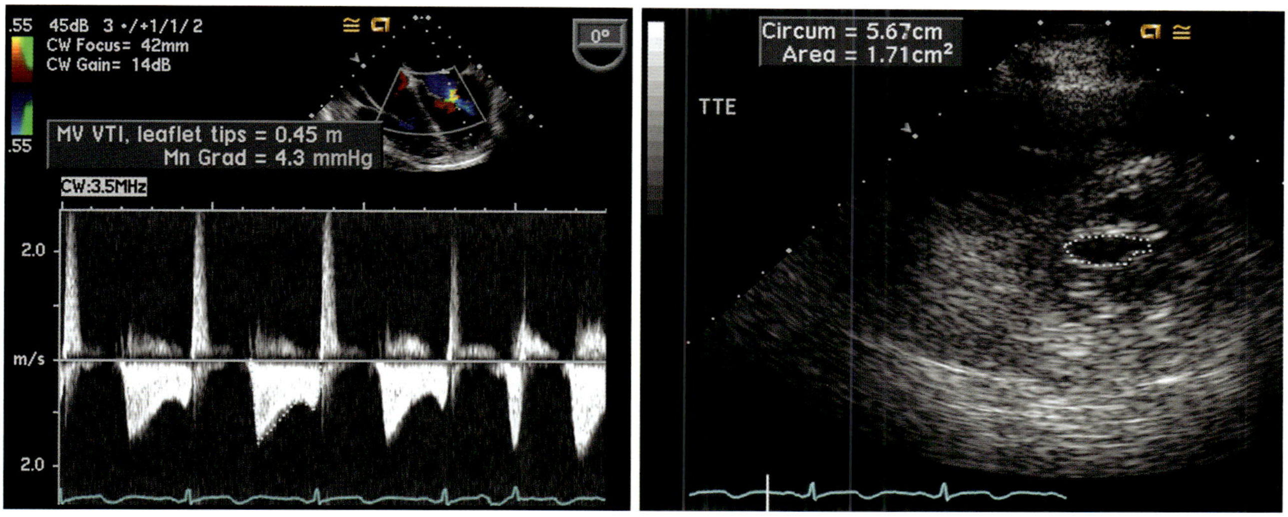

Fig 13.101 Transmitral mean gradient was reduced to 4.3 mmHg. Parasternal short imaging and planimetry with TTE showed a mitral valve area of 1.7 cm^2.

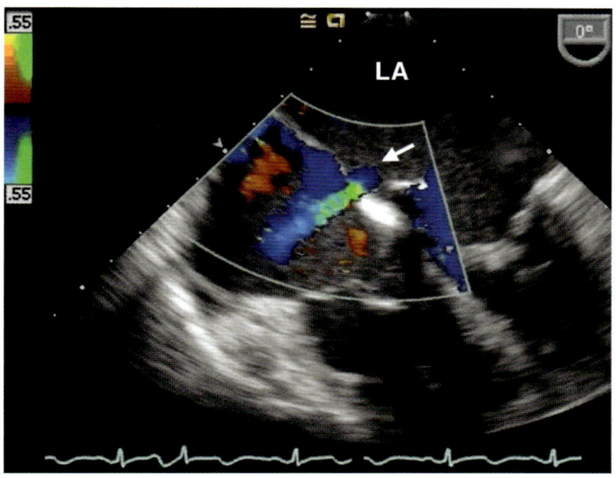

Fig 13.102 After removing the sheaths from the left atrium, an ASD was noted *(arrow)*. Because of its small size and left-to-right shunting only, no further action was taken. Fourteen weeks following the procedure, the patient underwent an uneventful Caesarian section, and delivered a healthy infant.

Comments

Balloon mitral commissurotomy (BMC) now is the preferred treatment for severe symptomatic mitral stenosis. Severe stenosis is defined as a valve area of 1.5 cm^2 or less because BMC is an effective durable procedure with low risk of adverse outcomes. BMC is most likely to benefit patients with commissural fusion resulting in a small orifice area but with thin flexible leaflets. The balloon dilation results in splitting of the fused commissures with a resultant increase in valve opening in diastole. Mitral stenosis severity is best evaluated by 3D imaging of the valve orifice, using the 3D image planes to identify and measure the minimal diastolic orifice at baseline and after the procedure. Recording Doppler data also is recommended but must be interpreted with caution, as the pressure gradient may fall because of a lower transmitral stroke volume with sedation and the pressure half-time may be an inaccurate result of changing ventricular and atrial compliances in the post-BMC period. TEE imaging is essential before BMC to ensure that no atrial thrombus is present and that MR is not significant. Echocardiography also can be used to evaluate MR severity after each balloon dilation and to detect other complications of the procedure.

Suggested Reading

1. Wunderlich NC, Beigel R, Siegel RJ: Management of mitral stenosis using 2D and 3D echo-Doppler imaging, JACC Cardiovasc Imaging 6(11):1191–1205, 2013.
2. Wilkins GT, Weyman AE, Abascal VM, et al: Percutaneous balloon dilatation of the mitral valve: An analysis of echocardiographic variables related to outcome and the mechanism of dilatation, Heart 60:299–308, 1988.

CASE 13-11
Transcatheter Mitral Valve Clip

The patient is an 83-year-old man with symptoms of progressive aortic stenosis and multiple admission for heart failure. His comorbidities included chronic obstructive pulmonary disease, chronic kidney disease, coronary disease with an LAD stent, and mitral valve prolapse with severe MR and elevated left atrial pressure. He underwent TAVR, and his postoperative course was complicated by colitis requiring 28 days of antibiotics. After discharge, his persistent symptoms were thought to be related to his severe MR and he was scheduled for MitraClip.

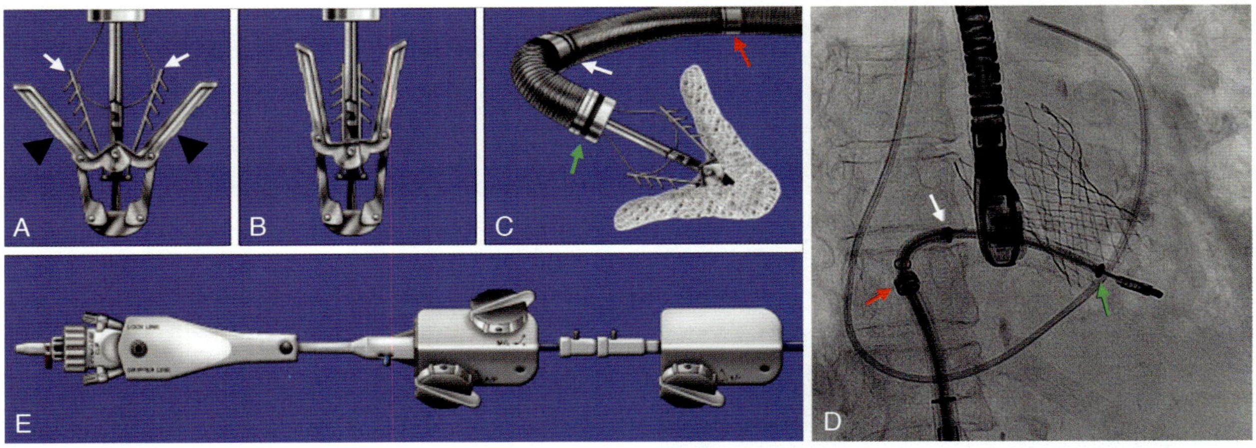

Fig 13.103 MitraClip system. **(A)** Partially open MitraClip (Abbott Laboratories, Abbott Park, Illinois) device is shown without its fabric covering. The MitraClip grasps the mitral leaflet between cobalt chromium grasper arms *(arrowheads)* and barbed gripper arms *(white arrows),* through which a fine wire (gripper wire) runs; this wire is used to raise the grippers. **(B)** Device in closed configuration. **(C,D)** MitraClip is attached to clip delivery system, which protrudes from end of steerable guide catheter *(red arrow).* White arrow indicates "sleeve radiopaque tip ring," the proximal point where delivery catheter meets up with the portion of the catheter where the Clip is attached. Green arrow indicates "delivery catheter radiopaque ring"; the Clip itself is mounted just beyond this visible marker. **(E)** Control knobs allow deflection of guide and clip delivery system to steer the system through left atrium and position MitraClip above mitral orifice. (From Feldman T, Young A, Percutaneous approaches to valve repair for mitral regurgitation, JACC 63:2057–2068, 2014. With permission.)

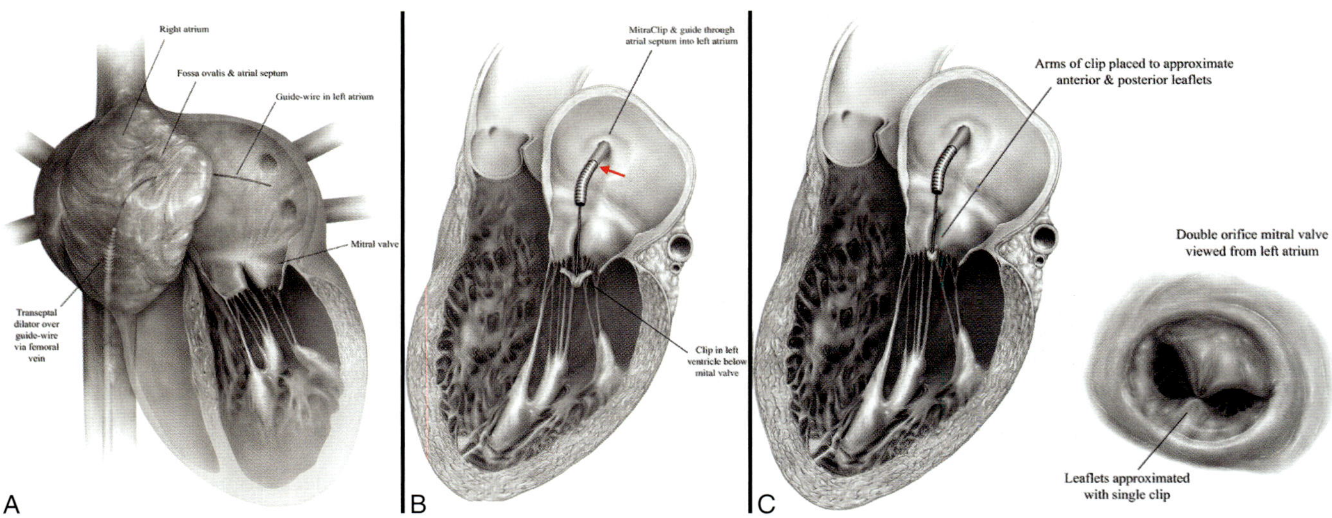

Fig 13.104 **(A)** Percutaneous access to right femoral vein is achieved. The fossa ovalis is crossed and guidewire is advanced into left atrium. Ideal transseptal location is posterior (away from aortic valve) with height above the plane of mitral valve coaptation of 3.5–4 cm. Steerable guide is placed from the femoral vein across the septum into left atrium. **(B)** TEE demonstrating MitraClip device across mitral valve. MitraClip is advanced under TEE guidance across mitral valve into left ventricle below the plane of coaptation and clip is closed to 120 degrees in preparation for leaflet capture. Red arrow indicates end of steerable catheter. **(C)** Capture of mitral leaflets is then accomplished by slow withdrawal of MitraClip with clip opened to 120 degrees and closing grippers. Partial closing allows assessment of leaflet insertion; MitraClip is fully closed, and following demonstration of adequate reduction of MR, clip is released. (From Pope NH, Ailawadi G: Transcatheter mitral valve repair, 19:219–237, 2014. With permission.)

TABLE 13-2 Procedural Steps in MitraClip Implantation
1. Obtaining femoral venous access
2. Puncture of interatrial septum
3. Advancement of steerable guide catheter into left atrium
4. Advancement of Clip Delivery System into left atrium through steerable guide
5. Steering and positioning MitraClip above mitral valve
6. Advancing MitraClip into left ventricle
7. Grasping of leaflets and assessment of proper leaflet insertion
8. Detachment of MitraClip

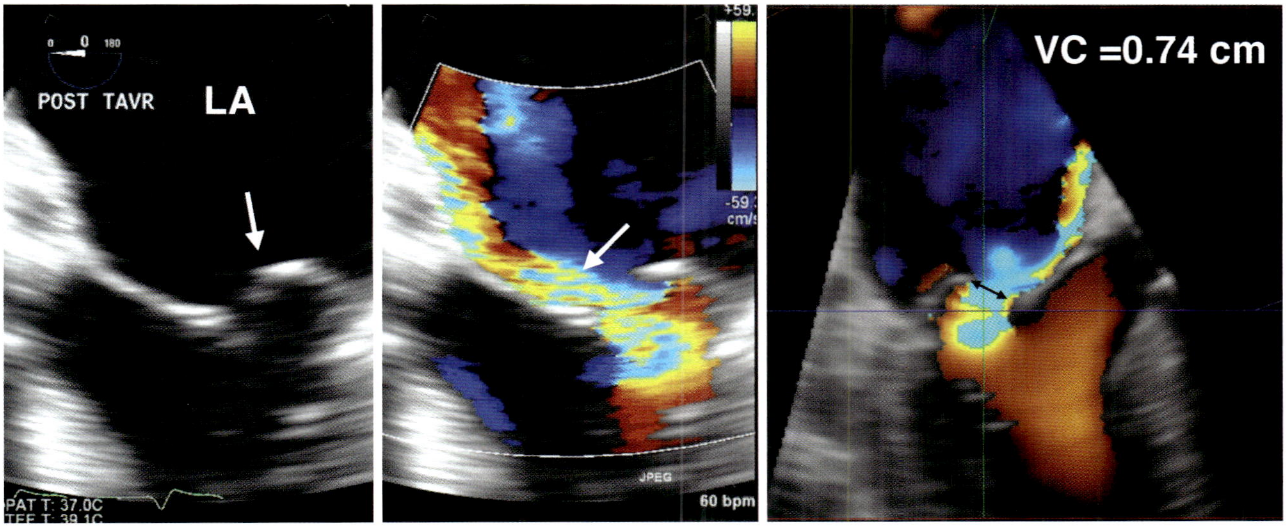

Fig 13.105 Midesophageal four-chamber imaging shows prolapsed portion of posterior leaflet *(left, arrow)* with dense jet of wall-hugging, anteriorly directed mitral regurgitation *(center, arrow)* vena contracta of 0.74 cm indicates severe MR *(right)*. Leaflets are thin and noncalcified, and coaptation point is close to level of annulus, both favorable for MitraClip.

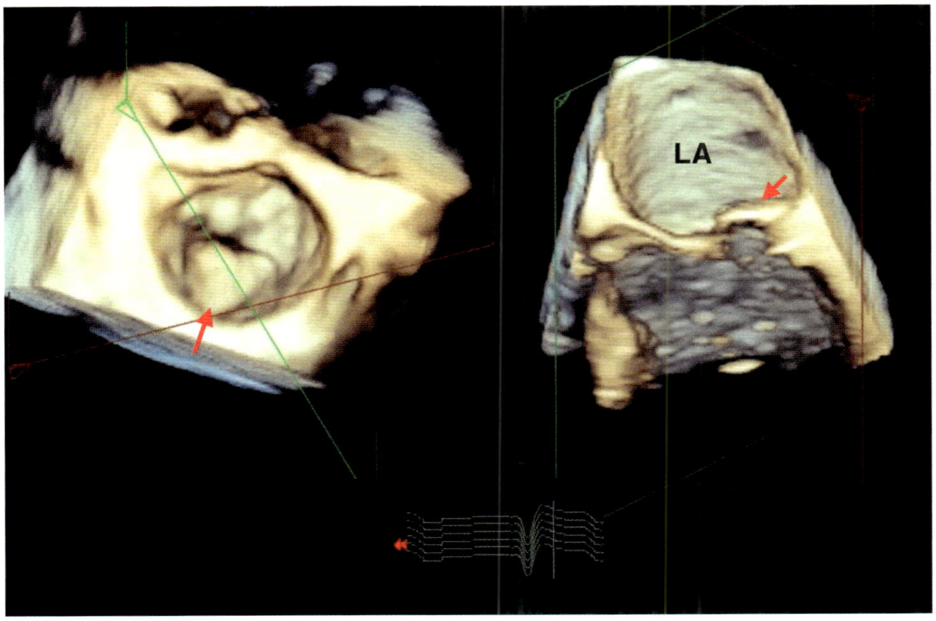

Fig 13.106 On left is an en face view of the mitral valve from left atrial perspective, and on right, the same image has been cropped from an anterolateral perspective. Arrows approximate the P2 segment. Both images are in systole.

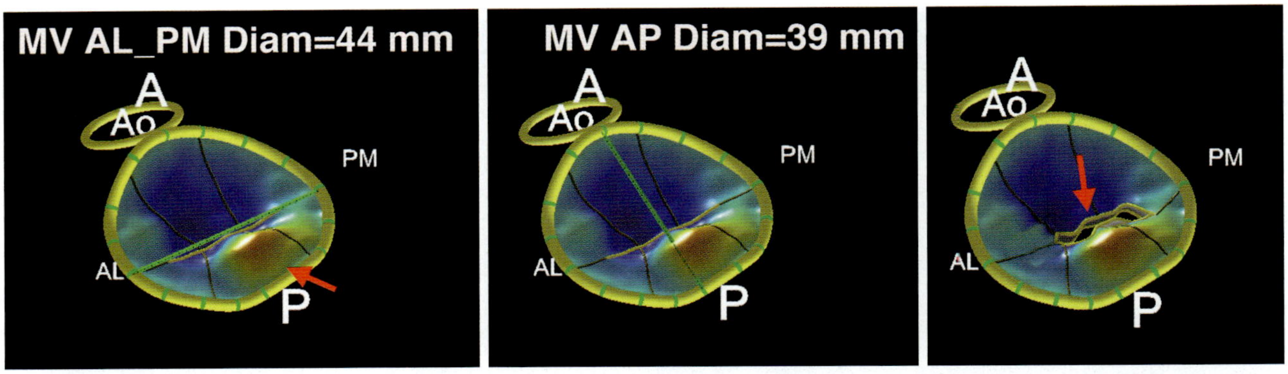

Fig 13.107 Mitral valve quantification (Phillips) shows a dilated mitral annulus, as well as prolapse, primarily of P2 *(arrow)*. At left, defect is seen primarily between A2 and P2 *(arrow)*.

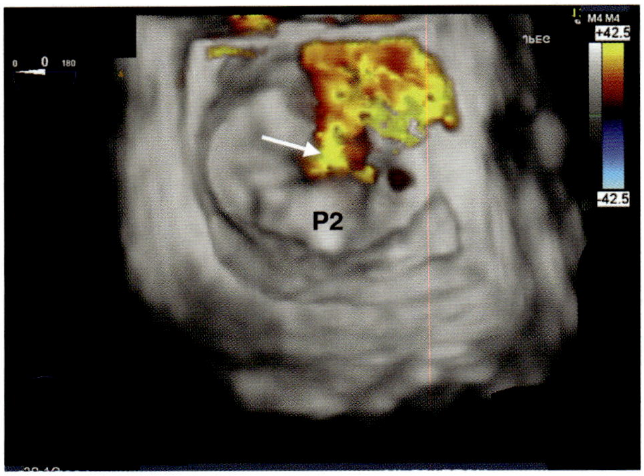

Fig 13.108 3D TEE en face view of mitral valve from left atrial perspective shows a broad anteriorly directed jet of mitral regurgitation.

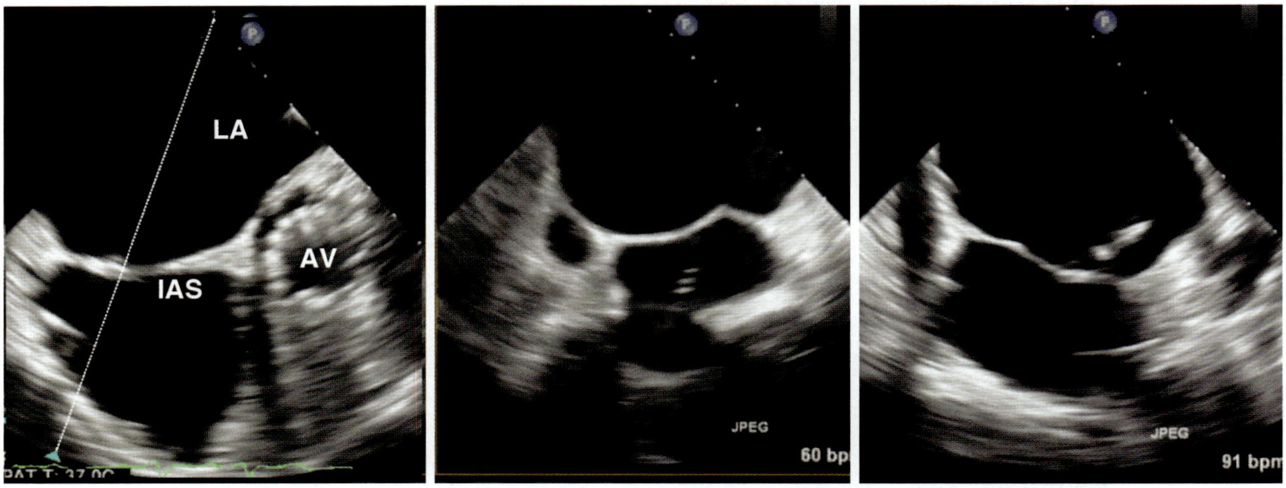

Fig 13.109 On left of this biplane image is a midesophageal view of approximately 80 degrees, with probe slightly turned to patient's left; this allows viewing of the previously placed TAVR. Cursor is shown intersecting the IAS. In middle, the orthogonal view shows tenting of the IAS, and at right, wire has passed through the IAS.

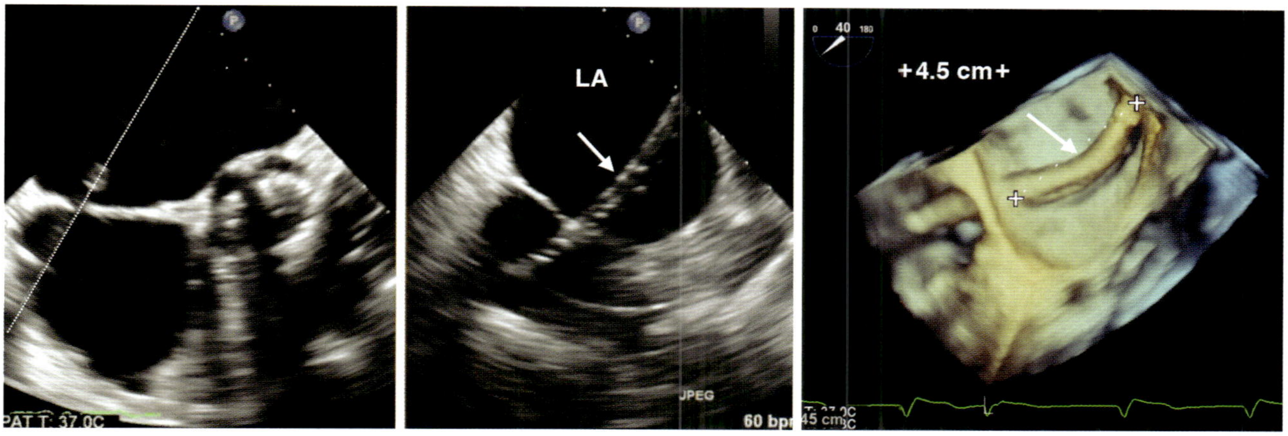

Fig 13.110 Following crossing of the IAS with a guidewire, the steerable guide catheter *(arrow)* is advanced into the left atrium *(center)*. On right is corresponding 3D TEE image that shows the steerable guide catheter a distance 4.5 cm into left atrium.

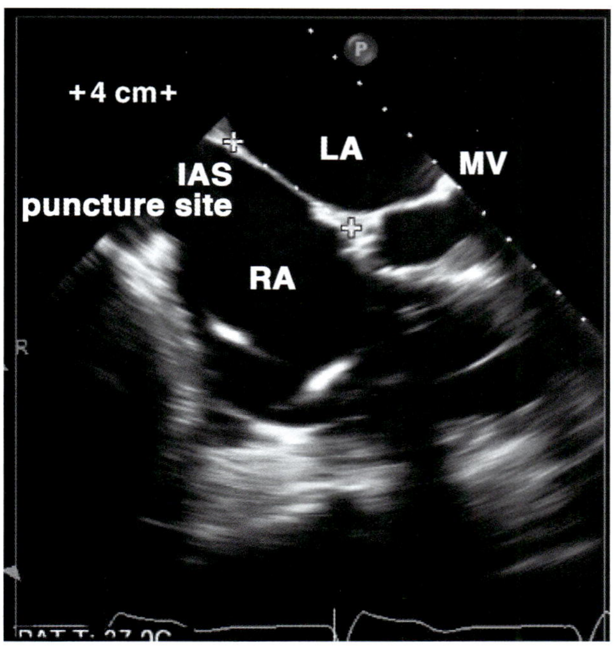

Fig 13.111 In this midesophageal view at 15 degrees, the IAS puncture is 4 cm above mitral annulus.

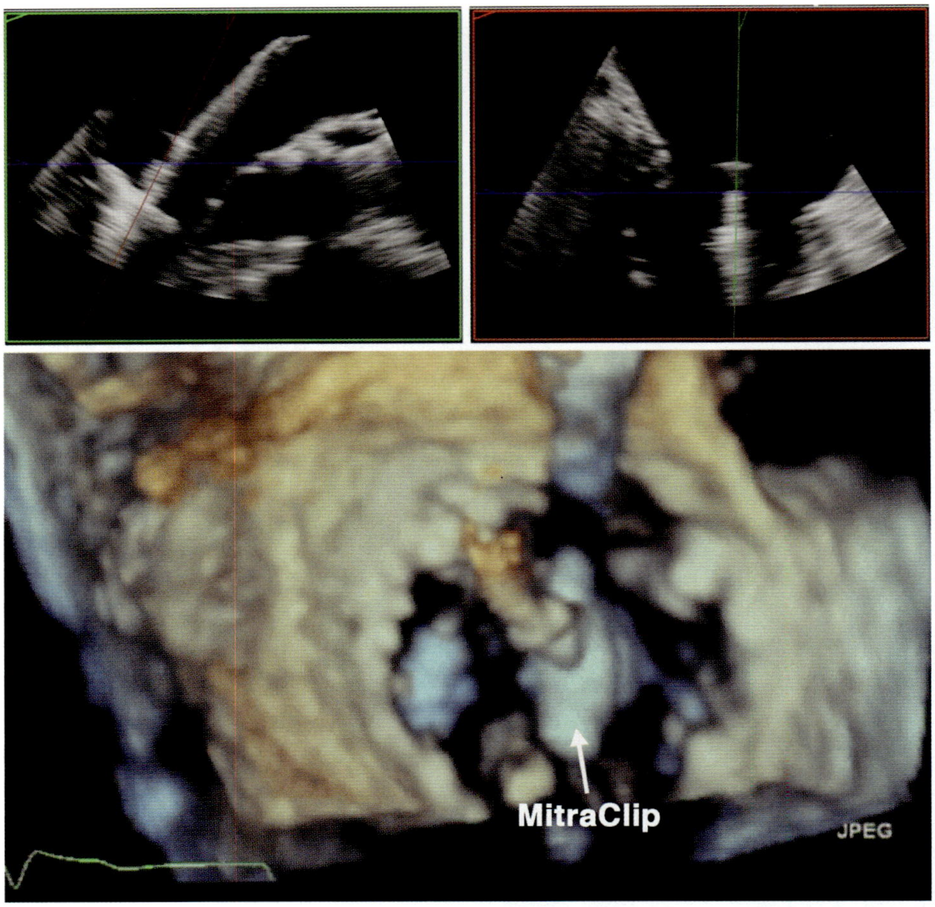

Fig 13.112 Top left and top right images are the midesophageal long-axis and commissural views, respectively. Clip has been advanced into left ventricle. 3D TEE en face view with gain turned way down shows clip in ventricle, with correct orientation.

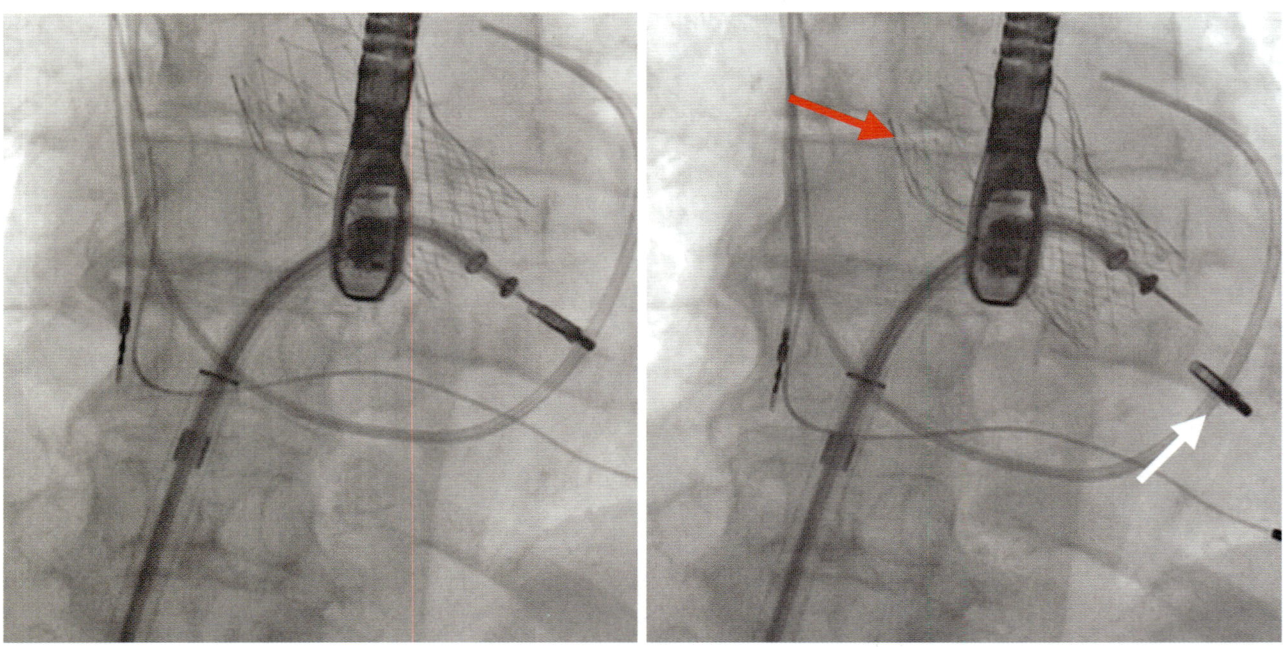

Fig 13.113 Fluoroscopy shows the release of clip *(white arrow)*. Red arrow indicates the CoreValve in aortic position.

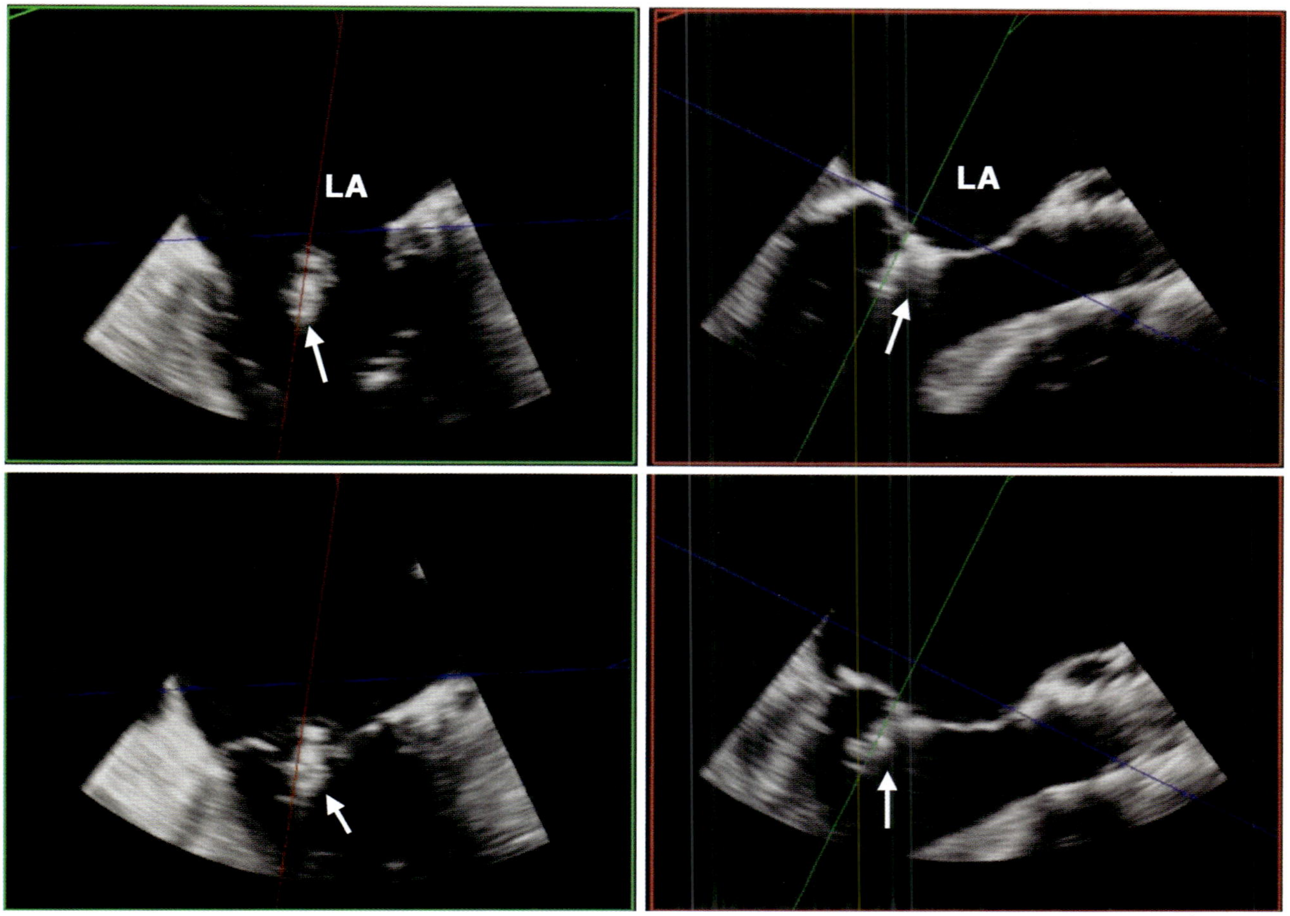

Fig 13.114 In top two frames in diastole, the clip *(arrow)* has been released and has created a double orifice in commissural view *(left)*. Midesophageal long-axis view on right shows no opening. In lower two frames in systole, both orifices are close in commissural view *(left)*, and remained closed in the midesophageal long-axis view at right.

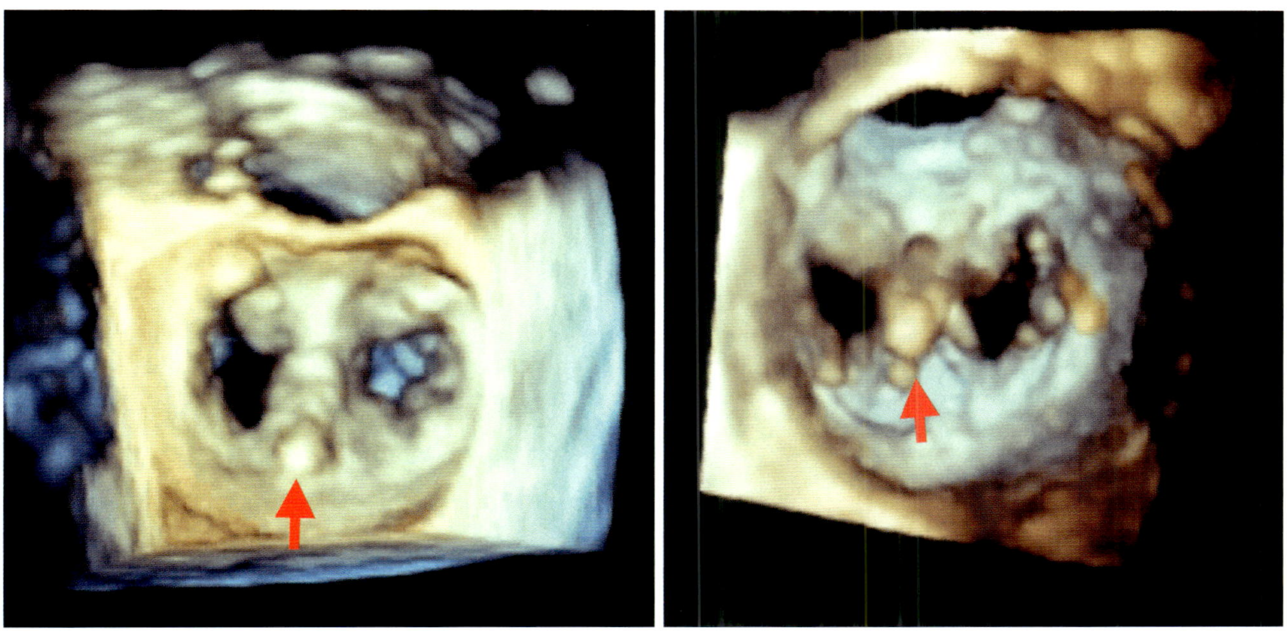

Fig 13.115 At left is an en face view from left atrial perspective, and on right from left ventricular perspective. During diastole, double orifice is appreciated, with clip *(arrow)* in middle.

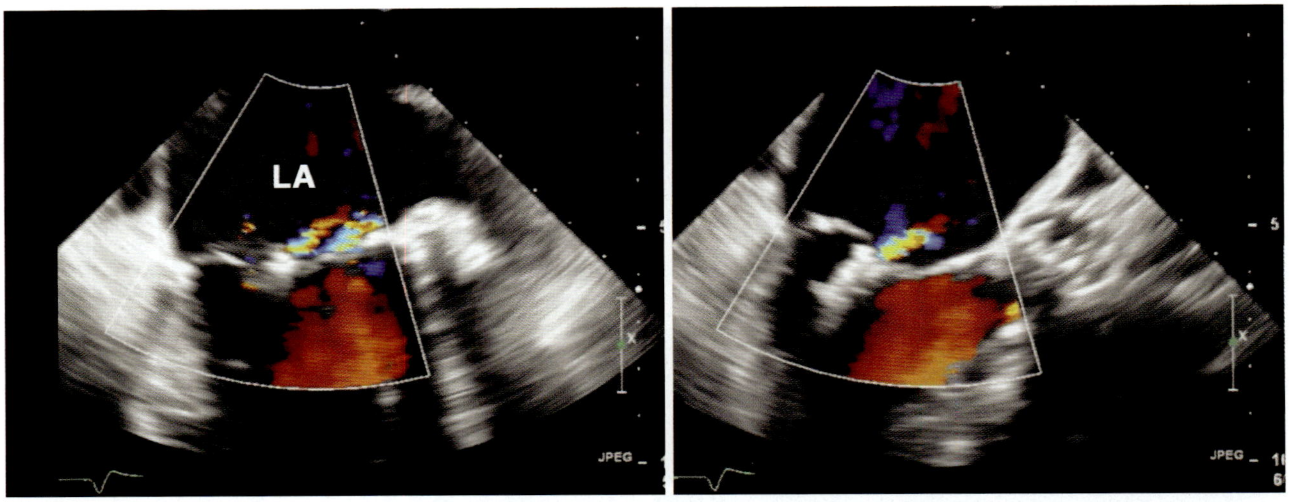

Fig 13.116 Color Doppler shows two small jets of mitral regurgitation in commissural view at left, and one in midesophageal long-axis view at right.

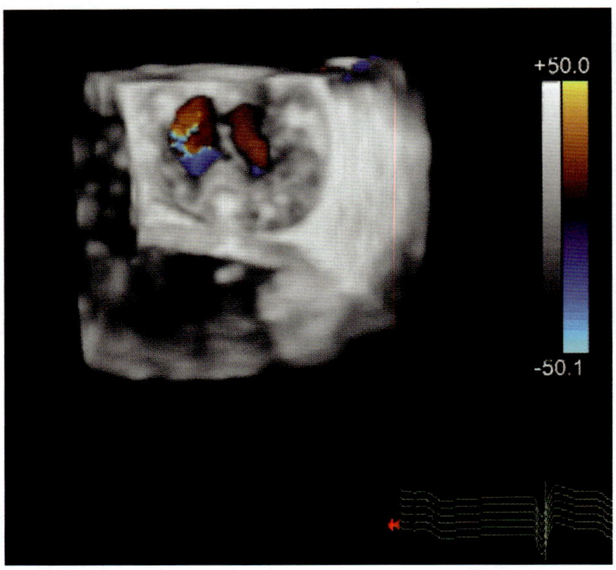

Fig 13.117 3D TEE color Doppler from left atrial en face view shows two small jets of mitral regurgitation.

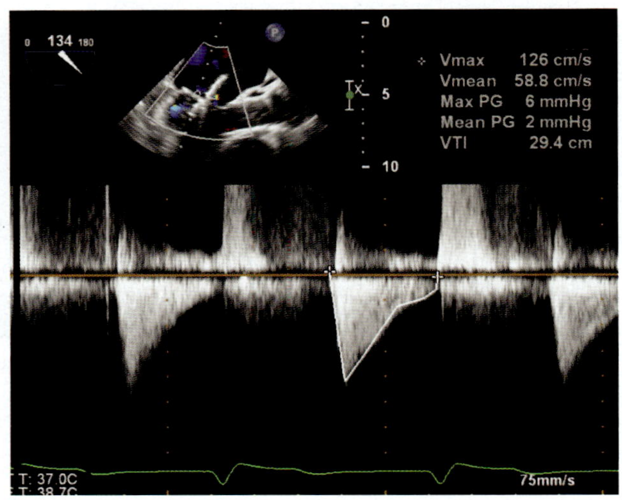

Fig 13.118 Mean pressure gradient across the repaired valve is estimated at 3 mmHg, which indicates a minimal degree of functional stenosis, unlikely to be clinically relevant.

Comments

In patients with severe mitral regurgitation and an indication for intervention, surgical valve repair is recommended whenever possible. When anatomy is not amendable to valve repair, surgical valve replacement is recommended in patients with an acceptable surgical risk. In patients with prohibitive surgical risk and severe symptomatic MR, transcatheter intervention may be reasonable. Although several other devices are in development, the most published clinical experience is with the approved mitral clip device, as in this case. The concept of this transcatheter approach is that clipping the anterior and posterior leaflets together will reduce the size of the regurgitant orifice, albeit at the expense of a slight reduction in the antegrade orifice area. TEE guidance is essential for this procedure both to identify the site of leaflet noncoaptation and to guide the placement of one (or more) clip devices.

Suggested Reading

1. González-Gómez A, Fernández-Santos S, Fernández-Golfín C, et al: Mitral valve anatomy: Preprocedural screening and imaging techniques, EuroIntervention 11 supplement W; W32-W36, 2015.
2. Munkholm-Larsen S, Wan B, Tian DH, et al: A systematic review on the safety and efficacy of percutaneous edge-to-edge mitral valve repair with the MitraClip system for high surgical risk candidates, Heart 100(6):473–478, 2014.

14 Transcatheter Closure Devices

Atrial Septum

CASE 14-1
Anatomy and Imaging of Atrial Septum

See Case 7-1 in Chapter 7, Adult Congenital Heart Disease.

CASE 14-2
PFO Device Closure for Recurrent Transient Neurological Events

About 3 years ago this 44-year-old female had an episode of transient dysarthria with a CT scan revealing evidence of a small cerebral infarct at that time. About 6 months ago, she had several brief episodes of right lower extremity paresthesias with the longest episode lasting several minutes in association with significant weakness in the right leg. She refused warfarin anticoagulation and has been managed with antiplatelet therapy. Transesophageal echocardiography demonstrated a patent foramen ovale, and after consenting, she was referred for transcatheter closure.

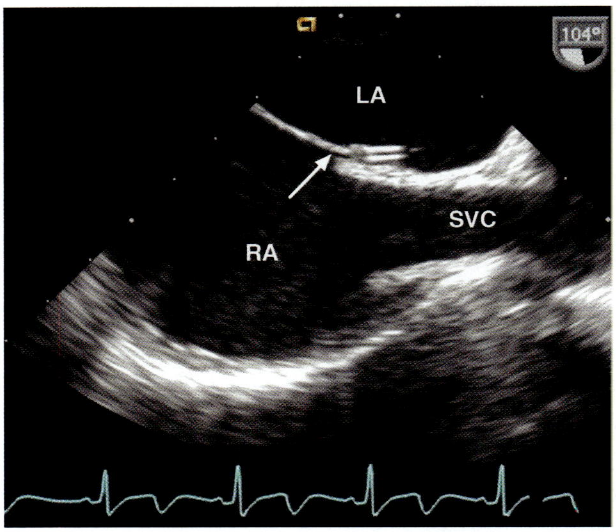

Fig 14.1 After placement of a sheath into the right femoral vein and a guidewire into the right atrium, a 6-French multipurpose diagnostic catheter was advanced to right atrium and the guidewire removed. Catheter as seen in this midesophageal bicaval view was used to gently probe across the patent foramen ovale *(arrow)*.

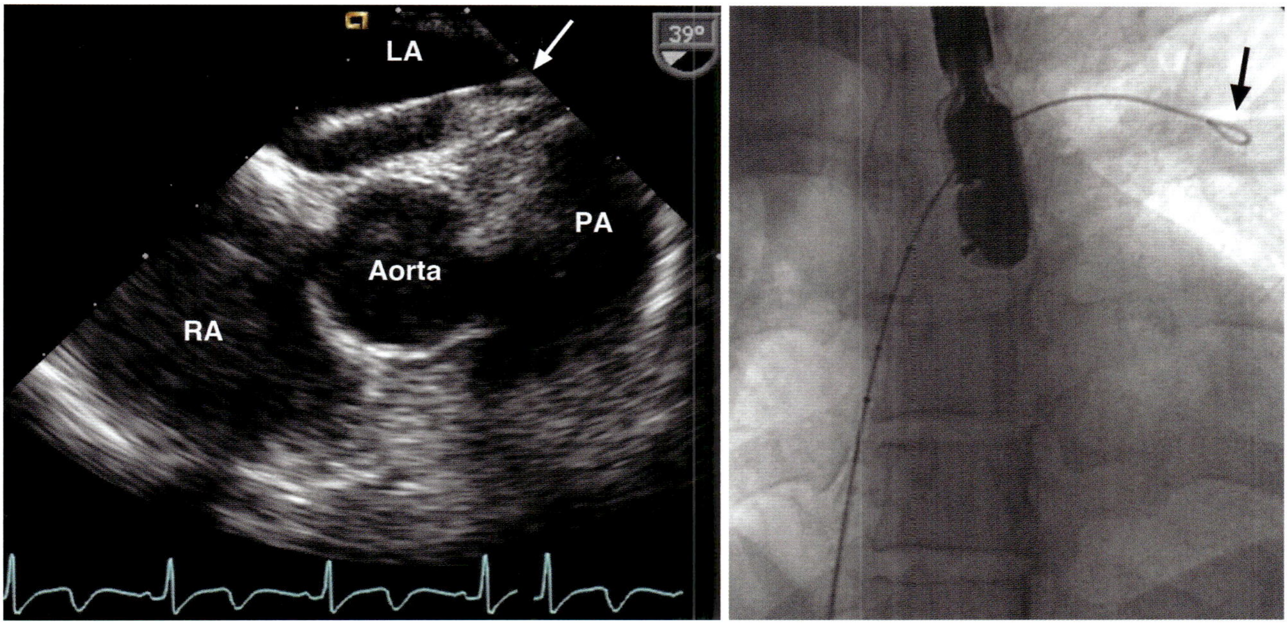

Fig 14.2 J-tipped wire was then reinserted into the catheter and advanced into left pulmonary vein as seen on TEE *(left)* and fluoroscopy *(right, arrows)*.

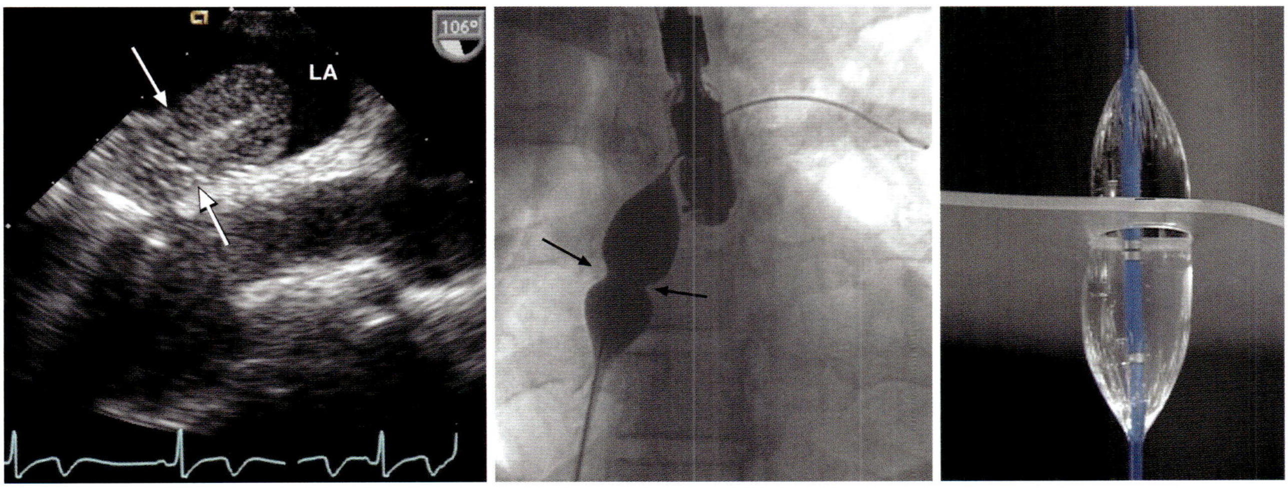

Fig 14.3 Using transesophageal echo *(left)* and fluoroscopic guidance *(middle)*, a 20-mm diameter NMT sizing balloon (NMT Medical, Inc., Boston, Massachusetts) was inserted over the wire and advanced across the atrial septum. By measurement of waist in balloon *(arrows)*, patent foramen ovale was measured at between 10 mm and 11 mm. Based on this measurement, a 28-mm CardioSeal device (NMT Medical, Inc., Boston, Massachusetts) was selected. Measurement is graphically depicted on right.

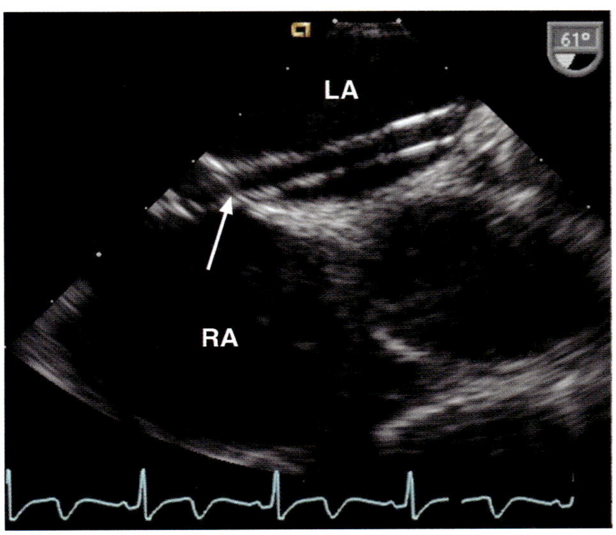

Fig 14.4 14-French transseptal catheter and dilator was advanced to the left atrium *(arrow)*. Dilator and wire were removed and the catheter was carefully aspirated and flushed to ensure that there was no air in the system.

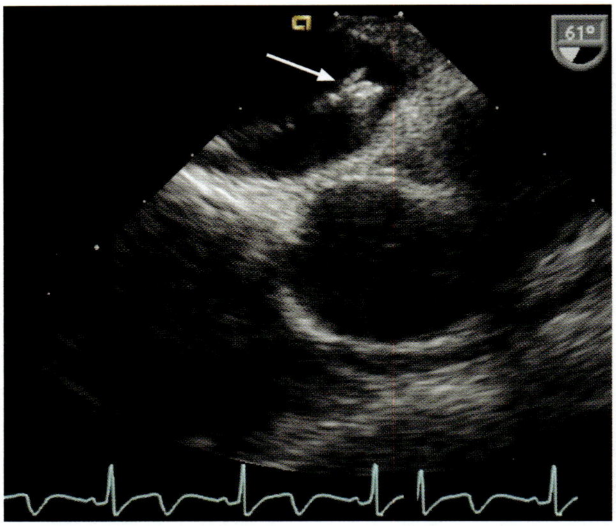

Fig 14.5 CardioSeal device was then loaded into the delivery catheter and advanced into left atrium *(arrow)*.

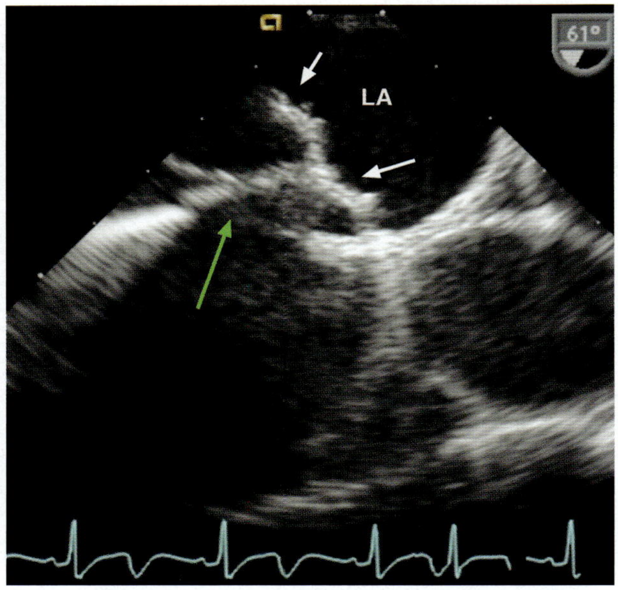

Fig 14.6 Transseptal sheath was pulled back to allow left atrial arms to unfold *(white arrows)*. This was then pulled back across atrial septum *(green arrow)* and was seen to be well placed by fluoroscopy and by transesophageal echo.

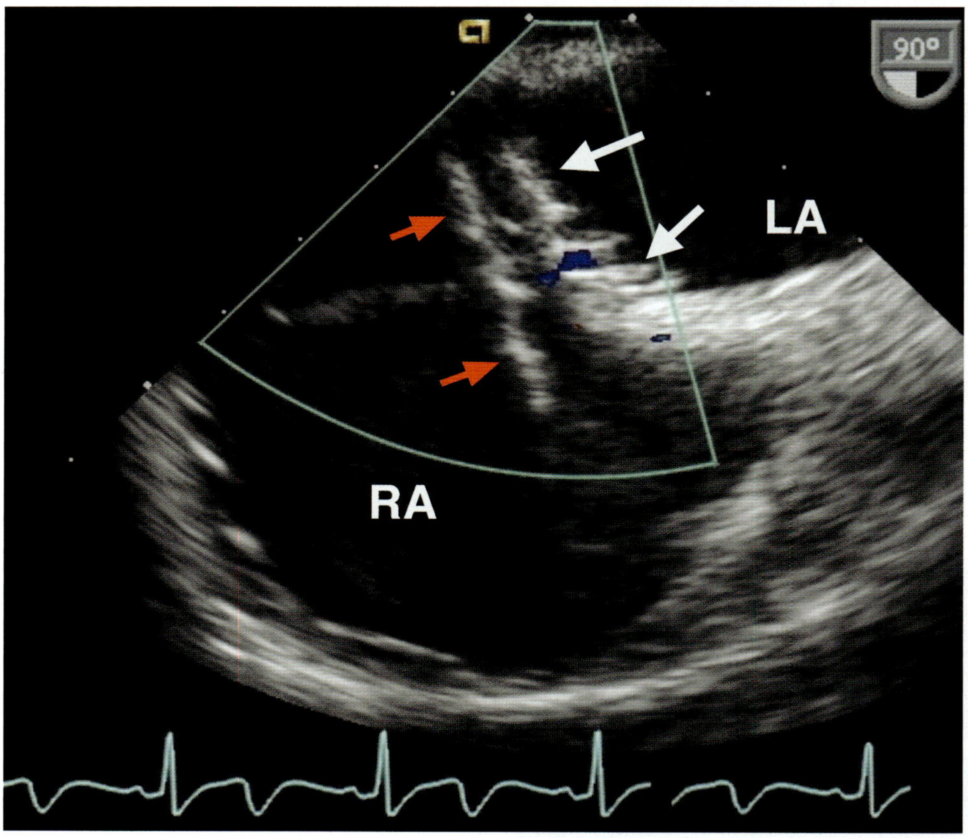

Fig 14.7 Transseptal catheter was then pulled back further until right atrial arms *(red arrows)* were released and the device could be seen to be in good position across patent foramen ovale *(white arrows indicate left atrial arms)*.

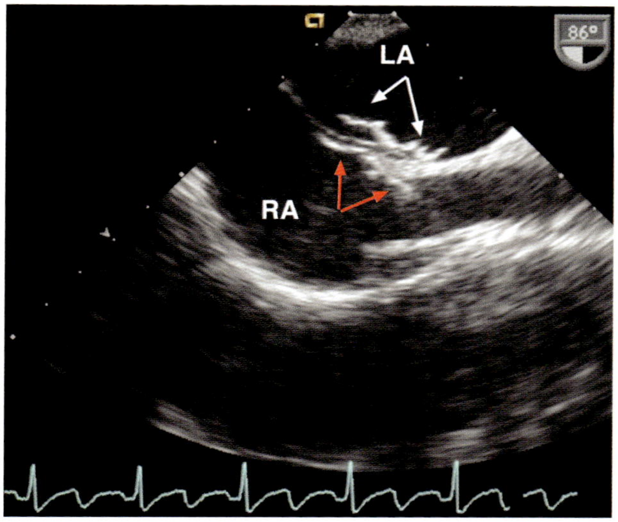

Fig 14.8 Device was then released from the delivery system and transesophageal echo was performed revealing good closure. Double arrows indicate the arms in each atrium.

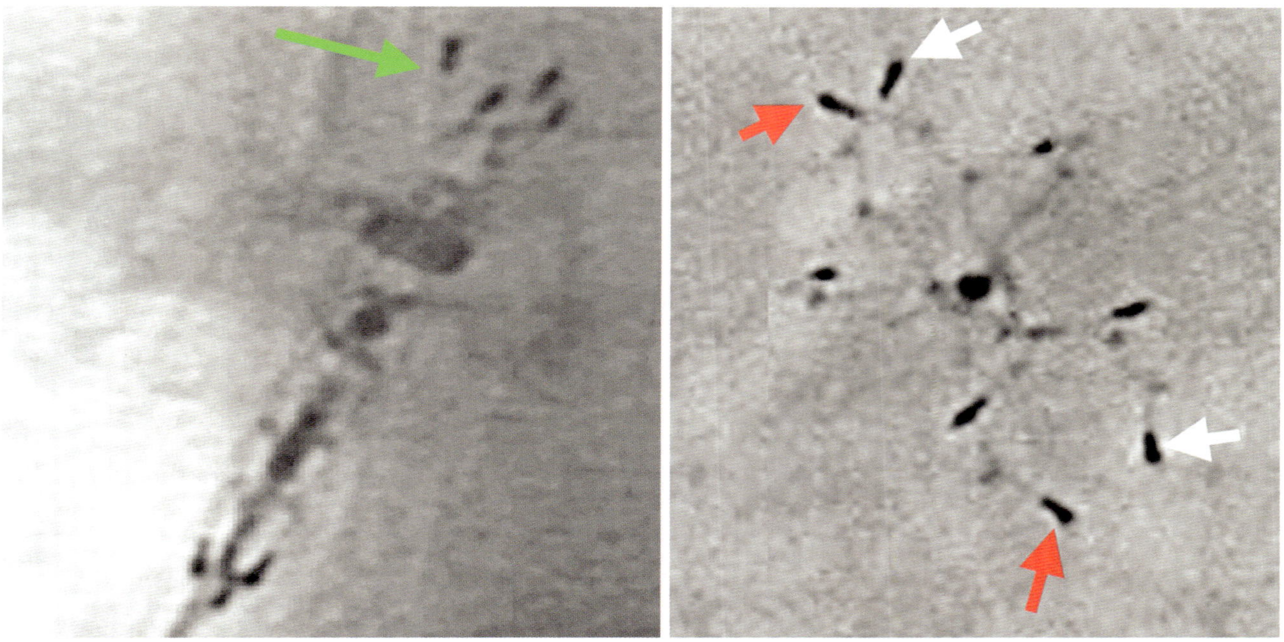

Fig 14.9 Fluoroscopy of device deployment. In the left frame, the device has been advanced into left atrium *(green arrow)*. On the right, the left atrial arms *(white arrows)* as well as the right atrial arms *(red arrows)* have also been deployed.

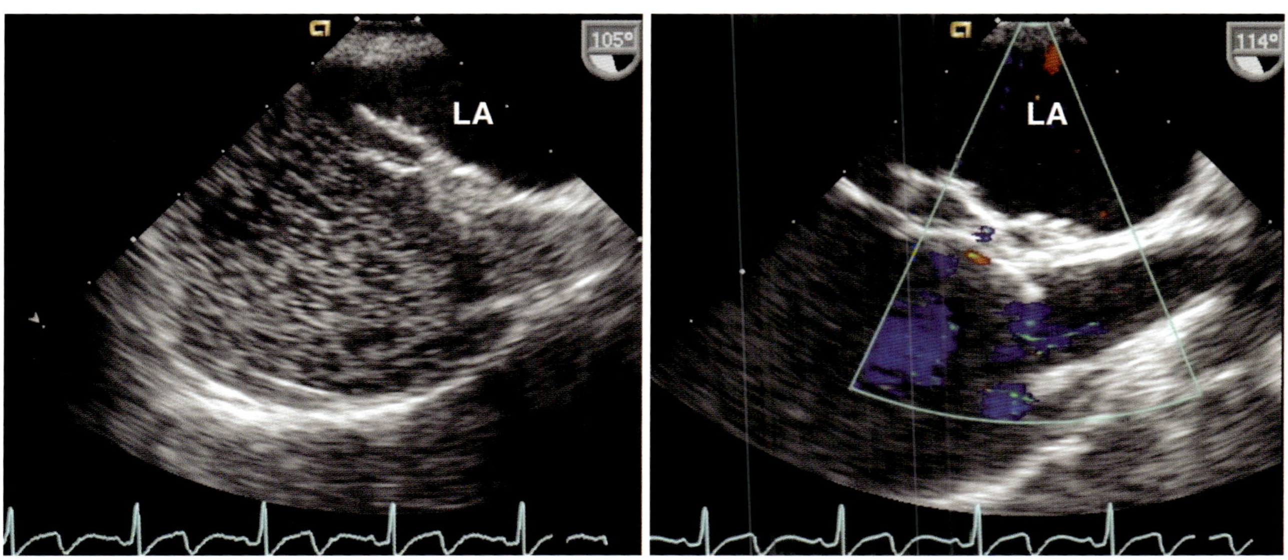

Fig 14.10 Both saline contrast and color Doppler imaging confirmed closure of the PFO with no residual resting shunt.

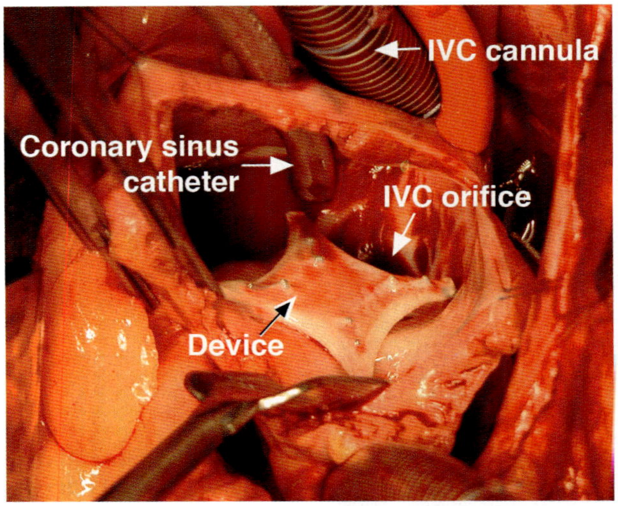

Fig 14.11 Another patient with similar device subsequently underwent mitral valve replacement. Upon opening the right atrium, the device is seen in good position.

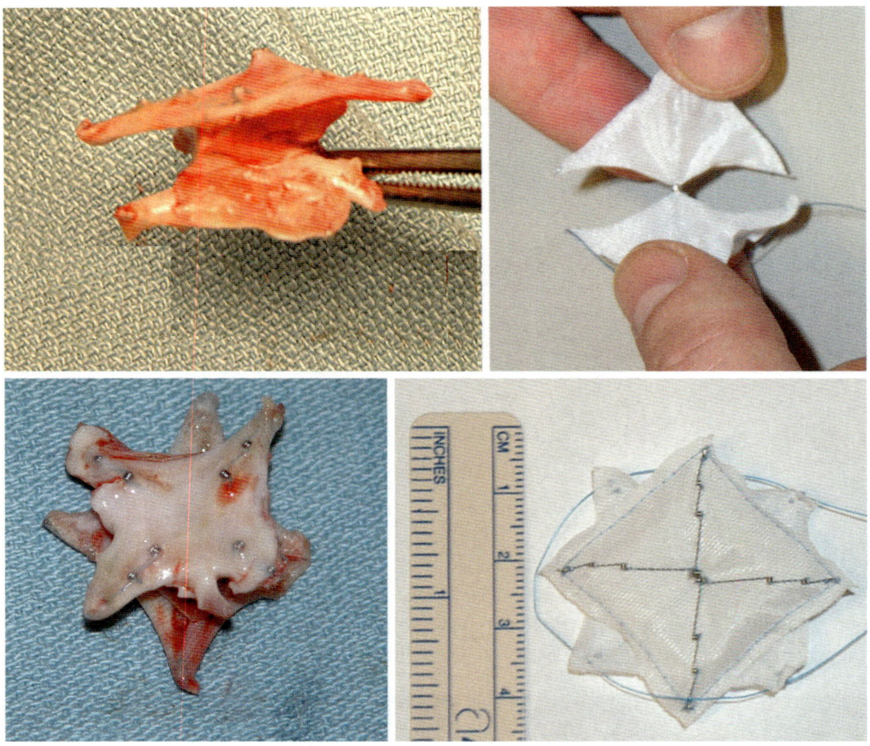

Fig 14.12 Device was removed as part of the valvular procedure. In top frames, the device is seen from the side, with an unused device for comparison. In lower frames, the device is seen from front.

Comments

TEE or intracardiac echocardiography (ICE) is an essential for transcatheter closure of atrial septal defects or a patent foramen ovale. As illustrated by these cases, the echo images allow visualization of the atrial septum including identification of the size, location, and shape of the atrial septal defect. During the procedure, imaging allows guidance of catheter position and correct placement of the device in the atrial septum. After device deployment, color Doppler and saline contrast imaging allow diagnosis of any residual shunt flow.

Suggested Reading

1. Tobis J, Shenoda M: Percutaneous treatment of patent foramen ovale and atrial septal defects, J Am Coll Cardiol 60:1722–1732, 2012.
2. Saric M, Perk G, Purgess JR, et al: Imaging atrial septal defects by real-time three-dimensional transesophageal echocardiography: Step-by-step approach, J Am Soc Echocardiogr 23:1128–1135, 2010.
3. Faletra FF, Nucifora G, Yen S: Imaging the atrial septum using real-time three-dimensional transesophageal echocardiography: Technical tips, normal anatomy, and its role in transseptal puncture, J Am Soc Echocardiogr 24:593–599, 2011.
4. Silvestry FE, Cohen MS, Armsby LB, et al: Guidelines for the echocardiographic assessment of atrial septal defect and patent foramen ovale, J Am Soc Echocardiogr 28:910–958, 2015.

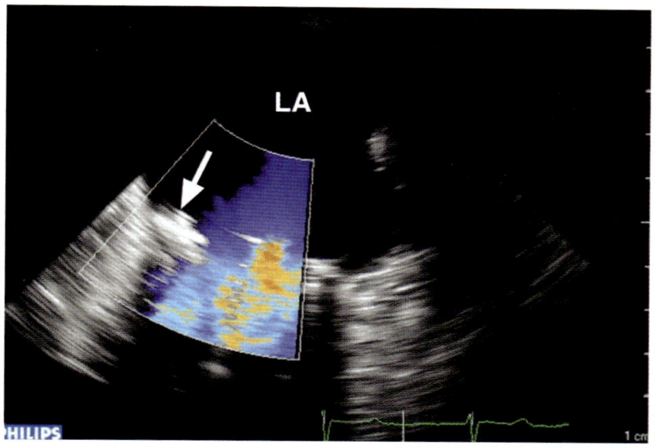

Fig 14.41 In midesophageal two-chamber view, 10-mm occluder has been deployed and color Doppler shows no flow into left atrium.

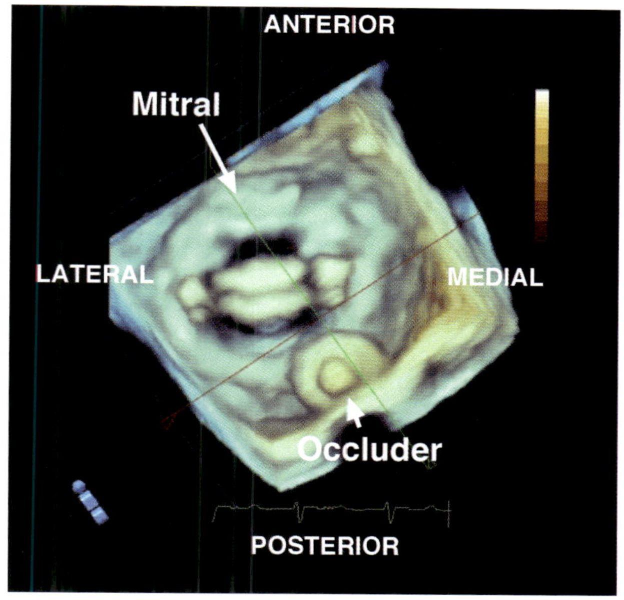

Fig 14.42 In 3D image from left atrial perspective, occluder is seen to be in good position.

CASE 14-8
Dislodgement of Paraprosthetic Occluder Device

The patient, a 51-year-old woman had, some 20 years previously undergone aortic and mitral valve replacements with bileaflet mechanical valves. She presented with severe right and left heart failure, hemolysis, and severe pulmonary hypertension, and was discovered on echocardiography to have a large prosthetic mitral paravalvular leak (PVL).

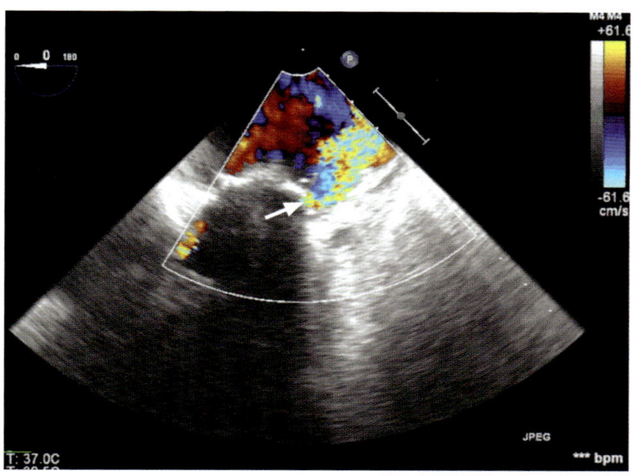

Fig 14.43 Midesophageal four-chamber view with color Doppler demonstrated large posterior paravalvular leak *(arrow)*.

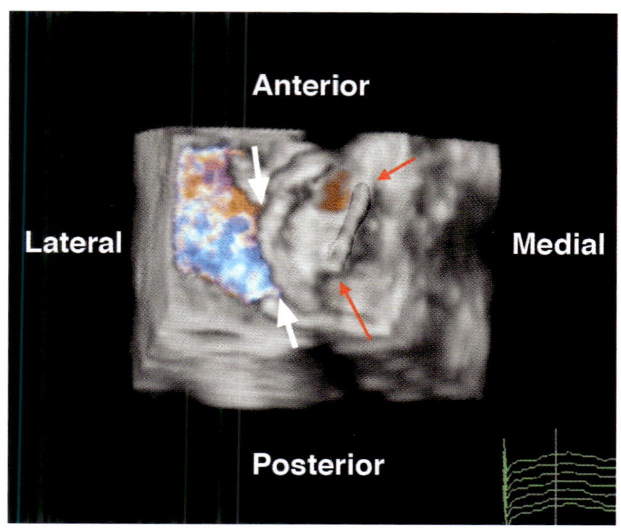

Fig 14.44 3D TEE with color Doppler revealed broad postero-lateral jet of paravalvular MR *(white arrows)*. The red arrows indicate the hinges of the bileaflet mechanical valve.

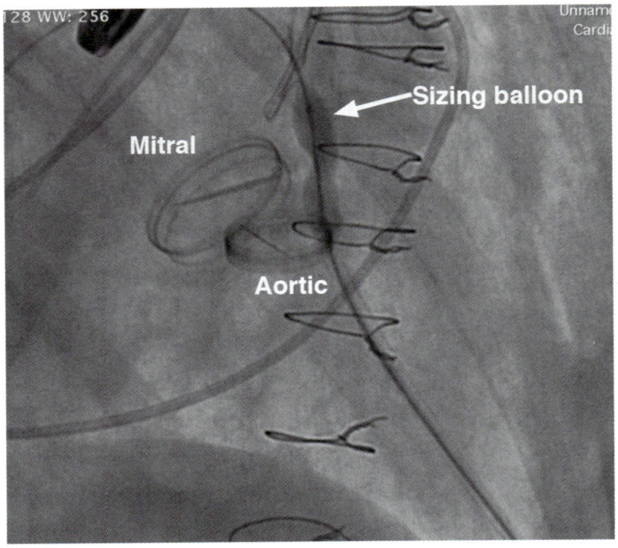

Fig 14.45 Defect was approached via trans-left ventricular apical approach. Defect was sized with balloon passed via femoral artery, through prosthetic aortic valve, and retrograde through paravalvular leak.

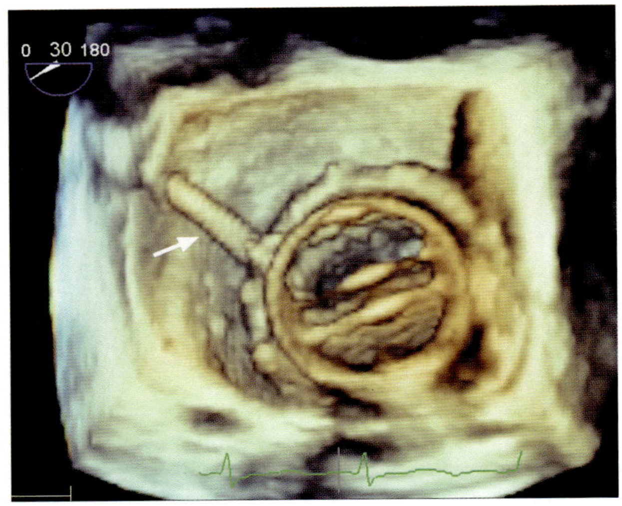

Fig 14.46 Using TEE and fluoroscopic guidance, a number of guidewire facilitated exchanges were performed, and a sheath was eventually passed through the defect *(arrow)* as seen on this 3D TEE from left atrial perspective.

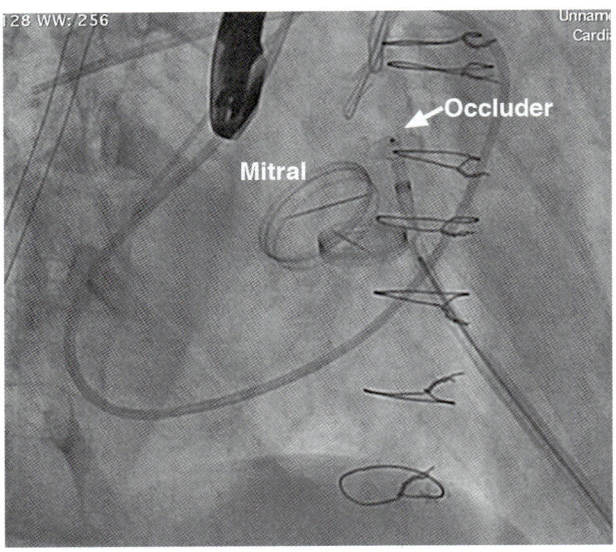

Fig 14.47 Fluoroscopy demonstrates deployment of first occluder.

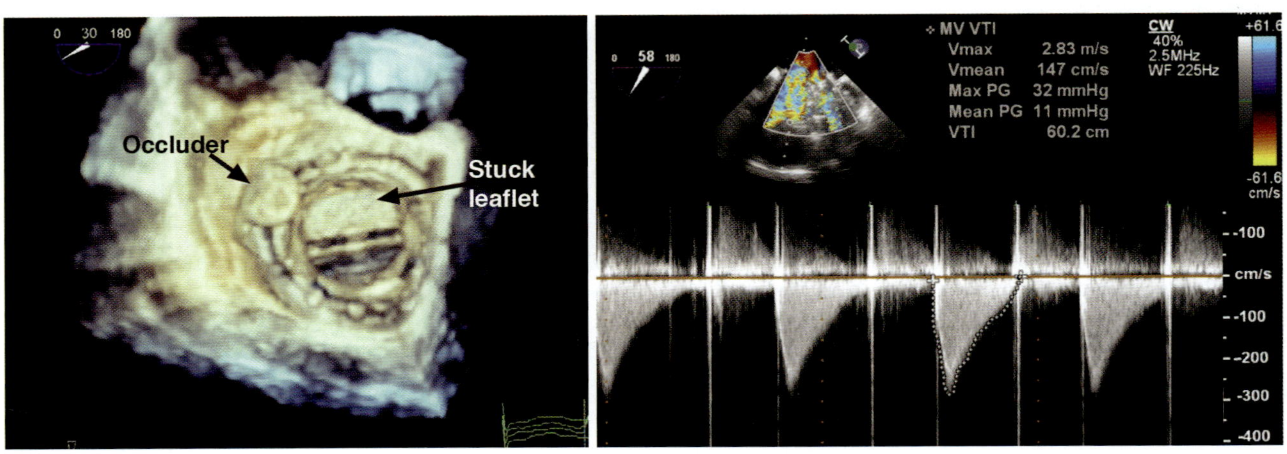

Fig 14.48 Unfortunately the ventricular side of occluder interfered with motion of anterior mitral prosthetic leaflet resulting in mean gradient of 11 mm Hg.

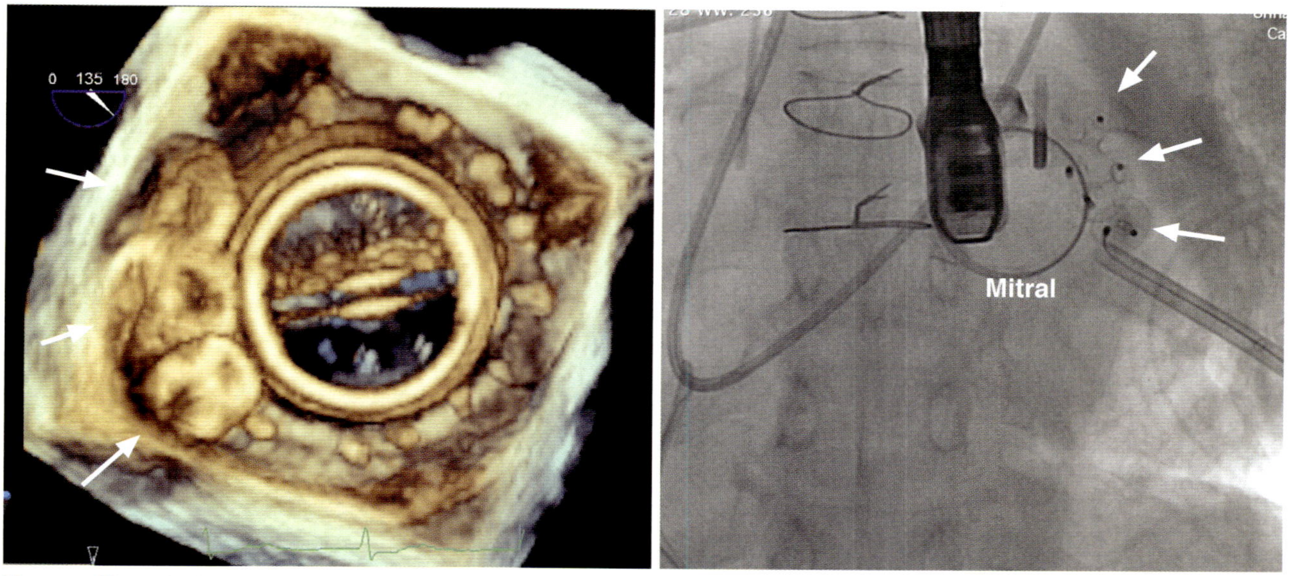

Fig 14.49 Occluder was removed and replaced. A total of three occluders were placed as seen on fluoroscopy, and 3D TEE from the left atrial perspective *(white arrows)*.

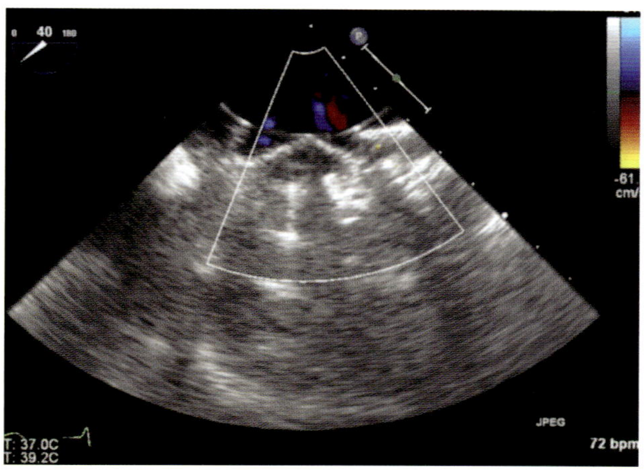

Fig 14.50 No regurgitation is seen on midesophageal 2D TEE with color Doppler.

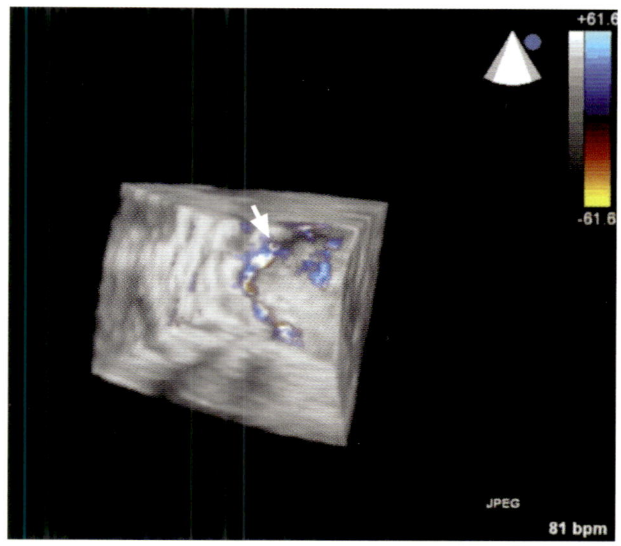

Fig 14.51 Similarly, no regurgitation is seen on 3D TEE with color Doppler from left atrial perspective.

The day after surgery, she was noted to be hemodynamically unstable and a TEE performed revealed that one of the closure devices had become dislodged and was free floating the left atrium. The remaining two previously placed devices stayed in their original positions across the PVL. She presents today for percutaneous retrieval of the embolized device and another attempt at percutaneous PVL closure using a transseptal approach.

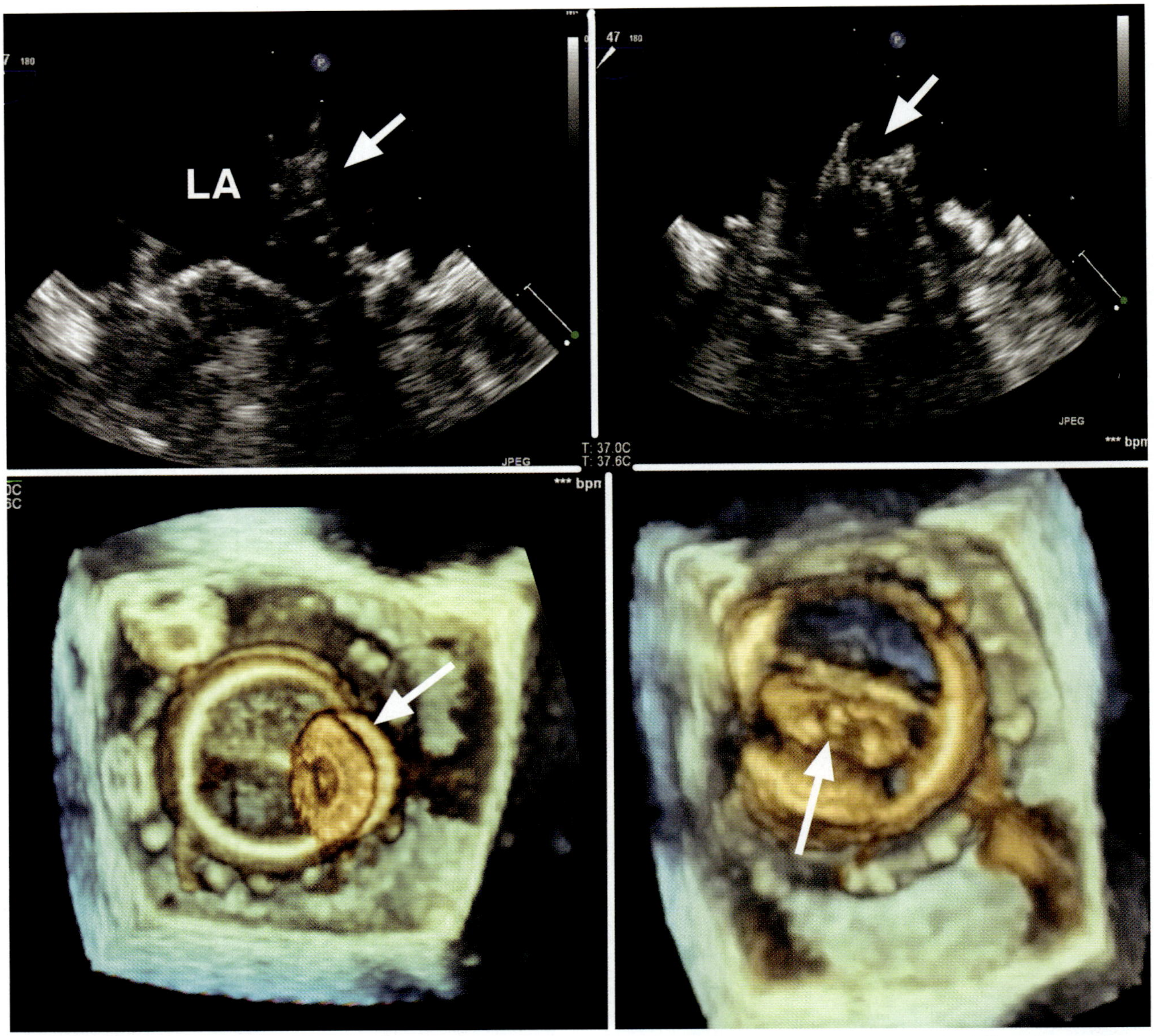

Fig 14.52 In top two frames, 2D representation shows the loose occluder free in the left atrium *(systole, left)* and engaging mitral prosthesis during diastole *(right)*. In lower two frames, corresponding 3D TEE images are seen. White arrows indicate free occluder.

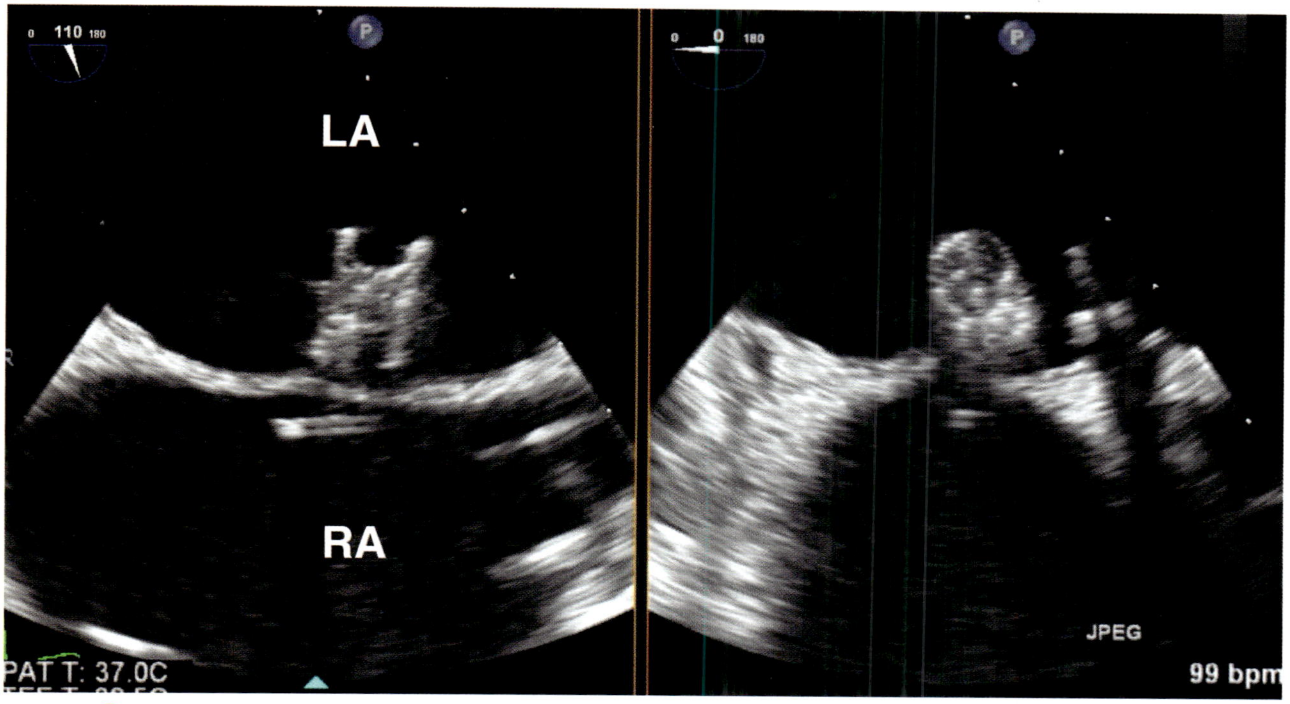

Fig 14.53 Mobile occluder is seen in biplane view of the atrial septum.

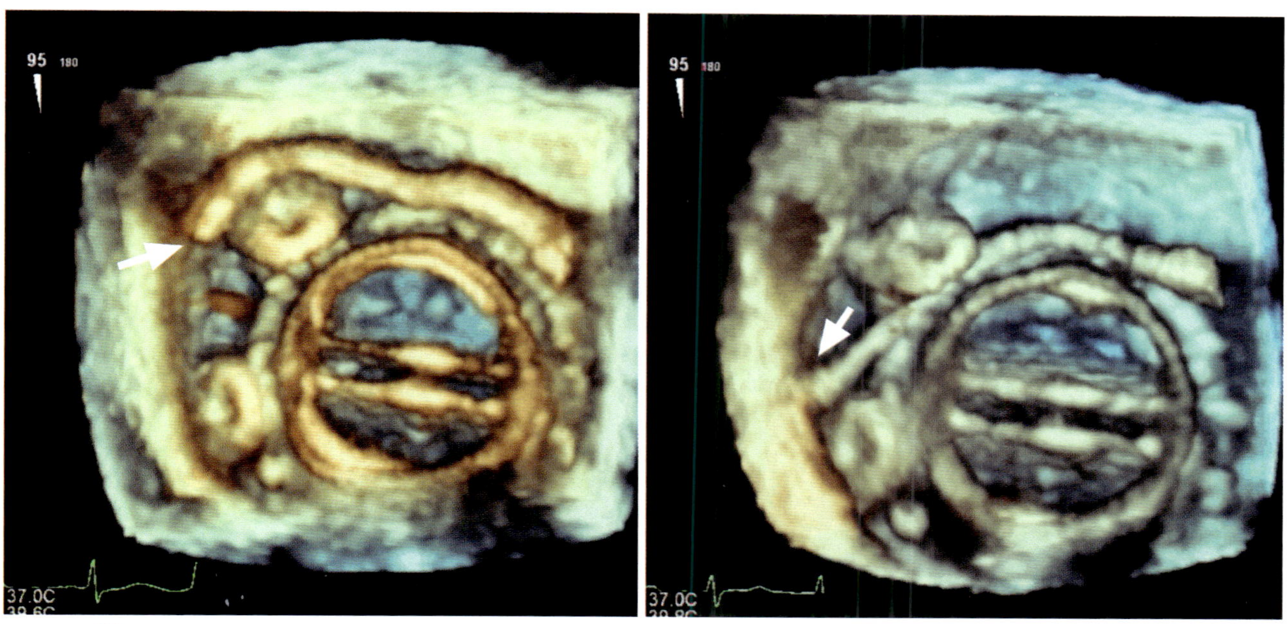

Fig 14.54 In 3D TEE views from the left atrial perspective, a sheath that has been passed in the left atrium transseptally *(arrow)* is moving toward the remaining defect *(left)* and engaging it *(right)*.

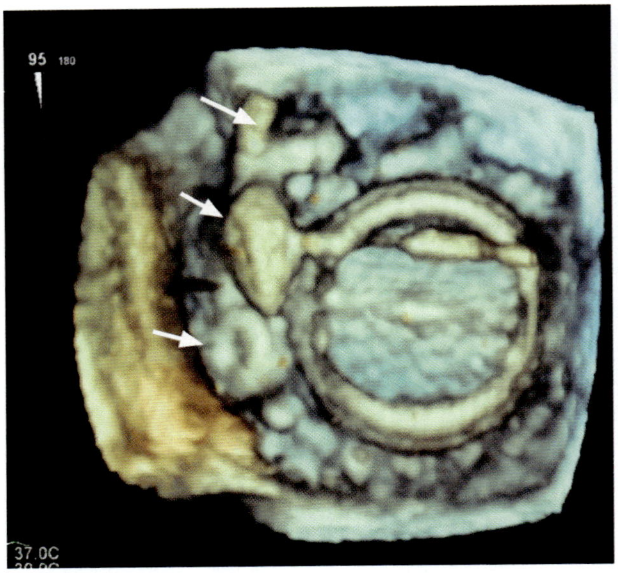

Fig 14.55 Three occluders are again present.

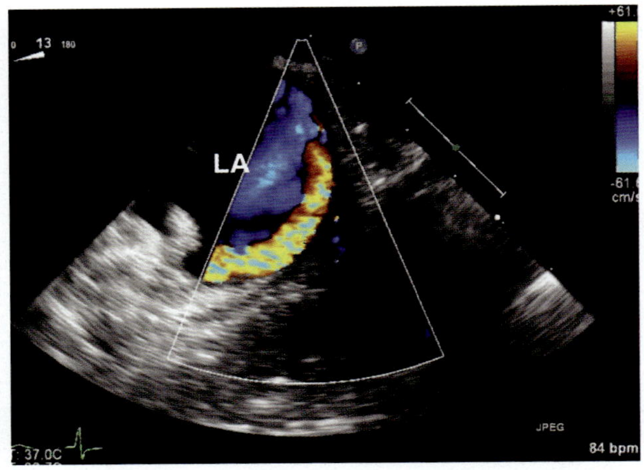

Fig 14.56 Large residual jet of laterally directed paravalvular MR is observed.

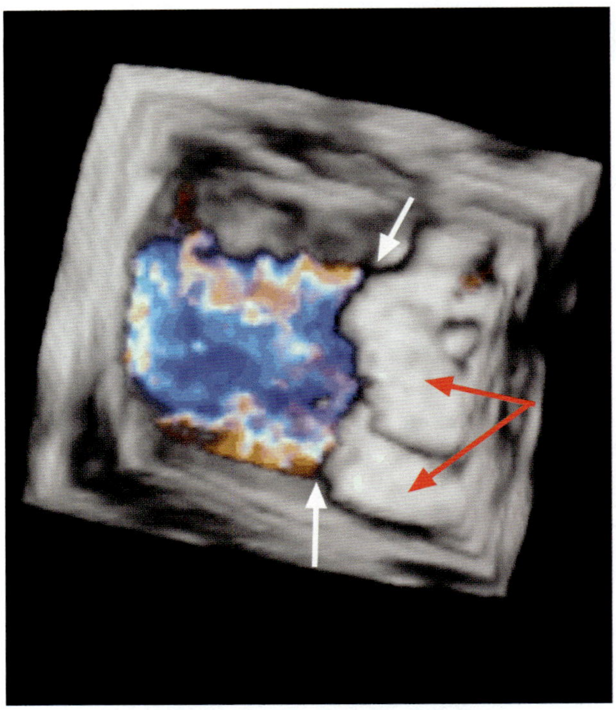

Fig 14.57 Red arrows indicate two occluders. White arrows describe the broad-based jet of paravalvular MR.

CASE 14-9
Regurgitation Posterior to Mitral Annuloplasty Ring

Two similar cases are presented with different therapies employed. The first patient, a 75-year-old man underwent a mitral valve repair 12 years before the current admission, and 9 years before the current admission underwent a redo mitral valve repair. Recent TTEs showed progressive reduction in left ventricular function and severe mitral regurgitation.

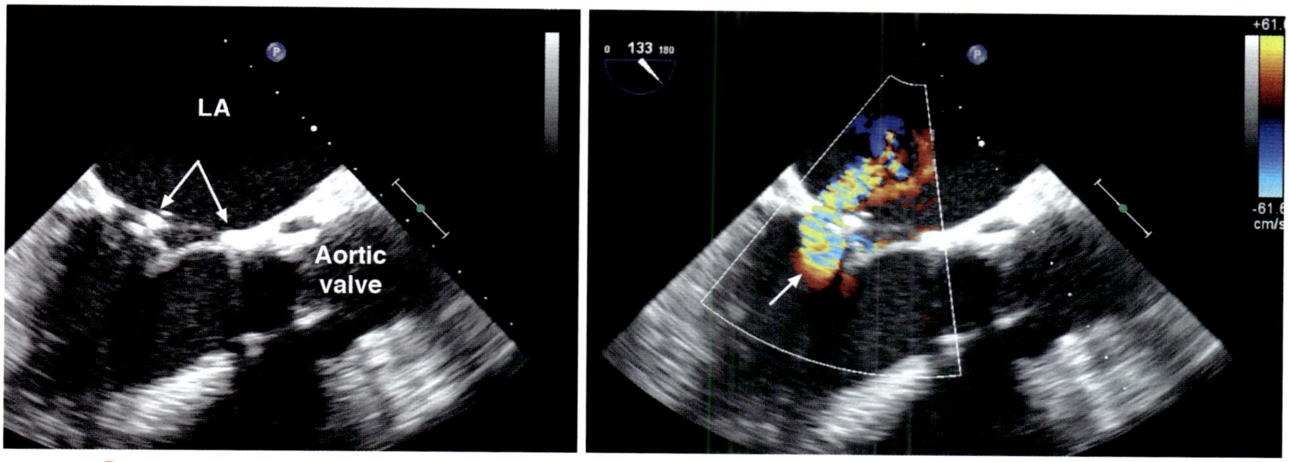

Fig 14.58 Midesophageal long-axis imaging showed a jet of mitral regurgitation *(arrow)* posterior to annuloplasty ring *(double arrows)*. No regurgitation is seen through native valve.

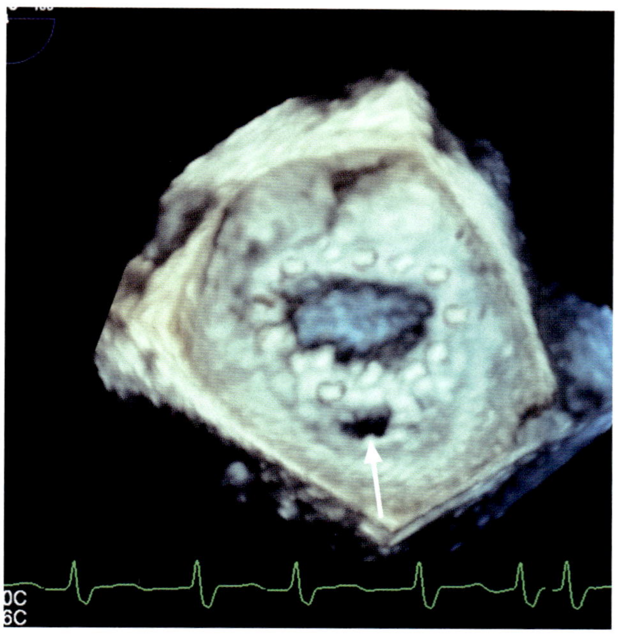

Fig 14.59 3D TEE from the left atrial perspective shows the annuloplasty ring and defect posterior to it that corresponds to area of dehiscence.

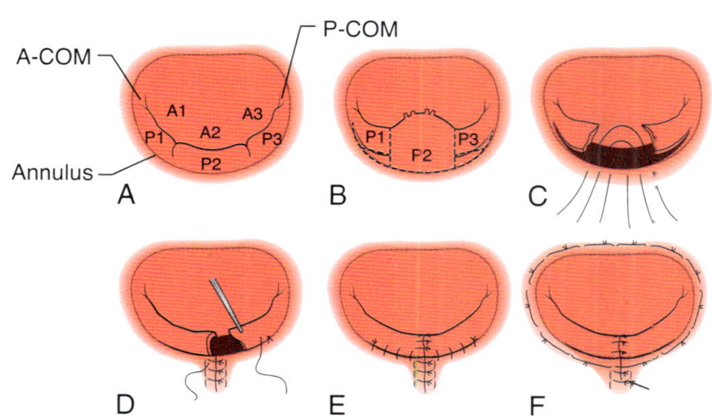

Fig 14.60 Image describes patient's original procedure, posterior leaflet quadrangular resection, and sliding plasty. **(A)** Normal mitral valve. **(B)** Limits of resection are identified, quadrangular resection is performed, and P1 and P3 are also detached to shorten their height. **(C)** Sutures are placed in order to vertically plicate posterior annulus. **(D)** Leaflet segments are reattached to annulus. **(E)** Leaflet edges are reapproximated before remodeling annuloplasty. **(F)** Annuloplasty is placed. Arrow in **(F)** is where suture breakdown led to defect posterior to annuloplasty ring. (Modified from Carpentier A, Adams DH, Filsoufi F: Carpentier's Reconstructive Valve Surgery, Philadelphia: W.B. Saunders, 2010.)

In the OR, the valve and ring were resected and a bileaflet mechanical prosthesis placed.

Eleven years before this admission, the second patient, a 65-year-old woman, underwent a mitral valve repair with a quadrangular resection and a #30 annuloplasty ring, with no mitral regurgitation seen postoperatively. She now presents with increasing shortness of breath, more peripheral edema, and an echocardiogram that showed worsening of mitral regurgitation.

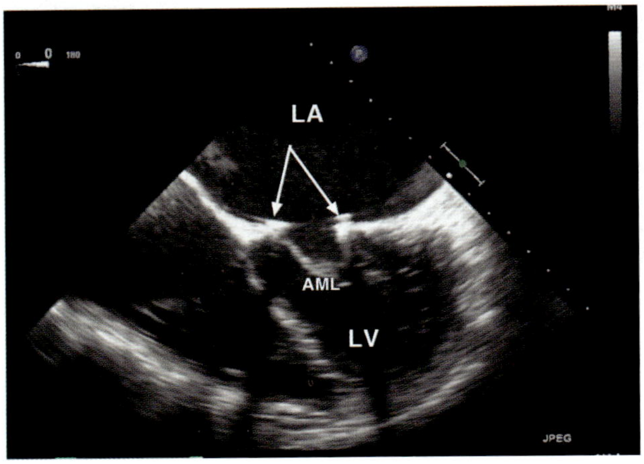

Fig 14.61 Midesophageal four-chamber view shows annuloplasty ring *(white arrows)*.

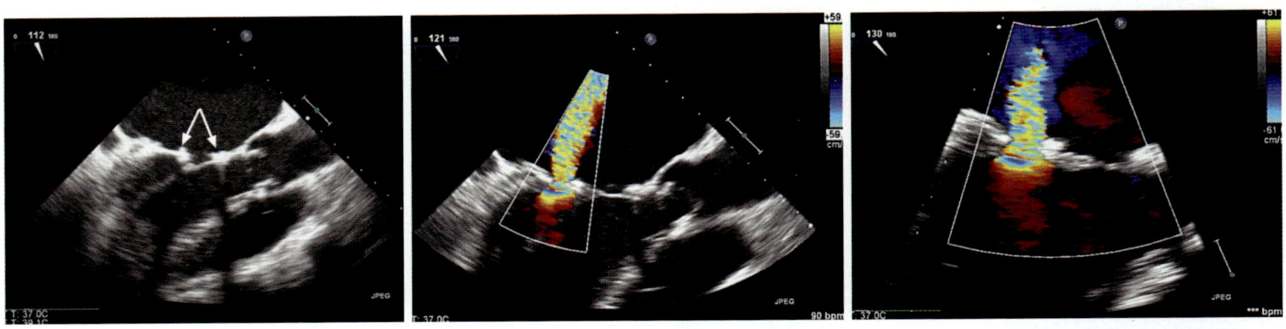

Fig 14.62 In left frame, midesophageal long-axis view, annuloplasty ring is again identified by white arrows. In corresponding color Doppler image, jet of regurgitation is seen posterior to annuloplasty ring. In zoom mode, same jet is seen and no regurgitation is seen traversing the valve leaflets.

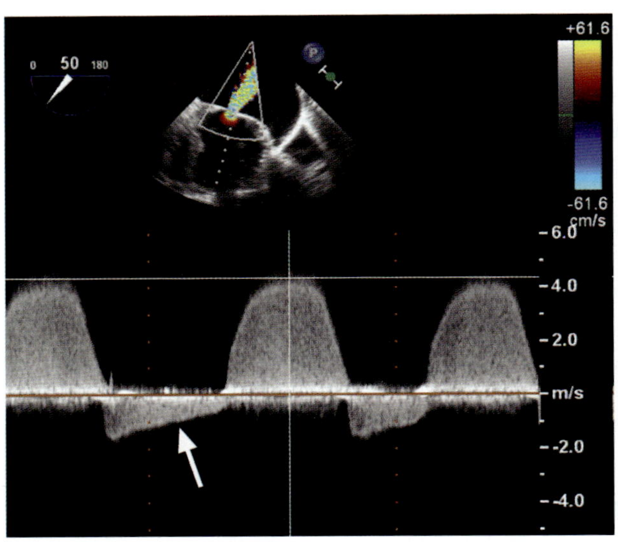

Fig 14.63 Continuous wave Doppler shows regurgitant jet, as well as an antegrade signal during diastole *(arrow)*.

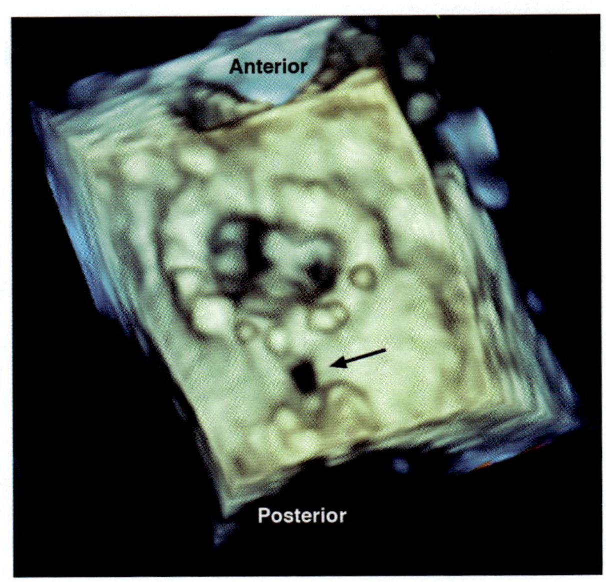

Fig 14.64 This 3D TEE of mitral valve seen from the left atrial perspective, shows a defect *(arrow)* posterior to annuloplasty ring.

Although the working diagnosis was initially thought to be intrinsic leaflet disease, intraoperative TEE demonstrated an etiology similar to that in the first vignette. The surgery was aborted, and after discussions, the patient opted for catheter-based occlusion of the defect, which was undertaken 1 month later.

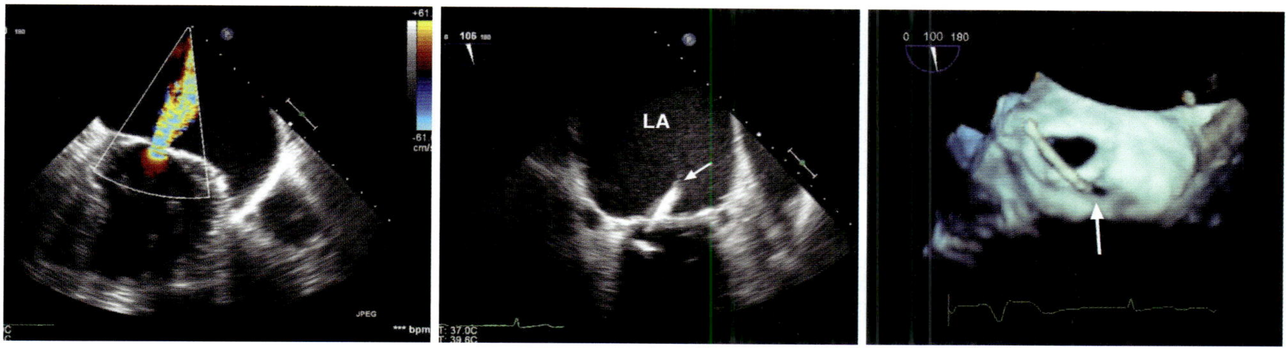

Fig 14.65 At left, color Doppler imaging is used to identify the defect. In middle frame, wire can be seen traversing the defect; at right is the image in 3D from left atrial perspective.

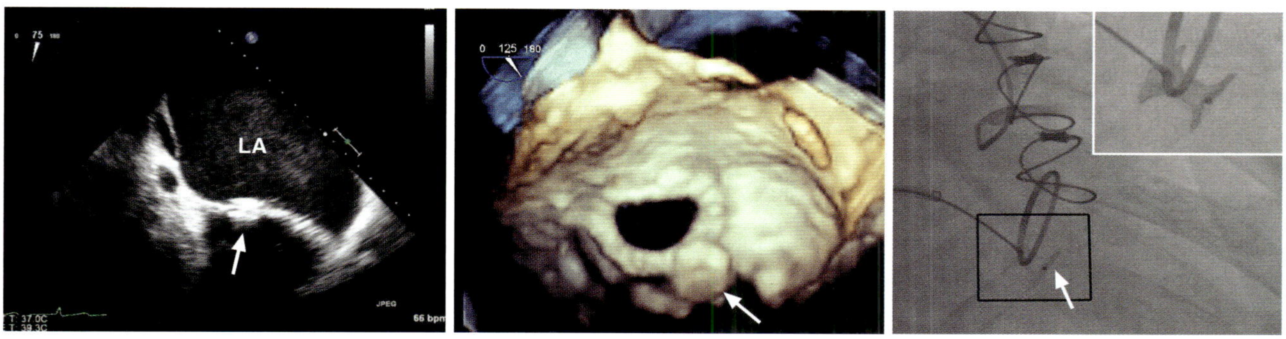

Fig 14.66 With 2D and 3D imaging, occluder device *(arrow)* is seen traversing the defect. At right, occlude is seen with fluoroscopy and is adjacent to annuloplasty ring.

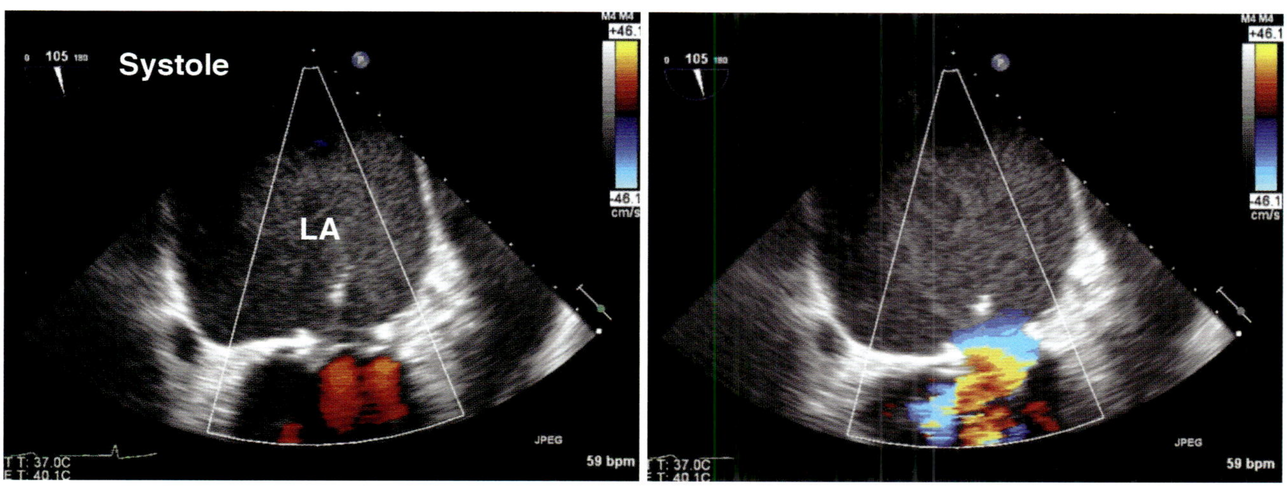

Fig 14.67 Color Doppler shows the absence of any regurgitation.

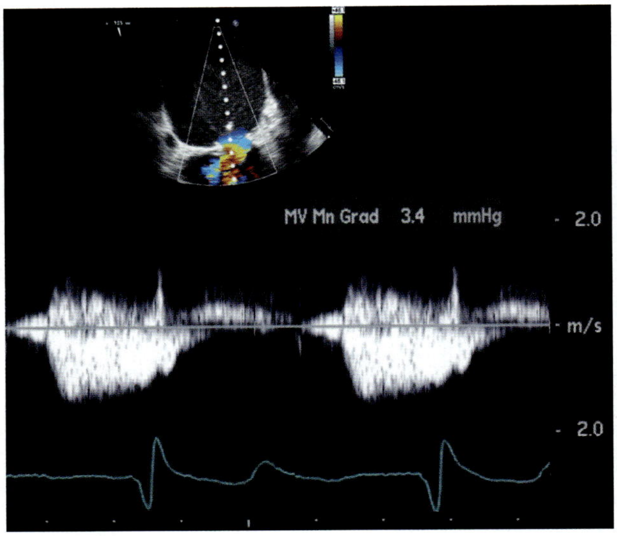

Fig 14.68 Mitral inflow gradient was 3.4 mm Hg, indicating absence of mitral stenosis.

Hemodynamics are Presented in Table 1:

	RA Mean Pressure (mmHg)	RA v-waves (mmHg)	LA Mean Pressure (mmHg)	LA v-waves (mmHg)
Baseline	16	20	29	38
Post intervention	11	12	14	16

Comments

New onset paravalvular prosthetic regurgitation raises the concern for endocarditis so that clinical evaluation and blood cultures are appropriate in these patients. However, most cases of chronic paravalvular regurgitation appear to be due to suture dehiscence related to chronic wear-and-tear, particularly in patients with annular fibrosis or calcification. Many patients with mild paravalvular regurgitation can be managed medically with closure indicated for intractable heart failure, progressive left ventricular dilation, or significant hemolytic anemia. Surgical closure may be considered but there is increasing interest in transcatheter closure using occluder devices, as in these four cases. Procedural success rates are 80% to 85%, at experienced centers. Complications occur in <5% of cases, including vascular injury, bleeding, heart block, cardiac perforation, and device embolization.

Suggested Reading

1. Franco E, Almería C, de Agustín JA, et al: Three-dimensional color Doppler transesophageal echocardiography for mitral paravalvular leak quantification and evaluation of percutaneous closure success, J Am Soc Echocardiogr 27(11):1153–1163, 2014.
2. Reed GW, Tuzcu EM, Kapadia SR, et al: Catheter-based closure of paravalvular leak, Exp Rev Cardiovasc Ther 12:681, 2014.
3. Bartel T, Müller S: Intraprocedural guidance: Which imaging technique ranks highest and which one is complementary for closing paravalvular leaks? Cardiovasc Diagn Ther 4(4):277–278, 2014.

Left Ventricular Pseudoaneurysm

CASE 14-10
Percutaneous Closure of Left Ventricular Pseudoaneurysm

The patient is a 73-year-old man, who 25 years previously had undergone a three-vessel bypass graft. A month before admission here, when he presented with bilateral arm pain and chest pain at work and on coronary angiography was found to have an occluded saphenous vein graft to the obtuse marginal and complete occlusion of his native circumflex artery. On echocardiography the patient was found to have severe postero-lateral akinesia with a pseudoaneurysm; the anatomical issue for treating this lesion, both for open and for percutaneous intervention, is proximity to the papillary muscles. Given his high surgical risk, the patient was offered an interventional approach.

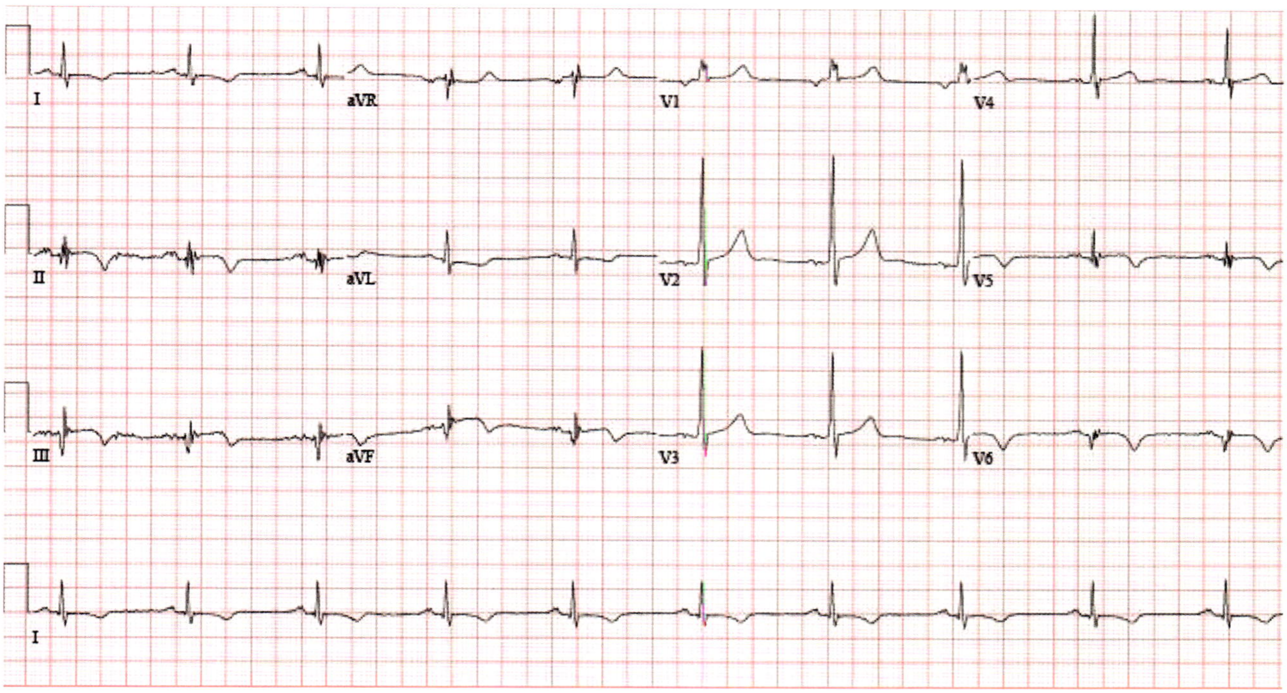

Fig 14.69 Preprocedural ECG shows evidence of myocardial infarction in the lateral and infero-posterior distributions.

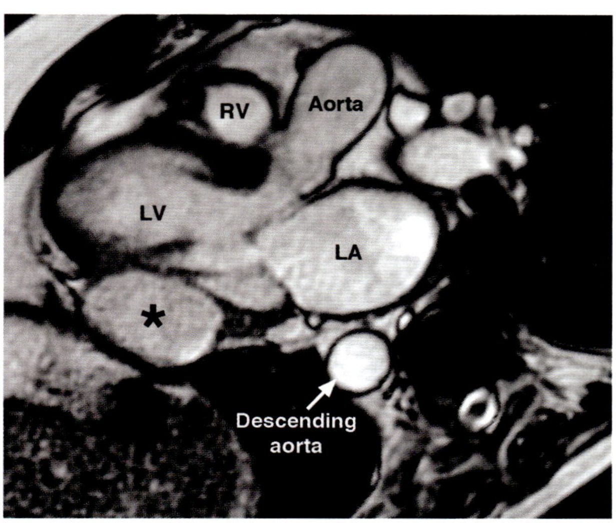

Fig 14.70 MRI has been rotated to assume the same relationships as a transthoracic parasternal long-axis echocardiographic view. Pseudoaneurysm *(asterisk)* originates from the midposterior wall of the LV. In real time, flow into the pseudoaneurysm during systole can be appreciated.

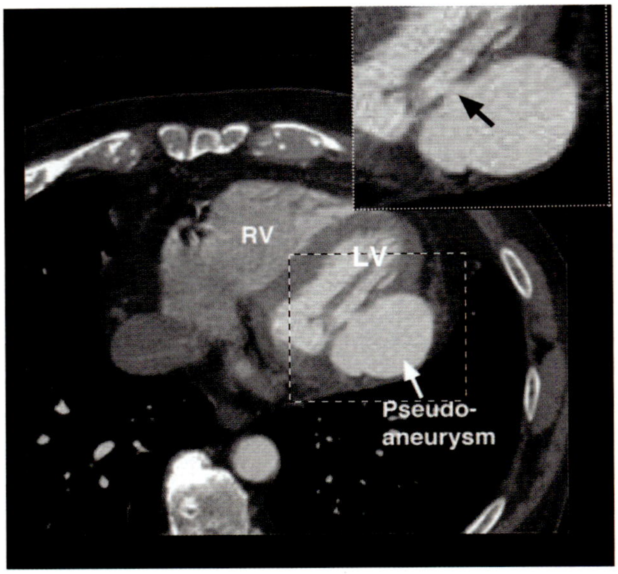

Fig 14.71 CT shows origin of the pseudoaneurysm; black arrow in the inset shows opening into pseudoaneurysm from LV.

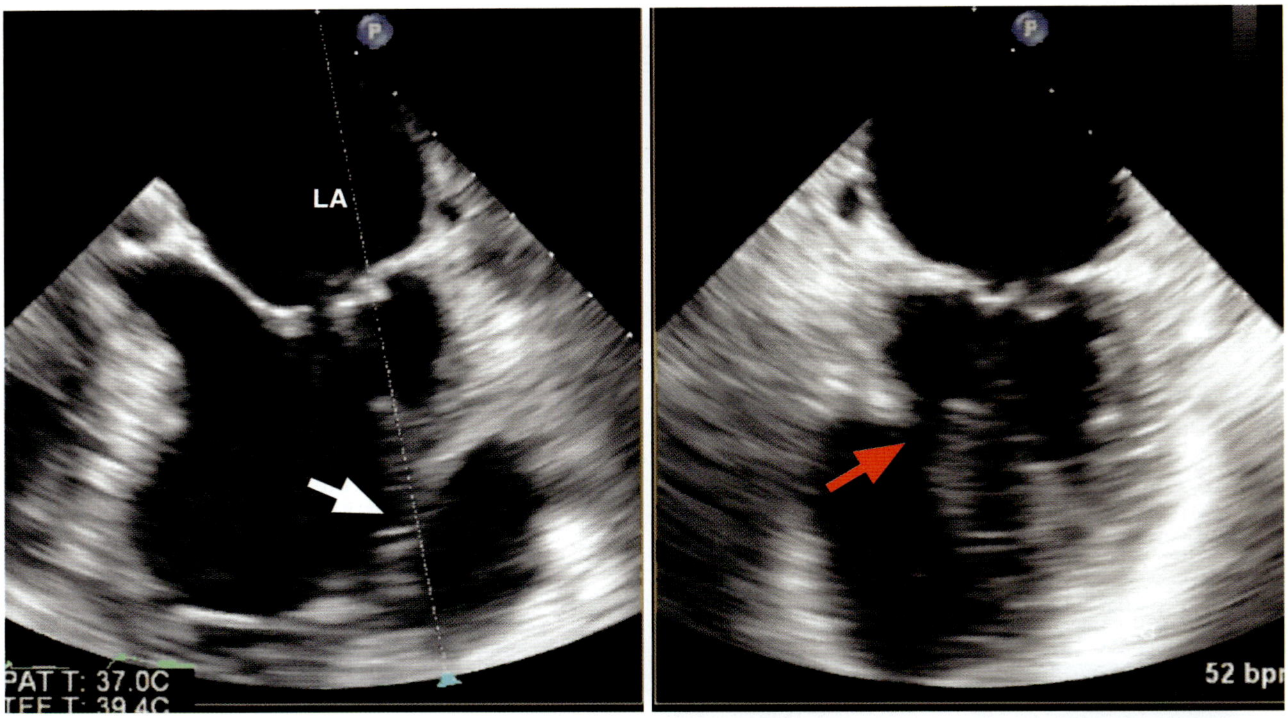

Fig 14.72 In this midesophageal view, four-chamber image on left shows the defect in the lateral wall *(white arrow)*. Orthogonal view at right shows the pseudoaneurysm's proximity to inferior wall *(red arrow)*.

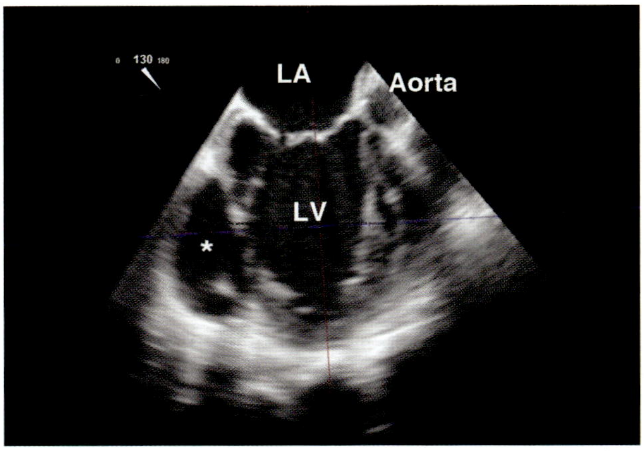

Fig 14.73 In this midesophageal long-axis view, the pseudoaneurysm *(asterisk)* can been seen adjacent to the posterior wall of the LV.

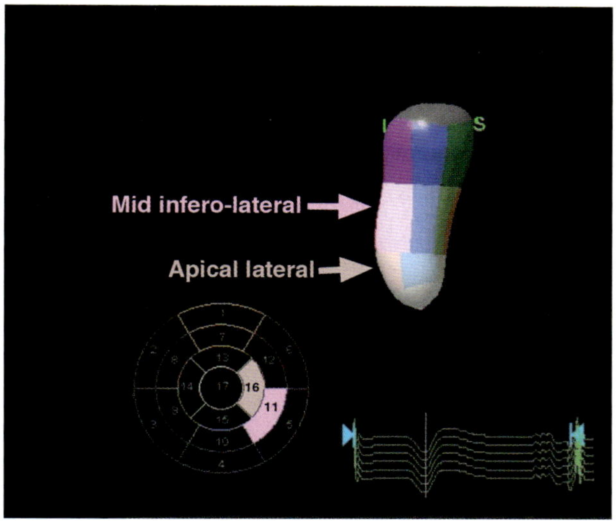

Fig 14.74 17-segment motion analysis. In real time, it shows paradoxical motion during systole of the segments subtending the pseudoaneurysm.

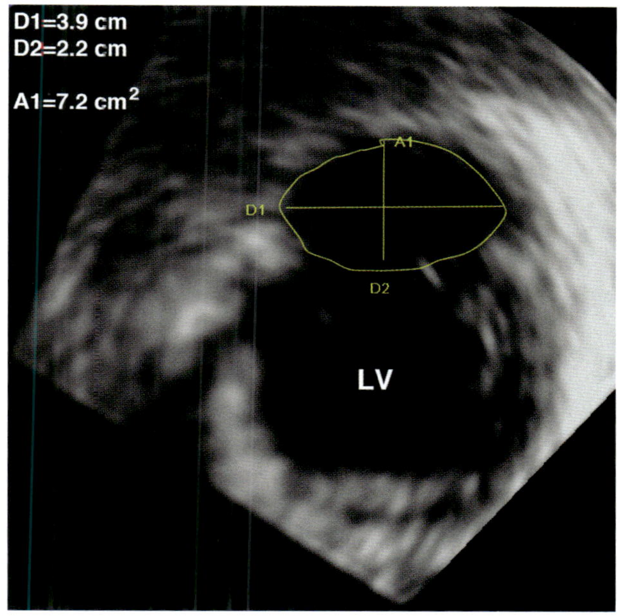

Fig 14.75 Using multiplanar reconstruction, measurements of the major and minor axis of the aneurysm and area were made.

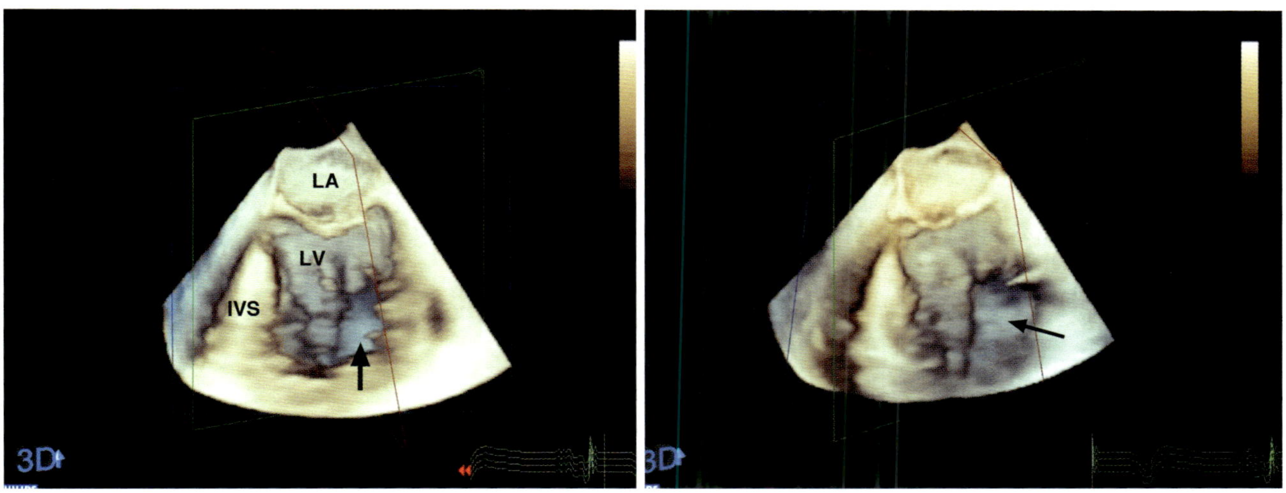

Fig 14.76 From full-volume acquisition, anterior wall has been cropped, revealing the pseudoaneurysm posteriorly *(left, arrow)*. As more of anterior wall is cropped, a greater extent of the pseudoaneurysm is seen *(right, arrow)*.

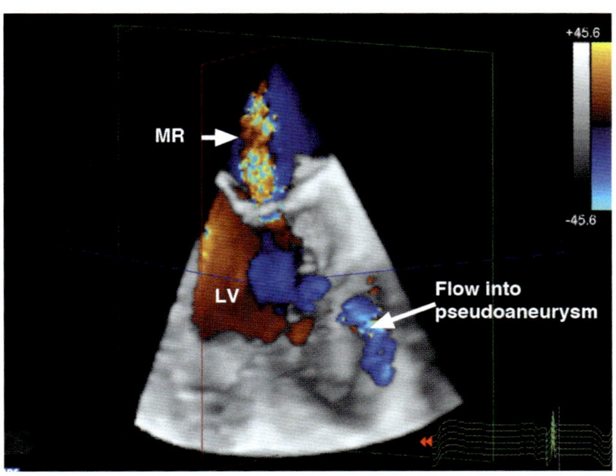

Fig 14.77 3D color Doppler during systole shows jet of MR as well as flow into pseudoaneurysm.

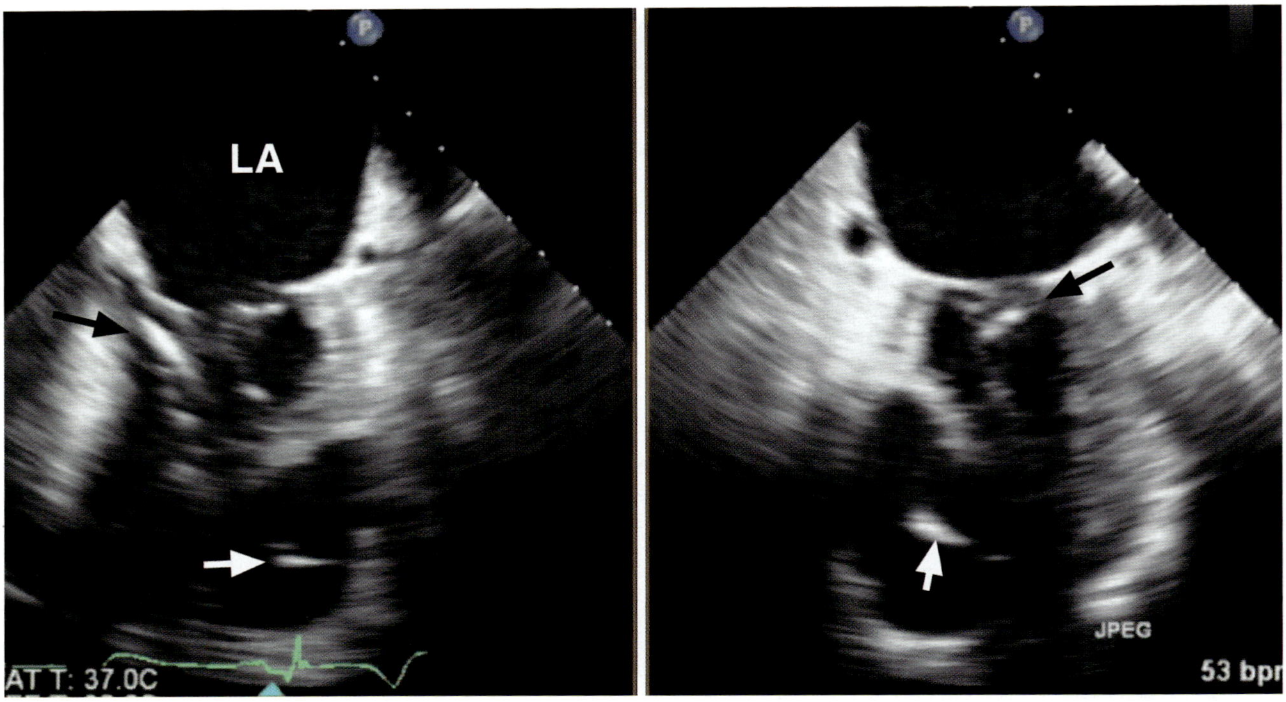

Fig 14.78 In this midesophageal four-chamber image *(left)*, guidewire is seen coming through the LVOT *(black arrow)* and entering pseudoaneurysm *(white arrow)*. Orthogonal view on right shows similar findings.

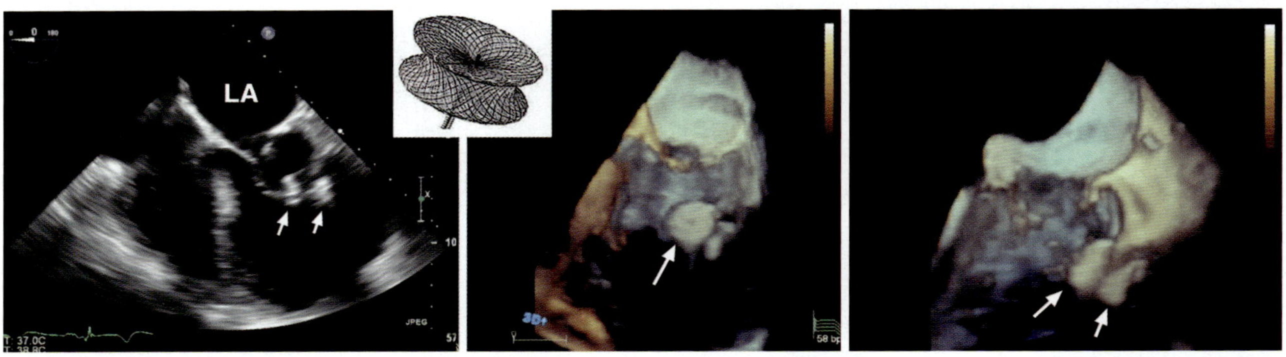

Fig 14.79 Wire was exchanged for sheath through which an Amplatzer device was introduced *(white arrows)*, successfully closing entry to the pseudoaneurysm. This is seen in 2D *(left)*, 3D en face *(center)*, and 3D from side *(right)*. Inset is artistic rendition of device.

Comments

A left ventricular pseudoaneurysm is a myocardial rupture that has been contained by adherent pericardium. Echocardiographic features include a narrow neck and an abrupt transition from normal myocardium to the thin-walled pseudoaneurysm cavity, which may be lined by thrombus. Long-term outcomes are poor without surgical intervention because the pseudoaneurysm can rupture further at any time, resulting in cardiac tamponade and death. Surgery is the recommended treatment but there has been recent interest in the possibility of transcatheter closure in selected high-risk patients on humanitarian grounds, although in the USA, this device is not approved for this purpose.

Suggested Reading

1. Narayan RL, Vaishnava P, Goldman ME, et al: Percutaneous closure of left ventricular pseudoaneurysm, Ann Thorac Surg 94(5):e123–e125, 2012.
2. Moriarty J, Harris TJ, Vorobiof G, et al: Direct percutaneous repair of left ventricular pseudoaneurysm via transthoracic deployment of a ventricular septal defect closure device, Tex Heart Inst J 42(4):362–366, 2015.
3. Moreno R, Gordillo E, Zamorano J, et al: Long term outcome of patients with postinfarction left ventricular pseudoaneurysm, Heart 89(10):1144–1146, 2003.

Left Atrial Appendage

CASE 14-11
Left Atrial Appendage Occlusion Device

This 76-year-old man with chronic atrial fibrillation was referred for placement of a Watchman® left atrial appendage occlusion device. Standard anticoagulation presented a high risk of complications in this patient because of a history of recurrent significant gastrointestinal bleeding.

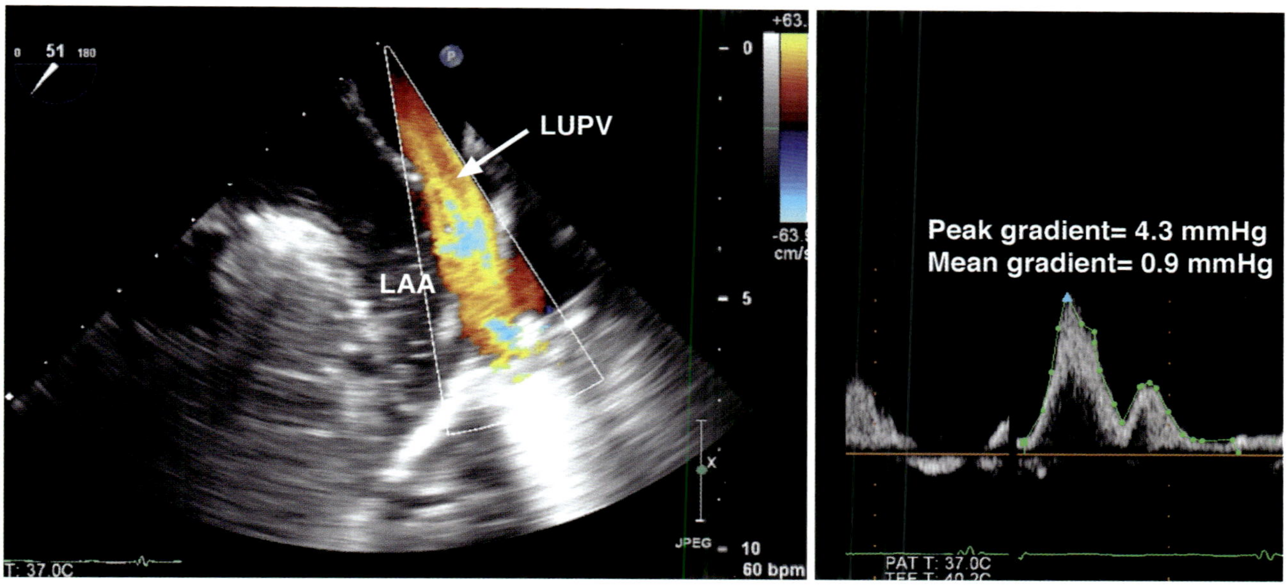

Fig 14.80 Imaging of left upper pulmonary vein with color and spectral Doppler showed no evidence of stenosis.

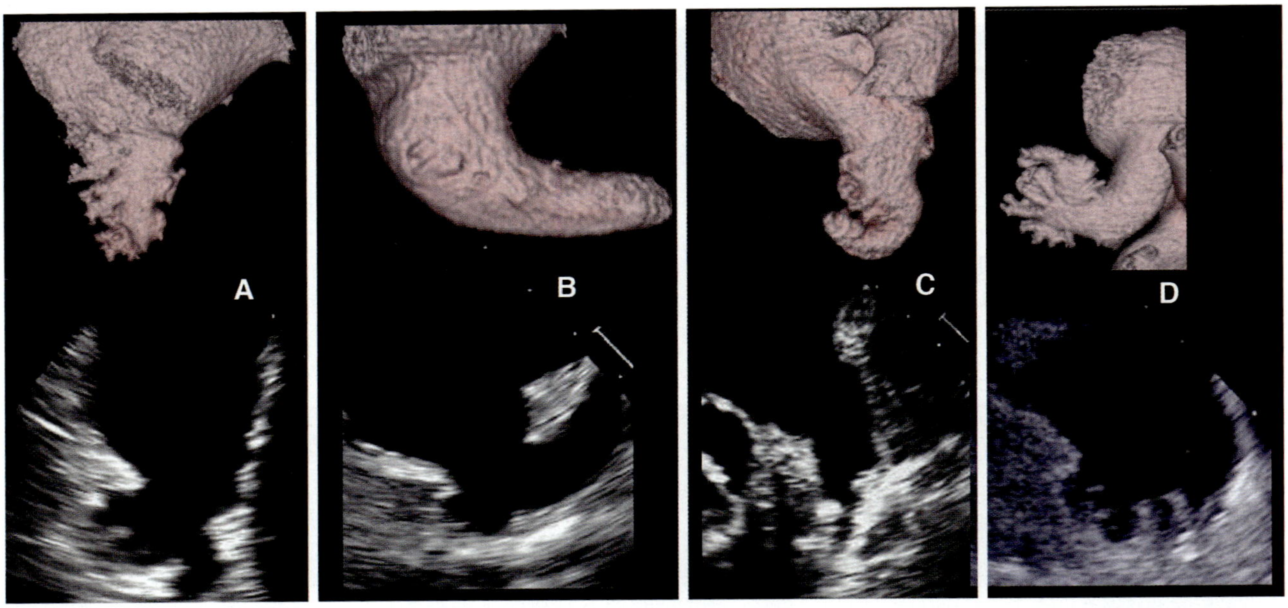

Fig 14.81 CT scans and 2D TEE images of LAA morphology from several different patients demonstrating range of atrial appendage anatomy. **(A)** "Cactus" LAA morphology presents dominant central lobe with secondary lobes extending from central lobe in both superior and inferior directions. CT = computed tomography. **(B)** "Chicken wing" LAA morphology presents obvious bend in proximal or middle part of the dominant lobe, or folding back of the LAA anatomy on itself at some distance from perceived LAA ostium. This type of LAA may have secondary lobes or twigs. **(C)** "Windsock" LAA morphology presents one dominant lobe of sufficient length as primary structure. Variations of this LAA type arise with location and number of secondary or even tertiary lobes arising from the dominant lobe. **(D)** "Cauliflower" LAA morphology presents limited overall length with more complex internal characteristics. Variations of this LAA type have more irregular shape of the LAA ostium (oval vs round) and variable number of lobes with lack of dominant lobe. LAA = left atrial appendage. (CT images from Di Biase L, Santangeli P, Anselmino M, et al: Does the left atrial appendage morphology correlate with risk of stroke in patients with atrial fibrillation? Results from a multicenter study, J Am Coll Cardiol 60:531–538, 2012. 2D TEE images from Beigel R, Wunderlich NC, Ho SY, et al: The left atrial appendage: Anatomy, function, and noninvasive evaluation, J Am Coll Cardiol Imaging 7:1251–2165, 2014. With permission.)

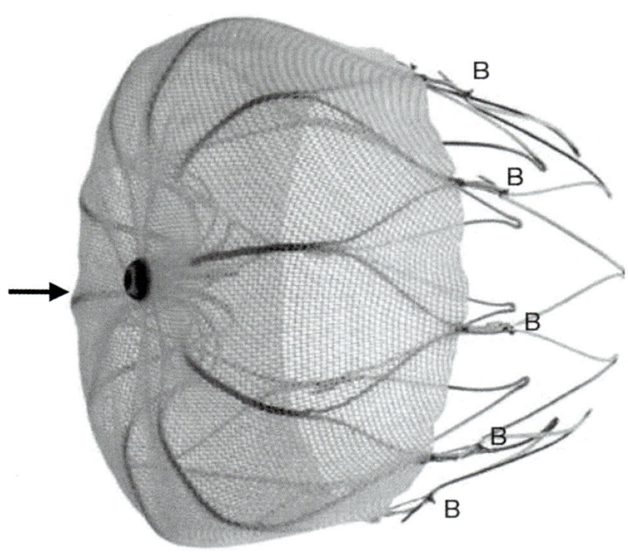

Fig 14.82 Watchman® occlusion device. Barbs *(B)* on outer edge of the wires help to fix this device to the musculature of left atrial appendage. Arrow shows which side faces left atrium when device is deployed. (From Block PC: Percutaneous left atrial appendage closure in a patient with atrial fibrillation, Nature Clin Pract Cardiovasc Med 3:456–459, 2006. With permission.)

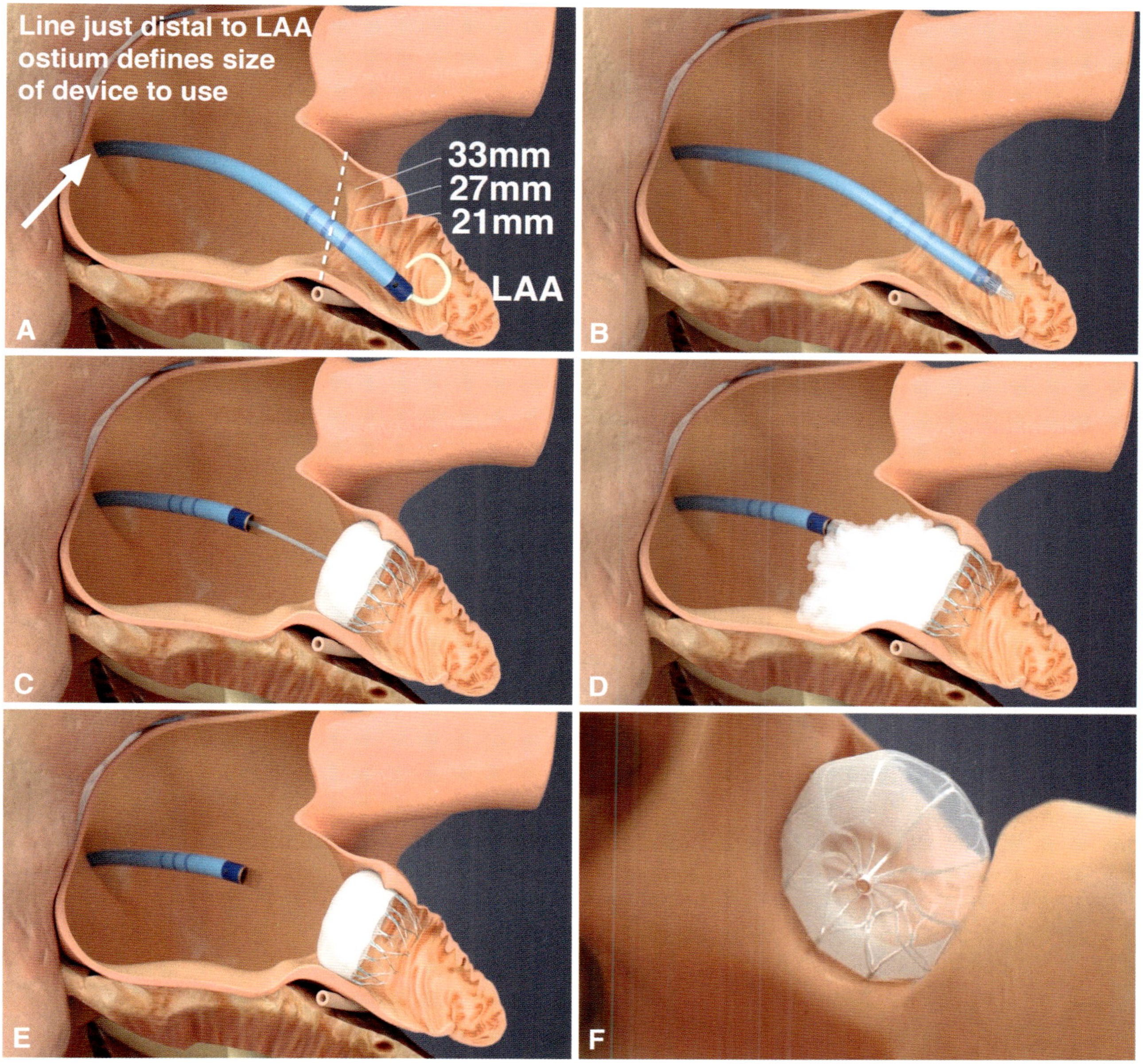

Fig 14.83 Procedural steps in placing the occlusion device are illustrated. **(A)** After transseptal puncture, left atrial appendage is sized in order to select appropriate occluder, based on the recommendations of the manufacturer. **(B,C)** Device is advanced into appendage and deployed. **(D)** Dye injection under fluoroscopic guidance is used to demonstrate absence of dye in body of appendage. **(E)** Delivery catheter is separated from occluder. **(F)** Final position of occluder as seen en face. (From Boston Scientific, Marlborough, Massachusetts.)

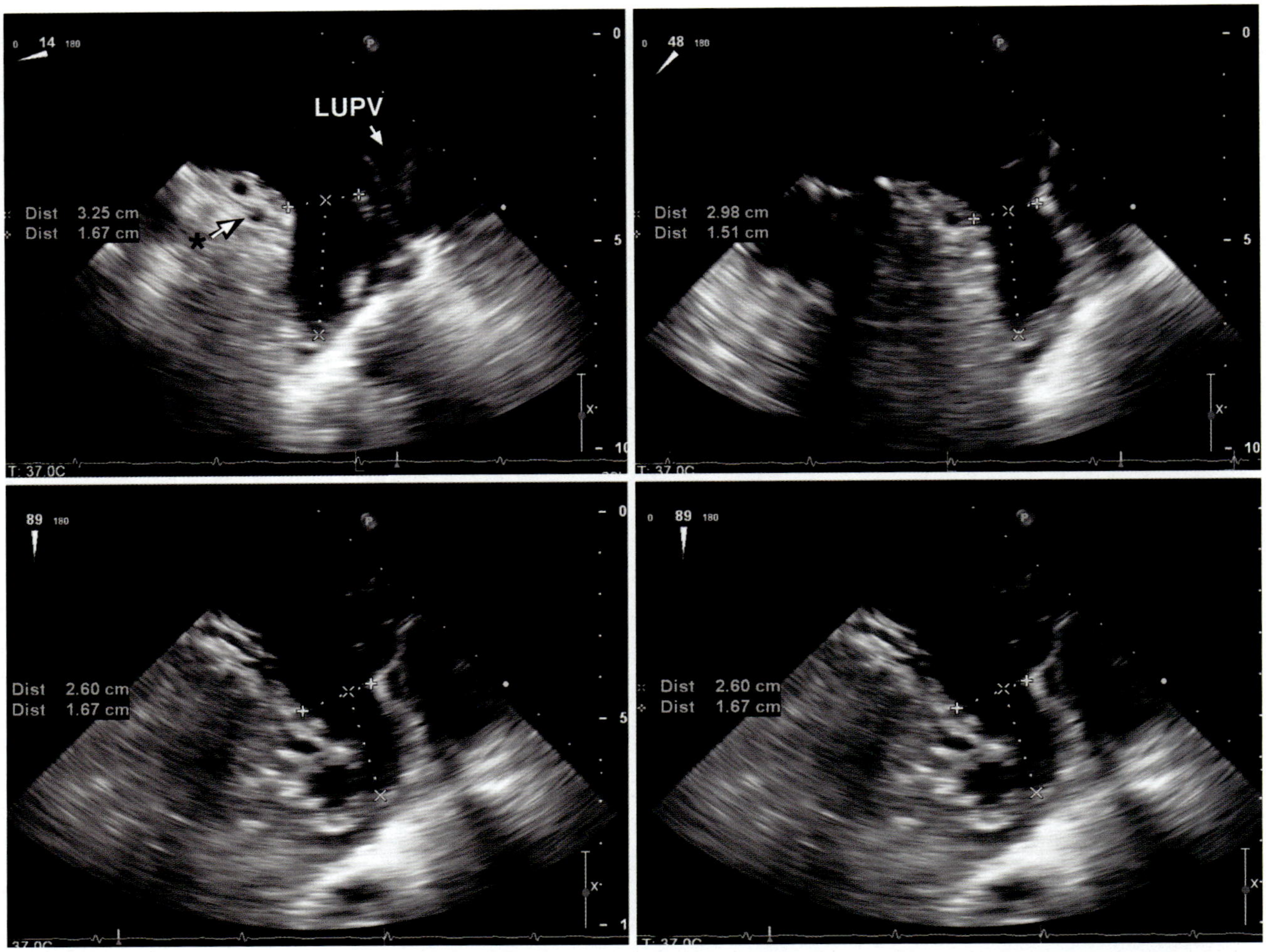

Fig 14.84 In our patient, LAA was imaged at approximately 0°, 45°, 90°, and 130° by TEE. The LAA width is measured in a plane from left coronary artery *(arrow)* to 1–2 cm from tip of left upper pulmonary vein (LUPV) limbus.

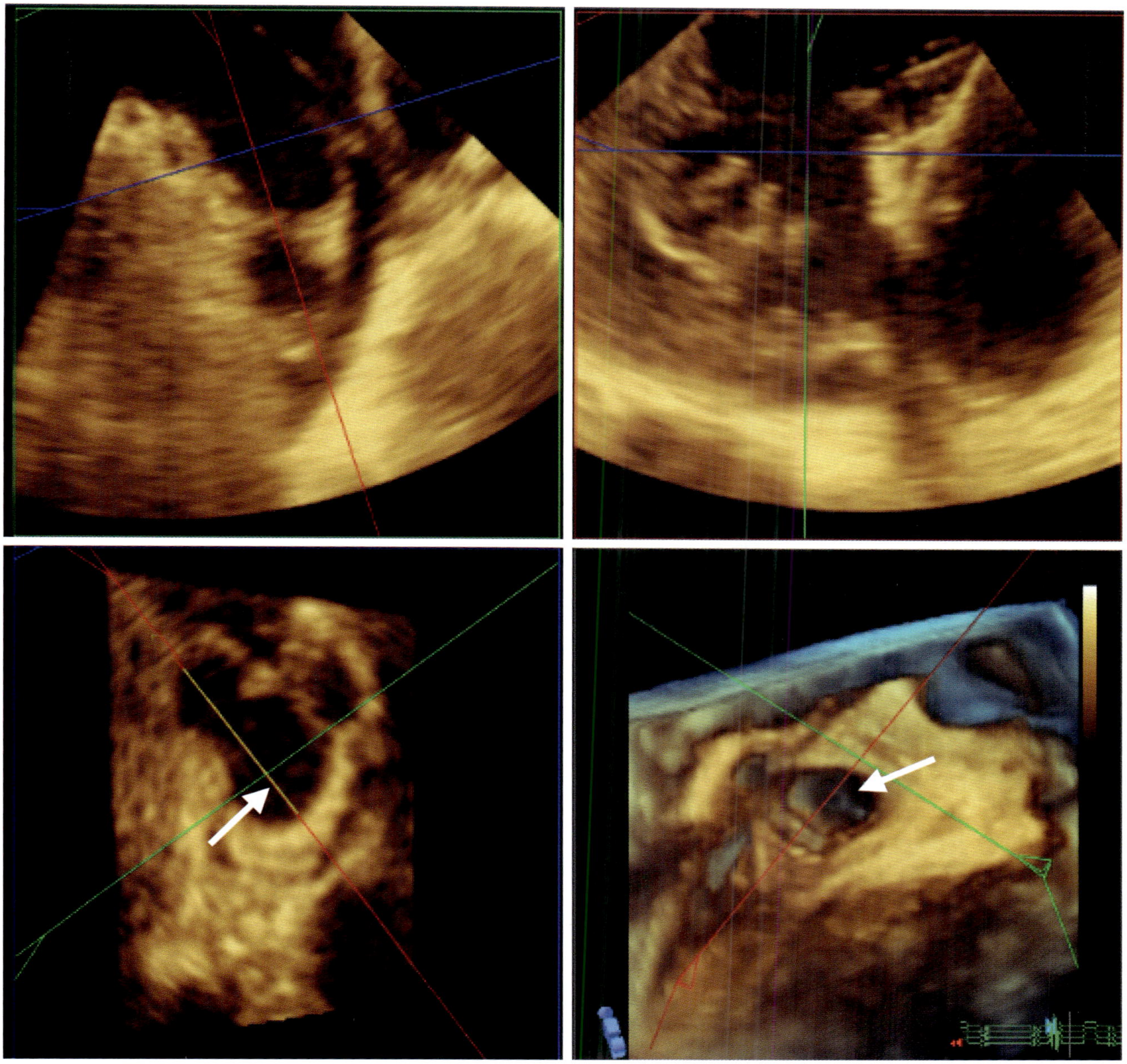

Fig 14.85 Multiplanar reconstruction, which demonstrates complex 3D shape of LAA. In both lower quadrants, appendage orifice is seen *(arrows)*.

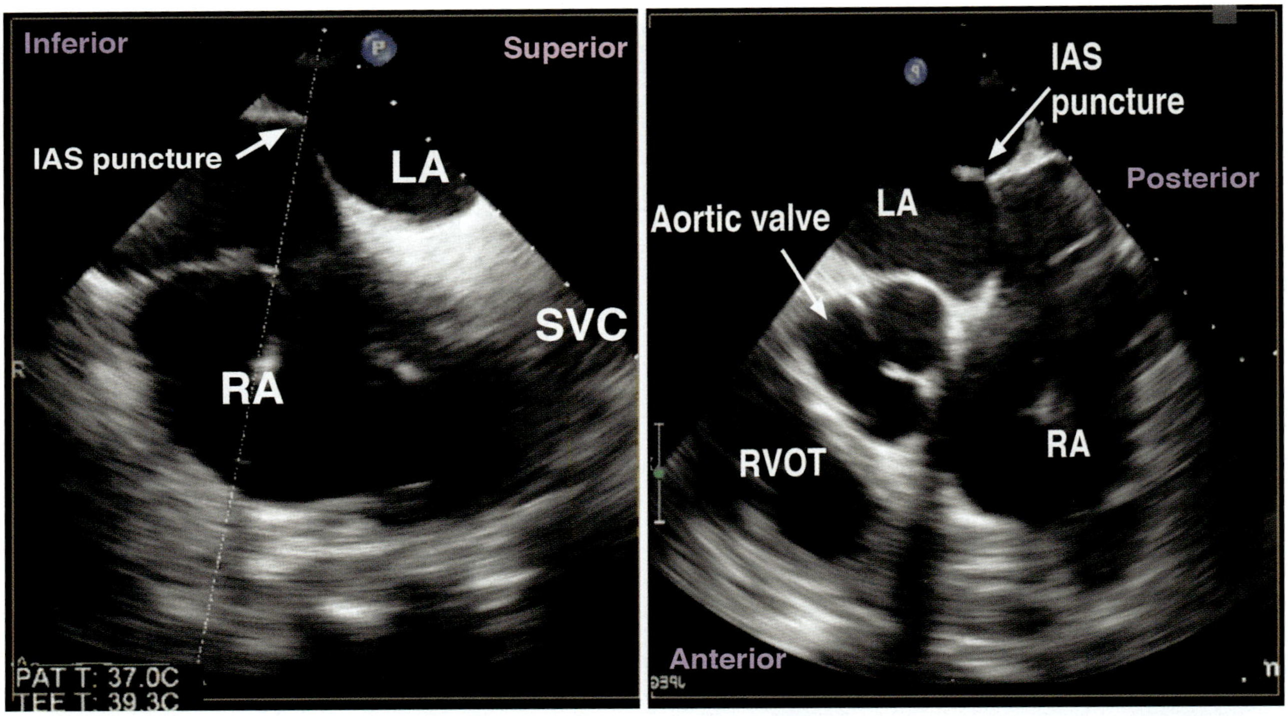

Fig 14.86 In preparation for device delivery, transseptal puncture is performed. In this biplane image, puncture site is chosen to be inferior *(left)* and posterior *(right)*, thus preventing entry into aorta, and allowing for proper trajectory of device toward LAA.

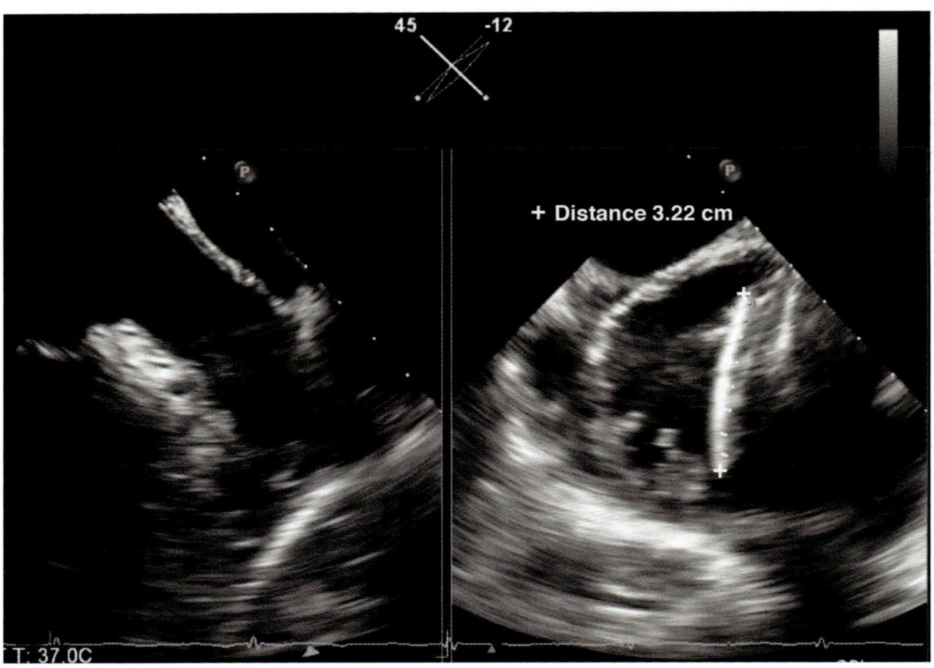

Fig 14.87 Sheath has been advanced into LAA as seen on biplane imaging; measurement from the orifice of LAA to its distal margin allows selection of correctly sized device.

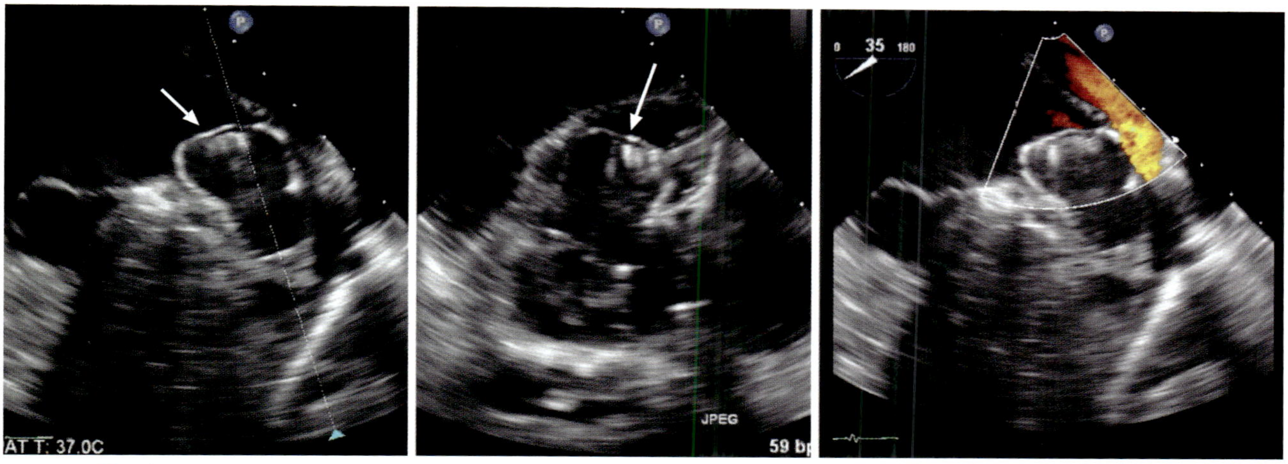

Fig 14.88 After exchange, the delivery device was advanced into the LAA and the device deployed *(arrows, left and center frames).* At right, flow is seen in LUPV, but none is seen going past device.

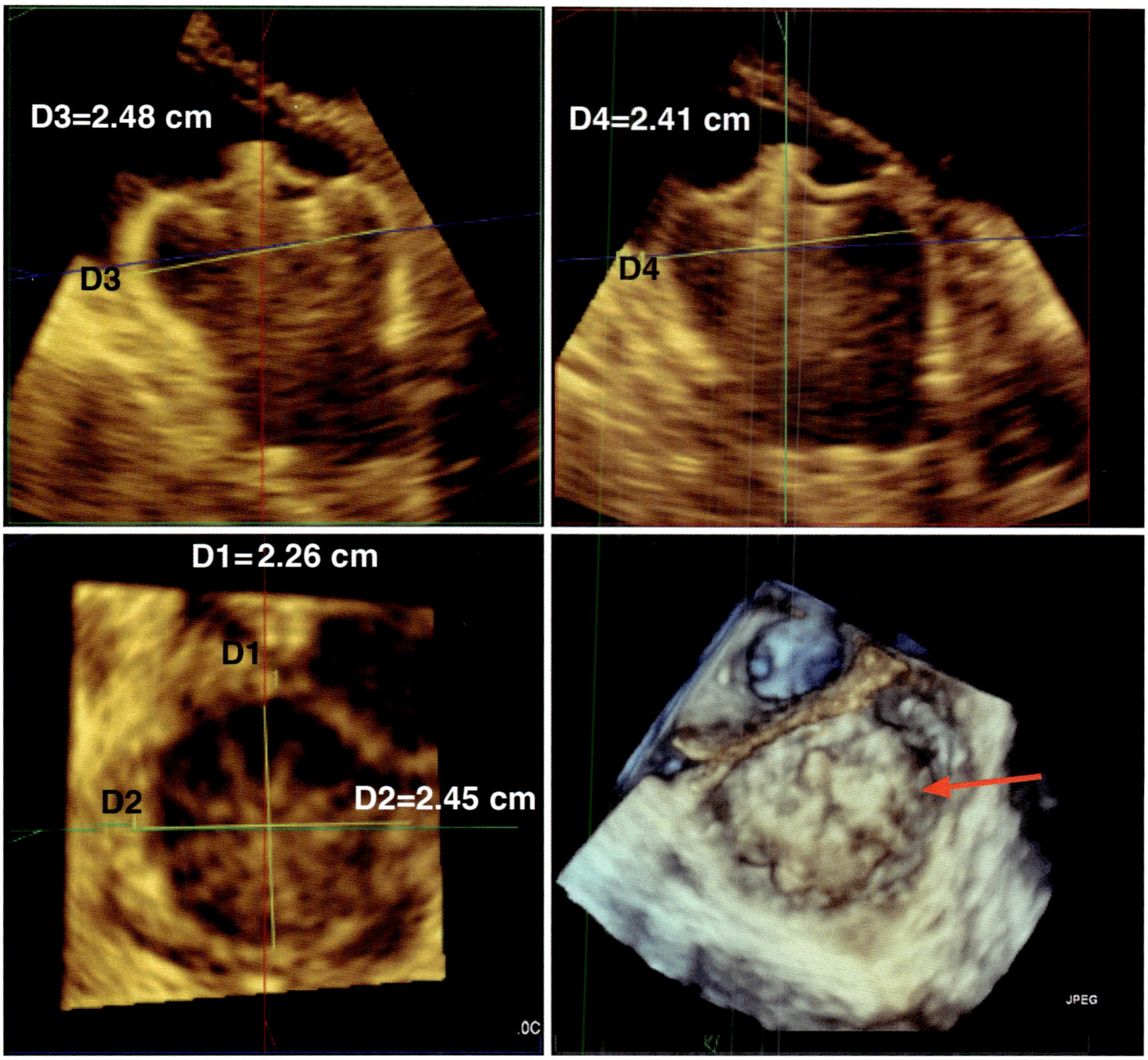

Fig 14.89 In this postdeployment multiplanar reconstruction, device is well seated and fully deployed. Measurements are made at LAA orifice. In bottom right, 3D image shows device *(red arrow)* protruding slightly past orifice.

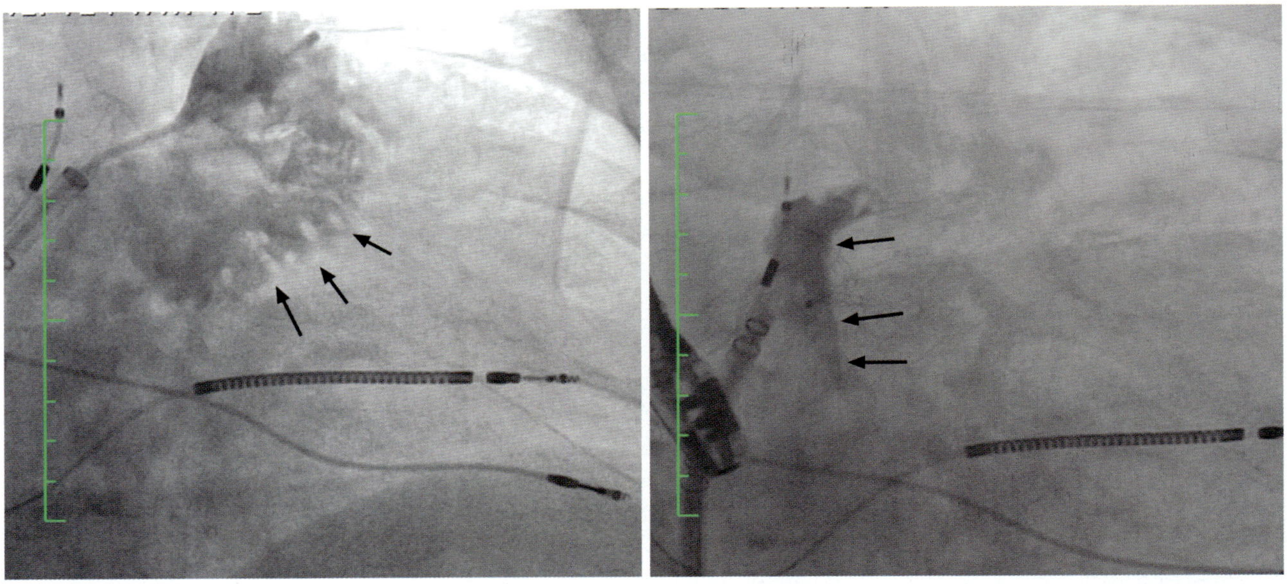

Fig 14.90 Using fluoroscopy, appendage is imaged predeployment *(left)*. Black arrows indicate pectinate muscles. At right, injection of contrast into the left atrium post-deployment fails to opacify LAA. Arrows indicate interface between left atrial contrast and proximal end of device.

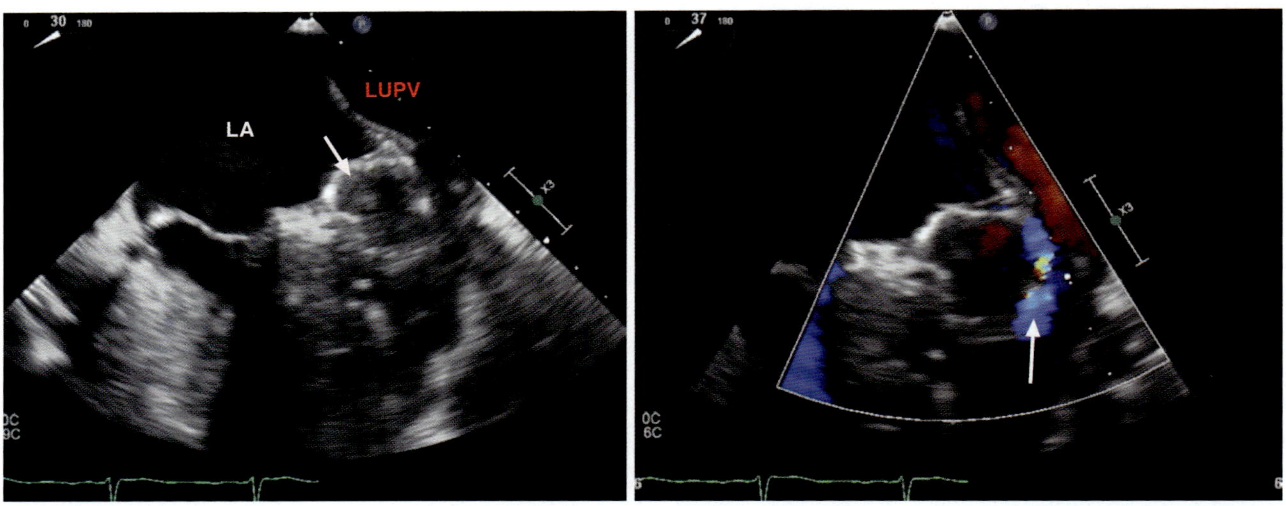

Fig 14.91 TEE was performed 5 weeks after implantation. Although the device appears well seated *(right, arrow)*, a small amount of color Doppler flow into the appendage is visible.

Comments

TEE guidance is essential during transcatheter occlusion of the left atrial appendage as illustrated by this case. Baseline imaging focuses on identification of potential contraindications to placement of a device in the left atrial appendage (LAA). These contraindications include LAA thrombus, and anatomical issues such as a multiorifice appendage. In addition, any contraindications to TEE or concerns with contrast angiography would preclude the procedure. During the procedure, TEE is used to ensure correct placement of the device and assess any residual leak. At follow-up, TEE imaging is used to identify and measure any residual leaks around the device that may affect decisions about anticoagulation therapy and long-term management.

Suggested Reading

1. Beigel R, Wunderlich NC, Ho SY, et al: The left atrial appendage: Anatomy, function, and noninvasive evaluation, J Am Coll Cardiol Imaging 7:1251–1265, 2014.
2. Lockwood SM, Alison JF, Obeyesekere MN, et al: Imaging the left atrial appendage prior to, during, and after occlusion, J Am Coll Cardiol Imaging 4:303–306, 2011.
3. Sommer M, Roehrich A, Boen F: Value of 3D TEE for LAA morphology, J Am Coll Cardiol Imaging 8:1107–1110, 2015.
4. Wunderlich NC, Beigel R, Swaans MJ, Ho SY, et al: Percutaneous interventions for left atrial appendage exclusion: options, assessment, and imaging using 2D and 3D echocardiography, JACC: Cardiovascular Imaging 8:472–488, 2015.

INDEX

D

E

F

G

H

I

L

M

N

O

P